DTT	dithiothreitol
EACA	epsilon aminocaproic acid
EBAA	Eye Bank Association of America
ECMO	extracorporeal membrane oxygenation
ECV	extracorporeal volume
EDTA	ethylenediaminetetraacetic acid
EIA	enzyme immunoassay
ELBW	extremely low birthweight
ELISA	enzyme-linked immunosorbent assay
EPO	erythropoietin
FACT	Foundation for the Accreditation of Cellular Therapy
FcR	Fc gamma receptor
FDA	Food and Drug Administration
FFP	Fresh Frozen Plasma
FMH	fetomaternal hemorrhage
FNAIT	fetal/neonatal alloimmune thrombocytopenia
FNHTR	febrile nonhemolytic transfusion reaction
FTA-ABS	fluorescent treponemal antibody absorption test
G-CSF	granulocyte colony-stimulating factor
GalNAc	N-acetylgalactosamine
GM-CSF	granulocyte-macrophage colony-stimulating factor
GMP	good manufacturing practice
GPIa	glycoprotein Ia
GPA	glycophorin A
GPB	glycophorin B
GPC	glycophorin C
GPD	glycophorin D
GTP	good tissue practice
GVHD	graft-vs-host disease
Gy	Gray
HAV	hepatitis A virus
HAZMAT	hazardous material
Hb	hemoglobin
HBc	hepatitis B core antigen
HBsAg	hepatitis B surface antigen
HBV	hepatitis B virus
Hct	hematocrit
HCT/Ps	human cells, tissues, and cellular and tissue-based products
HCV	hepatitis C virus
HDFN	hemolytic disease of the fetus and newborn
HES	hydroxyethyl starch

HHS	(US) Department of Health and Human Services
HIT	heparin-induced thrombocytopenia
HIV	human immunodeficiency virus
HNA	human neutrophil antigen
HPA	human platelet antigen
HPC	hematopoietic progenitor cell
HPC(A)	HPCs from apheresis (HPC, Apheresis)
HPC(C)	HPCs from cord blood (HPC, Cord Blood)
HPC(M)	HPCs from marrow (HPC, Marrow)
HSC	hematopoietic stem cell
HSCT	hematopoietic stem cell transplantation
HTLV-I	human T-cell lymphotropic virus, type I
HTR	hemolytic transfusion reaction
HUS	hemolytic uremic syndrome
IAT	indirect antiglobulin test
IATA	International Air Transport Association
ICAM-1	intercellular adhesion molecule-1
ID	identification or individual donation
Ig	immunoglobulin
IL-1α	interleukin-1 alpha
IL-1β	interleukin-1 beta
IL-2	interleukin-2
IM	intramuscular
IND	investigational new drug
INR	international normalized ratio
iPSCs	induced pluripotent stem cells
IRL	immunohematology reference laboratory
IS	immediate spin
ISBT	International Society of Blood Transfusion
ISO	International Organization for Standardization
ITP	immune thrombocytopenia
IU	international unit
IV	intravenous
IVIG	intravenous immune globulin
LDH	lactate dehydrogenase
LDL	low-density lipoprotein
LISS	low-ionic-strength saline
LN$_2$	liquid nitrogen
LR	leukocyte-reduced
MAC	membrane attack complex
2-ME	2-mercaptoethanol
MF	mixed field

MHC	major histocompatibility complex	RBCs	Red Blood Cells (blood donor unit)
MNC	mononuclear cell	RFLP	restriction fragment length polymorphism
MoAb	monoclonal antibody		
MPHA	mixed passive hemagglutination assay	rFVIIa	recombinant Factor VIIa
mRNA	messenger ribonucleic acid	Rh	Rhesus factor
MSC	mesenchymal stem cell	RHAG	Rh-associated glycoprotein
MSDS	material safety data sheet	RhIG	Rh Immune Globulin
MSM	male who has sex with another male	RIBA	recombinant immunoblot assay
NAIT	neonatal alloimmune thrombocytopenia	RIPA	radioimmunoprecipitation assay
NAN	neonatal alloimmune neutropenia	RNA	ribonucleic acid
NAT	nucleic acid testing	RPR	rapid plasma reagin (serologic test for syphilis)
NHLBI	National Heart, Lung, and Blood Institute		
		RT	room temperature or reverse transcriptase
NIH	National Institutes of Health		
NIPA	nonimmunologic protein adsorption	SCF	stem cell factor
NK	natural killer	SD	standard deviation or solvent/detergent
NMDP	National Marrow Donor Program	SNP	single nucleotide polymorphism
NRC	Nuclear Regulatory Commission	SOP	standard operating procedure
NRF	National Response Framework	SPRCA	solid-phase red cell adherence
OSHA	Occupational Safety and Health Administration	TA	transfusion-associated
		TACO	transfusion-associated circulatory overload
p	probability		
PAD	preoperative autologous (blood) donation	TCR	T-cell receptor
		TMA	transcription-mediated amplification
PBM	patient blood management	TNCs	total nucleated cells
PBS	phosphate-buffered saline	TNF-α	tumor necrosis factor alpha
PCH	paroxysmal cold hemoglobinuria	TPE	therapeutic plasma exchange
PCR	polymerase chain reaction	TPO	thrombopoietin
PEG	polyethylene glycol	TRALI	transfusion-related acute lung injury
PF24	Plasma Frozen Within 24 Hours After Phlebotomy	TSE	transmissible spongiform encephalopathy
PF24RT24	Plasma Frozen Within 24 Hours After Phlebotomy Held at Room Temperature Up to 24 Hours After Phlebotomy	TTP	thrombotic thrombocytopenic purpura
		UCB	umbilical cord blood
		UDP	uridine diphosphate
PPE	personal protective equipment	UNOS	United Network for Organ Sharing
PRA	panel-reactive antibody	USC	United States Code
PRCA	pure red cell aplasia	vCJD	variant Creutzfeldt-Jakob disease
PRP	platelet-rich plasma	VLBW	very low birthweight
PRT	pathogen reduction technology	vWD	von Willebrand disease
PT	prothrombin time or proficiency testing	vWF	von Willebrand factor
PTP	posttransfusion purpura	WAIHA	warm autoimmune hemolytic anemia
PTT	partial thromboplastin time	WB	whole blood or Western blot
PVC	polyvinyl chloride	WBC	white blood cell
QA	quality assessment or quality assurance	WHO	World Health Organization
QC	quality control	WNV	West Nile virus
QSE	Quality System Essential	ZIKV	Zika virus

Technical Manual

●

19TH EDITION

Other related publications available from the AABB:

Transfusion Therapy: Clinical Principles and Practice, 3rd edition
Edited by Paul D. Mintz, MD

Transfusion Medicine: Self-Assessment and Review, 3rd edition
By Douglas P. Blackall, MD, MPH, and Justin D. Kreuter, MD

Blood Transfusion Therapy: A Physician's Handbook, 12th edition
Edited by Nicholas Bandarenko, MD, and Karen King, MD

Judd's Methods in Immunohematology, 3rd edition
By John W. Judd, FIBMS; Susan T. Johnson, MSTM, MT(ASCP)SBB; and Jill Storry, PhD, FIBMS

Antibody Identification: Art or Science? A Case Study Approach
By Janis R. Hamilton, MS, MT(ASCP)SBB; Susan T. Johnson, MSTM, MT(ASCP)SBB;
and Sally V. Rudmann, PhD, MT(ASCP)SBB

Concise Guide to Transfusion Medicine
By Minh-Ha Tran, DO; Marissa Li, MD; Suchitra Pandey, MD; and
Erica Antell, MT(ASCP)SBB

To purchase books or to inquire about other book services, including digital downloads and large-quantity sales, please contact our sales department:

- 866.222.2498 (within the United States)
- +1 301.215.6499 (outside the United States)
- +1 301.951.7150 (fax)
- www.aabb.org>Resources>Marketplace

AABB customer service representatives are available by telephone from 8:30 am to 5:00 pm ET, Monday through Friday, excluding holidays.

Technical Manual

●

19TH EDITION

Edited by

Mark K. Fung, MD, PhD
University of Vermont
Burlington, VT

Anne F. Eder, MD, PhD
Food and Drug Administration
Rockville, MD

Steven L. Spitalnik, MD
Columbia University
New York, NY

Connie M. Westhoff, PhD, SBB
New York Blood Center
New York, NY

AABB
4550 Montgomery Avenue
Suite 700, North Tower
Bethesda, Maryland 20817

ISBN No. 978-1-56395-947-9
Printed in the United States

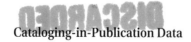

Cataloging-in-Publication Data

Technical manual / editor, Mark K. Fung—19th ed.
        p. ; cm.
    Including bibliographic references and index.
ISBN 978-1-56395-947-9
1. Blood Banks—Handbooks, manuals, etc. I. Fung, Mark K. II. AABB.
[DNLM: 1. Blood Banks-laboratory manuals. 2. Blood Transfusion-
laboratory manuals. WH 25 T2548 2017]
RM172.T43 2017
615'.39—dc23
DNLM/DLC

Technical Manual Authors

Chester Andrzejewski Jr, PhD, MD

J. Wade Atkins, MS, MT(ASCP)SBB, CQA(ASQ)

Debra J. Bailey, MT(ASCP)SBB

P. Dayand Borge Jr, MD, PhD

Scott A. Brubaker, CTBS

Brian R. Curtis, PhD, D(ABMLI), MT(ASCP)SBB

Melissa M. Cushing, MD

Robertson D. Davenport, MD

Meghan Delaney, DO, MPH

Gregory A. Denomme, PhD, FCSMLS(D)

Nancy M. Dunbar, MD

Arthur B. Eisenbrey III, MD, PhD

Susan A. Galel, MD

James D. Gorham, MD, PhD

Janis R. Hamilton, MS, MT(ASCP)SBB

Sarah K. Harm, MD

Jeanne E. Hendrickson, MD

Eldad A. Hod, MD

Orieji Illoh, MD

Eapen K. Jacob, MD

Melanie Jorgenson, RN, BSN, LSSGB

Cassandra D. Josephson, MD

Richard M. Kaufman, MD

Debra A. Kessler, RN, MS

Scott A. Koepsell, MD, PhD

Patricia M. Kopko, MD

Kevin J. Land, MD

Regina M. Leger, MSQA, MT(ASCP)SBB, CMQ/OE(ASQ)

Lani Lieberman, MD, MSc

Christine Lomas-Francis, MSc, FIBMS

Irina Maramica, MD, PhD, MBA

Martin L. Olsson, MD, PhD

Kathleen E. Puca, MD, MT(ASCP)SBB

Rowena C. Punzalan, MD

Eva D. Quinley, MS, MT(ASCP)SBB

Susan N. Rossmann, MD, PhD

William J. Savage, MD, PhD

Annette J. Schlueter, MD, PhD

Joseph Schwartz, MD, MPH

Nadine Shehata, MD, FRCP

Ira A. Shulman, MD

Jill R. Storry, PhD, FIBMS

Susan L. Stramer, PhD

Annika M. Svensson, MD, PhD

Leslie P. Taylor, CQA(ASQ)

Lynne Uhl, MD

Ralph R. Vassallo, MD, FACP

Stephen J. Wagner, PhD

Julia S. Westman, PhD

Barbee I. Whitaker, PhD

Edward C.C. Wong, MD

Acknowledgments

THE 19TH EDITION OF the *Technical Manual* is the collaborative result of many dedicated volunteers. My thanks go out to all the chapter authors, and my three Associate Editors for this edition—Anne Eder, Steve Spitalnik, and Connie Westhoff. This was a team effort, and I greatly appreciate their guidance in the subjects covered, and the many hours spent reviewing and revising each chapter with the authors.

We, in turn, would like to thank the many members of the following AABB committees and task forces who reviewed every word of the chapters, methods, and appendices in the 19th edition. Their participation makes this volume unique in the literature and contributes to its excellent reputation.

REVIEWING GROUPS

AABB Representative to ASFA

AABB Representative to ISBT Working Party for Transfusion Transmitted Infectious Disease

AATB Representative

Cellular Therapy Section Coordinating Committee – Subgroup, Cellular Therapy Product Collection and Clinical Practices

Cellular Therapy Section Coordinating Committee – Subgroup, Product Manufacturing and Testing

Circular of Information Task Force

Clinical Transfusion Medicine Committee

Donor History Task Force

FDA Liaison Committee

Immunohematology Reference Laboratories Accreditation Program Unit

Immunohematology Reference Laboratories Standards Program Unit

Interorganizational Task Force on Domestic Disasters and Acts of Terrorism

Molecular Testing Laboratories Standards Program Unit

Patient Blood Management Education Committee

Patient Blood Management Standards Committee

Quality Systems Accreditation Committee

Relationship Testing Standards Program Unit

Transfusion Medicine Section Coordinating Committee – Subgroup, Donor and Blood Component Management

Transfusion Medicine Section Coordinating Committee – Subgroup, Pediatric Transfusion

Transfusion Medicine Section Coordinating Committee – Subgroup, Technical Practices and Serology

Transfusion Medicine Section Coordinating Committee – Subgroup, Transfusion Safety and Patient Blood Management

Transfusion-Transmitted Disease Committee

We would be remiss if we did not also mention the valuable material drafted by contributors to the 18th and earlier editions that we included in this new edition. The selected tables, figures, methods, and narrative that we kept could not have been improved. Finally, we would like to thank AABB staff who supported our efforts.

Mark K. Fung, MD, PhD
Editor in Chief

Preface

●

O N BEHALF OF the 100+ contributors to this book, it is my pleasure to introduce you to the 19th edition of the AABB *Technical Manual*. To assure readers of a continuously renewed and refreshed approach to the contents, approximately one third of the chapters for each edition are written by a new lead author, with lead authors generally serving for no more than two editions. Similarly, the editors (including myself) rotate on a staggered basis. Therefore, this will be the second and last edition for Dr. Connie Westhoff and me serving as editors. I am very pleased to introduce both Drs. Steven Spitalnik and Anne Eder as editors for this edition, and very grateful for the guidance and support of my three colleagues. While we strive to keep the contents and writing of the *Technical Manual* fresh and up to date, one thing that remains consistent is the tremendous level of peer review by members of the transfusion medicine community. Numerous AABB committee members reviewed and provided feedback on the drafts of these chapters. This extra step results in a longer production cycle, but the review by these experts makes for a better resource. No other textbook on transfusion medicine is subject to as great a level of scrutiny for accuracy and clarity of content, and consistency with both professional (AABB) and regulatory requirements.

Before starting work on this edition of the *Technical Manual*, we surveyed readers and users to determine their preferences on content, format, value in day-to-day operations, and value as a teaching tool. Respondents told us their most used, most favorite, least used, and least favorite chapters. As a reflection of this feedback, we have refocused the content on cellular therapies, retaining the chapter on transfusion support of stem cell transplantation, and having one other chapter on stem cell transplantation for a broader audience. Also a result of survey feedback, we consolidated some transfusion service topics that had appeared in multiple overlapping chapters. In the case of massive transfusion, however, we expanded coverage to address increased interest in this area. We have also added a new chapter on hemovigilance, highlighting the ever-increasing emphasis on national and international systems that recognize and identify the scope of transfusion recipient and blood donor complications, and categorize errors in both component manufacturing and transfusion processes.

Consistent with AABB being an international leader in transfusion medicine and cellular therapies, we tried where possible to provide content in this edition that is more inclusive of practices outside of the United States. We have also reorganized the presentation of content, so that chapters are grouped together as much as possible based on use in a blood collection center vs in a hospital setting. The chapters related to patient blood management have been placed among those related to "mainstream" transfusion activities, rather than among those on special patient populations.

Writing on behalf of the editors, authors, AABB committee members, and AABB office personnel, it is a tremendous privilege and honor to have produced this edition of the *Technical Manual* for the members of the transfusion medicine/blood banking community.

Mark K. Fung, MD, PhD
Editor in Chief

Contents in Print

●

Preface ix

QUALITY AND RELATED ISSUES

1. Quality Management Systems: Principles and Practice 1

    Eva D. Quinley, MS, MT(ASCP)SBB

    Background 1
    Concepts in Quality 2
    Quality Management Systems Approach 4
    Evaluation of the Quality Management System 5
    The Quality Management System in Practice 6
    Key Points 23
    References 24
    Appendix 1-1. Glossary of Commonly Used Quality Terms.............. 26
    Appendix 1-2. *Code of Federal Regulations* Quality-Related References.... 28
    Appendix 1-3. Suggested Quality Control Performance Intervals for
        Equipment and Reagents 29

2. Facilities, Work Environment, and Safety 33

    *J. Wade Atkins, MS, MT(ASCP)SBB, CQA(ASQ), and
        Leslie P. Taylor, CQA(ASQ)*

    Facilities 34
    Safety Program 36
    Fire Prevention 39
    Electrical Safety 40
    Biosafety 41
    Chemical Safety 49
    Radiation Safety 53
    Shipping Hazardous Materials 56
    General Waste Management 57
    Key Points 57
    References 58
    Appendix 2-1. Safety Regulations and Recommendations Applicable to
        Health-Care Settings 61

Appendix 2-2. General Guidelines for Safe Work Practices,
   Personal Protective Equipment, and Engineering Controls. 63
Appendix 2-3. Biosafety Level 2 Precautions 66
Appendix 2-4. Sample List of Hazardous Chemicals that May Be
   Encountered in a Blood Bank 67
Appendix 2-5. Chemical Categories and How to Work Safely with Them . . . 69
Appendix 2-6. Incidental Spill Response. 71
Appendix 2-7. Managing Hazardous Chemical Spills. 74

3. Regulatory Considerations in Transfusion Medicine and
    Cellular Therapies 77

Joseph Schwartz, MD, MPH, and Orieji Illoh, MD

FDA Oversight of Blood Establishments 78
Medical Laboratory Laws and Regulations 84
Local Laws, Hospital Regulations, and Accreditation 85
Human Cells, Tissues, and Cellular and Tissue-Based Products
   (HCT/Ps) 86
Key Points. 89
References 90

4. National Hemovigilance: The Current State 93

Kevin J. Land, MD; Barbee I. Whitaker, PhD; and Lynne Uhl, MD

International Hemovigilance 94
US Hemovigilance 97
Recipient Hemovigilance in the United States 98
Blood Donor Hemovigilance in the United States 102
Conclusion 105
Key Points. 107
References 108

BLOOD COLLECTION AND TESTING

5. Allogeneic and Autologous Blood Donor Selection 111

Debra A. Kessler, RN, MS, and Susan N. Rossmann, MD, PhD

Overview of Blood Donor Screening 111
Selection of Allogeneic Blood Donors 112
Blood-Center-Defined Donor Eligibility Criteria 117
Abbreviated DHQ for Frequent Donors 119
Recipient-Specific "Designated" or "Directed" Blood Donation 120
Key Points. 121
References 122

6.   Whole Blood and Apheresis Collections for Blood
     Components Intended for Transfusion 125

     Stephen J. Wagner, PhD

     Donor Preparation 125
     Blood Collection Process 127
     Adverse Donor Reactions 129
     WB for Component Preparation or Transfusion 131
     Descriptions of Major Blood Components 133
     Blood Component Modification 148
     Quarantine 152
     Labeling 152
     Key Points 153
     References 154

7.   Infectious Disease Screening 161

     Susan L. Stramer, PhD, and Susan A. Galel, MD

     Historical Overview of Blood Donor Screening 161
     Donor Screening Tests 165
     Residual Infectious Risks of Transfusion 177
     Screening for Specific Agents 179
     Pathogen Inactivation Technology 193
     Summary 195
     Key Points 196
     References 197

BLOOD   GROUPS

8.   Molecular Biology and Immunology in Transfusion
     Medicine 207

     James D. Gorham, MD, PhD

     Analysis of DNA 207
     Analysis of Protein 215
     Basic Immunology 220
     Key Points 227
     References 227

9.   Blood Group Genetics 229

     Christine Lomas-Francis, MSc, FIBMS

     Basic Principles of Genetics 230
     Inheritance of Genetic Traits 239
     Population Genetics 248
     Relationship Testing 250
     Blood Group Gene Mapping 251

Chimerism 252
Blood Group Terminology 252
Blood Group Genomics 253
Key Points. 261
References 262

10. ABO and Other Carbohydrate Blood Group Systems 265

Julia S. Westman, PhD, and Martin L. Olsson, MD, PhD

The ABO System 265
The H System 278
The Lewis System 281
The I Blood Group System and Ii Collection 283
P1PK and Globoside Blood Group Systems and the GLOB Collection 286
The FORS Blood Group System 290
Key Points. 291
References 292

11. The Rh System 295

Gregory A. Denomme, PhD, FCSMLS(D)

Historical Perspective 295
Terminology 298
Rh Locus 299
RHD Genotype 299
Antigens 302
Rh Genotyping 310
Rh_{null} Syndrome and RhAG Blood Group System 311
Rh Antibodies 311
Technical Considerations for Rh Typing 312
Key Points. 314
References 314

12. Other Blood Group Systems and Antigens 319

Jill R. Storry, PhD, FIBMS

The MNS System 319
M (MNS1), N (MNS2), S (MNS3), and s (MNS4) 323
The Lutheran System 326
The Kell and KX Systems 327
The Duffy System 330
The Kidd System 332
The Diego System 334
The Yt System 335
The Xg System 335
The Scianna System 336
The Dombrock System 336
The Colton System 337
The Landsteiner-Wiener System 337

The Chido/Rodgers System 338
The Gerbich System 338
The Cromer System 339
The Knops System 339
The Indian System 340
The Ok System 340
The RAPH System 340
The John Milton Hagen System 341
The Gill System 341
The RHAG System 341
The FORS System 341
The Jr System 341
The Lan System 342
The Vel System 342
The CD59 System 342
The Augustine System 342
Antigens that Do Not Yet Belong to a Blood Group System 343
Erythroid Phenotypes Caused by Mutations in Transcription
    Factor Genes 344
Key Points 345
References 345

13. Identification of Antibodies to Red Cell Antigens 349

*Janis R. Hamilton, MS, MT(ASCP)SBB, and
    Debra J. Bailey, MT(ASCP)SBB*

Basic Concepts in Red Cell Antigen Expression 350
Initial Antibody Identification Considerations 351
Basic Antibody Identification 353
Complex Antibody Identification 359
Selected Procedures 371
Considerations Following Antibody Identification 377
Immunohematology Reference Laboratories 380
Key Points 381
References 382
Suggested Readings 384

14. The Positive Direct Antiglobulin Test and Immune-Mediated Hemolysis 385

*Regina M. Leger, MSQA, MT(ASCP)SBB, CMQ/OE(ASQ), and
    P. Dayand Borge Jr, MD, PhD*

The DAT 386
Autoimmune Hemolytic Anemia 391
Drug-Induced Immune Hemolytic Anemia 401
Key Points 405
References 406
Appendix 14-1. Drugs Associated with Immune Hemolytic Anemia...... 409

15. Platelet and Granulocyte Antigens and Antibodies 413

Ralph R. Vassallo, MD, FACP, and
Brian R. Curtis, PhD, D(ABMLI), MT(ASCP)SBB

Platelet Antigens and Antibodies 413
Granulocyte Antigens and Antibodies 425
Key Points... 429
References 429

16. The HLA System 435

Arthur B. Eisenbrey III, MD, PhD, and Patricia M. Kopko, MD

Biochemistry, Tissue Distribution, and Structure 436
Genetics of the MHC 440
Identification of HLA Antigens and Alleles 444
Crossmatching and Detection of HLA Antibodies 447
The HLA System and Transfusion 447
HLA Testing and Transplantation 450
Other Clinically Significant Aspects of HLA 452
Summary 453
Key Points... 454
References 454

ESSENTIALS OF TRANSFUSION PRACTICE

17. Transfusion-Service-Related Activities: Pretransfusion
     Testing and Storage, Monitoring, Processing,
     Distribution, and Inventory Management of
     Blood Components 457

Sarah K. Harm, MD, and Nancy M. Dunbar, MD

Samples and Requests 457
Pretransfusion Testing of Recipient Blood 458
Blood and Blood Component Storage and Monitoring 463
Pretransfusion Processing 471
Distribution 474
Issuing of Components 476
Inventory Management 479
Key Points... 481
References 482
Appendix 17-1. Sources of False-Positive Results in Antiglobulin
     Testing 485
Appendix 17-2. Sources of False-Negative Results in Antiglobulin
     Testing 486
Appendix 17-3. Causes of Positive Pretransfusion Test Results 487

18. Administration of Blood Components 489

Melanie Jorgenson, RN, BSN, LSSGB

Events and Considerations Before Dispensing Components 489
Blood Component Transportation and Dispensing 494
Administration 495
Documentation of the Transfusion 499
Unique Transfusion Settings 500
Conclusions 501
Key Points 501
References 502

19. Hemotherapy Decisions and Their Outcomes 505

Richard M. Kaufman, MD, and Nadine Shehata, MD, FRCP

Red Blood Cell Transfusion 505
Platelet Transfusion 511
Plasma Transfusion 516
Cryoprecipitate Transfusion 518
Granulocyte Transfusion 519
Key Points 520
References 521

20. Patient Blood Management 527

Kathleen E. Puca, MD, MT(ASCP)SBB

Definition and Scope of Patient Blood Management 527
The Rationale for PBM 528
Basic Elements of a PBM Program 529
Key Points 540
References 540
Appendix 20-1. Pharmacologic Therapies for Supporting Patient
    Blood Management 546
Appendix 20-2 . Responsibilities for Activity Levels 1, 2, and 3
    PBM Programs... 555

21. Approaches to Blood Utilization Auditing 557

Irina Maramica, MD, PhD, MBA, and Ira A. Shulman, MD

The Auditing Process 558
Types of Blood Utilization Review 559
Blood Utilization Review of Transfusions to High-Risk Patients 562
The Role of a Computerized Provider Order Entry System in
    Blood Utilization Review 563
Use of "Big Data" to Assess Performance and Progress Measures in
    Transfusion Medicine 564
Key Points 565
References 566

22. Noninfectious Complications of Blood Transfusion 569

William J. Savage, MD, PhD, and Eldad A. Hod, MD

Hemovigilance 569
Recognition and Evaluation of a Suspected Transfusion Reaction 569
Acute or Immediate Transfusion Reactions 576
Delayed Transfusion Reactions 588
Fatality Reporting Requirements 592
Key Points 593
References 594

SPECIAL PATIENTS AND SITUATIONS

23. Perinatal Issues in Transfusion Practice 599

*Meghan Delaney, DO, MPH; Annika M. Svensson, MD, PhD;
    Lani Lieberman, MD, MSc*

Hemolytic Disease of the Fetus and Newborn 599
Thrombocytopenia 605
Key Points 608
References 608

24. Neonatal and Pediatric Transfusion Practice 613

Edward C.C. Wong, MD, and Rowena C. Punzalan, MD

Transfusion in Infants Younger than 4 Months 613
Transfusion in Infants Older than 4 Months and Children 628
Prevention of Adverse Effects of Transfusion in the Pediatric
    Population 632
Key Points 634
References 634

25. Therapeutic Apheresis 641

Chester Andrzejewski Jr, PhD, MD, and Robertson D. Davenport, MD

General Principles 641
Device Modalities 642
Patient Evaluation and Management 643
Vascular Access 645
Anticoagulation 646
Adverse Effects 646
Therapeutic Apheresis Indications 648
Therapeutic Apheresis Procedure Documentation, Payment, and
    Provider Credentialing 663
Key Points 663
References 664

26. The Collection and Processing of Hematopoietic
    Progenitor Cells 667

    Eapen K. Jacob, MD, and Scott A. Koepsell, MD, PhD

    Clinical Utility 667
    Determination of Graft Source 670
    Collection/Sources of HPCs 672
    Processing HPCs 674
    Specialized Cell-Processing Methods 675
    Cryopreservation 676
    QC 676
    Shipping and Transporting HPC Cellular Products 677
    Patient Care 677
    Other Regulatory Considerations 678
    Conclusion 678
    Key Points 679
    References 679

27. Transfusion Support for Hematopoietic Stem Cell
    Transplant Recipients 683

    Melissa M. Cushing, MD, and Jeanne E. Hendrickson, MD

    ABO- and Non-ABO-Red-Cell-Antigen-Incompatible Transplantation ... 684
    Blood Component Considerations 685
    Neutropenic Patients with Infections Unresponsive to
        Antimicrobial Therapy 689
    Special Processing of Blood Components for Recipients of HSCT 689
    Special Considerations for Transfusing Pediatric HSCT Recipients 690
    Information Portability for HSCT Recipients 690
    Key Points 691
    References 691

28. Human Tissue Allografts and the Hospital
    Transfusion Service 695

    *Annette J. Schlueter, MD, PhD; Cassandra D. Josephson, MD; and
    Scott A. Brubaker, CTBS*

    Tissue Donation and Transplantation 695
    Federal Regulations, State Laws, and Professional Standards 700
    Hospital Tissue Services 701
    Key Points 706
    References 707

Index 709

Contents on USB Flash Card

METHODS

1. General Laboratory Methods—Introduction

Method 1-1. Shipping Hazardous Materials
Method 1-2. Monitoring Temperature During Shipment of Blood
Method 1-3. Treating Incompletely Clotted Specimens
Method 1-4. Solution Preparation Procedure
Method 1-5. Serum Dilution Procedure
Method 1-6. Dilution of Percentage Solutions Procedure
Method 1-7. Preparing a 3% Red Cell Suspension
Method 1-8. Preparing and Using Phosphate Buffer
Method 1-9. Reading and Grading Tube Agglutination

2. Red Cell Typing Methods—Introduction

Method 2-1. Determining ABO Group of Red Cells—Slide Test
Method 2-2. Determining ABO Group of Red Cells and Serum—Tube Test
Method 2-3. Determining ABO Group of Red Cells and Serum—Microplate Test
Method 2-4. Initial Investigation of ABO Grouping Discrepancies Procedure
Method 2-5. Detecting Weak A and B Antigens and Antibodies by Cold
   Temperature Enhancement
Method 2-6. Confirming Weak A and B Antigens Using Enzyme-Treated Red Cells
Method 2-7. Confirming Weak A or B Subgroup by Adsorption and Elution
Method 2-8. Testing Saliva for A, B, H, Le^a, and Le^b Antigens
Method 2-9. Confirming Anti-A$_1$ in an A$_2$ or Weak A Subgroup
Method 2-10. Resolving ABO Discrepancies Caused by Unexpected Alloantibodies
Method 2-11. Determining Serum Group Without Centrifugation
Method 2-12. Determining Rh(D) Type—Slide Test
Method 2-13. Determining Rh(D) Type—Tube Test
Method 2-14. Determining Rh(D) Type—Microplate Test
Method 2-15. Testing for Weak D
Method 2-16. Preparing and Using Lectins
Method 2-17. Removing Autoantibody by Warm Saline Washes
Method 2-18. Using Sulfhydryl Reagents to Disperse Autoagglutination
Method 2-19. Using Gentle Heat Elution to Test Red Cells with a Positive DAT Result
Method 2-20. Dissociating IgG by Chloroquine for Antigen Testing of Red Cells
   with a Positive DAT Result
Method 2-21. Using Acid Glycine/EDTA to Remove Antibodies from Red Cells
Method 2-22. Separating Transfused from Autologous Red Cells by Simple
   Centrifugation
Method 2-23. Separating Transfused from Autologous Red Cells in Patients with
   Hemoglobin S Disease

3.   Antibody Detection, Identification, and Compatibility Testing—
      Introduction

Method 3-1. Using Immediate-Spin Compatibility Testing to Demonstrate ABO
      Incompatibility
Method 3-2. Saline Indirect Antiglobulin Test Procedure
Method 3-3. Albumin or LISS-Additive Indirect Antiglobulin Test Procedure
Method 3-4. LISS-Suspension Indirect Antiglobulin Test Procedure
Method 3-5. PEG Indirect Antiglobulin Test Procedure
Method 3-6. Prewarming Procedure
Method 3-7. Detecting Antibodies in the Presence of Rouleaux—Saline
      Replacement
Method 3-8. Preparing Ficin Enzyme Stock, 1% w/v
Method 3-9. Preparing Papain Enzyme Stock, 1% w/v
Method 3-10. Standardizing Enzyme Procedures
Method 3-11. Evaluating Enzyme-Treated Red Cells
Method 3-12. One-Stage Enzyme Procedure
Method 3-13. Two-Stage Enzyme Procedure
Method 3-14. Performing a Direct Antiglobulin Test
Method 3-15. Antibody Titration Procedure
Method 3-16. Using Sulfhydryl Reagents to Distinguish IgM from IgG Antibodies
Method 3-17. Using Plasma Inhibition to Distinguish Anti-Ch and -Rg from
      Other Antibodies with Similar Characteristics
Method 3-18. Treating Red Cells Using DTT or AET
Method 3-19. Neutralizing Anti-Sd^a with Urine
Method 3-20. Adsorption Procedure
Method 3-21. Using the American Rare Donor Program

4.   Investigation of a Positive DAT Result—Introduction

Method 4-1. Cold-Acid Elution Procedure
Method 4-2. Glycine-HCl/EDTA Elution Procedure
Method 4-3. Heat Elution Procedure
Method 4-4. Lui Freeze-Thaw Elution Procedure
Method 4-5. Cold Autoadsorption Procedure
Method 4-6. Determining the Specificity of Cold-Reactive Autoagglutinins
Method 4-7. Cold Agglutinin Titer Procedure
Method 4-8. Adsorbing Warm-Reactive Autoantibodies Using Autologous Red
      Cells
Method 4-9. Adsorbing Warm-Reactive Autoantibodies Using Allogeneic Red Cells
Method 4-10. Polyethylene Glycol Adsorption Procedure
Method 4-11. Performing the Donath-Landsteiner Test
Method 4-12. Detecting Drug Antibodies by Testing Drug-Treated Red Cells
Method 4-13. Detecting Drug Antibodies by Testing in the Presence of Drug

5.   Hemolytic Disease of the Fetus and Newborn—Introduction

      Method 5-1. Testing for Fetomaternal Hemorrhage—The Rosette Test
      Method 5-2. Testing for Fetomaternal Hemorrhage—Modified Kleihauer-Betke
          Test
      Method 5-3. Using Antibody Titration Studies to Assist in Early Detection of
          Hemolytic Disease of the Fetus and Newborn

6.   Blood Collection, Component Preparation, and Storage—
          Introduction

      Method 6-1. Screening Female Donors for Acceptable Hemoglobin Level—
          Copper Sulfate Method
      Method 6-2. Preparing the Donor's Arm for Blood Collection
      Method 6-3. Collecting Blood and Samples for Processing and Testing
      Method 6-4. Preparing Red Blood Cells from Whole Blood
      Method 6-5. Preparing Prestorage Red Blood Cells Leukocytes Reduced from
          Whole Blood
      Method 6-6. Using High-Concentration Glycerol to Cryopreserve Red Cells—
          Meryman Method
      Method 6-7. Using High-Concentration Glycerol to Cryopreserve Red Cells—
          Valeri Method
      Method 6-8. Checking the Adequacy of Deglycerolization of Red Blood Cells
      Method 6-9. Preparing Fresh Frozen Plasma from Whole Blood
      Method 6-10. Preparing Cryoprecipitated AHF from Whole Blood
      Method 6-11. Thawing and Pooling Cryoprecipitated AHF
      Method 6-12. Preparing Platelets from Whole Blood
      Method 6-13. Removing Plasma from Platelets (Volume Reduction)

7.   Transplantation of Cells and Tissue—Introduction

      Method 7-1. Infusing Cryopreserved Hematopoietic Cells
      Method 7-2. Processing Umbilical Cord Blood
      Method 7-3. Investigating Adverse Events and Infections Following Tissue
          Allograft Use

8.   Quality Control Methods—Introduction

      Method 8-1. Validating Copper Sulfate Solution
      Method 8-2. Calibrating Liquid-in-Glass Laboratory Thermometers
      Method 8-3. Calibrating Electronic Oral Thermometers
      Method 8-4. Testing Refrigerator Alarms
      Method 8-5. Testing Freezer Alarms
      Method 8-6. Calibrating Centrifuges for Platelet Separation
      Method 8-7. Calibrating a Serologic Centrifuge for Immediate Agglutination
      Method 8-8. Calibrating a Serologic Centrifuge for Washing and Antiglobulin
          Testing
      Method 8-9. Testing Automatic Cell Washers

Method 8-10. Monitoring Cell Counts of Apheresis Components
Method 8-11. Counting Residual White Cells in Leukocyte-Reduced Blood and
    Components—Manual Method

APPENDICES

Appendix 1. Normal Values in Adults
Appendix 2. Selected Normal Values in Children
Appendix 3. Typical Normal Values in Tests of Hemostasis and Coagulation
    (Adults)
Appendix 4. Coagulation Factor Values in Platelet Concentrates
Appendix 5. Approximate Normal Values for Red Cell, Plasma, and Blood
    Volumes
Appendix 6. Blood Group Antigens Assigned to Systems
Appendix 7. Examples of Gene, Antigen, and Phenotype Symbols in
    Conventional and International Society of Blood Transfusion Terminology
Appendix 8. Examples of Correct and Incorrect Terminology
Appendix 9. Distribution of ABO/Rh Phenotypes by Race or Ethnicity
Appendix 10. Example of a Maximum Surgical Blood Order Schedule

Chapter 1

Quality Management Systems: Principles and Practice

• ● •

Eva D. Quinley, MS, MT(ASCP)SBB

A QUALITY MANAGEMENT system (QMS) is a collection of business processes focused on achieving quality while meeting customer requirements. It is expressed as the organizational structure, policies, procedures, processes, and resources needed to implement quality management. Why is this important in the fields of transfusion medicine and cellular therapies? The answer to this is simple—the customers served, whether they are other health-care providers or patients, depend on the assurance that the products and services produced and provided are safe and effective for their intended use. A QMS is the framework for continual improvement by enhancing customer satisfaction. In a QMS, customer requirements are defined, processes are designed to meet those requirements, and processes are in place to manage and improve the level of service that is provided.

It is also the expectation of regulators that organizations have processes in place to ensure that products and services are safe and successful in producing the desired results. The implementation of an effective QMS will help to ensure these outcomes.

Finally, with decreases in utilization and increased costs of operations, it is also important that organizations involved in transfusion medicine and cellular therapies operate in the most cost-effective manner possible. A good QMS will reduce rework, waste, and inefficiencies; thus, an organization will spend fewer resources to achieve the same operational and quality outcomes. An effective QMS provides confidence to the customer, the organization, and other interested parties that the organization will provide products and services that consistently meet or exceed requirements or customer expectations, and it increases efficiencies, thus reducing costs.

BACKGROUND

Quality has been central to transfusion medicine from its inception, the opening of the first blood bank in the United States at the Cook County Hospital in Chicago in 1937. Continuous scientific progress in many aspects of transfusion medicine has contributed to the quality and safety of blood components and transfusion services, and now cellular therapies. During the 1990s, after the advent of

Eva D. Quinley, MS, MT(ASCP)SBB, Chief Operating Officer, MEDIC Regional Blood Center, Knoxville, Tennessee and Regional Executive Director, LifeSource, Chicago, Illinois
E. Quinley has disclosed a financial relationship with Velico Medical.

AIDS and the human immunodeficiency virus (HIV), a very sensitized and informed public demanded that the highest level of quality be achieved and maintained in all processes involved in the provision of all blood components and services. The Food and Drug Administration (FDA) introduced the concept of a "zero risk blood supply" as the industry goal, a goal to strive for but in reality one that cannot be totally achieved. Regulatory agencies such as the FDA, the Centers for Medicare and Medicaid Services (CMS), state departments of health, and accrediting organizations such as AABB, the College of American Pathologists (CAP), The Joint Commission, and the Foundation for the Accreditation of Cellular Therapies (FACT) require facilities operating in transfusion medicine and cellular therapies to establish and follow a quality control (QC) and quality assurance program as part of their licensing, certification, and/or accreditation programs. Every laboratory must comply with the Clinical Laboratory Improvement Amendments of 1988 (CLIA), quality requirements implemented by CMS. In 1995, the FDA released its *Guideline for Quality Assurance in Blood Establishments*. This guideline, along with other FDA-issued guidelines, assists facilities in compliance with the current good manufacturing practice (cGMP) requirements found in the *Code of Federal Regulations* (CFR), Title 21, Parts 200 and 600. Title 21 CFR Part 820 provides regulations applicable to manufacturers of medical devices, including blood establishment computer systems (BECS). Formerly known as the GMP requirements for medical devices, the regulations found in Part 820 are known as the quality system regulation.

The AABB's Quality System Essentials (QSEs), minimum requirements for blood banking and cellular therapy operations, are based on all of these specifications and provide additional guidance in implementing practices that ensure quality and compliance with cGMP and current good tissue practice (cGTP) regulations. AABB and CAP are granted "deemed status" as accrediting organizations under the CLIA '88 program by CMS, as well as The Joint Commission and some state regulatory bodies. The International Organization for Standardization (ISO) has established international standards in most fields, which represent minimal requirements. These standards are generic in content and can be applied to any organization, large or small, whatever its product may be. The United States is represented in ISO by the American National Standards Institute (ANSI). The Clinical and Laboratory Standards Institute (CLSI), formerly the National Committee for Clinical Laboratory Standards (NCCLS), a global organization headquartered in the United States, is a member of ANSI. The FDA and AABB incorporate many ISO principles into their regulations and standards. For example, AABB's QSEs are rooted in the 20 clauses of the ISO 9000 series and are compatible with ISO standards.

CONCEPTS IN QUALITY

Quality Assurance

The concept of quality assurance is broad, and the goals of quality assurance are to significantly decrease errors; ensure the credibility of results; implement safe and effective manufacturing processes and system controls; and ensure continued product safety and quality. A quality assurance program is defined as a system designed and implemented to ensure that manufacturing is consistently performed in such a way as to yield a product of consistent quality.[1] A good quality assurance program includes ways to detect, investigate, assess, prioritize, and correct errors, with the ultimate goal of error prevention. Quality assurance activities also include retrospective reviews and analyses of operational performance data to determine whether the overall process is in a state of control and to detect shifts or trends that require attention. Quality assurance provides information to process managers regarding levels of performance that can be used in setting priorities for process improvement.

Quality Control

QC is one aspect of a quality assurance program. Its purpose is to determine, through testing or observation, if a process or particular task within a process is working as expected at a given time. QC involves sampling and testing. Historically, transfusion services and donor centers have used many QC measures as standard practices in their operations. Examples include reagent QC; product QC; clerical checks; visual inspections; and regular measurements, such as temperature readings on refrigerators and volume or cell counts on finished blood components. If QC is not within specifications, it may indicate a problem, either with the process itself or with how the process is being executed. Trends in QC may indicate the potential for a problem in the future.

Quality Management

Quality management considers interrelated processes in the context of the organization and its relations with customers and suppliers. It addresses the leadership role of executive management in creating a commitment to quality throughout the organization, the understanding of suppliers and customers as partners in quality, the management of human and other resources, and quality planning. An important goal in quality management is to establish a set of controls that ensure process and product quality but are not excessive. Controls that do not add value should be eliminated to conserve limited resources and allow staff to focus attention on those controls that are critical to the operation.

Statistical tools, such as process capability measurement and control charts, allow a facility to evaluate process performance during the planning stage and in operations. These tools help determine if a process is stable (ie, in statistical control) and if it is capable of meeting product and service specifications.

Quality Systems

A system is defined as an organized, purposeful structure that consists of interrelated and interdependent elements (components, processes, entities, factors, members, parts, etc). These elements continually influence one another (directly or indirectly) to maintain their activity and the existence of the system, in order to achieve the goal of the system. The quality system is made up of a set of interrelated processes that work together to ensure quality. (See Fig 1-1.)

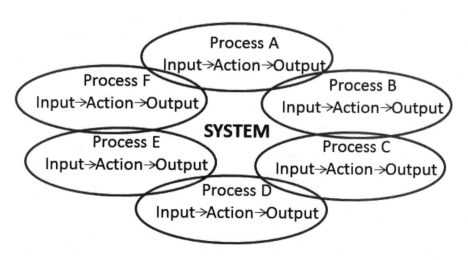

FIGURE 1-1. Systems and processes.

It is important to understand what a process is. Basically, a process can be defined as a set of activities that uses resources to transform inputs to outputs. The whole blood collection process, for example, has many inputs, such as a trained phlebotomist, an approved collection set, an approved arm-scrub solution, and phlebotomy standard operating procedures (SOPs), all working together to produce the output, a unit of whole blood. The quality of the output is determined by the quality and control that is in place with the inputs and with the process itself. Validation of a process is key in ensuring the process is consistent and produces the desired output. Validation is discussed more fully later in this chapter.

Control of the Process

Strategies for managing a process should address all of its components, including its interrelated activities, inputs, outputs, and resources. Supplier qualification, formal agreements, supply verification, and inventory control are strategies for ensuring that the inputs to a process meet specifications. Personnel training and competency assessment, equipment maintenance and control, management of documents and records, and implementation of appropriate in-process controls provide assurance that the process will operate as intended. End-product testing and inspection, customer feedback, and outcome measurement provide data to evaluate product quality and improve the process. These output measurements and quality indicators are used to evaluate the effectiveness of the process and process controls.

To manage a system of processes effectively, the facility must understand how its processes interact and what cause-and-effect relationships exist between them. As an example, the consequences of accepting a donor who is not eligible reach into almost every other process in the facility. For example, if a donor with a history of high-risk behavior is not identified as such during the selection process, the donated unit(s) may return positive test results for one of the viral marker assays, trigger-

ing follow-up testing, look-back investigations, and donor deferral and notification procedures. Components must be quarantined and their discard documented. Personnel involved in collecting and processing the unit(s) are at risk of exposure to infectious agents. Part of quality planning is to identify these relationships so that quick and appropriate corrective action can be taken when process controls fail.

It is important to remember that operational processes include not only product manufacture or service creation, but also the distribution of a product or service. Distribution generally involves interaction with the customer. The quality of that transaction is critical to customer satisfaction and should not be overlooked in the design and ongoing assessment of the QMS.

Quality Planning

A necessary activity to ensure success of the QMS is quality planning. This is defined as "a systematic process that translates quality policy into measurable objectives and requirements, and lays down a sequence of steps for realizing them within a specified time frame."[2] A written quality plan provides the framework for implementing and maintaining an effective QMS. This should be a living document that is reviewed and edited as needed.

QUALITY MANAGEMENT SYSTEMS APPROACH

To develop and implement a QMS, it is important for organizations to follow a planned path. The steps of this path include:

1. Determining the needs and expectations of the customer and other interested parties.
2. Establishing a quality policy and quality objectives.
3. Determining the processes needed to obtain those quality objectives and who is responsible for those processes.
4. Ensuring adequate resources are available to execute those processes.

5. Determining and applying methods to evaluate those processes, including making a determination of the effectiveness and efficiency of each process.

6. Designing ways to prevent nonconformances and ways to correct nonconformances that are not prevented.

7. Establishing a process for continual improvement of the QMS.

Such an approach can be used to develop a QMS or to maintain and improve an existing QMS. The needs and expectations of the customer or interested parties must be defined and documented as fully as possible. The voice of the customer is critical to success. Once an organization understands what customers want, a quality policy and quality objectives should be developed with that information in mind. It is important to consider those who regulate or accredit the organization in the development of the policy and objectives. Although some do not consider these bodies as customers, they certainly have a vested interest in an organization that operates in transfusion medicine or cellular therapies. Resources to achieve the objectives must be determined, and then there must be a way to ensure that they are adequate. As described further in the next section, once the policy, objectives, and procedures are in place, methods to evaluate the effectiveness and efficiency of these are necessary. A major goal is to find ways to prevent nonconformances from happening in the first place, but because of the nature of the work, nonconformances will occur. When they do, it is imperative to have a method that not only corrects nonconformances but prevents them from happening again. Finally, because a quality system is somewhat dynamic, a philosophy of continual improvement needs to be developed and executed.

EVALUATION OF THE QUALITY MANAGEMENT SYSTEM

It is important to evaluate the QMS routinely to determine if it is working as expected. The evaluation should include the following items:

- Engagement of the stakeholders.
- Purpose of the evaluation.
- Audience for the evaluation.
- Information needed for the evaluation.
- Sources for information related to the evaluation.
- Tools.

Evaluation begins with the engagement of those who have vested interest in the results of the evaluation. In blood establishments and cellular therapy facilities, stakeholders most often include quality, operations, and management but might include other areas such as recruitment and even human resources depending upon what processes are being evaluated. The purpose of the evaluation should be aligned with issues of greatest concern. For example, one area of concern to blood establishments and to their customers is product availability. An evaluation of product availability would provide information as to whether the right product is available at the right time, and opportunities to improve where this falls short. The audience for the evaluation is determined by the stakeholders and usually would include senior management and perhaps regulators or those groups that accredit the organization.

Information needed for the evaluation depends on the purpose and the audience. Once these are decided, then information can be gathered to support decision-making or to simply inform. The information may come from a number of sources: production reports, error reports, audits or inspections, and customer feedback, to name a few.

A number of tools exist to evaluate the information. A tool is any chart, device, software, strategy, or technique that supports quality management efforts. Many of the tools are easy to use, but it is important that the audience be considered when choosing which tools to use. A number of software vendors produce software that is designed specifically to monitor and evaluate the QMS.

THE QUALITY MANAGEMENT SYSTEM IN PRACTICE

Several elements comprise a QMS, and the application of those elements in transfusion medicine and cellular therapies is described in the text that follows. Basic elements of the QMS include:

- Organization and leadership.
- Customer focus.
- Human resources.
- Equipment management.
- Suppliers and materials management.
- Process control and management.
- Documents and records.
- Information management.
- Management of nonconforming events.
- Monitoring and evaluation.
- Process improvement.
- Facilities, work environment, and safety.

Organization and Leadership

An organization must be structured such that the QMS can be well implemented. The structure should facilitate communication throughout the organization. It is also important that clear descriptions of authority and the responsibilities of each role are defined in writing. The role of senior management is fundamental to the success of any QMS. It is the responsibility of leadership to create an environment where individuals are fully engaged in the QMS and to monitor it to ensure that the system operates effectively. Specific duties assigned to top management include:

- Establishing, implementing, and maintaining a quality policy and associated quality goals and quality objectives.
- Providing adequate resources to carry out the operations of the facility and the QMS.
- Ensuring appropriate design and effective implementation of new or modified processes and procedures.
- Participating in the review and approval of policies, processes, and procedures.
- Enforcing adherence to operational and quality policies, processes, and procedures.

- Overseeing operations and regulatory and accreditation compliance.
- Periodically reviewing and assessing QMS effectiveness.
- Identifying designees and defining their responsibilities when assisting executive management in carrying out these duties.

The individual who is assigned to oversee an organization's quality activities should report to top management. This individual may perform some of the tasks but does not have to personally perform all the quality functions. It is desirable for this individual to operate totally separate from operations, although in smaller organizations the individual may be involved in operational activities as well. The key here is that the individual should never review his or her own work. Quality functions include the following:

- Review and approval of SOPs.
- Review and approval of training plans.
- Review and approval of validation protocols and results.
- Review, validation, and approval of QMS software.
- Audit of operational functions.
- Development of evaluation criteria for systems.
- Review and approval of suppliers and maintenance of an approved supplier list.
- Review of product specifications.
- Review of reports of adverse reactions, error reports, and complaints.
- Determination of the suitability of products.
- Monitoring and trending.
- Inspection oversight and management.
- Reporting to regulators, accrediting bodies, customers, or others as necessary.

Although traditionally the quality department has had responsibility for the majority of these activities, it may be wise to have operations participate in some of these activities, again with the caveat that one does not review one's own work. This takes some of the burden from the quality department and reinforces the concept that quality is everyone's responsibility.

Customer Focus

To obtain true quality, it is imperative for an organization to understand the needs and requirements of the customer. Organizations that provide blood components or other cellular products and services have a variety of customers, and each should be considered. Processes and services should be designed and developed with the customer requirements in mind. Customer requirements need to be documented; oftentimes the documentation is contained in a supplier agreement or contract. Once the requirements are established, there should be a mechanism to receive feedback from the customer at regular intervals to determine if the requirements are being met. Such feedback may be obtained from an analysis of key metrics developed in conjunction with the customer or may be gleaned from customer surveys.

Human Resources

The human resources department is focused on activities relating to employees. These activities normally include recruiting and hiring of new employees, orientation and training of current employees, ongoing staffing needs, employee benefits, and retention. Staffing must be adequate to perform the work and to support the QMS.

Job Descriptions

Organizations should have well-written job descriptions for all personnel. The job descriptions should identify the key role and responsibilities of a particular position, as well as educational and experiential requirements. In some cases, the job description also contains physical requirements such as lifting a certain amount of weight or the ability to stand for long hours. Certain requirements in a job description may be the result of regulatory requirements or industry standards. For example, in some states individuals must have certain licenses to perform laboratory testing.

Such requirements should be well defined within each job description. Job descriptions should be periodically reviewed to ensure that they are truly reflective of what an individual does in a particular job. Employees should sign their initial job descriptions and any revisions to those job descriptions to indicate they are aware of what their job entails. Often, regulators or accrediting agencies request to see current signed job descriptions during their inspections or assessments of an organization. An additional benefit of a well-written job description is that it serves as an aid to the development of a training curriculum.

Hiring

Human resources oversees the hiring process, which includes activities such as contacting candidates, setting up interviews, and ensuring new employees are oriented. It may also include preemployment screening such as drug testing. During the hiring process, job qualifications are matched against applicant qualifications, and individuals are selected for hire based on their ability to meet those job qualifications, including training, education, and experience.

Orientation and Training

Orientation is critical for a new employee to get the right start. Each employee needs to understand not only his or her role but also how that role fits in the organization. Orientation training generally will include an overview of the organization and its customers, benefits training, an introduction to cGMP and/or cGTP regulations, and safety training.

Specific training for tasks that are performed as part of an individual's actual job usually occurs in the operational department where the individual is hired. Training on SOPs that the individual will need to perform those tasks is required. Additionally, each employee needs to fully understand the cGMP/cGTP requirements applicable in the performance of a job. All training must be documented, and initial and ongoing assessments of competence are required.

Competency Assessments

To ensure that staff maintain the ability to perform their jobs well, routine competency assessments should be conducted to determine their level of competence in performing the work. Organizations need to have a written plan for the conduct of competency assessments, and that plan must include what should be done if an individual does not pass the assessment. CMS has specific requirements for competency assessments of testing personnel. The following six procedures are the minimal regulatory requirements for assessment of competency for such individuals:

1. Direct observations of routine patient test performance, including patient preparation, if applicable, specimen handling, processing, and testing.
2. Monitoring the recording and reporting of test results.
3. Review of intermediate test results or worksheets, QC records, proficiency testing results, and preventive maintenance records.
4. Direct observations of the performance of instrument maintenance and function checks.
5. Assessment of test performance through testing previously analyzed specimens, internal blind testing samples, or external proficiency testing samples.
6. Assessment of problem-solving skills.

Competency assessment, which includes the six procedures, must be performed for testing personnel for each test the individual is approved to perform by the laboratory director.[3]

The competency program should be documented and administered fairly to all staff as required. There should be a defined schedule for the administration of the assessments. Documentation of the results of competency assessments should be available for inspection by regulatory or accrediting bodies.

Equipment Management

Equipment used in processes must be installed as directed by the manufacturer and qualified to ensure that it is working as the manufacturer states it should work. This qualification should be accomplished according to written procedures and should be documented. Qualification is necessary as part of validation activities, including installation qualification. (See the section on validation later in this chapter.) Organizations must ensure that they operate equipment in line with manufacturers' recommendations. Manufacturers may have requirements for temperature, humidity, surrounding space, or other environmental conditions for operation, which must be considered.

Equipment must be maintained to ensure proper working conditions. Organizations should have written programs for equipment cleaning and maintenance, again in line with manufacturers' recommendations. Preventive maintenance should be established and well documented. Records of this work must be available for inspectors or assessors to view.

For equipment used in measurement, routine calibration is required. Calibration involves comparing a measurement device to a known standard and then adjusting it, if necessary, to measure the same as the standard. Routine calibration is a requirement for some equipment. An organization should have a written program for calibration that lists what should be calibrated, the frequency of calibration, and procedures for performing the calibration. The manufacturer should recommend the frequency of calibration, and regulations can be found in the CFR.[4] However, if no guidance is available, the organization should follow standard practice in the industry or, if none exists, should establish a reasonable frequency based on the criticality of the measurement.

The actual performance of calibration can be outsourced to an approved outside vendor, but it is the organization's responsibility to maintain calibration records and to ensure that the vendor performs the activities in compliance with applicable regulations and standards. Calibration records and procedures need to be available during inspections and assessments.

Equipment QC, performed routinely, is also important in ensuring that equipment is operating as expected. Documentation of any QC that is performed should be evaluated in a timely manner, and the results should be evaluated to determine if there are trends over time that may indicate the equipment is beginning to fail. The frequency of QC again is dependent on the criticality of the function of the equipment. Equipment used in determining donor eligibility, for example, may require daily QC because of the criticality of its use. Review of QC records needs to be timely to limit the scope of investigation should the review reveal a problem.

Selection of Equipment

Organizations should select equipment based on its ability to meet preestablished and documented specifications. Other factors that should be considered are cost, service, history with others in the industry, and support. Usually, organizations have several vendors from which to choose, and thus the additional factors become even more important. It is key that organizations establish criteria on the front end of the selection process; the equipment should fit the organization's needs. Workflow should be well defined before selection of equipment. The organization should not have to alter its process to fit the equipment unless there is only one supplier and no other choice. The manufacturer of the equipment should be qualified according to the organization's supplier qualification process.

Equipment Identification

Equipment should be identified, and a list of equipment should be maintained. This list should be kept up to date, and when equipment is moved from one location to another or removed from service, the action taken should be recorded. Because of the amount of equipment in an organization that performs blood banking, transfusion medicine, or cellular therapy activities, tracking equipment can be a daunting task. Software vendors have developed automated solutions to assist organizations with this, but even if it must be done manually, the tracking of equipment is necessary. Equipment that is out of service should be removed from operational areas, if at all possible, and clearly labeled as out of service so it will not be used in the manufacturing process.

Suppliers and Materials Management

Ensuring that a supplier can provide what is needed to perform the work and that the supplies meet preestablished specifications is a critical aspect of the QMS. Organizations must determine and document requirements and seek suppliers, through the process of supplier qualification, that meet those requirements.

Supplier Qualification

Supplier qualification is a process whereby an organization determines whether or not a supplier can meet its requirements. Such requirements usually include the ability to meet regulations, the availability of supply, the timeliness of delivery, responsiveness to issues and problems, cost, and support. Other requirements may be specific to the organization. It is a common practice for organizations to participate in buying groups that perform qualification of suppliers for those participating in the group.

Supplier qualification may include surveys to the supplier, surveys to customers that the supplier currently serves, and onsite audits of the supplier. Surveys may be more cost-effective, but on-site audits are generally considered best if the supplier is providing materials or services that are critical to operations. In fact, the more critical the materials supplied, the more stringent the qualification should be. See Table 1-1 for a list of factors that may be considered during supplier qualification.

An organization should maintain a list of approved suppliers. This list should be reviewed routinely for each supplier's ability to consistently meet the needs of the organization. Suppliers can be added or removed from the list as necessary. Management of the list

TABLE 1-1. Factors to Consider in Supplier Qualification

Factor	Examples
Licensure, certification, or accreditation	FDA, ISO, EU
Supplier-relevant quality documents	Quality manual, complaint handling methodology
Results of audits or inspections	Previous FDA inspections, supplier qualification audit
Supply or product requirements	Ability to meet functional requirements
Cost of materials and services	Product cost, maintenance fees, parts costs
Delivery arrangements	Standing orders, turnaround time for stat
Financial security and market position	How long the organization has been in business, IRS 990
Support after sale	Training, validation guidance, contract/agreement review meetings

FDA = Food and Drug Administration; ISO = International Organization for Standardization; EU = European Union; IRS 990 = Internal Revenue Service Form 990.

usually falls to the quality department, although it could be placed in an area such as purchasing, with quality oversight.

Contracts and Agreements

It is common practice to develop a written contract or agreement with a supplier that stipulates the organization's requirements and expectations. The document should define the role of both the organization and the supplier in the relationship and should also stipulate the manner in which the supplier will operate to meet the organization's needs. It is a good idea to establish and document metrics that can be monitored on a regular basis. If metrics indicate that there is a problem, corrective actions should be taken. If the problem cannot be corrected, it may mean that the supplier should be removed from the approved list.

AABB standards stipulate that organizations should monitor their agreements. Other organizations have similar requirements. For example, The Joint Commission requires that hospital blood banks establish metrics with their blood suppliers that are evaluated routinely, with documentation of the results of that evaluation as well as any corrective actions required by the supplier as a result of failure to meet those metrics.

Receipt and Inspection of Incoming Supplies

When supplies are initially received, it is important that they are physically separated from supplies that are in use until they can be inspected for suitability of use. Some organizations have caged areas where incoming supplies are quarantined until inspected; others use shelving and labeling, often with color coding, to quarantine incoming supplies. The incoming inspection and release is most commonly performed by the quality department, but in some instances, operations may conduct the inspection for quality.

Organizations should develop criteria for acceptance, and incoming supplies should be inspected against such criteria. Supplies not meeting the preestablished criteria should remain in quarantine, and the supplier should be notified of the issue. The inspection should be conducted according to a written procedure, and there should be documentation of the suitability of the supplies or their disposition, if found unsuitable. Most often these supplies are returned to the supplier, but they may be discarded if the supplier does not need them for further investigation. Both external packaging and the contents of that packaging should be inspected for acceptance. If there is something wrong with the product or packaging, the product must be quarantined, either physically or with clear labeling, until disposition is determined by the quality department.

Process Control and Management

Process control is the sum of activities involved in ensuring a process is predictable, stable, and consistently operating at the target level of performance with only normal variation. Important aspects of process control include:

- SOPs.
- Process validation.
- Computer system validation.
- Test method validation.
- QC.
- Training.
- Tracking and trending.

Standard Operating Procedures

SOPs provide instruction on how to perform a task and are key to achieving consistency and control in operations. A full discussion of SOPs is found in the "Documents and Records" section.

Process Validation

One of the most important aspects of process control is the initial establishment that a process consistently works to produce a desired result; the validation of the process. Process validation is defined as the collection and evaluation of data, from the process design stage through commercial production, which establish scientific evidence that a process is capable of consistently delivering quality product.[5] Validation establishes that a process has consistent results that meet predetermined requirements. Validations should be performed for all critical processes according to a written validation protocol. The protocol should contain the following:

- System description.
- Purpose of the validation.
- Risk assessment.
- Responsibilities.

- Test cases.
- Acceptance criteria.
- Problem-reporting mechanism.
- Approval signature.
- Supporting documentation.

The system description identifies the components of the system used for the process and includes a description of how those components work together during the process. It should also include environmental conditions under which the system operates, as applicable, and any utility specifications.

The purpose of the validation is usually straightforward. Validations may be conducted because a process is new or something significant has changed within the process, and assurance is needed that the process still remains in a validated state. A process validation has three phases: installation qualification, operational qualification, and performance qualification. Installation qualification ensures that any equipment used within the process is installed appropriately and is qualified to perform as the manufacturer states, and that the environment, including utilities, is appropriate for its operation as defined by the manufacturer. It also ensures that necessary SOPs are written, training is developed, and staff are trained in the execution of related SOPs. Operational qualification demonstrates that the process operates as intended, and it focuses on the process capability (worst-case challenges). The final phase, performance qualification, demonstrates that the process works as expected in a normal working environment.

Although a manufacturer usually does a significant amount of validation work before bringing equipment or software to market, the end user still has to perform the user's own validation. For example, computer software vendors do a tremendous amount of testing of the software to determine limitations, etc; yet, the user of that software must validate the software in the user's environment with the user's staff and SOPs. Consultants may be used to assist with validation, but final validation and the results of that validation are the responsibility of the end user. The amount of validation work needed is dependent on the process, its criticality, and the ability to test the end result 100% of the time or not. (See Fig 1-2.)

A risk assessment aids in the determination of how much testing must be done. The more risk a process introduces, the more testing an organization normally does. This is especially important when there is no way to test the end result of a process other than to destroy good product. If the process is not a high-risk or critical process, then less testing may be done as the organization is willing to take the risk should the process not work as expected.

Within a validation there are multiple roles. The individual who writes the validation protocol is responsible for ensuring it is complete and contains all the necessary information and sufficient test cases to obtain the degree of assurance desired. Those who execute the validation protocol must have training in the process and may often be individuals who will perform the process routinely, although this is not always the case. The quality department and others, as appropriate, approve the validation protocol and the final results of the validation before a process is implemented.

Test cases should be developed to test the various parameters of the process and to challenge the process as much as reasonable. The more testing that is performed, the more assurance that the process works consistently, but it is not always possible to perform enough tests to get 100% assurance. Usually an organization seeks a comfort level of testing that is reasonable and in line with industry standards. Each test case should have expected results. If those results are not obtained, a problem report must be executed, and there should be a resolution before proceeding. Failure of a test case could be the result of improper installation qualification, a poorly written test case, an unrealistic expected result, or poor execution of the test case itself. If investigation does not produce a cause and a resolution for the issue, then the process itself may have to be changed, or the process may be implemented with limitations that are documented within the validation summary.

The acceptance criteria for a validation must be documented before the validation work begins. This criteria should not be changed in the middle of a validation unless

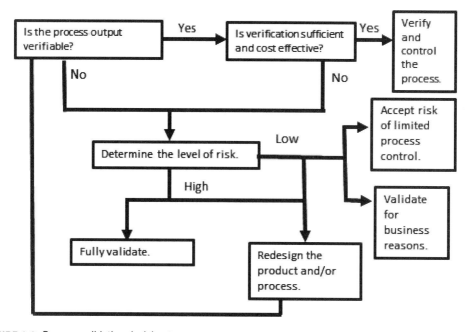

FIGURE 1-2. Process validation decision tree.

there is a good reason to change it, and if change does occur, the validation protocol must be amended, and the amended protocol must be approved again.

Once the validation protocol is completed, it needs approval from operations and quality, at a minimum. In a CLIA laboratory setting, the medical director must also serve as an approver of validation work. Approval must occur before any execution of test cases. As stated above, if there is good reason to modify the protocol, it is necessary to amend it and have it approved again. The protocol may include supporting documentation such as user manuals or pertinent technical articles.

The validation proves the process is consistent and produces an end result that meets specifications. During the validation an organization may uncover the following:

- Design flaws.
- Inadequate requirements.
- Errors in SOPs.
- Errors in user manuals.
- Training deficiencies.
- Incompatibilities with interfaces.
- Incompatibilities with the physical environment.
- Misconceptions about process capabilities.

Following completion of the test cases, a validation summary is normally written. This summary describes the expected and observed results and whether or not those results are acceptable. It also delineates any problems encountered during the validation and what was done to resolve those problems. It defines any process limitations, either known before beginning the validation or discovered during the validation. Finally, it contains a conclusion based on the results. Before implementing the process, the validation summary should be reviewed and approved, again by operations, quality, and the medical director, as appropriate. Supporting documentation may accompany the summary as well as a timeline for implementation of the process, although this is often a separate document. It is important to remember that while a validation gives an organization confidence in its processes and significantly reduces the need for end-product testing, no validation, no matter how extensive, can test every possibility or control the human element. Continual process monitoring is needed to ensure the process remains in a validated state.

Computer System Validation

A computer system is composed of hardware, software, peripheral devices, networks, personnel, and documentation. Validation of the computer system in the environment where it will be used by those who will use it is required. This also includes validation of interfaces between systems. For example, a blood establishment would need to validate the interface between its BECS and a testing instrument. Although much work is done by the vendors who develop software, the end user must still perform a validation and may even repeat work that the vendor has already done. An important part of validating a computer system is to ensure that the system can still operate when stressed. The FDA has issued guidance to assist organizations in the performance of computer system validation.[6]

Test Method Validation

When laboratories wish to implement a non-waived test using an FDA-approved or -cleared test system, CLIA requires that the performance specifications established by the manufacturer be verified by the laboratory before it reports patient results.[7] At a minimum, the laboratory must demonstrate that it can obtain performance specifications comparable to those of the manufacturer for accuracy, precision, reportable range, and reference intervals (normal values).

If the laboratory develops its own method, introduces a test system not subject to FDA approval or clearance, or makes modifications to an FDA-approved or -cleared test system, or if the manufacturer does not provide performance specifications, then the laboratory must establish the test system performance specifications before reporting patient results.[7] At a minimum, the following must be established for the test system:

- Accuracy.
- Precision.
- Reportable range of test results for the test system.
- Reference intervals (normal values).
- Analytical sensitivity.
- Analytical specificity, including interfering substances.
- Any other performance characteristic required for test performance (eg, specimen or reagent stability).

Based on performance specifications, the laboratory must also establish calibration and control procedures and document all activities for test method validation. Title 42 CFR Part 493.1253.1 provides additional information on this.

Quality Control

QC is an important aspect of process control. It ensures the proper functioning of materials, reagents, equipment, and methods. QC is an event that is different from validation in that it is not repeated to gain assurance of consistency, but rather it is repeated at a given frequency to ensure results are within acceptable ranges, and also over time to determine if any trends are developing that might indicate something is eventually going to fail. The frequency of QC testing is usually determined by the criticality of what is being tested. Some QC frequency is dictated by regulatory or accrediting bodies such as the FDA.[4] Additional information on QC frequency is found in Appendix 1-3. All QC should be well documented to include who did the testing, the date it was done, the results, and whether or not the testing was acceptable. Documentation should be concurrent with the performance of the testing, and records should be available for future inspections or assessments.

Unacceptable QC results should be evaluated, and the process should not continue until the issue is resolved. Corrective actions may be necessary before acceptable QC can be obtained. Items that fail QC should be marked "not for use" until the issue is resolved. Because QC is performed on a schedule, if a fail-ure occurs, it may be necessary to assess product produced since the last acceptable QC result. This is clearly why determining the criticality of what is being tested is important; the more frequent the QC, the less product is involved in the evaluation.

Training

Orientation training is critical for new employees, and is discussed along with specific job training and competency assessment in the section on "Human Resources." Workplace safety training is detailed in Chapter 2.

Tracking and Trending

Tracking is an integral part of record-keeping and is noted in the following section on "Documents and Records." Trending is a concept embodied in many quality system activities. Identifying and analyzing trends is discussed in the "Monitoring and Evaluation" section below.

Documents and Records

Documentation is important in that it provides evidence of what was done, as well as details about what was done. Good documentation can provide full traceability (details) and trackability (a logical sequence of steps) in the execution of processes. Organizations involved in the production of blood and cellular products create many documents and records. These include:

- Quality manuals.
- Policies and process documents.
- SOPs.
- Work instructions.
- Job aids.
- Forms.
- Labels.

Document Creation

Documents should be created in a consistent manner. An SOP should be in place to define the format of documents as well as the review and approval process, both initially and at routine intervals. Documents should have a numbering system, and changes to documents should be made in a controlled manner (change control). Document control is a key element of process control. Many organizations now have computerized document control systems that are validated for activities such as document development, document routing for review and approval, controlled document printing, and editing documents, when necessary. Some organizations have become completely paperless.

Quality Manual

The quality manual is one of the most important documents in a blood or cellular therapy establishment. The quality manual describes the organization's quality policy, quality objectives, and overall approach to quality in all aspects of the business. It defines how the organization is structured to ensure implementation of the quality system and defines the roles of staff, including line staff all the way up to senior management. It points out how the quality system integrates with operational tasks and how those tasks are monitored to ensure quality outcomes.

Policies and Process Documents

Policies describe the manner in which an organization operates. They are high-level documents describing the position that an organization takes on a particular topic. Not all policies are regulated. For example, a dress code policy or a tobacco use policy are not required by any regulatory or accrediting bodies, but if an organization wants staff to dress a particular way or to avoid the use of tobacco in the work place, a policy is a good way to document this. As necessary, policies are supported by other forms of documentation within an organization, such as SOPs and forms.

Process documents are also high level and describe the inputs for a process, the conversion that takes place, and the output of a process. A process document provides the big picture and may take the form of a flow chart.

This is particularly helpful when trying to understand a process at a high level.

Standard Operating Procedures and Work Instructions

SOPs describe who does what and when (in sequence or order); they describe the steps of a process. Well-written SOPs provide the "how" in performing a process. They should be detailed enough for a trained individual to perform the task but not so detailed that they are unnecessarily restrictive. SOPs should be written with input from subject-matter experts and should be validated to ensure that they are effective. SOP validation usually involves an individual performing the task using the SOP as written. The individual notes whether the steps in the SOP make sense and whether the steps can be performed as written. Finalized SOPs should be reviewed and approved by the appropriate department personnel and the medical director, as appropriate, and then approved by quality before becoming effective and released. Staff should receive training in all SOPs applicable to their jobs, and SOPs must be accessible at all times to staff performing the work.

SOPs need to be periodically reviewed to ensure that they are current and are reflective of the work as it is being done. Some organizations review a portion of their SOPs each quarter to ensure that the entire collection of SOPs is reviewed each year.

Work instructions provide step-by-step instructions for how a task is performed. They are more specific and more detailed than procedures. Not all organizations have work instructions; some organizations choose to just use the term *procedure* for all step-by-step documents. Whatever term an organization chooses, the documents describing how the work is done still need to be controlled and managed in a consistent manner. Changes to SOPs and/or work instructions need to be made in a controlled manner that allows for the changes to be made, validated, and communicated to all stakeholders before implementation.

Job Aids

A job aid is an excerpt from an approved procedure or work instruction. These are often used when a portion of the SOP has a table or information that must be frequently referenced. Job aids must be controlled just as procedures and work instructions, and there should be a way to reference a job aid to the procedure it represents. Uncontrolled job aids should not be allowed.

Forms

Blank forms provide templates for the capture of information. Forms should be managed within document control and should be designed by individuals with experience; it is not true that anyone can design a form. Often mistakes can be avoided by careful form design. If the form is not self-explanatory, instructions on how to complete it should be available, and individuals should receive training on completion of the form. This will reduce the likelihood of errors.

Labels

Although not always thought of as a document, labels need to be created and maintained within the document control system to ensure that the label is correct, meets regulatory requirements, and is current. Changes to labels need to be managed just as changes to documents are, within a controlled system, reviewed for accuracy and compliance, and approved. Certain labels must be submitted to the FDA for approval.[8] Organizations must maintain a current master set of labels for reference.

Document Maintenance

As previously stated, documents should be created and maintained in a controlled manner. Version control is critical. Organizations also need to have a mechanism whereby changes to documents can be requested and communicated once those changes have occurred. A document history that records changes to a document should be developed and maintained. When a document is revised, and the revised copy is approved and released, an archived copy of the original version should be retained for future reference.

Organizations should prepare a master list of all the various types of documents in use. This list should define the most current version, how many copies are out, and where those copies are. This aids in document control; when revisions occur, it helps to ensure that all old copies of the documents are removed and replaced with the revised version.

Records

Records are the evidence of what was done and prove that procedures were followed and documentation of the work performed was captured. Records should be created concurrent with the performance of the work, documenting each critical step. Good records provide the details (traceability—who, what, when, where, how) and a logical sequence of steps taken (trackability). It is also important that records are permanent, which means that indelible ink should be used, and any corrections should be made in a manner that allows one to see what the error was. Records should be managed so that the following aspects are addressed:

- Creation and identification of records.
- Confidentiality.
- Protection of the integrity of records.
- Protection from inadvertent destruction.
- Protection from damage from rodents, fire, and water.
- Storage and retrieval.
- Retention.
- Destruction.

Policies, process documents, procedures, and completed forms are also examples of records found in an organization involved in transfusion medicine and/or cellular therapy, and describe how the work was being performed at any particular time in the organization's history. The records may be in paper or electronic form and must be easily identified. There should also be information as to who created the record. Because organizations may use both signatures and initials, it is necessary to maintain a current signature sample and list of initials for all employees. If the identity of the record creator is captured electronically by entry into the computer system or by electronic badge swipe, this needs to be in compliance with electronic record-keeping rules.

Because of the nature of the records created by transfusion medicine or cellular therapy organizations, many records are confidential, especially those containing donor or patient information. Records should never be left where they can be viewed by individuals who have no need to view them. If records containing confidential information are made available to those outside the organization, any confidential information should be redacted.

Records, whether in paper or electronic form, must be protected from unauthorized changes, from inadvertent destruction, and from damage caused by rodents, fire, or water. Record storage should be designed to accomplish these goals. It also should allow the records to be retrieved easily. Access to records should be restricted, particularly if the records contain confidential information.

Organizations need to have a written record-retention policy that is compliant with regulations and standards; records should be retained in accordance with that policy. Once a record has reached its "end of life," it should be discarded in a manner that protects any confidential information. Such destruction methods include shredding or burning.

Many organizations outsource record storage, retrieval, retention, and destruction to off-site vendors. Such vendors should be qualified, and organizations need to ensure timely access to their records for inspections and assessments.

If records are stored electronically, an organization must ensure that the integrity of the electronic data is protected from unauthorized changes. Additionally, the data must be stored in a manner that would not cause inadvertent loss of data from overwriting, physical damage, or system crashes. Data integrity should be assessed periodically.

Organizations must have a documented mechanism for error correction for paper documents and for electronic documents. In both cases, it is important that the error is not obliterated. The common industry practice for correcting errors on paper documents is to draw a single line through the error, write the correction above it and then initial and date the correction. If an explanation for the correction is needed, this can be written alongside the correction. If there is insufficient room, an asterisk can be used and the explanation written elsewhere on the document, even on the back. Electronic document maintenance should allow an audit trail to show what the error was, what correction was made, who made it, and when it was made.

Information Management

Organizations have a tremendous amount of information that must be managed as part of the quality system, and much of that information, as previously stated, must be confidentially maintained. Access to information should be limited to those who need the information for work purposes. Unauthorized copying of information, whether paper or electronic, should not be allowed. If documents are maintained in a paper state and contain highly confidential information, they should be in locked file cabinets, and if stored electronically, they should be protected by access rights. Although the topic is not within the scope of this chapter, organizations that store personal health information must be compliant with the Health Insurance Portability and Accountability Act (HIPAA). More information on HIPAA may be found at www.hhs.gov/hipaa.

Backup of critical electronic information is important. Backups should be routinely run, and there should be written procedures to restore any data that may be inadvertently lost.

Management of Nonconforming Events

The QMS should contain processes and procedures to detect, document, investigate, correct, and follow up on nonconforming events such as the production of a product that does not meet specifications. Such processes and procedures must be in line with regulations and applicable standards and should include the following:

- Documentation of the event, either electronically or on paper, with some sort of classification.
- Determination of the effect, if any, on the quality of products or services.
- Evaluation of the effect on interrelated activities.
- Investigation and root cause analysis.
- Selection of appropriate corrective action.
- Implementation of corrective action, as appropriate.
- Notification and recall.
- Implementation of appropriate preventive action.
- Reporting to external agencies when required.
- Evaluation of the effectiveness of the corrective actions and preventive actions (CAPA) taken.

Staff should be trained to find and report nonconformances, which include errors and accidents, and adverse reactions in donors and recipients. It is important to capture the facts of the event in sufficient detail to allow a complete and thorough investigation.

It is critically important, once a nonconformance is discovered, to determine the impact of that nonconformance on products and/or services. If the nonconformance negatively impacts product quality, it may be necessary to quarantine the product(s) or to perform a recall if the product has been distributed. The sooner an organization can gain control of the affected product, the better. Organizations should always consider the impact on their products and/or services as soon as possible after discovery of a nonconformance.

It is also a good idea to determine if the nonconformance has impact on other areas of the organization's operations. It may be necessary to involve more than one department in the investigation to fully understand what occurred and its impact.

Not all nonconformances require a full investigation, but there is normally some level of investigation required for most nonconformances. A thorough investigation may involve interviewing staff, reviewing training records, and reviewing SOPs. Also, investigations may involve other record review or review of data to determine the extent of the nonconformance.

Root cause analysis is a collective term that describes a wide range of approaches, tools, and techniques used to uncover causes of problems. A root cause analysis to determine the cause or causes of the nonconformance is often necessary. It is important to continue to ask why to determine the true root cause(s). Without finding the true cause of a nonconformance, it is possible that the problem will recur. If the root cause is fixed, the problem should not recur. Although there is substantial debate on the definition of *root cause*, the following are considered true[9]:

- Root causes are specific underlying causes.
- Root causes are those that can reasonably be identified.
- Root causes are those management has control to fix.
- Root causes are those for which effective recommendations for preventing recurrences can be generated.

There are several tools that are useful in performing a root cause analysis. These include brainstorming, useful in generating potential causes; a fishbone diagram, useful in determining causes and contributing factors; a failure mode effects analysis (FMEA), a step-by-step approach for identifying all possible failures in a design, a manufacturing or assembly process, or a product or service; and the five whys, useful for drilling down to the true cause. For the last one, there is no magic to the number five; one may ask 3 or 7 or 10 whys to get to the true cause of a nonconformance. (See Fig 1-3.)

Once the root cause has been identified, it is then important to select an appropriate corrective action. The action should fix the issue,

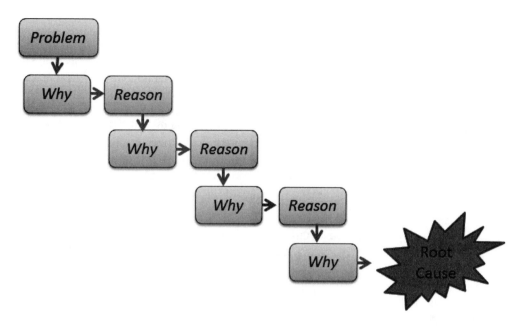

FIGURE 1-3. The five whys. Note: There is no magic to asking five times; it may take more or less to get to the root cause.

but at the same time, the corrective action must be reasonable. For example, if the true fix for a problem is a new computer system to capture specific data accurately, this cannot be accomplished quickly, so a more reasonable alternative may need to be chosen until the new computer system can be implemented. Also, although it seems intuitive, it should be noted that an organization must ensure the corrective action actually addresses the true issue and is not merely addressing a symptom of the problem. In the example given, the organization may choose to implement a newly designed form to reduce the likelihood of error or may implement a second review for accuracy. A note of caution here, however, is that simply adding more review seldom fixes the problem. In fact additional review can sometimes make things worse.

As part of corrective action, notification of customers about the nonconformance may be necessary, and it may be necessary to recall additional product, depending on the scope of the issue and the results of the investigation.

The organization should have a documented process for these actions.

Correcting the nonconformance is important, but equally important is determining if there are actions that can be taken to prevent the issue from recurring ever again. There are short-term corrective actions, which fix the problem temporarily, and long-term corrective actions, which normally include preventive action and permanently fix the problem. Finding the best way to minimize the likelihood of the problem recurring while maintaining the ability to operate within the constraints of limited resources is key.

Preventive actions should be implemented whenever possible. For example, proper training might be considered a preventive action if it is determined that a nonconformance resulted from a lack of training. In this instance, training might be considered both a corrective and a preventive action. It fixes the current problem, and it prevents future occurrences at the same time.

Depending on the nature of the nonconformance, regulatory bodies or accrediting agencies may need notification as well. Processes and procedures should include information on whom to notify and when. A voluntary recall is instituted for nonconforming product that has been distributed. In-house products can be dealt with directly.

Fatalities related to blood collection or transfusion or to cellular therapy products must be reported as soon as possible to the FDA Center for Biologics Evaluation and Research (CBER). (See 21 CFR 606.170(b) and 1271.350(a)(i), respectively.) Instructions for reporting to CBER are available in published guidance[10] and on the FDA website.[11] A written follow-up report must be submitted within 7 days of the fatality and should include a description of any new procedures implemented to avoid recurrence. AABB *Association Bulletin #04-06* provides additional information on these reporting requirements, including a form for reporting donor fatalities.[12]

Regardless of their licensure and registration status with the FDA, all donor centers, blood banks, and transfusion services must promptly report biological product deviations (BPDs)—and information relevant to these events—to the FDA[13,14] using Form FDA 3486 when the event 1) is associated with manufacturing (ie, collecting, testing, processing, packing, labeling, storing, holding, or distributing); 2) represents a deviation from cGMP, established specifications, or applicable regulations or standards or that is unexpected or unforeseen; 3) may affect the product's safety, purity, or potency; 4) occurs while the facility had control of, or was responsible for, the product; and 5) involves a product that has left the facility's control (ie, has been distributed).

Using the same form, facilities must also promptly report BPDs associated with a distributed cellular therapy product if the event represents a deviation from applicable regulations, standards, or established specifications that relate to the prevention of communicable disease transmission or contamination of the product. This requirement pertains to events that are unexpected or unforeseeable but may relate to the transmission or potential transmission of a communicable disease or may lead to product contamination.[15] More infor-mation concerning BPD reporting can be found on the FDA website.[16]

There must also be a mechanism to report medical device adverse events to the FDA and the device manufacturer.[17] The Joint Commission encourages reporting of sentinel events, including hemolytic transfusion reactions involving the administration of blood or components having major blood group incompatibilities.[18,19]

Hemoviligilance reporting provides an opportunity to detect, investigate, and respond to adverse transfusion reactions and events that result in nonconformances. A number of organizations monitor such data, including AABB and the Centers for Disease Control and Prevention (CDC).

Monitoring and Evaluation

Organizations should have a system for monitoring and evaluating the effectiveness of the organization's processes. This system should be defined as part of the QMS. Monitoring can occur at various levels: the level of input to the process, the in-process activities, the results, or the process, or even the system in which the process resides. While record review and analysis is an ongoing form of monitoring, the use of internal and external assessments of the processes is very useful. Assessments may include comparison of actual to expected results and can consist of quality assessments, peer reviews, self-assessments, and proficiency testing.

Organizations should have a process that describes how internal assessments are conducted. Each assessment should be well planned and conducted according to the plan. Assessors may look at data such as quality indicators and other quality records or observe processes as they are performed. The assessment should cover the QMS and, at a minimum, processes that are critical to the organization's operations. When issues are found during the assessment, the process should include a mechanism to respond to those issues, ensuring that important stakeholders are aware of the issues and what corrective actions, if any, are planned. The quality department should take responsibility for oversight of these assessments and to ensure that actions are taken as warranted.

Quality Indicators

Quality indicators are statistical measures that give an indication of output quality. They are useful in the evaluation of customer requirements, personnel, inventory management, and process control and stability (this list is not all inclusive). Quality indicators may be based on outcomes such as quantity-not-sufficient (QNS) rates, or they may be based on the process's ability to deliver an expected result consistently. As an example of a process quality indicator, if a customer requires stat deliveries to arrive within 1 hour, the percentage of deliveries that meet the customer's requirement is a measurement of the ability of the process to deliver within the required time frame. Organizations should establish alert limits for quality indicators; involving the customer is important in making sure that alert limits are appropriately set.

Organizations should communicate quality indicator results frequently so stakeholders are aware of how the organization is performing. Customers may want to be included in this reporting. Run charts, control charts, and bar charts are often useful in displaying quality indicator data. Control charts allow an organization to see if the process is operating as expected, and if not, corrective actions are indicated.

Blood Utilization

In recent years, organizations have become even more focused on blood utilization patterns. This is driven by the desire to decrease costs and to provide better patient care. Patient blood management (PBM) as a discipline has come to the forefront; many organizations now have a staff member devoted to transfusion safety: the transfusion safety officer, or TSO. Utilization committees review physician ordering and transfusion practices routinely. The committees also review sample collection and labeling, adverse events in patients, near-miss events, outdates, discard, appropriateness of use, and compliance. Many hospitals have set up order alerts in the hospital computer system when physicians order outside of established guidelines. AABB has published clinical practice guidelines for red cell and platelet transfusion.[20,21]

Alternatives to red cell transfusion such as preoperative anemia treatment are under study or have been incorporated into routine practice in efforts to decrease the need for transfusions. Physicians are asked to use data to determine if a second transfusion is warranted instead of issuing a blanket order for transfusion of 2 units, a common practice among transfusing physicians. (See Fig 1-4 for an example of this kind of improvement seen as a result of the implementation of a PBM program in a large teaching hospital.) The use of thromboelastography (TEG) or thromboelastometry (TEM) to guide physicians on

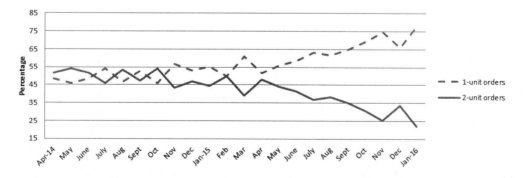

FIGURE 1-4. Results of patient blood management in reducing 2-unit blanket transfusions (lower line) at the University of Tennessee Medical Center Blood Bank, Knoxville, Tennessee. Provided courtesy of Dr. Chris Clark and Anna Rains.

when to transfuse to correct coagulation factor levels is now common practice. In addition to providing better patient care, PBM limits needless transfusions, thereby saving dollars and ensuring components are available for those who need them most.

External Assessments

External assessments are those that are conducted by agencies and organizations that are not affiliated with the facility being assessed. They may be voluntary, as in the case of AABB assessments, or mandatory, as in the case of FDA inspections. Organizations that assess or inspect blood banks, transfusion services, and cellular therapy facilities include the following:

- AABB.
- College of American Pathologists (CAP).
- Commission on Office Laboratory Accreditation (COLA).
- Centers for Medicare and Medicaid Services (CMS).
- The Joint Commission.
- Foundation for the Accreditation of Cellular Therapy (FACT).
- Food and Drug Administration (FDA).
- State health departments.

The list includes both accrediting organizations and regulatory entities. Other agencies such as the Department of Transportation (DOT) and the Nuclear Regulatory Commission (NRC) may assess the organization as well.

Accreditation is voluntary, whereas regulation is the law. The external assessments conducted by these entities are usually against standards or regulations promulgated by the organization that is performing the assessment. Although with any assessment or inspection there is some level of angst, these assessments are usually beneficial to the facility and are opportunities for learning and improving operations. It is important that staff are trained on how to conduct themselves during an assessment or inspection, both to decrease their anxiety and to ensure they un-

derstand what the assessor or inspector can and cannot do.

If issues are discovered during an external assessment or inspection, these are usually documented and provided to the facility in an exit meeting. The facility should perform root cause analysis and implement corrective actions as required. Normally the facility will submit a written response to the entity performing the external assessment. Just as with internal assessments, management needs to be well informed of the findings and corrective actions related to those findings.

Proficiency Testing

Proficiency testing (PT) is the testing of samples previously unknown to a laboratory that are sent by a CMS-approved PT program. There are a number of organizations that provide PT samples; AABB, for example, provides PT for immunohematology reference laboratories. Normally a facility will perform at least three testing events each year. PT samples should be managed as any other samples that the laboratory tests, and the testing should be rotated among staff so that different individuals are tested. Submitted results are compared to other laboratories, and a pass/fail determination is assigned. Accrediting organizations monitor the PT results for facilities they accredit. When failures occur, it is expected that the facility will conduct an investigation, try to find the root cause of the issue, and implement any CAPA that are needed.

Process Improvement

Continuous improvement is a tenet of any quality program, and organizations that manufacture blood components or cellular therapy products should have processes in place that allow for continuous improvement in operations and in patient safety. Information gleaned from the nonconformance management system should be used to improve operations. This is a primary benefit of an effective nonconformance management process. Other sources of improvement opportunities include:

TABLE 1-2. DMAIC Process

● **D**efine the problem, improvement activity, opportunity for improvement, project goals, and customer (internal and external) requirements.
● **M**easure process performance.
● **A**nalyze the process to determine root causes of variation, poor performance (defects).
● **I**mprove process performance by addressing and eliminating the root causes.
● **C**ontrol the improved process and future process performance.

- Customer-supplier established metrics.
- Complaints.
- QC records.
- Proficiency testing.
- Internal audits.
- Quality indicators.
- External assessments.
- Financial analysis of operations.

Many organizations combine the principles of lean manufacturing and Six Sigma as part of their continuous improvement processes. Lean Six Sigma is "a managerial approach that combines Six Sigma methods and tools of the lean manufacturing/lean enterprise philosophy, striving to eliminate waste of physical resources, time, effort, and talent, while assuring quality in production and organizational processes."[22] Lean Six Sigma has two objectives: 1) a focus on eliminating non-value-added steps in processes, and 2) eliminating defects and improving the overall process. Lean Six Sigma uses the define, measure, analyze, improve, and control (DMAIC) methodology—a five-step approach to process improvement. (See Table 1-2.) This approach can be used not only for problem-solving but also for process improvement. Organizations that have implemented Lean Six Sigma have

made significant improvements in their processes while saving valuable resources.

Facilities, Work Environment, and Safety

Facilities must be adequate for the work performed and must be maintained to provide a safe environment for staff, patients, donors, and visitors. The facility itself must be clean and orderly so as not to jeopardize staff or product safety. Sufficient space is necessary within the facility to prevent mix-ups during the performance of processes, and building utilities, ventilation, sanitation, trash, and hazardous substance disposal must support the organization's operations. Safety concerns include general safety components such as the use of nonslip surfaces and proper lifting techniques, as well as fire safety, biologic and chemical safety, radiation safety, and disaster preparedness, response, and recovery. A written disaster plan is crucial for the organization, addressing what to do in the event of a disaster to maintain safety for staff and to maintain business continuity as much as possible. Staff must have training in safety and on the disaster plan itself. A routine test of the disaster plan, including the various scenarios that might produce disaster situations, needs to be exercised under the oversight of management.

KEY POINTS

1. **Organization and Leadership.** A defined organizational structure in addition to top management's support and commitment to the quality policy, goals, and objectives is key to ensuring the success of the quality management system.

2. **Customer Focus.** Quality organizations should understand and meet or exceed customer needs and expectations. These needs and expectations should be defined in a contract, agreement, or other document developed with regular feedback from the customer.

3. **Human Resources.** Quality management of all personnel addresses adequate staffing levels and staff selection, orientation, training, and competency assessment, as well as specific regulatory requirements.

4. **Equipment Management.** Critical equipment may include instruments, measuring devices, and computer hardware and software. This equipment must be uniquely identified and operate within defined specifications, as ensured by qualification, calibration, maintenance, and monitoring.

5. **Suppliers and Materials Management.** Suppliers of critical materials and services (ie, those affecting quality) should be qualified, and these requirements should be defined in contracts or agreements. All critical materials should be qualified and then inspected and tested upon receipt to ensure that specifications are met.

6. **Process Control and Management.** A systematic approach to developing new policies, processes, and procedures and controlling changes to them includes process validation, test method validation, computer system validation, equipment validation, and QC. Validation must be planned and results reviewed and accepted.

7. **Documents and Records.** Documents include policies, process descriptions, procedures, work instructions, job aids, forms, and labels. Records provide evidence that the process was performed as intended and allow assessment of product and service quality.

8. **Information Management.** Unauthorized access to, or modification or destruction of, data and information must be prevented, and confidentiality of patient and donor records maintained. Data integrity should be assessed periodically, and backup devices, alternative systems, and archived documents maintained.

9. **Management of Nonconforming Events.** Deviations from facility-defined requirements, standards, and regulations must be addressed by documenting and classifying occurrences, assessing effects on quality, implementing remedial actions (CAPA), and reporting to external agencies as required.

10. **Monitoring and Evaluation.** Assessment of facility processes includes internal and external assessments, monitoring of quality indicators, blood utilization assessment, proficiency testing, and analysis of data.

11. **Process Improvement.** Opportunities for improvement may be identified from deviation reports, nonconforming products and services, customer complaints, QC records, proficiency testing results, internal audits, quality indicator monitoring, and external assessments. Process improvement includes determination of root causes, implementation of corrective and preventive actions, and evaluation of the effectiveness of these actions. The implementation of Lean Six Sigma can significantly increase efficiencies and reduce opportunities for error.

12. **Facilities, Work Environment, and Safety.** Procedures related to general safety; biologic, chemical, and radiation safety; fire safety; and disaster preparedness are required. Space allocation, building utilities, ventilation, sanitation, trash, and hazardous substance disposal must support the organization's operations.

REFERENCES

1. Food and Drug Administration. Guideline for quality assurance in blood establishments. (July 11, 1995) Silver Spring, MD: CBER Office of Communication, Outreach, and Development, 1995.

2. Business Dictionary. Quality planning. Fairfax, VA: WebFinance, Inc., 2017. [Available at http://www.businessdictionary.com/definition/quality-planning.html (accessed March 7, 2017).]

3. Centers for Medicare and Medicaid Services. What do I need to do to assess personnel competency? Baltimore, MD: CMS, 2012. [Available at https://www.cms.gov/Regulations-and-Guidance/Legislation/CLIA/Downloads/CLIA_CompBrochure_508.pdf (accessed March 7, 2017).]

4. Code of federal regulations. Title 21, CFR Part 606.60. Washington, DC: US Government Publishing Office, 2017 (revised annually).

5. Food and Drug Administration. Guidance for industry: Process validation: General principles and practices. (January 2011) Silver Spring, MD: CBER Office of Communication, Outreach, and Development, 2011.

6. Food and Drug Administration. General principles of software validation; final guidance for industry and FDA staff. (January 11, 2002) Silver Spring, MD: CBER Office of Communication, Outreach, and Development, 2002.

7. Code of federal regulations. Title 42, CFR Part 493. Washington, DC: US Government Publishing Office, 2017 (revised annually).

8. Food and Drug Administration. Guidance for industry: Changes to an approved application: Biological products: Human blood and blood components intended for transfusion or for further manufacture. (November 2014) Silver Spring, MD: CBER Office of Communication, Outreach, and Development, 2014. [Available at http://www.fda.gov/BiologicsBloodVaccines/GuidanceComplianceRegulatoryInformation/Guidances/Blood/ucm354559.htm (accessed March 7, 2017).]

9. Rooney JJ, Vanden Heuvel LN. Root cause analysis for beginners. Quality Progress 2004; 37:45-53.

10. Food and Drug Administration. Guidance for industry: Notifying FDA of fatalities related to blood collection or transfusion. (September 2003) Silver Spring, MD: CBER Office of Communication, Outreach, and Development, 2003.

11. Food and Drug Administration. Transfusion/donation fatalities: Notification process for transfusion related fatalities and donation related deaths. Silver Spring, MD: CBER Office of Communication, Outreach, and Development, 2016. [Available at http://www.fda.gov/BiologicsBloodVaccines/SafetyAvailability/ReportaProblem/TransfusionDonationFatalities/default.htm (accessed March 7, 2017).]

12. Reporting donor fatalities. Association bulletin #04-06. Bethesda, MD: AABB, 2004.

13. Code of federal regulations. Title 21, CFR Parts 606, 610, 630, and 640. Washington, DC: US Government Publishing Office, 2017 (revised annually).

14. Food and Drug Administration. Guidance for industry: Biological product deviation reporting for blood and plasma establishments. (October 2006) Silver Spring, MD: CBER Office of Communication, Outreach, and Development, 2006.

15. Code of federal regulations. Title 21, CFR Parts 1270 and 1271. Washington, DC: US Government Publishing Office, 2017 (revised annually).

16. Food and Drug Administration. Biological product deviations: Includes human tissue and cellular and tissue-based product (HCT/P) deviation reporting. Silver Spring, MD: CBER Office of Communication, Outreach, and Development, 2016 [Available at http://www.fda.gov/BiologicsBloodVaccines/SafetyAvailability/ReportaProblem/BiologicalProductDeviations/default.htm (accessed March 7, 2017).]

17. Code of federal regulations. Title 21, CFR Part 803. Washington, DC: US Government Publishing Office, 2017 (revised annually).

18. Hospital accreditation standards. Oakbrook Terrace, IL: Joint Commission Resources, 2017.

19. Laboratory accreditation standards. Oakbrook Terrace, IL: Joint Commission Resources, 2017.

20. Carson JL, Grossman BJ, Kleinman S, et al. Red blood cell transfusion: A clinical practice guideline from AABB. Ann Intern Med 2012; 157;49-58.

21. Kaufman M, Djulbegovic B, Gernsheimer T, et al. Platelet transfusion: A clinical practice guideline from the AABB. Ann Intern Med 2015;162:205-14.

22. Investopedia. Lean Six Sigma. New York: Investopedia LLC, 2017. [Available at http://www.investopedia.com/terms/l/lean-six-sigma.asp (accessed March 7, 2017).]

APPENDIX 1-1
Glossary of Commonly Used Quality Terms

Biovigilance	Collection and analysis of adverse event data for the purpose of improving outcomes in the collection and use of blood components, organs, tissues, and cellular therapies.
Calibration	Comparison of measurements performed with an instrument to those made with a more accurate instrument or standard for the purpose of detecting, reporting, and eliminating errors in measurement.
Change control	Established procedures for planning, documenting, communicating, and executing changes to infrastructure, processes, products, or services. Such procedures include the submission, analysis, approval, implementation, and postimplementation review of the change and decisions made about the change. Formal change control provides a measure of stability and safety and avoids arbitrary changes that might affect quality.
Control chart	A graphic tool used to determine whether the distribution of data values generated by a process is stable over time. A control chart plots a statistic vs time and helps to determine whether a process is in control or out of control according to defined criteria (eg, a shift from a central line or a trend toward upper or lower acceptance limits).
End-product test and inspection	Verification through observation, examination, or testing (or a combination) that the finished product or service conforms to specified requirements.
Near-miss event	An unexpected occurrence that did not adversely affect the outcome but could have resulted in a serious adverse event.
Process	An action that takes input(s) and transforms it into output.
Process control	Activities intended to minimize variation within a process to produce a predictable output that meets specifications.
Qualification	Demonstration that an entity is capable of fulfilling specified requirements, and verification of attributes that must be met or complied with for a person or thing to be considered fit to perform a particular function. For example, equipment may be qualified for an intended use by verifying performance characteristics, such as linearity, sensitivity, or ease of use. An employee may be qualified on the basis of technical, academic, and practical knowledge and skills developed through training, education, and on-the-job performance.
Quality assurance	Activities involving quality planning, control, assessment, reporting, and improvement necessary to ensure that a product or service meets defined quality standards and requirements.
Quality control	Operational techniques and activities used to monitor and eliminate causes of unsatisfactory performance at any stage of a process; involves sampling and testing.
Quality indicators	Measurable aspects of processes or outcomes that provide an indication of the condition or direction of performance over time. Quality indicators are used to monitor progress toward stated quality goals and objectives.
Quality management	The organizational structure, processes, and procedures necessary to ensure that the overall intentions and direction of an organization's quality program are met and that the quality of the product or service is ensured. Quality management includes strategic planning, allocation of resources, and other systematic activities, such as quality planning, implementation, and evaluation.

● APPENDIX 1-1
Glossary of Commonly Used Quality Terms (Continued)

Quality planning	A systematic process that translates quality policy into measurable objectives and requirements, and lays down a sequence of steps for realizing them within a specified time frame.
Requirement	A stated or obligatory need or expectation that can be measured or observed and that is necessary to ensure quality, safety, effectiveness, or customer satisfaction. Requirements can include things that the system or product must do, characteristics that it must have, and levels of performance that it must attain.
Specification	Description of a set of requirements to be satisfied by a product, material, or process indicating, if appropriate, the procedures to be used to determine whether the requirements are satisfied. Specifications are often in the form of written descriptions, drawings, professional standards, and other descriptive references.
System	An organized, purposeful structure that consists of interrelated and interdependent elements (components, processes, entities, factors, members, parts, etc).
Validation	Demonstration through objective evidence that the requirements for a particular application or intended use have been met. Validation provides assurance that new or changed processes and procedures are capable of consistently meeting specified requirements before implementation.
Verification	Confirmation, by examination of objective evidence, that specified requirements have been met.

● **APPENDIX 1-2**
Code of Federal Regulations Quality-Related References

Code of Federal Regulations, Title 21			
Topic	**Biologics, Blood**	**Drugs**	**Tissues, HCT/Ps**
Personnel	600.10, 606.20	211.25, 211.28	1271.170
Facilities	600.11, 606.40	211.42-58	1271.190
Environmental control and monitoring		211.42	1271.195
Equipment	606.60	211.63-72, 211.105, 211.182	1271.200
Supplies and reagents	606.65	211.80	1271.210
Standard operating procedures	606.100	211.100-101	1270.31, 1271.180
Process changes and validation		211.100-101	1271.225, 1271.230
Quality assurance/quality control unit		211.22	
Label controls	610.60-68, 606.120-122	211.122-130	1271.250, 1271.370
Laboratory controls	606.140	211.160	
Records and record reviews	600.12, 606.160	211.192, 211.194, 211.196	1270.33, 1271.55, 271.270
Receipt, predistribution, and distribution	606.165	211.142, 211.150	1271.265
Adverse reactions	606.170	211.198	1271.350
Tracking		211.188	1271.290
Complaints	606.170-171	211.198	1271.320
Reporting deviations	600.14, 606.171		1271.350
Storage	640.2, 640.11, 640.25, 640.34, 640.54, 640.69	211.142	1271.260

HCT/Ps = human cells, tissues, and cellular and tissue-based products.

● APPENDIX 1-3
Suggested Quality Control Performance Intervals for Equipment and Reagents*

Equipment or Reagent	Frequency of Quality Control
Refrigerators/freezers/platelet storage	
Refrigerators	
● Recorder	Daily
● Manual temperature	Daily
● Alarm system board (if applicable)	Daily
● Temperature charts	Daily (review and change weekly)
● Alarm activation	Quarterly
Freezers	
● Recorder	Daily
● Manual temperature	Daily
● Alarm system board (if applicable)	Daily
● Temperature charts	Daily (review and change weekly)
● Alarm activation	Quarterly
Platelet Incubators	
● Recorder	Daily
● Manual temperature	Daily
● Temperature charts	Daily (review and change weekly)
● Alarm activation	Quarterly
● Ambient platelet storage	Every 4 hours
Laboratory equipment	
Centrifuges/cell washers	
● Speed	Quarterly
● Timer	Quarterly
● Function	Yearly
● Tube fill level (serologic)	Day of use
● Saline fill volume (serologic)	Weekly
● Volume of antihuman globulin dispensed (if applicable)	Monthly
● Temperature check (refrigerated centrifuge)	Day of use
● Temperature verification (refrigerated centrifuge)	Monthly

(Continued)

● **APPENDIX 1-3**
Suggested Quality Control Performance Intervals for Equipment and Reagents*
(Continued)

Equipment or Reagent	Frequency of Quality Control
Heating blocks/waterbaths/view boxes	
● Temperature	Day of use
● Quadrant/area checks	Periodically
Component thawing devices	Day of use
pH meters	Day of use
Blood irradiators	
● Calibration	Yearly
● Turntable (visual check each time of use)	Yearly
● Timer	Monthly/quarterly
● Source decay	Dependent on source type
● Leak test	Twice yearly
● Dose delivery check (with indicator)	Each irradiator use
● Dose delivery verification	
– Cesium-137	Yearly
– Cobalt-60	Twice yearly
– Other source	As specified by manufacturer
Thermometers (vs NIST-certified or traceable thermometer)	
● Liquid-in-glass	Yearly
● Electronic	As specified by manufacturer
Timers/clocks	Twice yearly
Pipette recalibration	Quarterly
Sterile connecting device	
● Weld check	Each use
● Function	Yearly
Blood warmers	
● Effluent temperature	Quarterly
● Heater temperature	Quarterly
● Alarm activation	Quarterly

● **APPENDIX 1-3**
Suggested Quality Control Performance Intervals for Equipment and Reagents*
(Continued)

Equipment or Reagent	Frequency of Quality Control
Blood collection equipment	
Whole blood equipment	
● Agitators	Day of use
● Balances/scales	Day of use
● Gram weight (vs NIST-certified)	Yearly
Microhematocrit centrifuge	
● Timer check	Quarterly
● Calibration	Quarterly
● Packed cell volume	Yearly
Cell counters/hemoglobinometers	Day of use
Blood pressure cuffs	Twice yearly
Apheresis equipment	
● Checklist requirements	As specified by manufacturer
Reagents	
Red cells	Day of use
Antisera	Day of use
Antiglobulin serum	Day of use
Transfusion-transmissible disease marker testing	Each test run
Miscellaneous	
Copper sulfate	Day of use
Shipping containers for blood and component transport (usually at temperature extremes)	Twice yearly

*The frequencies listed are suggested intervals, not requirements. For any new piece of equipment, installation, operational, and performance qualifications must be performed. After the equipment has been suitably qualified for use, ongoing QC testing should be performed. Depending on the operational and performance qualification methodology, the ongoing QC may initially be performed more often than the ultimately desired frequency. Once a record of appropriate in-range QC results has been established (during either equipment qualification or the ongoing QC), the frequency of testing can be reduced. At a minimum, the frequency must comply with the manufacturer's suggested intervals; if no such guidance is provided by the manufacturer, the intervals given in this table are appropriate to use.
NIST = National Institute of Standards and Technology, QC = quality control.

Facilities, Work Environment, and Safety

• ● •

J. Wade Atkins, MS, MT(ASCP)SBB, CQA(ASQ), and
Leslie P. Taylor, CQA(ASQ)

THE PHYSICAL WORK environment can have a significant impact on the safety, efficiency, and effectiveness of work processes and on the quality of work. It should be designed and managed in a way that meets operational needs and provides for the safety of staff and visitors. The layout of the physical space; management of utilities; flow of personnel, materials, and waste; and ergonomic factors should all be considered in the facility management plan.

In addition to providing adequate facilities, the organization should develop and implement a safety program that defines policies and procedures for safe work practices and emergency responses. Such a program also includes requirements for training, hazard communication, use of engineering controls, and protective equipment. All employees are responsible for protecting their own safety and the safety of others by adhering to policies and procedures set forth in the facility safety program.

The AABB requires its accredited facilities to plan, implement, and maintain a program to minimize risks to the health and safety of donors, patients, volunteers, and employees from biological, chemical, and radiological hazards.[1,2] Other professional and accrediting organizations, including the College of American Pathologists (CAP), the Clinical and Laboratory Standards Institute, and The Joint Commission, have similar or more detailed safety program requirements.[3-6]

US federal regulations and recommendations intended to protect the safety of workers and the public in health-care settings are listed in Appendix 2-1. Appendix 2-1 also lists relevant safety recommendations of trade and professional associations. The contents of these regulations and guidelines are discussed in more detail in each section of this chapter. US state and local government regulations may have additional safety requirements, including architectural and construction safety considerations.

J. Wade Atkins, MS, MT(ASCP)SBB, CQA(ASQ), Quality Assurance Specialist, National Institutes of Health, Bethesda, Maryland; and Leslie P. Taylor, CQA(ASQ), Lead Technologist, National Institutes of Health, Bethesda, Maryland
The authors have disclosed no conflicts of interest.

FACILITIES

Facility Design and Workflow

Effective design and maintenance of facilities along with the physical organization of work activities can help reduce or eliminate many potential hazards. Facility design, workflow, and maintenance also affect process efficiency, productivity, error rates, employee and customer satisfaction, and the quality of products and services.

During the design phase for a new or renovated space, the location and flow of personnel, materials, and equipment should be considered in the context of the processes to be performed. Adequate space must be allotted for personnel movement, location of supplies and large equipment, and private or distraction-free zones for certain manufacturing tasks (eg, donor interviewing, record review, and blood component labeling). The facility must offer designated "clean" and "dirty" spaces and provide for controlled movement of materials and waste in and out of these areas. Chemical fume hoods and biological safety cabinets (BSCs) should be located away from drafts and high-traffic areas. The number and location of eyewash stations and emergency showers must also be considered in planning. In some cases, additional special water sources for reagent preparation must be provided. The location of very heavy equipment, such as irradiators, should be taken into account to ensure that the flooring has sufficient load-bearing capacity.

Laboratories must be designed with adequate illumination and electrical power and conveniently located electrical outlets. Emergency backup power sources, such as uninterruptible power supplies and backup generators, should be considered to ensure that blood components, cellular therapy products, and critical reagents are not compromised during power failures. The National Electrical Code is routinely used as a national guideline for the design of essential electrical distribution systems, with modifications approved by the local building authority that has jurisdiction.[7]

Heating, ventilation, and air handling must be adequate for the needs of the facility. Environmental monitoring systems should be considered for laboratories that require positive or negative air pressure differentials or where air filtration systems are used to control particle levels. The nationally accepted specifications for ventilation are published by the American Society of Heating, Refrigerating, and Air-Conditioning Engineers.[8]

Housekeeping

The workplace should be kept clean and free of clutter. Work surfaces and equipment should be regularly cleaned and disinfected. Items that may be hazardous or may accumulate dust and debris should not be stored above clean supplies or work surfaces. Exits and fire safety equipment must not be blocked or obstructed in any way. Receptacles and disposal guidelines for nonhazardous solid waste and biohazard, chemical, and radiation waste should be clearly identified. Housekeeping responsibilities, methods, and schedules should be defined for every work area. Written procedures, initial training, continuing education of personnel, and ongoing monitoring of housekeeping effectiveness are essential to safe operations.

Clean Rooms

Clean-room facilities should be considered for open processing activities that cannot be accommodated in a BSC. Laboratories that process cellular therapy products may choose to adopt clean-room specifications and maintenance practices to meet the requirements of the Food and Drug Administration (FDA) current good tissue practice regulations.[9]

International standards for clean rooms are published by the International Organization for Standardization and provide specifications for general manufacturing applications to limit airborne particulates, contaminants, and pollutants.[10] These standards also provide guidance for pharmaceutical and biotechnology applications that include methods to assess, monitor, and control biocontamination.[11]

Restricted Areas

Hazardous areas should be clearly and uniformly identified with warning signs in accordance with federal Occupational Safety and Health Administration (OSHA) and Nuclear Regulatory Commission (NRC) standards so that personnel entering or working around them are aware of existing biological, chemical, or radiation dangers.[12-15] Staff members not normally assigned to these areas should receive adequate training to avoid endangering themselves. Risk areas can be stratified. For example, high-risk areas might include those that contain chemical fume hoods, BSCs, and storage areas for volatile chemicals or radioisotopes. Technical work areas might be considered moderate risk and restricted to laboratory personnel. Administrative and clerical areas are generally considered low risk and not restricted. Guidelines for restricted access based on biosafety levels are published by the US Department of Health and Human Services (HHS).[16]

Organizations should consider establishing specific safety guidelines for visitors with business in restricted areas and verifying that safety guidelines have been reviewed before the visitors enter the area. Casual visitors should not be allowed in restricted areas. Children should not be allowed in areas where they could be exposed to hazards and should be closely supervised in those areas where their presence is permitted.

Mobile Sites

Mobile blood-collection operations can present special challenges. An advance safety survey of the proposed collection site helps ensure that hazards are minimized.

Responsibility for site safety should be assigned to an individual with adequate knowledge to recognize safety concerns and the authority to address them in a timely manner. All mobile personnel should be trained to recognize unsafe conditions and understand how to effectively implement infection-control policies and procedures in a variety of settings.

Hand-washing access is essential at collection sites. Carpeted or difficult-to-clean surfaces may be covered using an absorbent overlay with waterproof backing to protect them from possible blood spills. Portable screens and crowd-control ropes are helpful in directing traffic flow to maintain safe work areas. Food-service areas should be physically separated from areas for blood collection and storage. Blood-contaminated waste must be either returned to a central location for disposal or packaged and decontaminated in accordance with local regulations for medical waste.

Ergonomics

Consideration in physical design should be given to ergonomics and to accommodations for individuals covered under the Americans with Disabilities Act [42 United States Code (USC), Sections 12101-12213, 1990]. Several factors may contribute to employee fatigue, musculoskeletal disorder syndromes, or injury, including the following[17]:

- Awkward postures—positions that place stress on the body, such as reaching overhead, twisting, bending, kneeling, or squatting.
- Repetition—performance of the same motions continuously or frequently.
- Force—the amount of physical effort used to perform work.
- Pressure points—pressing of the body against hard or sharp surfaces.
- Vibration—continuous or high-intensity hand/arm or whole-body vibration.
- Other environmental factors—extreme high or low temperatures or lighting that is too dark or too bright.

Actions to correct problems associated with ergonomics may include the following:

- Engineering improvements to reduce or eliminate the underlying cause, such as making changes to equipment, workstations, or materials.
- Administrative improvements, such as providing variety in tasks; adjusting work schedules and work pace; providing recovery or relaxation time; modifying work

practices; ensuring regular housekeeping and maintenance of work spaces, tools, and equipment; and encouraging exercise.

- Provision of personal protective equipment (PPE), such as gloves, knee and elbow pads, protective footwear, and other items that employees wear to protect themselves against injury.

SAFETY PROGRAM

An effective safety program starts with a well-thought-out safety plan. This plan identifies the applicable regulatory requirements and describes how they will be met. A safety plan includes procedures to:

- Provide a workplace free of recognized hazards.
- Evaluate all procedures for potential exposure risks.
- Evaluate each job duty for potential exposure risks.
- Identify hazardous areas or materials with appropriate labels and signs.
- Educate staff; document training; and monitor compliance.
- Apply standard precautions (including universal and blood and body fluid precautions) to the handling of blood, body fluids, and tissues.
- Dispose of hazardous waste appropriately.
- Report incidents and accidents; provide treatment and follow-up.
- Provide ongoing review of safety policies, procedures, operations, and equipment.
- Develop facility-specific plans for disaster preparedness and response: test these plans at defined intervals.
- Develop facility-specific plans for response to threats to personal safety such as active shooters or bomb threats.

Safety programs should consider the needs of all persons affected by the work environment. Most obvious is the safety of technical staff members, but potential risks for blood donors, ancillary personnel, volunteers, visitors, housekeeping staff, and maintenance and repair workers must also be evaluated.

Laboratories should consider appointing a safety officer who can provide general guidance and expertise.[4] Typical duties of a safety officer are to develop the safety program, oversee orientation and training, perform safety audits, survey work sites, recommend changes, and serve on or direct the activities of safety committees. Facilities using hazardous chemicals and radioactive materials often assign specially trained individuals to oversee chemical and radiation protection programs as needed.[12,15] Five basic elements must be addressed for each type of hazard covered in the safety program:

- Training.
- Hazard identification and communication.
- Engineering controls and PPE.
- Safe work practices, including waste disposal.
- Emergency response plan.

Management controls should be established to ensure that these elements are implemented and maintained and that they are effective. Management is responsible for the following:

- Developing and communicating the written plan.
- Ensuring implementation and providing adequate resources.
- Providing access to employee health services related to prevention strategies and treatment of exposures.
- Monitoring compliance and effectiveness.
- Evaluating and improving the safety plan.

Basic Elements of a Safety Program

Training

Employees must be trained to recognize the hazards in their workplace and take appropriate precautions. Supervisors are responsible for assessing and documenting each employee's understanding of and ability to apply safety precautions before independent work is permitted. Safety training must precede even temporary work assignments if significant potential for exposure exists. Staff members who do not demonstrate the requisite understanding and skills must receive additional training. Training should be provided not only to laboratory staff but also to housekeeping and other personnel who may come into contact with hazardous substances or waste. Table 2-1 lists topics to cover in work safety training programs.

Hazard Identification and Communication

Employers are required to provide information about workplace hazards to their staff to help reduce the risk of occupational illnesses and injuries. Staff need to know what hazardous substances they are working with and where those materials are located in the facility. This communication is achieved by means of signage, labels on containers, written information, and training programs.

Engineering Controls and PPE

If the physical work space cannot be designed to eliminate the potential for exposure to hazards, appropriate protective gear must be provided. Engineering controls are physical plant controls or equipment, such as sprinkler systems, chemical fume hoods, and needleless systems that isolate or remove the hazard from the workplace.

PPE is specialized clothing or equipment, such as gloves, masks, and laboratory coats,

TABLE 2-1. Topics to Cover in a Work Safety Training Program

Work safety training programs should ensure that all personnel:
● Have access to a copy of pertinent regulatory texts and an explanation of the contents.
● Understand the employer's exposure control plan and how to obtain a copy of the written plan.
● Understand how hepatitis and human immunodeficiency virus (HIV) are transmitted and how often; be familiar with the symptoms and consequences of hepatitis B virus (HBV), hepatitis C virus (HCV), and HIV infection.
● Know that they are offered vaccination against HBV.
● Recognize tasks that pose infectious risks, and distinguish them from other duties.
● Know what protective clothing and equipment are appropriate for the procedures they will perform and how to use them.
● Know and understand the limitations of protective clothing and equipment (eg, different types of gloves are recommended according to the permeability of the hazardous material to be used).
● Know where protective clothing and equipment are kept.
● Become familiar with and understand all requirements for work practices specified in standard operating procedures for the tasks they perform, including the meaning of signs and labels.
● Know how to remove, handle, decontaminate, and dispose of contaminated material.
● Know the appropriate actions to take and the personnel to contact if exposed to blood or other biologic, chemical, or radiologic hazards.
● Know the corrective actions to take in the event of spills or personal exposure to fluids, tissues, and contaminated sharp objects; appropriate reporting procedures; and medical monitoring recommended when parenteral exposure may have occurred.
● Know their right to access to medical treatment and medical records.
● Know fire safety procedures and evacuation plans.
● Recognize facility-specific verbal announcements and how to respond.

worn by employees for protection against a hazard. Employees should remove their PPE, such as gloves and laboratory coats, and should wash their hands with soap and water when leaving a laboratory area. General guidance on the use of engineering controls and PPE is included in Appendix 2-2.

Safe Work Practices

Employees must be trained in how to work with hazardous materials in ways that protect themselves, their coworkers, and the environment. Safe work practices are defined as tasks performed in a manner that reduces the likelihood of exposure to workplace hazards. General recommendations for safe work practices are included in Appendix 2-2.

Emergency Response Plan

When engineering and work practice controls fail, employees must know how to respond promptly and appropriately. The purpose of advance planning is to control a hazardous situation as quickly and safely as possible. Regular testing of the emergency response plan identifies areas for improvement and builds staff confidence in their ability to respond effectively in a real emergency. OSHA requires facilities with more than 10 employees to have a written emergency response plan. Verbal communication of the plan is acceptable for facilities with 10 or fewer employees.[18]

Management Controls

Supervisory personnel must monitor safety practices in their areas of responsibility. Continuing attention to safety issues should be addressed in routine staff meetings and training sessions. Periodic audits performed by a safety professional increases safety awareness. Management should seek staff input on the design and improvement of the facility's safety plan.

The safety program policies, procedures, guidelines, and supporting references should be documented in writing and made available to all personnel at risk. These documents should be reviewed on a regular basis and updated as technology evolves and new informa-

tion becomes available. Risk mitigation studies should be conducted periodically. Strategies or other safety provisions should be updated or implemented with safety improvements. Work sites and safety equipment should be inspected regularly to ensure compliance and response readiness. Checklists may be helpful for documenting safety inspections and assessing safety preparedness.[3,4,19]

Employee Health Services

Hepatitis Prophylaxis

All employees routinely exposed to blood must be offered hepatitis B virus (HBV) vaccine if they do not already have HBV-protective antibodies (ie, anti-HBs). OSHA requires that the vaccine be offered at no cost to all employees and, if any employee refuses the vaccine, that the refusal be documented.[14]

Monitoring Programs

Employers must provide a system for monitoring exposure to certain substances as defined in the OSHA standard if there is reason to believe that exposure levels routinely exceed the recommended action level.[20]

Medical First Aid and Follow-Up

When requested by a worker who has sustained known or suspected blood exposure, monitoring for HBV, hepatitis C virus (HCV), and human immunodeficiency virus (HIV) infection should be provided with appropriate counseling. In some states, consent is required for this voluntary testing; rejection of offered testing must be documented. The usual schedule includes immediate tests of the worker and the source of the potentially infectious material, with follow-up testing of the worker at intervals after exposure.[13,14] All aspects of accident follow-up should be appropriately documented.

The Centers for Disease Control and Prevention (CDC) has published recommendations for both preexposure and postexposure prophylaxis if the contaminating material is HBV positive or if this information is unknown.[21] HBV immune globulin is usually given concurrently with HBV vaccine in cases of penetrating injuries. Postexposure prophylaxis for HIV is continually evolving; policies are generally based on Public Health Service recommendations and current standards of practice.

Reporting Accidents and Injuries

When an injury occurs, relevant information should be documented, including the date and time of injury and the place where it occurred; the nature of the injury; descriptions of what happened from the injured person and any witnesses; and first aid or medical attention provided. The supervisor should complete any accident reports and investigation forms required by the institution's insurer and worker's compensation agencies. Employers must report fatalities and injuries resulting in the hospitalization of three or more employees to OSHA within 8 hours of the accident.[22]

OSHA requires health-service employers with 11 or more workers to maintain records of occupational injuries and illnesses requiring a level of care that exceeds the capabilities of a person trained in first aid.[23] Initial documentation must be completed within 6 days of the incident. Records of first aid provided by a nonphysician for minor injuries, such as cuts or burns, do not need to be retained. All logs, summaries, and supplemental records must be preserved for at least 5 years beyond the calendar year of occurrence. Medical records of employees should be preserved for the duration of employment plus 30 years, with few exceptions.[24]

Latex Allergies

Adverse reactions associated with latex, powdered gloves, or both include contact dermatitis, allergic dermatitis, urticaria, and anaphylaxis. Medical devices that contain latex must bear a caution label. The National Institute for Occupational Safety and Health (NIOSH) offers the following recommendations to prevent these allergic reactions[25]:

- Make latex-free gloves available as an alternative to latex, and encourage the use of latex-free gloves for activities and work environments where there is minimal risk of exposure to infectious materials.
- If latex gloves are used, consider providing reduced-protein and powder-free gloves.
- Use good housekeeping practices to remove latex-containing dust from the workplace.
- Use work practices that reduce the chance of reaction, such as hand washing and avoiding oil-based hand lotions.
- Educate workers about latex allergy.
- Evaluate current prevention strategies.
- Periodically screen high-risk workers for latex allergy symptoms.
- If symptoms develop, have workers avoid direct contact with latex and consult a physician about allergy precautions.

FIRE PREVENTION

Fire prevention relies on a combination of facility design that is based on the National Fire Protection Association (NFPA) Life Safety Code, which identifies processes to maintain fire protection systems in good working order, and fire safe-work practices.[26] The Life Safety Code includes both active and passive fire-protection systems (eg, alarms, smoke detectors, sprinklers, exit lights in corridors, and fire-rated barriers).

Training

Fire safety training is recommended at the start of employment and at least annually thereafter. Training should emphasize prevention and an employee's awareness of the work environment, including how to recognize and report unsafe conditions, how to report fires, where the nearest alarm and fire-containment equipment are located and how to use it, and what the evacuation policies and routes are.

All staff members in facilities accredited by CAP or The Joint Commission are required to participate in fire drills at least annually.[3,5] In areas where patients are housed or treated, The Joint Commission requires quarterly drills on each shift. Staff participation and understanding should be documented.

Hazard Identification and Communication

Emergency exits must be clearly marked with an exit sign. Additional signage must be posted along the exit route to show the direction of travel if it is not immediately apparent. All flammable materials should be labeled with appropriate hazard warnings, and flammable storage cabinets should be clearly marked.

Engineering Controls and PPE

Laboratories storing large volumes of flammable chemicals are usually built with 2-hour fire separation walls, or with 1-hour separation walls if there is an automatic fire-extinguishing system.[4] Fire detection and alarm systems should be provided in accordance with federal, state, and local regulations. All fire equipment should be inspected on a regular basis to ensure that it is in good working order. Fire extinguishers should be readily available, and the staff should be trained to use them properly. Housekeeping and inventory management plans should be designed to control the accumulations of flammable and combustible materials stored in the facility. In areas where sprinkler systems are installed, all items should be stored at least 18 inches below the sprinkler heads. Facilities should consult local fire codes, which may require greater clearance.

Safe Work Practices

Emergency exit routes must be clear of anything that would obstruct evacuation efforts. Exit doors must not be locked in such a way as to impede egress. Permanent exit routes must be designed to allow free and unobstructed exit from all parts of the facility to an area of safety. Secondary exits may be required for areas larger than 1000 square feet; facilities should consult local safety authorities with jurisdiction, such as the local fire marshal and NFPA, for guidance on secondary exits.

Emergency Response Plan

The fire emergency response plan should encompass both facility-wide and area-specific situations. It should describe reporting and alarm systems; location and use of emergency equipment; roles and responsibilities of the staff during the response; "defend-in-place" strategies; and conditions for evacuation, evacuation procedures, and exit routes.[5,18]

When a fire occurs, the general sequence for immediate response should be to 1) rescue anyone in immediate danger; 2) activate the fire alarm system and alert others in the area; 3) confine the fire by closing doors and shutting off fans or other oxygen sources if possible; and 4) extinguish the fire with a portable extinguisher if the fire is small, or evacuate if it is too large to manage.

ELECTRICAL SAFETY

Electrical hazards, including fire and shock, may arise from the use of faulty electrical equipment; damaged receptacles, connectors, or cords; or unsafe work practices. Proper use of electrical equipment, periodic inspection and maintenance, and hazard recognition training are essential to help prevent accidents that may result in electric shock or electrocution. The severity of shock depends on the path that the electrical current takes through the body, the amount of current flowing through the body, and the length of time that current is flowing through the body. Even low-voltage exposures can lead to serious injury.[27]

Training

Safety training should be designed to make employees aware of electrical hazards associated with receptacles and connectors. This training should also help them recognize potential problems, such as broken receptacles and connectors, improper electrical connections, damaged cords, and inadequate grounding.

Hazard Identification and Communication

The safety plan should address the proper use of receptacles and connectors. Equipment that does not meet safety standards should be marked to prevent accidental use.

Engineering Controls and PPE

OSHA requires that electrical systems and equipment be constructed and installed in a way that minimizes the potential for workplace hazards. When purchasing equipment, the facility should verify that it bears the mark of an OSHA-approved independent testing laboratory, such as Underwriters Laboratories.[28] Adequate working space should be provided around equipment to allow easy access for safe operation and maintenance. Ground-fault circuit interrupters should be installed in damp or wet areas.

Safe Work Practices

Electrical safety practices focus on two factors: 1) proper use of electrical equipment and 2) proper maintenance and repair of this equipment. Staff should not plug equipment into or unplug equipment from an electrical source with wet hands. Overloading circuits with too many devices may cause the current to overheat the wiring and potentially generate a fire. Damaged receptacles and faulty electrical equipment must be tagged and removed from service until they have been repaired and checked for safety. Flexible cords should be secured to prevent tripping and should be protected from damage from heavy or sharp objects. Flexible cords should be kept slackened to prevent tension on electrical terminals, and cords should be checked regularly for cut, broken, or cracked insulation. Extension cords should not be used in lieu of permanent wiring.

Emergency Response Plan

In case of an emergency in which it is not possible to decrease the power or disconnect equipment, the power supply should be shut off from the circuit breaker. If it is not possible to interrupt the power supply, a nonconductive material, such as dry wood, should be used to pry a victim from the source of current.[27] Victims must not be touched directly. Emergency first aid for victims of electrical shock must be sought. Water-based fire extinguishers should not be used on electrical fires.

BIOSAFETY

The facility must define and enforce measures to minimize the risk of exposure to biohazard materials in the workplace. Requirements published by OSHA (Blood-Borne Pathogens Standard) and recommendations published by the US HHS provide the basis for an effective biosafety plan.[13,14,16]

Blood-Borne Pathogens Standard

The OSHA Blood-Borne Pathogens Standard is intended to protect employees in all occupations where there is a risk of exposure to blood and other potentially infectious materials. It requires the facility to develop an exposure control plan and describes appropriate engineering controls, PPE, and work practice controls to minimize the risk of exposure. The standard also requires employers to provide HBV vaccinations to any staff members with occupational exposure, provide medical follow-up care in case of accidental exposure, and keep records related to accidents and exposures.

Standard Precautions

Standard precautions represent the most current recommendations by the CDC to reduce the risk of transmission of blood-borne pathogens and other pathogens in hospitals. Standard precautions apply to all patient-care activities, regardless of diagnosis, in which there is a risk of exposure to 1) blood; 2) all body fluids, secretions, and excretions, *except sweat*, regardless of whether or not they contain visible blood; 3) nonintact skin; or 4) mucous membranes.

The OSHA Blood-Borne Pathogens Standard refers to the use of universal precautions. However, OSHA recognizes the more recent guidelines from the CDC and, in Directive CPL 02-02-069, allow hospitals to use acceptable alternatives, including standard precautions, as long as all other requirements in the standard are met.[29]

Biosafety Levels

Recommendations for biosafety in laboratories are based on the potential hazards pertaining to specific infectious agents and the activities performed.[16] Biosafety recommendations include guidance on both engineering controls and safe work practices. The four biosafety levels are designated in ascending order, with increasing protection for personnel, the environment, and the community:

- Biosafety Level 1 (BSL-1) involves work with agents of no known or of minimal potential hazard to laboratory personnel and the environment. Activities are usually conducted on open surfaces, and no containment equipment is needed.
- BSL-2 work involves agents of moderate potential hazard to personnel and the environment, usually from contact-associated exposure. Most blood bank laboratory activities are considered BSL-2.
- BSL-3 includes work with indigenous or exotic agents that may cause serious or potentially lethal disease as a result of exposure to aerosols (eg, *Mycobacterium tuberculosis*) or by other routes (eg, HIV) that would result in grave consequences to the infected host. Recommendations for BSL-3 work are designed to contain aerosols and minimize the risk of surface contamination.
- BSL-4 applies to work with dangerous or exotic agents that pose high individual risk of life-threatening disease from aerosols (eg, agents of hemorrhagic fevers or filoviruses). BSL-4 is not applicable to routine blood-bank-related activities.

The precautions described in this section focus on BSL-2 requirements. Laboratories should consult the CDC or National Institutes of Health guidelines for precautions appropriate for higher levels of containment.

Training

OSHA requires annual training for all employees whose tasks increase their risk of infectious exposure.[14,29] Training programs must be tailored to the target group both in level and content. General background knowledge of biohazards, understanding of control procedures, or work experience cannot meet the requirement for specific training, although an assessment of such knowledge is a first step in planning program content. Workplace volunteers require at least as much safety training as paid staff members who perform similar functions.

Hazard Identification and Communication

The facility's exposure control plan communicates the risks present in the workplace and describes controls to minimize exposure. BSL-2 through BSL-4 facilities must have a biohazard sign posted at the entrance when infectious agents are in use. The sign notifies personnel and visitors of the presence of infectious agents, provides a point of contact for the area, and indicates any special protective equipment or work practices required.

Biohazard warning labels must be placed on containers of regulated waste; refrigerators and freezers containing blood or other potentially infectious material; and other containers used to store, transport, or ship blood or other potentially infectious materials. Blood components that are labeled to identify their contents and have been released for transfusion or other clinical use are exempted.

Engineering Controls and PPE

OSHA requires that hazards be controlled by engineering or work practices whenever possible.[14] Engineering controls for BSL-2 laboratories include limited access to the laboratory when work is in progress and BSCs or other containment equipment for work that may involve infectious aerosols or splashes. Hand-washing sinks and eyewash stations must be available. The work space should be designed so that it can be easily cleaned, and bench tops should be impervious to water and resistant to chemicals and solvents.

To help prevent exposure or cross-contamination, work area telephones can be equipped with speakers to eliminate the need to pick up the receiver. Computer keyboards and telephones can be covered with plastic. Such equipment should be cleaned on a regular basis and when visibly soiled.

BSCs are primary containment devices for handling moderate-risk and high-risk organisms. There are three types—Classes I, II, and III—with Class III providing the highest protection to workers. In addition to protecting personnel during the handling of biohazard materials, a BSC may be used to prevent contamination of blood and cellular therapy products during open processing steps. A comparison of the features and applications of the three classes of cabinets is provided in Table 2-2.

BSCs are not required by standard precautions, but centrifugation of open blood samples or manipulation of units known to be positive for HBV surface antigen or HIV are examples of blood bank procedures for which a BSC could be useful. The effectiveness of the BSC is a function of directional airflow inward and downward through a high-efficiency filter. Efficacy is reduced by anything that disrupts the airflow pattern. Care should be taken not to block the front intake and rear exhaust grills. Performance of the BSC should be certified annually.[31]

In 2001, OSHA revised the Blood-Borne Pathogens Standard and required that employers implement appropriate control technologies and safer medical devices in exposure control plans and that employers solicit input from their employees to identify, evaluate, and select engineering and work practice controls. Examples of safer devices are needleless systems and self-sheathing needles in which the sheath is an integral part of the device.

Decontamination

Reusable equipment and work surfaces that may be contaminated with blood require daily cleaning and decontamination. Obvious spills on equipment or work surfaces should be cleaned up immediately; routine wipe-downs with disinfectant should occur at the end of each shift or on a different frequency that provides equivalent safety. Equipment that is exposed to blood or other potentially infectious material must be decontaminated before it is serviced or shipped. When decontamination of all or a portion of the equipment is not feasible, a biohazard label stating which portions remain contaminated should be attached before the equipment is serviced or shipped.

Choice of Disinfectants

The Environmental Protection Agency (EPA) maintains a list of chemical products that have been shown to be effective hospital antimicrobial disinfectants.[32] The Association for Professionals in Infection Control and Epidemiology also publishes a guideline to assist health-care professionals with decisions involving judicious selection and proper use of specific disinfectants.[33] For facilities covered under the Blood-Borne Pathogens Standard, OSHA allows the use of EPA-registered tuberculocidal disinfectants, EPA-registered disinfectants that are effective against both HIV and HBV, a diluted bleach solution to decontaminate work surfaces, or a combination of these.[29]

Before selecting a disinfectant product, several factors should be considered. Among them are the type of material or surface to be treated and the hazardous properties of the disinfectant product, such as corrosiveness and the level of disinfection required. After a product has been selected, procedures need to be written to ensure effective and consistent cleaning and treatment of work surfaces. Some factors to consider for effective decontamination include contact time, type of microorganisms, presence of organic matter, and concentration of the chemical agent. Laboratory personnel should review the basic information on decontamination and follow the manufacturer's instructions.

TABLE 2-2. Comparison of Classes I, II, and III Biological Safety Cabinets*

Category	Main Features	Intended Use	Common Applications
Class I	Unfiltered room air is drawn into the cabinet. Inward airflow protects personnel from exposure to materials inside the cabinet. Exhaust is high-efficiency particulate air (HEPA) filtered to protect the environment. It maintains airflow at a minimum velocity of 75 linear feet per minute (lfpm) across the front opening (face velocity).	Personal and environmental protection	To enclose equipment (eg, centrifuges) or procedures that may generate aerosols
Class II (general—applies to all types of Class II cabinets)	Laminar flow (air moving at a constant velocity in one direction along parallel lines) is used. Room air is drawn into the front grille. HEPA-filtered air is forced downward in a laminar flow to minimize cross-contamination of materials in the cabinet. Exhaust is HEPA filtered.	Personal, environmental, and product protection	Work with microorganisms assigned to Biosafety Levels 1, 2, or 3
			Handling of products for which prevention of contamination is critical, such as cell culture propagation or manipulation of blood components in an open system
Class II, A	Approximately 75% of air is recirculated after passing through a HEPA filter. Face velocity = 75 lfpm.	See Class II, general	See Class II, general
Class II, B1	Approximately 70% of air exits through the rear grille, is HEPA filtered, and is then discharged from the building. The other 30% is drawn into the front grille, is HEPA filtered, and is recirculated. Face velocity = 100 lfpm.	See Class II, general	Allows for safe manipulation of small quantities of hazardous chemicals and biologics

Class II, B2	All air is exhausted, and none is recirculated. A supply blower draws air from the room or outside and passes it through a HEPA filter to provide the downward laminar flow. Face velocity = 100 lfpm.	See Class II, general	Provides both chemical and biological containment; is more expensive to operate because of the volume of conditioned room air being exhausted
Class II, B3	Although similar in design to Type A, the system is ducted and includes a negative pressure system to keep any possible contamination within the cabinet. Face velocity = 100 lfpm.	See Class II, general	Allows for safe manipulation of small quantities of hazardous chemicals and biologics
Class III	Cabinet is airtight. Materials are handled with rubber gloves attached to the front of the cabinet. Supply air is HEPA filtered. Exhaust air is double HEPA filtered or may have one filter and an air incinerator. Materials are brought in and out of the cabinet either through a dunk tank or a double-door passthrough box that can be decontaminated. Cabinet is kept under negative pressure.	Maximum protection to personnel and environment	Work with Biosafety Level 4 microorganisms

*Data from the US Department of Health and Human Services.[30]

Storage

Hazardous materials must be segregated, and areas for different types of storage must be clearly demarcated. Blood must be protected from unnecessary exposure to other materials and vice versa. If transfusion products cannot be stored in a separate refrigerator from reagents, specimens, and unrelated materials, areas within the refrigerator must be clearly labeled and extra care must be taken to reduce the likelihood of spills and other accidents. Storage areas must be kept clean and orderly; food or drink is never allowed where biohazard materials are stored.

PPE

When hazards cannot be eliminated, OSHA requires employers to provide appropriate PPE and clothing and to clean, launder, or dispose of PPE at no cost to their employees.[14] Standard PPE and clothing include uniforms, laboratory coats, gloves, face shields, masks, and safety goggles. Indications and guidelines for their use are discussed in Appendix 2-2.

Safe Work Practices

Safe work practices appropriate for standard precautions include the following:

- Wash hands after touching blood, body fluids, secretions, excretions, and contaminated items, whether or not gloves are worn.
- Wear gloves when touching blood, body fluids, secretions, excretions, and contaminated items, and change gloves between tasks.
- Wear a mask and eye protection or a face shield during activities that are likely to generate splashes or sprays of blood, body fluids, secretions, and excretions.
- Wear a gown during activities that are likely to generate splashes or sprays of blood, body fluids, secretions, or excretions.
- Handle soiled patient-care equipment in a manner that prevents exposure; ensures that reusable equipment is not used for another patient until it has been cleaned and reprocessed appropriately; and en-

sures that single-use items are discarded properly.
- Ensure that adequate procedures are defined and followed for the routine care, cleaning, and disinfection of environmental surfaces and equipment.
- Handle soiled linen in a manner that prevents exposure.
- Handle needles, scalpels, and other sharp instruments or devices in a manner that minimizes the risk of exposure.
- Use mouthpieces, resuscitation bags, or other ventilation devices as an alternative to mouth-to-mouth resuscitation methods.

Laboratory Biosafety Precautions

Several factors need to be considered when assessing the risk of blood exposures among laboratory personnel. Some of these factors include the number of specimens processed, personnel behaviors, laboratory techniques, and types of equipment.[34] The laboratory director may wish to institute BSL-3 practices for procedures that are considered to be higher risk than BSL-2. When there is doubt whether an activity is BSL-2 or BSL-3, the safety precautions for BSL-3 should be followed. BSL-2 precautions that are applicable to the laboratory setting are summarized in Appendix 2-3.

Considerations for the Donor Room

The Blood-Borne Pathogens Standard acknowledges a difference between hospital patients and healthy donors, in whom the prevalence of infectious disease markers is significantly lower. The employer in a volunteer blood donation facility may determine that routine use of gloves is not required for phlebotomy as long as the following conditions exist[14]:

- The policy is periodically reevaluated.
- Gloves are made available to those who want to use them, and their use is not discouraged.
- Gloves are required when an employee has cuts, scratches, or breaks in skin; when there is a likelihood that contamination will occur; while an employee is drawing

autologous units; while an employee is performing therapeutic procedures; and during training in phlebotomy.

Procedures should be assessed for risks of biohazard exposures and risks inherent in working with a donor or patient during the screening and donation processes. Some techniques or procedures are more likely to cause injury than others, such as using lancets for finger puncture, handling capillary tubes, crushing vials for arm cleaning, handling any unsheathed needles, cleaning scissors, and giving cardiopulmonary resuscitation.

In some instances, it may be necessary to collect blood from donors known to pose a high risk of infectivity (eg, collection of autologous blood or source plasma for the production of other products, such as vaccines). The FDA provides guidance on collecting blood from such "high-risk" donors.[35,36] The most recent regulations and guidelines should be consulted for changes or additions.

Emergency Response Plan

Table 2-3 lists steps to take when a spill occurs. Facilities should be prepared to handle both small and large blood spills. Good preparation for spill cleanup includes several elements:

- Work areas designed so that cleanup is relatively simple.
- A spill kit or cart containing all necessary supplies and equipment with instructions for their use. It should be placed near areas where spills are anticipated.
- Responsibility assigned for kit or cart maintenance, spill handling, record-keeping, and review of significant incidents.
- Personnel trained in cleanup procedures and procedures for reporting significant incidents.

Biohazard Waste

Medical waste is defined as any waste (solid, semisolid, or liquid) generated in the diagnosis, treatment, or immunization of human

TABLE 2-3. Blood Spill Cleanup Steps

Evaluate the spill.
Wear appropriate protective clothing and gloves. If sharp objects are involved, gloves must be puncture resistant, and a broom or other instrument should be used during cleanup to avoid injury.
Remove clothing if it is contaminated.
Post warnings to keep the area clear.
Evacuate the area for 30 minutes if an aerosol has been created.
Contain the spill if possible.
If the spill occurs in the centrifuge, turn the power off immediately and leave the cover on for 30 minutes. The use of overwraps helps prevent aerosolization and contain the spill.
Use absorbent material to mop up most of the liquid contents.
Clean the spill area with detergent.
Flood the area with disinfectant and use it as described in the manufacturer's instructions. Allow adequate contact time with the disinfectant.
Wipe up residual disinfectant if necessary.
Dispose of all materials safely in accordance with biohazard guidelines. All blood-contaminated items must be autoclaved or incinerated.

beings or animals in related research, production, or testing of biologics. Infectious waste includes disposable equipment, articles, or substances that may harbor or transmit pathogenic organisms or their toxins. In general, infectious waste should be either incinerated or decontaminated before disposal in a sanitary landfill.

If state law allows, blood and components, suctioned fluids, excretions, and secretions may be carefully poured down a drain connected to a sanitary sewer. Sanitary sewers may also be used to dispose of other potentially infectious wastes that can be ground and flushed into the sewer. State and local health departments should be consulted about laws and regulations pertaining to disposal of biologic waste into the sewer.

In the blood bank, all items contaminated with liquid or semi-liquid blood are to be considered hazardous materials. Items contaminated with dried blood are considered hazardous if there is potential for the dried material to flake off during handling. Contaminated sharp objects are always considered hazardous because of the risk for percutaneous injury. However, items such as used gloves, swabs, plastic pipettes with excess liquid removed, or gauze contaminated with small droplets of blood may be considered nonhazardous if the material is dried and will not be released into the environment during handling.

Guidelines for Biohazard Waste Disposal

Employees must be trained before handling or disposing of biohazard waste, even if it is packaged. The following disposal guidelines are recommended[37]:

- Identify biohazard waste consistently; red seamless plastic bags (at least 2 mm thick) or containers carrying the biohazard symbol are recommended.
- Place bags in a protective container with closure upward to avoid breakage and leakage during storage or transport.
- Prepare and ship waste transported over public roads according to US Department of Transportation (DOT) regulations.

- Discard sharps (eg, needles, broken glass, glass slides, and wafers from sterile connecting devices) in rigid, puncture-proof, leak-proof containers.
- Put liquids in leak-proof, unbreakable containers only.
- Do not compact waste materials.

Storage areas for infectious material must be secured to reduce accident risk. Infectious waste must never be placed in the public trash collection system. Most facilities hire private carriers to decontaminate and dispose of infectious or hazardous waste. The facility should disclose all risks associated with the waste in their contracts with private companies. The carrier is responsible for complying with all federal, state, and local laws for biohazard (medical) waste transport, treatment, and disposal.

Treating Infectious or Medical Waste

Facilities that incinerate hazardous waste must comply with EPA standards of performance for new stationary sources and emission guidelines for existing sources.[38] In this regulation, a hospital/medical/infectious waste incinerator is any device that combusts any amount of hospital waste or medical/infectious waste.

Autoclaving is another common method for decontamination of biohazard waste, used for blood samples and blood components. The following elements are considered in determining processing time for autoclaving:

- Size of load being autoclaved.
- Type of packaging of item(s) being autoclaved.
- Density of items being autoclaved.
- Number of items in a single autoclave load.
- Placement of items in the autoclave to allow for steam penetration.

It is useful to place a biologic indicator in the center of loads that vary in size and contents to evaluate optimal steam penetration times. The EPA provides detailed information about choosing and operating such equipment.[37]

For decontamination, material should be autoclaved for a minimum of 1 hour. For sterilization, longer treatment times are needed. A general rule for decontamination is to process for 1 hour for every 10 pounds of waste. Usually, decontaminated laboratory wastes can be disposed of as nonhazardous solid wastes. The staff should check with the local solid-waste authority to ensure that the facility is in compliance with regulations for the area. Waste containing broken glass or other sharp items should be disposed of using a method consistent with policies for the disposal of other sharp or potentially dangerous materials.

CHEMICAL SAFETY

One of the most effective preventive measures that a facility can take to reduce hazardous chemical exposure is to choose alternative nonhazardous chemicals whenever possible. When the use of hazardous chemicals are required, purchasing these supplies in small quantities reduces the risks associated with storing excess chemicals and then dealing with their disposal.

OSHA requires that facilities using hazardous chemicals develop a written chemical hygiene plan (CHP) and that the plan be accessible to all employees. The CHP should outline procedures, equipment, PPE, and work practices that are capable of protecting employees from hazardous chemicals used in the facility.[15,20] The CHP must also provide assurance that equipment and protective devices are functioning properly and that criteria to determine implementation and maintenance of all aspects of the plan are in place. Employees must be informed of all chemical hazards in the workplace and be trained to recognize chemical hazards, protect themselves when working with these chemicals, and know where to find information about particular hazardous chemicals. Safety audits and annual reviews of the CHP are important control steps to help ensure that safety practices comply with the policies set forth in the CHP and that the CHP is up to date.

Establishing a clear definition of what constitutes hazardous chemicals is sometimes difficult. Generally, hazardous chemicals pose a significant health risk if an employee is exposed to them or a significant physical risk, such as fire or explosion, if handled or stored improperly. Categories of health and physical hazards are listed in Tables 2-4 and 2-5. The *NIOSH Pocket Guide to Chemical Hazards* provides a quick reference for many common chemicals.[39]

The facility should identify a qualified chemical hygiene officer to be responsible for developing guidelines for hazardous materials.[20] The chemical hygiene officer is also accountable for monitoring and documenting accidents and for initiating process change as needed.

Training

Employees who may be exposed to hazardous chemicals must be trained before they begin work in an area in which hazards exist. If a new employee has received prior training, it may not be necessary to retrain the individual, depending on the employer's evaluation of the new employee's level of knowledge. New employee training is likely to be necessary regarding such specifics as the location of each relevant safety data sheet (SDS), details on chemical labeling, PPE to be used, and site-specific emergency procedures.

Training must be provided for each new physical or health hazard when it is introduced into the workplace but not for each new chemical that falls within a particular hazard class.[15] For example, if a new solvent is brought into the workplace and the solvent has hazards similar to existing chemicals for which training has already been conducted, then the employer need only make employees aware of the new solvent's hazard category (eg, corrosive or irritant). However, if the newly introduced solvent is a suspected carcinogen and carcinogenic hazard training has not been provided, then new training must be conducted for employees with potential exposure. Retraining is advisable as often as necessary to ensure that employees understand the hazards linked to

TABLE 2-4. Categories of Health Hazards

Hazard	Definition
Carcinogens	Cancer-producing substances
Irritants	Agents causing irritation (eg, edema or burning) to skin or mucous membranes upon contact
Corrosives	Agents causing destruction of human tissue at the site of contact
Toxic or highly toxic agents	Substances causing serious biologic effects following inhalation, ingestion, or skin contact with relatively small amounts
Reproductive toxins	Chemicals that affect reproductive capabilities, including chromosomal damages and effects on fetuses
Other toxins	Hepatotoxins; nephrotoxins; neurotoxins; agents that act on the hematopoietic system; and agents that damage the lungs, skin, eyes, or mucous membranes

TABLE 2-5. Categories of Physical Hazards

Hazard	Definition
Combustible or flammable chemicals	Chemicals that can burn (including combustible and flammable liquids, solids, aerosols, and gases)
Compressed gases	Gases or mixtures of gases in a container under pressure
Explosives	Unstable or reactive chemicals that undergo violent chemical changes at normal temperatures and pressure
Unstable (reactive) chemicals	Chemicals that could be self-reactive under certain conditions (shocks, pressure, or temperature)
Water-reactive chemicals	Chemicals that react with water to release a gas that either is flammable or presents a health hazard

the materials with which they work, particularly any chronic and specific target-organ health hazards.

Hazard Identification and Communication

Hazard Communication

Employers must prepare a comprehensive hazard communication program for all areas in which hazardous chemicals are used to complement the CHP and "ensure that the hazards of all chemicals produced or imported are classified, and that information concern-

ing the classified hazard is transmitted to employers and employees."[15] The program should include labeling of hazardous chemicals, instructions on when and how to post warning labels for chemicals, directions for managing SDS reports for hazardous chemicals in the facilities, and employee training. Safety materials made available to employees should include the following:

- The facility's written CHP.
- The facility's written program for hazard communication.
- Identification of work areas where hazardous chemicals are located.

- Required list of hazardous chemicals and the relevant SDSs. (It is the responsibility of the facility to determine which chemicals may present a hazard to employees. This determination should be based on the quantity of chemical used; physical properties, potency, and toxicity of the chemical; manner in which the chemical is used; and means available to control the release of, or exposure to, the chemical.)

Hazardous Chemical Labeling and Signs

The Hazard Communication Standard requires manufacturers of chemicals and hazardous materials to provide the user with basic information about the hazards of these materials through product labeling and the SDS.[15] Employers are required to provide employees who are expected to work with these hazardous materials with information about what the hazards of the materials are, how to read the labeling, how to interpret symbols and signs on the labels, and how to read and use the SDS.

SDS forms typically include the following:

- Identification.
- Hazard(s) identification.
- Composition/information on ingredients.
- First-aid measures.
- Fire-fighting measures.
- Accidental release measures.
- Handling and storage considerations.
- Exposure controls/personal protection information.
- Physical and chemical properties.
- Stability and reactivity.
- Toxicology information.
- Ecologic information.
- Disposal considerations.
- Transport information.
- Regulatory information.
- Other information.

At a minimum, hazardous-chemical container labels must include the name of the chemical, name and address of the manufacturer, hazard warnings, symbols, designs, and other forms of warning to provide visual reminders of specific hazards. The label may refer to any SDS for additional information. Labels applied by the manufacturer must remain on containers. The user may add storage requirements and dates of receipt, opening, and expiration. If chemicals are aliquoted into secondary containers, the secondary container must be labeled with the name of the chemical and appropriate hazard warnings. Additional information, such as precautionary measures, concentration if applicable, and date of preparation, are helpful but not mandatory.

It is a safe practice to label all containers with their content, even water. Transfer containers used for temporary storage need not be labeled if the person performing the transfer retains control and intends the containers to be used immediately. Information regarding acceptable standards for hazard communication labeling is provided by the NFPA[40] and the National Paint and Coatings Association.[41]

Signs meeting OSHA requirements must be posted in areas where hazardous chemicals are used. Decisions about where to post warning signs are based on the manufacturer's recommendations regarding the chemical hazards, the quantity of the chemical in the room or laboratory, and the potency and toxicity of the chemical.

Safety Data Sheet

The SDS identifies the physical and chemical properties of a hazardous chemical (eg, flash point or vapor pressure), its physical and health hazards (eg, potential for fire, explosion, and signs and symptoms of exposure), and precautions for the chemical's safe handling and use. Specific instructions in an individual SDS take precedence over generic information in the hazardous materials program.

Employers must maintain copies of each required SDS in the workplace for each hazardous chemical and ensure that SDS copies are readily accessible during each work shift to employees when they are in their work areas. When household consumer products are used in the workplace in the same manner that a consumer would use them (ie, when the duration and frequency of use, and therefore exposure, are not greater than those that the typical consumer would experience), OSHA does not require that an SDS be provided to purchasers. However, if exposure to such products exceeds that normally found in consumer applications, employees have a right to know about the properties of such hazardous chemicals. OSHA does not require or encourage employers to maintain an SDS for nonhazardous chemicals.

Engineering Controls and PPE

Guidelines for laboratory areas in which hazardous chemicals are used or stored must be established. Physical facilities, and especially ventilation, must be adequate for the nature and volume of work conducted. Chemicals must be stored according to chemical compatibility (eg, corrosives, flammables, and oxidizers) and in minimal volumes. Bulk chemicals should be kept outside work areas. NFPA standards and others provide guidelines for proper storage, sometimes in storage cabinets.[4,40,42]

Chemical fume hoods are recommended for use with organic solvents, volatile liquids, and dry chemicals with a significant inhalation hazard.[4] Although constructed with safety glass, most fume hood sashes are not designed to serve as safety shields. Hoods should be positioned in an area where there is minimal foot traffic to avoid disrupting the airflow and compromising the containment field.

PPE that may be provided, depending on the hazardous chemicals used, includes chemical-resistant gloves and aprons, shatterproof safety goggles, and respirators.

Emergency showers should be accessible to areas where caustic, corrosive, toxic, flammable, or combustible chemicals are used.[4,43] There should be unobstructed access, within 10 seconds, to the showers from the areas where hazardous chemicals are used. Safety showers should be periodically flushed and tested for function, and associated floor drains should be checked to ensure that drain traps remain filled with water.

Safe Work Practices

Hazardous material should not be stored or transported in open containers. Containers and their lids or seals should be designed to prevent spills or leakage in all reasonably anticipated conditions. Containers should be able to safely store the maximum anticipated volume and be easy to clean. Surfaces should be kept clean and dry at all times.

When an employee is working with a chemical fume hood, all materials should be kept at least six inches behind the face opening. The vertical sliding sash should be positioned at the height specified on the certification sticker. The airfoil baffles and rear ventilation slots must not be blocked. Appendix 2-5 lists suggestions for working safely with specific chemicals.

Emergency Response Plan

The time to prepare for a chemical spill is before it occurs. A comprehensive employee training program should provide each employee with all tools necessary to act responsibly at the time of a chemical spill. The employee should know response procedures, be able to assess the severity of a chemical spill, know or be able to quickly look up the basic physical characteristics of the chemicals, and know where to find emergency response telephone numbers. The employee should be able to assess, stop, and confine the spill; either clean up the spill or call for a spill cleanup team; and follow procedures for reporting the spill. The employee must know when to ask for assistance, when to isolate the area, and where to find cleanup materials.

Chemical spills in the workplace can be categorized as follows[44]:

- *Incidental releases* are limited in quantity and toxicity and pose no significant safety or health hazard to employees. They may be safely cleaned up by employees familiar with the hazards of the chemical involved in the spill. Waste from the cleanup may be classified as hazardous and must be disposed of in the proper fashion. Appendix

2-6 describes appropriate responses to incidental spills.

- *Releases that may be incidental or may require an emergency response* may pose an exposure risk to employees depending on the circumstances. Considerations such as the hazardous substance properties, circumstances of release, and mitigating factors play a role in determining the appropriate response. The facility's emergency response plan should provide guidance on how to determine whether a spill is incidental or requires an emergency response.
- *Emergency response releases* pose a threat to health and safety regardless of the circumstances surrounding their release. These spills may require evacuation of the immediate area. The response typically comes from outside the immediate release area by personnel trained as emergency responders. These spills include those that involve immediate danger to life or health, serious threat of fire or explosion, and high levels of toxic substances.

Appendix 2-7 addresses the management of hazardous chemical spills. Spill cleanup kits or carts tailored to the specific hazards present should be available in each area. The kits or carts may contain rubber gloves and aprons, shoe covers, goggles, suitable aspirators, general absorbents, neutralizing agents, a broom, a dust pan, appropriate trash bags or cans for waste disposal, and cleanup directions. Chemical absorbents, such as clay absorbents or spill blankets, can be used for cleaning up a number of chemicals and thus may be easier for employees to use in spill situations.

With any spill of a hazardous chemical, but especially of a carcinogenic agent, it is essential to refer to the SDS and contact a designated supervisor or designee trained to handle these spills and hazardous waste disposal.[4] Facility environmental health and safety personnel can also offer assistance. The employer must assess the extent of the employee's exposure. After an exposure, an employee must be given an opportunity for medical consultation to determine the need for a medical examination.

Another source of workplace hazards is the unexpected release of hazardous vapors into the environment. OSHA has set limits for exposure to hazardous vapors from toxic and hazardous substances.[45] The potential risk associated with a chemical is determined by the manufacturer and listed on the SDS.

Chemical Waste Disposal

Most laboratory chemical waste is considered hazardous and is regulated by the EPA through the Resource Conservation and Recovery Act (42 USC §6901 et seq, 1976). This regulation specifies that hazardous waste can be legally disposed of only at an EPA-approved disposal facility. Disposal of chemical waste into a sanitary sewer is regulated by the Clean Water Act (33 USC §1251 et seq, 1977), and most US states have strict regulations concerning disposal of chemicals in the water system. Federal and applicable state regulations should be consulted when a facility is setting up and reviewing its waste disposal policies.

RADIATION SAFETY

Radiation can be defined as energy in the form of waves or particles emitted and propagated through space or a material medium. Gamma rays are electromagnetic radiation, whereas alpha and beta emitters are examples of particulate radiation. The presence of radiation in the blood bank, such as self-contained blood irradiators, requires additional precautions and training.[4,46]

Radiation Measurement Units

The measurement unit quantifying the amount of energy absorbed per unit mass of tissue is the gray (Gy) or radiation absorbed dose (rad); 1 Gy = 100 rad.

Dose equivalency measurements are more useful than simple energy measurements because dose equivalency measurements take into account the ability of different types of radiation to cause biologic effects. The ability of radiation to cause damage is assigned a number, called a quality factor (QF). For example, exposure to a given amount of alpha particles (QF = 20) is far more damaging than exposure to an equivalent amount of gamma rays (QF = 1). The common unit of measurement for dose equivalency is the roentgen or rad equivalent man (rem). Rem is the dose from any type of radiation that produces biologic effects in humans equivalent to 1 rad of x-rays, gamma rays, or beta rays. To obtain the dose from a particular type of radiation in rem, the number of rad should be multiplied by the QF (rad × QF = rem). Because the QF for gamma rays, x-rays, and most beta particles is 1, the dose in rad is equal to the dose in rem for these types of radiation.

Biologic Effects of Radiation

Any harm to tissue begins with the absorption of radiation energy and subsequent disruption of chemical bonds. Molecules and atoms become ionized or excited (or both) by absorbing this energy. The direct action path leads to radiolysis or formation of free radicals that, in turn, alter the structure and function of molecules in the cell.

Molecular alterations can cause cellular or chromosomal changes, depending on the amount and type of radiation energy absorbed. Cellular changes can be manifested as a visible somatic effect (eg, erythema). Changes at the chromosome level may be manifested as leukemia or other cancers or possibly as germ-cell defects that are transmitted to future generations.

Several factors influence the level of biologic damage from exposure, including the type of radiation, part of the body exposed, total absorbed dose, and dose rate. The total absorbed dose is the cumulative amount of radiation absorbed in the tissue. The greater the dose, the greater the potential for biologic damage. Exposure can be acute or chronic. The low levels of ionizing radiation likely to occur in blood banks should not pose any detrimental risk.[47-50]

Regulations

The NRC controls the use of radioactive materials by establishing licensure requirements. States and municipalities may also have requirements for inspection, licensure, or both. The type of license for using radioisotopes or irradiators depends on the scope and magnitude of the use of radioactivity. US facilities should contact the NRC and appropriate state agencies for information on license requirements and applications as soon as such activities are proposed.

Each NRC-licensed establishment must have a qualified radiation safety officer who is responsible for establishing personnel protection requirements and for ensuring proper disposal and handling of radioactive materials. Specific radiation safety policies and procedures should address dose limits, employee training, warning signs and labels, shipping and handling guidelines, radiation monitoring, and exposure management. Emergency procedures must be clearly defined and readily available to the staff.

In 2005, the NRC imposed additional security requirements for high-risk radioactive sources, including those used in blood irradiators. The purpose of the increased controls is to reduce the risk of unauthorized use of radioactive materials that may pose a threat to public health and safety. These 2005 measures include controlled access, approval in writing of individuals deemed trustworthy and reliable to have unescorted access, a system of monitoring to immediately detect and respond to unauthorized access, and documentation of authorized personnel and monitoring activities.[51] In 2007, a requirement for fingerprinting was added.[52]

Exposure Limits

The NRC sets standards for protection against radiation hazards arising from licensed activities, including dose limits.[12] Such limits, or maximal permissible dose equivalents, are a measure of the radiation risk over time and serve as standards for exposure. The occupational total effective-dose-equivalent limit is 5 rem/year, the shallow dose equivalent limit (skin) is 50 rem/year, the extremity dose equivalent limit is 50 rem/year, and the eye dose equivalent limit is 15 rem/year.[12,47] Dose limits for an embryo or fetus must not exceed 0.5 rem during pregnancy.[12,47,53] Employers are expected not only to maintain radiation exposure below allowable limits, but also to keep exposure levels as far below these limits as can reasonably be achieved.

Radiation Monitoring

Monitoring is essential for early detection and prevention of problems resulting from radiation exposure. Monitoring is used to evaluate the facility's environment, work practices, and procedures and to comply with regulations and NRC licensing requirements. Monitoring is accomplished with the use of dosimeters, bioassays, survey meters, and wipe tests.[4]

Dosimeters, such as film or thermoluminescent badges, rings, or both, measure personnel radiation doses. The need for dosimeters depends on the amount and type of radioactive materials in use; the facility radiation safety officer determines individual dosimeter needs. Film badges must be changed at least quarterly and in some instances monthly, be protected from high temperature and humidity, and be stored at work away from sources of radiation.

Bioassays, such as thyroid and whole body counting or urinalysis, may be used to determine whether there is radioactivity inside the body and if so, how much. If necessary, bioassays are usually performed quarterly and after an incident where accidental intake may have occurred.

Survey meters are sensitive to low levels of gamma or particulate radiation and provide a quantitative assessment of radiation hazard. Survey meters can be used to monitor storage areas for radioactive materials or wastes, testing areas during or after completion of a procedure, and packages or containers of radioactive materials. Survey meters must be calibrated annually by an authorized NRC licensee. Selection of appropriate meters should be discussed with the radiation safety officer.

In areas where radioactive materials are handled, all work surfaces, equipment, and floors that may be contaminated should be checked regularly with a wipe test. In the wipe test, a moistened absorbent material (the wipe) is passed over the surface and then measured for radiation.

Training

Personnel who handle radioactive materials or work with blood irradiators must receive radiation safety training before beginning work. This training should address the presence and potential hazards of radioactive materials in the employee's work area, general health protection issues, emergency procedures, and radiation warning signs and labels in use. Instruction in the following areas is also suggested:

- NRC regulations and license conditions.
- The importance of observing license conditions and regulations and of reporting violations or conditions of unnecessary exposure.
- Precautions to minimize exposure.
- Interpretation of results of monitoring devices.
- Requirements for pregnant workers.
- Employees' rights.
- Documentation and record-keeping requirements.

The need for refresher training is determined by the license agreement between the NRC and the facility.

Engineering Controls and PPE

Although self-contained blood irradiators present little risk to laboratory staff and film badges are not required for routine operation, blood establishments with irradiation programs must be licensed by the NRC.[48]

The manufacturer of the blood irradiator usually accepts responsibility for radiation safety requirements during transportation, installation, and validation of the unit as part of the purchase contract. The radiation safety officer can help oversee the installation and validation processes and should confirm that appropriate training, monitoring systems, procedures, and maintenance protocols are in place before use and that they reflect the manufacturer's recommendations. Suspected malfunctions must be reported immediately so that appropriate actions can be initiated.

Blood irradiators should be located in secure areas so that only trained individuals have access. Fire protection for the unit must also be considered. Automatic fire detection and control systems should be readily available in the immediate area. Blood components that have been irradiated are not radioactive and pose no threat to the staff or the general public.

Safe Work Practices

Each laboratory should establish policies and procedures for the safe use of radioactive materials. These policies and procedures should include requirements for following general laboratory safety principles, appropriate storage of radioactive solutions, and proper disposal of radioactive wastes. Radiation safety can be improved with the following procedures:

- Minimizing the time of exposure by working as efficiently as possible.
- Maximizing the distance from the source of the radiation by staying as far from the source as possible.
- Maximizing shielding (eg, by using a self-shielded irradiator or wearing a lead apron) when working with certain radioactive materials. These requirements are usually stipulated in the license conditions.
- Using good housekeeping practices to minimize the spread of radioactivity to uncontrolled areas.

Emergency Response Plan

Radioactive contamination is the dispersal of radioactive material into or onto areas in which it is not intended—for example, the floor, work areas, equipment, personnel clothing, or personnel skin. The NRC regulations state that gamma or beta radioactive contamination cannot exceed 2200 disintegrations per minute (dpm) per 100 cm^2 in the posted (restricted) area or 220 dpm/100 cm^2 in an unrestricted area, such as a corridor. For alpha emitters, these values are 220 dpm/100 cm^2 and 22 dpm/100 cm^2, respectively.[54]

If a spill occurs, employees' contaminated skin surfaces must be washed several times, and the radiation safety officer must be notified immediately to provide further guidance. Others must not be allowed to enter the area until emergency response personnel arrive.

Radioactive Waste Management

Policies for the disposal of radioactive waste, whether liquid or solid, should be established with input from the radiation safety officer.

Liquid radioactive waste may be collected into large sturdy bottles labeled with an appropriate radiation waste tag. The rules for separation by chemical compatibility apply. Bottles must be carefully stored to protect against spillage or breakage. Dry or solid waste may be sealed in a plastic bag and tagged as radiation waste. The isotope, its activity, and the date on which the activity was measured should be recorded on the bag. Radioactive waste must never be discharged into the facility's drain system without prior approval by the radiation safety officer.

SHIPPING HAZARDOUS MATERIALS

Hazardous materials commonly shipped by transfusion medicine, cellular therapy, and clinical diagnostic services include infectious substances, biologic substances, liquid nitrogen, and dry ice.

The US DOT regulations for transportation of hazardous materials are harmonized with the international standards published annually by the International Air Transport Association (IATA).[55,56] These regulations provide instructions for identifying, classifying, packaging, marking, labeling, and documenting hazardous materials to be offered for shipment on public roadways or by air.

Specimens are classified as Category A if they are known or likely to contain infectious substances in a form that is capable of causing permanent disability or life-threatening or fatal disease in otherwise healthy humans or animals when an exposure occurs. The proper shipping name for Category A specimens is "infectious substances, affecting humans" (UN2814) or "infectious substances, affecting animals only" (UN2900).

Specimens that may contain infectious substances but do not have the level of risk described above are classified as Category B, and the proper shipping name is "biological substance, Category B" (UN3373). HIV or HBV in culture are classified as Category A infectious substances, but these viruses present in a patient blood specimen are classified as Category B.

Patient specimens with minimal likelihood of containing pathogens are exempt from hazardous materials regulations if the specimens are properly packaged and marked. Blood components, cellular therapy products, and tissue for transfusion or transplantation are not subject to hazardous material regulations. Method 1-1 provides additional shipping instructions for safe transport of these materials. However, the most recent revision of the IATA or US DOT regulations should be consulted for the most current classification, packaging, and labeling requirements as well as for limitations on the volumes of hazardous materials that can be packaged together in one container.

GENERAL WASTE MANAGEMENT

Those responsible for safety at a facility must be concerned with protecting the environment as well as all staff members. Every effort should be made to establish facility-wide programs to reduce solid wastes, including nonhazardous and, especially, hazardous wastes (ie, biohazard, chemical, and radioactive wastes).

A hazardous-waste-reduction program instituted at the point of use of the material achieves several goals. It reduces the institutional risk for occupational exposures to hazardous agents, reduces "cradle-to-grave" liability for disposal, and enhances compliance with environmental requirements to reduce pollution generated from daily operations of the laboratory.[37,57,58]

Facilities can minimize pollution of the environment by practicing the "three R's": reduce, reuse, and recycle. Seeking suitable alternatives to materials that create hazardous waste and separating hazardous waste from nonhazardous waste can reduce the volume of hazardous waste and decrease costs for its disposal.

Changes in techniques or materials to reduce the volume of infectious waste or render it less hazardous should be carefully considered, and employees should be encouraged to identify safer alternatives whenever possible.

Facilities should check with state and local health and environmental authorities about current requirements for storage and disposal of a particular multihazardous waste before creating that waste. If creating the multihazardous waste cannot be avoided, the volume of waste generated should be minimized. In some states, copper sulfate contaminated with blood is considered a multihazardous waste. The disposal of this waste poses several problems with transportation from draw sites to a central facility for disposal of the final containers. State and local health departments must be involved in reviewing transportation and disposal practices where this is an issue, and procedures must be developed in accordance with state and local regulations as well as those of the US DOT.

KEY POINTS

1. Facilities should be designed and maintained in a way that supports the work being done in the physical space. Designing the space to accommodate planned work flow, the need to restrict certain areas, the movement of materials and waste, equipment location, special air-handling requirements, and other critical aspects of the operation help ensure safety for staff and visitors as well as the quality of products and services.

2. A facility's safety program should: a) strive to reduce hazards in the workplace; b) ensure that staff are trained to handle known hazards and potential risks; c) ensure that known hazards are clearly identified and marked; and d) describe policies and procedures for workplace safety and emergency response.

3. Safety programs should address fire, electrical, biologic, chemical, and radioactive hazards that may be found in the facility.

4. For each type of hazard, five basic elements that must be covered are: a) training; b) hazard identification and communication; c) engineering controls and PPE; d) safe work practices, including waste disposal; and e) an emergency response plan.

5. Management controls ensure that the safety program is implemented, maintained, and effective. Management is responsible for: a) developing and communicating the written plan; b) ensuring implementation of the plan and providing adequate resources for this implementation; c) providing access to employee health services for prevention strategies and treatment of exposures; d) monitoring compliance and effectiveness; and e) evaluating and improving the safety plan.

REFERENCES

1. Ooley PW, ed. Standards for blood banks and transfusion services. 30th ed. Bethesda, MD: AABB, 2016.

2. Haspel RL, ed. Standards for cellular therapy services. 8th ed. Bethesda, MD: AABB, 2017.

3. Laboratory Accreditation Program laboratory general checklist. Northfield, IL: College of American Pathologists, 2017.

4. Clinical laboratory safety: Approved guideline. 3rd ed. NCCLS Document GP17-A3. Wayne, PA: Clinical and Laboratory Standards Institute, 2012.

5. Hospital accreditation standards. Oakbrook Terrace, IL: The Joint Commission, 2017.

6. Laboratory accreditation standards. Oakbrook Terrace, IL: The Joint Commission, 2017.

7. NFPA 70—National electrical code. Quincy, MA: National Fire Protection Association, 2017.

8. ANSI/ASHRAE Standard 62.1-2016. Ventilation for acceptable indoor air quality. Atlanta, GA: American Society of Heating, Refrigerating, and Air-Conditioning Engineers, Inc., 2016.

9. Code of federal regulations. Title 21, CFR Part 1271.190. Washington, DC: US Government Publishing Office, 2017 (revised annually).

10. ISO-14644: Cleanrooms and associated controlled environments, Parts 1-9. ISO/TC 209. Geneva, Switzerland: International Organization for Standardization, 1999-2012.

11. ISO-14698: Cleanrooms and associated controlled environments—bio-contamination control, Part 1: General principles and methods. ISO/TC 209. Geneva, Switzerland: International Organization for Standardization, 2003.

12. Code of federal regulations. Title 10, CFR Part 20. Washington, DC: US Government Publishing Office, 2017 (revised annually).

13. Siegel JD, Rhinehart E, Jackson M, et al. 2007 Guideline for isolation precautions: Preventing transmission of infectious agents in healthcare settings. Atlanta, GA: Centers for Disease Control and Prevention (Healthcare Infection Control Practices Advisory Committee), 2007. [Available at http://www.cdc.gov/hicpac/pdf/isolation/Isolation2007.pdf (accessed January 15, 2017).]

14. Code of federal regulations. Title 29, CFR Part 1910.1030. Washington, DC: US Government Publishing Office, 2017 (revised annually).

15. Code of federal regulations. Title 29, CFR Part 1910.1200. Washington, DC: US Government Publishing Office, 2017 (revised annually).

16. US Department of Health and Human Services. Biosafety in microbiological and biomedical laboratories. 5th ed. Washington, DC: US Government Publishing Office, 2009.

17. Bernard B, ed. Musculoskeletal disorders and workplace factors: A critical review of epide-

miologic evidence for work-related musculo-skeletal disorders of the neck, upper extremity, and low back. NIOSH publication no. 97-141. Washington, DC: National Institute for Occupational Safety and Health, 1997.

18. Code of federal regulations. Title 29, CFR Part 1910.38. Washington, DC: US Government Publishing Office, 2017 (revised annually).

19. Wagner KD, ed. Environmental management in healthcare facilities. Philadelphia: WB Saunders, 1998.

20. Code of federal regulations. Title 29, CFR Part 1910.1450. Washington, DC: US Government Publishing Office, 2017 (revised annually).

21. Centers for Disease Control and Prevention. Public Health Service guidelines for the management of occupational exposures to HBV, HCV, and HIV and recommendations for post-exposure prophylaxis. MMWR Morb Mortal Wkly Rep 2001;50:1-52.

22. Code of federal regulations. Title 29, CFR Part 1904.39. Washington, DC: US Government Publishing Office, 2017 (revised annually).

23. Code of federal regulations. Title 29, CFR Part 1904.1, Part 1904.7. Washington, DC: US Government Publishing Office, 2017 (revised annually).

24. Code of federal regulations. Title 29, CFR Part 1910.1020. Washington, DC: US Government Publishing Office, 2017 (revised annually).

25. NIOSH Alert: Preventing allergic reactions to natural rubber latex in the workplace. (June 1997) NIOSH Publication No. 97-135. Washington, DC: National Institute for Occupational Safety and Health, 1997. [Available at http://www.cdc.gov/niosh/docs/97-135/ (accessed January 15, 2017).]

26. NFPA 101: Life safety code. Quincy, MA: National Fire Protection Association, 2012.

27. Fowler TW, Miles KK. Electrical safety: Safety and health for electrical trades student manual. (January 2002) NIOSH Publication No. 2002-123. Washington, DC: National Institute for Occupational Safety and Health, 2002.

28. OSHA technical manual: TED 1-0.15A. Washington, DC: US Department of Labor, 1999.

29. Enforcement procedures for the occupational exposure to bloodborne pathogens. Directive CPL 02-02-069. Washington, DC: US Department of Labor, 2001.

30. US Department of Health and Human Services. Primary containment for biohazards: Selection, installation, and use of biological safety cabinets. Washington, DC: US Govern-

ment Publishing Office, 2009. [Available at http://www.cdc.gov/biosafety/publications (accessed January 15, 2017).]

31. Richmond JY. Safe practices and procedures for working with human specimens in biomedical research laboratories. J Clin Immunoassay 1988;11:115-19.

32. US Environmental Protection Agency. Pesticide registration: Selected EPA-registered disinfectants. Washington, DC: EPA, 2016. [Available at https://www.epa.gov/pesticide-registration/selected-epa-registered-disinfectants (accessed January 15, 2017).]

33. Rutala WA. APIC guideline for selection and use of disinfectants. Am J Infect Control 1996;24:313-42.

34. Evans MR, Henderson DK, Bennett JE. Potential for laboratory exposures to biohazardous agents found in blood. Am J Public Health 1990;80:423-7.

35. Food and Drug Administration. Memorandum: Guideline for collection of blood products from donors with positive tests for infectious disease markers ("high risk" donors). (October 26, 1989) Silver Spring, MD: CBER Office of Communication, Outreach, and Development, 1989.

36. Food and Drug Administration. Memorandum: Revision to 26 October 1989 guidelines for collection of blood or blood products from donors with positive tests for infectious disease markers ("high-risk" donors). Silver Spring, MD: CBER Office of Communication, Outreach, and Development, 1991. [Available at http://www.fda.gov/BiologicsBloodVaccines/GuidanceComplianceRegulatoryInformation/OtherRecommendationsforManufacturers/MemorandumtoBloodEstablishments/default.htm (accessed January 24, 2017).]

37. US Environmental Protection Agency. EPA guide for infectious waste management. EPA/530-SW-86-014. NTIS #PB86-199130. Washington, DC: National Technical Information Service, 1986.

38. Code of federal regulations. Title 40, CFR Part 264. Washington, DC: US Government Publishing Office, 2017 (revised annually).

39. NIOSH pocket guide to chemical hazards. Washington, DC: National Institute for Occupational Safety and Health, 2010. [Available at http://www.cdc.gov/niosh/npg (accessed January 15, 2017).]

40. NFPA 704—Standard for the identification of the hazards of materials for emergency re-

sponse. Quincy, MA: National Fire Protection Association, 2012.

41. Hazardous Materials Identification System. HMIS implementation manual. 3rd ed. Neenah, WI: JJ Keller and Associates, Inc., 2001.

42. Lisella FS, Thomasston SW. Chemical safety in the microbiology laboratory. In: Fleming DO, Richardson JH, Tulis JJ, Vesley D, eds. Laboratory safety, principles, and practices. 2nd ed. Washington, DC: American Society for Microbiology Press, 1995:247-54.

43. American national standards for emergency eyewash and shower equipment. ANSI Z358.1-2009. New York: American National Standards Institute, 2009.

44. Inspection procedures for 29 CFR 1910.120 and 1926.65, paragraph (q): Emergency response to hazardous substance releases. OSHA Directive CPL 02-02-073. Washington, DC: Occupational Safety and Health Administration, 2007.

45. Code of federal regulations. Title 29, CFR Part 1910.1000. Washington, DC: US Government Publishing Office, 2017 (revised annually).

46. Cook SS. Selection and installation of self-contained irradiators. In: Butch S, Tiehen A, eds. Blood irradiation: A user's guide. Bethesda, MD: AABB Press, 1996:19-40.

47. Beir V. Health effects of exposure to low levels of ionizing radiation. Washington, DC: National Academy Press, 1990:1-8.

48. Regulatory guide 8.29: Instruction concerning risks from occupational radiation exposure. Washington, DC: Nuclear Regulatory Commission, 1996.

49. NCRP report no. 115: Risk estimates for radiation protection: Recommendations of the National Council on Radiation Protection and Measurements. Bethesda, MD: National Council on Radiation Protection and Measurements, 1993.

50. NCRP report no. 105: Radiation protection for medical and allied health personnel: Recommendations of the National Council on Radiation Protection and Measurements. Bethesda, MD: National Council on Radiation Protection and Measurements, 1989.

51. EA-05 090. Enforcement action: Order imposing increased controls (licensees authorized to possess radioactive material quantities of concern). (November 14, 2005) Rockville, MD: US Nuclear Regulatory Commission, 2005.

52. RIS 2007-14. Fingerprinting requirements for licensees implementing the increased control order. (June 5, 2007) Rockville, MD: US Nuclear Regulatory Commission, 2007.

53. US Nuclear Regulatory Commission regulatory guide 8.13: Instruction concerning prenatal radiation exposure. Washington, DC: NRC, 1999.

54. Nuclear Regulatory Commission regulatory guide 8.23: Radiation surveys at medical institutions. Washington, DC: NRC, 1981.

55. Code of federal regulations. Title 49, CFR Parts 171.22. Washington, DC: US Government Publishing Office, 2017 (revised annually).

56. Dangerous goods regulations manual. 54th ed. Montreal, PQ, Canada: International Air Transport Association, 2017 (revised annually).

57. United States Code. Pollution prevention act. 42 USC §§13101 and 13102 et seq.

58. Clinical laboratory waste management. Approved guideline. 3rd ed. GP05-A3. Wayne, PA: Clinical and Laboratory Standards Institute, 2011.

● **APPENDIX 2-1**

Safety Regulations and Recommendations Applicable to Health-Care Settings

Agency/Organization	Reference	Title
Federal Regulations and Recommendations		
Nuclear Regulatory Commission	10 CFR 20	Standards for Protection Against Radiation
	10 CFR 36	Licenses and Radiation Safety Requirements for Irradiators
	Guide 8.29	Instructions Concerning Risks from Occupational Radiation Exposure
Occupational Safety and Health Administration	29 CFR 1910.1030	Occupational Exposure to Bloodborne Pathogens
	29 CFR 1910.1020	Access to Employee Exposure and Medical Records
	29 CFR 1910.1096	Ionizing Radiation
	29 CFR 1910.1200	Hazard Communication Standard
	29 CFR 1910.1450	Occupational Exposure to Hazardous Chemicals in Laboratories
Department of Transportation	49 CFR 171-180	Hazardous Materials Regulations
Environmental Protection Agency (EPA)		EPA Guide for Infectious Waste Management
Centers for Disease Control and Prevention		Guideline for Isolation Precautions in Hospitals
Food and Drug Administration	21 CFR 606.3-606.171	Current Good Manufacturing Practice for Blood and Blood Components
	21 CFR 630.6	General Requirements for Blood, Blood Components, and Blood Derivatives
	21 CFR 640.1-640.130	Additional Standards for Human Blood and Blood Products
	21 CFR 211.1-211.208	Current Good Manufacturing Practice for Finished Pharmaceuticals
	21 CFR 1270	Human Tissue Intended for Transplantation
	21 CFR 1271	Human Cells, Tissues, and Cellular and Tissue-Based Products

(Continued)

● **APPENDIX 2-1**
Safety Regulations and Recommendations Applicable to Health-Care Settings (Continued)

Agency/Organization	Reference	Title
Trade and Professional Organizations		
National Fire Protection Association (NFPA)	NFPA 70	National Electrical Code
	NFPA 70E	Electrical Safety Requirements for Employee Workplaces
	NFPA 101	Life Safety Code
	NFPA 99	Standards for Health Care Facilities
	NFPA 704	Standard for Identification of the Hazards of Materials for Emergency Response
National Paint and Coatings Association		Hazardous Materials Identification System Implementation Manual
International Air Transport Association		Dangerous Goods Regulations

CFR = Code of Federal Regulations.

● APPENDIX 2-2
General Guidelines for Safe Work Practices, Personal Protective Equipment, and Engineering Controls

UNIFORMS AND LABORATORY COATS

Personnel should wear closed laboratory coats or full aprons over long-sleeved uniforms or gowns when they are exposed to blood, corrosive chemicals, or carcinogens. The material of required coverings should be appropriate for the type and amount of hazard exposure. Plastic disposable aprons may be worn over cotton coats when there is a high probability of large spills or splashing of blood and body fluids; nitrile rubber aprons may be preferred when caustic chemicals are poured.

Protective coverings should be removed before the employee leaves the work area and should be discarded or stored away from heat sources and clean clothing. Contaminated clothing should be removed promptly, placed in a suitable container, and laundered or discarded as potentially infectious. Home laundering of garments worn in Biosafety Level 2 areas is not permitted because unpredictable methods of transportation and handling can spread contamination and home laundering techniques may not be effective.[1]

GLOVES

Gloves or equivalent barriers should be used whenever tasks are likely to involve exposure to hazardous materials.

Types of Gloves

Glove type varies with the task:

- Sterile gloves: for procedures involving contact with normally sterile areas of the body.

- Examination gloves: for procedures involving contact with mucous membranes, unless otherwise indicated, and for other patient care or diagnostic procedures that do not require the use of sterile gloves.

- Rubber utility gloves: for housekeeping chores involving potential blood contact, instrument cleaning and decontamination procedures, and handling concentrated acids and organic solvents. Utility gloves may be decontaminated and reused but should be discarded if they show signs of deterioration (eg, peeling, cracks, or discoloration) or if they develop punctures or tears.

- Insulated gloves: for handling hot or frozen material.

Indications for Glove Use

The following guidelines should be used to determine when gloves are necessary[1]:

- For donor phlebotomy when the health-care worker has cuts, scratches, or other breaks in his or her skin.

- For phlebotomy of autologous donors or patients (eg, therapeutic apheresis procedures or intraoperative red cell collection).

- For persons who are receiving training in phlebotomy.

- When handling open blood containers or specimens.

- When collecting or handling blood or specimens from patients or donors known to be infected with a blood-borne pathogen.

- When examining mucous membranes or open skin lesions.

- When handling corrosive chemicals and radioactive materials.

- When cleaning up spills or handling waste materials.

(Continued)

● **APPENDIX 2-2**
General Guidelines for Safe Work Practices, Personal Protective Equipment, and Engineering Controls (Continued)

● When the likelihood of exposure cannot be assessed because of lack of experience with a procedure or situation.
The Occupational Safety and Health Administration (OSHA) does not require the routine use of gloves by phlebotomists working with healthy prescreened donors or the changing of unsoiled gloves between donors if gloves are worn.[1,2] Experience has shown that the phlebotomy process is low risk because donors typically have low rates of infectious disease markers. Also, exposure to blood is rare during routine phlebotomy, and other alternatives can be used to provide barrier protection, such as using a folded gauze pad to control any blood flow when the needle is removed from the donor's arm.
Employers whose policies and procedures do not require routine gloving should periodically reevaluate the potential need for gloves. Employees should never be discouraged from using gloves, and gloves should always be available.

Guidelines for Use

Guidelines for the safe use of gloves by employees include the following[3,4]:
● Securely bandage or cover open skin lesions on hands and arms before putting on gloves.
● Change gloves immediately if they are torn, punctured, or contaminated; after handling high-risk samples; or after performing a physical examination (eg, on an apheresis donor).
● Remove gloves by keeping their outside surfaces in contact only with outside and by turning the glove inside out while taking it off.
● Use gloves only when needed, and avoid touching clean surfaces such as telephones, doorknobs, or computer terminals with gloves.
● Change gloves between patient contacts. Unsoiled gloves need not be changed between donors.
● Wash hands with soap or other suitable disinfectant after removing gloves.
● Do not wash or disinfect surgical or examination gloves for reuse. Washing with surfactants may cause "wicking" (ie, enhanced penetration of liquids through undetected holes in the glove). Disinfecting agents may cause deterioration of gloves.
● Use only water-based hand lotions with gloves, if needed; oil-based products cause minute cracks in latex.

FACE SHIELDS, MASKS, AND SAFETY GOGGLES

Where there is a risk of blood or chemical splashes, the eyes and mucous membranes of the mouth and nose should be protected.[5] Permanent shields fixed as a part of equipment or bench design are preferred (eg, splash barriers attached to tubing sealers or centrifuge cabinets). All barriers should be cleaned and disinfected on a regular basis.
Safety glasses alone provide impact protection from projectiles but do not adequately protect eyes from biohazard or chemical splashes. Full-face shields or masks and safety goggles are recommended when permanent shields cannot be used. Many designs are commercially available; eliciting staff input on comfort and selection can increase use.
Masks should be worn whenever there is danger from inhalation. Simple, disposable dust masks are adequate for handling dry chemicals, but respirators with organic vapor filters are preferred for areas where noxious fumes are produced (eg, for cleaning up spills of noxious materials). Respirators should be fitted to their wearers and checked annually.

● **APPENDIX 2-2**
General Guidelines for Safe Work Practices, Personal Protective Equipment, and
Engineering Controls (Continued)

HAND WASHING

Frequent, thorough hand washing is the first line of defense in infection control. Blood-borne pathogens generally do not penetrate intact skin, so immediate removal reduces the likelihood of transfer to a mucous membrane or broken skin area or of transmission to others. Thorough washing of hands (and arms) also reduces the risks from exposure to hazardous chemicals and radioactive materials.

Employees should always wash their hands before leaving a restricted work area or using a biosafety cabinet, between medical examinations, immediately after becoming soiled with blood or hazardous materials, after removing gloves, or after using the toilet. Washing hands thoroughly before touching contact lenses or applying cosmetics is essential.

OSHA allows the use of waterless antiseptic solutions for hand washing as an interim method.[2] These solutions are useful for mobile donor collections or in areas where water is not readily available for cleanup purposes. If such methods are used, however, hands must be washed with soap and running water as soon as possible thereafter. Because there is no listing or registration of acceptable hand-wipe products similar to the one that the Environmental Protection Agency maintains for surface disinfectants, consumers should request data from the manufacturer to support advertising claims.

EYEWASHES

Laboratory areas that contain hazardous chemicals must be equipped with eyewash stations.[3,6] Unobstructed access within a 1-second walk from the location of chemical use must be provided for these stations. Eyewashes must operate so that both of the user's hands are free to hold open the eyes. Procedures and indications for use must be posted, and routine function checks must be performed. Testing eyewash fountains weekly helps ensure proper function and flushes out stagnant water. Portable eyewash systems are allowed only if they can deliver flushing fluid to the eyes at a rate of at least 1.5 liters per minute for 15 minutes. They should be monitored routinely to ensure the purity of their contents.

Employees should be trained in the proper use of eyewash devices, although prevention—through consistent and appropriate use of safety glasses or shields—is preferred. If a splash occurs, the employee should be directed to keep his or her eyelids open and to use the eyewash according to procedures, or the employee should go to the nearest sink and direct a steady, tepid stream of water into his or her eyes. Solutions other than water should be used only in accordance with a physician's direction.

After eyes are adequately flushed (many facilities recommend 15 minutes), follow-up medical care should be sought, especially if pain or redness develops. Whether washing the eyes is effective in preventing infection has not been demonstrated, but it is considered desirable when accidents occur.

1. Code of federal regulations. Title 29, CFR Part 1910.1030.
2. Occupational Safety and Health Administration. Enforcement procedures for the occupational exposure to bloodborne pathogens. OSHA Instruction CPL 02-02-069. Washington, DC: US Government Printing Office, 2001. [Available at https://www.osha.gov/pls/oshaweb/owadisp.show_document?p_table=DIRECTIVES&p_id=2570 (accessed January 28, 2017).]
3. Clinical laboratory safety: Approved guideline. 3rd ed (GP17-A3). Wayne, PA: Clinical and Laboratory Standards Institute, 2012.
4. CAP accreditation checklists: Laboratory general. Chicago: College of American Pathologists, 2017.
5. American national standards for emergency eyewash and shower equipment. ANSI Z358.1-2009. New York: American National Standards Institute, 2009.

● APPENDIX 2-3
Biosafety Level 2 Precautions

Biosafety Level 2 precautions as applied in the blood establishment setting include at least the following[1,2]:

- High-risk activities are appropriately segregated from lower-risk activities, and the boundaries are clearly defined.

- Bench tops are easily cleaned and are decontaminated daily with a hospital disinfectant approved by the Environmental Protection Agency.

- Laboratory rooms have closable doors and sinks. An air system with no recirculation is preferred but not required.

- Workers are required to perform procedures that create aerosols (eg, opening evacuated tubes, centrifuging, mixing, or sonication) in a biological safety cabinet or equivalent or to wear masks and goggles in addition to gloves and gowns during such procedures. (Note: Open tubes of blood should not be centrifuged. If whole units of blood or plasma are centrifuged, overwrapping is recommended to contain leaks.)

- Gowns and gloves are used routinely and in accordance with general safety guidelines. Face shields or their equivalents are used where there is a risk from splashing.

- Mouth pipetting is prohibited.

- No eating, drinking, smoking, applying cosmetics, or manipulating contact lenses occurs in the work area. All food and drink are stored outside the restricted area, and laboratory glassware is never used for food or drink. Personnel are instructed to avoid touching their face, ears, mouth, eyes, or nose with their hands or other objects, such as pencils and telephones.

- Needles and syringes are used and disposed of in a safe manner. Needles must never be bent, broken, sheared, replaced in a sheath, or detached from a syringe before being placed in puncture-proof, leak-proof containers for controlled disposal. Procedures are designed to minimize exposure to sharp objects.

- All blood specimens are placed in well-constructed containers with secure lids to prevent leaking during transport. Blood is packaged for shipment in accordance with regulatory agency requirements for etiologic agents or clinical specimens, as appropriate.

- Infectious waste is not compacted and is decontaminated before its disposal in leak-proof containers. Proper packaging includes double, seamless, tear-resistant, orange or red bags that are enclosed in protective cartons. Both the cartons and the bags inside display the biohazard symbol. Throughout delivery to an incinerator or autoclave, waste is handled only by suitably trained persons. If a waste management contractor is used, the agreement should clearly define the respective responsibilities of the staff and the contractor.

- Equipment to be repaired or submitted for preventive maintenance, if potentially contaminated with blood, must be decontaminated before its release to a repair technician.

- Accidental exposure to suspected or actual hazardous material is reported to the laboratory director or responsible person immediately.

1. Clinical laboratory safety: Approved guideline. 3rd ed (GP17-A3). Wayne, PA: Clinical and Laboratory Standards Institute, 2012.
2. Fleming DO. Laboratory biosafety practices. In: Fleming DO, Richardson JH, Tulis JJ, Vesley DD, eds. Laboratory safety, principles, and practices. 2nd ed. Washington, DC: American Society for Microbiology Press, 1995:203-18.

● **APPENDIX 2-4**
Sample List of Hazardous Chemicals that May Be Encountered in a Blood Bank

Chemical	Hazard
Ammonium chloride	Irritant
Bromelin	Irritant, sensitizer
Calcium chloride	Irritant
Carbon dioxide, frozen (dry ice)	Corrosive
Carbonyl iron powder	Oxidizer
Chloroform	Toxic, suspected carcinogen
Chloroquine	Irritant, corrosive
Chromium-111 chloride hexahydrate	Toxic, irritant, sensitizer
Citric acid	Irritant
Copper sulfate (cupric sulfate)	Toxic, irritant
Dichloromethane	Toxic, irritant
Digitonin	Toxic
Dimethyl sulfoxide	Irritant
Dry ice (carbon dioxide, frozen)	Corrosive
Ethidium bromide	Carcinogen, irritant
Ethylenediaminetetraacetic acid	Irritant
Ethyl ether	Highly flammable and explosive, toxic, irritant
Ficin (powder)	Irritant, sensitizer
Formaldehyde solution (34.9%)	Suspected carcinogen, combustible, toxic
Glycerol	Irritant
Hydrochloric acid	Highly toxic, corrosive
Imidazole	Irritant
Isopropyl (rubbing) alcohol	Flammable, irritant
Liquid nitrogen	Corrosive
Lyphogel	Corrosive
2-Mercaptoethanol	Toxic, stench
Mercury	Toxic
Mineral oil	Irritant, carcinogen, combustible
Papain	Irritant, sensitizer
Polybrene	Toxic
Sodium azide	Toxic, irritant, explosive when heated

(Continued)

● **APPENDIX 2-4**
Sample List of Hazardous Chemicals That May Be Encountered in a Blood Bank
(Continued)

Chemical	Hazard
Sodium ethylmercurithiosalicylate (thimerosal)	Highly toxic, irritant
Sodium hydrosulfite	Toxic, irritant
Sodium hydroxide	Corrosive, toxic
Sodium hypochlorite (bleach)	Corrosive
Sodium phosphate	Irritant, hygroscopic
Sulfosalicylic acid	Toxic, corrosive
Trichloroacetic acid	Corrosive, toxic
Trypsin	Irritant, sensitizer
Xylene	Highly flammable, toxic, irritant

● **APPENDIX 2-5**
Chemical Categories and How to Work Safely with Them

Chemical Category	Hazard	Precautions	Special Treatment
Acids, alkalis, and corrosive compounds	Irritation, severe burns, tissue damage	During transport, protect large containers with plastic or rubber bucket carriers. During pouring, wear eye protection and chemical-resistant-rated gloves and gowns as recommended. Always add acid to water; never add water to acid. When working with large jugs, have one hand on the neck and the other hand at the base, and position them away from the face.	Store concentrated acids in acid safety cabinets. Limit volumes of concentrated acids to 1 liter per container. Post cautions for materials in the area. Report changes in appearance to chemical safety officer. (Perchloric acid may be explosive if it becomes yellowish or brown.)
Acrylamide	Neurotoxic, carcinogenic, absorbed through the skin	Wear chemically rated gloves. Wash hands immediately after exposure.	Store in a chemical cabinet.
Compressed gases	Explosive	Label contents. Leave valve safety covers on until use. Open valves slowly for use. Label empty tanks.	Transport using hand trucks or dollies. Place cylinders in a stand or secure them to prevent tipping over. Store in well-ventilated separate rooms. Do not store oxygen close to combustible gas or solvents. Check connections for leaks using soapy water.

(Continued)

● **APPENDIX 2-5**
Chemical Categories and How to Work Safely with Them (Continued)

Chemical Category	Hazard	Precautions	Special Treatment
Flammable solvents	Classified according to flash point—see material safety data sheet, classified according to volatility	Use extreme caution when handling. Post "No Smoking" signs in working area. Keep a fire extinguisher and solvent cleanup kit in the room. Pour volatile solvents under a suitable hood. Use eye protection and chemical-resistant neoprene gloves when pouring. No flame or other source of possible ignition should be in or near areas where flammable solvents are being poured. Label as "flammable."	Make every attempt to replace hazardous materials with less hazardous materials. Store containers larger than 1 gallon in a flammable solvent storage room or a fire safety cabinet. Ground metal containers by connecting the can to a water pipe or ground connection. If the recipient container is also metal, it should be electrically connected to the delivery container during pouring.
Liquid nitrogen	Freeze injury, severe burns to skin or eyes	Use heavy insulated gloves and goggles when working with liquid nitrogen.	The tanks should be securely supported to avoid being tipped over. The final container of liquid nitrogen (freezing unit) must be securely supported to avoid being tipped over.

● **APPENDIX 2-6**
Incidental Spill Response*

Chemicals	Hazards	PPE	Control Materials

Acids
  Acetic
  Hydrochloric
  Nitric
  Perchloric
  Sulfuric
  Photographic chemicals (acidic)
	If inhaled, causes severe irritation.
	Contact causes burns to skin and eyes.
	Spills are corrosive.
	Fire or contact with metal may produce irritating or poisonous gas.
	Nitric, perchloric, and sulfuric acids are water-reactive oxidizers.
		Acid-resistant gloves
		Apron and coveralls
		Goggles and face shield
		Acid-resistant foot covers
			Acid neutralizers or absorbent material
			Absorbent boom
			Leak-proof containers
			Absorbent pillow
			Mat (cover drain)
			Shovel or paddle

Bases and caustics
  Potassium hydroxide
  Sodium hydroxide
  Photographic chemicals (basic)
	Spills are corrosive.
	Fire may produce irritating or poisonous gas.
		Gloves; impervious apron or coveralls
		Goggles or face shield; impervious foot covers
			Base control/neutralizer
			Absorbent pillow
			Absorbent boom
			Drain mat
			Leak-proof container
			Shovel or paddle

Chlorine
  Bleach
  Sodium hypochlorite
	Inhalation can cause respiratory irritation.
	Liquid contact can produce irritation of the eyes or skin.
	Toxicity is caused by alkalinity, possible chlorine gas generation, and oxidant properties.
		Gloves (double set of 4H undergloves and butyl or nitrile overgloves); impervious apron or coveralls
		Goggles or face shield
		Impervious foot covers (neoprene boots for emergency response releases)
		Self-contained breathing apparatus (emergency response releases)
			Chlorine control powder
			Absorbent pillow
			Absorbent material
			Absorbent boom
			Drain mat
			Vapor barrier
			Leak-proof container
			Shovel or paddle

Cryogenic gases
  Carbon dioxide
  Nitrous oxide
  Liquid nitrogen
	Contact with liquid nitrogen can produce frostbite.
	Release can create an oxygen-deficient atmosphere.
	Nitrous oxide has anesthetic effects.
		Full face shield or goggles; neoprene boots; gloves (insulated to provide protection from the cold)	Hand truck (to transport cylinder outdoors if necessary)
			Soap solution (to check for leaks)
			Putty (to stop minor pipe and line leaks)

(Continued)

● **APPENDIX 2-6**
Incidental Spill Response* (Continued)

Chemicals	Hazards	PPE	Control Materials
Flammable gases Acetylene Oxygen gases Butane Propane	Simple asphyxiant (displaces air). Inhaled vapors have an anesthetic potential. Flammable gases pose an extreme fire and explosion hazard. Release can create an oxygen-deficient atmosphere.	Face shield and goggles; neoprene boots; double set of gloves; coveralls with hood and feet	Hand truck (to transport cylinder outdoors if needed) Soap solution (to check for leaks)
Flammable liquids Acetone Xylene Methyl alcohol toluene Ethyl alcohol Other alcohols	Vapors are harmful if inhaled (central nervous system depressants). Liquid is harmful if absorbed through the skin. Substances are extremely flammable. Liquid evaporates to form flammable vapors.	Gloves (double set of 4H undergloves and butyl or nitrile overgloves); impervious apron or coveralls; goggles or face shield; impervious foot covers	Absorbent material Absorbent boom Absorbent pillow Shovel or paddle (nonmetal, nonsparking) Drain mat Leak-proof container
Formaldehyde and glutaraldehyde 4% formaldehyde 37% formaldehyde 10% formalin 2% glutaraldehyde	Vapors are harmful if inhaled; liquids are harmful if absorbed through skin. Substances are irritants to skin, eyes, and respiratory tract. Formaldehyde is a suspected human carcinogen. 37% formaldehyde should be kept away from heat, sparks, and flames.	Gloves (double set of 4H undergloves and butyl or nitrile overgloves); impervious apron or coveralls; goggles; impervious foot covers	Aldehyde neutralizer or absorbent Absorbent boom Absorbent pillow Shovel or paddle (nonsparking) Drain mat Leak-proof container

● **APPENDIX 2-6**
Incidental Spill Response* (Continued)

Chemicals	Hazards	PPE	Control Materials

Mercury
  Cantor tubes
  Thermometers
  Barometers
  Sphygmomanometers
  Mercuric chloride
	Mercury and mercury vapors are rapidly absorbed in respiratory tract, gastrointestinal (GI) tract, or skin. Short-term exposure may cause erosion of respiratory or GI tracts, nausea, vomiting, bloody diarrhea, shock, headache, or metallic taste. Inhalation of high concentrations can cause pneumonitis, chest pain, dyspnea, coughing, stomatitis, gingivitis, and salivation. Avoid evaporation of mercury from tiny globules by quick and thorough cleaning.	Gloves (double set of 4H undergloves and butyl or nitrile overgloves); impervious apron or coveralls; goggles; impervious foot covers	Mercury vacuum or spill kit
			Scoop
			Aspirator
			Hazardous waste containers
			Mercury indicator powder
			Absorbent material
			Spatula
			Disposable towels
			Sponge with amalgam
			Vapor suppressor

*This list of physical and health hazards is not intended as a substitute for the material safety data sheet (SDS) information. In case of a spill or if any questions arise, always refer to the chemical-specific SDS for more complete information.

● **APPENDIX 2-7**
Managing Hazardous Chemical Spills

Actions	Instructions for Hazardous Liquids, Gases, and Mercury
Deenergize.	Liquids: For 37% formaldehyde, deenergize and remove all sources of ignition within 10 feet of spilled hazardous material. For flammable liquids, remove all sources of ignition.
	Gases: Remove all sources of heat and ignition within 50 feet for flammable gases.
	Remove all sources of heat and ignition for nitrous oxide release.
Isolate, evacuate, and secure the area.	Isolate the spill area and evacuate everyone from the area surrounding the spill except those responsible for cleaning up the spill. (For mercury, evacuate within 10 feet for small spills or 20 feet for large spills.) Secure the area.
Have the appropriate personal protective equipment (PPE).	See Appendix 2-2 for recommended PPE.
Contain the spill.	Liquids or mercury: Stop the source of spill if possible.
	Gases: Assess the scene; consider the circumstances of the release (quantity, location, and ventilation). If circumstances indicate that it is an emergency response release, make appropriate notifications; if the release is determined to be incidental, contact the supplier for assistance.
Confine the spill.	Liquids: Confine the spill to the initial spill area using appropriate control equipment and material. For flammable liquids, dike off all drains.
	Gases: Follow the supplier's suggestions or request outside assistance.
	Mercury: Use appropriate materials to confine the spill (see Appendix 2-6). Expel mercury from the aspirator bulb into a leak-proof container, if applicable.
Neutralize the spill.	Liquids: Apply appropriate control materials to neutralize the chemical (see Appendix 2-6).
	Mercury: Use a mercury spill kit if needed.
Clean up the spill.	Liquids: Scoop up solidified materials, booms, pillows, and any other materials. Put used materials into a leak-proof container. Label the container with the name of the hazardous materials. Wipe up residual material. Wipe the spill area surface three times with a detergent solution. Rinse the areas with clean water. Collect the supplies used (eg, goggles or shovels) and remove gross contamination; place equipment to be washed and decontaminated into a separate container.
	Gases: Follow the supplier's suggestions or request outside assistance.
	Mercury: Vacuum up the spill using a mercury vacuum, or scoop up mercury paste after neutralization and collect the paste in a designated container. Use a sponge and detergent to wipe and clean the spill surface three times to remove absorbent. Collect all contaminated disposal equipment and put it into a hazardous waste container. Collect supplies and remove gross contamination; place equipment that will be thoroughly washed and decontaminated into a separate container.

● **APPENDIX 2-7**
Managing Hazardous Chemical Spills (Continued)

Actions	Instructions for Hazardous Liquids, Gases, and Mercury
Dispose.	Liquids: Dispose of material that was neutralized as solid waste. Follow the facility's procedures for disposal. For flammable liquids, check with the facility safety officer for appropriate waste determination.
	Gases: The manufacturer or supplier will instruct the facility about disposal if applicable.
	Mercury: Label with appropriate hazardous waste label and Department of Transportation diamond label.
Report.	Follow appropriate spill documentation and reporting procedures. Investigate the spill; perform a root cause analysis if needed. Act on opportunities for improving safety.

Chapter 3

Regulatory Considerations in Transfusion Medicine and Cellular Therapies

• ● •

Joseph Schwartz, MD, MPH, and Orieji Illoh, MD

THE FIELDS OF transfusion medicine and cellular therapy are highly regulated disciplines. Over the years, different regulatory bodies have provided oversight at both the state and federal levels in the United States. The Food and Drug Administration (FDA) and the Centers for Medicare and Medicaid Services (CMS) are the primary regulatory bodies providing federal oversight. In addition, state health departments and other agencies may provide some degree of regulatory oversight. Individuals and establishments involved with transfusion medicine and cellular therapies should be familiar with the different requirements of these agencies.

It is important to distinguish between regulation and accreditation. Regulations have the force of law, while accreditation standards are not legally binding. Blood banks, transfusion services, and cellular therapy facilities must follow the rules set by regulatory agencies. In contrast, accreditation organizations such as AABB or The Joint Commission publish specific sets of standards that need to be met in order for accreditation to be granted. Some regulatory agencies will grant deeming authority to select accreditation organizations. For example, CMS regulates laboratory testing through the Clinical Laboratory Improvement Amendments (CLIA). CMS accepts certain accreditation organization inspections, meaning that the organizations have been approved by CMS as having standards and an inspection process that meet or exceed the CMS requirements. Table 3-1 summarizes agencies and organizations involved in regulation and accreditation of blood bank, transfusion medicine, and cellular therapy facilities. The scope of their regulatory oversight and/or accreditation is detailed on these organizations' respective websites.

Joseph Schwartz, MD, MPH, Director, Transfusion Medicine and Cellular Therapy, Columbia University Medical Center and New York Presbyterian Hospital, and Professor of Pathology and Cell Biology, Columbia University, New York, New York; and Orieji Illoh, MD, Director, Division of Blood Components and Devices, Office of Blood Research and Review, Center for Biologics Evaluation and Research, Food and Drug Administration, Silver Spring, Maryland

The authors have disclosed no conflicts of interest.

TABLE 3-1. Regulatory and Accreditation Bodies Involved in Blood Banking and Cellular Therapies

Regulatory Agencies	Accreditation Organizations
Food and Drug Administration (FDA)	AABB
Centers for Medicare and Medicaid Services (CMS)	College of American Pathologists (CAP)
Department of Homeland Security	The Joint Commission
Nuclear Regulatory Commission (NRC)	Foundation for the Accreditation of Cellular Therapy (FACT)
Environmental Protection Agency (EPA)	National Marrow Donor Program (NMDP)
Occupational Safety and Health Administration (OSHA)	World Marrow Donor Association (WMDA)
Local state departments of health	American Association for Laboratory Accreditation (A2LA)
US Department of Transportation (US DOT)	
National Fire Protection Association (NFPA)	

FDA OVERSIGHT OF BLOOD ESTABLISHMENTS

In the United States, when federal laws are enacted by Congress, they are published as statutes and placed into the appropriate subject areas (titles) of the United States Code (USC).[1] Regulations created by federal agencies to enforce laws are placed (by title) in the *Code of Federal Regulations* (CFR). The Food and Drug Administration (FDA) is the federal agency that enforces the federal laws related to drugs and biologics, which include blood and blood components, related devices, and manufacturing facilities.

Section 351 of the Public Health Service (PHS) Act (USC Title 42, Section 262) and the Food, Drug, and Cosmetic (FD&C) Act (21 USC 301-399d) are two statutes that govern the regulation of blood and blood components. The PHS Act defines blood and blood components as biological products. This law was first established in 1944 as an expansion of the Biologics Control Act. In addition to requiring that biological products be manufactured in a manner to ensure the safety, purity, and potency of the product, the PHS Act requires a manufacturer to obtain a biologics license before placing a product in interstate commerce.[2] In addition, the US Department of Health and Human Services (DHHS) has broad authority to prevent communicable disease transmission under Section 361 of the PHS Act (42 USC 264).

The FDA regulates drugs and medical devices under the FD&C Act, which was first passed in 1938 and amended in 1976. Under this act, blood and blood components are defined as drugs because they are intended to cure, mitigate, treat, or prevent disease in humans. Manufacturers of drugs and certain devices must demonstrate to the FDA the safety and efficacy of a product before it can be marketed. The FD&C Act requires blood product manufacturers to register with the FDA, obtain biologics licenses and follow current good manufacturing practice regulations. It also prohibits adulteration and misbranding of products, authorizes inspection of manufacturing facilities, and defines civil and criminal penalties for violations. The act provides requirements for the use of unapproved drugs and devices in their investigational phases and in public health emergencies.[3]

Within the FDA, the Center for Biologics Evaluation and Research (CBER) regulates blood products and most other biological therapies.[4] CBER uses multiple overlapping safeguards to ensure that recipients of blood products or cellular therapies are protected. This FDA blood-safety system includes measures in the following areas: donor screening, donor testing, donor deferral lists, quarantine, and investigation of deficiencies. The Center for Devices and Radiological Health (CDRH) regulates most medical devices, but CBER retains primary jurisdiction over medical devices used with blood donation, transfusion, and cellular products. The FDA's Office of Regulatory Affairs (ORA) has responsibility for all field operations, which include inspections and investigations of blood and device manufacturers.[5]

FDA promulgates applicable regulations for blood and blood components and related devices under both the PHS and FD&C Acts. Regulations for blood products are found in Parts 210, 211, and 600-680 of CFR Title 21.[6] These regulations are intended to ensure blood donor safety, and the safety, purity, and potency of blood and blood components. In addition, blood establishments are required to report deaths associated with blood donation or transfusion to the FDA. Table 3-2 provides a summarized list of relevant regulations applicable to blood establishments. On May 22, 2015, the FDA published "Requirements for Blood and Blood Components Intended for Transfusion or for Further Manufacturing Use," codified under Part 600 of Title 21 of the CFR.[7] This rule updated FDA's previous requirements. The new requirements include a determination of donor eligibility and donation suitability, as well as regulations to help protect donor health.

Manufacturers of blood and blood components may submit written requests to the FDA for approval of exceptions or alternative procedures to any requirement in the regulations [21 CFR 640.120 (a)]. When the FDA grants approvals of exceptions or alternative procedures, the circumstances for these approvals may not necessarily apply to other facilities. These approvals are periodically published on FDA's website.[8]

In addition to regulations, which are legally binding, the FDA may publish recommendations in guidance documents. These guidance documents generally explain FDA's current thinking on an issue. The guidance may clarify or explain how manufacturers may comply with the statute or regulations, or establish good manufacturing standards for blood products. FDA guidance documents generally do not establish legally enforceable responsibilities unless specific regulatory or statutory requirements are cited. Alternative approaches to the recommendations stated in guidance documents may be used if such approaches satisfy the requirements of the applicable law or statute.[9]

As part of the development process for FDA regulations and guidance documents, several forums are offered for input from the public and regulated industry. Proposed rules and draft guidance documents are published with an invitation for written comments, which are filed in public dockets. When final rules are published in the *Federal Register*, the accompanying preamble responds to key questions and comments submitted by the public. The FDA also receives petitions to write or change regulations. Expert opinions on current issues are sought from several advisory committees, including the FDA Blood Products Advisory Committee (BPAC); its Cellular, Tissue, and Gene Therapies Advisory Committee (CTGTAC); and the DHHS Advisory Committee on Blood and Tissue Safety and Availability (ACBTSA). Public meetings and workshops hosted by the FDA on selected topics provide an additional opportunity for input.

Registration of Blood Establishments and Device Manufacturers

The FDA has promulgated regulations that require blood establishments (21 CFR 607) and device manufacturers (21 CFR 807) to register their manufacturing facilities and list the products they manufacture. All establishments that manufacture blood products are required to register with the FDA, unless they are exempt under 21 CFR 607.65. Registrants must provide a list of every blood product manufactured, prepared, or processed for commercial distribution. Manufacturers must register and list their products within 5 days of beginning operations and annually. Blood establishments include blood and plasma donor centers, blood banks, transfusion services, other blood product manufacturers, and independent laboratories that engage in

TABLE 3-2. Regulations of Interest in Title 21 of the CFR (Food and Drugs)

Topic	Section	Topic	Section
FDA general		Donor eligibility	630.10, 630.15
Enforcement	1-19	Donation suitability	630.30
Research and development	50-58	Donor notification	630.40
cGMP for drugs	210-211	Blood product standards	640
Biological products	600-680	Blood collection	640.4
General	600	Blood testing	640.5, 610.40
Licensing	601	Red Blood Cells	640.10-.17
cGMP for blood components	606	Platelets	640.20-.25, 606.145
Personnel, resources	606.20-.65	Plasma	640.30-.34
Standard operating procedures	606.100	Cryoprecipitated AHF	640.50-.56
Labeling	606.120-.122	Exceptions, alternatives	640.120
Compatibility testing	606.151	Medical devices	800-898
Records	606.160-.165	Device adverse events	803
Adverse reactions	606.170	Hematology and pathology	864
Product deviations	606.171	Tissues	
Establishment registration	607	Human cells, tissues, and cellular and tissue-based products	1271*
General standards	610	General provisions	1271.1-.20
Donor testing	610.40	Procedures for registration and listing	1271.21-.37
Donor deferral	610.41	Donor eligibility	1271.45-.90
Look-back	610.46-.47	cGTP	1271.145-.320
Dating periods	610.53	Additional requirements and inspection and enforcement	1271.330-.440

*The following citations represent Subparts A, B, C, D, and E-F, respectively.
CFR = Code of Federal Regulations; FDA = Food and Drug Administration; cGMP = current good manufacturing practice; AHF = antihemophilic factor; cGTP = current good tissue practice.

testing of donors and blood and blood components.[10]

Facilities that routinely collect blood (including autologous units) or perform such procedures as irradiation; washing; prestorage leukocyte reduction; pooling; or freezing, deglycerolization, and rejuvenation must register with the FDA. Transfusion services acting as depots for forwarding products to other hospitals must register as distribution centers. If blood irradiation is performed outside the blood bank or transfusion service, such as in a nuclear medicine department, that facility must register as well.

Transfusion services that do not collect or process blood and blood components are exempt from the registration requirement in 21 CFR 607. In order to be exempt, they must be part of a facility certified under CLIA (1988; 42 USC 263a and 42 CFR 493) or certified for reimbursement by CMS.[11] Their manufacturing activities are basic, such as compatibility tests, preparing Red Blood Cells from whole blood, converting unused plasma to recovered plasma, pooling certain blood components immediately before transfusion, reducing leukocytes in blood components with bedside filters, or collecting blood only in emergency situations. Under the memorandum of understanding in 1980 between the FDA and CMS, the responsibility for routine inspections of these transfusion services was assigned to CMS.[12] The FDA, however, still has jurisdiction over transfusion services and may conduct its own inspections if warranted.

Licensure of Blood and Blood Component Manufacturers

Blood and blood component manufacturers who distribute blood products in interstate commerce must be registered and licensed. The blood establishment obtains licensure by submitting a Biologics License Application (BLA) to the FDA. The FDA's review of BLAs typically includes the review of supporting documents, such as standard operating procedures, labels, quality control data, and a prelicense facility inspection. Once a license is issued, the license number is placed on the label for those products approved to be distributed in interstate commerce. In addition, licensed manufacturers are required to inform the FDA of changes in the manufacturing process described in their approved BLA.[13] The reporting category for such changes depends on the potential of the change to adversely impact the safety, purity, and potency of the product.

The FDA has published specific guidance ("Changes to an Approved Application: Biological Products: Human Blood and Blood Components Intended for Transfusion or for Further Manufacture," December 2014) to assist blood establishments in determining the appropriate reporting mechanism.[14] As described in the guidance, the three reporting categories into which a change to an approved application may be placed are defined in 21 CFR 601.12 and are as follows:

- *Major Change:* A change that has a substantial potential to have an adverse effect on the safety or effectiveness of the product. Major changes require the submission of a Prior Approval Supplement (PAS) to the FDA, which the FDA must approve before the product is distributed in interstate commerce [21 CFR 601.12(b)].
- *Moderate Change:* A change that has a moderate potential to have an adverse effect on the safety or effectiveness of the product. Moderate changes require the submission of a Changes Being Effected in 30 Days Supplement (CBE30) to the FDA at least 30 days before interstate distribution of the product made using the change [21 CFR 601.12(c)]. In certain circumstances, the FDA may determine that the product made using the change may be distributed immediately upon receipt of the Changes Being Effected Supplement (CBE) by the FDA [21 CFR 601.12(c)(5)].
- *Minor Change:* A change that has a minimal potential to have an adverse effect on the safety or effectiveness of the product. Minor changes do not need prior approval from the FDA and must be described by the manufacturer in an annual report [21 CFR 601.12(d)].

Blood-Related Devices

CBER has the lead responsibility for devices marketed for transfusion and the collection and processing of blood products and hematopoietic progenitor cells (HPCs). These devices include apheresis machines; devices and reagents used for compatibility testing; blood establishment computer software; and blood and human cells, tissues, and cellular and tissue-based product (HCT/P) screening tests for infectious diseases.

The medical device classifications are based on the risks the device poses to the patient and the user or on the level of controls that may be necessary to ensure the device can be operated safely and effectively[15]:

- Class I medical devices represent the lowest-level risks to the patient or user. Such devices are subject to a comprehensive set of regulatory authorities called general controls. General controls are applicable to all classes of devices. Examples of Class I devices include copper sulfate solutions for hemoglobin screening, blood grouping view boxes, and heat sealers.
- Class II medical devices carry greater patient or user risks than Class I devices. These are devices for which general controls alone are insufficient to provide reasonable assurance of the safety and effectiveness of the device, and for which there is sufficient information to establish special controls to provide such assurance. Most blood-related devices are in Class II and cleared through the 510(k) pathway, where a device is found to show equivalence to a predicate.
- Class III medical devices carry the greatest risk of the three device classifications. These are devices for which general controls, by themselves, are insufficient and for which there is insufficient information to establish special controls to provide reasonable assurance of their safety and efficacy. Tests used to determine red cell antigen type by molecular methods are regulated as Class III devices.

The FDA approves some blood-related devices under the PHS Act and therefore requires the submission of BLAs or related supplements. These devices include reagents used for immunohematology testing by serologic methods and most donor-screening infectious disease assays [eg, tests for human immunodeficiency virus (HIV), hepatitis B virus (HBV), and hepatitis C virus (HCV)].

The FDA requires device manufacturers to register and list the products they manufacture (21 CFR 807). Each device category is assigned a code, and all cleared or approved manufacturers and products for that code are searchable in the Establishment Registration and Device Listing database on the CDRH website.[16]

Manufacturers and importers of medical devices must report deaths and serious injuries related to medical devices to the FDA (21 CFR 803).[17] User facilities must report deaths and serious injuries in which a device was or may have been a factor. Serious injury is defined as being life threatening, causing permanent impairment or damage, or needing medical or surgical intervention. For user facilities, reports of serious injuries are sent to the device manufacturer using FDA MedWatch Form 3500A within 10 working days of the event, or to the FDA if the device manufacturer is unknown. Deaths must be reported to both the manufacturer and the FDA. In years when a Form 3500A report is submitted, the user facility must send an annual user facility report (Form 3419) to the FDA by January 1 of the following year.[18] Users may voluntarily report other device-related adverse events or malfunctions to the FDA (Form 3500). All possible adverse events, whether reported or not, must be investigated, and these records must be kept on file for a minimum of 2 years.

FDA Inspections

The FDA inspects regulated facilities to determine compliance with regulations.[19] These inspections can be classified as one of the following:

- Prelicense or preapproval inspection after a manufacturer submits an application to the FDA for a biologics license or to market a new device or product.
- Routine inspection of a regulated facility.
- "For-cause" inspection, which involves investigation of a specific problem that has

come to the FDA's attention, such as a complaint or fatality.

The FDA's ORA and CBER oversee inspection activities related to transfusion medicine and blood banking. The inspection of a blood establishment is to ensure manufacturers meet the standards described in applicable provisions of the regulations intended to protect donors and ensure the safety and efficacy of the products they make. These include regulations for blood components in CFR Title 21, Parts 600, 601, 606, 607, 610, 630, and 640, as well as the process and production controls, equipment regulations, and quality control requirements in 21 CFR 211. (See Table 3-2.) The licensed manufacturers must also meet any additional conditions of licensure incorporated in their approved BLA.[20]

When a blood establishment applies for a BLA, the facility is generally inspected by a team from CBER and ORA. Subsequent routine inspections are generally performed by ORA every 2 years or sooner depending on the facility's compliance history.

ORA provides and publishes policies and instructions for FDA investigators. There is a specific *Compliance Program Guidance Manual (CPGM)* for inspections of licensed and unlicensed blood banks. The foundations for blood establishment inspections are in the general FDA regulations for current good manufacturing practice and drugs, and the specific requirements for blood components. All inspections address the FDA's five layers of blood safety. Investigators review the following operational systems that are associated with the layers of safety: quality assurance, donor eligibility, product testing, quarantine/inventory management, and production and processing. Within each system, the investigators review standard operating procedures, personnel and training, facilities, equipment calibration and maintenance, and records. Specific requirements for individual systems and processes are discussed in detail in their respective chapters of the *CPGM*.[20]

Full inspections of all systems are designated Level I. After two favorable inspection profiles, facilities with only four or five systems

sometimes have streamlined Level II inspections of three systems. Prelicense and preapproval inspections or for-cause investigations for complaints or fatalities need not follow these formats because they are more focused on a specific issue.

If the FDA investigator observes that significant objectionable practices, violations, or conditions are present that could result in a drug or device being adulterated or injurious to health, these observations are written and presented to the facility on FDA Form 483. The FDA Form 483 serves to notify the manufacturer of the objectionable conditions and does not constitute a final determination of whether a violation has occurred. Investigators are instructed to seek and record the manufacturer's intentions to make corrections. The investigator documents observations and discussions in an Establishment Inspection Report (EIR). The FDA reviews and considers all the information provided in a Form 483, EIR, and any responses from the manufacturer and then determines what further action, if any, is appropriate to protect public health.

The FDA can take a number of enforcement actions in response to a violation.[21] Enforcement actions are categorized as advisory, administrative, or judicial. Under advisory actions, the FDA issues a warning or an untitled letter, informing the manufacturer of noncompliant activities that could impact donor safety or result in the distribution of an unsafe biological product. The letters provide the facility with the opportunity for voluntary compliance. Administrative actions include product recalls, withdrawals of product approvals, formal citations of violation, and—for licensed facilities—suspension or revocation of a license. Judicial actions range from seizures of products to court injunctions, civil monetary penalties, and criminal prosecution.

Biological Product Deviation Reporting

When blood establishments discover after distribution that a blood product was in violation of rules, standards, or specifications, they must report the biological product deviation

(BPD) to the FDA [21 CFR 606.171, 21 CFR 1271.350(b)]. BPD events are ones in which the safety, purity, or potency of a distributed blood product may be affected, and may involve any event associated with manufacturing a product, including collection, testing, processing, packing, labeling, or storing and distributing. Licensed and unlicensed manufacturers, registered blood establishments, and transfusion services that are exempt from registration are required to report BPDs in distributed products. Blood establishments must report a BPD as soon as possible, not to exceed 45 calendar days from the date the manufacturer became aware of the reportable event.[22] CBER publishes an annual summary of reported BPDs.[23] Most of the reports from blood establishments fall into the category of postdonation information (information provided by the donor after a blood product has been collected but would have been a cause for deferral). Blood establishments should have procedures to investigate a BPD and determine if the product should be recalled or withdrawn.

Managing Recalls and Withdrawals

The FDA's requirements for monitoring and investigating problems with drugs extend to the time after a product's release.

A recall is defined as the removal or correction of a marketed product that is in violation of the law (21 CFR 7.3 and 7.40). Recalls may be initiated by the manufacturers, requested by the FDA, or ordered by the FDA under statutory authority. The FDA classifies recalls by severity.[24] Recalls are classified as Class I, II, or III. Most blood component recalls are in Class III, not likely to cause adverse health consequences. Class II recalls are for products that may cause temporary adverse effects or remotely possible serious problems. Class I recalls involve a reasonable probability of serious or fatal adverse effects. All recalls are published by the FDA.[25,26]

Market withdrawals occur when a product has a minor violation that would not be subject to FDA legal action.[24] The manufacturer voluntarily removes the product from the market or corrects the violation. In collection establishments, problems such as postdonation information are often in this category. Withdrawals are not published.

In some blood guidance documents on infectious diseases, the FDA has included recommendations on whether to notify the recipient's physician about transfused units. In cases of possible recent infectious disease exposure in donors or transfusion recipients, the seroconversion window periods for the agent and test kits should be consulted for scheduling prospective testing or reviewing retrospective results, such as for a donor who has been retested after an exposure.[27]

"Look-back" investigations on units from donors found after donation to have HIV or HCV are discussed in Chapter 7.

MEDICAL LABORATORY LAWS AND REGULATIONS

CMS regulates all US medical laboratories under CLIA [42 USC 263(a) and 42 CFR 493] and Section 353 of the PHS Act.[28,29] The law and regulations establish the requirements and procedures for laboratories to be certified under CLIA as both a general requirement and a prerequisite for receiving Medicare and Medicaid reimbursement. They provide minimal standards for facilities, equipment, and personnel. Furthermore, they require participation in a proficiency testing (PT) program.

To be certified, laboratories must have adequate facilities and equipment, supervisory and technical personnel with training and experience appropriate to the complexity of testing, a quality management system (see Chapter 1), and successful ongoing performance in CMS-approved PT.[30] All laboratories must register with CMS, submit to inspection by CMS or one of its "deemed status" partners, and obtain recertification every 2 years.

All laboratory tests are rated for complexity by the FDA for CMS as waived or moderate or high complexity. Waived tests are simple and easily performed with limited technical training. Examples include over-the-counter tests, urinalysis dipsticks, copper sulfate specific-gravity hemoglobin screens, microhematocrits, and some simple devices for measuring hemoglobin. Laboratories that perform only waived tests register with CMS for a certificate of waiver. The Centers for Disease Control and Prevention provides technical and advisory support to CMS for laboratory regulation and has published practice recommendations for waived-testing sites.[31]

Nonwaived tests are classified as being of moderate or high complexity based on a scoring system of needs for training, preparation, interpretive judgment, and other factors (42 CFR 493.17).[28] The "Medical Devices" section of the FDA website provides a searchable CLIA database that provides the complexity levels of specific tests.[32] Compatibility testing with manual reagents and infectious disease testing are generally considered high-complexity testing.

Blood banks and transfusion services have three pathways to obtain a CLIA certificate to perform testing: 1) certificate of compliance: approval via state health department inspections using CMS requirements; 2) certificate of accreditation: approval via a CMS-approved accrediting organization; and 3) CMS-exempt status: licensure programs for nonwaived laboratories in New York and Washington states that are accepted by CMS.[33]

The CLIA regulations delineate general requirements for facilities; quality systems, including quality assurance and quality control systems; and management and technical personnel qualifications. High-complexity tests require more stringent personnel qualifications. Immunohematology laboratories have standards for blood supply agreements, compatibility testing, blood storage and alarms, sample retention, positive identification of blood product recipients, investigation of transfusion reactions, and documentation (42 CFR 493.1103 and 493.1271).[28] Viral and syphilis serologic tests are part of the immunology requirements. CMS has published guidelines for conducting surveys (inspections).[34]

CMS has approved six laboratory accreditation organizations with requirements that meet CMS regulations: AABB, the American Osteopathic Association, the American Society for Histocompatibility and Immunogenetics (ASHI), the College of American Pathologists (CAP), COLA (formerly the Commission on Office Laboratory Accreditation), and The Joint Commission.[35] The Joint Commission has cooperative agreements with ASHI, CAP, and COLA to accept their laboratory accreditations in facility surveys.[36] CMS may perform its own follow-up surveys to validate those of the accreditation organizations.

CMS requires successful PT for ongoing laboratory certification of nonwaived testing. Within each laboratory section, CMS regulations specify tests and procedures (regulated analytes) that must pass approved PT if the laboratory performs them. The CMS website has a list of approved PT providers.[37] (PT is discussed in Chapter 1.) CMS can remove certification or impose fines for failure to comply with its regulations.

LOCAL LAWS, HOSPITAL REGULATIONS, AND ACCREDITATION

Facilities also should be familiar with all relevant state and local laws and regulations, including professional licensure requirements for medical and laboratory personnel, as many states have regulations that apply to blood banks and transfusion services. Furthermore, in some situations, facilities providing products or services in other states must comply with local regulations in the customer's location.

CMS approves hospitals for Medicare reimbursement through state surveys or accreditation programs from The Joint Commission, the American Osteopathic Association, and DNV Healthcare. These inspections cover CMS regulations for blood administration and the evaluation of transfusion reactions found within "Basic Hospital Functions" regulations [42 CFR 482.23(c)].[38] The Joint Commission has standards for preventing misidentification of laboratory specimens and transfusion recipients (National Patient Safety Goal section—NPSG.01.01.01, .01.03.01), checking blood products in the "Universal Protocol" preprocedure verification process ("timeout"—UP.01.01.01), and assessing transfusion appropriateness (MS.05.01.01).[39] The Joint Commission also addresses utilization review of blood components in the Performance Improvement (PI) section of the hospital accreditation requirements. Furthermore, in the same section of standards, The Joint Commission directs hospitals to collect data on all reported and confirmed transfusion reactions, and directs that these areas should "be measured regularly." The Joint Commission includes hemolytic transfusion reactions in its Sentinel Events reporting program.[40]

AABB and CAP have both developed standards for transfusion services. The AABB *Standards for Blood Banks and Transfusion Services* is updated every 2 years.[41] The CAP transfusion medicine checklist TRM[42] is updated periodically. AABB- and CAP-accredited facilities need to be physically surveyed every 2 years to receive reaccreditation. AABB and CAP can coordinate joint surveys of facilities seeking both types of accreditation.

HUMAN CELLS, TISSUES, AND CELLULAR AND TISSUE-BASED PRODUCTS (HCT/Ps)

HCT/Ps are defined as articles containing or consisting of human cells or tissues that are intended for implantation, transplantation, infusion, or transfer into a human recipient.[43] HCT/Ps can be derived from deceased or living donors (Table 3-3). The FDA has established a comprehensive, tiered, risk-based regulatory framework applicable to HCT/Ps.

These regulations, which were published in three parts (referred to as the "tissue rules") and contained in 21 CFR 1271, became fully effective on May 25, 2005. They apply to all HCT/Ps, including HPCs, that are recovered on or after this date.[44,45]

Under this tiered, risk-based regulatory framework, some HCT/Ps (referred to as "361" HCT/Ps) are regulated solely under Section 361 of the PHS Act (42 USC 264), which authorizes the FDA to establish and enforce regulations necessary to prevent the introduction, transmission, or spread of communicable diseases.[46] For an HCT/P to be regulated solely under Section 361 of the PHS Act and the regulations in 21 CFR 1271, it must meet *all* of the following criteria in 21 CFR 1271.10(a):

1. The HCT/P is minimally manipulated (relates to the extent of processing).
2. The HCT/P is intended for homologous use only. (The product performs the same basic function or functions in the donor as in the recipient.)
3. The HCT/P is not combined with another regulated article (with some exceptions).
4. The HCT/P does not have a systemic effect and is not dependent on the metabolic activity of living cells for its primary function unless the HCT/P is for autologous use; for allogeneic use in a first-degree or second-degree blood relative; or for reproductive use.

TABLE 3-3.   Examples of HCT/Ps

From Deceased Donors*	From Living Donors*
▪ Skin	▪ Hematopoietic stem/progenitor cells from peripheral or cord blood
▪ Dura mater	▪ Other cellular therapy products (eg, pancreatic islets, mesenchymal stem/stromal cells, fibroblasts)
▪ Cardiovascular tissues	
▪ Ocular tissues	▪ Reproductive cells and tissues
▪ Musculoskeletal tissues	

*In general, but there are exceptions.

Manufacturers of 361 HCT/Ps must comply with the requirements in 21 CFR 1271, which include 1) establishment registration and product listing; 2) donor eligibility, including screening and testing for relevant communicable disease agents or diseases; and 3) current good tissue practice (cGTP); and are not subject to the requirements for premarket review and approval. FDA guidance documents related to these requirements can be found on the agency's website.[45]

If an HCT/P does not meet one or more of the criteria listed in 21 CFR 1271.10(a), it will be regulated as a drug, device, and/or biological product under the FD&C Act and/or Section 351 of the PHS Act (referred to as a "351" HCT/P) and applicable regulations, including 21 CFR 1271. Premarket review to obtain an FDA license will be required. During the development phase, an Investigational New Drug (IND) or Investigational Device Exemption (IDE) application must be submitted to the FDA before studies involving humans are initiated. Manufacturers of such HCT/Ps are required to comply with the regulations in 21 CFR 1271 and all the regulations for drugs, devices, or biological products, as applicable (Table 3-4).

Regarding HPCs, peripheral blood stem cells (PBSCs) or cord blood for use in a first- or second-degree blood relative or for autologous use that meet all the other criteria in 21 CFR 1271.10(a) are regulated as 361 HCT/Ps. PBSCs from unrelated donors are regulated as 351 products; however, for some clinical indications of PBSCs, these regulations remain under a period of delayed implementation. For clarification on regulatory expectations for specific uses, it may be prudent to contact the agency directly. Since October 20, 2011, minimally manipulated, unrelated umbilical cord blood intended for hematopoietic or immunologic reconstitution in patients with disorders affecting the hematopoietic system must be FDA licensed or used under an IND protocol. Minimally manipulated marrow that is not combined with another regulated article (with some exceptions) and is intended for homologous use is not considered an HCT/P.

The Health Resources and Services Administration (HRSA) within DHHS oversees the CW Bill Young Cell Transplantation Program and the National Cord Blood Inventory for marrow and cord blood donations and transplant procedures coordinated by the National Marrow Donor Program (NMDP) in the United States.

The *Circular of Information for the Use of Cellular Therapy Products* is jointly written by AABB and multiple organizations involved in cellular therapy for users of certain minimally manipulated unlicensed cellular therapy products.[47] AABB and the Foundation for the Accreditation of Cellular Therapy (FACT) set voluntary standards covering the collection, processing, and administration of cellular therapy products.[48,49] AABB and FACT have standards review cycles of 2 and 3 years, respectively. (See Table 3-5.) The CAP transfusion medicine checklist[42] includes cellular therapy requirements. The World Marrow Donor Association (WMDA) fosters international collaboration to facilitate the exchange of high-quality hematopoietic stem cells for clinical transplantation worldwide and to promote the interests of donors. WMDA also accredits and qualifies donor registries that follow its global standards covering all aspects of unrelated hematopoietic stem cell registry operations. The NMDP standards set forth basic guidelines and requirements for programs working with the NMDP. The standards encompass network participation criteria with requirements for transplant centers, recruitment centers, and product collection centers. The NMDP standards are designed to ensure that donors and patients receive high-quality care and that government standards are met (Table 3-5).

The Alliance for Harmonisation of Cellular Therapy Accreditation (AHCTA), which is under the umbrella of the Worldwide Network for Blood and Marrow Transplantation (WBMT), encompasses all the above-mentioned accreditation organizations. AHCTA is working to harmonize standards that cover all aspects of the process, from assessment of donor eligibility to transplantation and clinical outcome for hematopoietic stem cells and related cellular

TABLE 3-4. US Regulations for Manufacturers of Hematopoietic Progenitor Cells

Type of HPC Product	Oversight/Regulatory Category	Key Regulations (21 CFR except as noted)	FDA Premarket Licensure, Approval, or Clearance?
Minimally manipulated marrow, not combined with another article (with some exceptions) and for homologous use	Health Resources and Services Administration oversight	42 US Code 274(k)	Not applicable
Autologous or allogeneic related-donor (first- or second-degree blood relative) HPCs	PHS Act Section 361: HCT/Ps*	1271.10(a)† (must meet all criteria); 1271 Subparts A-F	No
Minimally manipulated unrelated-donor peripheral blood HPCs, not combined with another article (with some exceptions) and for homologous use	PHS Act Sections 361 and 351: HCT/Ps regulated as drugs and/or biological products	1271 Subparts A-D Applicable biologics/ drug regulations	Delayed implementation
Minimally manipulated unrelated-donor umbilical cord blood cells	PHS Sections 361 and 351: HCT/Ps regulated as drugs and/or biological products	1271 Subparts A-D	Yes (after October 20, 2011): BLA or IND application
HPCs that don't meet all the criteria in 21 CFR 1271.10(a)	PHS Sections 361 and 351: HCT/Ps regulated as drugs and/or biological products	1271 Subparts A-D Applicable drugs/biologics regulations	Yes: IND and BLA

*As defined by 2005 tissue regulations [21 CFR 1271.3(d)].
†21 CFR 1271.10(a) as applied to PHS Act Section 361 requires that HPCs be: 1) minimally manipulated, 2) for homologous use only, 3) not combined with another article (except water; crystalloids; or sterilizing, preserving, or storage agents with no new safety concerns), and 4) for autologous use or for allogeneic use in a first- or second-degree blood relative. (See full rule for details.)
HPC = hematopoietic progenitor cell; CFR = Code of Federal Regulations; FDA = Food and Drug Administration; PHS = Public Health Service; HCT/Ps = human cells, tissues, and cellular and tissue-based products; BLA = Biologics License Application; IND = Investigational New Drug.

TABLE 3-5. Cellular Therapy Accreditation

Organization	Standards Review Cycle
AABB	2 years
FACT-JACIE (Foundation for the Accreditation of Cellular Therapy and the Joint Accreditation Committee of ISCT and EBMT)	3 years
National Marrow Donor Program (NMDP)	2 years
World Marrow Donor Association (WMDA)	5 years
College of American Pathologists (CAP)	Not set (publishes updated checklist annually)

therapies. AHCTA provides helpful documents to navigate the different sets of participating organizations' standards. Moreover, crosswalk documents comparing the different set of cellular therapy standards were created and are available on the AHCTA website.[50]

Of note, the FDA regulations in 21 CFR 1271 require HCT/P manufacturers to have a tracking and labeling system that allows for tracking each product from the donor to the recipient and from the recipient back to the donor. HCT/P manufacturers are also required to inform the facilities that receive the products of the tracking system that they have established. However, FDA's regulations for HCT/Ps, including the requirements for tracking, do not apply to facilities that receive, store, and administer cells or tissues but do not perform any manufacturing steps. The Joint Commission has hospital standards for receiving, handling, and tracing tissues and investigating adverse events (TS.03.01.01 to TS.03.03.01).[39] (See Chapter 28 for information on these standards.)

KEY POINTS

1. The fields of transfusion medicine and cellular therapy are highly regulated, involving multiple regulatory agencies and accreditation organizations.

2. FDA regulates biological products including blood and blood components, HCT/Ps and related devices through established laws and regulations. In addition to the legally binding regulations, FDA may periodically publish recommendations in guidance documents. The FDA website provides links to blood and HCT/Ps-related regulations and relevant guidance documents.

3. Blood establishments and device manufacturers must register their manufacturing facilities and list the products they manufacture. Some blood establishments eg, transfusion services that do not collect or process blood and blood components are exempt from registration but must be CLIA certified.

4. Blood establishments that manufacture or participate in the manufacture of blood and blood components are inspected by the FDA to determine compliance with regulations. Observations of significant noncompliance activities are reported to the facility in writing for its response and correction. FDA determines if further enforcement action is appropriate.

5. The FDA requires drug (and blood) manufacturers to conduct recalls or market withdrawals when noncompliance is found after products are distributed, such as for post-donation information.

6. CMS regulates all US medical laboratories under CLIA. CLIA regulations establish requirements for certification. This includes the use of adequate facilities, qualified personnel commensurate with the complexity of testing, and ongoing successful performance in proficiency testing by CMS-approved vendors. Laboratory approval by CMS is granted via inspections performed by CMS-approved accrediting organizations or state health departments.

7. Health-care facilities also have CMS regulations for their activities, and The Joint Commission and other organizations accredit many hospitals for CMS compliance. CMS and The Joint Commission have requirements for monitoring transfusion practices, evaluating adverse transfusion reactions, and preventing mistransfusions.

8. HCT/Ps are regulated by the FDA under a tiered risk-based framework. The FDA website provides links to HCT/Ps-related regulations and relevant guidance documents. The FDA has a licensure process for unrelated-donor umbilical cord blood HPCs.

REFERENCES

1. Office of the Law Revision Council. Search the United States Code. Washington, DC: US House of Representatives, 2017. [Available at http://uscode.house.gov/ (accessed January 18, 2017).]

2. Food and Drug Administration. Regulatory information: §262 Regulation of biological products. Silver Spring, MD: FDA, 2009. [Available at http://www.fda.gov/RegulatoryInformation/Legislation/ucm149278.htm (accessed January 18, 2017).]

3. Food and Drug Administration. Regulatory information: Federal Food, Drug, and Cosmetic Act (FD&C Act). Silver Spring, MD: FDA, 2015. [Available at http://www.fda.gov/RegulatoryInformation/Legislation/FederalFoodDrugandCosmeticActFDCAct/default.htm (accessed January 18, 2017).]

4. Food and Drug Administration. Blood and blood products. Silver Spring, MD: CBER Office of Communication, Outreach, and Development, 2016. [Available at http://www.fda.gov/BiologicsBloodVaccines/BloodBloodProducts/default.htm (accessed January 18, 2017).]

5. Food and Drug Administration. About the Office of Regulatory Affairs. Silver Spring, MD: FDA, 2016. [Available at http://www.fda.gov/aboutfda/centersoffices/officeofglobalregulatoryoperationsandpolicy/ora/default.htm (accessed January 18, 2017).]

6. Electronic code of federal regulations. Washington, DC: US Government Publishing Office, 2017. [Available at http://www.ecfr.gov/cgi-bin/ECFR (accessed January 18, 2017).]

7. Food and Drug Administration. Requirements for blood and blood components intended for transfusion or for further manufacturing use; final rule. (May 22, 2015) Fed Regist 2015;80:29841-906. [Available at https://www.federalregister.gov/articles/2015/05/22/2015-12228/requirements-for-blood-and-blood-components-intended-for-transfusion-or-for-further-manufacturing (accessed January 18, 2017).]

8. Food and Drug Administration. Exceptions and alternative procedures approved under 21 CFR 640.120. Silver Spring, MD: CBER Office of Communication, Outreach, and Development, 2016. [Available at http://www.fda.gov/BiologicsBloodVaccines/BloodBloodProducts/RegulationoftheBloodSupply/ExceptionsandAlternativeProcedures/default.htm (accessed January 18, 2017).]

9. Food and Drug Administration. Guidance, compliance and regulatory information (biologics). Silver Spring, MD: CBER Office of Communication, Outreach, and Development, 2015. [Available at http://www.fda.gov/BiologicsBloodVaccines/GuidanceComplianceRegulatoryInformation/default.htm (accessed January 18, 2017).]

10. Code of federal regulations. Title 21, CFR Part 607.3. Washington, DC: US Government Publishing Office, 2017 (revised annually).

11. Code of federal regulations. Title 21, CFR Part 607.65. Washington, DC: US Government Publishing Office, 2017 (revised annually).

12. MOU 225-80-4000. Memorandum of understanding between the Health Care Financing Administration and the Food and Drug Administration. (June 6, 1983) Silver Spring, MD: FDA, 1983. [Available at http://www.fda.gov/AboutFDA/PartnershipsCollaborations/MemorandaofUnderstandingMOUs/DomesticMOUs/ucm116313.htm (accessed January 18, 2017).]

13. Code of federal regulations. Title 21, CFR Part 601.12. Changes to an approved application. Washington, DC: US Government Publishing Office, 2017 (revised annually). [Available at https://www.gpo.gov/fdsys/pkg/CFR-2011-title21-vol7/xml/CFR-2011-title21-vol7-sec601-12.xml (accessed January 18, 2017).]

14. Food and Drug Administration. Changes to an approved application: Biological products: Human blood and blood components intended for transfusion or for further manufacture; guidance for industry. (November 2014) Silver Spring, MD: CBER Office of Communication, Outreach, and Development, 2014. [Available at http://www.fda.gov/BiologicsBloodVaccines/GuidanceComplianceRegulatoryInformation/Guidances/Blood/ucm354559.htm#Recommendations (accessed January 18, 2017).]

15. Food and Drug Administration.Classify your medical device. Silver Spring, MD: CDRH, 2014. [Available at http://www.fda.gov/MedicalDevices/DeviceRegulationandGuidance/Overview/ClassifyYourDevice/ucm2005371.htm (accessed January 18, 2017).]

16. Food and Drug Administration. Medical devices: Search registration and listing. Silver

Spring, MD: CDRH, 2014. [Available at http://www.fda.gov/MedicalDevices/DeviceRegulationandGuidance/HowtoMarketYourDevice/RegistrationandListing/ucm053199.htm (accessed January 18, 2017).]

17. Code of federal regulations. Title 21, CFR Part 803. Washington, DC: US Government Publishing Office, 2017 (revised annually). [Available at http://www.accessdata.fda.gov/scripts/cdrh/cfdocs/cfcfr/CFRSearch.cfm?CFRPart=803 (accessed January 18, 2017).]

18. Food and Drug Administration. Mandatory reporting requirements: Manufacturers, importers and device user facilities. Silver Spring, MD: CDRH, 2016. [Available at http://www.fda.gov/MedicalDevices/DeviceRegulationandGuidance/PostmarketRequirements/ReportingAdverseEvents/default.htm#1 (accessed January 18, 2017).]

19. Food and Drug Administration. What does FDA inspect? Silver Spring, MD: FDA, 2016. [Available at http://www.fda.gov/AboutFDA/Transparency/Basics/ucm194888.htm (accessed January 18, 2017).]

20. Food and Drug Administration. Blood and blood components. Inspection of licensed and unlicensed blood banks, brokers, reference laboratories, and contractors—7342.001. In: Compliance Program guidance manual. Silver Spring, MD: CBER Office of Compliance and Biologics Quality, 2016. [Available at http://www.fda.gov/downloads/BiologicsBloodVaccines/GuidanceComplianceRegulatoryInformation/ComplianceActivities/Enforcement/CompliancePrograms/UCM337001.pdf (accessed January 18, 2017).]

21. Food and Drug Administration. FDA compliance and enforcement information. Silver Spring, MD: FDA, 2014. [Available at http://www.fda.gov/AboutFDA/Transparency/TransparencyInitiative/ucm254426.htm (accessed January 18, 2017).]

22. Code of federal regulations. Title 21, CFR Part 606.171. Washington, DC: US Government Publishing Office, 2017 (revised annually). [Available at https://www.gpo.gov/fdsys/pkg/CFR-2001-title21-vol7/xml/CFR-2001-title21-vol7-sec606-171.xml (accessed January 18, 2017).]

23. Food and Drug Administration. Biological product deviation reports annual summaries. Silver Spring, MD: CBER Office of Communication, Outreach, and Development, 2016. [Available at http://www.fda.gov/BiologicsBloodVaccines/SafetyAvailability/ReportaProblem/BiologicalProductDeviations/ucm129757.htm (accessed January 18, 2017).]

24. Food and Drug Administration. Safety. Silver Spring, MD: FDA, 2009. [Available at http://www.fda.gov/Safety/Recalls/ucm165546.htm (accessed January 18, 2017).]

25. Food and Drug Administration. Recalls (biologics). Silver Spring, MD: CBER Office of Communication, Outreach, and Development, 2016. [Available at http://www.fda.gov/BiologicsBloodVaccines/SafetyAvailability/Recalls/default.htm (accessed January 18, 2017).]

26. Food and Drug Administration. Enforcement reports. Silver Spring, MD: FDA, 2016. [Available at http://www.fda.gov/safety/recalls/enforcementreports/default.htm (accessed January 18, 2017).]

27. Food and Drug Administration. Blood guidances. Silver Spring, MD: CBER Office of Communication, Outreach, and Development, 2017. [Available at http://www.fda.gov/BiologicsBloodVaccines/GuidanceComplianceRegulatoryInformation/Guidances/Blood/default.htm (accessed January 18, 2017).]

28. Code of federal regulations. Laboratory requirements. Title 42, CFR Part 493. Washington, DC: US Government Publishing Office, 2017 (revised annually).

29. United States code. Certification of laboratories. Title 42, USC Part 263a.

30. Rauch CA, Nichols JH. Laboratory accreditation and inspection. Clin Lab Med 2007;27:845-58.

31. Howerton D, Anderson N, Bosse D, et al. Good laboratory practices for waived testing sites: Survey findings from testing sites holding a certificate of waiver under the Clinical Laboratory Improvement Amendments of 1988 and recommendations for promoting quality testing. MMWR Recomm Rep 2005;54(RR-13):1-25.

32. Food and Drug Administration. Medical device databases. Silver Spring, MD: CDRH, 2016 (revised monthly). [Available at http://www.fda.gov/medicaldevices/deviceregulationandguidance/databases/default.htm (accessed January 18, 2017).]

33. Clinical Laboratory Improvement Amendments (CLIA): How to obtain a CLIA certificate. (March 2006) Baltimore, MD: Centers for Medicare and Medicaid Services, 2006. [Available at https://www.cms.gov/Regulations-and-Guidance/Legislation/CLIA/downloads/

howobtaincliacertificate.pdf (accessed January 18, 2017).]

34. Interpretive guidelines for laboratories. Appendix C. Survey procedures and interpretive guidelines for laboratories and laboratory services. Baltimore, MD: Centers for Medicare and Medicaid Services, 2016. [Available at https://www.cms.gov/Regulations-and-Guidance/Legislation/CLIA/Interpretive_Guidelines_for_Laboratories.html (accessed January 18, 2017).]

35. List of approved accreditation organizations under the Clinical Laboratory Improvement Amendments (CLIA). Baltimore, MD: Centers for Medicare and Medicaid Services, 2013. [Available at https://www.cms.gov/Regulations-and-Guidance/Legislation/CLIA/Downloads/AOList.pdf (accessed January 18, 2017).]

36. Laboratory services. Facts about the cooperative accreditation initiative. Oakbrook Terrace, IL: The Joint Commission, 2015. [Available at http://www.jointcommission.org/facts_about_the_cooperative_accreditation_initiative/ (accessed January 18, 2017).]

37. CLIA approved proficiency testing programs - 2017. Baltimore, MD: Centers for Medicare and Medicaid Services, 2017. [Available at https://www.cms.gov/Regulations-and-Guidance/Legislation/CLIA/downloads/ptlist.pdf. (accessed January 18, 2017).]

38. Code of federal regulations. Condition of participation: Nursing services. Title 42, CFR Part 482.23(c). Washington, DC: US Government Publishing Office, 2017 (revised annually).

39. 2016 Hospital accreditation standards. Oakbrook Terrace, IL: The Joint Commission Resources, 2016.

40. Sentinel event. Oakbrook Terrace, IL: The Joint Commission, 2017. [Available at http://www.jointcommission.org/topics/hai_sentinel_event.aspx (accessed January 18, 2017).]

41. Ooley P, ed. Standards for blood banks and transfusion services. 30th ed. Bethesda, MD: AABB, 2016.

42. College of American Pathologists, Commission on Laboratory Accreditation. Transfusion medicine checklist. July 28, 2015 ed. Northfield, IL: CAP, 2015.

43. Code of federal regulations. Title 21, CFR Part 1271.3(d). Washington, DC: US Government Publishing Office, 2017 (revised annually). [Available at http://www.accessdata.fda.gov/scripts/cdrh/cfdocs/cfcfr/cfrsearch.cfm?fr=1271.3 (accessed January 18, 2017).]

44. Code of federal regulations. Title 21, CFR Part 1271. Washington, DC: US Government Publishing Office, 2017 (revised annually). [Available at http://www.accessdata.fda.gov/scripts/cdrh/cfdocs/cfcfr/CFRSearch.cfm?CFRPart=1271 (accessed January 18, 2017).]

45. Food and Drug Administration. Tissue guidances. Silver Spring, MD: CBER Office of Communication, Outreach, and Development, 2016. [Available at http://www.fda.gov/BiologicsBloodVaccines/GuidanceComplianceRegulatoryInformation/Guidances/Tissue/ (accessed January 18, 2017).]

46. United States code. Regulations to control communicable diseases. Title 42, USC Part 264.

47. AABB, America's Blood Centers, American Association of Tissue Banks, American Red Cross, American Society for Apheresis, American Society for Blood and Marrow Transplantation, College of American Pathologists, Foundation for the Accreditation of Cellular Therapy, ICCBBA, International Society for Cellular Therapy, Joint Accreditation Committee of ISCT and EBMT, National Marrow Donor Program, Netcord. Circular of information for the use of cellular therapy products. Bethesda, MD: AABB, 2016. [Available at http://www.aabb.org/aabbcct/coi/Pages/default.aspx (accessed January 18, 2017).]

48. Haspel RL, ed. Standards for cellular therapy services. 8th ed. Bethesda, MD: AABB, 2017.

49. International standards for hematopoietic cellular therapy: Product collection, processing and administration. 6th ed. Omaha, NE: Foundation for Accreditation for Cellular Therapy, 2015.

50. Alliance for Harmonisation of Cellular Therapy Accreditation. Comparison of cellular therapy standards: Crosswalk documents. AHCTA, 2016. [Available at http://www.ahcta.org/documents.html (accessed January 18, 2017).]

Chapter 4

National Hemovigilance: The Current State

• ● •

Kevin J. Land, MD; Barbee I. Whitaker, PhD; and Lynne Uhl, MD

4

ALTHOUGH THIS IS a new chapter for the *Technical Manual*, the concept of vigilance in relation to donor and recipient safety within AABB and its membership has existed for a number of years.[1-4] The term *hemovigilance* has been defined as "[a] set of surveillance procedures of the whole transfusion chain intended to minimize adverse events or reactions in donors and recipients and to promote safe and effective use of blood components."[5] Hemovigilance, though, will have limited utility if the data are shared and compared only within a single institution. As implied by the phrase "the whole transfusion chain," hemovigilance is considered to be a national-level activity and has been since its inception, when countries were struggling with the (primarily infectious) complications of blood component therapy. Today, hemovigilance increasingly includes not merely the collection of data across many institutions and geopolitical entities at state, regional, national,

and multinational levels, but also the analysis of shared data and best practices. This is encouraging progress, for donor and recipient safety are global concerns and benefit most from lessons learned next door, across the country, and around the world.

Hemovigilance programs are broadly implemented systems based on Deming-style process improvement management, which in turn is based on the scientific method. Dr. Edward Deming, a statistician during the World War II era, espoused a management philosophy whereby organizations increase overall quality while reducing costs through a practice of continual improvement. He is credited with the Plan-Do-Check-Act (PDCA)-cycle iterative management method, which became popularized in Japan's "just-in-time" lean manufacturing systems of the 1940s through 1970s.[6] Mature process improvement programs combine elements of strategic business planning, quality systems, data gathering, and proactive

Kevin J. Land, MD, Adjunct Professor of Pathology, University of Texas Health Science Center at San Antonio, San Antonio, Texas, and Vice President of Clinical Services, Blood Systems, Inc., Scottsdale, Arizona; Barbee I. Whitaker, PhD, Senior Director, Research and AABB Center for Patient Safety, AABB, Bethesda, Maryland; and Lynne Uhl, MD, Vice Chair for Laboratory and Transfusion Medicine, Beth Israel Deaconess Medical Center, and Division Director, Laboratory and Transfusion Medicine, Beth Israel Deaconess Medical Center, and Associate Professor of Pathology, Harvard Medical School, Boston, Massachusetts
The authors have disclosed no conflicts of interest.

surveillance with data analysis, hypothesis generation, and active process improvement. Hemovigilance takes this process one step further by structuring the data and subsequent analysis using standardized definitions and conventions, allowing data to be widely shared and compared in order to identify and influence best practices. Hemovigilance is the ultimate benchtop-to-bedside collaboration, where stakeholders (researchers, policymakers, blood establishments, and hospitals) share data and ideas, implement potential solutions, and then evaluate the results and further refine hypotheses based on real-world data.

This chapter is the culmination of a decade of efforts within the United States to encourage the collaboration between public and private organizations to improve donor and patient outcomes by standardizing terms used to describe key parts of the transfusion chain from blood donation to manufacturing of components to transfusion of the recipient. This chapter is not an exhaustive review of international hemovigilance efforts or a treatise on how to set up a national hemovigilance system; others have already accomplished these tasks well.[5,7] Instead, this chapter focuses on *what* is being done in various countries and what can be done with the increased transparency and collaboration across organizations and nationally to improve donor and recipient outcomes.

INTERNATIONAL HEMOVIGILANCE

Early Efforts

Hemovigilance has more than two decades of history in the international arena, with many programs having been established as a consequence of concern over transfusion-transmitted viral infections and their sequelae [eg, transfusion-transmitted human immunodeficiency virus (HIV), hepatitis B, and hepatitis C]. The architecture and oversight of these hemovigilance programs varies widely, reflecting management and control by various organizations, including blood establishments,

governmental regulators, national medical societies, and departments of public health.[8] Hemovigilance has been implemented on a country-by-country basis, with early adopters now having the more robust systems, as expected with experience. In January of 1993, the Japanese Red Cross Society began aggregating information on adverse reactions and infectious diseases at a national level.[9] In 1994, France became the first European country to develop a formal national hemovigilance system in response to HIV transfusion-transmissions in that country. Since then, many other hemovigilance systems have been developed and regularly provide annual reports (Table 4-1).

In 1998, those practicing hemovigilance in Europe established the European Haemovigilance Network (EHN) and its annual seminar to bring practitioners together to exchange ideas for improving not only patient safety but also hemovigilance reporting. Eventually, national hemovigilance programs were required by the 2002 and 2005 European Blood Directives (2002/98/EC, 2005/61/EC),[10,11] which mandated implementation of hemovigilance systems with minimum common donor and recipient elements in all European Union (EU) member states and subsequent reporting of results to EU authorities. The EHN was reinvented as the International Haemovigilance Network (IHN) in 2009, when the interest and membership of non-EU countries made it clear that the desire to develop robust hemovigilance systems and share critical experiences was truly global.

International Resources

Recognition of the importance of sharing aggregated data between and among countries led to the development of the International Surveillance of Transfusion-Associated Reactions and Events (ISTARE) database in 2008, whose stated mission is to unify the collection and sharing of donor and recipient hemovigilance information with the intent of harmonizing best practices among hemovigilance systems around the world. As of 2016, 23 countries and two regions have reported data

TABLE 4-1. Hemovigilance Reports Throughout the World (not exhaustive)

Country	Year Reporting Began	Public Website (if available)
Australia	2007	http://www.blood.gov.au/haemovigilance-reporting
Austria	2003	http://www.basg.gv.at/en/medicines/blood/
Brazil	2010	http://portal.anvisa.gov.br/contact-us?
Canada	2007	http://www.phac-aspc.gc.ca/hcai-iamss/ttiss-ssit/index-eng.php
(Québec)	2000	http://msssa4.msss.gouv.qc.ca/santpub/sang_en.nsf/vdocdate?Open View
Denmark	1999	http://dski.dk/
France	1994	http://ansm.sante.fr/Declarer-un-effet-indesirable/Hemovigilance/L-hemovigilance-et-son-organisation/(offset)/0 (available only in French)
Germany	1997	http://www.pei.de/EN/information/pharmacists-physicians/haemovigilance/haemovigilance-node.html (available only in German)
Greece	1995	http://www.keelpno.gr/en-us/structurefunction.aspx
Hong Kong SAR, China	2000	--
India	2012	http://nib.gov.in/haemovigilance.html
Ireland	1999	http://www.giveblood.ie/Clinical_Services/Haemovigilance/
Japan	1993	http://www.jrc.or.jp/mr/english/
Kingdom of Saudi Arabia	2007	--
Namibia	2010	--
The Netherlands	2003	http://www.tripnet.nl/pages/en/
New Zealand	2005	http://www.nzblood.co.nz/clinical-information/haemovigilance-programme/
Norway	2004	http://www.hemovigilans.no/ (available only in Norwegian)
Republic of Korea	2007	--
Singapore	2003	http://www.hsa.gov.sg/content/hsa/en/Blood_Services/Transfusion_Medicine/Blood_Safety.html
Slovenia	2002	https://www.jazmp.si/en/blood/haemovigilance/
South Africa	2010	http://www.sanbs.org.za http://www.wpblood.org.za/?q=clinical/haemovigilance-reports
Spain	2004	http://www.msc.es/profesionales/saludPublica/medicinaTransfusional/home.htm (available only in Spanish)
Switzerland	2004	https://www.swissmedic.ch/marktueberwachung/00138/00186/index.html?lang=en
United Kingdom	1996	http://www.shotuk.org/
United States	2006	http://www.cdc.gov/nhsn/acute-care-hospital/bio-hemo/index.html

into ISTARE, including countries in Europe, Asia and Oceania, Africa, and the Americas.[12]

The World Health Organization (WHO) is active in promoting development of hemovigilance efforts,[13] offering several resources, including draft guidelines for adverse event reporting and learning systems. One of its more recent resources is the Project Notify Library, a website where international experts collaborate to share didactic, peer-reviewed documentation on adverse outcomes associated with the application of human organs, blood, tissue, and cells (www.notifylibrary.org).

In all hemovigilance systems, there is a reliance on hospital surveillance of transfusion-associated adverse events occurring in recipients and the reporting of them into a central data repository. In contrast, the detailed donor information that blood establishments have collected for years has only recently begun to be compiled on a national level.[14-15] There are challenges common to all newly introduced hemovigilance programs, including 1) the significant delays between data submission and release of a final annual report; 2) the lack of sufficiently granular data to understand many observations; 3) the concern that systems do not adequately capture new, rapidly evolving, or unusual diseases; 4) the reality that systems do not capture all events from all potential institutions; and 5) financial pressures that constantly expect systems to provide more and increasingly sophisticated results with fewer resources.

For example, a review of annual hemovigilance reporting by the UK reporting system Serious Hazards of Transfusion (SHOT) shows that at program inception, the number of reports was low; however, with education and involvement of key stakeholders and recognition of the program having an impact, the observed number of reports increased while the number of transfusion-associated fatalities declined (Fig 4-1). Today, UK's SHOT program is widely acknowledged for its impact on global hemovigilance and transfusion safety. Most notable are the SHOT reports heralding the association of transfusion-related acute lung injury (TRALI) with plasma and platelet transfusions derived from female donors in the early 2000s.[16] The observation and reporting of this association promoted far-reaching changes in the management of donor collections and product manufacturing around the world.

Equally important are the SHOT data on lapses in safe transfusion practice, including

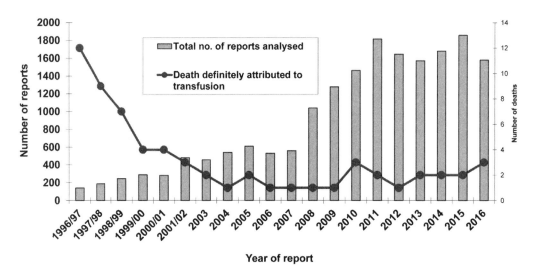

FIGURE 4-1. Total reports submitted to the United Kingdom's Serious Hazards of Transfusion (SHOT) between 1996 and 2016, and total deaths determined as definitely due to transfusion. Used with permission from P. Bolton-Maggs.

inadequate patient identification at the time of specimen acquisition and blood component administration.[17] These data have prompted public campaigns engaging patients to actively participate in their care as a means to mitigate risks of misidentification and transfusion errors. In 2011 in Great Britain, an 18-minute video was produced with the help of actors Hugh Laurie and Imelda Staunton about the importance of proper procedures to ensure the safety of blood. The video, titled "The Strange Case of Penny Allison," was an excellent example of the benefits of collaboration on a national scale. Other resources can be found on the Joint UK Blood Transfusion and Tissue Transplantation Services Professional Advisory Committee website.[18]

Eventually, as hemovigilance programs evolved, it became increasingly clear that proper analysis of hemovigilance events requires standardization of data structures and harmonization of terminology with simple and objective definitions that lend themselves to comparison (eg, expressing adverse events per transfusion or per 1000 donations, etc), and extensive use of subject matter experts to aid in interpretation.[19,20]

US HEMOVIGILANCE

In 2009, US hemovigilance was described as a "patchwork of reporting processes"[21] with significant but limited programs to collect specific donor and recipient data and where only fatal transfusion reactions, donation-related deaths, and product deviations were reported at a national level to the US Food and Drug Administration (FDA). However, some programs, while not national in scale in the United States, are still robust in that they capture more data than reported to the FDA, can retrospectively review and capture supplemental data, and can more readily validate their data.

Hospitals and transfusion services are required to perform an investigation of all adverse reactions associated with blood transfusion and to report complications that may be related to the blood donor or to the manufacture of the blood components to the collection facility. [See the *Code of Federal Regulations* (CFR), Title 21 Part 606.170.] Transfusion-related fatalities must also be reported directly to the FDA by the transfusing facility. Mandatory reporting of product deviations by licensed manufacturers, unlicensed registered blood establishments, and transfusion services has also been defined by the FDA (21 CFR 606.171). These requirements will likely continue even if a more formal US national hemovigilance system is eventually required because hemovigilance reports are retrospective, while reporting to the FDA following an adverse event or for product deviations must occur closer to real time, as outlined in the CFR.

There has been no nationwide, systematic assessment either of transfusion reactions that were not fatal or of nonfatal donor-related reactions. However, comprehensive data including work on emerging infectious diseases, noninfectious complications of transfusion, and donation-related reactions have been generated from a few very strong investigator-led or collaborative research initiatives [the American Red Cross (ARC); Blood Systems Research Institute; and National Heart, Lung, and Blood Institute (NHLBI)-sponsored collaborations such as the Retrovirus Epidemiology Donor Study (REDS), REDS-II, and the Recipient Epidemiology and Donor Evaluation Study-III (REDS-III)]. Another contributing source of data was the work that began in the mid-1990s on the medical event reporting system for transfusion medicine (MERS-TM) in blood centers and hospitals by Drs. Harold Kaplan and James Battles.[22] The successful launch of a voluntary system of hemovigilance in the United States has required collaboration among all stakeholders and many organizations. Specific acknowledgment is given to the strategic partnership, resources, financial support, and guidance provided by the US Department of Health and Human Services (DHHS), including the FDA and the Centers for Disease Control and Prevention (CDC).

Task Force on Biovigilance

In early 2006, a number of prominent individuals in transfusion medicine recognized the need for a more cohesive and coordinated approach, termed *biovigilance*, that encompassed not only blood recipient and blood donor hemovigilance but also tissues, organs, and cellular therapy (CT) components.[8] AABB established an Interorganizational Task Force on Biovigilance, inviting key governmental thought leaders and representatives from the private sector to initiate the development of a national hemovigilance program as a first step. Amid concerns of additional oversight by governmental agencies, including a perception that such oversight could result in punitive actions that might interfere with patient care, hemovigilance was established in the United States within a framework of a public-private partnership.[23] Through the efforts of the task force and an international working group of advisors representing established hemovigilance systems, recipient and donor hemovigilance programs were designed based on the important tenets of voluntary reporting: confidentiality, a just culture (nonpunitive data analysis), and efficient data reporting with a focus on improvements to patient and donor safety.[4]

Elements of Biovigilance

Efficient reporting for recipient hemovigilance was achieved through leveraging an existing hospital event reporting system, the CDC's National Healthcare Safety Network (NHSN). (See Recipient Hemovigilance, below.) Donor hemovigilance required building a new and effective infrastructure to capture national reporting by US blood establishments. (See Blood Donor Hemovigilance, below.) Other areas essential to comprehensive biovigilance in the US include tissue and organ surveillance and CT biovigilance. CT adverse event and outcome monitoring occurs through national and international registries, including the Center for International Blood and Marrow Transplant Registry (CIBMTR), the National Marrow Donor Program (NMDP), and the World Marrow Donor Association (WMDA). A centralized tissue and organ surveillance system was piloted in 2008 and awaits additional funding to proceed. In ongoing efforts to promote hemovigilance ideals, AABB's *Standards for Blood Banks and Transfusion Services* requires accredited blood banks, transfusion services, and blood centers to adopt standardized terminology for adverse reactions associated with blood donation and the transfusion of blood and blood components.[24]

RECIPIENT HEMOVIGILANCE IN THE UNITED STATES

CDC's NHSN is a secure, web-based surveillance system. Originally developed to capture data on hospital-acquired infections (HAI), it is now currently used by more than 12,000 US health-care facilities to report on a variety of infection-related and other patient safety issues.[25] The Hemovigilance Module of the NHSN affords hospital transfusion services the ability to report on transfusion-related adverse events. Additionally, transfusion services can report on transfusion activity, including annual transfusion volumes and discards by component type. The module allows hospitals to monitor their own transfusion activity as well as to share data with external groups (governmental and nongovernmental) at the individual hospital's discretion, for mandatory or voluntary reporting activities.[25]

The NHSN modules were established as data repositories for surveillance of adverse events and reactions of interest. To be useful, data must be reported using common definitions for all aspects of data element reporting. Ideally, reporting thresholds would be as similar as possible between different hospitals. To this end, the components of the NHSN Hemovigilance Module and the terms and definitions employed were developed and thoroughly vetted by subject matter experts. The major components of the module include: 1) demographic and utilization data, which permit classification of facilities for comparisons in aggregate data analyses; 2) reports on transfusion-related adverse events in accordance with case definition criteria (Table 4-2); and 3) incident reporting (ie, mistakes or adverse events associated with transfusion). Reporting of incidents is not mandatory for participation. As of 2016, 277 transfusion services were enrolled in the NHSN Hemovigilance Module, 135 of which are actively reporting data to NHSN.[25] Of note, the state of Massachusetts, as of June 2014, mandated participation in the NHSN Hemovigilance Module by all blood banks and transfusion services in the state as a means to comply with state regulatory reporting requirements on transfusion activity and transfusion-related adverse events.[27] Other state departments of health have expressed interest, but whether they will mandate reporting has yet to be determined.

Getting Connected

Nearly every US hospital uses the CDC's NHSN for HAI reporting, as this centralized HAI reporting is required for reimbursement from the DHHS Centers for Medicare and Medicaid Services (CMS). In order for a hospital to begin using the Hemovigilance Module, the hospital's NHSN administrator must activate the Biovigilance Component and invite someone from the blood bank or transfusion service to join for the purposes of setting up the module and hemovigilance reporting. Each person who has access to the system must establish an individual account and acquire a Secure Access Management Services (SAMS) card in order to access the CDC system. Once access has been attained and the module initiated, the Annual Hospital Survey must be completed before any data submission may begin. This includes a significant number of data elements that describe the demographics of the hospital. Following completion of the survey, the hospital can begin to submit data using the web forms to complete monthly reporting plans and then report monthly denominators, adverse reactions, and incidents. Monthly denominator reports should include the components transfused each month and are reported in the month following the reporting month (eg, March reporting for February transfusions). Adverse events (reactions and incidents) should be reported upon completion of their investigation.

Transfusion-Related Adverse Reaction Reporting

Adverse reactions should be investigated and categorized according to the CDC protocol[25] into 12 different reaction types, and coded according to the degree to which each reaction conforms to the surveillance definition (criteria), the severity or grade of the reaction, and the reaction's imputability to the transfusion (Table 4-2). Imputability is an important concept for hemovigilance; it is the degree to which the reaction was caused by the transfusion.

Transfusion Incident Reporting

Mistakes or incidents associated with transfusion can be reported on a detailed incident form or summarized on a monthly incident summary report. The CDC requires reporting only of incidents that result in a transfusion reaction on the detailed form. However, incident review and more detailed reporting can be a valuable activity if conducted regularly and compared with other transfusion services using harmonized event codes incorporated into the CDC system that were based on the adverse event coding developed in MERS-TM.[28]

Using Recipient Data via the AABB Patient Safety Organization

The timing of the launch of the US hemovigilance system at the CDC was fortuitous in that it followed an important effort within the United States to recognize the impact of error on health-care quality.[29] Implementation of the Patient Safety and Quality Improvement Act of 2005 (PSQIA)[30] and the regulations that followed allowed the establishment of Patient Safety Organizations (PSOs) through the DHHS Agency of Healthcare Research and Quality (AHRQ), which has the mission to produce evidence to make health care safer, of higher quality, and more accessible, equitable, and affordable. The PSQIA established a voluntary reporting system designed to enhance

TABLE 4-2. NHSN Hemovigilance Module Adverse Reaction Codes, Severity Codes, and Imputability*†

Case Definition	Severity	Imputability
Definitive: The adverse reaction fulfills all of the case definition criteria. *Probable:* The adverse reaction meets some of the clinical signs of symptoms or radiologic, laboratory evidence, and/or available information but does not meet all definitive case definition criteria.	*Nonsevere:* Medical intervention (eg, symptomatic treatment) is required but there is minimal risk of permanent damage to the transfusion recipient. *Severe:* Inpatient hospitalization or prolonged hospitalization is directly attributable to the transfusion reaction, persistent or significant disability or incapacity of the patient as a result of the reaction, or a medical or surgical intervention is necessary to preclude permanent damage or impairment of a body function. *Life-threatening:* Major intervention was required after the transfusion reaction (eg, vasopressors, intubation, transfer to intensive care) to prevent death. *Death:* The recipient died as a result of the transfusion reaction. *Not determined:* The severity of the adverse reaction is unknown or not stated.	*Definite:* There is conclusive evidence that the reaction can be attributed to the transfusion. *Probable:* There are other potential causes present that could explain the recipient's symptoms, but transfusion is the most likely cause of the reaction. *Possible:* There are other potential causes that are most likely; however, transfusion cannot be ruled out.

Optional	Optional	Optional
Possible: The reported clinical signs or symptoms, radiologic or laboratory evidence, and available information are not sufficient to meet definitive or probable case definition criteria.		*Doubtful:* There is evidence clearly in favor of a cause other than the transfusion, but transfusion cannot be excluded.
		Ruled out: There is conclusive evidence beyond reasonable doubt of a cause other than the transfusion.
		Not determined: The relationship between the reaction and transfusion is unknown or not stated.

*Used with permission from Chung et al.[26]

†The NHSN Hemovigilance Module protocol specifies the case definition for 12 adverse transfusion reactions based on the presence of signs, symptoms, and laboratory and radiologic data. Reactions are reported with a severity designation based on clinical outcomes. Imputability designations that specify the likelihood that reaction was associated with the transfusion event are also reported.

the data available to assess and resolve patient safety and health-care quality issues, provided federal privilege and confidentiality protections for patient safety information (by designating certain data as patient safety work product), and established PSOs. AHRQ established common formats for harmonized event reporting, including specific reporting forms for blood safety events.[31]

A PSO is an entity whose workforce has expertise in analyzing patient safety events and whose primary activity is to improve patient safety and health-care quality by reducing errors. These organizations are regulated under the DHHS Office of Civil Rights [Health Insurance Portability and Accountability Act (HIPAA) Privacy Rule] and are subject to civil monetary penalties for violations of patient safety confidentiality. They are required to report to AHRQ annually, to renew listing with AHRQ review every 2 years, and to be subject to audit by AHRQ. Other changes in health-care law, notably the Affordable Care Act of 2010, have solidified the standing of PSOs and require qualified health plans in insurance exchanges to contract with hospitals (of greater than 50 beds) that report data to a PSO (effective January 1, 2017) or other like-quality organizations. The job of the PSO is to be involved in patient safety activities, including engaging in efforts to improve patient safety and the quality of health-care delivery; collecting and analyzing patient safety data; and developing and disseminating information regarding patient safety (recommendations, protocols, and best practices).

To this end, AABB established the AABB Center for Patient Safety (CPS) as a component PSO of AABB, separate from its accreditation and other functions. This allows the AABB CPS access to hospital data—such as hemovigilance reports—while retaining the ability to keep reports confidential and maintain HIPAA protections for patient information. AABB established CPS so that hospitals reporting to NHSN may share their data and maintain confidentiality and protections; these strong privacy and confidentiality protections are intended to encourage greater participation by providers in the examination of patient safety events. Providers may engage in detailed discussions about the causes of adverse events without the fear of liability from information shared and/or analyses generated from those discussions.

The AABB CPS is the only transfusion safety PSO. Using the CDC NHSN infrastructure, it offers additional services and analyses based on the shared reported hemovigilance data, as well as through additional data submitted directly to the CPS. Upon joining, hospitals receive full data protection and access to benefits, including quarterly hemovigilance benchmark reports, quarterly blood utilization benchmark reports, feedback and sharing through quarterly "Safe Table" conference calls with members to review data and address coding and system differences, and other offerings to improve patient safety through hemovigilance.

BLOOD DONOR HEMOVIGILANCE IN THE UNITED STATES

Part of maintaining a safe and adequate blood supply involves vigilance over donor safety and well-being. The donor expects some discomfort (needle, time, etc) for the good that they are performing, but no real harm. Blood donors are healthy volunteers, not patients and not research subjects. Blood centers have an obligation and responsibility to minimize the risks associated with collection. Potential donors perform their own risk-vs-benefit analysis when considering blood donation. When the risks outweigh the benefits, they do not donate. Hospitals are expected to constantly improve patient care by transforming their entire operations (and not just their clinical practice) through implementation of solid quality systems, listening to the experience of others, and basing the design of their policies and therapies on evidence-based medicine.[32] Blood establishments can do no less for donor safety if they are to be the stewards donors expect them to be. "Because it has always been done that way," is not an acceptable reason for how donors are recruited and units are collected, manufactured, distributed, and transfused; hence the need for a donor hemovigilance system.

Blood establishments collect a wealth of data every day centered on donor-related activities. They are driven to maximize the efficiency of collecting each donation type while also reducing donor reactions. Blood-center-based donor hemovigilance systems and collaborative research have evolved primarily to capture adverse reaction rates and have been used in donor safety studies to mitigate adverse events.[33-37] Such programs within large blood systems have demonstrated their utility in identifying and implementing measures that improved donation safety for young donors.[33,34] Blood center data have also been analyzed to help identify donation deterrents and motivators and to increase overall donor satisfaction.[38,39] Improvements in donor safety can occur through a variety of methods, such as avoiding high-risk donors (eg, potential donors with low estimated blood volume), educating donors and staff on hydration and salt-loading of donors, improving the ability to predict donors at risk for vasovagal reactions with loss of consciousness (especially off-site), and developing strategies to decrease deferrals (eg, iron replacement) and increase donor return rates. Blood establishments, through a mature donor hemovigilance system, utilize the collected data not only to improve donor safety and satisfaction but also to inform decisions about complex business and operational issues.

Building a New Program for Donor Hemovigilance

Like the recipient hemovigilance system in the United States, US donor hemovigilance emerged through a public-private partnership, which developed out of the AABB Interorganizational Task Force on Biovigilance. A Donor Hemovigilance Working Group was established with representation from blood establishments, including hospital-based collection programs, the US Armed Services Blood Program, Canadian Blood Services, the Plasma Protein Therapeutics Association (PPTA), and

international liaisons with the International Society of Blood Transfusion (ISBT) and IHN in partnership with representatives from DHHS. The Donor Hemovigilance Working Group was charged to develop and implement a national monitoring program on donor safety issues. Tasks included developing a US common definition set for donor hemovigilance based on existing models, and providing subject matter expertise for the development of software that would gather donor data and provide a systematic and standard mechanism to calculate and compare rates. The working group also provided the necessary subject matter expertise for the Donor Hemovigilance Analysis and Reporting Tool (DonorHART) software, developed by Knowledge Based Systems, Incorporated (KBSI, College Station, TX), with funding from DHHS. It contains a robust set of reporting and graphing tools designed to greatly simplify initial data reporting and analysis.

Many organizations (ISBT, IHN, ARC, America's Blood Centers, Blood Systems, Inc., etc) have a long-standing interest in donor hemovigilance activities, which has made it easy to adopt many preexisting terms and ideas. Where needed, the working group developed or adapted objective, evidence-based definitions to aid in the collection of highly reliable and reproducible data. Once completed, the system was piloted and validated successfully by one small, one medium, and one large blood center (defined as annual red cell collections of ~30,000, ~150,000, and >1 million units, respectively). Observed variation in reaction rates led to changes in practice in one blood center that likely reduced reaction rates among donors less than 30 years old.[40,41]

In 2013, AABB published its first Hemovigilance Report, based on 2012 data reported by five blood centers.[14] The first report highlighted that, unfortunately, not all data elements of interest in hemovigilance are readily available electronically from current blood establishment computer systems (BECS). Fortunately, though, sufficient data elements were electronically available for several calculations, including reaction rates per 1000 donations, with 95% confidence intervals, for the most common donor reactions for all donations among the five centers (Table 4-3).[14] Univariate aggregate denominator data, such as donor age and gender, were also analyzed. For example, a graph from the 2016 AABB Hemovigilance Report (2014 data) comparing the reaction rates of vasovagal reactions and hematoma/bruise reactions demonstrated that although these reactions are present in all age groups, they are each more common on opposing ends of the donor age spectrum (Fig 4-2).[15]

A Global Standard

The 2008 ISBT "Standard for Surveillance of Complications Related to Blood Donation" was foundational to the development of surveillance definitions for US donor hemovigi-lance. Although very useful, the definitions were internationally felt to be 1) insufficiently specific to permit standard classification and comparison across different programs, and 2) difficult to apply in all countries because of a lack of the required information. Eventually, a formal revision group made up of representatives from the ISBT Working Party on Haemovigilance, the IHN, and the AABB US Donor Hemovigilance Working Group was created to address both issues. The group reconciled the differences between the AABB and ISBT surveillance terms and on December 11, 2014, published the first internationally harmonized AABB-ISBT standard definitions for complications related to blood donation. The Alliance of Blood Operators, the European Blood Alliance, and the IHN have formally endorsed

TABLE 4-3. Reaction Rates per 1000 Donations, from the AABB Donor Hemovigilance 2012 Report[14]

	Reaction Rate	Odds Ratio	Lower 95% CI	Upper 95% CI
Overall Reaction Rate	13.41			
Vasovagal	9.65			
Prefaint, No LOC, uncomplicated or minor	7.33	1.00	1.00	1.00
LOC, any duration, uncomplicated	1.87	0.25	0.24	0.27
LOC, any duration, complicated	0.40	0.05	0.05	0.06
Injury	0.06	0.01	0.01	0,01
Local Injury Related to Needle	2.48			
Nerve Irritation	0.23	0.10	0.09	0.12
Hematoma/Bruise	2.23	1.00	1.00	1.00
Arterial Puncture	0.03	0.01	0.01	0.02
Apheresis Related	0.83			
Citrate	0.05	0.06	0.05	0.08
Hemolysis	0.00	0.01	0.00	0.01
Air Embolism	0.00	0.00	0.00	0.01
Infiltration	0.77	1.00	1.00	1.00
Allergic	0.22			
Local	0.18	1.00	1.00	1.00
Systemic	0.04	0.20	0.14	0.28
Anaphylaxis	0.00	0.00		
Other	0.23			

CI = confidence interval; LOC = loss of consciousness.

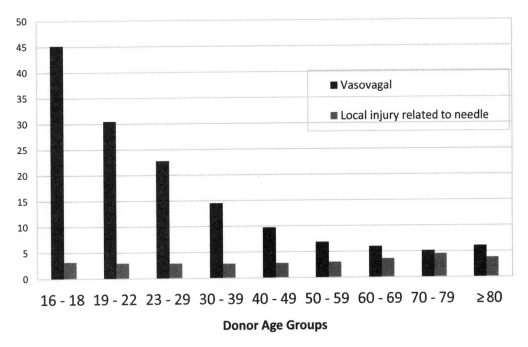

FIGURE 4-2. Reaction rate by donor age and reaction type (2014 data). Used with permission from the AABB Donor Hemovigilance 2016 Report.[15]

these definitions.[42] A copy of the document is available on the donor hemovigilance section of the AABB website.[43]

CONCLUSION

A 2009 DHHS report on the critical gaps in US biovigilance[21] identified 16 gaps in total for blood, tissue, and organ national vigilance programs, eight of which were focused on blood-related activities (Table 4-4). The key deficiencies seen in the US hemovigilance system were notably the absence of: common definitions, multicenter design, active use of document practice improvement, broad data access and sharing, national scope, real-time data availability, and long-term stability. Eight years later, some of the gaps have been addressed, but many of the gaps are still present. Gaps 4 and 6 (see Table 4-4) are largely closed, with precise recipient and donor definitions and identified denominator data; however, the system is still very fragmented (Gap 1) with

only some centers voluntarily providing detailed data on donor serious events (Gap 5) through DonorHART beyond the FDA-required fatality reporting. Some of the key deficiencies mentioned above also should still be considered as potential discrepancies in the current US hemovigilance system: active use of data to document practice improvement; broad data access and sharing; and long-term stability.

Although reporting institutions technically should have always had access to their own data, the complexities of hospital information systems and BECS have not lent themselves to easy accessibility and analysis of data. Fortunately, this is beginning to be addressed in broad terms with the successful completion of national repository databases, the publishing of annual reports, and (limited) access to composite data for researchers and analysts (addressing the deficiencies above regarding active use of data and broad data access). Short of a formal revamping of the current reporting system and increasing what is required to be

TABLE 4-4. Gaps Identified in US Biovigilance, 2009[21]

Blood	Gap 1	Patchwork and sometimes fragmented system of various adverse event reporting.
	Gap 2	Likely underreporting of transfusion adverse events.
	Gap 3	Challenges with FDA-required reporting.
	Gap 4	Need for accurate recipient denominator data, precise definitions, and training.
	Gap 5	No national surveillance of donor serious adverse events other than fatalities.
	Gap 6	Need for accurate donor denominator data, precise definitions, and training.
	Gap 7	Need for accurate tracking of all donor infectious disease test data.
	Gap 8	Need for timely analysis of reported data.
Tissues	Gap 9	Limited information on the potential for HCT/Ps to transmit infectious disease.
	Gap 10	Ability is limited to ascertain that reported infections in HCT/P recipients can be attributed to the tissue.
	Gap 11	Regulations concerning HCT/P adverse reaction reporting do not extend to the level of the health-care facility or health-care provider.
	Gap 12	Current mechanisms are limited for tracking HCT/P grafts to the level of the recipient.
	Gap 13	Adverse reaction reporting is limited to infectious diseases for HCT/Ps regulated solely under Section 361 of the PHS Act.
	Gap 14	Information may not be readily available about adverse reactions in other recipients of HCT/Ps from an implicated donor.
Organs	Gap 15	Lack of nationwide common organ/tissue donor network system for real-time reporting, data collection, communication, and analysis of donor-transmitted diseases in organ and tissue transplant recipients, including a common donor identifier necessary for linkage back to implicated donor of both organs and tissues.
	Gap 16	No requirement to retain donor and recipient samples.

HCT/Ps = human cells, tissues, and cellular and tissue-based products; PHS = Public Health Service.

reported, Gaps 2, 3, and 5 will likely remain. Real-time data availability (Gap 8) is also a difficult issue, but steps are being made to shorten the reporting window.

As the blood banking community and the threats to it continue to evolve, so do the tools needed to evaluate risk and the impact of decisions. Because of ongoing concerns about the need for real-time assessment of postmarket recipient risk and as a result of a congressional mandate (Food and Drug Administration Amendments Act of 2007), the FDA developed the Sentinel BloodSCAN Program in 2011 as an active surveillance system to monitor the safety of FDA-regulated medical products, including blood components.[44,45] (See www.sentinelinitiative.org for more information.) It is a distributed database composed of data from 18 data partners, covering more than 193 million individuals (about 60% of the US population). The project's aim is to help the FDA work with public, academic, and private entities to collect quality data, provide a rapid response (days to weeks) to safety questions, and make the results accessible to the public domain. This pilot project goes a long way toward addressing several of the key hemovigilance deficiencies, including real-time data availability. Assessment of TRALI after platelet, plasma, or red cell transfusion is a current focus. Although such data mining may speed up discovery of emerging events, there is also an inherent risk of inaccurate and/or incomplete data, resulting in false signals.

With the constant threat of existing (eg, HIV, West Nile virus) and emerging infectious diseases (eg, Zika virus), it is no wonder that improved infectious disease surveillance and rapid alert systems are still considered primary parts of any national hemovigilance program (Gap 7). In early 2015, FDA's Center for Biologics Evaluation and Research and NHLBI announced a joint program to develop a Transfusion-Transmissible Infections Monitoring System (TTIMS), by leveraging existing and successful programs (REDS-II) to establish a framework for transfusion-transmissible infection surveillance to include known pathogens and emerging infectious disease agents. Such programs are invaluable to objectively assess the value of new blood safety initiatives, such as the FDA's recent policy change involving deferral for men who have sex with men (MSM), from a lifetime deferral to a deferral of 1 year since the last MSM sexual contact. Programs such as Sentinel BloodSCAN and TTIMS are needed for the FDA to have the objective, national data necessary for other policy changes, such as dropping syphilis or other infectious disease testing requirements for components treated using pathogen inactivation technology.

Unfortunately, the final key discrepancy of the US hemovigilance system, long-term stability, is still largely unmet, outside of perhaps the CDC's NHSN Hemovigilance Module. The availability of long-term funding for many programs, such as DonorHART, Sentinel BloodSCAN, and TTIMS is still unknown. To be successful, these systems must continue to provide stakeholders with quality data to drive new safety hypotheses and objective analytics to demonstrate outcomes. Future directions for hemovigilance, therefore, must include a stable long-term financial model before attention can be turned to important donor and recipient safety issues, such as the impact of pathogen inactivation technology and mitigating donation-related iron deficiency.

KEY POINTS

1. Hemovigilance is a set of surveillance procedures of the whole transfusion chain intended to minimize adverse events or reactions in donors and recipients and to promote safe and effective use of blood components.
2. Since inception over two decades ago, hemovigilance has been considered a national-level activity that has its roots in Deming-style process improvement management.
3. The earliest hemovigilance efforts in Japan and France arose out of concerns over transfusion-transmitted viral infections and their sequelae (eg, transfusion-transmitted HIV, hepatitis B, and hepatitis C) for recipients of blood component therapy.
4. National monitoring of emerging infectious agents (such as Zika virus) and surveillance of known transfusion-transmissible pathogens are still important today. Such programs are invaluable, in part as they offer an opportunity to assess the value of new blood safety initiatives, such as the FDA's recent policy change for men who have sex with men (MSM) from lifetime deferral to a 1-year deferral since last MSM contact.
5. There are challenges common to all newly introduced surveillance programs—including a) the significant delays between data submission and release of a final annual report; b) the lack of sufficiently granular data to understand many observations; c) the concern that systems do not adequately capture new, rapidly evolving, or unusual diseases; d) the reality that systems do not capture all events from all potential institutions; and e) financial pressures that constantly impact the ability of systems to provide more and increasingly sophisticated results, often with fewer resources.
6. *Biovigilance* has been used as an all-encompassing term that captures surveillance efforts in not only blood donor and transfusion recipient programs but also donors and transplant recipients of cellular therapies, tissues, and organs.
7. In the United States, national hemovigilance has lagged behind other countries. Currently, it consists of a patchwork of reporting processes with significant but limited programs to

collect specific and high-level donor and recipient data at a national level. Some individual programs, however, while not national in scale, are very robust in their ability to capture and validate their data.

8. Recipient hemovigilance in the United States is handled through CDC's National Healthcare Safety Network (NHSN), a secure, web-based surveillance system. The Hemovigilance Module of the NHSN affords hospital transfusion services the ability to report on transfusion-related adverse events using standardized nomenclature. The module allows hospitals to monitor their own data as well as share data with governmental and nongovernmental groups as needed.

9. Blood establishments have an obligation to minimize the risks of blood collection. The rise in formal donor hemovigilance efforts over the past decade culminated in December 2014 in the first internationally harmonized AABB-ISBT standard definitions for complications related to blood donation.

10. Hemovigilance is the ultimate benchtop-to-bedside collaboration, where stakeholders (researchers, policymakers, blood establishments, and hospitals) share data and ideas, implement potential solutions, and then evaluate the results and further refine hypotheses based on real-world data.

ACKNOWLEDGMENT

The authors wish to thank Paula Bolton-Maggs, DM, FRCP, FRCPath, Medical Director, SHOT for her contribution of the cumulative SHOT data in Fig 4-1.

REFERENCES

1. Busch MP, Lee LL, Satten GA, et al. Time course of detection of viral and serological markers preceding human immunodeficiency virus type 1 seroconversion: Implications for screening of blood and tissue donors. Transfusion 1995;35:91-7.

2. Jennings ER, Hindman WM, Zak B, et al. The thymol turbidity test in screening of blood donors. Am J Clin Pathol 1957;27:489-502.

3. Keating LJ, Gorman R, Moore R. Hemoglobin and hematocrit values of blood donors. Transfusion 1967;7:420-4.

4. AuBuchon JP, Whitaker BI. America finds hemovigilance! Transfusion 2007;47:1937-42.

5. De Vries RRP, Faver J-C, eds. Hemovigilance: An effective tool for improving transfusion safety. 1st ed. West Sussex, UK: Wiley-Blackwell, 2012.

6. Walton M. The Deming management method. New York: Berkley Publishing Group, 1986.

7. Strengers PFW. Haemovigilance—Why? [Available at http://www.ztm.si/uploads/publication/990/1009.pdf (accessed January 20, 2017).]

8. HHS Advisory Committee on Blood and Tissue Safety and Availability meeting minutes, April 30-May 1 and November 19-20, 2009 (transcripts). Silver Spring, MD: HHS, 2016. [Available at http://wayback.archive-it.org/3919/20160728222436/http://www.hhs.gov/ash/bloodsafety/advisorycommittee/pastmeetings/pastmeetings.html, (accessed January 20, 2017).]

9. Japanese Red Cross Society. Haemovigilance annual report 2001 and 1993-2001. Tokyo: Japanese Red Cross Central Blood Center, 2003. [Available at http://www.jrc.or.jp/mr/english/ (accessed January 20, 2017).]

10. European Union. Directive 2002/98/EC of the European Parliament and of the Council of 27 January 2003 setting standards of quality and safety for the collection, testing, processing, storage and distribution of human blood and blood components and amending Directive 2001/83/EC. Official Journal of the European Union 2003;L33:30-40. [Available at http://eur-lex.europa.eu/legal-content/EN/TXT/?uri=CELEX%3A32002L0098 (accessed January 20, 2017).]

11. European Commission. Commission Directive 2005/61/EC of 30 September 2005 implementing Directive 2002/98/EC of the European

Parliament and of the Council as regards traceability requirements and notification of serious adverse reactions and events (text with EEA relevance). Official Journal of the European Union 2005;L256:350-8. [Available at http://eur-lex.europa.eu/legal-content/EN/ALL/?uri=CELEX%3A32005L0061 (accessed January 20, 2017).]

12. Politis C, Wiersum JC, Richardson C, et al. The International Haemovigilance Network Database for the Surveillance of Adverse Reactions and Events in Donors and Recipients of Blood Components: Technical issues and results. Vox Sang 2016;111:409-17.

13. World Health Organization. Haemovigilance. Geneva, Switzerland: WHO, 2017. [Available at http://www.who.int/bloodsafety/haemovigilance/en/ (accessed January 20, 2017).]

14. Land KJ, Whitaker BI, eds, for the AABB US Donor Hemovigilance Working Group. 2012 AABB donor hemovigilance report. Bethesda, MD: AABB, 2013. [Available at http://www.aabb.org/research/hemovigilance/Pages/donor-hemovigilance.aspx (accessed January 20, 2017).]

15. Rajbhandary S, Stubbs JR, Land KJ, Whitaker BI, for the AABB US Donor Hemovigilance Working Group. AABB donor hemovigilance report: 2012-2014. Bethesda, MD: AABB, 2016.

16. Serious Hazards of Transfusion. TRALI tables. Manchester, UK: SHOT, 2010. [Available at www.shotuk.org/shot-reports/trali-tables/ (accessed January 20, 2017).]

17. Bolton-Maggs P, Wood EM, Wiersum-Osselton JC. Wrong blood in tube - potential for serious outcomes: Can it be prevented? Br J Haematol 2015;168:3-13.

18. Joint United Kingdom (UK) Blood Transfusion and Tissue Transplantation Services Professional Advisory Committee. 2012/2013 Transfusion Awareness Campaign: "Do you know who I am?" [Available at http://www.transfusionguidelines.org/uk-transfusion-committees/national-blood-transfusion-committee/transfusion-awareness/do-you-know-who-i-am (accessed January 20, 2017).]

19. Zins C. Conceptual approaches for defining data, information, and knowledge. J Am Soc Inf Sci Technol 2007;58:479-93.

20. Strehlow RA. Content analysis of definitions. In: Wright SE, Strehlow RA, eds. Standardizing and harmonizing terminology: Theory and practice. ASTM STP 1223. Philadelphia: American Society for Testing and Materials, 1994:53-62.

21. Public Health Service Biovigilance Task Group. Biovigilance in the United States: Efforts to bridge a critical gap in patient safety and donor health. Washington, DC: HHS, 2009. [Available at https://wayback.archive-it.org/3922/20140403203201/http://www.hhs.gov/ash/bloodsafety/biovigilance/ash_to_acbsa_oct_2009.pdf (accessed January 20, 2017).]

22. Kaplan HS, Battles JB, Van der Schaaf TW, et al. Identification and classification of the causes of events in transfusion medicine. Transfusion 1998;38:1071-81.

23. Strong DM, AuBuchon J, Whitaker B, Kuehnert MJ. Biovigilance initiatives. ISBT Science Series 2008;3:77-84.

24. Ooley PW, ed. Standards for blood banks and transfusion services. 30th ed. Bethesda, MD: AABB, 2016.

25. Centers for Disease Control and Prevention. National Healthcare Safety Network (NHSN): Blood safety surveillance. Atlanta, GA: CDC, 2016. [Available at http://www.cdc.gov/nhsn/acute-care-hospital/bio-hemo/ (accessed January 20, 2017).]

26. Chung KW, Harvey A, Basavaraju SV, Kuehnert MJ. How is national recipient hemovigilance conducted in the United States? Transfusion 2015;55:703-7.

27. Cumming M, Osinski A, O'Hearn L, et al. Hemovigilance in Massachusetts and the adoption of statewide hospital blood bank reporting using the National Healthcare Safety Network. Transfusion 2017;57:478-83.

28. Callum JL, Kaplan HS, Merkley LL, et al. Reporting of near-miss events for transfusion medicine: Improving transfusion safety. Transfusion 2001;41:1204-11.

29. Institute of Medicine (US) Committee on Quality of Health Care in America; Kohn LT, Corrigan JM, Donaldson MS, eds. To err is human: Building a safer health system. Washington, DC: National Academy Press, 2000.

30. Patient Safety and Quality Improvement Act of 2005. Pub. L. No.109-41, §§ 921-26, 119 Stat. 424 (2005). Rockville, MD: Agency for Healthcare Research and Quality, 2005. [Available at http://www.gpo.gov/fdsys/pkg/PLAW-109publ41/pdf/PLAW-109publ41.pdf (accessed January 20, 2017).]

31. PSO Privacy Protection Center. Rockville, MD: Agency for Healthcare Research and Quality, 2017. [Available at https://www.psoppc.org/

psoppc_web/publicpages/commonFormatsOverview, (accessed January 20, 2017).]

32. Roubinian NH, Escobar GJ, Liu V, et al. Trends in red blood cell transfusion and 30-day mortality among hospitalized patients. Transfusion 2014;54(10 Pt 2):2678-86.

33. Eder AF, Dy BA, Kennedy JM, et al. Improved safety for young whole blood donors with new selection criteria for total estimated blood volume. Transfusion 2011;51:1522-31.

34. Tomasulo P, Kamel H, Bravo M, et al. Interventions to reduce the vasovagal reaction rate in young whole blood donors. Transfusion 2011; 51:1511-21.

35. Custer B, Bravo M, Bruhn R, et al. Predictors of hemoglobin recovery or deferral in blood donors with an initial successful donation. Transfusion 2014;54:2267-75.

36. Wieling W, France CR, van Dijk N, et al. Physiologic strategies to prevent fainting responses during or after whole blood donation. Transfusion 2011;51:2727-38.

37. Eder AF. Current efforts to reduce the risk of syncope among young blood donors. Curr Opin Hematol 2012;19:480-5.

38. Kamel HT, Bassett MB, Custer B, et al. Safety and donor acceptance of an abbreviated donor history questionnaire. Transfusion 2006; 46:1745-53.

39. Bednall TC, Bove LL. Donating blood: A meta-analytic review of self-reported motivators and deterrents. Transfus Med Rev 2011;25:317-34.

40. Townsend M, Land KJ, Whitaker B, et al. US donor hemovigilance system: Mechanism for nationwide reporting (abstract 3A-S1-02). Vox Sang 2001;101(Suppl 1):11-12.

41. Land KJ. Update on donor hemovigilance. HHS Advisory Committee on Blood and Tissue Safety and Availability meeting minutes, November 4-5, 2010 (transcripts). [Available at http://wayback.archive-it.org/3919/20160728222436/http://www.hhs.gov/ash/bloodsafety/advisorycommittee/pastmeetings/pastmeetings.html (accessed January 20, 2017).]

42. Goldman M, Land K, Wiersum-Osselton J. Development of standard definitions for surveillance of complications related to blood donation. Vox Sang 2016;110:185-8.

43. Working Group on Donor Vigilance of the International Society of Blood Transfusion Working Party on Haemovigilance; The International Haemovigilance Network; The AABB Donor Haemovigilance Working Group. Standard for surveillance of complications related to blood donation. December 11, 2014. [Available at http://www.aabb.org/research/hemovigilance/Documents/Donor-Standard-Definitions.pdf (accessed January 29, 2017).]

44. Menis M, Izurieta HS, Anderson SA, et al. Outpatient transfusions and occurrence of serious noninfectious transfusion-related complications among US elderly, 2007-2008: Utility of large administrative databases in blood safety research. Transfusion 2012;52:1968-76.

45. Menis M, Anderson SA, Forshee RA, et al. Transfusion-related acute lung injury and potential risk factors among the inpatient US elderly as recorded in Medicare claims data, during 2007 through 2011. Transfusion 2014; 54:2182-93.

Chapter 5

Allogeneic and Autologous Blood Donor Selection

• ● •

Debra A. Kessler, RN, MS, and Susan N. Rossmann, MD, PhD

T
HE FOREMOST RESPONSIBILITY of blood collection facilities is to maintain a safe and adequate blood supply. The selection of appropriate blood donors is essential to protect donors' health during and following donation and to ensure the safety, quality, identity, purity, and potency of the donated blood components to protect the transfusion recipient. Key elements of the selection process, as part of the overall approach to blood safety, are education; a donor history questionnaire; a focused physical examination; infectious disease testing (see Chapter 7); management of all information about the donation, including subsequent postdonation information; and the donation itself in accordance with current good manufacturing practice.

This chapter describes the current federal regulations, accreditation requirements, and medical considerations related to screening blood donors before their blood is collected and tested for various blood-borne diseases.[1-3]

OVERVIEW OF BLOOD DONOR SCREENING

The blood collection facility must determine donor eligibility in accordance with federal and state regulations and AABB's voluntary accreditation standards. Specific criteria used to select donors are established by Food and Drug Administration (FDA) regulations and recommendations in guidance and memoranda. In addition, AABB has developed professional standards for donor selection with which accredited blood collection facilities must comply.[1]

Blood collection facilities provide prospective blood donors with information on the donation process and potential donation-related adverse effects and instruct them not to donate if they may be infected with blood-borne pathogens. The donor screening process includes a focused physical examination and direct questioning about specific risk behaviors, medications, travel, and other factors that potentially affect transfusion recipient or

Debra A. Kessler, RN, MS, Director, Special Donor Services, New York Blood Center, New York, New York; and Susan N. Rossmann, MD, PhD, Chief Medical Officer, Gulf Coast Regional Blood Center, Houston, Texas
The authors have disclosed no conflicts of interest.

donor safety. The donor screening questions address risks related to relevant transfusion-transmitted infections (RTTIs) for which sensitive tests are currently performed [eg, human immunodeficiency virus (HIV)], for which tests are not universally used (eg, *Babesia*), and for which licensed screening tests are not yet available (eg, sporadic and variant Creutzfeldt-Jacob diseases and malaria). Facilities must establish donor eligibility on the day of donation and before collection. If a donor's responses to the screening questions are incomplete or unclear, the collector may clarify the responses within 24 hours of donation and remain compliant with the "day of collection" requirement [Code of Federal Regulations (CFR), Title 21, Part 630.10(c)].

If individuals are instructed not to donate blood for others because of their health history, reactive test results, behavioral risks, or medical reasons, they must be added to a confidential deferral list at the blood center to prevent future donations [21 CFR 606.160(e)(1) and (2); and 630.10(d)(1)]. Depending on the causative reason, deferrals may be for a defined interval of time, an indefinite period (for which there may be the possibility of reinstatement to the donor pool), or permanent with no potential for reinstatement as a blood donor in the future.[1] In addition, collection facilities are required to manage information received after the donation (ie, postdonation information) that could affect the safety, purity, and potency of the blood components from the current donation and any previous donations, and affect the future eligibility of the donor.[2]

The criteria to evaluate individuals who are donating blood for their own use (ie, autologous donation) may be less stringent than those for people who donate for use by others (allogeneic donation). However, the focus remains on providing the safest possible blood for transfusion to the donor-patient and on evaluating the risks that the collection procedure poses to his or her health.[3]

The AABB Donor History Questionnaire (DHQ) is currently used by most blood collection facilities in the United States.[4-7] The references in this chapter are to DHQ Version 2.0 (February 2016), which was officially recognized in the May 2016 FDA guidance as acceptable for use.

A precautionary approach attempts to reduce the risk of known or potential RTTIs but also results in the deferral of a significant proportion of the healthy population. Medical directors of blood collection facilities are responsible for determining donor eligibility policies on issues that are not covered by regulations or standards.[3,8-11] Consequently, medical decisions regarding the same issue may differ among facilities or even among physicians at the same facility. Considerable variability exists in national and international practices for determining donor eligibility, which reveals the inherent uncertainty in risk assessment.[9] The facility's collection staff should be able to explain to donors the intended purpose of AABB and FDA requirements, as well as their center-specific eligibility screening practices.

Answers to the most frequently asked questions about federal regulations defining blood donor eligibility are available to the public in the "Questions about Blood" section of the FDA website.[12] Frequently asked questions about the interpretation or underlying rationale of AABB *Standards for Blood Banks and Transfusion Services (Standards)* can be found through the AABB Standards Portal,[13] or questions may be directed to the AABB Standards Department (standards@aabb.org); responses and discussion of selected issues are posted on the AABB website.

SELECTION OF ALLOGENEIC BLOOD DONORS

Registration and Donor Identification

In the United States, blood components for allogeneic transfusion are typically collected from volunteer, nonremunerated donors; otherwise, components must be labeled as being from paid donors [21 CFR 606.121(c)(8)(v)].

Prospective blood donors should provide an acceptable form of identification. Acceptable forms of identification include government-issued documents, such as a driver's license or passport, or a blood-center-issued donor card with a unique alphanumeric code, or other forms of identification as determined by the blood collection facility. Many facilities no longer use Social Security numbers for donor identification because of donor privacy concerns.

Accurate records are essential to identify all prior donations from any given donor, including whether the donor has ever given blood under a different name, so that the link with all prior donations within the blood system is maintained. Accurate records are also essential to ensure that the donor can be contacted following the donation and informed of test results or other relevant information from the current donation, if necessary. Facilities must make reasonable attempts to notify the donor within 8 weeks of the donation if any test results disqualify the individual from continued donation.[2] FDA regulations posted in the CFR require facilities to ask donors to provide an address and telephone number where they can be reached during this interval for counseling or other follow-up, if necessary. Accurate donation records must be kept by the facility for the requisite amount of time, according to current regulations and standards (21 CFR 606.160; AABB Reference Standards 6.2A-6.2E).[1]

Individual blood collection facilities or systems must maintain a list of deferred donors, but, notably, there is currently no national registry of deferred blood donors in the United States. Individuals who are deferred by one blood center may be eligible in another blood system. The available evidence suggests that national deferral registries are not necessary because they do not contribute to blood safety and do not prevent the release of unsuitable components.[14] In addition, national registries have raised privacy concerns.

Educational Materials and Donor Consent

US blood collection facilities provide all prospective blood donors with information about blood donation via educational materials and informed consent. The AABB DHQ Blood Donor Educational Material incorporates all necessary elements required by federal regulations and AABB *Standards*, and facilities may add elements to protect both blood donors and transfusion recipients.[1,2,4] At each encounter, the donor must be informed about the collection procedure in terms that the donor understands, and the donor's consent or acknowledgment must be documented. It must also be documented that the donor has read the educational material and has had an opportunity to ask questions.[1] The setting used for the donor screening process should provide adequate privacy for donors to be comfortable discussing confidential information. The donor should be informed about possible adverse reactions to the collection procedure and the tests that will be performed for RTTIs on his or her donated blood. The donor should also be informed of the notification process for positive test results, any reporting requirements to public health authorities, and the possibility of inclusion in the facility's deferral registry and subsequent deferral from future donation. The individual should agree not to donate if his or her blood could pose a risk to the blood supply. Donors should also be informed if investigational tests or other research may be performed on samples or information collected during the blood donation. Finally, the limitations of the tests to detect early infections and the possibility that a test may not be performed if samples are not adequate should be explained to the donor. The Blood Donor Educational Material instructs the donor not to donate blood for the purpose of receiving free infectious disease testing. Blood collection facilities must comply with applicable state laws to obtain permission from parents or guardians for minors (ie, 16- or 17-year-olds).[1] Moreover, AABB Standard 5.2.2 requires that blood collection facilities have a process to provide information about the donation process to parents or legally authorized representatives of donors when parental permission is required.[1]

Blood collection facilities should also establish policies on accommodating individuals who are not fluent in English or are illiterate, are vision or hearing impaired, or have other physical disabilities. Many facilities try to make reasonable accommodations for donors' special needs. However, facilities must also ensure that the collection procedure does not pose undue risk to donors or staff members, that an accurate health history can be obtained, and that the informed consent process is not compromised. The final authority for decisions on such issues rests with the facility's physician who supervises donor qualification and phlebotomy.[1]

Donor Qualification by Focused Physical Examination and Hemoglobin or Hematocrit Measurement

Qualification screening procedures for blood donation include a focused physical examination and a hemoglobin or hematocrit measurement.[1,2] The donor eligibility regulations define not only the specific physical requirements, but also the level of medical supervision required for the assessment (21 CFR 630.5; 21 CFR 630.10). This evaluation has potential implications for the potency or safety of the collected component or the well-being of the donor. Additional requirements apply to apheresis donors, who must meet the weight and hemoglobin or hematocrit requirements approved by the FDA for the automated collection device. The collector must weigh the donor and not rely on self-reported weight for donation of any plasma product collected by apheresis.

The donor must have his or her blood pressure measured, and it must be in the range of 90 to 180 mm Hg for systolic and 50 to 100 mm Hg for diastolic measures. If the measurement falls outside of these ranges, the donor must be seen in person by a physician to assess the safety of performing a collection. For pulse, the rate must be between 50 and 100 beats per minute without irregularities in rhythm. A physician may approve rates outside this range or irregularities in rhythm using his or her judgment of the safety, for the donor, of performing a collection. This approval may be in person or by telephone. Approval for blood pressure or pulse outside the stated ranges cannot be delegated to a nonphysician.

In general, neither the FDA nor AABB specifies the test method, specimen type [capillary (finger stick) or venous blood], or acceptable performance characteristics for tests used for hemoglobin/hematocrit screening. One exception is that a capillary sample collected from an earlobe puncture is not an acceptable specimen for hemoglobin/hematocrit screening for allogeneic or autologous donors because of its poor accuracy.[1] Most US blood collection facilities use finger stick samples for hemoglobin/hematocrit determination. These samples tend to give slightly higher values than venous samples.[15]

The methods to measure hemoglobin or hematocrit are generally selected for their ease of use in the mobile blood collection setting. The copper sulfate density method (Method 6-1) is still an acceptable screening tool in blood centers in the United States but has been largely replaced by methods such as spectrophotometric measurement of hemoglobin with portable devices or hematology analyzers to measure hematocrit. The point-of-care methods that use portable devices yield quantitative hemoglobin results, with a coefficient of variation (CV) of 1.5%. A typical automated analyzer measures hemoglobin levels in a venous sample with a CV ≤1.2%.[16] Most quantitative methods currently in use reliably measure hemoglobin levels within approximately 0.2 to 0.5 g/dL, and the vast majority of deferred donors have hemoglobin or hematocrit values near the cutoff value. For capillary-sample-based methods, the most likely source of preanalytical error is the sampling technique, and testing must be performed in compliance with the manufacturer's instructions. Noninvasive measurements, not involving a blood sample but using measurements through the skin, have also been approved.

Donor hemoglobin screening may help ensure a minimum content of hemoglobin in a unit of Red Blood Cells (RBCs), but currently neither the FDA nor AABB define potency standards for RBC units prepared from whole blood collection. If a donor's hemoglobin level is 12.5 g/dL, a 500-mL whole blood collection is expected to yield about 62.5 g of hemoglobin per unit of RBCs, but determining the final content of hemoglobin in an RBC unit prepared from whole blood is not required. AABB *Standards* requires apheresis RBC units to be prepared using a method known to ensure a final component containing a mean hemoglobin level of ≥60 g of hemoglobin, with 95% of the units sampled containing >50 g of hemoglobin.[1]

As of May 2016, FDA regulations define the minimum acceptable hemoglobin concentration for male donors as 13.0 g/dL or the essentially equivalent hematocrit of 39% [21 CFR 630.10(f)(3)]. For females, the acceptable hemoglobin concentration is 12.5 g/dL or 38% hematocrit. Hemoglobin or hematocrit screening may help prevent collection of blood from a donor with significant anemia, but it is clear that many donors do not have adequate iron stores even though they meet donor hemoglobin requirements.[17] This could have implications for the health of the donor as well as the potency of the collected component. If the organization wishes to collect blood from female donors with hemoglobin levels of 12.0 to 12.5 g/dL, or 36% to 38% hematocrit, they may do so if additional steps are followed to ensure that the health of the donor will not be adversely affected by the donation, in accordance with a procedure that has been found acceptable for this purpose by the FDA [21 CFR 630.10(f)(3)(i)(A)]. At the time of this writing, the procedures the FDA will approve to accept female donors with hemoglobin values of 12.0 to 12.5 g/dL are not clear. The strategies might involve extended intervals between donations, iron supplementation, and/or ferritin testing (using a predonation sample). Unfortunately, no point-of-care tests for assessing iron stores are available at this time.

Low hemoglobin/hematocrit is the most common reason for blood donor deferral at most donor centers. The various strategies to mitigate iron deficiency in blood donors address the concern that has arisen about possible health effects of low iron, particularly among teens, females of childbearing age, and repeat donors of either gender.[18-22] Both physical issues and impaired cognitive functions have been suggested in individuals with low iron stores, even in the absence of anemia.[23]

Donors, particularly frequent donors, may develop iron-deficient erythropoiesis or advance to frank absence of iron stores.[20] Without iron supplementation, two-thirds of donors may not recover iron stores even after 168 days (24 weeks).[24] Recent studies have shown the benefit of iron supplementation in improving iron stores and hemoglobin in these donors. The amount of elemental iron found in an over-the-counter daily multivitamin is typically 19 mg; iron tablets available over the counter may contain 38 mg of elemental iron. Either can be an effective supplement for blood donors. Another successful approach is to perform ferritin testing and to notify donors who have low levels, offering them the option of iron supplementation or delaying further donation.[20-25] Simple notification of donors of their low iron status was shown to be essentially as effective as providing iron supplements.[25] Various methods can be used to encourage iron replacement with blood donors, including providing iron tablets to the donor at the donation site, providing coupons for iron products, and/or informing donors of the need for supplemental iron. Low ferritin levels can also serve as the basis for an extended deferral from donations that include red cell components. Extended deferrals without providing information about ferritin or iron supplementation will not restore iron levels in a reasonable time. Donors with an abnormally low or high ferritin level should be referred to their health-care provider for evaluation as appropriate.

Finally, before phlebotomy, the collection staff inspect the donor's antecubital skin, to determine that it is free of lesions and evidence of injection drug use, such as multiple needle punctures (eg, small scars lined up in "tracks") and that the veins are adequate for donation. Scars or pitting on the forearm associated with frequent blood donation should not be mistaken for evidence of injection drug use. Common and mild skin disorders (eg, poison ivy rash) are not a cause for deferral unless there are signs of localized bacterial superinfection or the condition interferes with proper skin disinfection in the antecubital site before phlebotomy.

Health History Assessment—AABB DHQ

The AABB DHQ is now used by most blood centers in the United States. The DHQ includes the information required for compliance with both AABB *Standards* and the FDA. Its use is not mandated by the FDA,[6,7] but alternative procedures for collecting required information from blood donors must be submitted for FDA approval in a Prior Approval Supplement under 21 CFR 601.12(b). In addition, the FDA acknowledges that the DHQ documents contain questions related to the following issues not addressed by any FDA requirement or recommendation: cancer; certain organ, tissue, or marrow transplants; and bone or skin grafts. However, AABB recommends that blood collection facilities implement the DHQ materials, including the following documents, as approved by FDA and in their entirety:

- Blood Donor Educational Material.
- Full-Length DHQ.
- User Brochure, including glossary and references.
- Medication Deferral List.

The use of the DHQ flowcharts as a resource is optional, and facilities may implement an equivalent method to evaluate responses to the DHQ. The current FDA-recognized DHQ and accompanying materials, Version 2.0, are available on the AABB website.[6]

The wording, order, and text of the DHQ questions must not be changed because FDA has accepted the Version 2.0 DHQ as presented. The User Brochure for the DHQ details the purpose and limitations for the use of the DHQ and related materials. A blood collection facility may make minor changes to a question on the DHQ only if the changes make the question more restrictive. Facilities may choose to include additional questions as long as they are placed in the designated area for additional questions at the end of the DHQ. The DHQ documents are intended to be self-administered by the donor, but facilities may choose to use direct oral questioning, or a combination of both methods to administer the DHQ.

If AABB standards or FDA regulations do not address specific medical conditions that a blood collection facility has chosen to include in the DHQ, the facility must develop standard operating procedures (SOPs) for determining the criteria for acceptance or deferral of a donor. A rational approach to donor health history assessment attempts to balance the need to take appropriate precautions to protect the blood supply with avoiding unnecessarily restrictive policies that disqualify large segments of the population without contributing to either recipient or donor safety.[3] Decisions about donor eligibility should be based on available evidence regarding the risk that the medical condition or history poses to the blood donor and the transfusion recipient.

If a potential risk exists for the transfusion recipient or donor, the effectiveness and incremental benefit of screening donors by questioning should be evaluated, especially in light of other safeguards that protect the donor or other transfusion practices that mitigate potential risks to the recipient. If the facility receives postdonation information that should have been cause for deferral had it been reported at the time of donation, then any subsequent actions, such as product quarantine, retrieval, market withdrawal, or consignee notification, should be commensurate with the potential hazard and likelihood of possible harm to the recipient. The facility's approach to developing donor deferral criteria should take into account evidence as it becomes available to modify those decisions. Some of these issues that allow for medical judgment and for which questions exist in the DHQ can be explored further with the donor, but each donor center must develop and follow its own procedures.[3]

Emergency Measures

In some cases, measures must be immediately taken to reduce risk from an emerging or re-emerging RTTI. Donor screening may play a particularly important role if testing is not available or used, or if the agent has not been shown to be reduced by available pathogen-inactivation measures. Donor information materials requesting self-deferral can be implemented quickly, asking prospective donors not to donate if, for example, they have traveled to certain regions where the RTTI is common or there is an outbreak. Donor screening questions may also be added, dealing with travel risks or exposure to others who may have been infected. The interval before such screening questions are implemented will vary with the length of time it takes to modify a blood collection facility's operational methods, including its blood establishment computer system (BECS), involved in donor screening. It may be necessary to temporarily stop collections entirely in locations where the risk otherwise cannot be effectively managed. The FDA, other authorities, and/or AABB will provide guidance in emergency situations, to which blood collection facilities should remain alert and flexible to meet such emergencies. Depending on the situation, measures such as donor education information and screening questions may become a permanent part of donor screening or may be discontinued as the risk recedes.

BLOOD-CENTER-DEFINED DONOR ELIGIBILITY CRITERIA

Unlike questions about potential risks to transfusion recipients, most selection criteria directed primarily at protecting donor safety are left to the discretion of the blood center's medical director. Consequently, practice varies at different blood centers.[3,9] AABB *Standards* requires that prospective donors appear to be in good health and be free of major organ disease (eg, diseases of the heart, liver, or lungs), cancer, or abnormal bleeding tendency, unless determined eligible by the medical director.[1] The rationale for each deferral for medical conditions should be carefully considered because even temporary deferrals adversely affect the likelihood that individuals will return to donate blood.[26]

Cancer

Each year in the United States, blood collection facilities receive hundreds of reports of cancer in individuals who had donated blood. Direct transmission of cancer through blood transfusion—although biologically plausible—has not yet been documented to occur even though people with cancer frequently donate blood before discovering their diagnosis.[27] A retrospective study examined the incidence of cancer among patients in Denmark and Sweden who received blood from donors with subclinical cancer at the time of donation. Of the 354,094 transfusion recipients, 12,012 (3%) were exposed to blood components from precancerous donors, yet there was no excess risk of cancer among these recipients compared with recipients of blood from donors without cancer.[28] A similar study indicated no risk for recipients of blood from donors who were later demonstrated to have chronic lymphocytic leukemia.[29] These data indicate that cancer transmission by blood collected from blood donors with incident cancer, if it occurs at all, is so rare that it could not be detected in a large cohort of transfusion recipients that included the total blood experience of two countries over several years.

In considering the future eligibility of donors with cancer, some degree of caution is warranted to allow sufficient time for donors to recover after chemotherapy or other treatment. There are currently no US federal regulations or professional standards regarding the criteria that should be used to evaluate donors with a history of cancer. For this reason, a blood center's medical director has considerable flexibility in determining donor eligibility policies.

Almost all licensed blood collection facilities currently accept donors who report localized cancers after treatment, with no deferral period. These cancers include skin cancer (eg, basal cell or superficial squamous cell carcinoma) and carcinoma in situ (eg, cervical) that have been fully excised and are considered cured. Most facilities defer individuals with a history of a solid organ or nonhematologic malignancy for a defined period after completion of treatment, provided that the donor remains symptom free without recurrence. The deferral period following completion of treatment for nonhematologic cancer ranges from 1 to 5 years.[28] Hematologic malignancy typically results in permanent deferral from allogeneic blood donation, although some US blood centers reportedly accept adults if they have been successfully treated for childhood leukemia or lymphoma. These various deferral policies are currently defensible but should be reevaluated if new information becomes available about the potential for cancer transmission through blood transfusion.

Bleeding Conditions or Blood Diseases

Bleeding conditions and blood diseases have the potential to affect donor safety, as well as product potency, and blood collection facilities must define SOPs for handling donors with hematologic disorders. In general, prospective donors should be evaluated for bleeding conditions or blood diseases that 1) place the donors at risk of bleeding or thrombosis as a result of the collection procedure or 2) may affect the hemostatic efficacy of their blood and its suitability for transfusion to others.[3]

Plasma components and cryoprecipitated antihemophilic factor should contain adequate amounts of functional coagulation factors and should not contain significant inhibitory or prothrombotic factors. Similarly, platelet components intended as the sole source for patients should contain platelets that have adequate function and are not irreversibly impaired by the presence of inhibitors.

Individuals with a history of significant bleeding complications are usually counseled to avoid blood donation. However, screening donors for such a history does not prevent the rare but serious thrombotic or hemorrhagic complications in otherwise healthy blood donors. Individuals with hemophilia, clotting factor deficiencies, or clinically significant inhibitors—all of which are manifested by variable bleeding tendencies—require deferral for both donor safety and product potency considerations. The exception is Factor XII defi-

ciency, which is not associated with either bleeding or thrombosis.

Carriers of autosomal-recessive or sex-linked recessive mutations in clotting factors usually are not at risk of bleeding. They typically have decreased factor levels but are accepted by most facilities because of the normal, wide variability in clotting factor activity levels (50% to 150%) compared to the much lower relative activity that is necessary to maintain hemostasis (5% to 30%).[3] Individuals with von Willebrand disease are typically deferred by most facilities, although some may allow individuals with mild disease and no history of bleeding to donate red cells. Antithrombotic medications are discussed below.

Heart and Lung Conditions

Cardiovascular disease is common in the United States, affecting an estimated 86 million (more than 1 in 3) adults.[30] Prospective blood donors are asked if they have ever had problems with their heart or lungs as a donor safety measure, but the criteria for accepting donors with a history of heart or lung disease are defined by each blood center.

The collective, published experience with autologous donation by patients scheduled for cardiac procedures has demonstrated that adverse effects are not more frequent than in donors without a history of cardiac disease.[31-35] Despite the relative frequency of cardiovascular disease in the adult population, vasovagal reactions occur in only about 2% to 5% of whole blood donations by healthy donors and are actually more likely to occur among young, healthy adolescents than older adults.[36-37]

A rational approach to screening donors with a history of cardiac disease allows the acceptance of donors who are asymptomatic on the day of donation, have been medically evaluated, and report no functional impairment or limitations on daily activity after being diagnosed or treated for cardiac disease. Some donor centers advise individuals to wait at least 6 months after a cardiac event, procedure, or diagnosis. These centers then allow these individuals to donate if they have been asymptomatic and able to perform their usual daily activities during this interval. Indications for deferral may include recent symptoms, limitations on activity or functional impairment resulting from unstable angina, recent myocardial infarction, left main coronary disease, ongoing congestive heart failure, or severe aortic stenosis.[3]

Medications

The DHQ and Medication Deferral List contain the requirements for deferrals for specific medications as stipulated by the FDA and AABB. These requisite medication deferrals fall into five broad categories:

1. Potent teratogens that pose potential harm to unborn children (although there have been no documented cases of adverse fetal outcomes related to transfusions from donors taking these medications).
2. Antibiotics or antimicrobials to treat an infection that could be transmitted through blood transfusion (excluding preventive antibiotics for acne, rosacea, and other chronic conditions with a low risk of bacteremia).
3. Anticoagulants and antiplatelet agents that affect component potency (plasma or platelet components only).
4. Potential variant Creutzfeldt-Jakob disease risk from bovine insulin manufactured in the United Kingdom (although there have been no documented cases of transfusion transmission from donors taking bovine insulin).
5. Human pituitary-derived growth hormone, which theoretically increases the risk of Creutzfeldt-Jakob disease (although there have been no documented cases of transfusion transmission from donors who are taking these growth hormones). Human pituitary-derived growth hormone has been prohibited for use in the United States since 1985.

Although blood collection facilities may add medications whose use requires local donor deferral to the Medication Deferral List, many have chosen to use the Medication Deferral List as developed by the FDA and AABB or have added only a few drugs. The Donor History Task Force (DHTF) has encouraged facilities to fully consider the reasons behind each local deferral and avoid unnecessary deferral practices.[3] The recent explosion in the number of drugs affecting platelet function or clotting, such as the direct Factor X inhibitors, which are increasingly used instead of warfarin, are often encountered as a cause for deferral [21 CFR 630.10(e); 21 CFR 640.21(b) and (c)].

FDA's older pregnancy-risk categories, which are designed to assess the benefit-vs-risk ratio if drugs are taken during pregnancy, are often inappropriately used for blood donor selection. For example, categories D and X include some commonly used drugs (eg, oral contraceptives and anticholesterol agents) that may be contraindicated in pregnancy but pose negligible, if any, risk to any transfusion recipient. In 2016, FDA eliminated the risk categories and introduced a new descriptive approach to prescription drug labeling for risk to pregnant or breastfeeding women, which may also make inappropriate application to blood donor eligibility less of a problem.[38]

Local medication deferrals are often based on concerns about the reason for the potential donor's use of the medication and his or her underlying medical condition rather than on any inherent threat posed by residual medication in the collected blood component. Most drugs used by donors pose no harm to recipients, and many factors should be considered when evaluating the potential risk of a drug's use by a donor (eg, the medication's half-life, mean and peak plasma concentration, residual concentration in a blood component, and dilution when transfused to a recipient).

ABBREVIATED DHQ FOR FREQUENT DONORS

Blood collection facilities have recognized for years that frequent and repeat donors, notably platelet and plasma donors, must answer the same questions at every donation about remote risk factors that are not likely to change—a situation that leaves many dedicated donors dissatisfied with the donation experience. The FDA allows the administration of the AABB's Abbreviated DHQ (aDHQ) for frequent donors who qualify by successfully completing the Full-Length DHQ on at least two separate occasions, with one or more donations within the past 6 months. The User Brochure for the aDHQ details the purpose and limitations on the use of the aDHQ. The AABB Version 2.0 aDHQ, which was developed and validated by the DHTF along with the Full-Length DHQ, has been officially recognized in FDA guidance as "acceptable" and can be implemented by blood collection facilities using the corresponding Full-Length DHQ.[7] In the aDHQ, two "capture questions" about new diagnoses or treatments since the last donation replace 17 previous questions about remote risks (eg, blood transfusion, Chagas disease, and babesiosis). An abbreviated questionnaire for frequent donors may improve donors' experience.

RECIPIENT-SPECIFIC "DESIGNATED" OR "DIRECTED" BLOOD DONATION

Exceptional Medical Need

In certain limited clinical circumstances, a patient may benefit from blood components collected from a specific donor, such as a patient with multiple antibodies or with antibodies to high-incidence antigens who requires units from donors whose red cells are negative for the corresponding antigens. Frequent donation by a specific donor for a specific patient with a medical need requires that the blood collection facility have a procedure that typically calls for both a request from the patient's physician and approval by the donor center's physician. The donor must meet all allogeneic donor selection requirements, with the exception of donation frequency, provided that they are examined and certified by a physician [21 CFR 630.15(a)(1)(ii)(B)]. In emergency medical situations, blood components can be released before test results for RTTIs are available pro-

vided that the units are labeled and managed in accordance with the CFR. Testing on the units must be completed as soon as possible after release or shipment, and results must be promptly reported to the hospital or transfusion service.[2]

Directed Blood Donations

The use of directed donors, that is, when patients ask the blood center if they can designate their own blood donors (usually relatives or friends) for their anticipated transfusion needs, has decreased in recent years, but there is still ongoing demand. The concern likely reflects an inaccurate perception continuing among the general public of the risk for RTTIs associated with blood transfusion from the general inventory. Most facilities and hospitals accommodate the associated collection, storage, tracking, payment, and logistical difficulties to provide a directed donation service.

Directed donations have higher viral marker rates than volunteer donations, mostly but not entirely reflecting the higher prevalence of first-time donors among the former group.[39] There is no evidence that directed donations are safer to use than donations from volunteer community donors. On the contrary, some concerns persist that directed donors may feel unduly pressured to give blood, which could compromise blood safety. The confidentiality of directed donors with positive test results may be difficult to maintain. Nevertheless, directed donations are sometimes sought by patients and their families, particularly for neonatal and other pediatric patients.

Directed donors must meet the same criteria as voluntary donors, and their blood can be used for other patients if not needed by the individual for whom the donations were initially intended. The facility should clearly communicate its directed-donation procedures so that the expectations regarding availability of directed-donor units are known to the hospital, ordering physician, and patient. The communication required includes defining the mandated interval between collection of the blood and its availability to the patient, mentioning the possibility that the patient will identify donors who are not ABO compatible or not otherwise acceptable blood donors, and defining the policy for release of donor-directed units for transfusion to other patients.

Autologous Blood Donations

Autologous donations have declined dramatically in the United States since the 1990s. Waning interest in autologous donations may reflect the decline in viral risk associated with allogeneic blood transfusion, the lower rate of surgical transfusion generally, and, consequently, the minimal medical benefit and increased cost of autologous blood.[40-42] The most appropriate candidates are alloimmunized donors for whom compatible blood is hard to collect, who are undergoing elective surgery for which transfusion will likely be required, and who have adequate time before the procedure to replace the hemoglobin lost via phlebotomy.

In general, the use of preoperative autologous blood donation alone provides only a relatively small benefit in reducing the probability of allogeneic transfusion and may actually increase the risk of lower postoperative hematocrits. Preoperative autologous donations may still be used in conjunction with other blood conservation methods, such as acute normovolemic hemodilution, perioperative blood recovery, and pharmacologic strategies. (See further discussion in Chapter 20.)

Patients identified as candidates for autologous donation are evaluated by the donor center as well as the referring physician. The following criteria for autologous donations are specified by the FDA, AABB, or both:

- A prescription or order from the patient's physician.
- Minimum hemoglobin concentration of 11 g/dL or hematocrit of 33%.
- Collection at least 72 hours before the anticipated surgery or transfusion.
- Absence of conditions presenting a risk of bacteremia.
- Use only for the donor-patient if labeled "autologous use only."

Contraindications to autologous blood donation should be defined by the blood center and may include medical conditions associated with the greatest risk from blood donation, such as 1) unstable angina, 2) recent myocardial infarction or cerebrovascular accident, 3) significant cardiac or pulmonary disease with ongoing symptoms but without an evaluation by the treating physician, or 4) untreated aortic stenosis.[42] Both the ordering physician and the donor center physician need to carefully balance the risks of the collection procedure against any perceived benefit to the patient-donor. The FDA has issued guidance on the process by which autologous donations may be collected, making it clear that rules for allogeneic donors may not necessarily be applied.[43]

ACKNOWLEDGMENT

The authors would like to thank Anne Eder for laying such an excellent foundation for this chapter.

KEY POINTS

1. The AABB DHQ and associated documents, including an abbreviated form for frequent donors, were developed by AABB's DHTF, and their use is recognized by the FDA as an adequate process to determine the eligibility of volunteers for allogeneic blood donation.
2. The current version of the DHQ and associated documents, Version 2.0, are available on the AABB website, and the May 2016 FDA guidance formally recognizing all DHQ documents is available on the FDA website.[6,7]
3. Prospective blood donors are informed of the risks of blood donation, clinical signs and symptoms associated with HIV infection, behavioral risk factors for transmission of RTTIs,

and importance of refraining from blood donation if they are at increased risk of carrying an RTTI.

4. There are possible negative health effects of low iron levels (even in the absence of anemia) in donors who are in their teens, who are females of childbearing potential, or who are repeat donors (of either gender).

5. To be accepted for allogeneic blood donation, individuals must feel healthy and well on the day of donation and must meet all AABB and FDA requirements, as well as medical criteria defined by the blood collection facility.

6. The ongoing demand from patients to choose specific donors to provide blood for their transfusions during scheduled surgeries in the absence of a defined medical need has dramatically decreased in recent years but persists despite the lack of evidence of improved safety with directed donations.

REFERENCES

1. Ooley P, ed. Standards for blood banks and transfusion services. 30th ed. Bethesda, MD: AABB, 2016.

2. Code of federal regulations. Title 21, CFR Parts 600 to 799. Washington, DC: US Government Publishing Office, 2017 (revised annually).

3. Eder A, Bianco C, eds. Screening blood donors: Science, reason, and the donor history questionnaire. Bethesda, MD: AABB Press, 2007.

4. Zou S, Eder AF, Musavi F, et al. ARCNET Study Group. Implementation of the uniform donor history questionnaire across the American Red Cross Blood Services: Increased deferral among repeat presenters but no measurable impact on blood safety. Transfusion 2007;47:1990-8.

5. Fridey JL, Townsend M, Kessler D, Gregory K. A question of clarity: Redesigning the AABB blood donor history questionnaire—a chronology and model for donor screening. Transfus Med Rev 2007;21:181-204.

6. Blood donor history questionnaires. Version 2.0. Bethesda, MD: AABB, 2016. [Available at http://www.aabb.org/tm/questionnaires/Pages/dhqaabb.aspx (accessed January 23, 2017).]

7. Food and Drug Administration. Guidance for industry: Implementation of acceptable full-length and abbreviated donor history questionnaires and accompanying materials for use in screening donors of blood and blood components. (May 2016) Rockville, MD: CBER Office of Communication, Outreach, and Development, 2016. [Available at http://www.fda.gov/BiologicsBloodVaccines/GuidanceComplianceRegulatoryInformation/Guidances/Blood/default.htm (accessed January 23, 2017).]

8. Eder AF. Evidence-based selection criteria to protect the blood donor. J Clin Apher 2010;25:331-7.

9. Eder A, Goldman M, Rossmann S, et al. Selection criteria to protect the blood donor in North America and Europe: Past (dogma), present (evidence), and future (hemovigilance). Transfus Med Rev 2009;23:205-20.

10. Strauss RG. Rationale for medical director acceptance or rejection of allogeneic platelet-pheresis donors with underlying medical disorders. J Clin Apher 2002;17:111-17.

11. Reik RA, Burch JW, Vassallo RR, Trainor L. Unique donor suitability issues. Vox Sang 2006;90:255-64.

12. Food and Drug Administration. Questions about blood. Rockville, MD: CBER Office of Communication, Outreach, and Development, 2016. [Available at http://www.fda.gov/biologicsbloodvaccines/bloodbloodproducts/questionsaboutblood/default.htm (accessed January 23, 2017).]

13. Standards portal. Bethesda, MD: AABB, 2017. [Available at http://www.aabb.org/sa/Pages/Standards-Portal.aspx (accessed January 23, 2017).]

14. Cable R, Musavi F, Notari E, Zou S. ARCNET Research Group. Limited effectiveness of donor deferral registries for transfusion-transmitted disease markers. Transfusion 2008;48:34-42.

15. Cable RG, Steele WR, Melmed RS, et al for the NHLBI Retrovirus Epidemiology Donor Study-II (REDS-II). The difference between finger-stick and venous hemoglobin and hematocrit varies by sex and iron stores. Transfusion 2012;52:1031-40.

16. Cable RG. Hemoglobin determination in blood donors. Transfus Med Rev 1995;9:131-44.

17. Cable RG, Glynn SA, Kiss JE, et al for the NHL-BI Retrovirus Epidemiology Donor Study-II (REDS-II). Iron deficiency in blood donors: Analysis of enrollment data from the REDS-II Donor Iron Status Evaluation (RISE) study. Transfusion 2011;51:511-22.

18. Beutler E, Waalen J. The definition of anemia: What is the lower limit of normal of the blood hemoglobin concentration? Blood 2006;107:1747-50.

19. Simon TL, Garry PJ, Hooper EM. Iron stores in blood donors. JAMA 1981;245:2038-43.

20. Cable RG, Glynn SA, Kiss JE, et al. Iron deficiency in blood donors: The REDS-II Donor Iron Status Evaluation (RISE) study. Transfusion 2012;52:702-11.

21. Updated strategies to limit or prevent iron deficiency in blood donors. Association bulletin #17-02. Bethesda, MD: AABB, 2017. [Available at http://www.aabb.org/programs/publications/bulletins/Pages/default.aspx (accessed May 18, 2017).]

22. Bialkowski W, Bryant BJ, Schlumpf KS, et al. The strategies to reduce iron deficiency in blood donors randomized trial: Design, enrollment and early retention. Vox Sang 2015;108:178-85.

23. Eder AF, Kiss JE. Adverse reactions and iron deficiency after blood donation. In: Simon TL, McCullough J, Snyder EL, et al, eds. Rossi's principles of transfusion medicine. 5th ed. Chichester, UK: John Wiley and Sons, 2016:43-57.

24. Kiss JE, Brambilla D, Glynn SA, et al for the National Heart, Lung, and Blood Institute (NHLBI) Recipient Epidemiology and Donor Evaluation Study–III (REDS-III). Oral iron supplementation after blood donation: A randomized clinical trial. JAMA 2015;313:575-83.

25. Mast AE, Bialkowski W, Bryant BJ, et al. A randomized, blinded, placebo-controlled trial of education and iron supplementation for mitigation of iron deficiency in regular blood donors. Transfusion 2016;56:1588-97.

26. Custer B, Schlumpf KS, Wright D, et al. NHLBI Retrovirus Epidemiology Donor Study-II. Donor return after temporary deferral. Transfusion 2011;51:1188-96.

27. Eder AF. Blood donors with a history of cancer. In: Eder AF, Bianco C, eds. Screening blood donors: Science, reason, and the donor history questionnaire. Bethesda, MD: AABB Press, 2007:77-92.

28. Edgren G, Hjalgrim H, Reilly M, et al. Risk of cancer after blood transfusion from donors with subclinical cancer: A retrospective cohort study. Lancet 2007;369:1724-30.

29. Hjalgrim H, Rostgaard K, Vasan SK, et al. No evidence of transmission of chronic lymphocytic leukemia through blood transfusion. Blood 2015;126:2059-61.

30. AHA Statistics Committee and Stroke Statistics Subcommittee. Heart disease and stroke statistics—2016 Update: A report from the American Heart Association. Circulation 2016;133:e38-360.

31. Kasper SM, Ellering J, Stachwitz P, et al. All adverse events in autologous blood donors with cardiac disease are not necessarily caused by blood donation. Transfusion 1998;38:669-73.

32. Mann M, Sacks HJ, Goldfinger D. Safety of autologous blood donation prior to elective surgery for a variety of potentially high risk patients. Transfusion 1983;23:229-32.

33. Klapper E, Pepkowitz SH, Czer L, et al. Confirmation of the safety of autologous blood donation by patients awaiting heart or lung transplantation: A controlled study using hemodynamic monitoring. J Thorac Cardiovasc Surg 1995;110:1594-9.

34. Dzik WH, Fleisher AG, Ciavarella D, et al. Safety and efficacy of autologous blood donation before elective aortic valve operation. Ann Thorac Surg 1992;54:1177-80.

35. Popovsky MA, Whitaker B, Arnold NL. Severe outcomes of allogeneic and autologous blood donation: Frequency and characterization. Transfusion 1995;35:734-7.

36. Eder AF, Dy BA, Kennedy J, et al. The American Red Cross donor hemovigilance program: Complications of blood donation reported in 2006. Transfusion 2008;48:1809-19.

37. Wiltbank TB, Giordano GF, Kamel H, et al. Faint and prefaint reactions in whole-blood donors: An analysis of predonation measurements and their predictive value. Transfusion 2008;48:1799-808.

38. Food and Drug Administration. Content and format of labeling for human prescription drug and biological products; requirements for pregnancy and lactation labeling; final rule. Title 21, CFR Part 201. (December 4, 2014) Fed Regist 2014;79:72063-103. [Available at https://www.federalregister.gov/documents/2014/12/04/2014-28241/content-and-format-

of-labeling-for-human-prescription-drug-and-biological-products-requirements-for (accessed January 23, 2017).]

39. Dorsey KA, Moritz ED, Steele WR, et al. A comparison of human immunodeficiency virus, hepatitis C virus, hepatitis B virus and human T-lymphotropic virus marker rates for directed versus volunteer blood donations to the American Red Cross during 2005 to 2010. Transfusion 2013;53:1250-6.

40. Brecher ME, Goodnough LT. The rise and fall of preoperative autologous blood donation. Transfusion 2002;42:1618-22.

41. Schved JF. Preoperative autologous blood donation: A therapy that needs to be scientifically evaluated. Transfus Clin Biol 2005;12:365-9.

42. Goodnough LT. Autologous blood donation. Anesthesiol Clin North Am 2005;23:263-70.

43. Food and Drug Administration. Guidance for industry: Determining donor eligibility for autologous donors of blood and blood components intended solely for autologous use—compliance policy. (August 2016) Rockville, MD: CBER Office of Communication, Outreach, and Development, 2016. [Available at http://www.fda.gov/downloads/Biologics BloodVaccines/GuidanceComplianceRegula toryInformation/Guidances/Blood/UCM 514072.pdf (accessed January 23, 2017).

Chapter 6

Whole Blood and Apheresis Collections for Blood Components Intended for Transfusion

• ● •

Stephen J. Wagner, PhD

THE COLLECTION OF whole blood (WB) from the donor and subsequent processing of blood into components requires careful attention to techniques to ensure the optimal care of both the donor and recipient. This chapter describes manual and newer innovations for automating component preparation from WB collections, as well as fully automated apheresis collections. "Hemapheresis" and all of the various terms used to refer to automated blood component collection procedures are derived from the Greek word "aphairos," meaning "to take from." Specifically, WB is separated into components during collection, the desired component is removed/modified, and the remaining components are returned to the donor or patient. Centrifugal and membrane-based apheresis techniques were under development in the late 19th and early 20th centuries, and by the 1970s, apheresis processes advanced rapidly.

DONOR PREPARATION

Donor Consent

Potential donors must be provided predonation information, counseling about the blood donation process, and an opportunity to have their questions answered before every blood donation. The *Code of Federal Regulations* (CFR) requires blood centers to obtain donors' written acknowledgment of the following elements [21 CFR Part 630.10(g)(2)][1]:

- The donor has reviewed the educational material regarding relevant transfusion-transmitted infections.
- The donor agrees not to donate if the donation could result in a potential risk to recipients as described in the educational material.
- A sample of the donor's blood will be tested for specified relevant transfusion-transmitted infections.

Stephen J. Wagner, PhD, Senior Director, American Red Cross Holland Laboratory, Transfusion Innovation Department, Rockville, Maryland

S. Wagner has disclosed financial relationships with NanoEnTek, Fenwal, and Cerus Corporation.

- If the donation is determined to be unsuitable or if the donor is deferred from donation as required by regulations, the donor's record will identify the donor as ineligible to donate, and the donor will be notified of the basis for the deferral and the period of deferral.
- The donor has been provided and has reviewed information regarding the risks and hazards of the specific donation procedure.
- The donor has the opportunity to ask questions and withdraw from the donation procedure.

In addition, the CFR requires the blood center's responsible physician or appropriate designee to obtain donors' informed consent for plasmapheresis and plateletpheresis collections. The physician or appropriate designee should explain the risk of the procedure to the donor, provide opportunity for the donor to ask questions, and give the donor a chance to refuse to donate. The informed consent process for plateletpheresis must be performed before the first donation and annually thereafter [21 CFR Parts 640.21(g) and 630.5]. Likewise, the informed consent process for plasmapheresis stipulates these requirements as well as that the process be repeated if more than 6 months elapse between plasmapheresis collections (21 CFR 630.15).

Donor Eligibility and Identification

Phlebotomy must be performed only after the donor has been found to be eligible for blood donation and the following items have been properly labeled using a unique donation identification number (DIN) label: the blood donor record, primary and satellite containers, and sample tubes. Identification of blood components and maintaining test results linked to the donor are critical to ensure recipient safety by permitting look-back investigations and product withdrawals if indicated. The blood component identification process uniformly uses both a bar-coded and an eye-readable, unique DIN that is assigned to each

sample tube and each component prepared from the donation. The donor history questionnaire and blood sample tubes are similarly labeled with the unique number for each donation. Electronic records of the donation are also assigned the same number. The DIN should be verified on the donation record, collection set primary and secondary containers, and sample tubes before blood collection can proceed, as well as during and after the collection. A final check of appropriate labeling before phlebotomy helps to ensure that the donor history data, laboratory data, and other manufacturing data are associated with the correct blood components.

Vein Selection and Disinfection Methods for Venipuncture Site

The phlebotomist inspects both arms of the donor to select an appropriate vein. The phlebotomist checks for a prominent, large, firm vein in the antecubital fossa to permit a single, readily accessible phlebotomy site that is devoid of scarring or skin lesions.

Specific instructions in the package insert for the use of approved agents should be followed for arm and phlebotomy site preparation (Method 6-2). These methods provide surgical cleanliness, but none of the methods can achieve an absolutely aseptic site. Approximately 50% of donors have no bacterial colonies in studies using a contact plate culture of the venipuncture site after disinfection with povidone iodine or isopropyl alcohol plus iodine tincture; low colony numbers (1 to 100) were found in the other donors. More than 100 colonies is rare (1%).[2] Bacteria residing deep within skin layers are not accessible to disinfectants and may contribute to contamination. In one study, pigskin epidermal cells were detectable in the lavage fluid in 1 out of 150 punctures.[3] AABB *Standards for Blood Banks and Transfusion Services (Standards)*[4(p22)] requires collection containers that divert the first few milliliters of blood into a special pouch, which reduces the proportion of platelet components containing viable bacteria.[5]

BLOOD COLLECTION PROCESS

Method 6-3 describes steps for blood and sample collection for processing and compatibility tests. The average time to collect 500 mL of blood is <10 minutes. A draw time longer than 15 to 20 minutes may not be suitable for collecting platelets or plasma for transfusions, as determined by blood center policy. The collection bag should be periodically mixed during the collection to ensure uniform distribution of anticoagulant. Devices are available to automatically mix the unit during collection.

If insufficient volume is available for test samples obtained from the diversion pouch, a second phlebotomy may be performed immediately after the blood collection.

Volume of Blood Collected

AABB *Standards* permits collection of 10.5 mL of blood per kilogram of the donor's weight for each donation, including the blood unit and all samples for testing.[4(p60)] In North America and Europe, the volume of blood collected during routine phlebotomy is typically either 450 ± 10% (405-495 mL) or 500 mL ± 10% (450-550 mL). The volume may be different in other regions and may be as low as 200 to 250 mL. For general blood banking applications, the volume of blood collected can be determined from the net weight in grams collected divided by the density of WB (1.053 g/mL).

Collection volumes must be within the manufacturer's specified range to ensure the correct anticoagulant-to-WB ratio. Volumes exceeding the manufacturer's specifications for allogeneic collections should be discarded. Low-volume allogeneic collections should be relabeled as "RBCs Low Volume" (Table 6-1). The evidence indicates that the volume in undercollected and overcollected units (275-600 g) does not affect in-vivo red cell recovery even after 21 to 35 days of storage.[6,7] Plasma and platelets from low-volume units should be discarded. Low-volume autologous collections may be retained if they are approved by a physician.

Volumes of other components may also be determined gravimetrically by dividing the net weight in grams by the appropriate density in g/mL. Table 6-2 provides generally accepted densities and, for some, a specific value as provided by applicable regulatory documents.[8-11]

Donor Care after Phlebotomy

Immediately after collection, the needle is withdrawn into a protective sleeve to prevent accidental injuries. Local pressure is applied by hand to the gauze placed directly over the venipuncture site while the donor's arm is kept elevated. Pressure is applied until hemostasis is achieved and a bandage or tape may be applied. For donors who are taking anti-

TABLE 6-1. Weight and Volumes of Routine-Volume, Low-Volume, and Overweight Whole Blood Collections*

		450-mL Collection Bag		500-mL Collection Bag
Low-volume collection	Volume	300-404 mL	Volume	333-449 mL
	Weight	316-425 g	Weight	351-473 g
Routine-volume collection	Volume	405-495 mL	Volume	450-550 mL
	Weight	427-521 g	Weight	474-579 g
Overweight collection	Volume	>495 mL	Volume	>550 mL
	Weight	>521 g	Weight	>579 g

*A density of 1.053 g/mL was used for conversion calculations. The volume and weight of anticoagulant and bag(s) are not accounted for in this table. Low-volume Red Blood Cell (RBC) components must be labeled as low-volume components.

TABLE 6-2. Density of Principal Blood Cells and Components

Blood Cell or Component	Specific Gravity*	Source
Cell		Council of Europe[8]
Platelet	1.058	
Monocyte	1.062	
Lymphocyte	1.070	
Neutrophil	1.082	
Red cell	1.100	
Components		
Red cells collected by automated methods with additive solution	1.06	FDA guidance[9]
Red cells collected by automated methods without additive solution	1.08	FDA guidance[9]
Apheresis platelets	1.03	FDA guidance[10]
Plasma		Dependent on manufacturer of plasma or plasma derivatives
Octapharma AG[†]	1.026	
CSL Plasma[‡]	1.027	
Fenwal (Amicus Cell Separator)[§]	1.027	
Whole blood	1.053[†]	FDA guide for inspection of blood banks[11]

*Specific gravity (SG) is the density relative to water. Assuming a density of water of 1000 g/mL, the values of SG and density are equal.
[†]Octapharma AG, Lachen, Switzerland.
[‡]CSL (previously ZLB) Plasma, Boca Raton, FL.
[§]Fenwal, Lake Zurich, IL.
FDA = Food and Drug Administration.

coagulants or antiplatelet drugs, more time may be required for hemostasis.

AABB *Standards* requires blood centers to provide donors with written postdonation instructions.[4(p16)] Postphlebotomy care includes observing the donor for signs or symptoms of reactions. If the donor tolerates a sitting position without problems, he or she may proceed to a recovery area and should be encouraged to drink fluids and have light snacks and remain in the recovery area for about 15 minutes or until he or she feels comfortable to leave. In addition, blood centers may encourage the donor to drink more fluid and refrain from heavy lifting or vigorous exercise or activities that might put him or her or others at risk for several hours after blood donation. The donor is also instructed to apply local pressure to the phlebotomy site if any bleeding recurs and to call the blood center if the bleeding does not stop with pressure. A telephone number is provided so that the donor can report if he or she feels that the donated unit should not be used, has any reactions, or experiences any signs or symptoms of infection.

ADVERSE DONOR REACTIONS

Adverse reactions occur at the time of donation or are reported later in about 3.5% of donations. The American Red Cross observed[12] a rate of 4.91% (491 per 10,000 donations) in approximately 5 million WB donations in 2014. (See Table 6-3.) Reactions that need medical care after the donor has left the donation site occur in 1 in 3700 donors. A population-based European study found the rate of complications leading to long-term morbidity or disablement to be 5 in 100,000 donations and 2.3 in 100,000, respectively.[13] Donor hemovigilance programs instituted by the American Red Cross recorded a lower rate of complications for WB collections than for apheresis methods for platelets and 2-unit red cell collection, with minor presyncopal reactions and small hematomas representing most of the reactions. Major reactions were slightly more common for WB collection (7.4/10,000) compared with plateletpheresis (5.2/10,000) and 2-unit red cell apheresis (3.3/10,000).[14] Serious reactions occur less often among apheresis donors than WB donors.[15] All adverse reactions occurring during collection procedures must be documented along with the results of thorough investigations.

Needle-Related Injuries

Bruise or Hematoma

In donor follow-up surveys, minor reactions, such as small (<2 inches by 2 inches) hematomas at the phlebotomy site, are reported by as many as one-third of all donors.[16] Bruises and hematomas are common after phlebotomy but generally do not prevent donors from donating again.

Local Nerve Injury

Phlebotomy-related nerve injuries are relatively uncommon but still inevitably occur even with good phlebotomy technique because of anatomic variation and the close association of nerves with veins. In 40% of cases of nerve injuries, phlebotomy was performed without difficulty.[16] Donors may complain of sensory changes away from the phlebotomy site, such as in the forearm, wrist, hand, upper arm, or shoulder. These injuries are usually transient, and recovery almost always occurs; however, in 7% of injured donors, recovery may take 3 to 9 months.[16] In severe cases, referral to a neurologist may be indicated.

Arterial Puncture

Presence of bright red blood, rapid collection (within 4 minutes), and a pulsating needle suggest arterial puncture, although not all signs might be present. Hematomas are more likely to occur with arterial puncture. When puncture is recognized early, the needle should be pulled out immediately, and local pressure should be applied for an extended period. Most donors recover quickly and completely, but some might present with waxing and waning hematomas and should be evaluated for pseudoaneurysm by ultrasound studies.

Systemic Reactions

Vasovagal reactions (also referred to as prefaint or presyncope) include dizziness, sweating, nausea, vomiting, weakness, apprehension, pallor, hypotension, and bradycardia. The reaction might progress to syncope (loss of consciousness), and convulsions and loss of bladder and bowel function might occur. Syncope can also result from orthostatic blood pressure changes after donation. Vasovagal reactions are distinguished by a low pulse rate, whereas reactions related to volume depletion are associated with an increased pulse rate. Typically, however, this difference has no practical value and both mechanisms are treated similarly. Some donors with severe reactions or with prolonged recovery times may need short-term observation, intravenous fluid administration in the emergency room, or both. A protocol for telephone follow-up of donors who have experienced severe reactions is helpful to assess the donors for any residual

TABLE 6-3. Adverse Reactions after Allogeneic Whole Blood and Apheresis Donations in the American Red Cross, 2014*

Reaction Category and Description†		Whole Blood Donations				Automated Procedures‡			
		All Reactions		Outside Medical Care		All Reactions		Outside Medical Care	
		n	Rate§	n	Rate§	n	Rate§	n	Rate§
Systemic (syncopal)	Presyncope (prefaint)	134,710	285.96	123	2.23	11,401	147.72	17	0.22
	LOC (<1 minute)	7,300	15.50	51	0.52	542	7.02	3	0.04
		Major (includes callbacks)							
	LOC (>1 minute)	687	1.46	182	1.46	62	0.61	13	0.17
	Prolonged recovery◊	1,792	3.80	456	3.80	138	1.17	34	0.44
	LOC in injury	1,131	2.40	412	2.40	46	0.47	18	0.23
Phlebotomy	Small hematoma¶	80,432	170.74	68	1.88	35,560	460.73	10	0.13
		Major (includes callbacks)							
	Large hematoma¶	2,287	0.64	350	4.85	1,003	8.03	106	1.37
	Suspected nerve injury	2,252	1.09	430	5.35	269	0.69	55	0.71
	Suspected arterial puncture	828	0.89	70	1.76	28	0.21	1	0.01
Citrate reactions	Citrate (minor)	-	-	-	-	6,920	89.66	15	0.19
	Citrate (major) (includes callbacks)	-	-	-	-	143	1.81	24	0.31
Allergic reactions	Local (minor) allergic reactions	64	0.14	29	0.48	21	0.27	26	0.34
	Systemic allergic reactions (major) (includes callbacks)	12	0.01	9	0.03	7	0.03	4	0.05
TOTAL		**231,495**	**491.42**	**2,180**	**4.63**	**56,140**	**727.37**	**326**	**4.22**

*2014 data from the American Red Cross Hemovigilance Program. (For information on this program, see Eder et al.[12])

†Minor reactions (eg, presyncope, small hematoma) are documented at the collection site. Major reactions are documented at the collection site or reported after donation, require follow-up with the donor, and are reviewed by a blood center physician.

‡Automated collections include plateletpheresis, plateletpheresis with concurrent plasma or other co-component, 2-unit red cell collections, and plasmapheresis procedures.

§Rate per 10,000 donations.

◊Prolonged recovery: more than 30 minutes after presyncope.

¶Small hematoma: 2 × 2 inches or less; large hematoma: more than 2 × 2 inches.

LOC = loss of consciousness; Outside medical care = treatment provided by someone other than blood center staff after a blood-related adverse event.

symptoms. Donor reactions after WB donation do not predict accurately the possibility of recurrent syncope in returning donors, although they reduce the likelihood of future donations.[17]

Most reactions occur at the collection site in the canteen or recovery area. The main predictors of immediate and delayed vasovagal and presyncopal reactions are young age, low estimated blood volume, and first-time donation status.[18,19] Ingestion of antihypertensive medications does not appear to be a risk factor.[20] Approximately 15% of reactions occur away from the donation site, usually within 1 hour of donation.[17] In donors experiencing a reaction, an injury to head, face, or extremity may occur. The staff should be vigilant to detect reactions early and prevent injuries as much as possible. Deferral strategies for young donors with estimated low blood volume (<3.5 liters) and physiologic strategies to minimize donor reactions in young donors are aimed at improving donor safety.[18] Donor education, environmental controls, instructions to donors to drink fluid before and soon after donation, distraction, and muscle tension have been identified as strategies to reduce reactions in young donors.[21]

In case of a vasovagal reaction, phlebotomy should be stopped, and the donor should be placed in a recumbent position as soon as the reaction is suspected. Applying cold wet towels to the donor's neck and shoulder area and loosening the donor's clothes can assist in symptom management.

Vasovagal and hypovolemic reactions are rare in apheresis donors but may occur. Paresthesias (tingling sensations) and other reactions to citrate anticoagulant are not uncommon. (Similar citrate toxicity reactions in recipients are discussed along with WB transfusions in Chapter 22.)

The Food and Drug Administration (FDA) requires blood establishments to report deaths caused by blood donation. For fiscal years 2012 through 2014, the FDA received 45 reports of postdonation fatalities for automated and manual collections, of which only 11 followed WB donation. After medical review, two cases were ruled out and in eight cases, there was no evidence of a causal relationship between blood donation and the donors' demise.[22] Most deaths that take place after blood donation are coincidentally related to the donation rather than caused by it. However, in one case in which a donor was managed conservatively with fluids and rest after complaining of lightheadedness, the donor fell after walking a short distance, resulting in tramatic brain injury and death.[22]

WB FOR COMPONENT PREPARATION OR TRANSFUSION

WB is most often separated into components and is rarely used for transfusion directly. Severe hemorrhage cases, such as those resulting from trauma, may benefit from fresh WB transfusions when platelets are not available.[23] Labile coagulation factor activities diminish in WB during storage, and platelets may activate and develop a storage lesion.

WB units are collected in sterile, plasticized polyvinyl chloride (PVC) bags containing anticoagulant—typically citrate-phosphate-dextrose (CPD), citrate-phosphate-dextrose-dextrose (CP2D), or citrate-phosphate-dextrose-adenine (CPDA-1). (See Tables 6-4 and 6-5.) WB in acid-citrate-dextrose (ACD), CPD, or CP2D has an expiration date of 21 days when stored at 1 to 6 C; the maximum storage time for units in CPDA-1 is 35 days. A single WB collection contains either 450 mL (±10%) or 500 mL (±10%) of blood collected from allogeneic blood donors with a minimum hematocrit for females between 36% and 38%, and for males, 39%, depending on the collection system used. For autologous adult blood donors, a hematocrit as low as 33% is acceptable. Occasionally, units with other volumes are collected, and those volumes are stated on the label. WB collection containers must be approved by the appropriate regulatory body within a country. Blood collection and processing sets are generally latex free. The containers should be sterile, pyrogen free, and identified by a lot number. They should also list an expiry date and include other label data

TABLE 6-4. Anticoagulant-Preservative Solutions for Collection of 450-mL Whole Blood*

Variable	CPD	CP2D	CPDA-1
pH	5.0-6.0	5.3-5.9	5.0-6.0
Ratio (mL solution to blood)	1.4:10	1.4:10	1.4:10
FDA-approved shelf life (days)	21	21	35
Content (mg in 63 mL)			
Sodium citrate, dehydrate	1660	1660	1660
Citric acid, anhydrous	188	206	188
Dextrose, monohydrate	1610	3220	2010
Monobasic sodium phosphate, monohydrate	140	140	140
Adenine	0	0	17.3

*Data were supplied and verified by manufacturers.
CPD = citrate-phosphate-dextrose; CP2D = citrate-phosphate-dextrose-dextrose; CPDA-1 = citrate-phosphate-dextrose-adenine; FDA = Food and Drug Administration.

TABLE 6-5. Anticoagulant-Preservative Solutions for Collection of 500-mL Whole Blood*

Variable	CPD	CP2D	CPDA-1
pH	5.0-6.0	5.3-5.9	5.0-6.0
Ratio (mL solution to blood)	1.4:10	1.4:10	1.4:10
FDA-approved shelf life (days)	21	21	35
Content (mg in 70 mL)			
Sodium citrate dehydrate	1840	1840	1840
Citric acid, anhydrous	209	229	300
Dextrose, monohydrate	1780	3570	2230
Monobasic sodium phosphate, phosphate, monohydrate	155	155	155
Adenine	0	0	19.3

*Data were supplied and verified by manufacturers.
CPD = citrate-phosphate-dextrose; CP2D = citrate-phosphate-dextrose-dextrose; CPDA-1 = citrate-phosphate-dextrose-adenine; FDA = Food and Drug Administration.

required by regulatory authorities. Sterile collection systems can contain integrally attached tubing to allow aseptic fluid transfer to satellite containers for component preparation, as well as integral access ports for open connection of infusion sets or other spike entry. Open spiked access accelerates outdate from the time of entry. Innovations in WB collection include scales for monitoring the collection volume plus automatic mixing and devices to add anticoagulant at a fixed ratio as the blood is withdrawn from the vein.

The acceptable temperature during short-term storage, transport and handling of WB immediately after collection is determined by processing requirements for component preparation. In some cases, this may mean that collections at mobile blood drives or fixed collection sites should be transported as soon as possible to the central component preparation laboratory. With other processing methods, transportation may not be as urgent. Requirements for cooling and transportation methods are quite variable, and the specifications of the appropriate device manufacturer should be carefully followed. By the time phlebotomy is completed, the blood has air cooled to about 30 C.[24] If such units are left at the ambient temperature, the cooling rate is quite slow, and about 6 hours more are needed for units to reach 25 C.[24] To cool blood more rapidly, units are typically placed in specific storage environments. Some centers use cooling plates that provide rate-controlled cooling toward 20 C. These cooling plates contain 1,4-butanediol, which has a melting temperature of 20 C and serves as a heat absorber. With the cooling plates, about 2 hours are needed for the collected blood to reach 20 C.[24]

Tests for ABO group, Rh type, unexpected alloantibodies, and transfusion-transmitted diseases are performed. Each unit must be tested unless the donor is undergoing repeated procedures to support a specific patient—for example in some apheresis procedures, in which case testing for infectious disease markers needs to be repeated only at 30-day intervals.[25]

WB may be reconstituted by combining Red Blood Cells (RBCs) with thawed plasma to achieve a desired hematocrit level—for example, when used for neonatal exchange transfusions. Additional information about the preparation of reconstituted WB is provided in Chapter 17.

DESCRIPTIONS OF MAJOR BLOOD COMPONENTS

Blood Collection Systems

Descriptions of the various blood components can be found in the *Circular of Information for the Use of Human Blood and Blood Components* (*Circular of Information*).[26] Blood collection systems may be designed in different configurations for manual and mechanical methods (eg, centrifugation, manual bag transfers, and manual expression of contents) or used in a fully automated system, such as in modern apheresis devices. Satellite bags and integrally attached tubing that are hermetically sealed allow component manufacturing to take place in a closed system. The blood container should not be entered before issue except for the purposes of blood collection or transfer of components to a different container. Components prepared with an open system require a reduction in their expiration time from the time that the system was opened to reduce the risk of bacterial sepsis. This period may range from 24 hours (RBCs at 1-6 C) to 4 hours (RBCs and platelets held at room temperature; thawed cryoprecipitate and plasma). The use of approved sterile connecting devices maintains a functionally closed system when various connections are performed, such as pooling or sampling, thereby maintaining the component's original expiry date.

The collection of components by apheresis follows many of the same rules and guidelines that apply to WB donation. Although the apheresis collection and preparation processes differ from those used for WB-derived components, the storage and transportation requirements and several quality-control steps are the same for both processes.

The facility must maintain written procedures and protocols for all types of collections used and must keep records of each procedure as required by AABB *Standards.*[4(pp68-74)] Records of all laboratory findings and collection data must be periodically reviewed by a knowledgeable physician and must be found to be within acceptable limits.

Red Blood Cells

Blood containers for RBC storage often are composed of PVC plasticized by di-(2-ethylhexyl) phthalate (DEHP). DEHP not only imparts flexibility to the PVC but also has been shown to protect red cells against hemolysis during storage. Because of concerns over possible toxicity of DEHP, alternative plasticizers, such as butyryl-trihexyl-citrate (BTHC) and 1,2-cyclohexane dicarboxylic acid diisononyl ester (DINCH), have been made available in some collection sets. Because of the protective effect of DEHP on red cells, finding an equally effective substitute for DEHP has been challenging. This has recently been reviewed by Simmchen.[27]

The preparation of RBC components is described in Methods 6-4 and 6-5. RBCs from WB in anticoagulant-preservative CPD or CP2D have a shelf life of 21 days at 1 to 6 C with a hematocrit of 65% to 85%, or 35 days in CPDA-1 with a hematocrit of <80%. Additive solution (Table 6-6) reduces the hematocrit to approximately 55% to 65%. The use of additive solutions enables extension of RBC shelf life to 42 days in the United States and to 56 days in some other jurisdictions. Four additive solutions are currently approved in the United States; others are approved in other regions (Table 6-6).[28] RBCs stored for less than 7 to 10 days are often issued for neonatal or pediatric transfusions, although practice varies both with regard to freshness and preferred anticoagulant or additive solution at different institutions, with sparse evidence to suggest the optimal approach. (See Chapter 24.) Approved anticoagulants used for apheresis collections include ACD formula A (ACD-A) or formula B (ACD-B), and RBCs collected by apheresis instruments include the use of additive solutions. For RBCs collected by either WB or apheresis methods, hemolysis at the end of storage should be <1% in the United States or <0.8% in the European Union (EU). RBCs may be subject to several secondary processing steps—for example, leukocyte reduction, or gamma or x-ray irradiation to prevent graft-vs-host disease (GVHD).

Segments are made from tubing from the RBC container, which is marked with repeating serial numbers and may be sealed at several locations with either a dielectric (heat) sealer or a metal clip (grommet) to prepare approximately 13 to 15 segments containing a unique imprinted number. These segments may be used later for ABO/Rh typing, crossmatching, antigen typing, investigation of adverse transfusion reactions, or other laboratory tests. Hemolysis identified by visual inspection of a segment often does not correlate with hemolysis in the unit. In one study, approximately three-fourths of the visual assessments did not agree with the hemoglobin levels measured by chemical methods, indicating a high false-positive rate with visual assessment.[29]

Visual inspection of RBC units can detect abnormal color caused by bacterial contamination, hemolysis, and clots. Abnormal color caused by bacterial contamination may be observed in the bag, while some uncontaminated segments appear to be lighter than the color of the bag because of oxygen consumption by bacteria in the bag.[30] The bag content may look purple with or without hemolysis, and large clots may be evident. The unit can be centrifuged to facilitate inspection of the supernatant in the case of suspected bacterial contamination, and visual inspection of the supernatant may reveal murky, brown, or red fluid.[30] However, visual inspection will not detect all contaminated units.

Blood clots in RBC units are often too small to be detected by visual inspection. Clots are sometimes revealed during transfusion when they clog the filter, or in the component laboratory when the units are filtered through a leukocyte reduction filter. Units that fail visual inspection or are otherwise observed to have clots should not be released for transfusion.

TABLE 6-6. RBC Additive Solutions Currently in Routine Use around the World*†

Constituents (mM)	SAGM	AS-1 Adsol Fresensius Kabi (Fenwal)	AS-3 Nutricel Haemon-etics	AS-5 Optisol Terumo-BCT	AS-7 SOLX Haemon-etics	MAP	PAGGSM MacoPharma
NaCl	150	154	70	150	-	85	72
NaHCO$_3$	-	-	-	-	26	-	-
Na$_2$HPO$_4$	-	-	-	-	12	-	16
NaH$_2$PO$_4$	-	-	23	-	-	6	8
Citric acid			2			1	
Na$_3$-citrate	-	-	23	-	-	5	-
Adenine	1.25	2	2	2.2	2	1.5	1.4
Guanosine	-	-	-	-	-	-	1.4
Dextrose (glucose)	45	111	55	45	80	40	47
Mannitol	30	41	-	45.5	55	80	55
pH	5.7	4.6 - 7.2	5.8	5.5	8.5	5.7	5.7
Density (g/mL)	1.02	1.012	1.005	‡	1.01	‡	1.02
Osmolality (mOsm)	347 - 383	462	418	393	237	‡	270 - 310
Anticoagulant	CPD	CPD	CP2D	CPD	CPD	ACD	CPD
FDA-licensed	No	Yes	Yes	Yes	Yes	No	No
Where used	Europe United Kingdom Australia Canada New Zealand	United States	United States Canada	United States	United States Europe	Japan	Germany

*Adapted from Sparrow.[28]
†Data were supplied and verified by manufacturers. Brand names and primary sources are listed for each solution. Formulations may be available through other sources.
‡Not reported.
SAGM = saline, adenine, glucose, and mannitol; AS = additive solution; MAP = mannitol-adenine-phosphate; PAGGSM = phosphate-adenine-glucose-guanosine-saline-mannitol; NaCl = sodium chloride; NaHCO$_3$ = sodium bicarbonate; Na$_2$HPO$_4$ = sodium hydrogen phosphate; NaH$_2$PO$_4$ = monosodium phosphate; Na$_3$-citrate = trisodium citrate; FDA = Food and Drug Administration.

Red Blood Cells Prepared from WB

WB that will not be used to prepare platelets should be cooled to refrigerator temperature as soon as possible; this is often accomplished by placing the unit on wet ice or other appropriate cooling media. All current methods for separation and preparation of the three major blood components—RBCs, platelets, and plasma—rely on one or more centrifugation steps. Centrifuges should be properly validated, maintained, and calibrated, or checked in a systematic manner to verify the processing conditions. The major variables that affect the recovery of cells from WB by differential centrifugation are rotor size, centrifuge speed, duration of centrifugation, and acceleration/deceleration protocol. Published papers often refer to relative centrifugal force (g-force), which is derived from the radius of the centrifuge rotor and its revolutions.

Following separation by centrifugation, components must be carefully divided into separate containers for further processing. Many laboratories use manual expressers for this purpose, in which case the component laboratory staff identifies when the red cell interface approaches the tubing and stops expression using a hemostat. Blood component extractors are available for making components in an automated manner and are capable of automatically detecting the red cell interface and clamping. After primary centrifugation, WB is placed in the extractor, and a pressure plate creates an outflow of components from the container. Outflow can occur from the top and/or bottom of the container, depending on the device.

Automated expression may improve the standardization of components, but it is not widely used in the United States. Automated devices control the rate of expression, detect an interface with an optical sensing device for clamping and sealing tubing, monitor component weights, add storage solutions, and perform other useful functions that assist in the consistent preparation of blood components. Some systems also combine nearly all of these functions, including centrifugation, without relying on operator interventions.

Hemoglobin content per unit varies because of differences between donors and between processing specifics. For example, more hemoglobin is generally lost with buffy-coat preparation methods than with platelet-rich plasma (PRP)-type methods. Hemoglobin content per unit may be more precisely controlled with automated collections. Total hemoglobin content is not directly regulated in the United States but has a lower limit of 45 g per unit or 40 g per unit for leukocyte-reduced RBCs in the EU.[31] Some experts have advocated for standardizing the amount of hemoglobin per RBC unit at 50 g.[32]

RBCs that are labeled as low-volume units are made available for transfusion when 300 to 404 mL of WB is collected into an anticoagulant volume calculated for 450 ± 45 mL, or when 333 to 449 mL of WB is collected into an anticoagulant volume calculated for 500 ± 50 mL. Although the resulting RBCs may be transfused, other components, such as platelets, plasma, and cryoprecipitate, should not be prepared from low-volume units.

Apheresis Red Blood Cells (Red Blood Cells Pheresis) and Multicomponent Donations

Apheresis RBCs contain at least 60 g of hemoglobin (or 180 mL red cell volume) per unit.[4(p27)] As apheresis technology continued to evolve and equipment, disposables, and software became increasingly sophisticated, the collection of various combinations of components became possible. (See Table 6-7.) Both AABB *Standards* and FDA guidance documents address the removal of red cells by automated apheresis methods.[4,9] A guidance document issued in 2001 by the FDA finalized recommendations for the use of automated apheresis equipment to collect the following[9]:

- Single units of RBCs and plasma.
- Single units of RBCs and platelets.
- Single units of RBCs, platelets, and plasma.
- Double units of RBCs only.

The guidance document includes FDA regulations requiring that equipment perform

TABLE 6-7. Components That Can Be Collected with Various Instruments

Instrument	GRAN	PLT	cRBC*	2-RBC	PLASMA	cPLASMA*
Fenwal ALYX			X	X		X
Fenwal Amicus		X	X			X
Fenwal Autopheresis C†					X	
Fresenius AS104	X					
TerumoBCT (COBE) Spectra	X	X				X
TerumoBCT Spectra Optia	X					
TerumoBCT Trima V-4		X	X	X		X
TerumoBCT Trima Accel		X	X	X		X
Haemonetics Cymbal				X		
Haemonetics MCS+ LN9000	X	X				X
Haemonetics MCS+ LN8150			X	X		X
Haemonetics PCS-2†					X	

*Concurrent collection refers to the ability to collect more than one type of component.
†Open system.
GRAN = granulocytes; PLT = plateletpheresis (single, double, triple); cRBC = concurrent 1 unit of Red Blood Cells (RBCs); 2-RBC = double unit of RBCs; PLASMA = 1 unit of plasma; cPLASMA = concurrent plasma; V-4 = software version 4.

and be used in the manner for which it was designed to collect or process blood and components. It includes sections on donor selection and monitoring, including ensuring that donor red cell loss does not exceed acceptable limits, as well as quality control (QC) issues and record requirements. Some of these requirements have also been described in previous editions of the *Technical Manual*.[33]

Devices for Red Cell Collection by Apheresis

TerumoBCT Trima and Trima Accel. The Trima (TerumoBCT, Lakewood, CO) can collect a single unit of RBCs concurrently with platelets.[34-36] A kit is available to collect a double unit of RBCs with or without concurrent plasma, depending on the donor's size and hema-

tocrit. The Trima uses the single-stage channel for the double-RBC collection, and saline is returned to the donor during the collection. The addition of the preservative solution and leukocyte reduction by filtration are performed manually and offline after the collection is complete for both the single and double RBC units.

Fenwal ALYX. The ALYX (Fenwal, Lake Zurich, IL) is capable of collecting 2 units of RBCs or 1 unit of RBCs and concurrent plasma at the same time, depending on donor size and hematocrit.[34,36,37] The ALYX uses a rigid, cylinder-shaped chamber in the centrifuge to separate the plasma from the cells. During reinfusion, the plasma and saline are returned to the donor. When the collection is complete, the ALYX automatically adds the preservative solution and pumps the red cells through an in-line leukocyte reduction filter into the final storage bags. The ALYX uses a single-access kit only, and its extracorporeal volume (ECV) is approximately 110 mL.

Fenwal Amicus. The Fenwal Amicus can collect a single unit of RBCs concurrently with plateletpheresis, but only with the single-access kit.[34,38] The addition of the preservative solution and leukocyte reduction by filtration are performed manually and offline after the collection is complete.

Haemonetics Cymbal. The Cymbal (Haemonetics, Braintree, MA) is a collection system that uses an expanding, variable-volume bowl. The system has a relatively small ECV when compared to the Haemonetics MCS+ LN8150 and collects a double-RBC unit.[39]

Haemonetics MCS+ LN8150. The Haemonetics MCS+ LN8150 uses the blow-molded bowl that is also used for plasma collection. It uses a single-access kit and its ECV varies, depending on the donor's hematocrit, from 542 mL (38% hematocrit) to 391 mL (54% hematocrit). The LN8150 is capable of collecting a single or double unit of RBCs with or without concurrent plasma, depending on the donor's size and hematocrit.[34,36,40] The addition of preservative and leukocyte reduction by filtration are performed manually and offline after the collection is complete.[41]

Frozen Red Blood Cells

Glycerol is the most commonly used cryopreservative agent and is added in either high or low concentration to RBCs within 6 days of collection. Two commonly used protocols for the high-glycerol method are described in Methods 6-6 and 6-7.

Frozen RBCs must be stored at temperatures colder than –65 C and expire after 10 years. Rare frozen units may be used beyond the expiration date, but only after medical review and approval based on the patient's needs and availability of other rare compatible units. The units should be handled with care because the containers may crack during shipment or if they are bumped or handled roughly.

The units should be thawed at 37 C, taking about 10 minutes to thaw completely.

Glycerol must be removed after thawing by instruments that allow the addition and removal of sodium chloride solutions. In most cases, addition and removal of glycerol (deglycerolization) is performed in an open system; thus, thawed and deglycerolized units can be stored only for 24 hours at 1 to 6 C. The final solution in which cells are suspended is 0.9% sodium chloride and 0.2% dextrose. Dextrose provides nutrients and has been shown to support satisfactory posttransfusion viability for 4 days of storage after deglycerolization.[42] For QC, determining the volume of red cells in the unit after deglycerolization and examining the last wash for hemolysis are recommended. (See Method 6-8.)

Recently, automated addition of glycerol to RBCs and removal from RBCs in a closed system has become possible. With this system, glycerol is added within 6 days of WB collection. Postthaw red cells prepared in this manner are suspended in additive solution formula 3 (AS-3) and can be stored for 14 days at 4 C.[41] Postwash units have a hematocrit of 51% to 53% and contain a mean of about 9.0×10^6 leukocytes per unit.[43]

Plasma Components

Plasma preparations are defined and regulated through extensive combinations of differences in collection methods, storage temperatures, freezing methods, secondary processing, timing, and storage after thawing. These specifications are covered in an array of standards, rules, and guidelines overlaid with various requirements of the country where the plasma is prepared and/or used. Major, although not exhaustive, sources of this information include the US CFR, FDA guidance documents, the US *Circular of Information*,[26] the AABB *Standards*, and EU directives. The definitions and requirements of the country where the plasma is prepared should always be consulted.

Plasma from WB and apheresis collections is generally frozen to maintain factor activity and provide an extended shelf life. Frozen plasma is thawed for clinical use and may be maintained at 1 to 6 C for some time before use. Frozen plasma is also the source of cryoprecipitate and cryoprecipitate-reduced plasma. There are several methods available for pathogen reduction of plasma that may be applied depending on national regulatory approvals. Plasma may be used for preparation of specific plasma protein products through fractionation processes. The descriptions below are based on the *Circular of Information*.

Fresh Frozen Plasma

In the United States, Fresh Frozen Plasma (FFP) is plasma collected either from a single-unit WB collection or by apheresis. WB in the United States is routinely collected in volumes (eg, 500 mL) that maximize plasma collections from the smallest donor (10.5 mL/kg for a donor of 110 lb). A unit from WB on average contains 200 to 250 mL, but apheresis units may contain as much as 400 to 600 mL of plasma. The preparation of FFP from WB is described in Method 6-9. FFP contains normal amounts of all coagulation factors, antithrombin, and ADAMTS13. FFP must be placed in the freezer within 8 hours of collection; within 6 hours if anticoagulated with ACD; or as directed by the manufacturer's instructions for use of the blood collection, processing, and storage system. FFP has a shelf life of 12 months when stored at –18 C or colder and, with FDA approval, may be stored longer than 12 months at –65 C.[4(p56)] The glass-transition temperature of PVC bags is about –25 C to –30 C. At and below these temperatures, the container is brittle and should be treated as if it were made of glass and fragile enough to break during transport and handling. Rapid freezing of plasma can be accomplished using a blast freezer, dry ice, or a mixture of dry ice with either ethanol or antifreeze. Plasma should be thawed at 30 to 37 C in a waterbath or by using an FDA-cleared device. When a waterbath is used, the component should be placed in a protective plastic overwrap. Thawing of larger units of FFP collected by apheresis may require more time. FFP, once thawed, has a shelf life of 24 hours at 1 to 6 C. Thawed plasma held longer than 24 hours must be relabeled as Thawed Plasma, and can be stored for an additional 4 days at 1 to 6 C.

AABB requires[4(p17)] interventions to reduce the risk of transfusion-related acute lung injury (TRALI) from apheresis platelets, plasma products, and WB transfusion.[44] These components should be collected from males, never-pregnant females, or parous female donors who test negative for HLA antibodies, to minimize the risk of exposing patients to HLA alloantibodies that could cause TRALI.

The Council of Europe defines "plasma, fresh frozen" as prepared from either WB or plasma collected by apheresis. Plasma freezing must be initiated within 6 hours of collection, within 18 hours if the WB is held at 1 to 6 C, or within 24 hours if WB or apheresis plasma is rapidly conditioned to 20 to 22 C following collection. Freezing must be completed within 1 hour to less than –30 C. Plasma, fresh frozen has an expiry time of 36 months if held at less than –25 C, or 3 months if held at –18 C to –25 C.[8] The Council of Europe does not address specific thawing methods or treatment of the plasma following thawing, including expiry dating.

Quarantine plasma was introduced to increase the viral safety of plasma. The Council of Europe notes that quarantine FFP can be released from quarantine after the donor returns to the blood center and has repeatedly negative test results for, at a minimum, hepatitis B and C viruses, human immunodeficiency virus, type 1 (HIV-1), and HIV-2 beyond a minimum quarantine period that is greater than the diagnostic window period for viral infection (typically 6 months). With the use of nucleic acid tests for viral screening, this window period for quarantine FFP may be reduced.[45]

Plasma Frozen Within 24 Hours After Phlebotomy

The FDA defines plasma (collected by manual or automated methods) that is frozen within 24 hours of collection as Plasma Frozen Within 24 Hours After Phlebotomy (PF24). Once thawed, PF24 has a shelf life of 24 hours at 1 to 6 C. Thawed plasma held longer than 24 hours must be relabeled as Thawed Plasma, which can be stored for an additional 4 days at 1 to 6 C.

Plasma Frozen Within 24 Hours After Phlebotomy Held At Room Temperature Up To 24 Hours After Phlebotomy

The FDA defines Plasma Frozen Within 24 Hours After Phlebotomy Held At Room Temperature Up To 24 Hours After Phlebotomy (PF24RT24) as plasma (collected by manual or automated methods) that is held for up to 24 hours after collection at room temperature and then stored at less than –18 C. Once thawed, PF24 and PF24RT24 have a shelf life of 24 hours at 1 to 6 C. Thawed plasma held for longer than 24 hours must be relabeled as Thawed Plasma and can be stored for an additional 4 days at 1 to 6 C. A similar component prepared from WB held at room temperature for more than 8 hours (ie, overnight hold) may be defined in the future if FDA approves an overnight-hold WB process.

Plasma Cryoprecipitate Reduced

Plasma Cryoprecipitate Reduced (United States) or plasma, fresh frozen cryoprecipitate depleted (Europe) is a byproduct of cryoprecipitate preparation. In the United States, Plasma Cryoprecipitate Reduced must be refrozen within 24 hours at <–18 C. The storage temperatures and expiration that apply to FFP apply to this component in both the United States and Europe. The component contains a normal level of Factor V (85%), Factor I, Factor VII, Factor X, antiplasmin, antithrombin, protein C, and protein S. Even after the removal of cryoprecipitate, the component has a fibrinogen level of about 200 mg/dL.[46] Levels of Factor VIII, the von Willebrand factor (vWF) antigen, vWF activity, fibrinogen, and Factor XIII are decreased.[47]

Thawed Plasma

Thawed Plasma (which is not licensed by the FDA) is FFP, PF24, or PF24RT24 that has been thawed and held at 1 to 6 C for >24 hours.[26] Thawed Plasma may be held at 1 to 6 C for up to 4 days after the initial 24-hour postthaw period has elapsed. Stable Factor II and fibrinogen and reduced amounts of other factors have been observed in Thawed Plasma.

Thawed Plasma prepared from FFP and stored for 4 days after the initial 24-hour postthaw period contains reduced levels of Factor V (>60%) and Factor VIII (>40%). ADAMTS13 levels are well maintained for 5 days at 1 to 6 C in Thawed Plasma.

Liquid Plasma

In the United States, liquid plasma for transfusion can be separated from WB at any time during storage and stored at 1 to 6 C for up to 5 days after the WB's expiration date.

Recovered Plasma

Blood centers often convert plasma and liquid plasma to an unlicensed component, "recovered plasma (plasma for manufacture)," which is usually shipped to a fractionator and processed into derivatives, such as albumin and/or immune globulins. To ship recovered plasma, the collecting facility must have a "short supply agreement" with the manufacturer. Because recovered plasma has no expiration date, records for this component should be retained indefinitely. Storage conditions for recovered plasma are established by the fractionator. FFP used as human plasma for fractionation in Europe must comply with the applicable *European Pharmacopoeia* guidelines.

Plasma Collected by Apheresis

Apheresis devices can be used to collect plasma for transfusion (eg, FFP) or use as Source Plasma for subsequent manufacturing. Recently, the FDA approved apheresis devices for the collection of plasma held at 1 to 6 C within 8 hours and frozen within 24 hours after phlebotomy (PF24) and plasma held at room temperature for up to 24 hours and frozen within 24 hours after phlebotomy (PF24RT24).

The FDA has provided guidance with regard to the volume of plasma that may be collected using automated devices. A distinction is made between infrequent plasmapheresis, in which the donor undergoes plasmapheresis no more frequently than once every 4 weeks, and serial plasmapheresis (or Source Plasma collection, the process to collect plasma for fractionation into plasma components), in which the donation is more frequent than once every 4 weeks. For donors in infrequent plasmapheresis programs, donor selection and monitoring requirements are the same as those for WB donation. Plasma obtained by these processes is intended for direct transfusion.

For serial plasma (Source Plasma) collection using automated instruments or manual techniques, the following principles apply[48]:

1. Donors must give consent for the procedure, and they must be observed closely during the procedure. Emergency medical care must always be available.

2. Red cell losses related to the procedure, including samples collected for testing, should be monitored so that no more than 200 mL of red cells are removed in 8 weeks. If the donor's red cells cannot be returned during an apheresis procedure, hemapheresis or WB donation should be deferred for 8 weeks.

3. For manual collection systems, a mechanism must exist to ensure safe reinfusion of the autologous red cells.

4. In manual procedures for donors weighing 110 to 175 lb, no more than 500 mL of WB should be removed at one time or no more than 1000 mL during a phlebotomy session or within a 48-hour period. The limits for donors who weigh ≥175 lb are 600 mL and 1200 mL, respectively. For automated procedures, the allowable volume has been determined for each instrument by the FDA.

5. At least 48 hours should elapse between successive procedures. Donors should not undergo more than two procedures within a 7-day period.

6. At the time of initial plasmapheresis and at 4-month intervals for donors undergoing serial (large-volume) plasmapheresis, serum or plasma must be tested for total protein and for serum protein electrophoresis or for quantitative immunoglobulins. Results must be within normal limits.

7. A qualified licensed physician, knowledgeable about all aspects of hemapheresis, must be responsible for the program.

For manual apheresis collection systems, a process that is rarely used in the United States at present, requirements are outlined in the CFR[48] and have been summarized in previous editions of this *Technical Manual*.[33]

Devices for the Collection of Apheresis Plasma

Two apheresis devices for the sole collection of plasma use open systems. Other closed-system apheresis devices are available for collection of plasma concurrent with red cell or platelet collections (Table 6-7).

Fenwal Autopheresis C. The Autopheresis C uses a rotating cylindrical filter to separate the plasma from the cellular elements of blood. Because of the high efficiency of the rotating filter, the filter is small and the system's ECV is approximately 200 mL. The Autopheresis C is a single-access system, and saline replacement can be administered. It is considered an open system and can collect several units of plasma. According to the FDA definition, an open system requires that plasma outdates 4 hours after thawing. Variances can be granted that allow 24-hour outdates, but these units cannot be relabeled as Thawed Plasma.

Haemonetics PCS-2. The PCS-2, a simplified version of the Haemonetics MCS Plus, is designed for plasma collection.[49] The PCS-2 uses a blow-molded (grenade-shaped) centrifuge bowl to separate plasma from cellular elements. Depending on the degree of cell reduction required, one of three versions of the PCS-2 bowl can be used: standard, filter core, or high-separation core. The standard bowl uses centrifugal force to remove the plasma from the top of the bowl. To increase cell reduction, the filter core and high-separation core bowls allow plasma to pass through the core, which is covered with a filter membrane.[50-52] The ECV of the PCS-2 is variable depending on the hematocrit of the donor and ranges from 491 mL

(38% hematocrit) to 385 mL (50% hematocrit). The PCS-2 is a single-access system, and saline replacement can be administered. It is considered an open system. As noted for the Autopheresis C, a variance can be granted allowing 24-hour outdates of plasma processed with this device, but these units may not be relabeled as Thawed Plasma. The PCS-2 can collect several units of plasma at a time.

Cryoprecipitated Components

Cryoprecipitated antihemophilic factor (AHF), or simply "cryoprecipitate" in Europe, is prepared from FFP. Cold-insoluble protein that precipitates when FFP is thawed to 1 to 6 C is collected by centrifugation; supernatant plasma is transferred into a satellite container; the precipitate is resuspended in a small amount of residual plasma, generally 15 mL; and the precipitate is refrozen as described in Method 6-10. FFP can be thawed to prepare Cryoprecipitated AHF by placing the FFP in a refrigerator (at 1 to 6 C) overnight or in a circulating waterbath at 1 to 6 C. An alternate method that uses microwaves for thawing has been described. The Cryoprecipitated AHF is placed in a freezer within an hour of removal from the refrigerated centrifuge and can be stored at –18 C for 12 months from the original collection date. In Europe, thawing is to be performed at 2 to 6 C, and the component can be stored for up to 36 months below –25 C and for 3 months at –18 to –25 C.

AABB *Standards*[4(pp28-29)] requires that Cryoprecipitated AHF contain at least 80 international units (IU) of Factor VIII and 150 mg of fibrinogen per unit, although the average fibrinogen content is generally 250 mg.[53] European standards require at least 70 IU of Factor VIII, 140 mg of fibrinogen, and 100 IU of vWF per unit. Currently, preparations are reported to have much higher amounts of fibrinogen (median: 388 mg/unit).[54] Cryoprecipitated AHF also contains the vWF ristocetin cofactor activity (approximately 170 units/bag), Factor XIII (approximately 60 units/bag), and fibronectin. Rapid freezing of FFP is found to increase the Factor VIII yield in Cryoprecipitated AHF.[55] ADAMTS13 levels are normal in Cryo-

precipitated AHF.[56] Anti-A and anti-B are known to be present in Cryoprecipitated AHF, but the combined amount of these antibodies from the unit of plasma is only 1.15% of the total.[57]

Thawed Cryoprecipitated AHF should be used as soon as possible but may be held at room temperature (20-24 C) for 6 hours as single units or a pool prepared as a closed system using an approved sterile connecting device, or for 4 hours if pooling was with an open system. Pooling may be accomplished with the aid of a diluent, such as 0.9% sodium chloride (USP), to facilitate removal of material from individual bags.

At room temperature, the mean declines of Factor VIII levels at 2, 4, and 6 hours are approximately 10%, 20%, and 30%, respectively.[58] Cryoprecipitated AHF from blood groups A and B has higher levels of Factor VIII compared to that derived from blood group O donors (about 120 vs 80 IU per bag, respectively).[59] Thawed cryoprecipitate should not be refrozen.

Platelet Components

Platelets are stored and shipped at 20 to 24 C in plastic containers that have greater gas permeability than those for red cells or plasma and must be agitated during storage to adequately support platelet metabolism and ensure adequate in-vivo recovery.[10,60] Agitation supports platelet metabolism by ensuring effective exchange of oxygen, carbon dioxide, and lactic acid between the platelets and the suspending media. Modern platelet containers with high gas permeability are composed of PVC plasticized with BTHC or tri(2-ethylhexyl)trimellitate or, alternatively, composed of ethylvinylacetate, polyolefins (polyethylene or polypropylene), or fluoropolymers. Long periods of static storage of platelets disrupt oxidative metabolism and enhance glycolysis, resulting in increased lactic acid production and decreases in pH.[61] If pH levels decline to ≤6.2, platelets will have unacceptably low in-vivo recoveries.[62] During transport to hospitals from the blood center or long-distance air transport, or when components are exchanged between blood centers, platelets are not agitated. In-vitro studies have shown that platelets are not damaged when they are stored without agitation for 24 hours.[61,63] However, longer periods without agitation can lead to unacceptable pH decline.[63]

With 20 to 24 C storage, contaminating bacteria can proliferate during storage and result in septic transfusion reactions, some of which are fatal. Therefore, platelet shelf life is limited to 5 days in the United States, 3 days in Japan, 4 days in Germany, and up to 7 days in most EU and other countries. These limits are primarily determined by regulatory risk assessments of the likelihood of septic transfusion reactions.

In order to limit the chance of bacteria entering the collection container, collection systems intended for platelet preparation by WB or apheresis methods include a diversion pouch immediately after the access needle.[4(p22)] Diversion of the first few milliliters of blood into a pouch has been shown to reduce the risk of bacterial contamination of the blood unit by capturing bacteria from the skin.[64] The diversion pouch should be isolated by a heat seal or metal clip before any collection into the primary collection container, and then blood in the pouch may be used for donor testing. Other practices to prevent and detect bacterial contamination such as optimal methods of arm cleansing and bacterial culture have been effectively implemented. Pathogen inactivation technologies are anticipated by many to be the best general protection. Updates on technologies obtaining regulatory approval in the United States are listed on the FDA website.

Visual inspections of platelets after they are prepared have shown an absence of visible red cells in the vast majority of units, which implies that the units contain fewer than 0.4×10^9 red cells. Generally, the number of red cells in a unit of platelets does not exceed 1.0×10^9, although occasionally WB-derived platelets contain more red cells.[65] If red cells are visible in a component, the hematocrit should be determined. AABB *Standards* states that if the component contains >2 mL of red cells, the red cells must be ABO compatible with the recipient's plasma and be crossmatched.[4(pp37-38)] In such cases, a sample of do-

nor blood is attached to the container for compatibility testing.

On the day of preparation, some WB-derived platelet units as well as apheresis platelet units may contain clumps composed of platelet aggregates.[65] In routine practice, visual inspection is adequate to determine the degree of clumping subjectively and ensure that units with excessive clumping are not released for labeling. Most of the clumps seen on day 0 disappear on day 1 of storage with continuous agitation, particularly those units showing light to moderate clumping.[65] The temperature at which WB platelets are prepared may influence clumping; platelets prepared at 24 C appear to show the least amount of clumping compared to those prepared at less than 24 C.[66]

Occasionally because of adverse shipping conditions, temporary equipment failures, or power outages, platelets cannot be maintained at 20 to 24 C. One study indicated that platelets can maintain their in-vitro properties after exposure to 37 C for 6 hours followed by room-temperature storage without agitation for an additional 18 hours.[67] However, two studies have demonstrated negative effects on in-vivo platelet recovery and survival when platelets are stored at temperatures <20 C.[68,69] Thus, proper steps should be taken to maintain the required range of temperatures during storage at the blood center and during transport.

WB-Derived Platelets

WB destined for platelet preparation should not be cooled to <20 C. In the United States, platelets must be separated from WB within 8 hours of collection to prepare platelets from PRP. For preparation of platelets from WB, two primary methods are available (Method 6-12): preparation from PRP and preparation from buffy coats. Both methods involve centrifugation, and conditions must be tailored for the blood bag system and the method of platelet preparation. Centrifuge speed and duration can be altered in a stepwise fashion in a simplex strategy to determine the optimal conditions for preparing PRP.[70] The simplex strategy can also be used to identify the optimal conditions of centrifugation for platelet concentrates when QC data show that the platelet counts in platelet concentrates are not satisfactory. Method 8-6 describes a process of functional calibration of the centrifuge to maximize platelet yield. The device manufacturer should be consulted for recommendations on validating the performance of automated systems.

One unit of platelets prepared from WB usually contains $\geq 5.5 \times 10^{10}$ platelets suspended in 40 to 70 mL of plasma, although studies have shown good recovery and survival rates when platelets are stored in plasma volumes of 35 to 40 mL.[71,72] Four to 6 units of platelets are typically pooled, labeled, and stored in an approved container[73] or stored as individual units and pooled within 4 hours of transfusion for one therapeutic dose. In the United States, no platelet additive solutions are approved for use with platelets prepared from WB. Platelets prepared by the PRP or buffy-coat methods can be further processed to reduce leukocytes in the PRP or platelet concentrate stage by using a leukocyte reduction filter as described in Method 6-12.

Preparation of platelets from PRP begins with a soft spin of the WB to separate red cells from PRP, followed by separation and hard spin of the PRP to concentrate platelets. This is done either manually or using an automated sequence of steps in recently developed systems. Plasma for further processing is removed from the platelet pellet, which is held undisturbed for 30 to 60 minutes before being resuspended.[74]

The buffy-coat method is employed in many regions but is not currently cleared in the United States. In short, non-leukocyte-reduced WB units are first centrifuged under a high g-force (ie, hard or heavy spin), and plasma, red cells, and buffy coats are removed for further processing. Buffy coats from 4 or 5 units are pooled with 1 unit of plasma and then centrifuged under a low g-force (ie, soft or light spin) to separate the platelet concentrate for additional processing, such as leukocyte reduction. These processes are often associated with extended holding of the WB and buffy coats for 8 to 24 hours at 20 to 24 C.[75] Hold times are generally adjusted to ease the operational logistics for the blood center. Compared to the PRP preparation method, the buffy-coat method yields more plasma, greater red cell loss, better initial white blood cell (WBC) reduction before filtration, and moderate reduction in viable bacteria in the platelets that interact with leukocytes. An automated system is available in Europe that performs multiple functions to prepare pooled platelet concentrates derived from WB by the buffy-coat method. Steps that are automated include pooling, rinsing, centrifugation, transfer, filtration, and sealing.

Apheresis Platelets

Apheresis is used to obtain platelets from volunteer donors, patients' family members, or donors with HLA- or platelet-antigen-compatible phenotypes. By design, apheresis procedures are intended to collect large numbers of platelets from an individual, thereby providing a more potent product with fewer donor exposures for the patient. AABB *Standards* requires that an apheresis platelet component contain at least 3×10^{11} platelets in 90% of sampled units.[4(p30)]

With newer technology and more efficient processes, higher yields of platelets may be obtained from one donor, and the original apheresis unit may be split into multiple units, each of which must meet minimum standards. Some instruments are programmed to calculate the platelet yield based on the donor's hematocrit, platelet count, height, and weight. For apheresis collections, FDA guidelines require a periodic review of donor records to monitor platelet counts.[10]

For alloimmunized patients who do not respond to WB-derived allogeneic platelets, transfusions of platelets from an apheresis donor selected by a compatible platelet crossmatch or HLA match may be the only way to achieve a satisfactory posttransfusion platelet increment. In the United States, the use of apheresis platelets has been steadily increasing over the past 25 years. It is estimated that 93% of platelets transfused in the United States are apheresis platelets.[76]

Apheresis platelets can also be volume reduced during the collection. In early trials, collection of apheresis platelets in approximately 60-mL volumes showed good in-vitro platelet characteristics and function. In-vivo autologous recovery was at least equivalent to that of control apheresis platelets at standard concentrations when the storage time of 1, 2, or 5 days was adjusted based on the platelet concentration.[77,78] A volume reduction from 250 mL to 90 mL by centrifugation has been shown to cause a mild increase in platelet activation and an impaired aggregation response to adenosine diphosphate but not to collagen. In these experiments, the platelet count before the volume reduction was 1.0×10^9/mL, and after reduction, 1.9×10^9/mL.[79]

Recent developments include refinements in collection protocols for apheresis instruments that result in the collection of platelets in a high concentration, which may, therefore, obviate the need for volume reduction. Platelet collections have reached concentrations as high as 3.0 to 4.0×10^9/L.[77,79] Furthermore, the highly concentrated platelets may be suspended in a platelet additive solution with autologous plasma at a ratio of 5:1 to 3:1. Platelet units prepared in this manner contain much lower amounts of plasma compared to standard apheresis platelets.[80] Recently, the FDA has approved platelet additive solutions for apheresis platelets, decreasing the amount of plasma.

Donor Selection and Monitoring

Plateletpheresis donors may donate more frequently than WB donors but must meet all of the other criteria for WB donation. The interval between donations should be at least 2 days, and donors should not undergo plateletpheresis more than twice in a week or 24 times in a rolling 12-month period.[4(p20)] If a unit of WB is collected or if it becomes impossible to return the donor's red cells during plateletpheresis, at least 8 weeks should elapse before a subsequent plateletpheresis procedure unless the red cell ECV is <100 mL. Platelets may be collected more frequently from donors if there is exceptional medical need for a specific

recipient and the blood center's responsible physican determines that the health of the donor will not be adversely affected by the collection. Donors who have taken antiplatelet medications that irreversibly inhibit platelet function are deferred for specific intervals before donation (48 hours for aspirin/aspirin-containing medications and piroxicam, 14 days for clopidogrel and ticlopidine) because apheresis platelets are often the sole source of platelets given to a patient.[4(p61)]

A platelet count is not required before the first apheresis collection; however, triple collections of platelets may not be drawn from first-time donors unless a qualifying platelet count is obtained on a sample collected before the procedure. AABB *Standards* permits qualification of a donor with a platelet count from a sample collected immediately before the procedure or one obtained either before or after the previous procedure.[4(p21)] Exceptions to these laboratory criteria should be approved in writing by the apheresis program physician based on documented medical need.

It is possible to collect plasma concurrently with platelets. The FDA specifies that the total volume of plasma collected should be no more than 500 mL (or 600 mL for donors weighing more than 175 lb) or the volume described in the labeling of the automated blood cell separator device (which may be more or less than the 500-mL or 600-mL volume previously mentioned). The platelet count of each unit should be kept on record but need not be written on the component label. Units containing <3.0×10^{11} platelets should be labeled with the actual platelet count.[10]

Devices for Platelet Apheresis Collection

TerumoBCT (COBE) Spectra. The Spectra uses a dual-stage (different radius) channel to collect leukocyte-reduced platelets. Leukocyte reduction to <5×10^6 WBCs can be obtained in approximately 80% of the collections for software versions that are lower than 5.0.[81] Use of software versions 5.0 and 7.0 can more consistently result in the collection of components containing <1.0×10^6 WBCs with the leukocyte-reduction system (LRS), which uses a cone in the centrifuge and saturated, fluidized, particle-bed filter technology to remove residual WBCs leaving the second stage of the channel.[82-86] The Spectra is capable of single- or double-access procedures. The ECV of the single-access kit is 361 mL, and that of the double-access kit is 272 mL. The Spectra is being replaced by the more efficient Trima or Trima Accel.[34]

TerumoBCT Trima and Trima Accel. The TerumoBCT Trima (version 4) uses a smaller, modified, dual-stage channel and LRS cone to consistently collect leukocyte-reduced platelets ($<1.0 \times 10^6$ WBCs). To increase platelet yields, the Trima Accel (versions 5.0, 5.01, and 5.1) uses a single-stage, doughnut-shaped channel and larger LRS cone to consistently collect leukocyte-reduced platelets.[87] The Trimas use single-access kits only. The ECV of the Trimas is 182 to 196 mL. They are capable of collecting single, double, or triple units of apheresis platelets as well as concurrent plasma and red cells, depending on donor size, platelet count, and hematocrit.[36,87,88]

Fenwal Amicus. The Amicus is capable of collecting single, double, or triple apheresis platelets as well as concurrent plasma and red cells (single-access kit only), depending on the donor's size, platelet count, and hematocrit.[82,83,88,89] The Amicus uses centrifugal force and a double compartment belt wrapped around a spool to separate the platelets. Platelets accumulate in the collection chamber and are transferred to the final collection bags at the end of the procedure. The Amicus is capable of single- or double-access procedures. The ECV of the single- and double-access kits is approximately 210 mL. The ECV of the WB bag is adjustable. Consistent leukocyte reduction is accomplished without external filtration, and this process is approved by the FDA for submission of a Prior Approval Supplement.

Haemonetics MCS+ LN9000. The Haemonetics MCS+ LN9000 system uses the Latham conical bowl, plasma-controlled hematocrit, and plasma surge technique to accumulate platelets and float them off the bowl with rapid plasma infusion. Although this technique results in leukocyte-reduced platelets, the use of an inline leukocyte reduction filter ensures consistency in leukocyte reduction.[41,82,90-92] The LN9000 uses a single-access kit, and the ECV ranges from 480 mL (38% hematocrit) to 359 mL (52% hematocrit). The LN9000 is capable of collecting single, double, or triple units of apheresis platelets as well as concurrent plasma, depending on donor size and platelet count.[41,82,90-92]

Granulocytes

The use of granulocyte transfusions has been controversial for a number of years. Analysis of randomized controlled trials of granulocyte transfusions in adults and children has indicated that there is insufficient evidence to determine whether granulocyte transfusions affect all-cause mortality.[93]

Agents Administered to Increase Yields

AABB *Standards* requires that 75% of granulocyte components contain at least 1×10^{10} granulocytes,[4(p30)] although the optimal therapeutic dose in adult patients is unknown. For infants and children, a dose of 10 to 15 mL/kg may provide an adequate number of granulocytes per dose. To collect this number of cells in a unit of granulocytes, drugs or sedimenting materials are typically administered to the donor. Sedimenting agents enhance granulocyte harvest by increasing sedimentation of the red cells, thereby enhancing the interface in the collection device and resulting in minimal red cell content in the final product. The donor's consent to the procedure must provide permission for any of these drugs or sedimenting agents to be used.

Hydroxyethyl Starch. A common sedimenting agent, hydroxyethyl starch (HES) causes red cells to aggregate, thereby sedimenting them more completely. Because HES can be detected in donors as long as a year after infusion, AABB *Standards* requires facilities performing granulocyte collections to have a process to control the maximum cumulative dose of any sedimenting agent administered to a donor within a given interval.[4(p23)] HES is a colloid that acts as a volume expander. Donors who receive HES may experience headaches or peripheral edema because of expanded circulatory volume. A boxed warning from the FDA exists for its use, as a result of increased mortality and severe renal injury in certain patient populations, although HES has a low-risk adverse-event profile for granulocyte donors, and only a few adverse events that were minor in intensity have been attributed to HES in recipients.[94,95]

Corticosteroids. Corticosteroids can double the number of circulating granulocytes by mobilizing granulocytes from the marginal pool. The common protocol is to use 60 mg of oral prednisone in a single or divided dose before donation to collect large numbers of granulocytes with minimal systemic steroid activity. Another protocol uses 8 mg of oral dexamethasone. Donors should be questioned about their relevant medical history before they use systemic corticosteroids. Hypertension, diabetes, cataracts, or peptic ulcers can be relative or absolute contraindications to corticosteroid use.

Growth Factors. Although not a licensed indication, granulocyte colony-stimulating factor (G-CSF) can effectively increase granulocyte yields. Hematopoietic growth factors given alone can result in the collection of up to 4 to 8 × 10^{10} granulocytes per apheresis procedure. Typical doses of G-CSF are 5 to 10 µg/kg given 8 to 12 hours before granulocyte collection. Preliminary evidence suggests that invivo recovery and survival of these granulocytes are excellent and that growth factors are well tolerated by donors.

Laboratory Testing

Testing for ABO group, Rh type, red cell antibodies, and infectious disease markers is required on a sample drawn at the time of phlebotomy. Red cell content in granulocyte components is inevitable; the red cells should be ABO compatible with the recipient's plasma. If >2 mL of red cells are present, the component should be crossmatched for Rh and HLA compatibility.[4(pp37-38),26(p27)]

Storage and Infusion

Granulocyte function deteriorates rapidly during storage, and concentrates should be transfused as soon as possible after preparation. AABB *Standards* mandates a storage temperature of 20 to 24 C for no longer than 24 hours.[4(p55)] Agitation during storage is undesirable. Irradiation is required for components to be administered to immunodeficient recipients and is indicated for nearly all recipients because their primary diseases are likely to involve deficiencies in their immune systems. Use of a microaggregate or leukocyte reduction filter is contraindicated because it removes the collected granulocytes.

Apheresis Devices for Granulocyte Collection

TerumoBCT (COBE) Spectra. The Spectra is capable of collecting granulocytes.[34,96,97] It uses a doughnut-shaped, single-stage channel in the centrifuge to isolate the granulocytes that are continuously collected in the final storage bag. It uses a double-access kit only, and its ECV is 285 mL.

TerumoBCT Spectra Optia. The Spectra Optia system (not to be confused with the Spectra system above), used mainly for therapeutic apheresis procedures, has recently been approved for granulocyte collections.[98] Its ECV is 191 mL, as it is modified from the mononuclear cell (MNC) protocol.

Fresenius AS 104. The Fresenius AS 104 (Fresenius Kabi, Bad Homburg, Germany) is capable of collecting several components, including granulocytes.[34,99] It uses a doughnut-shaped, single-stage channel to separate the granulocytes. The granulocytes build up in the centrifuge and are harvested into the final collection bag intermittently. The AS 104 uses a double-access kit, and its ECV is 175 mL.

Haemonetics MCS+ LN9000. The LN9000 can also be used to collect granulocytes. It uses the conical Latham bowl for separation, and the buffy coat is then transferred to one of two bags. The red cells settle to the bottom of the bag before being returned to the donor. The LN9000 switches from one bag to another to return the red cells. A single- or double-access kit can be used for granulocyte collection, and the ECV ranges, based on the hematocrit of the donor, from 480 mL (38% hematocrit) to 359 mL (52% hematocrit).

BLOOD COMPONENT MODIFICATION

Methods and devices are available to process WB or components in a variety of manners for leukocyte reduction, irradiation to prevent GVHD, and pathogen reduction.

Container System Modification by Sterile Connecting Device

Blood containers may be modified by using a sterile connecting device cleared or approved by the appropriate regulatory body for that purpose.[100] The use of approved sterile connecting devices maintains a functionally closed system when various connections are performed, such as pooling or sampling, thereby maintaining the component's original expiry date. FDA-approved indications for the use of a sterile connecting device are presented in Table 6-8. Sterile connecting devices are primarily used to obtain an apheresis platelet sample for bacteria detection, to attach a leukocyte reduction filter to prepare prestorage leukocyte-reduced (LR) RBCs and platelets, to prepare prestorage pooled platelets and pooled cryoprecipitate, and to aid in splitting triple platelet apheresis units. Recently available computer software permits tracking of lot numbers (eg, for wafers, bags, and filters) and product codes, as well as other steps that involve the scanning of bar codes.

Prestorage Leukocyte Reduction by Filtration

Blood collection systems may also include in-line filters for removal of leukocytes from WB, RBC units, and/or platelets. Many WB leuko-

TABLE 6-8. Use of Sterile Connecting Devices for Modification of Collection Containers[100]

Use	Comment
To add a new or smaller needle to a blood collection set	If a needle is added during the procedure, an approved device to weld liquid-filled tubing should be used.
To prepare components	Examples include adding a fourth bag to make cryoprecipitate, adding solution to the RBC unit, or adding an in-line filter.
To pool blood products	Appropriate use of a sterile connecting device to pool platelets prepared from whole blood collection may obviate potential contamination from the spike and port entries commonly used.
To prepare an aliquot for pediatric use and divided units	FDA provides specific guidance if this activity is considered to involve manufacturing of new products.
To connect additional saline or anticoagulant lines during an automated plasmapheresis procedure	SOPs are required, although prior approval from the FDA is not required.
To attach processing solutions	Examples include washing and freezing RBCs.
To add an FDA-cleared leukocyte reduction filter	The purpose is to prepare prestorage leukocyte-reduced RBCs.
To remove samples from blood product containers for testing	The label may need revision if the product's cell count is affected.

RBC = Red Blood Cell; FDA = Food and Drug Administration; SOPs = standard operating procedures.

cyte reduction systems allow filtration at ambient temperature beginning soon after collection and lasting up to 24 hours. WB filtration may also be started and/or completed at refrigerator temperatures. The FDA requires that there be <5.0 × 10⁶ residual leukocytes per unit for LR RBCs. The Council of Europe requires that the residual number be <1 × 10⁶ per unit. In the United States, leukocyte reduction by filtration of RBCs should result in a component that contains at least 85% of the original red cell content. The Council of Europe's standards require a minimum of 40 g of hemoglobin to be present in each unit after leukocyte reduction.[8]

Prestorage leukocyte reduction is generally performed soon after WB collection and is always performed within 5 days of collection. In-line WB filters are available in collection sets that permit preparation of LR RBCs and FFP. WB filters that spare platelets are now available as well. If WB is collected without the in-line leukocyte reduction filter, a filter can be attached to the tubing by an FDA-cleared sterile connecting device. The number of platelets in LR platelet concentrates is generally lower than in non-LR platelet concentrates.

Sickle cell trait in red cells is the most common cause of filter failure. Approximately 50% of the RBC units with sickle cell trait fail to filter. Although the other 50% pass through the filter, the residual leukocyte content may be higher than allowable limits.[101]

AABB *Standards* requires that 95% of LR platelet units contain <8.3 × 10⁵ leukocytes, at least 75% of units contain ≥5.5 × 10¹⁰ platelets, and at least 90% of units have a pH ≥6.2 at the end of the allowable storage period.[4(p29)] The number in the Council of Europe's standards is <0.2 × 10⁶ residual leukocytes per unit of platelets from WB.[8]

Methods that measure residual leukocytes include Nageotte hemocytometry and flow cytometry. In a multicenter study, flow cytometry gave better results than Nageotte hemocytometry when freshly prepared samples (within 24 hours) were tested. In general, Nageotte hemocytometry tends to underestimate the number of white cells compared to flow cytometry.[102] A new semiautomated methodology offers to reduce the technical burden associated with both Nageotte and flow cytometry methods.[103]

Irradiation

Cellular blood components can be irradiated for prevention of transfusion-associated GVHD. The irradiation sources in use include gamma rays—from either cesium-137 or cobalt-60 sources—or x-rays produced by radiation therapy linear accelerators or standalone units. Both sources achieve satisfactory results in rendering T lymphocytes inactive. Freestanding irradiators are commercially available for blood bank use. The US Nuclear Regulatory Commission requires increased security measures to reduce the risk of unauthorized use of radioactive materials for gamma irradiators.[104] The licensee is required to secure any area where radioactive source is present and limit access to irradiations to only approved individuals.

In the United States, the radiation dose targeted to the midplane of the container must be at least 25 gray (Gy) [2500 centigray (cGy)] and no more than 50 Gy (5000 cGy).[105] Moreover, the minimum delivered dose to any portion of the blood components must be at least 15 Gy in a fully loaded canister.[4(p25)] The European standard requires a higher dose, with no part of the component receiving <25 Gy and a maximum dose to any part of the component of 50 Gy.[8] Both US and European standards are effective for prevention of GVHD.

Each instrument must be routinely monitored to ensure that an adequate dose is delivered to the container that houses the blood components during irradiation. Dose mapping using irradiation-sensitive films or badges that monitor the delivered dose are used for QC of the irradiators.[104] FDA regulations require verification of the delivered dose annually for the cesium-137 source and semiannually for the cobalt-60 source. For x-ray irradiators, the dosimetry should be performed in accordance with the manufacturer's recommendations. Dose verification is also required after major repairs or relocation of the irradiator. For gamma irradiators, the turntable opera-

tion, timing device, and lengthening of irradiation time caused by source decay should also
be monitored periodically.

Another important quality assurance step
is the demonstration that the component that
was irradiated received the desired amount of
irradiation. For that reason, irradiation-
sensitive labels are used to demonstrate that
irradiation of each batch of units was accomplished; this is a requirement in Europe.[8]

In the United States, RBCs may be irradiated up to the end of their storage shelf life.
The postirradiation expiration date is 28 days
or the original expiration date, whichever is
earlier. In Europe, RBCs may be irradiated only
up to day 28 following collection, and irradiated cells may not be stored longer than the earlier of 14 days after irradiation or 28 days after
collection. Platelets may be irradiated until
their expiration date, and their postirradiation
expiration date is the same as the original expiration date.

Irradiation of RBCs followed by storage
does result in a decrease in the percentage of
recovery after transfusion. In addition, an increased efflux of potassium from red cells
causes the potassium levels to rise approximately twofold compared to nonirradiated
units. For most adult and child recipients, the
increased potassium in irradiated RBC units
poses no risk. However, with neonatal and rapid transfusions of small children, high potassium levels may cause heartbeat complications,[106,107] prompting the usage of shorter-
stored or washed irradiated RBCs. Platelets are
not damaged by an irradiation dose as high as
50 Gy.[108]

Pooling

Platelets that are pooled have an expiration
time of 4 hours from when the system was
opened for pooling. A closed system for
prestorage pooling of platelets has been licensed by the FDA. This system permits the
storage of pooled platelets for up to 5 days
from the time of WB collection. Four to 6 LR or
non-LR platelet units that are ABO identical
can be pooled using a set consisting of a mul-
tilead tubing manifold for sterile connection.

If non-LR units are pooled, they are then filtered as part of the pooling process. The short-
est expiration date of the pooled units determines the expiration date of the pool.

In the United States, each pool prepared
from LR platelets must have $<5.0 \times 10^6$ residual
leukocytes. The approved pooling set also allows sampling of the pool for bacteria detection. A record of the unique DIN for each individual member of the pool must be available.
The pool must be labeled with the approximate total volume, ABO/Rh type of the units in
the pool, and number of units in the pool. An
Rh-positive unit in a pool containing Rh-
negative units is labeled as Rh positive.

Many countries in Europe prepare
prestorage pools of buffy-coat platelets that
are preserved in platelet additive solution or in
the plasma from one of the units from which
platelets are prepared.[109] Instruments that au-
tomate the pooling process are increasingly
used in Europe. In a few countries in Europe,
systems for prestorage pooling of buffy-coat-
derived platelets followed by pathogen inactivation treatment have become available. The
latter systems are not yet licensed by the FDA.

Cryoprecipitated AHF units may be
pooled immediately before transfusion in an
"open" system; the pool has an expiration time
of 4 hours at 20 to 24 C storage. Prestorage
pools can also be prepared in an "open" system and stored for 12 months at –18 C as described in Method 6-11. After thawing, the
component expires in 4 hours. Prestorage
pools prepared with the use of an FDA-cleared
sterile connecting device are stored for 12
months at –18 C; postthaw expiration time is 6
hours. The number of units pooled may vary
and can consist of 4, 5, 6, 8, or 10 units.
Prestorage pools must be placed in a freezer
within 1 hour. The potency of the pool is calculated by assuming that each unit in the pool
contains 80 IU of coagulation Factor VIII and
150 mg of fibrinogen multiplied by the number of units in the pool. If normal saline is used
to rinse the bags during preparation of the
pool, the amount of saline in the pool must be
stated on the label.

Volume Reduction (WB Platelets)

Volume-reduced platelets may be needed for patients in whom a reduced amount of plasma is desired to prevent cardiac overload, to minimize ABO antibody infusion, or for intrauterine transfusion. Method 6-13 describes volume reduction by centrifugation. Platelet concentrate volume can be reduced to 10 to 15 mL/unit just before transfusion. In-vitro properties such as platelet morphology, mean volume, hypotonic shock response, synergistic aggregation, and platelet factor 3 activity appear to be maintained when volume reduction is performed on storage day 5, and platelet increments after transfusion have been satisfactory.[110] The in-vitro recovery rate of platelets is about 85% after the volume-reduction step. Platelets from WB that are volume reduced by centrifugation ($580 \times g$ for 20 minutes) from an approximate volume of 60 mL to between 35 and 40 mL yield a high platelet count ($>2.3 \times 10^9$/L).[111] Lowering the pH of platelets prepared from WB avoids platelet aggregates visible to the unaided eye (macroaggregates).[112] The addition of 10% ACD-A to platelets to lower the pH before centrifugation can help with resuspension of high-concentration platelets and avoid aggregation. If an open system is used, the maximum allowable storage time is 4 hours. The maximum allowable storage time has not been established for closed systems. However, the overall in-vivo survival data for volume-reduced platelets are limited.

Pathogen Inactivation

Plasma

Plasma can be treated to inactivate microbial agents by pathogen inactivation. Two methods have been cleared by the FDA [solvent/detergent and amotosalen/ultraviolet A (UVA) light], and four methods are CE (Council of Europe)-marked in Europe [methylene blue, psoralen (amotosalen), riboflavin, and solvent/detergent].

Methylene blue (approximately 0.085 mg/unit of plasma) can be added to thawed FFP, followed by activation using white light. After removal of methylene blue with a filter (residual concentration: 0.3 µM), plasma can be refrozen. Methylene-blue-treated plasma contains approximately 15% to 20% less Factor VIII and fibrinogen than untreated plasma.

Plasma prepared from WB or by apheresis can be treated with 150 µM amotosalen followed by illumination with 3.0 J/cm^2 UVA light (320-400 nm). After amotosalen is removed by exposing treated plasma to an adsorption device, the unit is frozen for storage at –18 C. Average activity values for coagulation and antithrombotic factors are reported to be within reference ranges for untreated plasma.

Plasma prepared by apheresis or from single WB units (volume range 170-360 mL) can be treated with the Mirasol system by adding 35 mL of riboflavin (vitamin B2) followed by illumination for 6 to 10 minutes. Immediately after illumination, the plasma can be released or frozen below –30 C for 2 years. Residual red cell levels up to 15×10^9 per liter have been qualified to result in successful pathogen and leukocyte inactivation. Coagulation and anticoagulation proteins are well preserved in plasma treated with the Mirasol system.[113,114]

Solvent/detergent-treated plasma (SD plasma) is prepared from a pool of plasma from many donors (630-1520) that is tested for parvovirus B19 DNA and hepatitis E virus RNA, and undergoes treatment with 1% tri-n-butyl phosphate and 1% Triton X-100 for pathogen inactivation. This treatment has been shown to significantly inactivate lipid-enveloped viruses. SD plasma is manufactured in facilities that can manage large-scale production rather than in blood centers. Each unit contains 200 mL of plasma that is stored frozen at –18 C with an expiration date of 12 months.[115] Most coagulation factors are reduced by approximately 10% in SD plasma, except for Factor VIII, which is reduced by 20%.[116] Also, levels of protein S and alpha$_2$-antiplasmin, which are labile to SD treatment, are controlled to ensure levels within the range of normal human plasma (≥0.4 IU/mL).[117] The product is labeled with the ABO blood group and, once thawed, should be used within 24 hours. SD plasma is available in Europe and has been recently approved in the United States.[118]

Platelets

Two photochemical methods and one light-alone platelet pathogen-inactivation method are currently CE-marked and used in some countries in Europe: 1) amotosalen and UVA light, 2) riboflavin and UV light, and 3) UVC illumination. The use of amotosalen and UVA light for pathogen inactivation of apheresis platelets suspended in additive solution has recently been cleared by the FDA. All methods target the nucleic acids of viruses, bacteria, and parasites, preventing their replication. Because platelets do not contain genomic nucleic acid, and intact mitochondrial DNA is not required for successful platelet storage, these techniques primarily target pathogens, although there is some evidence of small losses of platelet in-vitro properties and function.[119]

QUARANTINE

All units of blood collected should be immediately placed in quarantine in a designated area until donor information and donation records have been reviewed, the current donor information has been compared to the previous information, the donor's previous deferrals have been examined, and all laboratory testing has been completed.[120] Because of the limited amount of time after collection that is available for component separation, WB units may be separated into components before all of the earlier processes have been completed. Separated components are quarantined at the appropriate temperature until all of the suitability steps have been completed and reviewed. Often, physical and electronic quarantine are used simultaneously.

Certain blood components from previous donations by donors whose more recent donations test positive for infectious disease also require quarantine and appropriate disposition, as do units identified as unsuitable for transfusion because of postdonation information. Other components may need to be quarantined so that QC samples can be taken and analyzed. For instance, if a sample is obtained for bacteria detection, the component is held

in quarantine for some preset time and then released if the test results remain negative.

A thorough understanding of the quarantine process is needed to prevent erroneous release of unsuitable blood components. Components may be removed from the quarantine area, labeled, and released for distribution if all of the donor information, previous donor records, and current test results are satisfactory.

Some blood components require emergency release because they have a very short storage time. Such is the case for granulocytes. Emergency release requires physician approval and a label or tie tag to indicate that testing was incomplete at the time of release.

Despite the widespread use of software to control manufacturing processes, instances of failure resulting in the distribution of unsuitable components continue to be reported to the FDA. For example, during fiscal year 2014, the FDA received 49,699 reports of blood and plasma product deviations, including some related to quarantine. Of these reports, 4460 (9.0%) involved QC and distribution errors.[121]

LABELING

The FDA requirements for labeling of blood and components are available in several publications. The "Guideline for the Uniform Labeling of Blood and Blood Components" was published in 1985.[122] The FDA approved the International Society of Blood Transfusion (ISBT) 128 symbology, Version 1.2.0, in 2000, and Version 2.0.0 in 2006.[123] Detailed requirements are described in the CFR (Title 21, CFR Parts 606.120, 606.121, and 606.122). AABB *Standards* requires that accredited facilities label blood and blood component containers in accordance with the most recent version of the "United States Industry Consensus Standard for the Uniform Labeling of Blood and Blood Components Using ISBT 128."[4(p12)] Base labels and any additional labels that are placed directly on the container must use approved adhesives. In accordance with the 1985 FDA guideline, only those substances that are FDA approved as "indirect food additives" may be used in adhesives and coating components for labels placed over the base label.[121] The FDA has additional standards for labels that are applied directly on plastic blood containers. Tie tags may be used as an extension of the label if there is insufficient label space, particularly for informational items that do not have to be directly affixed to the container. National regulatory requirements should be verified when selecting labels and establishing labeling policies.

The FDA rule that requires all blood components to be labeled with a bar-coded label became effective on April 26, 2006. The rule requires that, at a minimum, the label contain the following bar-coded information: 1) the unique facility identifier (eg, registration number), 2) lot number relating to the donor, 3) product code, and 4) ABO group and Rh type of the donor. These pieces of information must be present in eye-readable and machine-readable format. The rule applies to blood establishments that collect and prepare blood components, including hospital transfusion services that perform manufacturing steps such as preparation of pooled cryoprecipitate and/or divided units or aliquots of RBCs, platelets, and plasma for pediatric use.

Another major part of labeling in the United States is the *Circular of Information,*[26] which must be made available to everyone involved in the transfusion of blood components. The *Circular* is produced by AABB, America's Blood Centers, the American Red Cross, and the Armed Services Blood Program and is recognized as acceptable by the FDA. The *Circular* provides important information about each blood component and should be consulted for information not included in this chapter.

Special message labels may also be affixed to blood component containers. The labels may include one or more of the following indications: 1) hold for further manufacturing, 2) for emergency use only, 3) for autologous use only, 4) not for transfusion, 5) irradiated, 6) biohazard, 7) from a therapeutic phlebotomy, and 8) screened for special factors [eg, HLA type or cytomegalovirus (CMV) antibody status]. ISBT 128 allows incorporation of special attributes of the component, such as CMV antibody status.

As mentioned above, additional information on the container can be conveyed using a tie tag. Tie tags are especially useful for autologous and directed donations. Tie tags include the patient's identifying information, name of the hospital where the patient will be admitted for surgery, date of surgery, and other information that may be helpful to the hospital transfusion service.

Each component must also bear a unique DIN that can be traced back to the blood donor. If components are pooled, a pool number must allow tracing to the individual units within a pool.

ISBT 128 is a requirement by AABB *Standards.* An important source of information is ICCBBA (formerly known as the International Council for Commonality in Blood Banking Automation). The ICCBBA website (iccbba.org) features updates and a revised list of product codes. In the future, ISBT 128 is expected to permit information transfer by radiofrequency ID tags or other means of electronic data transmission.

KEY POINTS

1. Modern blood containers are composed of soft plastic and identified by a lot number. They should be pyrogen free, flexible yet tough, and both kink and scratch resistant. During frozen storage, each plastic container has a glass-transition temperature below which it becomes brittle and susceptible to breakage during transportation.

2. The initial 35 to 45 mL of blood drawn is collected into a diversion pouch. The pouch reduces bacterial contamination of collected blood by diverting bacteria from the skin plug that may have otherwise entered the collection. Blood in this pouch may be used for laboratory tests.

3. The average rate of adverse donor reactions after donation is 3.5% to 5%. Most reactions are mild and require no further medical care. These reactions can be systemic (eg, fainting) or local (eg, hematoma). About 1 in 3700 donors experience a reaction after leaving the donation site and may need medical care. Deferral of low-blood-volume (<3.5 L) donors may be helpful in reducing the risk of reactions, especially in young donors.

4. During centrifugation for component preparation, primary variables that affect cell separation and cell recovery are rotor size, centrifuge speed, and duration. The platelet-rich plasma method is used in the United States for platelet concentrate preparation, and the buffy-coat method is more common in Canada and Europe.

5. Plasma components for transfusion can be prepared from WB (by manual or apheresis methods) or from apheresis and are defined by the manufacturing process.

6. Apheresis components must meet the same basic regulatory requirements (eg, donor consent, storage conditions, and transportation requirements) as WB-derived components, although more specific requirements also apply to each type of apheresis component collection.

7. The majority of platelets collected and transfused in the United States are apheresis platelets.

8. Several instruments and systems have been developed and/or adapted for apheresis collection of blood components, using different technologies. Some are appropriate for the collection of only one type of component, while others can collect multiple component types.

9. In multicomponent donations, various combinations of components may be collected with apheresis technology. Regulations specific to this practice apply to donor selection and monitoring, QC, and records. Red cells can be removed concurrently with other components, or a double RBC unit may be collected.

10. Granulocyte collection differs from that of other components. Specific techniques should be used and certain factors must be taken into consideration for the optimal collection of granulocytes by apheresis.

11. LR RBCs and platelets are not to exceed 5.0×10^6 residual WBCs per transfusion dose in the United States or 1.0×10^6 residual WBCs per transfusion dose in Europe.

12. For irradiated components, the radiation dose must be 25 to 50 Gy with a minimum delivered dose to any portion of the blood components of 15 Gy in the United States. RBCs may be irradiated up until the end of their storage shelf life; the postirradiation expiration date is 28 days after irradiation or the original expiration date, whichever is sooner. The European standard requires that no part of the component receive <25 Gy, a maximum dose to any part of the component of 50 Gy, and irradiation of RBCs only until day 28, with storage for no longer than 14 days after irradiation or 28 days after collection, whichever is earliest. Platelet shelf life is not reduced after irradiation.

13. Bar-coded and eye-readable container labels now use the ISBT symbology (ISBT 128), which allows identification of the manufacturer throughout the world, more product codes, better accuracy as a result of reduced misreads during scanning, and enhanced conveyance of other labeling information.

REFERENCES

1. Food and Drug Administation. Requirements for blood and blood components intended for transfusion or for further manufacturing use; final rule. (May 22, 2015) Fed Regist 2015;80:29841-906. [Available at https:// www.federalregister.gov/articles/2015/05/22/2015-12228/requirements-for-blood-and-blood-components-intended-for-transfusion-or-for-further-manufacturing (accessed January 30, 2017).]

2. Goldman M, Roy G, Fréchette N, et al. Evaluation of donor skin disinfection methods. Transfusion 1997;37:309-12.

3. Buchta C, Nedorost N, Regele H, et al. Skin plugs in phlebotomy puncture for blood donation. Wien Klin Wochenschr 2005;117:141-4.

4. Ooley PW, ed. Standards for blood banks and transfusion services. 30th ed. Bethesda, MD: AABB, 2016.

5. deKorte D, Curvers J, deKort WLAM, et al. Effects of skin disinfection method, deviation bag, and bacterial screening on clinical safety of platelet transfusions in the Netherlands. Transfusion 2006;46:476-85.

6. Button LN, Orlina AR, Kevy SV, Josephson AM. The quality of over- and undercollected blood for transfusion. Transfusion 1976;16: 148-54.

7. Davey RJ, Lenes BL, Casper AJ, Demets DL. Adequate survival of red cells from units "undercollected" in citrate-phosphate-dextrose-adenine-one. Transfusion 1984;24:319-22.

8. European Directorate for the Quality of Medicines and HealthCare. Guide to the preparation, use and quality assurance of blood components. 17th ed. Strasbourg, France: Council of Europe Publishing, 2013.

9. Food and Drug Administration. Guidance for industry: Recommendations for collecting red blood cells by automated apheresis methods. (January 30, 2001) Silver Spring, MD: CBER Office of Communication, Outreach, and Development, 2001. [Available at http://www.fda.gov/downloads/BiologicsBloodVaccines/GuidanceComplianceRegulatoryInformation/Guidances/Blood/ucm080764.pdf (accessed January 30, 2017).]

10. Food and Drug Administration. Guidance for industry and FDA review staff: Collection of platelets by automated methods. (December 17, 2007) Silver Spring, MD: CBER Office of Communication, Outreach, and Development, 2007. [Available at http://www.fda.gov/BiologicsBloodVaccines/GuidanceComplianceRegulatoryInformation/Guidances/Blood/ucm073382.htm (accessed January 30, 2017).]

11. Food and Drug Administration. Blood and blood components. Inspection of licensed and unlicensed blood banks, brokers, reference laboratories, and contractors—7342.001. In: Compliance Program guidance manual. Silver Spring, MD: CBER Office of Compliance and Biologics Quality, 2016. [Available at http://www.fda.gov/downloads/biologicsbloodvac cines/guidancecomplianceregulatoryinformation/complianceactivities/enforcement/complianceprograms/ucm337001.pdf (accessed January 30, 2017).]

12. Eder AF, Ky BA, Kennedy JM, Benjamin RJ. The ARC Hemovigilance Program: Advancing the safety of blood donation and transfusion. Immunohematol 2009;25:179-85.

13. Sorensen BS, Johnsen SP, Jorgensen J. Complications related to blood donation: A population-based study. Vox Sang 2008;94: 132-7.

14. Eder AF, Dy BA, Kennedy JM, et al. The American Red Cross donor hemovigilance program: Complications of blood donation reported in 2006. Transfusion 2008;48:1809-19.

15. Wiltbank TB, Giordano GE. The safety profile of automated collections: An analysis of more than 1 million collections. Transfusion 2007; 47:1002-5.

16. Newman BH. Blood donor complications after whole-blood donation. Curr Opin Hematol 2004;11:339-45.

17. Eder AF, Notari IV EP, Dodd RY. Do reactions after whole blood donation predict syncope on return donation? Transfusion 2012;52: 2570-6.

18. Rios JA, Fang J, Tu Y, et al, NHLBI Retrovirus Epidemiology Donor Study-II. The potential impact of selective donor deferrals based on estimated blood volume on vasovagal reactions and donor deferral rates. Transfusion 2010;50:1265-75.

19. Kamel H, Tomasulo P, Bravo M, et al. Delayed adverse reactions to blood donation. Transfusion 2010;50:556-65.

20. Pisciotto P, Sataro P, Blumberg N. Incidence of adverse reactions in blood donors taking antihypertensive medications. Transfusion 1982; 22:530-1.

21. Eder AF, Kiss JE. Adverse reactions and iron deficiency after blood donation. In: Simon TL, McCullough J, Snyder EL, et al, eds. Rossi's principles of transfusion medicine. 5th ed. Chichester, UK: John Wiley and Sons, 2016:43-57.

22. Food and Drug Administration. Fatalities reported to FDA following blood collection and transfusion: Annual summary for Fiscal Year 2014. Silver Spring, MD: CBER Office of Communication, Outreach, and Development, 2015. [Available at http://www.fda.gov/downloads/BiologicsBloodVaccines/SafetyAvail ability/ReportaProblem/TransfusionDona

tionFatalities/UCM459461.pdf (accessed January 30, 2017).]

23. Nessen SC, Eastridge BJ, Cronk D, et al. Fresh whole blood use by forward surgical teams in Afghanistan is associated with improved survival compared to component therapy without platelets. Transfusion 2013;53(Suppl):107S-13S.

24. Högman CF, Knutson F, Lööf H. Storage of whole blood before separation: The effect of temperature on red cell 2,3-DPG and the accumulation of lactate. Transfusion 1999;39:492-7.

25. Code of federal regulations. Title 21, CFR Part 610.40. Washington, DC: US Government Publishing Office, 2017 (revised annually).

26. AABB, American Red Cross, America's Blood Centers, Armed Services Blood Program. Circular of information for the use of human blood and blood components. (September 2017) Bethesda, MD: AABB, 2017. [Available at https://www.aabb.org/tm/coi/Documents/coi0917.pdf.]

27. Simmchen J, Ventura R, Segura J. Progress in the removal of di-[2-ethylhexyl]-phthalate as plasticizer in blood bags. Transfus Med Rev 2012;26:27-37.

28. Sparrow RL. Time to revisit red blood cell additive solutions and storage conditions: A role for "omics" analyses. Blood Transfus 2012; 10(Suppl 2):s7-11.

29. Janatpour KA, Paglieroni TG, Crocker VL, et al. Visual assessment of hemolysis in red blood cell units and segments can be deceptive. Transfusion 2004;44:984-9.

30. Kim DM, Brecher ME, Bland LA, et al. Visual identification of bacterially contaminated red cells. Transfusion 1992;32:221-5.

31. European Union. Commission Directive 2004/33/EC of 22 March 2004 implementing Directive 2002/98/EC of the European Parliament and of the Council as regards certain technical requirements for blood and blood components. 30.3.2004. Official Journal of the European Union 2004;91:25-39. [Available at http://eur-lex.europa.eu/legal-content/EN/TXT/?qid=1485766671528&uri=CELEX:32004L0033 (accessed January 30, 2017).]

32. Högman CF, Meryman HT. Red blood cells intended for transfusion: Quality criteria revisited. Transfusion 2006;46:137-42.

33. Smith JW. Blood component collection by apheresis. In: Fung MK, Grossman BJ, Hillyer CD, Westhoff CM, eds. Technical manual. 18th ed. Bethesda, MD: AABB, 2014:167-78.

34. Burgstaler EA. Blood component collection by apheresis. J Clin Apher 2006;21:142-51.

35. Elfath MD, Whitley P, Jacobson MS, et al. Evaluation of an automated system for the collection of packed RBCs, platelets, and plasma. Transfusion 2000;40:1214-22.

36. Picker SM, Radojska SM, Gathof BS. Prospective evaluation of double RBC collection using three different apheresis systems. Transfus Apher Sci 2006;35:197-205.

37. Snyder EL, Elfath MD, Taylor H, et al. Collection of two units of leukoreduced RBCs from a single donation with a portable multiple-component collection system. Transfusion 2003;43:1695-705.

38. Moog R, Frank V, Müller N. Evaluation of a concurrent multicomponent collection system for the collection and storage of WBC-reduced RBC apheresis concentrates. Transfusion 2001;41:1159-64.

39. Nussbaumer W, Grabmer C, Maurer M, et al. Evaluation of a new mobile two unit red cell apheresis system (abstract). J Clin Apher 2006; 21:20.

40. Smith JW. Automated donations: Plasma, red cells, and multicomponent donor procedures. In: McLeod BC, Szczepiorkowski ZM, Weinstein R, Winters JL, eds. Apheresis: Principles and practice. 3rd ed. Bethesda, MD: AABB Press, 2010:125-40.

41. Rose C, Ragusa M, Andres M, et al. Evaluation of the MCS+ LN9000 in-line leukoreduction filter (abstract). Transfusion 1996;36(Suppl):85.

42. Valeri CR, Ragno G, Pivacek LE, et al. A multicenter study of in vitro and in vivo values in human RBCs frozen with 40-percent (wt/vol) glycerol and stored after deglycerolization for 15 days at 4°C in AS-3: Assessment of RBC processing in the ACP 215. Transfusion 2001;41:933-9.

43. Valeri CR, Pivacek LE, Cassidy GP, Ragno G. The survival, function, and hemolysis of human RBCs stored at 4°C in additive solution (AS-1, AS-3, or AS-5) for 42 days and then biochemically modified, frozen, thawed, washed, and stored at 4°C in sodium chloride and glucose solution for 24 hours. Transfusion 2000;40:1341-5.

44. TRALI risk mitigation for plasma and whole blood for transfusion. Association bulletin #14-02. Bethesda, MD: AABB, 2014.

45. Roth WK. Quarantine Plasma: Quo vadis? Transfus Med Hemother 2010;37:118-22.

46. Smak Gregoor PJH, Harvey MS, Briet E, Brand A. Coagulation parameters of CPD fresh-frozen plasma and CPD cryoprecipitate-poor plasma after storage at 4 C for 28 days. Transfusion 1993;33:735-8.

47. Yarraton H, Lawrie AS, Mackie IJ, et al. Coagulation factor levels in cryosupernatant prepared from plasma treated with amotosalen hydrochloride (S-59) and ultraviolet A light. Transfusion 2005;45:1453-8.

48. Code of federal regulations. Title 21, CFR Part 640, Subpart G. Washington, DC: US Government Publishing Office, 2017 (revised annually).

49. Hood M, Mynderup N, Doxon L. Evaluation of Haemonetics PCS-2 and Fenwal Auto-C plasmapheresis collection systems (abstract). J Clin Apher 1996;11:99.

50. Burkhardt T, Kappelsberger C, Karl M. Evaluation of a new combined centrifugation/filtration method for the collection of plasma via plasmapheresis (abstract). Transfusion 2001; 41(Suppl):50S.

51. Burnouf T, Kappelsberger C, Frank K, Burkhardt T. Protein composition and activation markers in plasma collected by three apheresis procedures. Transfusion 2003;43:1223-30.

52. Burnouf T, Kappelsberger C, Frank K, Burkhardt T. Residual cell content in plasma produced by three apheresis procedures. Transfusion 2003;43:1522-6.

53. Ness PM, Perkins HA. Fibrinogen in cryoprecipitate and its relationship to factor VIII (AHF) levels. Transfusion 1980;20:93-6.

54. Callum JL, Karkouti K, Yulia L. Cryoprecipitate: The current state of knowledge. Transfus Med Rev 2009;23:177-88.

55. Farrugia A, Prowse C. Studies on the procurement of blood coagulation factor VIII: Effects of plasma freezing rate and storage conditions on cryoprecipitate quality. J Clin Pathol 1985; 122:686-92.

56. Scott EA, Puca KE, Pietz BC, et al. Analysis of ADAMTS13 activity in plasma products using a modified FRETS-VWF73 assay (abstract). Blood 2005;106(Suppl):165a.

57. Smith JK, Bowell PJ, Bidwell E, Gunson HH. Anti-A haemagglutinins in factor VIII concentrates. J Clin Pathol 1980;33:954-7.

58. Pesquera-Lepatan LM, Hernandez FG, Lim RD, Chua MN. Thawed cryoprecipitate stored for 6 h at room temperature: A potential alternative to factor VIII concentrate for continuous infusion. Haemophilia 2004;10:684-8.

59. Variables involved in cryoprecipitate production and their effect on factor VIII activity. Report of a working party of the Regional Transfusion Directors Committee. Br J Haematol 1979;43:287-95.

60. Murphy S, Gardner FH. Platelet preservation. Effect of storage temperature on maintenance of platelet viability—Deleterious effect of refrigerated storage. N Engl J Med 1969;280: 1094-8.

61. Dumont LJ, Gulliksson H, van der Meer PF, et al. Interruption of agitation of platelet concentrates: A multicenter in vitro study by the BEST Collaborative on the effects of shipping platelets. Transfusion 2007;47:1666-73.

62. Dumont LJ, AuBuchon JP, Gulliksson H, et al. In vitro pH effects on in vivo recovery and survival of platelets: An analysis by the BEST Collaborative. Transfusion 2006;46:1300-5.

63. Wagner SJ, Vassallo R, Skripchenko A, et al. The influence of simulated shipping conditions (24- or 30-hr interruption of agitation) on the in vitro properties of apheresis platelets during 7-day storage. Transfusion 2008;48: 1072-80.

64. McDonald CP, Roy A, Mahajan P, et al. Relative values of the interventions of diversion and improved donor-arm disinfection to reduce the bacterial risk from blood transfusion. Vox Sang 2004;86:178-82.

65. Berseus O, Högman CF, Johansson A. Simple method of improving the quality of platelet concentrates and the importance of production control. Transfusion 1978;18:333-8.

66. Welch M, Champion AB. The effect of temperature and mode of agitation on the resuspension of platelets during preparation of platelet concentrates. Transfusion 1985;25:283-5.

67. Moroff G, George VM. The maintenance of platelet properties upon limited discontinuation of agitation during storage. Transfusion 1990;30: 427-30.

68. Gottschall JL, Rzad L, Aster RH. Studies of the minimum temperature at which human platelets can be stored with full maintenance of viability. Transfusion 1986;26:460-2.

69. Moroff G, Holme S, George VM, Heaton WA. Effect on platelet properties of exposure to temperatures below 20 degrees C for short periods during storage at 20 to 24 degrees C. Transfusion 1994;34:317-21.

70. Reiss RF, Katz AJ. Optimizing recovery of platelets in platelet-rich plasma by the Simplex strategy. Transfusion 1976;16:370-4.

71. Holme S, Heaton WA, Moroff G. Evaluation of platelet concentrates stored for 5 days with reduced plasma volume. Transfusion 1994;34:39-43.

72. Ali AM, Warkentin TE, Bardossy L, et al. Platelet concentrates stored for 5 days in a reduced volume of plasma maintain hemostatic function and viability. Transfusion 1994;34:44-7.

73. Food and Drug Administration. Pall Acrodose PL System. (January 26, 2006) Silver Spring, MD: CBER Office of Communication, Outreach, and Development, 2015. [Available at http://www.fda.gov/BiologicsBloodVaccines/BloodBloodProducts/ApprovedProducts/SubstantiallyEquivalent510kDeviceInformation/ucm080918.htm (accessed January 30, 2017).]

74. Levin E, Culibrk B, Gyongyossy-Issa MI, et al. Implementation of buffy coat platelet component production: Comparison to platelet-rich plasma platelet production. Transfusion 2008; 48:2331-7.

75. Pérez-Pujol S, Lozano M, Perea D, et al. Effect of holding buffy coats 4 or 18 hours before preparing pooled filtered PLT concentrates in plasma. Transfusion 2004;44:202-9.

76. Whitaker BI, Rajbhandary S, Harris A. The 2013 AABB blood collection, utilization, and patient blood management survey report. (December 18, 2015) Bethesda, MD: AABB, 2015. [Available at http://www.aabb.org/research/hemovigilance/bloodsurvey/Pages/default.aspx (accessed January 30, 2017).]

77. Dumont LJ, Krailadsiri P, Seghatchian J, et al. Preparation and storage characteristics of white-cell-reduced high-concentration platelet concentrates collected by an apheresis system for transfusion in utero. Transfusion 2000;40:91-100.

78. Dumont LJ, Beddard R, Whitley P, et al. Autologous transfusion recovery of WBC-reduced high-concentration platelet concentrates. Transfusion 2002;42:1333-9.

79. Schoenfeld H, Muhm M, Doepfmer UR, et al. The functional integrity of platelets in volume-reduced platelet concentrates. Anesth Analg 2005;100:78-81.

80. Ringwald J, Walz S, Zimmerman R, et al. Hyperconcentrated platelets stored in additive solution: Aspects of productivity and in vitro quality. Vox Sang 2005;89:11-18.

81. Valbonesi AM, Florio G, Venturino V, Bruni R. Plateletpheresis: What's new? Transfus Sci 1996;17:537-44.

82. Burgstaler EA. Current instrumentation for apheresis. In: McLeod BC, Szczepiorkowski ZM, Weinstein R, Winters JL, eds. Apheresis: Principles and practice. 3rd ed. Bethesda, MD: AABB Press, 2010:71-110.

83. Burgstaler EA, Pineda AA, Bryant SC. Prospective comparison of plateletapheresis using four apheresis systems on the same donors. J Clin Apher 1999;14:163-70.

84. Perseghin P, Mascaretti L, Riva M, et al. Comparison of plateletapheresis concentrates produced with Spectra LRS version 5.1 and LRS Turbo version 7.0 cell separators. Transfusion 2000;40:789-93.

85. Zingsem J, Glaser A, Weisbach V. Evaluation of a platelet apheresis technique for the preparation of leukocyte-reduced platelet concentrates. Vox Sang 1998;74:189-92.

86. Zingsem J, Zimmermann R, Weisbach V, et al. Comparison of COBE white cell-reduction and standard plateletpheresis protocols in the same donors. Transfusion 1997;37:1045-9.

87. McAteer M, Kagen L, Graminske S, et al. Trima Accel improved platelet collection efficiency with the merging of single stage separation technology with leukoreduction performance of the LRS chamber (abstract). Transfusion 2002;42(Suppl):37S.

88. Burgstaler EA, Winters JL, Pineda AA. Paired comparison of Gambro Trima Accel vs Baxter Amicus single-needle plateletapheresis. Transfusion 2004;44:1612-20.

89. Yockey C, Murphy S, Eggers L, et al. Evaluation of the Amicus separator in the collection of apheresis platelets. Transfusion 1999;38:848.

90. Valbonesi M, Florio G, Ruzzenenti MR, et al. Multicomponent collection (MCC) with the latest hemapheresis apparatuses. Int J Artif Organs 1999;22:511-15.

91. Paciorek L, Holme S, Andres M, et al. Evaluation of the continuous filtration method with double platelet products collected on the MCS+ (abstract). J Clin Apher 1998;13:87.

92. Ford K, Thompson C, McWhorter R, et al. Evaluation of the Haemonetics MCS+ LN9000 to produce leukoreduced platelet products (abstract). J Clin Apher 1996;11:104.

93. Estcourt LJ, Stanworth SJ, Hopewell S, et al. Granulocyte transfusions for treating infections in people with neutropenia or neutrophil

dysfunction. Cochrane Database Syst Rev 2016;4:CD005339.

94. Food and Drug Administration. Safety communication: Boxed warning on increased mortality and severe renal injury, and additional warning on risk of bleeding, for use of hydroxyethyl starch solutions in some settings. (November 25, 2013) Silver Spring, MD: CBER Office of Communication, Outreach, and Development, 2013. [Available at http://www.fda.gov/BiologicsBloodVaccines/SafetyAvailability/ucm358271.htm (accessed January 30, 2017).]

95. Ambruso DR. Hydroxyethyl starch and granulocyte transfusions: Considerations of utility and toxicity profile for patients and donors. Transfusion 2015;55:911-18.

96. Worel N, Kurz M, Peters C, Höcker P. Serial granulocyte apheresis under daily administration of rHuG-CSF: Effects on peripheral blood counts, collection efficiency, and yield. Transfusion 2001;41:390-5.

97. Dale DC, Lises WC, Llewellyn C, et al. Neutrophil transfusions: Kinetics and functions of neutrophils mobilized with granulocyte colony-stimulating factor and dexamethasone. Transfusion 1998;38:713-21.

98. Food and Drug Administration. Substantially equivalent 510(k) device information: BK130065 summary. TerumoBCT Spectra Optia. Silver Spring, MD: CBER Office of Communication, Outreach, and Development, 2013. [Available at http://www.fda.gov/BiologicsBloodVaccines/BloodBloodProducts/ApprovedProducts/SubstantiallyEquivalent510kDeviceInformation/ucm390957.htm (accessed January 30, 2017).]

99. Kretschmer V, Biehl M, Coffe C, et al. New features of the Fresenius blood cell separator AS104. In: Agishi T, Kawamura A, Mineshima M, eds. Therapeutic plasmapheresis (XII): Proceedings of the 4th International Congress of Apheresis of the World Apheresis Association and the 12th Annual Symposium of the Japanese Society for Apheresis, 3-5 June 1992, Sapporo, Japan. Utrecht, the Netherlands: VSP BV, 1993:851-5.

100. Food and Drug Administration. Guidance for industry: Use of sterile connecting devices in blood bank practices. (November 22, 2000) Silver Spring, MD: CBER Office of Communication, Outreach, and Development, 2000. [Available at http://www.fda.gov/BiologicsBloodVaccines/GuidanceComplianceRegulatoryInformation/Guidances/Blood/ucm076779.htm (accessed January 30, 2017).]

101. Schuetz AN, Hillyer KL, Roback JD, Hillyer CD. Leukoreduction filtration of blood with sickle cell trait. Transfus Med Rev 2004;18:168-76.

102. Dzik S, Moroff G, Dumont L. A multicenter study evaluating three methods for counting residual WBCs in WBC-reduced blood components: Nageotte hemocytometry, flow cytometry, and microfluorimetry. Transfusion 2000;40:513-20.

103. Whitley PH, Wellington M, Sawyer S, et al. A simple, new technology for counting low levels of white blood cells in blood components: Comparison to current methods. Transfusion 2012;52(Suppl):59A.

104. Nuclear Regulatory Commission. Memorandum to holders of material licenses authorized to possess radioactive material quantities of concern. Issuance of order for increased controls for certain radioactive materials licensees. (November 14, 2005) Rockville, MD: NRC, 2005. [Available at https://www.nrc.gov/docs/ML0531/ml053130183.pdf (accessed February 5, 2017).]

105. Moroff G, Leitman SF, Luban NLC. Principles of blood irradiation, dose validation, and quality control. Transfusion 1997;37:1084-92.

106. Strauss RC. Red blood cell storage avoiding hyperkalemia from transfusions to neonates and infants. Transfusion 2010;50:1862-5.

107. Fung MKI, Roseff SD, Vermoch KL. Blood component preferences of transfusion services supporting infant transfusions: A University HealSystem Consortium benchmarking study. Transfusion 2010;50:1921-5.

108. Voak D, Chapman J, Finney RD, et al. Guidelines on gamma irradiation of blood components for the prevention of transfusion-associated graft-versus-host disease. Transfus Med 1996;6:261-71.

109. Van der Meer PF, de Korte D. The buffy-coat method. In: Blajchman M, Cid J, Lozano M, eds. Blood component preparation: From benchtop to bedside. Bethesda, MD: AABB Press, 2011:55-81.

110. Moroff G, Friedman A, Robkin-Kline L, et al. Reduction of the volume of stored platelet concentrates for use in neonatal patients. Transfusion 1984;24:144-6.

111. Pisciotto P, Snyder EL, Napychank PA, Hopper SM. In vitro characteristics of volume-reduced platelet concentrate stored in syringes. Transfusion 1991;31:404-8.

112. Aster RH. Effect of acidification in enhancing viability of platelet concentrates: Current status. Vox Sang 1969;17:23.

113. Larrea L, Calabuig M, Roldán V, et al. The influence of riboflavin photochemistry on plasma coagulation factors. Transfus Apher Sci 2009; 41:199-204.

114. Rock G. A comparison of methods of pathogen inactivation of FFP. Vox Sang 2011;100:169-78.

115. Hellstern P, Haubelt H. Manufacture and composition of fresh frozen plasma and virus-inactivated therapeutic plasma preparations: Correlation between composition and therapeutic efficacy. Thromb Res 2002; 107(Suppl 1):S3-8.

116. Sharma AD, Sreeram G, Erb T, Grocott HP. Solvent-detergent-treated fresh frozen plasma: A superior alternative to standard fresh frozen plasma? J Cardiothorac Vasc Anesth 2000;14:712-17.

117. Octoplas package Insert. Hoboken, NJ: Octapharma USA, Inc. [Available at http:// www.fda.gov/downloads/BiologicsBloodVac cines/BloodBloodProducts/ApprovedProd ucts/LicensedProductsBLAs/UCM336161.pdf (accessed January 30, 2017).]

118. Food and Drug Administration. Octaplas. Silver Spring, MD: CBER Office of Communication, Outreach, and Development, 2014. [Available at http://www.fda.gov/BiologicsBloodVac cines/BloodBloodProducts/ApprovedProd ucts/LicensedProductsBLAs/ucm336140.htm (accessed January 30, 2017).]

119. Marks DC, Faddy HM, Johnson L. Pathogen reduction technologies. ISBT Science Series 2014;9:44-50.

120. Code of federal regulations. Title 21, CFR Part 606. Washington, DC: US Government Publishing Office, 2017 (revised annually).

121. Food and Drug Administration. Biological product and HCT/P deviation reports: Annual summary for Fiscal Year 2014. Silver Spring, MD: CBER Office of Communication, Outreach, and Development, 2015. [Available at http:// www.fda.gov/downloads/BiologicsBloodVac cines/SafetyAvailability/ReportaProblem/Bio logicalProductDeviations/UCM440635.pdf (accessed January 30, 2017).]

122. Food and Drug Administration. Guideline for the uniform labeling of blood and blood components. (August 1985) Silver Spring, MD: CBER Office of Communication, Outreach, and Development, 1985. [Available at http://www. fda.gov/downloads/BiologicsBloodVaccines/ GuidanceComplianceRegulatoryInformation/ Guidances/Blood/UCM080974.pdf (accessed January 30, 2017).]

123. Distler P, ed. United States industry consensus standard for the uniform labeling of blood and blood components using ISBT 128. Version 2.0.0, November 2005. San Bernardino, CA: IC-CBBA, 2013. [Available at http://www.fda.gov/ downloads/BiologicsBloodVaccines/Guidan ceComplianceRegulatoryInformation/Guid ances/Blood/UCM079159.pdf (accessed January 30, 2017).]

Chapter 7

Infectious Disease Screening

• ● •

Susan L. Stramer, PhD, and Susan A. Galel, MD

B LOOD COMPONENTS, LIKE all other medications in the United States, are regulated by the Food and Drug Administration (FDA). The FDA requires medication manufacturers to verify the suitability of every raw material in their products.[1] For biologic pharmaceuticals, the donor is the key ingredient whose suitability must be scrutinized.

Blood banks test a sample of blood from each donation with screening tests approved by the FDA to identify donors and donated components that might harbor infectious agents. This screening process is critically important because most blood components (eg, red cells, platelets, plasma, and cryoprecipitate) are infused without pasteurization, sterilization, or other treatments to inactivate infectious agents. Thus, infectious agents in a donor's blood at the time of donation that are not detected by the screening process can be transmitted directly to recipients.

HISTORICAL OVERVIEW OF BLOOD DONOR SCREENING

Table 7-1 shows the progression over time of donor testing for infectious diseases in the United States. Initially, donors were screened only for syphilis. In the 1960s, studies showed that >30% of patients who received multiple transfusions developed posttransfusion hepatitis (PTH).[2] Studies in the early 1970s found that the newly discovered hepatitis B virus (HBV) accounted for only 25% of PTH cases.[2] Both HBV and non-A, non-B (NANB) hepatitis occurred more frequently in recipients of blood from commercial (paid) blood donors than in recipients of blood from volunteer donors. By the mid-1970s, implementation of sensitive tests for hepatitis B surface antigen (HBsAg) and a nearly universal changeover to a volunteer donor supply resulted in a dramatic reduction in the incidence of both HBV and NANB PTH. Still, NANB PTH continued to

Susan L. Stramer, PhD, Vice President, Scientific Affairs, American Red Cross, Gaithersburg, Maryland; and Susan A. Galel, MD, Senior Director of Medical Affairs, Blood Screening, Roche Molecular Systems, Inc., Pleasanton, California, and Associate Professor Emeritus, Stanford University School of Medicine, Stanford, California

S. Stramer has disclosed no conflicts of interest. S. Galel has disclosed a conflict of interest with Roche Molecular Systems, Inc. The conclusions, findings, and opinions expressed in this chapter are solely those of the author and do not reflect or represent those of Roche Molecular Diagnostics.

TABLE 7-1. Changes in US Donor Testing for Infectious Diseases

Year First Implemented	Screening Test	Comments
1940s-1950s	Syphilis	The syphilis test was mandated by FDA in the 1950s.
1970s	HBsAg	The first-generation test was available in 1970, and a higher-sensitivity test was required in 1973.
1985	Antibody to HIV (anti-HTLV-III)	The initial name for HIV, the virus that causes AIDS, was HTLV-III. The first test for antibody to HIV was called "anti-HTLV-III."
1986-1987	ALT and anti-HBc	ALT and anti-HBc were recommended by AABB as surrogate tests for NANB hepatitis. These tests were initially not licensed by FDA for donor screening. AABB's recommendation for donor ALT testing was dropped in 1995 after antibody testing for HCV was in place. Anti-HBc was licensed and required by FDA in 1991.
1988	Anti-HTLV-I	Although HTLV-I infection is usually asymptomatic, a small percentage of infected individuals develop leukemia, lymphoma, or a neurologic disease.
1990	Antibody to HCV, Version 1 (anti-HCV 1.0)	HCV was identified as the cause of most cases of NANB hepatitis.
1991	Anti-HBc	Anti-HBc was previously recommended by AABB as a surrogate screen for NANB hepatitis. It was required by FDA in 1991 as an additional screen for HBV.
1992	Anti-HCV 2.0	This version had improved ability to detect antibody to HCV.
1992	Anti-HIV-1/2	The new HIV antibody tests had improved ability to detect early infection and an expanded range of detection that included HIV-2 in addition to HIV-1.
1996	HIV-1 p24 antigen test	This test was found to detect HIV-1 infection 6 days earlier than the antibody test. FDA permitted discontinuation of HIV-1 p24 antigen testing with the implementation of a licensed HIV-1 nucleic acid test.
1996	Anti-HCV 3.0	This version has improved ability vs anti-HCV 2.0 to detect antibody to HCV.

1997-1998	Anti-HTLV-I/II	The new HTLV antibody tests detected HTLV-II in addition to HTLV-I.
1999	HIV-1 and HCV nucleic acid tests to detect HIV and HCV RNA	These tests were implemented initially as investigational assays and were licensed by FDA in 2002. They detect infection earlier than antibody or antigen assays.
2003	West Nile virus nucleic acid test to detect WNV RNA	This test was implemented initially as an investigational assay and was licensed by FDA during 2005-2007. Testing of individual donations, rather than minipools, at times of increased WNV activity in a region was recommended by AABB in 2004 and FDA in 2009.
2004	Sampling of platelet components to detect bacterial contamination	Testing was recommended by AABB in 2004. Some tests are approved by FDA as quality-control tests. Since 2011, AABB has accepted only FDA-approved tests or those validated to have equivalent sensitivity.
2006-2007	Antibody to *Trypanosoma cruzi*	This test was approved by FDA as a donor screen late in 2006, and widespread testing was implemented in 2007. The rarity of seroconversion in US residents led to endorsement in FDA 2010 guidance of one-time donor screening.
2007-2008	HBV nucleic acid test to detect HBV DNA	This test was initially implemented as part of automated multiplex assays that detect HIV RNA, HCV RNA, and HBV DNA simultaneously. HBV DNA screening was explicitly recommended by FDA guidance issued in October 2012.
2016	Zika virus nucleic acid test to detect Zika virus RNA	Universal individual donation nucleic acid testing was recommended by FDA guidance issued in August 2016 in response to the epidemic in the Americas (with immediate implementation in Puerto Rico, 4-week implementation in high-risk Southern states and New York, and 12-week implementation in all other states).

FDA = Food and Drug Administration; HBsAg = hepatitis B surface antigen; HIV = human immunodeficiency virus; AIDS = acquired immune deficiency syndrome; HTLV = human T-cell lymphotropic virus; ALT = alanine aminotransferase; HBc = hepatitis B core antigen; NANB = non-A, non-B; HCV = hepatitis C virus; HBV = hepatitis B virus; RNA = ribonucleic acid; WNV = West Nile virus; DNA = deoxyribonucleic acid.

occur in approximately 6% to 10% of multi-transfused patients.[2,3]

In the absence of a specific test for the causative agent of NANB PTH, investigators searched for surrogate markers that could be used to identify donations associated with NANB hepatitis. The presence of antibody to hepatitis B core antigen (anti-HBc) and/or the presence of elevated alanine aminotransferase in blood donors was shown to be associated with an increased risk of NANB PTH.[4-7] However, concerns about the nonspecific nature of these tests led to a delay in their implementation for donor screening.

The concept of surrogate testing was revisited in the early 1980s when concerns arose about the transmission of AIDS by transfusions before the identification of its causative agent. In an effort to reduce the potential transmission of AIDS by transfusion, some blood banks implemented donor testing for anti-HBc (because this antibody was highly prevalent in populations at increased risk of AIDS) and/or donor screening for inverted CD4/CD8 T-cell ratio [an immune abnormality found both in AIDS patients and in people during the pre-AIDS incubation period of what was subsequently identified as human immunodeficiency virus (HIV) infection].[8] The leaders of most blood banks, however, believed that the risk of transmitting AIDS by transfusion was too low to warrant surrogate interventions.[9] After HIV was isolated and identified as the causative agent of AIDS, a donor screening test for antibody to this agent was rapidly developed and implemented in 1985.

Once the HIV antibody test became available and cases of HIV were recognized in both prior donors and transfusion recipients, it became clear that the risk of transmitting HIV via blood transfusion had been greatly underestimated.[10] The HIV experience highlighted the fact that an infectious agent associated with a lengthy asymptomatic carrier state could be present in the blood supply for years without being recognized.

In the wake of this realization, the approach to donor screening was extended beyond known agents. Current donor history evaluations include screening for and exclusion of donors with an increased risk of exposure to blood-borne or sexually transmitted infections. The intention is to reduce the likelihood that the blood supply will be subject to other as-yet-unidentified agents that are potentially transmissible by blood.

Transfusion transmission of HIV persisted even after implementation of donor testing because of a delay of weeks or months between the time a person is infected with HIV and the time the screening test for HIV antibody shows positive results.[11] Blood donated during this seronegative "window period" contains infectious HIV that is not detected by the donor screening tests.

The most straightforward means of protecting the blood supply from window-period donations is to exclude potential donors with an increased likelihood of exposure to HIV. The FDA initially recommended in 1983 that blood banks provide donors with informational materials listing HIV risk activities and requesting that individuals not donate if they had engaged in these behaviors. Experience from San Francisco clearly documented the efficacy of this approach.[12] In 1990, the FDA recommended asking each donor directly about each risk activity. In 1992, the FDA issued comprehensive guidance describing this questioning process.

In the years since the discovery of HIV, the risk of transfusion-transmitted disease has been progressively reduced through a variety of measures:

1. Use of donor education and questioning to minimize window-period donations, exclude donors at increased risk of blood-borne or sexually transmitted infections, and screen for infections for which no tests are available.

2. Shortening of the window period for specific agents by improving and/or adding tests to detect earlier stages of infection.

3. Adoption of current good manufacturing practice (cGMP) regulations to ensure that unsuitable units are not collected and/or distributed.

4. Surveillance for transfusion-transmissible diseases and implementation of new donor screening tests, when available.

The approach used to screen potential donors for an agent depends on whether specific risk factors are identifiable and whether donor screening tests are available. Table 7-2 lists the screening approaches used for different types of infectious agents.

DONOR SCREENING TESTS

The donor infectious disease tests required by the FDA are specified in Title 21, Part 610.40, of the *Code of Federal Regulations* (CFR).[1] In addition to the CFR, FDA communicates changes in its recommendations by issuing guidance publications. Although FDA guidance documents do not constitute legal requirements, they define the standard of practice in the United States, and many blood collectors consider them legal imperatives. AABB also issues (recommendations) and requirements to the blood banking community. These are communicated either by Association Bulletins or by inclusion in AABB *Standards for Blood Banks and Transfusion Services (Standards)*. AABB recommendations and standards do not have the force of law except in California, where some sets of AABB standards have been incorporated into state law.

AABB *Standards* are often considered throughout the United States as defining a standard of practice in the blood banking community and therefore are widely implemented. Since 1985, the FDA and AABB have issued a series of recommendations, regulations, and/or standards for additional screening tests in addition to the long-standing donor screens for syphilis and HBsAg. Table 7-1 summarizes the chronology of changes in donor infectious disease testing, and Table 7-3 lists the donor screening tests that are performed by US blood banks.

TABLE 7-2. Approaches to Donor Screening

Approach	Context for Use	Example(s)
Questioning only	Infectious agents with defined risk factors and no sensitive and/or specific test	Malaria, prions
Testing only	Donor test is available, but no question to distinguish individuals at risk of infection	West Nile virus
Questioning and testing	Agents for which there are both identified risk factors and effective tests	Human immunodeficiency virus, hepatitis B and C viruses
Use of blood components that test negative for specific recipients	Agents with a high prevalence in donors but for which an identifiable subset of recipients can benefit from blood components that test negative	Cytomegalovirus (universal leukocyte reduction of cellular blood components has nearly replaced the use of cytomegalovirus-seronegative blood except in selected patient populations)
Testing of blood components	Infectious agent not detectable in donor samples; detection in blood component (platelets) required	Bacteria

TABLE 7-3. Blood Donor Screening Tests Performed in the United States

Agent	Marker Detected	Screening Test Method	Supplemental Assays*
HBV	Hepatitis B surface antigen	ChLIA or EIA	Positive HBV DNA (FDA)[†] Neutralization (FDA)
	Total (IgM and IgG) antibody to hepatitis B core antigen	ChLIA or EIA	
	HBV DNA[‡]	TMA or PCR	
HCV	IgG antibody to HCV peptides and recombinant proteins	ChLIA or EIA	Positive HCV RNA (FDA)[†] RIBA (FDA),[§] line immunoblots (not FDA licensed)
	HCV RNA[‡]	TMA or PCR	
HIV-1/2	IgM and IgG antibody to HIV-1/2	ChLIA or EIA	Positive HIV RNA (FDA)[†] HIV-1: IFA or Western blot (FDA) HIV-2: EIA (FDA)
	HIV-1 RNA[‡]	TMA or PCR	
HTLV-I/II	IgG antibody to HTLV-I/II	ChLIA or EIA	Western blot (FDA), and line immunoblots (not FDA licensed)

Syphilis	IgG or IgG + IgM antibody to *Treponema pallidum* antigens or Nontreponemal serologic test for syphilis (eg, rapid plasma reagin)◊	Microhemagglutination or EIA Particle agglutination	Second FDA-cleared *T. pallidum* screening test *T. pallidum* antigen-specific immunofluorescence or agglutination assays
Trypanosoma cruzi	IgG antibody to *T. cruzi* (one time)◊	ChLIA or EIA	ESA (FDA)
WNV and ZIKV	WNV or ZIKV RNA¶	TMA or PCR	Repeat or alternate NAT and antibody (IgM, IgG)

*Supplemental assays with "(FDA)" are FDA-approved supplemental assays. Other supplemental assays listed are not required but may be useful for donor counseling.

†Positive results on some nucleic acid tests are approved by the FDA as providing confirmation for reactive HBsAg, HIV antibody, and HCV antibody serology tests. If a nucleic acid test result is negative, a serologic supplemental test(s) must be performed.

‡Screening for HIV, HCV, and HBV nucleic acid in the United States is usually performed on minipools of 6 to 16 donor samples.

§As of 2013, RIBA is not available. An FDA variance may be obtained to use a second licensed screening test as an alternative.

◊*T. cruzi* antibody testing may be limited to one-time testing of each donor.

¶ZIKV RNA testing may be performed with investigational assays. See WNV text for specific use of individual and minipool NAT.

HBV = hepatitis B virus; ChLIA = chemiluminescent immunoassay; EIA = enzyme immunoassay; HBsAg = hepatitis B surface antigen; HIV = human immunodeficiency virus; HCV = hepatitis C virus; FDA = Food and Drug Administration; Ig = immunoglobulin; TMA = transcription-mediated amplification; PCR = polymerase chain reaction; RIBA = recombinant immunoblot assay; HIV-1/2 = HIV types 1 and 2; IFA = immunofluorescence assay; HTLV-I/II = human T-cell lymphotropic virus, types I and II; WNV = West Nile virus; ZIKV = Zika virus; NAT = nucleic acid testing; ESA = enzyme strip assay.

Logistics of Testing

All infectious disease testing for blood donor qualification purposes is performed on samples collected at the time of donation and sent to the donor testing laboratory. In addition, most platelet components are tested for bacterial contamination typically by the component manufacturing facility.

Laboratories that perform donor testing mandated by the FDA must be registered with the FDA as biologics manufacturers because this "qualification of raw materials" is considered part of the blood component manufacturing process. The infectious disease tests and testing equipment used to screen donors must be approved (licensed or cleared) for this purpose by the FDA Center for Biologics Evaluation and Research. The FDA website maintains lists of assays approved for donor screening.[13] The tests must be performed exactly as specified in the manufacturers' package inserts. Tests and test platforms that are approved *only* for diagnostic use may *not* be used for screening blood donors.

Serologic Testing Process

Most of the serologic screening tests (assays for the detection of antibody or antigen) are enzyme immunosorbent assays or chemiluminescent immunoassays (ChLIAs). Typically, the process involves performing the required screening test once on each donor sample. If the screening test is nonreactive, the test result is considered negative (ie, there is no evidence of infection). If a test is reactive during the first round of testing ("initially reactive"), the package insert for the test typically requires that the test be repeated in duplicate. If both of the repeat results are nonreactive, the final interpretation is nonreactive or negative, and the unit may be used. If one or both of the repeat results are reactive, the donor sample is characterized as "repeatedly reactive," and the blood unit is not permitted to be used for allogeneic transfusion. (In the case of cellular therapy products, there are some circumstances in which repeatedly reactive donations may be used. (See "Considerations in Testing Donors

of Human Cells, Tissues, and Cellular and Tissue-Based Products" later in this chapter.)

The infectious disease tests that are approved for donor screening have performance characteristics chosen to make them highly sensitive. They are designed to detect almost all infected individuals and minimize false-negative results. However, to achieve this sensitivity, the assays also react with samples from some individuals who are not infected (false-positive results). Because the blood donor population is preselected by questioning to be at low risk of infection, the vast majority of repeatedly reactive results in donors do not represent true infections. To determine whether a repeatedly reactive screening result represents a true infection rather than a false-positive result, additional, more specific testing should be performed on the donor sample.

The FDA requires that repeatedly reactive donor specimens be further evaluated by FDA-approved supplemental assays when such assays are available.[1] The FDA has approved supplemental assays for HBsAg, HIV type 1 (HIV-1) antibodies, hepatitis C virus (HCV) antibodies, antibodies to human T-cell lymphotropic virus, types I and II (HTLV-I/II), and antibodies to *Trypanosoma cruzi*. The HCV antibody confirmatory test (the recombinant immunoblot assay) is no longer available, but blood centers can obtain FDA approval to use an alternate HCV supplemental testing pathway.[14] Table 7-3 displays the available supplemental assays. If no licensed supplemental assay is available, the FDA requires retesting of the donor sample using another FDA-licensed, -approved, or -cleared test to provide additional information for donor counseling; unlicensed supplemental testing may also provide useful information but cannot be used to requalify a donor or donation.

A donation that is repeatedly reactive on a screening test may not be used for allogeneic transfusion, regardless of the results of further testing. Syphilis is the only agent for which negative results on supplemental tests can, in some circumstances, enable use of a screening test-reactive unit. (This applies only to donations screened using a nontreponemal assay.)

This situation is discussed more fully in the "Syphilis" section.

Nucleic Acid Testing

Nucleic acid testing (NAT) was implemented to reduce the seronegative window periods described above. The process of screening donor samples for viral nucleic acid [ribonucleic acid (RNA) or deoxyribonucleic acid (DNA)] is somewhat different from the serologic screening process. NAT requires the extraction of nucleic acid from a donor plasma or serum sample followed by use of a nucleic acid amplification test to amplify and detect viral genetic sequences.

The test systems that were initially implemented in 1999 to screen donors for HIV and HCV RNA were semiautomated and had insufficient throughput to allow individual testing of each donor sample. Testing of seroconversion panels showed little loss of sensitivity if donor plasma samples were tested in small pools [minipools (MPs)] because levels of HIV and HCV RNA are typically high in the blood of infected individuals, and NAT assays are exquisitely sensitive.

Thus, in the initially approved NAT donor screening systems, MPs of 16 to 24 donor samples were prepared and tested together. Current systems use pools of six to 16. If a pool tested negative, all donations contributing to that pool were considered negative for HIV and HCV RNA. If a pool showed reactivity on the nucleic acid test, further testing of smaller pools and, ultimately, individual samples was performed to determine which donation was responsible for the reactive test result. Donations that were nonreactive on this additional testing could be released for transfusion. Donations that were reactive at the individual sample level were considered reactive for viral nucleic acid and could not be released for transfusion.

In recent years, fully automated NAT systems have been developed. The automated test platforms that are approved by the FDA for donor screening use multiplex assays that detect HIV RNA, HCV RNA, and HBV DNA in one reaction chamber. Some of the assays directly discriminate the reactive target during the initial screen; other assays require separate discriminatory testing to identify which virus is present. These systems are approved for testing of individual donations and pools of 6 to 16 donor samples, depending on the platform. The availability of fully automated NAT platforms creates the possibility of performing routine screening on individual donor samples [individual donation screening (ID-NAT)], rather than testing of pools (MP-NAT). However, the predicted frequency of reactive donations identified solely by ID-NAT as compared with MP-NAT at present does not justify this practice in the United States. It has been estimated that ID-NAT screening would minimally increase detection of infected donors, whereas the associated testing cost would be significantly higher than with MP-NAT.[15] Furthermore, it is not clear that ID-NAT screening of the entire US blood supply would be logistically feasible using the available platforms. An additional concern is that donors might be deferred for false-positive results more frequently with ID-NAT screening than with pooled screening.

In contrast to serologic testing policies, repeat testing is not permitted by the FDA for an individually reactive NAT sample to determine whether the initially reactive result represents a true-positive result. If an individual (unpooled) specimen is reactive on a NAT screen for HIV, HCV, or HBV, the FDA requires that the corresponding blood component be discarded and the donor be deferred indefinitely. FDA-approved donor reentry algorithms are available (see below). In countries where donor screening for HIV/HCV/HBV is routinely performed by ID-NAT, it is common practice for initially reactive specimens to be subjected to repeat testing. Practices vary regarding the management of donors and components in cases where initial testing is reactive and repeat testing is nonreactive; in many countries, such donations are discarded because these results would not rule out the presence of a low concentration of virus. Donor management for this scenario varies and may include a deferral and reentry algorithm.

ID-NAT screening rather than MP-NAT screening for West Nile virus (WNV) is recommended when WNV activity is high in a specific geographic area. Circulating levels of viral RNA are often low during WNV infection. When donor samples are combined into MPs, the RNA from a WNV-infected sample may become diluted to below the detectable level. It has been estimated that MP-NAT screening for WNV RNA may fail to detect 50% or more of infected donations.[16-18] Therefore, both the FDA and AABB have recommended ID-NAT screening for WNV RNA at times of high WNV activity in a region.[18,19]

Implications of Reactive Test Results

A repeatedly reactive result on a screening test (or individually reactive NAT result) typically results in mandatory discarding of the reactive donation. Linkage of laboratory information systems to blood bank computer systems prevents labeling and/or release of components from donations with reactive test results. A reactive test result may also indicate that the donor should be prohibited from making future donations, because many infections are persistent. Furthermore, past donations may also be considered suspect because the exact date of onset of a donor's infection cannot be determined.

Both the FDA and AABB have issued recommendations regarding whether reactive test results affect a donor's eligibility for future donations, whether components from prior donations should be retrieved (and if so, how far back in time), and whether patients who previously received components from that donor should be notified. These recommendations are often guided by the results of supplemental or confirmatory testing performed on the donor sample. Many of these recommendations have evolved over time.

Because these recommendations are complex, blood bank laboratories typically create checklists that list each of the actions to be performed after a specific reactive test result is obtained. Staff use these checklists to document completion of each action as they perform it.

Table 7-4[1,18-43] lists federal regulations, FDA guidance documents, AABB standards, and AABB Association Bulletins with recommendations regarding management of blood donors with reactive test results, retrieval of other components, and notification of prior recipients. These regulations and recommendations are described briefly below.

Donor Eligibility

FDA regulations in Title 21, CFR Part 610.41 address donors with reactive screening test results. FDA guidance documents and AABB Association Bulletins contain more detailed recommendations regarding additional testing, donor eligibility, and donor counseling for these and other tests. Donors must be notified of any test results that affect their eligibility or that could have important implications for their health. Blood banks should have systems that prevent future collections from ineligible donors and the release of any components inadvertently collected from such individuals.

For donors deferred for reactive screening tests, 21 CFR 610.41 provides for reinstatement by means of FDA-defined requalification algorithms. The FDA has issued guidance documents (listed in Table 7-4) that define reentry pathways for donors deferred for reactivity on HIV, HCV, HBsAg, and anti-HBc tests; serologic tests for syphilis; and HIV/HCV/HBV NAT tests. Most of the pathways require that the donor have negative results on specified tests after a defined waiting period. Blood banks that desire to reenter donors must follow the FDA-defined algorithms explicitly.

Retrieval of Prior Donations and Notification of Prior Recipients ("Look-Back")

The FDA and AABB offer guidance with regard to the appropriate management of previously collected blood components from donors whose current donation is repeatedly reactive (or, in the case of NAT, individually reactive) on an infectious disease screening test. These recommendations address the concern that at the time of the previous donation(s), the donor

TABLE 7-4. Regulations and Standards Related to Blood Donor Testing and Actions Following Reactive Test Results*

Agent/Test	Regulatory Document	Donor Testing	Donor Management	Product Retrieval	Recipient Notification	Donor Reentry
HIV-1/2	Title 21, CFR Part 610.40[1]	X				
	Title 21, CFR Part 610.41[1]		X			
	Title 21, CFR Part 610.46[1]			X	X	
	Title 42, CFR Part 482.27[20]			X	X	
	FDA guidance, October 2004[31]	X				
	FDA guidance, May 2010[26]	X	X	X	X	X
	AABB BB/TS Standard 5.8.5, 5.8.6[35]	X				
HIV-1 group O	FDA guidance, August 2009[28]	X	X			X
HBV	Title 21, CFR Part 610.40[1]	X				
	Title 21, CFR Part 610.41[1]		X			
	FDA guidance, October 2012[22]	X	X			X
	AABB BB/TS Standard 5.8.5, 5.8.6[35]	X				
HBsAg	FDA memorandum, December 1987[34]	X	X			X
HBsAg and anti-HBc†	FDA memorandum, July 1996[33]			X		
Anti-HBc	FDA guidance, May 2010[27]					X
HBV (vaccine)	FDA guidance, November 2011[23]					X

(Continued)

TABLE 7-4. Regulations and Standards Related to Blood Donor Testing and Actions Following Reactive Test Results* (Continued)

Agent/Test	Regulatory Document	Donor Testing	Donor Management	Product Retrieval	Recipient Notification	Donor Reentry
				Topics		
HCV	Title 21, CFR Part 610.40[1]	X				
	Title 21, CFR Part 610.41[1]		X			
	Title 21, CFR Part 610.47[1]			X	X	
	Title 42, CFR Part 482.27[20]			X	X	
	FDA guidance, October 2004[31]	X				
	FDA guidance, May 2010[26]	X	X	X	X	X
	FDA guidance, December 2010[24]			X	X	
	AABB BB/TS Standard 5.8.5, 5.8.6[35]	X				
HTLV-I/II	Title 21, CFR Part 610.40[1]	X				
	Title 21, CFR Part 610.41[1]		X			
	FDA guidance, August 1997[32]	X	X	X		
	AABB BB/TS Standard 5.8.5, 5.8.6[35]	X				
	Association Bulletin #99-9[39]	X	X			
Syphilis	Title 21, CFR Part 610.40[1]	X				
	Title 21, CFR Part 610.41[1]		X			
	FDA guidance, September 2014[21]	X	X			X
	AABB BB/TS Standard 5.8.5, 5.8.6[35]	X				

Trypanosoma cruzi	FDA guidance, December 2010[25]	X	X	X	X	
	FDA draft guidance, November 2016[40]					X
	AABB BB/TS Standard 5.8.5, 5.8.6[35]	X				
WNV	FDA guidance, June 2005[30]		X	X	X	
	FDA guidance, November 2009[19]	X	X	X		
	AABB BB/TS Standard 5.8.5, 5.8.6[35]	X				
	Association Bulletin #13-02[18]	X				
ZIKV	FDA guidance, February 2016 and August 2016[41,42]	X	X	X	X	X
ZIKV (and DENV and CHIKV)	Association Bulletin #16-07[43]	X	X	X	X	X
Bacteria	AABB BB/TS Standards 5.1.5.1, 5.1.5.2, 5.1.5.3[35]	X		X‡		
	Association Bulletin #05-02[37]		X			X
	Association Bulletin #12-04[36]	X				
	Association Bulletin #04-07[38]	X		X	X	
Parvovirus B19§	FDA guidance, July 2009[29]					

*Recommendations in effect as of February 2017. Blood centers may be bound by additional requirements, such as specifications in recovered plasma contracts.

†Memorandum also includes recommendations regarding HCV and HTLV, but these recommendations have been superseded by subsequent documents.

‡Co-components of current donation.

§Plasma for further manufacture only.

HIV-1/2 = human immunodeficiency virus, types 1 and 2; CFR = *Code of Federal Regulations*; FDA = Food and Drug Administration; BB/TS Standards = *Standards for Blood Banks and Transfusion Services*; HBV = hepatitis B virus; HBsAg = hepatitis B surface antigen; anti-HBc = antibody to hepatitis B core antigen; HCV = hepatitis C virus; HTLV-I/II = human T-cell lymphotropic virus, types I and II; WNV = West Nile virus; ZIKV = Zika virus; DENV = dengue viruses; CHIKV = chikungunya virus.

could have been in the window period of an early infection even though the screening test results were negative.

For HIV and HCV tests, the algorithms for managing prior donations and recipients of prior donations are spelled out in 21 CFR 610.46 and 610.47. These requirements are replicated in the Centers for Medicare and Medicaid Services regulations (Title 42, CFR Part 482.27) to ensure hospital transfusion service compliance with recipient notification requirements. For other agents, recommendations for the management of previously donated components may be found in the FDA guidance documents or AABB Association Bulletins (or both) listed in Table 7-4.

In most cases, the FDA and AABB recommend retrieval and quarantine of any remaining components from prior donations of that donor. It is essential that the retrieval of in-date components be initiated immediately after the repeatedly reactive result is obtained. This prevents transfusion of these components while confirmatory testing is performed. The FDA requires initiation of retrieval within 3 calendar days of a reactive HIV or HCV test and within 1 week of reactive HBsAg, anti-HBc, or anti-HTLV screening tests. If confirmatory test results on the current donation are negative, the FDA, in some circumstances, permits rerelease of the prior donations. In many cases, some or all of the components from prior donations will have been transfused. For some infectious agents, the FDA and AABB recommend that the recipients of prior donations from confirmed positive donors be notified of their possible exposure to the infectious agent.

Recommendations for notification of recipients of prior donations ("look-back") are usually issued by AABB, the FDA, or both at the time a new test is implemented, but these recommendations may evolve as confirmatory tests become available or medical treatments are developed for the infection in question. Look-back is required by law only for HIV and HCV tests (21 CFR 610.46 and 610.47). For an HIV look-back investigation involving a deceased prior recipient, the next of kin must be notified. The CFR spells out specific timelines

for component retrieval and recipient notification. It also specifies how far back in time (ie, to which donations) the retrieval and notification should extend. For other agents, such as WNV, Zika virus (ZIKV) and *T. cruzi*, recommendations regarding retrieval and recipient notification are included in FDA guidance documents and AABB Association Bulletins. Investigational protocols for unlicensed screening assays may also include these requirements (eg, assays for ZIKV and *Babesia microti*). Table 7-4 indicates which of these documents address product retrieval or recipient notification.

In the absence of published guidance, it is not always obvious whether or when it is appropriate to notify prior recipients of their possible exposure to infection. If there is no supplemental assay available or further testing performed, it is not possible to determine whether a repeatedly reactive screening test result for a donor represents a true infection. Furthermore, if there is no effective treatment for that infection, there may be no medical benefit to the recipient of being told that he or she might have been exposed. There could, however, be a public health benefit from such a notification. Specifically, a recipient who is alerted of a potential exposure can be tested and, if the results are positive, take precautions to avoid further spread of the infection.

Cytomegalovirus Testing of Components for Immunocompromised Recipients

Some common infections cause relatively innocuous illnesses in immunocompetent individuals but can cause severe disease in immunocompromised patients. Such is the case with cytomegalovirus (CMV).

CMV is a lipid-enveloped DNA virus in the *Herpesviridae* family. Like other herpesviruses, CMV causes lifelong infection, typically in a latent state, with the potential for reactivation. Primary CMV infection in immunologically competent individuals is mild, with symptoms ranging from none to an infectious mononucleosis-type syndrome. In immunocompromised patients, however, both primary infection and reactivation disease can be overwhelming and even fatal. CMV can be transmitted by blood transfusion, primarily through intact white cells contained in cellular blood components. Frozen/thawed plasma components do not appear to transmit CMV infection. Immunocompromised patients who are at increased risk of transfusion-transmitted disease include fetuses, low-birthweight premature infants who are born to CMV-seronegative mothers, and CMV-seronegative recipients of solid-organ or allogeneic hematopoietic cell transplants from seronegative donors.[44]

The majority of blood donors have had prior exposure to CMV, indicated by the presence of CMV antibodies. Therefore, it would not be possible to produce an adequate supply of blood if all CMV-antibody-positive donations were discarded.

It is possible, however, to minimize CMV transmission to patients at risk of severe CMV disease, such as those described above. These patients should be supported with cellular blood components that have a reduced risk of transmitting CMV. These reduced-risk options include using blood components from donors who are CMV antibody negative or components that have been effectively leukocyte reduced. The literature suggests that these two methods have similar but not identical efficacy, with an estimated transmission risk by seronegative components of 1% to 2% vs a risk of 2% to 3% with leukocyte-reduced components.[44-46] Recent studies, however, found no CMV transmissions among a total of 176 carefully monitored allogeneic hematopoietic cell transplant recipients who received CMV-untested, leukocyte-reduced components.[47,48] Because many at-risk patients receive leukocyte-reduced components and are monitored closely for CMV infection, treated early with anti-CMV drugs, or both, it is difficult to measure a benefit from also providing CMV-seronegative components to these patients. The use of leukocyte-reduced, anti-CMV-untested blood components expands the inventory available for their support.

Autologous Donations

The FDA requires infectious disease testing of autologous donations that are shipped from one facility to another. If the receiving facility does not permit autologous donations to be crossed over to the general inventory, the FDA requires testing of only the first donation in each 30-day period [21 CFR 610.40(d)]. The labeling of the unit must be consistent with its testing status. Units from donors with repeatedly reactive tests must be labeled with biohazard labels. Some hospitals have policies that prohibit acceptance of autologous units with positive results on some tests because there is a potential for an infectious unit to be transfused to the wrong patient. AABB has warned that refusal of test-positive units could be interpreted as violating the Americans with Disabilities Act.[49]

Considerations in Testing Donors of Human Cells, Tissues, and Cellular and Tissue-Based Products

Both the questions and tests required by the FDA to screen donors of human cells, tissues, and cellular and tissue-based products (HCT/Ps) differ from those for blood donors, and the requirements vary by type of tissue. The general requirements are spelled out in 21 CFR 1271 and an August 2007 FDA guidance document and are summarized in Table 7-5.[50,51] The FDA has issued additional guidance regarding testing of HCT/Ps for syphilis[52] and WNV,[53] as well as draft guidance documents on other infectious agents. An up-to-date list of FDA HCT/P guidance documents may be found on the Tissue Guidances page of the FDA website.[54]

The time frames for testing HCT/P donors are specified in 21 CFR 1271 and the August 2007 FDA guidance document.[50,51] In most cases, the samples for infectious disease testing must be obtained within 7 days before or after the tissue donation. Samples from donors of peripheral blood hematopoietic progenitor cells or marrow may be tested up to 30 days before donation; however, longer intervals between testing and transplantation may be

TABLE 7-5. FDA Testing Requirements for HCT/Ps (as of March 2017)

Tissue Type	Agent	Tests
All tissues	HIV	Antibody to HIV-1 and HIV-2* HIV-1 RNA*
	HBV	Hepatitis B surface antigen* Antibody to hepatitis B core antigen*
	HCV	Antibody to hepatitis C* HCV RNA*
	Treponema pallidum	FDA-licensed, -approved, or -cleared donor screening test
All living donors	WNV	WNV RNA*
For donors of viable leukocyte-rich HCT/Ps (eg, hematopoietic progenitor cells or semen), test for the following in addition to the above:	HTLV-I/II	Antibody to HTLV-I/II*
	CMV	FDA-cleared screening test for anti-CMV (total IgG and IgM)
For donors of reproductive tissues, test for the following in addition to the above:	*Chlamydia trachomatis*	FDA-licensed, -approved, or -cleared diagnostic test
	Neisseria gonorrhea	FDA-licensed, -approved, or -cleared diagnostic test

*These tests must be FDA licensed for donor screening.
FDA = Food and Drug Administration; HCT/Ps = human cells, tissues, and cellular and tissue-based products; HIV = human immunodeficiency virus; HBV = hepatitis B virus; HCV = hepatitis C virus; WNV = West Nile virus; HTLV = human T-cell lymphotropic virus; CMV = cytomegalovirus; Ig = immunoglobulin.

associated with transmission of infectious agents. Autologous tissues and reproductive tissues from recipients' sexually intimate partners may be exempt from some testing requirements.

Blood bank laboratories that test samples from HCT/P donors must be registered with the FDA and must use tests approved for testing of these donors, when such tests are available. HCT/P testing requirements and approved tests may be found on the FDA website.[55] Testing laboratories must take care to check package inserts for HCT/P testing methods; a package insert may require a different testing method for HCT/P donors than for blood donors. For example, NAT for most types of HCT/P donors must be performed on individual donor samples; MP-NAT is not permitted for most HCT/P donor categories.

In some cases, FDA regulations permit the use of HCT/P donations that are reactive on infectious disease screening tests. These exceptions are listed in 21 CFR 1271.65. FDA has issued specific labeling, storage, and notification requirements for these tissues.

Testing of HCT/P donors for antibody to *T. cruzi* is not required by the FDA as of March 2017.

International Variations in Donor Testing

Although this chapter focuses on infectious disease screening in the United States, the general approach to donor screening is similar in other countries. However, the specific donor questions and tests vary from country to country based on the regional epidemiology of infections and tests available. For example, most countries where WNV is not endemic do not test for this agent, although they may question donors and defer them for travel to WNV-affected countries. Countries where HBV is hyper-endemic cannot exclude donations from individuals who test positive for anti-HBc without adversely affecting the adequacy of their blood supply. The AABB Standards Interpretation Committee considers variance applications from facilities desiring accreditation in countries where national practices and available testing methods are different from those used in the United States. Some blood donations outside the United States are tested for agents not included in routine US donor testing. An example of this is hepatitis E virus, discussed later in this chapter.

RESIDUAL INFECTIOUS RISKS OF TRANSFUSION

Despite donor screening, blood components may still transmit infections. The residual risk of transmission varies according to the incidence of the infection in the donor population and the nature of the donor screening processes in place.

Agents for Which Blood Is Tested

Transfusion transmissions of HIV, HCV, and HBV are now so rare that the rates of transmission cannot be measured by prospective clinical studies. The risk can only be estimated by theoretical modeling.

One theoretical source of risk is a virus strain that the current test kits do not detect. The Centers for Disease Control and Prevention (CDC) and the test manufacturers conduct surveillance for such emerging strains. Over time, the FDA has required that test manufacturers expand their detection capabilities to include new strains. A second potential cause of transmission is a quarantine failure (ie, a blood bank's failure to quarantine a unit that tests positive). Quarantine errors are

thought to be rare in blood banks that use electronic systems to control blood component labeling and release because these systems are designed to prevent the labeling and subsequent release of any unit with incomplete testing or a reactive test result. Erroneous releases appear to occur more frequently in blood banks that rely on manual records and quarantine processes.[56]

The primary cause of residual transmissions is thought to be donations from individuals in the window period of early infection, before test results are positive. Figure 7-1 displays the sequence in which different types of donor screening tests demonstrate reactivity. Over time, the window periods have been shortened by the implementation of donor screening tests that detect earlier infections. However, because no test gives a positive result immediately after an individual acquires an infection, a window period remains. With MP-NAT, the average duration of the window period is estimated to be 9.0 to 9.1 days for HIV and 7.4 days for HCV.[15,57] The window period for HBV is longer, as discussed in the HBV section below.

The likelihood that a blood donation has been obtained from a donor in the window period can be estimated mathematically using the incidence/window-period model[57]:

Probability a donation was made during the window period = length of window period × incidence of infections in the donor population

The incidence of infections in repeat donors can be calculated from the observed number of donors with a negative test result on one donation but a positive result on a subsequent donation (ie, seroconverting donors). This method measures incidence rates only in repeat donors and does not permit assessment of the likelihood that first-time donors might be in the window period. This method also does not consider NAT-converting donors.

Other methods permit measurement of new infection rates in both first-time and repeat donors using tests that differentiate new from established infections. Such tests in-

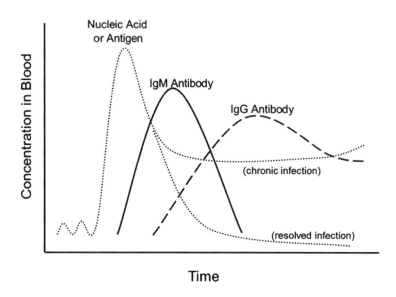

FIGURE 7-1. Time sequence of the appearance of various markers of infection.

clude NAT (ie, donor blood that contains HIV or HCV RNA, or HBV DNA, but not antibody most likely represents a very early infection) and "sensitive/less sensitive" or "detuned" antibody testing.[15,57-59] When these alternative methods have been used, new HIV and HCV infections were two to four times more common among first-time donors than among repeat donors.[57-59] However, both of these donor populations have significantly lower infection rates than the general population. The continued importance of using donor education and questioning to select donors with a low incidence of infection is explored in more detail in the HIV section below.

The current estimated risks of HIV, HCV, and HBV transmission in donors, based on window-period and incidence calculations, are shown in Table 7-6.[57,60]

Agents for Which No Donor Screening Tests Are Available

Essentially any infectious agent that can circulate in the blood of an apparently healthy person might be transmitted by transfusion. It is impossible to estimate the risk of transmission for each of the infectious agents for which do-

nors are not tested. The infections that are most likely to be recognized as transmitted by transfusion are those that have a distinctive clinical presentation and are otherwise rare in the United States. The likelihood that an infection will be recognized as transmitted by transfusion is enhanced if the infection is usually associated with a clinical or behavioral risk that the transfusion recipient lacks (eg, when malaria develops in a transfusion recipient who has not traveled outside the United States).

If a life-threatening agent is recognized as a potential threat to the blood supply, both AABB and the FDA typically consider whether a donor screening question could be used to exclude potentially exposed donors in the absence of a donor screening test. Donor questioning regarding travel to and residence in endemic areas is currently the only means of protecting the US blood supply from malaria and variant Creutzfeldt-Jakob disease (vCJD). Most infectious agents, however, do not have such clear geographic risk areas. In general, it is difficult to design donor questions that are both sensitive (ie, detect most infected individuals) and specific (ie, exclude only infected individuals).

TABLE 7-6. Estimated Risks of Transfusion-Transmitted Infection in the United States Based on the Incidence/Window-Period Model*

Study Period	Agent	Incidence per 10⁵ Person/Years	Infectious Window Period (days)	Residual Risk per Donated Unit
2007-2008[57]*	HIV	3.1	9.1	1:1,467,000
2007-2008[57]*	HCV	5.1	7.4	1:1,149,000
2009-2011[60]†	HBV	1.6	26.5-18.5	1:843,000 to 1:1,208,000

*HIV and HCV risk estimates are based on minipool nucleic acid testing in pools of 16.
†HBV risk estimates are based on minipool nucleic acid testing in pools of 16 using the Grifols Ultrio Plus assay. The range indicated for the HBV window period reflects uncertainty regarding the minimum infectious dose of HBV (1 copy in 20 mL plasma vs 10 copies in 20 mL).
HIV = human immunodeficiency virus; HCV = hepatitis C virus; HBV = hepatitis B virus.

An alternative method of protecting the blood supply from infectious agents is pathogen inactivation. Heat-inactivation, solvent/detergent (SD) treatment, nanofiltration, chromatography, cold ethanol fractionation, and other approaches have been used with remarkable success to inactivate or remove residual pathogens in plasma derivatives. Pathogen inactivation systems for platelets and transfusable plasma have been available outside the United States for several years, and one manufacturer's system was FDA approved for use in the United States in December 2015 (INTERCEPT Blood System, Cerus Corp., Concord, CA). SD-treated plasma (SD plasma) is also available for transfusion in the United States; Octaplas (Octapharma, Lachen, Switzerland) is manufactured from pools of human source plasma (630-1520 individual donors). Pathogen inactivation systems are discussed later in this chapter.

The AABB Transfusion-Transmitted Diseases Committee published an extensive review of infectious agents that are possible threats to the blood supply.[61] Potential mitigation strategies were discussed for each agent, including the documented or theoretical efficacy of pathogen inactivation processes. AABB periodically updates this information via its website, adding materials for new potential threats as they are identified.[62] The agents deemed to pose the highest threat from either a scientific or public perspective are briefly discussed in this chapter. (See the 2009 supplement to *TRANSFUSION* and updates on the AABB website for a more thorough review of these potential infectious risks.[61,62])

SCREENING FOR SPECIFIC AGENTS

Human Immunodeficiency Virus

HIV-1, a lipid-enveloped, single-stranded RNA spherical retrovirus containing two linear, positive-sense strands of RNA, was identified in 1984 as the causative agent of AIDS. Blood donation screening for antibodies to this virus was implemented in the United States in 1985. In 1992, donor screening tests were modified to include detection of antibodies to HIV-2, a closely related virus identified initially in West Africa, only rarely identified in the United States.[63]

HIV can be transmitted sexually, parenterally, and from infected mothers to their infants. Although heterosexual and vertical spread of HIV predominate in some parts of the world, new HIV cases in the United States continue to be concentrated in men who have sex with men (MSM) and individuals with high-risk heterosexual contact (defined as contact with an individual who is HIV positive or in an identified risk group for HIV, such as MSM or injection drug users).[64]

Current donation screening for HIV includes NAT for HIV-1 RNA and serologic testing for antibodies to HIV. The antibody tests approved for donor screening detect both immunoglobulin M (IgM) and IgG antibody to both HIV-1 and HIV-2. Current-generation assays also detect antibody to HIV-1 group O, a strain of HIV-1 found primarily in Central and West Africa. With this detection claim, donor centers no longer need to exclude individuals who have resided in, received medical treatment in, or had sex partners from HIV-1 group O endemic areas.[28]

The average window period after HIV-1 infection to test detection is currently estimated to be 9.0 to 9.1 days for MP-NAT.[15,57] Based on window-period and incidence-rate calculations, the current risk in the US of acquiring HIV from transfusion is estimated to be approximately 1 in 1.5 million units (Table 7-6).

In the United States, blood donor screening questions exclude very broadly defined populations at increased risk of HIV. Given the short delay of only days between infection and detection of infection by NAT, experts have questioned whether donor interviews and exclusion of donors with increased risk remain medically necessary. The continued importance of a low-risk donor population becomes evident if different HIV incidence figures are used for the blood safety calculation. For example, HIV incidence rates as high as 1% to 8% have been observed in some high-risk populations, such as young urban MSM.[65,66] If an individual from a population with a 1% incidence of HIV donates blood, the likelihood that this individual is in the window period and that the component will transmit HIV can be calculated as follows:

Risk that the donation is in window period = length of window period × incidence of infection in donor population = (9.0 days/365 days/year) × (1/100 person-years) = 1/4100.

This is the likelihood that a unit from this high-risk donor would harbor HIV but be missed by the current donor screening. This risk is clearly much higher than the estimated HIV transmission risk of 1 in 1.5 million for a unit of blood obtained from the current donor population. Thus, despite the short window period with current testing, inclusion of donors with a high risk of HIV would have a profoundly adverse impact on blood safety. Accordingly, questioning of donors for risk and temporarily excluding those at increased risk to minimize window-period donations continue to be critical for preserving blood safety.

Although there has been great interest in developing a more specific donor-screening algorithm for MSM that would exclude only individuals who are truly at increased risk of HIV, the FDA guidance issued in December 2015 indicates that the efficacy of a more specific algorithm has not yet been established.[67] This guidance lists the current definitions of potential risks for HIV exposure in the United States that require donor deferral. Most of these risk categories, including MSM behavior, now require a 12-month deferral.[67]

Hepatitis B Virus

HBV is a lipid-enveloped, spherical virus in the *Hepadnavirdiae* family. It is unique in that it has a partially double-stranded circular DNA genome with overlapping reading frames. Like HIV, HBV is transmitted parenterally, sexually, and perinatally. Jaundice is noted in only 25% to 40% of adult cases and in a smaller proportion of childhood cases. A large percentage of perinatally acquired cases result in chronic infection, but most HBV infections acquired in adulthood are cleared. HBV is highly prevalent in certain parts of the world, such as eastern Asia and Africa, where perinatal transmission and resultant chronic infection have amplified infection rates in the population. In the United States, the incidence of acute HBV infection has decreased by at least 80% with the implementation of routine vaccination programs. Perinatal screening and newborn prophylaxis have also been effective in reducing perinatal transmission.

During HBV infection, DNA and viral envelope material (HBsAg) are typically detectable in circulating blood. Antibody to the core antigen is produced soon after the appearance of HBsAg, initially in the form of IgM antibody, followed by IgG. As infected individuals produce antibody to the surface antigen (anti-HBsAg), the HBsAg is cleared.

The FDA requires donor screening for HBsAg, HBV DNA, and total anti-HBc (IgM and IgG antibody). Measurements of HBV incidence in donors have been complicated by the transience of HBsAg and false-positive results on the HBsAg test.[60] Published estimates of the infectious window have varied because of differences in the sensitivity of various HBV assays and lack of certainty regarding the level of virus in a blood component that is required for infectivity.[68,69] Recent publications provide window-period estimates for different potential infectious doses of virus (eg, 10 copies/20 mL of plasma vs 1 copy/20 mL of plasma). The infectious window before a positive result on the Abbott PRISM (Abbott Laboratories, Abbott Park, IL) HBsAg test has been estimated to be 30 to 38 days.[68] With the addition of HBV DNA testing in MPs of 16, the window period is estimated to have been reduced to 18.5 to 26.5 days.[60] Using these MP testing estimates, US HBV transfusion-transmission risk has been estimated to be between 1 in 843,000 donations and 1 in 1.2 million donations (Table 7-6).[60]

Donor screening for HBV DNA can be of value at a variety of points in infection. HBV DNA may be detected during the infectious window period before HBsAg detection; however, DNA levels may be low and could be below the limits of detection of MP-NAT assays.[68,69] Later in infection, following the clearance of HBsAg, HBV NAT may detect persistent (ie, "occult" HBV) infection.[68,69] Such infections are interdicted in the United States by the donor screening test for anti-HBc, with about 1% of anti-HBc repeat-reactive donations considered to be from donors with occult HBV infection due to the presence of HBV DNA in the absence of detectable HBsAg.[60] High sensitivity NAT is required to detect occult HBV infections because viral loads are typically low. HBV NAT can also detect acute HBV infections in individuals who have previously been vaccinated.[70,71] Such individuals may never develop detectable HBsAg, but they may have detectable DNA. The infectivity of such donations is not known because these units contain vaccine-induced antibodies to HBsAg in addition to the virus. Routine HBV DNA screening of US blood donations detects at least some of these infections.

Hepatitis C Virus

Hepatitis C is a small lipid-enveloped, single-stranded RNA virus in the family *Flaviviridae*. HCV was shown to be the cause of up to 90% of cases previously called NANB transfusion-related hepatitis.[72] The majority of HCV infections are asymptomatic. However, HCV infection is associated with a high risk of chronicity, which can result in liver cirrhosis, hepatocellular carcinoma, and a variety of extrahepatic syndromes.

HCV is thought to be transmitted primarily through blood exposure. In the United States, about 55% of HCV infections are associated with injection drug use or receipt of transfusion before donor screening in 1992, but the risk factors for the remainder of the infections are not clear.[73] Sexual and vertical transmissions are uncommon, although co-infection with HIV increases transmission rates by these routes.

Current donor screening for HCV includes NAT for HCV RNA and serologic testing for antibodies to HCV. The average window period between exposure and detection of infection by MP-NAT is estimated to be 7.4 days.[15] The serologic test detects only IgG antibody, a relatively late marker of infection. Therefore, there may be a significant lag (1.5 to 2 months) between detection of RNA and detection of antibody.[74] Donor questioning has limited potential to exclude individuals who may be harboring HCV infection because a large proportion of infected individuals are asymptomatic and admit to no risk factors or possible exposure. Despite this limitation, the current estimated US risk of HCV transmission by transfusion is extremely low—approximately 1 in 1.1 million (Table 7-6).[57]

Human T-Cell Lymphotropic Virus, Types I and II

HTLV-I is a lipid-enveloped RNA retrovirus. It was the first human retrovirus identified, isolated in 1978 from a patient with cutaneous T-cell lymphoma. A closely related virus, HTLV-II, was later isolated from a patient with hairy cell leukemia. Both viruses are highly cell associated, infect lymphocytes, and cause lifelong infections, but most of these infections remain asymptomatic. Approximately 2% to 5% of HTLV-I-infected individuals develop adult T-cell leukemia/lymphoma after a lag of 20 to 30 years. A smaller percentage develop a neurologic disease called HTLV-associated myelopathy or tropical spastic paraparesis. HTLV-II disease associations remain unclear. Both infections are thought to be spread through blood, sexual contact, and breast feeding.

HTLV-I infection is endemic in certain parts of the world, including regions of Japan, South America, the Caribbean, and Africa. In the United States, infections are found in immigrants from endemic areas, injection drug users, and the sexual partners of these individuals. Approximately one-half of the HTLV infections in US blood donors are with HTLV-II.[75,76]

The only FDA-approved donor tests for HTLV infection are screening assays for IgG antibody to HTLV-I and HTLV-II. Units that are reactive on the screening assay may not be released for transfusion. Until recently only screening assays were licensed by the FDA for HTLV-I/II antibody detection. The screening tests do not differentiate between HTLV-I and HTLV-II antibodies. A Western blot was licensed in December of 2014 [MP Biomedicals (Santa Ana, CA), version 2.4]; this assay uses recombinant and peptide antigens in addition to HTLV-I viral lysate to detect and differentiate between HTLV-I and HTLV-II antibodies. Risk estimates for transfusion-transmitted HTLV are somewhat uncertain, given the absence of well-defined window periods for the current HTLV antibody tests; however, there is no evidence of residual HTLV transfusion-transmission risk, which is estimated at <1 per several million. Because HTLV is cell associated, leukocyte reduction likely reduces infectivity; in addition, infectivity is reduced with increased refrigerated red cell storage. Like CMV, HTLV is thought to be transmitted only by white-cell-containing blood components and not by frozen/thawed plasma components.[75,76]

Hepatitis E Virus

One agent that has received recent attention globally is HEV, a small, nonenveloped, icosahedral, single-stranded RNA virus in its own family, *Hepeviridae*. HEV was first recognized in the 1980s in Afghanistan among soldiers with unexplained hepatitis. There is a single serotype but at least four genotypes with differing geographic distributions and epidemiologic patterns. Genotypes 1 and 2 are generally associated with large, water-borne (fecal-orally transmitted) outbreaks in less-developed tropical countries. Genotypes 3 and 4 appear to be animal viruses that result in zoonotic infection of humans, most often through consumption of inadequately cooked pork products. Genotype 3 is widely distributed and is present in developed countries, while genotype 4 seems to be more common in certain Asian countries.

The incubation period is 3 to 8 weeks with resulting illness that is generally self-limited but can result in fulminant hepatitis in those who are immunosuppressed or patients with chronic liver disease. Genotypes 1 and 2 can be lethal in pregnant women and their fetuses. Transfusion-related transmission, mostly of genotype 3, has been well-documented in Japan, France, England, the Netherlands, and Spain.[77] Recent studies suggest a wide range of seroprevalence rates in endemic areas of 20% to 40%, but some of the variability may be attributable to the differences in performance characteristics of the tests used, and some to dietary habits. Most studies indicate a cohort effect, with prevalence rates increasing with age. Transfusion infectivity is associated with the presence of viral RNA in plasma; reported frequencies of RNA prevalence in donations have ranged from 1 in 1000 to 1 in 10,000. In a large study in England, 225,000 donations were tested, and 79 (1 in 2848) were positive when tested for HEV RNA by an in-house NAT assay.[78] Tracing was possible for 43 recipients, of whom 18 (42%) showed evidence of transfusion-transmitted infection, with 10 having prolonged infection; three were immunosuppressed individuals requiring treatment to clear the virus, and another had clinical hepatitis. In contrast, in a smaller, blinded study in the United States, 7.7% of donors were anti-HEV positive and only two of approximately 19,000 were RNA positive (1:9500).[79] The current broader concern is the finding that highly immunosuppressed patients (such as solid-organ transplant recipients) do develop chronic HEV infections with long-term clinical sequelae, although these have not been specifically linked to infection via transfusion in the United States.

As a nonenveloped agent, HEV is not susceptible to SD treatment or to current-generation pathogen inactivation technologies. Some cases of breakthrough infection following inactivation methods have been documented. NAT donation screening has been implemented as a routine intervention in some European countries and areas of Japan with high HEV incidence, and other countries are evaluating such testing.

Syphilis

Syphilis is caused by the spirochete *Treponema pallidum*. Donor screening for syphilis has been performed for >60 years. Donors were initially screened by nontreponemal serologic tests that detect antibody to cardiolipin [eg, rapid plasma reagin (RPR)]. In recent years, however, most blood banks have begun using tests that detect specific antibodies to *T. pallidum* because these tests can be performed with automated testing instruments.

The vast majority of reactive donor test results do not represent active cases of syphilis. Most reflect either biologic false-positive results or persistent antibody in previously treated individuals (the former have negative and the latter have positive treponemal-specific antibody screening tests). FDA recommendations vary depending on whether the initial screening is performed using a nontreponemal test (eg, RPR) or a treponemal-specific test. If screening is performed with a nontreponemal test, additional testing with a treponemal-specific test can be used to guide donor and component management. The FDA permits release of units from donors who have reactive nontreponemal screening test results and negative treponemal-specific results if the units are labeled with both test results.[1,21] If screening is performed using a treponemal-specific test, the FDA recommends additional testing by a second FDA-cleared treponemal test. If the second test is nonreactive, the donor can be reentered, although the component cannot be released. If the result of the second treponemal-specific test is positive, the donor must be deferred for at least 12 months.

The current value of donor screening for syphilis is controversial.[80-82] Although numerous cases of transfusion-transmitted syphilis were reported before World War II, no cases have been reported in the United States for >40 years. The low transmission risk is probably related to a declining incidence of syphilis in donors as well as the limited survival of the *T. pallidum* spirochete during blood storage.

One issue that has been considered is whether the syphilis screen improves blood safety by serving as a surrogate marker of high-risk sexual activity. However, studies have demonstrated that donor screening for syphilis does not provide incremental value in detecting other blood-borne and sexually transmitted infections, such as HIV, HBV, HCV, or HTLV.[82]

Other Bacteria

Bacterial contamination of blood components (mainly platelets) continues to cause transfusion-related fatalities.[83,84] As defined by the FDA in March 2016 by draft guidance, platelets are associated with a higher risk of sepsis and related fatality than any other transfusable blood component and are the leading cause of infection from blood transfusion, with an associated rate of approximately 1 per 100,000 transfused apheresis platelet units.[84,85] Bacteria are currently detected in approximately 1 in 6000 apheresis platelet do-nations by routine quality-control culture, but some escape detection by current screening methods to cause septic transfusion reactions.[84-86] The source of the bacteria is most commonly the donor's skin but can also be asymptomatic bacteremia in the donor.

The level of bacteria in components just after collection is generally too low to detect or to cause symptoms in the recipient. However, bacteria can multiply during component storage, particularly in platelet components, which are kept at room temperature. Bacteria proliferate to a lesser extent in refrigerated red cells, and septic reactions occur much less commonly with these components. In rare cases, Red Blood Cell (RBC) units contaminated with bacteria capable of growth at cold temperatures during the storage period have caused life-threatening sepsis.[83,86] To reduce the risk of septic transfusion reactions associated with platelets, AABB implemented a requirement for facilities' processes to limit and detect bacterial contamination in all platelet components in 2004. AABB recognized in 2009 the availability in some countries of pathogen reduction methods, which can be used instead of bacteria detection methods for platelet components.[35(p11)]

To limit blood component contamination by bacteria from donor skin, two elements of the blood collection process are critical. Before venipuncture, the donor skin must be carefully disinfected using a method with demonstrated efficacy. Most of these methods involve iodophors, chlorhexidine, or alcohol.[86] Second, diversion of the first 10 mL to 40 mL of donor blood, which can contain contaminated skin and its appendages, away from the collection container (eg, into a sample pouch) further reduces the likelihood that skin contaminants will enter the component.[84-87] Since 2008, AABB has required that collection sets with diversion pouches be used for all platelet collections, including whole blood collections from which platelets are made.[35(p22)]

A variety of technologies are available for detection of bacteria in platelet components. AABB *Standards* requires blood centers to use a bacteria detection method that is approved by the FDA or validated to provide sensitivity equivalent to FDA-approved methods. None of these methods is sensitive enough to detect bacteria immediately after collection. All methods require a waiting time for bacteria contaminants to multiply before the component is sampled.

The process most commonly used in the United States to screen apheresis platelets is a culture-based system that requires waiting at least 24 hours after phlebotomy before sampling the platelet donation. After that time, a sample is withdrawn and inoculated into one or more culture bottles. The bottles are then incubated in the culture system. Some blood centers continue to hold the platelet components during the first 12 to 24 hours of culture and release it for use only if the culture is negative at the end of that time. In all cases, the culture is continued for the shelf life of the unit. If the culture becomes positive after the component is released, the blood center attempts to retrieve it. If the component has not been transfused, resampling of the component for culture is very informative because approximately two-thirds of the initially positive signals are caused by either contamination of the bottle (and not the component) or false signals from the culture system.[85,86] All positive cultures should be tested to determine the identity of the organism. If a true-positive result is related to an organism that is not a common skin contaminant but could indicate asymptomatic bacteremia, the donor should be notified and advised to seek medical consultation.[37]

Other methods approved in the United States for platelet quality control testing early in the storage period include a culture-based system with a one-time-point readout and an optical scanning system. All of the methods are approved for testing leukocyte-reduced apheresis platelets, and some are approved for testing pools of leukocyte-reduced, whole-blood-derived platelets.[88] These methods are not generally used for routine screening of individual (unpooled) whole-blood-derived platelet concentrates. Low-technology methods for screening platelets just before issue—such as visually inspecting the platelets for swirling or testing them for low glucose or pH—lack both sensitivity and specificity and do not fulfill the AABB standard for bacteria detection.[35,87] However, FDA-cleared point-of-issue assays can be used for bacteria detection testing of platelet concentrates that are pooled immediately before issue.

Since the implementation of routine bacteria screening of apheresis platelets, the frequency of FDA-reported fatalities from contaminated apheresis platelets has declined.[83] However, some contaminated apheresis platelets escape detection by this early testing, presumably because bacterial concentrations remain below limits of detection at the time of sampling; thus, septic, and even fatal, reactions do still occur. AABB has recommended consideration of policies to further reduce the risk of bacterially contaminated platelets, and the FDA has issued draft guidance.[84-87] The point-of-issue assays mentioned above are cleared by the FDA as adjunct (time-of-issue) tests for apheresis platelets that have been screened by another method. In a large clinical trial, one of these assays detected nine bacterially contaminated components among 27,620 apheresis platelet units (1 in 3069 components) that were negative by an early-storage culture-based assay.[89] There were also 142 false-positive results. As of March 2017, point-of-issue retesting of apheresis platelets had not been widely implemented in the United States.

The current approach provides incomplete assurance of bacteria detection. Pathogen inactivation methods, which impair proliferation of bacteria in the blood component, could theoretically be used to reduce the risk of septic reactions from bacteria in blood components, although none is yet available for red cells. Indeed, in some regions outside the United States, pathogen inactivation has replaced bacteria detection testing for platelets, but such replacement has not widely occurred in the United States. Draft FDA guidance for industry (March 2016) recommends interventions beyond those included in AABB *Standards*.[84] The guidance cites current surveillance data indicating that 95% of septic transfusion reactions and 100% of fatalities associated with platelets occur on storage days 4 and 5 (evenly between the two days, which are noted as the days when most platelets are used). Thus, these draft recommendations include: secondary testing with an FDA-cleared rapid test of previously cultured apheresis platelets or prestorage pooled platelets within 24 hours of transfusion, or reculture of platelets on day 4 with a hold for at least the first 12 hours after reculture. Alternately, bacteria testing could be substituted (as is the case in some areas outside of the United States) with an FDA-approved pathogen inactivation process within 24 hours of collection. The FDA draft guidance concludes that either pathogen inactivation or secondary testing of previously cultured but not pathogen-reduced platelets would provide adequate control of the risk of platelet bacterial contamination.

Infections Transmitted by Insect Vectors

Until recently, malaria was the only vector-transmitted disease that was widely recognized as having the potential for secondary transmission by transfusion in the United States. Vectorial transmission of malaria is rare in the United States, and the blood supply has been effectively protected by questions that exclude donors who have recently traveled to or resided in malaria-endemic regions. In the past decade, however, other vector-transmitted infections have been recognized as threats to the US blood supply, and these infections are targeted by the newest blood donor screening assays.

West Nile Virus

WNV is a lipid-enveloped RNA virus in the *Flaviviridae* family. The first WNV cases were identified in the West Nile district of Uganda in 1937. Afterward, outbreaks occurred in the Middle East, South Africa, and Europe. First detected in the United States in 1999, it subsequently spread throughout North America, appearing in annual epidemics every summer and autumn. It is transmitted primarily in a bird-to-bird transmission cycle by culicine mosquitoes, and human infections occur incidentally. WNV viral loads in humans are too low to reinfect mosquitoes. Approximately 80% of human cases are asymptomatic; 20% are associated with a self-limited febrile illness; and <1% are associated with severe neuroinvasive disease, such as meningoencephalitis or acute flaccid paralysis.

During the summer of 2002, a model suggesting a significant risk for WNV infection in blood donors was published,[90] and then four recipients of organ allografts from a single donor developed neuroinvasive WNV infection.[91] Infection of the organ donor was traced to donor blood transfused before death from trauma. Transfusion transmission was documented in 23 recipients in 2002 compared with a background of 2946 cases of WNV-meningoencephalitis in the general population.[91] A rapid multidisciplinary effort led to the implementation of WNV investigational screening assays by the following summer. Because RNA-positive units, not antibody-positive units, were considered to pose the greatest risk from this acute infection, NAT, rather than serologic testing, was required to protect the blood supply. Donor tests for WNV RNA are now approved by the FDA and required by both the FDA and AABB.[18,19,35] In retrospective cohort studies of blood donors with positive WNV RNA tests, 29% to 61% described symptoms before or after donation, compared to 3% to 20% of control uninfected donors, demonstrating that the donor history is neither sensitive nor specific enough to prevent transfusion transmission.[92]

To maximize efficiency, donation samples are tested by MP-NAT in pools of 6 to 16 donations, as is done for HCV, HBV, and HIV. However, because circulating levels of WNV RNA are low (the highest viral load documented has been 720,000 copies/mL), a donor sample may contain a low concentration of RNA that will not be detected by MP-NAT.[93] Therefore, both the FDA and AABB recommend testing by ID-NAT, not MP-NAT, when WNV activity is high in a particular collection region.[18,19] Regional WNV activity is monitored through active communications between neighboring blood collection agencies and includes monitoring RNA-reactive donations, public health reports of clinical WNV cases, and animal and mosquito surveillance in the area.

In total, following the 23 cases of transfusion-transmitted WNV documented before the initiation of donation NAT screening in 2003, an additional 14 cases have been reported, most related to donations having only low levels of RNA.[94] All implicated donations, except one in 2002, have been IgM negative.[93,94] Blood centers must remain vigilant to make the very rapid conversion from MP- to ID-NAT needed for this seasonal and localized strategy to be effective.

Zika Virus

ZIKV is a tropical arbovirus of the flavivirus group, very closely related to dengue viruses using the same *Aedes* mosquito vectors. ZIKV was first recognized in Africa in 1947, and more recently it began circulating in the Pacific islands. In 2007, the first human outbreak was recognized on the island of Yap in Micronesia, with subsequent spread to French Polynesia in 2013, to Brazil in May 2015, and to Puerto Rico in December 2015.[95] As of February 2016, 61 countries or areas have reported active transmission, including 50 countries or areas in the Americas. ZIKV infection has been proven to cause fetal loss, congenital ZIKV-related syndromes including microcephaly, and Guillain-Barré syndrome and other neurologic complications in adults.[95-101] However, in most cases (~80%) ZIKV infection is asymptomatic, although symptomatic case rates may be higher.[102]

ZIKV RNA can be recovered from blood donors, as demonstrated in the 2013-2014 ZIKV outbreak in French Polynesia, in which 2.8% of donors tested RNA positive by NAT, and subsequently in Martinique and Puerto Rico with rates of 1.8%.[102-105] As of March 2017, there have been four probable transfusion transmissions, all reported in Brazil.[106,107] These occurred from three donors who were identified by postdonation information reports of dengue/Zika-like symptoms. None of the recipients developed Zika-related symptoms following transfusion. In addition to mosquito-borne transmission and transfusion transmission, sexual transmission has also been documented.[95] Although the majority of sexually transmitted ZIKV cases have been from an infected male to his partner (male or female); a female-to-male sexual transmission has also been reported.[108]

The duration of ZIKV viremia as detected by diagnostic assays is believed to be 1 to 2 weeks, consistent with other mosquito-borne viruses. Viral clearance was estimated, using these assays, to be 19 days for 95% of affected patients (95% confidence interval of 13 to 80 days in a pooled analysis of published studies).[109] ZIKV has been reported to persist longer in whole blood, semen, vaginal fluid, and urine vs serum and plasma. One report found persistence of ZIKV RNA (as opposed to infectious virus) in whole blood for 5 to 58 days after symptom onset despite RNA-negative findings in corresponding serum samples; RNA positivity for 5 to 26 days occurred in urine from these same individuals.[110] Testing of urine is now recommended for diagnostic testing in the United States in patients with suspected Zika disease based on a study documenting that 5 days after symptom onset, 82% of Zika clinical cases remained RNA positive from urine but not serum. If diagnostic testing is performed <7 days after symptom onset, both urine and serum testing should be performed.[111,112] The longest persistence of ZIKV has been in semen. In one case, RNA was detected for 62 days, and in others for 92 to 93 days with the longest at 188 days, all in travelers returning from Zika-active or previously active areas.[113-115] ZIKV RNA duration was estimated from following 150 ZIKV polymerase chain reaction (PCR)-positive patients in Puerto Rico.[116] The medians and 95th percentiles (plus 95% confidence limits) for ZIKV RNA persistence in serum, urine, and semen, respectively, were 14 (11-17) and 54 (43-64) days, 8 (6-10) and 39 (31-47) days, and 34 (31-47) and 81 (64-98) days.

As of February 2017, there were 4780 travel-associated Zika cases in the continental United States reported to the CDC, 41 sexually transmitted cases, and 1 laboratory-acquired case.[117] In addition, a fatal, rapidly progressive

infection acquired outside of the United States resulted in a secondary local transmission in the absence of known ZIKV risk factors.[118] Local mosquito-borne transmission has been reported in two states: Florida (214 cases) and Texas (6 cases). In contrast, 36,498 locally transmitted cases of Zika clinical disease have been reported in the United States territories, mostly in Puerto Rico. An additional 13 cases of Guillain-Barré syndrome associated with ZIKV infection have been reported to the CDC in the continental United States, and 51 in US territories.[117]

Because of concern about severe disease associations, rapid virus spread in the Americas, recovery of RNA from blood of asymptomatic donors, and reports of transfusion transmission, blood centers initially asked donors about travel to or residence in Zika-active areas using a specific question with an associated 28-day deferral. In addition, donors who had sexual contact with an individual with a Zika diagnosis or symptoms, or who had traveled to Zika-active area(s), or who have symptoms or a diagnosis of Zika were asked to self-defer for 28 days. These recommendations were included by the FDA in guidance released on February 16, 2016.[41] However, because of increased concern about the probability of autochthonous transmission and travel-related and sexual transmission, the FDA revised its guidance on August 26, 2016, to require universal ZIKV ID-NAT or the use of approved pathogen inactivation technologies; three sets of timelines were included, which depended on the presence/threat of transmission in a given state or territory.[42,43] Donors are still requested to self-defer based on a Zika disease diagnosis. Donors testing NAT reactive and/or with a diagnosis are deferred for 120 days, with subsequent reinstatement allowed after that period.

Two NAT assays are being used under investigational new drug (IND) applications. One is manufactured by Roche Molecular Systems, Inc., and the other by Grifols, Inc.; these assays are used in the continental United States and in Puerto Rico. The donor screening NAT assays appear to be more sensitive than the diagnostic assays.[119] RNA has been detected in donor plasma samples as long as 71 and 97 days after donor return from Zika-endemic areas.[120,121] The FDA-approved pathogen inactivation process for platelets and plasma has been shown to be effective for reducing relevant arbovirus titers. Published data using the FDA-approved method demonstrate a >6 $\log_{10}$ reduction in ZIKV infectivity titers in plasma, with similar reductions observed for red cells, as well as SD plasma and other plasma-derived products.[122-125]

Other Arboviruses

There are many other vector-transmitted infections that could be secondarily transmitted by transfusion. These agents and potential intervention strategies are reviewed in the publicly available AABB emerging infectious disease resources.[61,62] Two of these agents, the dengue and chikungunya viruses (DENV and CHIKV), received attention because donations containing viral nucleic acid were documented during epidemics outside the continental United States.

Forty percent of the world's population lives in areas with risk for dengue, including many areas visited by US travelers. It has spread rapidly in Latin America and the Caribbean since the 1980s. Dengue is endemic in Puerto Rico, the US Virgin Islands, and American Samoa, and there have been outbreaks in Hawaii, Texas, and Florida during the last 10 years.[126] Dengue is caused by four related flaviviruses spread person to person by *Aedes aegypti* and *A. albopictus*. Most infections are asymptomatic, but illness ranges from undifferentiated fever to classic break-bone fever and severe dengue (dengue hemorrhagic fever and dengue shock syndrome). An approximately 7-day viremia is a feature of both asymptomatic and symptomatic infection, and asymptomatic blood donors from Hong Kong, Singapore, Brazil, and Puerto Rico have transmitted dengue to blood recipients in seven clusters. Although the number of reports of transfusion-transmitted infections is limited compared to the high rates of vector-borne infection, the lack of systematic surveillance for transfusion-transmitted DENV makes its rec-

ognition in the face of widespread outbreaks problematic.[127] RNA-positive, asymptomatic donors have been identified in Brazil, Central America, and Puerto Rico using NAT and antigen detection tests. Rates of donor RNA positivity in Puerto Rico are comparable to those found in US donors during the most active WNV seasons.[128,129] A study in Brazil documented transfusion transmission from RNA-positive donors; however, when the medical charts of infected recipients transfused from those donors were compared to control recipients who did not receive an RNA-positive unit, there was no measurable apparent clinical illness.[130] This further illustrates the difficulty in identifying transfusion-transmitted DENV among severely ill patients who are frequently transfused.

In the absence of sustained outbreaks of locally transmitted DENV in the continental United States, transfusion risk relates mainly to return of infected, asymptomatic or presymptomatic travelers. A 3- to 14-day incubation period precedes symptom onset. Deferral for travel to malarious areas (1 year for US residents) offers some protection, but a large proportion of dengue-affected areas frequently visited from the US are malaria free, and donor-travelers to those areas could potentially introduce the virus into the community and the blood supply. The conditions for sustained spread of DENV exist in large areas of the United States: a source of infection from travelers, a susceptible population, and competent vectors.

CHIKV is another tropical arbovirus transmitted by *Aedes* spp. mosquitoes. It is a togavirus of the alphavirus group first recognized in Africa. It has been responsible for explosive outbreaks in the islands of the Indian Ocean followed by spread to the Caribbean, where >1.7 million clinical cases were reported from the end of 2013 to the middle of 2015, including RNA positivity in blood donors.[131,132] There have been no reported cases of transmission by transfusion, but the similarity of early infection to that of dengue has resulted in significant concern. Notably, French authorities responded to the outbreak in the islands of the Indian Ocean by halting local collection of red cells (providing for the islands' needs by supplying blood from the French mainland) and by implementation of limited NAT and the use of pathogen inactivation for platelets.[132] Other precautions that have been used include strengthening requirements of postdonation information from donors [a process that is enhanced by the high (50%-80%) frequency of symptoms among infected subjects], along with deferrals for residence in affected areas. Chikungunya symptoms are similar to those of dengue, but without the impact on the circulatory system. Arthralgia is a prominent symptom and may be prolonged. Routine testing is not currently available. Rates of CHIKV RNA detection in unlinked blood donation samples reached 2.1% in Puerto Rico during the 2014 outbreak; viral titers in positive donations ranged from 10^4 to 10^9 RNA copies per mL.[133]

Trypanosoma cruzi

T. cruzi, the protozoan parasite that causes Chagas disease, is endemic in parts of Mexico, Central America, and South America. It is transmitted to humans most commonly by an insect vector, triatomine or reduviid bugs, but can also be transmitted by ingesting contaminated foods or beverages, by transfusion, and from mother to child. The insect vector is associated with a wide variety of mammalian hosts in rural areas of endemic countries that serve as the reservoir; human infections most commonly occur when the vector cannot find an alternative mammalian host from which to acquire a blood meal. Acute infection is usually self-limited, involving localized swelling at the bite site and fever, but may be severe in immunocompromised patients. Most infections become chronic but remain asymptomatic. Decades after the initial infection, 10% to 40% of infected individuals develop late-stage manifestations, including intestinal dysfunction or cardiac disease, which can be fatal. Transfusion transmission of *T. cruzi* from the blood of chronically infected, asymptomatic donors has been reported in endemic areas, although it has become uncommon with decreasing use

of fresh whole blood and implementation of donor serologic screening.

A blood donor screening enzyme immunoassay (EIA) (Ortho Diagnostics, Raritan, NJ) for antibodies to *T. cruzi*, using parasite lysate, was approved by the FDA for US use in December 2006. Although not initially required by the FDA, the test was widely implemented by US blood centers during 2007. Subsequently a second licensed screening test using ChLIA on the PRISM platform (Abbott Laboratories, Chicago, IL) was approved using recombinant antigens for antibody capture instead of epimastigote lysate as used for the EIA. Initially there was no FDA-approved supplemental assay, but additional testing of reactive donations using an unlicensed radioimmunoprecipitation assay (RIPA) was helpful for guiding donor counseling. Based on the results of the latter assay, about 25% of reactive US donors appear to be truly infected.[134,135] An enzyme strip assay (ESA) using the same *T. cruzi* recombinant antigens as used in the PRISM test is now approved by the FDA as a supplemental assay.

The vast majority of US donations with reactive *T. cruzi* screening test results and positive supplemental results are from donors born in *T. cruzi*-endemic areas. Other confirmed-positive donors appear mostly to have congenitally acquired infections (ie, the donor's mother is from a *T. cruzi*-endemic area), and only a small number of donor infections appear to have been acquired from vector exposure within the United States (autochthonous cases). In the first 2 years of universal donor screening in the United States, no donor seroconversions were identified.[135] In December 2010, the FDA issued guidance recommending one-time testing of each US donor for *T. cruzi*.[25] A draft amendment to the guidance has been released maintaining one-time donor screening, eliminating the Chagas disease screening question, and providing a donor reentry algorithm.[40]

Before implementation of donor screening, seven cases of transfusion-transmitted *T. cruzi* had been identified in the United States and Canada; all of the cases with available data were linked to platelet transfusion, and none was from a donor with recent infection. Twenty cases of transfusion transmission in the United States, Canada, and Spain have now been documented—again, all related to platelets from remotely infected donors who have resided in highly endemic areas.[136] Since the implementation of donor screening, confirmed-positive donors have been identified, and recipients of their prior donations have been notified and tested. Thus far, only two prior recipients (of platelets from one remotely infected donor born in a Chagas-endemic country) appear to have been infected by transfusion, which were identified only through look-back procedures.[137] Thus, despite historically reported transmission rates of 10% to 20% from whole blood from infected donors in endemic areas, no *T. cruzi* transmissions by red cells in the United States have been documented (one case in Belgium has been documented recently).[138] The lower infectivity of red cell components compared to platelets or fresh whole blood is likely attributable to the limited survival of the parasite in refrigerated components.

Babesia

Babesia are intraerythrocytic parasites that are the causative agent of babesiosis. Well over 100 species have been described worldwide. Human *Babesia* infections are zoonotic, usually acquired through the bite of an infected tick. In the northeastern and midwestern United States, the most common *Babesia* species is *B. microti*. The vector is *Ixodes scapularis*, the same tick that transmits Lyme disease. In the western United States, *Babesia* infections appear to be less common, and a different species, *B. duncani*, predominates. The vector for *B. duncani* has not been clearly defined. Reported human infections with *Babesia* are becoming more frequent, and in response in 2011, the CDC made babesiosis nationally notifiable, although not all states require reporting; 95% of cases occur in seven states considered to be endemic. Transfusion-transmitted babesiosis (TTB) is being identified with increasing frequency. There is no FDA-approved donor screening test for this infection.[139] The

FDA requires that donors be asked if they have had a history of babesiosis and are permanently deferred for affirmative responses; this is an insensitive (and nonspecific) intervention allowing continued TTB, with 162 TTB cases described from 1979 to 2009.[140] Investigational testing has been introduced regionally as an intervention, and pathogen inactivation technology is capable of significantly reducing *B. microti* infectivity.

Babesia infection is usually asymptomatic, even though parasites can circulate for months to years. In some individuals, however, *Babesia* infection presents as a severe malaria-like illness that can be fatal. Generally, fatalities range from 6% to 9% but may be as high as 21% in immunocompromised patients.[139,140] Immunocompromised, elderly, and asplenic patients are at increased risk of severe disease, but following a review of published TTB cases, it has become clear that any recipient is susceptible to infection and clinical illness.[141] Treatment with antibiotics is very effective, most commonly including oral atovaquone with azithromycin for 7 to 10 days; more severe cases often receive red cell exchange transfusion. The key is prompt recognition and diagnosis of infection.

Babesia infection is most commonly diagnosed when the intraerythrocytic parasites are seen on a blood smear; tetrads of parasites in infected red cells, referred to as a Maltese cross, are characteristic of *B. microti* (vs malaria) infection. If a patient is suspected of having acquired the infection by transfusion, donors of the patient's components can be recalled and tested for antibodies to *Babesia* using an immunofluorescence assay and by PCR; the presence of *B. microti* DNA or high-titer antibody in the donor is suggestive of recent infection. Most of the donors implicated in TTB cases have been residents of endemic areas, although rarely residents of nonendemic areas who were apparently exposed to *Babesia* during travel to endemic areas have been implicated in TTB cases.[139,140,142] The frequency of TTB from travelers is estimated at 1 per 10 million donations.[143]

The results of investigational blood donation screening describing the yield of the tests used, the duration of donor positivity, the relationship of test-negative units to transfusion transmission, the infectivity of test-positive units, and residual risks have been reported.[143] Approximately 90,000 donations from consenting donors were tested by two investigational assays: automated immunofluorescence for antibody detection and ID-NAT by PCR to detect the parasite's DNA. Donors reactive by either test were further tested to confirm infection. The frequency of infected donors in a highly endemic area where screening occurred was 1 per 300 donations with 1 per 10,000 donations in the PCR-positive, antibody-negative window period. The current risk of TTB from an unscreened RBC unit in endemic states is 1 per 100,000 but as high as 1 per 18,000 in highly endemic areas. Receipt of unscreened red cells in a highly endemic area was 9 times more likely to result in TTB than screened blood (screened blood was not associated with any case of TTB). DNA clearance in infected donors occurred after 1 year, but antibody clearance occurred in <10% during that interval. Overall from January 2010 through the end of August 2016, another 62 TTB cases from unscreened blood were reported, which can be added to the 162 cases previously documented.[140,143] These reported cases are an underestimate of the true number of transmissions because most infections are asymptomatic.

Malaria

Malaria is caused by an intraerythrocytic parasite of the genus *Plasmodium*. Infection is transmitted to humans through a mosquito bite. Five species account for most human infections: *P. falciparum, P. vivax, P. malariae, P. ovale*, and *P. knowlesi*. Disease symptoms most notably include periodic fever, rigors and chills, and hemolytic anemia.

The parasites are present in the circulation during a prolonged asymptomatic period and are readily transmitted by blood transfusion. Recognition of infected recipients, as is true of *Babesia* infection, may be complex and is achieved through a high index of suspicion and identification of the parasite in red cells from blood smear examination, detection of parasite DNA by PCR, or detection by antibody test methods. Transfusion transmission is common in tropical endemic areas and is of significant risk elsewhere because of travelers returning from endemic areas or residents of endemic areas who have partial or incomplete immunity traveling to nonendemic areas. No FDA-approved test is available to screen US blood donations for malaria infection. Screening is accomplished solely by donor questioning. Donors are excluded temporarily from donating blood after traveling to malaria-endemic areas, after residing in malaria-endemic countries, or after recovery from clinical malaria. Donor questioning has been remarkably effective at preventing transfusion-transmitted malaria (TTM) in the United States, with only six cases reported between 1999 and 2016. All six cases were linked to donors with a history of residence (as opposed to short-term travel) in Africa; on re-interview, five of the six donors were verified to have met acceptance criteria, but one had emigrated <3 years before donation.[144,145]

This level of transfusion safety has been achieved at a substantial cost in terms of donor loss; malaria-related questions have excluded hundreds of thousands of otherwise acceptable US donors annually. In 2013, the FDA issued guidance redefining malaria-endemic areas as only those for which chemoprophylaxis is recommended.[146] With this new definition, travel to many popular tourist locations is no longer considered a malarial risk; for example, in the past, Mexico has accounted for the largest proportion of deferred donors while having risk that is exceeding low.[147] However, this guidance adds a complex algorithm for evaluating travel by donors who have lived for >5 years in malaria-endemic countries because of a concern about the clinical impact of partial immunity in such donors.

Outside of the United States, some countries that exclude donors after travel to malaria-endemic areas permit reinstatement of these donors if they test negative for malaria antibodies 4 to 6 months after completion of travel. In the absence of an approved assay, such a "test-in" reinstatement strategy has not been accepted by the FDA.[148] Pathogen inactivation methods have been shown to be effective at reducing transfusion transmission in endemic areas.[149] A randomized clinical trial involved 214 patients in Africa (Kumasi, Ghana) who completed a blinded evaluation comparing the efficacy of pathogen-reduced vs untreated whole blood for prevention of TTM (107 treated and 107 untreated patients).[149] Overall, 65 nonparasitemic recipients (28 treated and 37 untreated) were exposed to parasitemic blood. The incidence of transfusion-transmitted malaria was significantly lower for the patients treated with pathogen-reduced blood [1 (4%) of 28 patients] than the untreated group [8 (22%) of 37 patients]. No adverse events could be attributed to the treated units compared to the control units.

Prions

Prions are proteinaceous infectious particles that induce disease by triggering conformational changes in naturally occurring protein counterparts. These agents cause fatal infections of the nervous system called transmissible spongiform encephalopathies (TSEs).

Classical Creutzfeldt-Jakob disease (CJD) is a TSE with both a sporadic form and familial forms and an incidence of about 1 per million population. Iatrogenic CJD has been transmitted by injection or implantation of products from infected central nervous system tissues. Blood components do not appear to transmit classical CJD. Nevertheless, blood donations are not accepted from donors who are at increased risk for this disease.[150]

Another TSE, variant CJD (vCJD), does appear to be transmissible by blood transfusion. This TSE is caused by the same prion that causes bovine spongiform encephalopathy (BSE), also known as "mad cow disease," with human infection occurring after ingesting tissues from infected animals. vCJD differs from CJD in that infected individuals are younger, present with psychiatric symptoms, and generally have a longer course from diagnosis to death. Postmortem diagnosis involves unusual florid plaques in the brain. Clinical cases have occurred primarily in the United Kingdom, but

cases have occurred in other areas worldwide as a result of the export of contaminated animal tissues. The number of cases reported have declined over the past 5 years; as of December 2014 (the last update as of March 2017), 229 cases have been reported worldwide, with 178 cases in the United Kingdom. Of those, four were cases of vCJD transmission by transfusion in the United Kingdom. Three of these four resulted in the development of vCJD; the fourth occurred in an individual who died of underlying disease but whose spleen and one lymph node were found to contain vCJD prions. In addition, one latent vCJD infection was identified in a patient with hemophilia in the United Kingdom who died of other causes. This patient had received UK-plasma-derived Factor VIII, including material from a donor who later developed vCJD, suggesting that vCJD might have been transmitted by clotting factor concentrates.[61,62] vCJD infection is extremely rare in the United States. The few reported cases have been in individuals who most likely acquired their infections elsewhere, and no US transfusion-transmitted cases have been reported.

There are no FDA-approved donor screening tests for prion infections. Blood donors in the United States are screened solely by questioning and are excluded if they have an increased risk of either CJD or vCJD. CJD exclusions are based on family history of the disease, receipt of human growth hormone derived from pituitary glands, or receipt of a dura mater tissue graft. vCJD exclusions are for residence in the United Kingdom or Europe during specified times when BSE was endemic, receipt of a transfusion in the United Kingdom or France, or receipt of UK bovine insulin.[150] It is thought that plasma-derivative manufacturing processes remove substantial amounts of TSE infectivity.[150]

Screening for Plasma Derivatives

Commercial plasma derivatives are prepared from large pools of plasma derived from thousands of donors. Before the incorporation of specific pathogen inactivation processes, contamination of these large pools with viral agents was common. Today, plasma-derivative manufacturing processes incorporate methods—such as prolonged heat or SD treatment—that remove or inactivate most known pathogens. SD treatment inactivates lipid-enveloped agents, such as HIV, HCV, and HBV. Pathogen infectivity may also be reduced by nanofiltration, chromatography, or cold ethanol fractionation, which are used in the production of certain products. Not all infectious agents, however, are removed or inactivated by these processes.

One agent that can persist in plasma-derivative products is human parvovirus B19. This small, nonenveloped DNA virus is extremely resistant to physical inactivation. Acute infection is typically mild and self-limited; clinical manifestations include "fifth disease" (erythema infectiosum) and polyarthropathy. Acute infection is associated with transient red cell aplasia that may be clinically significant in immunodeficient individuals and those with underlying hemolytic processes. The aplasia in immunodeficient individuals can be prolonged. Intrauterine infection is associated with severe fetal anemia and hydrops fetalis.

Parvovirus B19 infection is very common; most adults have antibodies to this agent, indicating previous exposure. Levels of viral DNA during acute infection may exceed 10^{12} IU/mL, decreasing over weeks to months in association with antibody production.

Viral DNA, mostly at low concentrations, has been detected in approximately 1% of blood donations and in essentially all lots of pooled plasma derivatives. Transmission of parvovirus B19 by transfusion has been linked only to blood components or plasma products that contain high concentrations of viral DNA; only one transmission has been documented with a product containing <10^4 IU/mL.[62]

Currently, there is no FDA-approved test to screen fresh blood donations for parvovirus B19 infection. However, plasma-derivative manufacturers require screening of incoming plasma units for the presence of high-titer parvovirus B19. This is accomplished by performing NAT on pools of samples from plasma units, with sensitivity adjusted to detect only units with a high concentration of virus. By excluding high-titer units from the plasma pools, the final titer in the plasma pool is kept below 10^4 IU/mL.

Other Agents

AABB maintains a publicly accessible electronic resource containing expert analyses of emerging infectious disease agents that have received attention as potential threats to the US or global blood supply.[62] This digital resource contains up-to-date fact sheets on a variety of agents. Each fact sheet includes information about clinical manifestations and epidemiology of infection, evidence of transfusion transmissibility, and analyses of the potential effectiveness of various mitigation strategies (eg, donor questioning, serologic testing or NAT, or pathogen inactivation). Readers are encouraged to use this rich resource.

PATHOGEN INACTIVATION TECHNOLOGY

Donor screening reduces, but cannot eliminate, the infectious risks of blood transfusion. The efficacy of blood donor testing is limited by a number of factors, including the following[151]:

1. It is not logistically feasible to test donors for every infection that is conceivably transmissible by transfusion.

2. For every test, there is a lag time (ie, window period) between when a person becomes infected and when the test detects infection.

3. Every test has limited sensitivity (concentration of the target marker that can be detected by the test).

4. Developing a donor test can be a long, multiphase process that includes identification of the infectious agent, selection of the type of test that would be effective in interdicting infectious donations (eg, serology vs NAT), development of a test suitable for donor screening, performance of clinical

trials of the test, and regulatory approval. During this development process, infections can be transmitted.

5. Testing cannot interdict unknown pathogens or pathogens not yet recognized or suspected to be transfusable.

Pathogen inactivation provides an attractive alternative to relying on donor questioning and testing to interdict infectious donations. Pathogen inactivation processes reduce the infectivity of residual pathogens in blood components. This approach could reduce the transmission of infectious agents for which there are no donor screening tests and further reduce the residual transmission risks of known agents. Once approved and implemented, pathogen inactivation could theoretically enable discontinuation of some testing that is currently performed (eg, CMV testing and bacteria testing of platelets, ID-NAT), and pathogen inactivation methods have been shown to obviate the need for irradiation, potentially offsetting some of its cost.

As discussed above, pathogen inactivation methods are an essential component of the plasma-derivative manufacturing process. An SD-treated pooled plasma product has been approved for transfusion in the United States [Octaplas (Octapharma)]. Because these methods used on plasma (SD treatment and methylene blue/visible light treatment) damage cell membranes, these methods are not used for platelets or red cells. The pooling of plasma products for use with these technologies results in an increased risk of transmitting an agent that lacks a lipid envelope and is particularly resistant to inactivation. Hence, incoming lots of plasma intended for manufacture of plasma derivatives are prescreened to eliminate the risk of contamination by these agents, such as parvovirus B19, HEV, and hepatitis A virus (another nonenveloped hepatitis agent rarely transfusion transmitted). Such prescreening also occurs for SD plasma lots used for transfusion in the United States.

One manufacturer's pathogen inactivation process is now approved in the United States for treatment of individual units of plasma and platelets (INTERCEPT) using amotosalen (a psoralen) and ultraviolet A (UVA) light. Additional technologies are in use outside the United States. Riboflavin (vitamin B2) and UVB and UVA light are being used for plasma and platelets (TerumoBCT, Lakewood, CO). The nucleic-acid-damaging pathogen inactivation technologies provide significant activity against all agents for which tests are performed currently: HIV, HBV, HCV, HTLV, WNV, CMV, ZIKV, and parasites, as well as syphilis and agents causing bacterial contamination of platelets. However, pathogen inactivation methods appear to differ greatly in their capacity. INTERCEPT treatment also inactivates white cells to prevent transfusion-associated graft-vs-host disease, decreases formation and release of cytokines during storage, reduces febrile nonhemolytic transfusion reactions, and abrogates white-cell-induced alloantibody (eg, HLA antibody) formation, mitigating alloimmune platelet refractoriness. Clinical trials are under way in the United States and internationally on pathogen-reduced red cells using amustaline plus glutathione (INTERCEPT, Cerus Corp.) and whole blood using riboflavin and UV light (TerumoBCT). Processes that are available or in development have been recently reviewed in detail and are summarized in Table 7-7.[152-154]

Pathogen inactivation technologies that target nucleic acids usually do so by generation of cross-linking, preventing pathogen replication. Platelets treated with these technologies have somewhat lower 1-hour posttransfusion corrected count increments.[154] In clinical trials, mild and moderate bleeding frequency is increased, but not severe bleeding complications; the time between transfusions and the total number of platelet transfusions have not generally been different. Pulmonary toxicity similar to transfusion-related acute lung injury (TRALI) has been reported in clinical trials and in animal model experiments. Previous clinical trials of one red cell inactivation method were halted because of asymptomatic immunoreactivity against the red cell neoantigens believed to be the result of treatment and are being resumed with a reformulated process (amustaline plus glutathione).

TABLE 7-7. Pathogen Inactivation Technologies for Transfusable Blood Components

Component	Technology	Manufacturer
Plasma: commercially prepared pools	Solvent/detergent treatment	Octapharma (FDA cleared)
Plasma: individual units	Amotosalen (psoralen) + UV light	Cerus (FDA cleared)
	Riboflavin (vitamin B2) + UV light	TerumoBCT
	Methylene blue + light	Macopharma
Platelets	Amotosalen (psoralen) + UV light	Cerus (FDA cleared)
	Riboflavin (vitamin B2) + UV light	TerumoBCT
	UV light	Macopharma
Red Blood Cells/Whole Blood	Amustaline and glutathione	Cerus
	Riboflavin (vitamin B2) + UV light	TerumoBCT

FDA = Food and Drug Administration; UV = ultraviolet.

Preliminary reports suggest riboflavin/UV causes functional impairment in red cells stored nearest the 42-day expiration. Although there have been discussions about the potential for adverse reactions to treated components, extensive reviews of European data on pathogen-reduced platelets and plasma do not support the additional concern. Nevertheless, the FDA required Phase IV postmarketing studies in the United States as part of the implementation of INTERCEPT-treated platelets, and this is likely for other methods approved in the future.

The benefit to be gained from pathogen inactivation in the United States is primarily the mitigation of emerging pathogens and platelet-associated bacterial sepsis. Currently, the quantifiable infectious risks of transfusion in the United States are low. Therefore, it is critically important to demonstrate that inactivating treatments do not introduce new hazards to patients. Rigorous preclinical and clinical studies are required for US regulatory approval. Extensive toxicology studies have been critical because most of the pathogen inactivation agents interact with nucleic acid, raising the theoretical potential of carcinogenicity and mutagenicity. Treated components should be assessed for neoantigen formation and the impact of the inactivating process on the final product's clinical efficacy. The evaluation processes required for approval of pathogen inactivation methods in North America have been reviewed.[152-154]

Interest in pathogen inactivation remains high because it has the potential to 1) reduce sepsis-related platelet transfusion complications and eliminate the need for complex testing procedures to reduce risk related to bacterially contaminated platelets; 2) inactivate parasites such as *B. microti* and *P. falciparum;* 3) mitigate risks associated with recognized emerging pathogens such as DENV, CHIKV, and ZIKV; and 4) proactively decrease threats from unknown, emerging pathogens. Again, it should be noted that inactivation capabilities differ greatly between the various technologies, and each must be evaluated for its intended use.

SUMMARY

The current level of safety of blood components is based on two critical elements of donor screening: donor education and questioning, which is the sole method of screening for certain agents, such as malaria and prions, and donor testing. Testing must be performed carefully and in accordance with manufacturers' instructions, FDA regulations, and AABB

Standards, and facilities must have robust systems for quarantining components of donations that test reactive and for retrieving prior donations from donors whose samples have tested positive.

Current quantifiable risks of infectious disease transmission are very low; the estimated risk of HIV transmission by transfusion in the United States is approximately 1 in 1.5 million units, the risk of HCV transmission is approximately 1 in 1.1 million units, and the risk of HBV transmission is approximately 1 in 800,000 to 1 in 1.2 million units.[57,60] However, it is critical to remain vigilant for evidence of new infectious agents and to implement mitigation measures as quickly as feasible, as often required.[41,42,155] Pathogen inactivation technologies have shown efficacy in providing protection against infectious agents for which no screening is in place or for which screening assays potentially may be replaced.

KEY POINTS

1. Infectious disease screening of donors is accomplished by a) questioning potential donors and excluding those with an increased risk of infection, and b) testing donated blood.
2. There is a delay between the time when an individual is exposed to an infection and the time when the donor screening test for the infection yields a positive result. Blood donated during this window period can transmit infections.
3. The estimated window period with MP-NAT of donor samples is <10 days for HIV and HCV and <28 days for HBV.
4. The residual risk of transfusion-transmitted infection is a function of the length of the window period and the incidence of infection in the donor population. Maintaining a donor population that has a low incidence of infection continues to play a key role in preserving blood safety.
5. Based on window-period and incidence calculations, the current risk of HIV transmission by transfusion in the United States is approximately 1 in 1.5 million units, the risk of HCV transmission is approximately 1 in 1.1 million units, and the risk of HBV transmission is approximately 1 in 800,000 to 1 in 1.2 million units.
6. There are no donor screening tests approved by the FDA for malaria or vCJD. Donor questioning about potential exposure is the sole means of protecting the US blood supply from these diseases.
7. AABB requires blood banks to have processes that limit and detect or inactivate bacteria in platelet components. Either pathogen inactivation or bacteria testing can satisfy this requirement.
8. Infections transmitted to humans by vectors are increasingly recognized as a potential source of transfusion-transmitted infection. These include WNV, *T. cruzi*, *Babesia* species, dengue viruses, potentially chikungunya virus, and most recently ZIKV.
9. Pathogen inactivation may reduce the transmission of infectious agents for which there are no donor screening tests and may further reduce the residual transmission risks of known agents. Pathogen-reduced products include commercially manufactured plasma derivatives and pooled solvent/detergent-treated plasma, as well as pathogen-reduced platelet and plasma components.
10. Blood banks must have processes in place to ensure that donations with positive test results are not released for transfusion. In some circumstances, 1) prior donations from those donors must also be retrieved and quarantined, and 2) recipients of prior donations must be notified of their possible exposure to infection.

REFERENCES

1. Code of federal regulations. Title 21, CFR Parts 211 and 610. Washington, DC: US Government Publishing Office, 2017 (revised annually).
2. Alter HJ, Klein HG. The hazards of blood transfusion in historical perspective. Blood 2008; 112:2617-26.
3. Seeff LB, Wright EC, Zimmerman HJ, McCollum RW. VA cooperative study of post-transfusion hepatitis, 1969-1974: Incidence and characteristics of hepatitis and responsible risk factors. Am J Med Sci 1975;270:355-62.
4. Alter HJ, Purcell RH, Holland PV, et al. Donor transaminase and recipient hepatitis. Impact on blood transfusion services. JAMA 1981; 246:630-4.
5. Aach RD, Szmuness W, Mosley JW, et al. Serum alanine aminotransferase of donors in relation to the risk of non-A, non-B hepatitis in recipients: The transfusion-transmitted viruses study. N Engl J Med 1981;304:989-94.
6. Alter HJ, Holland PV. Indirect tests to detect the non-A, non-B hepatitis carrier state. Ann Intern Med 1984;101:859-61.
7. Stevens CE, Aach RD, Hollinger FB, et al. Hepatitis B virus antibody in blood donors and the occurrence of non-A, non-B hepatitis in transfusion recipients. An analysis of the Transfusion-Transmitted Viruses Study. Ann Intern Med 1984;101:733-8.
8. Galel SA, Lifson JD, Engleman EG. Prevention of AIDS transmission through screening of the blood supply. Annu Rev Immunol 1995;13:201-27.
9. American Red Cross, AABB, Council of Community Blood Centers. Joint statement on directed donations and AIDS. (January 13,1983) Arlington, VA: AABB, 1983. (See Transfusion 1983;23:87.)
10. Busch MP, Young MJ, Samson SM, et al. Risk of human immunodeficiency virus (HIV) transmission by blood transfusions before the implementation of HIV-1 antibody screening. The Transfusion Safety Study Group. Transfusion 1991;31:4-11.
11. Ward JW, Holmberg SD, Allen JR, et al. Transmission of human immunodeficiency virus (HIV) by blood transfusions screened as negative for HIV antibody. N Engl J Med 1988;318:473-8.
12. Perkins HA, Samson S, Busch MP. How well has self-exclusion worked? Transfusion 1988; 28:601-2.
13. Food and Drug Administration. Infectious disease tests. Silver Spring, MD: CBER Office of Communication, Outreach, and Development, 2016. [Available at http://www.fda.gov/BiologicsBloodVaccines/BloodBloodProducts/ApprovedProducts/LicensedProducts BLAs/BloodDonorScreening/InfectiousDisease/default.htm (accessed March 4, 2017).]
14. Food and Drug Administration. Information for blood establishments: Unavailability of CHIRON® RIBA® HCV 3.0 SIA (RIBA). (December 18, 2012) Silver Spring, MD: CBER Office of Communication, Outreach, and Development, 2012.
15. Busch MP, Glynn SA, Stramer SL, et al. A new strategy for estimating risks of transfusion-transmitted viral infections based on rates of detection of recently infected donors. Transfusion 2005;45:254-64.
16. O'Brien SF, Scalia V, Zuber E, et al. West Nile virus in 2006 and 2007: The Canadian Blood Services' experience. Transfusion 2010;50:1118-25.
17. Dodd RY, Foster GA, Stramer SL. Keeping blood transfusion safe from West Nile virus: American Red Cross experience, 2003 to 2012. Transfus Med Rev 2015;29:153-61.
18. West Nile virus nucleic acid testing—revised recommendations. Association bulletin #13-02. Bethesda, MD: AABB, 2013.
19. Food and Drug Administration. Guidance for industry: Use of nucleic acid tests to reduce the risk of transmission of West Nile virus from donors of whole blood and blood components intended for transfusion. (November 2009) Silver Spring, MD: CBER Office of Communication, Outreach, and Development, 2009. [Available at http://www.fda.gov/downloads/BiologicsBloodVaccines/Guidance ComplianceRegulatoryInformation/Guidances/Blood/UCM189464.pdf (accessed March 4, 2017).]
20. Code of federal regulations. Title 42, CFR Part 482.27. Washington, DC: US Government Publishing Office, 2017 (revised annually).
21. Food and Drug Administration. Guidance for industry: Recommendations for screening,

testing, and management of blood donors and blood and blood components based on screening tests for syphilis. (September 2014) Silver Spring, MD: CBER Office of Communication, Outreach, and Development, 2014.

22. Food and Drug Administration. Guidance for industry: Use of nucleic acid tests on pooled and individual samples from donors of whole blood and blood components, including source plasma, to reduce the risk of transmission of hepatitis B virus. (October 2012) Silver Spring, MD: CBER Office of Communication, Outreach, and Development, 2012. [Available at http://www.fda.gov/BiologicsBloodVac cines/GuidanceComplianceRegulatoryInfor mation/Guidances/Blood/ucm327850.htm (accessed March 4, 2017).]

23. Food and Drug Administration. Guidance for industry: Requalification method for reentry of donors who test hepatitis B surface antigen (HBsAg) positive following a recent vaccination against hepatitis B virus infection. (November 2011) Silver Spring, MD: CBER Office of Communication, Outreach, and Development, 2011. [Available at http:// www.fda.gov/downloads/BiologicsBloodVac cines/GuidanceComplianceRegulatoryInfor mation/Guidances/Blood/UCM280564.pdf (accessed March 4, 2017).]

24. Food and Drug Administration. Guidance for industry: "Lookback" for hepatitis C virus (HCV): Product quarantine, consignee notification, further testing, product disposition, and notification of transfusion recipients based on donor test results indicating infection with HCV. (December 2010) Silver Spring, MD: CBER Office of Communication, Outreach, and Development, 2010. [Available at http://www.fda.gov/downloads/Biologics BloodVaccines/GuidanceComplianceRegula toryInformation/Guidances/Blood/ucm 238488.pdf (accessed March 4, 2017).]

25. Food and Drug Administration. Guidance for industry: Use of serological tests to reduce the risk of transmission of *Trypanosoma cruzi* infection in whole blood and blood components intended for transfusion. (December 2010) Silver Spring, MD: CBER Office of Communication, Outreach, and Development, 2010. [Available at http://www.fda.gov/down loads/BiologicsBloodVaccines/Guidance ComplianceRegulatoryInformation/Guid

ances/Blood/UCM235960.pdf (accessed March 4, 2017).]

26. Food and Drug Administration. Guidance for industry: Nucleic acid testing (NAT) for human immunodeficiency virus type 1 (HIV-1) and hepatitis C virus (HCV): Testing, product disposition, and donor deferral and reentry. (May 2010) Silver Spring, MD: CBER Office of Communication, Outreach, and Development, 2010. [Available at http://www.fda.gov/ downloads/BiologicsBloodVaccines/Guid anceComplianceRegulatoryInformation/ Guidances/Blood/UCM210270.pdf (accesssed March 4, 2017).]

27. Food and Drug Administration. Guidance for industry: Requalification method for reentry of blood donors deferred because of reactive test results for antibody to hepatitis B core antigen (Anti-HBc). (May 2010) Silver Spring, MD: CBER Office of Communication, Outreach, and Development, 2010. [Available at http://www.fda.gov/downloads/Biologics BloodVaccines/GuidanceComplianceRegula toryInformation/Guidances/Blood/UCM 210268.pdf (accessed March 4, 2017).]

28. Food and Drug Administration. Guidance for industry: Recommendations for management of donors at increased risk for human immunodeficiency virus type 1 (HIV-1) group O infection. (August 2009) Silver Spring, MD: CBER Office of Communication, Outreach, and Development, 2009. [Available at http:// www.fda.gov/BiologicsBloodVaccines/Guid anceComplianceRegulatoryInformation/ Guidances/Blood/ucm180817.htm (accessed March 4, 2017).]

29. Food and Drug Administration. Guidance for industry: Nucleic acid testing (NAT) to reduce the possible risk of parvovirus B19 transmission by plasma-derived products. (July 2009) Silver Spring, MD: CBER Office of Communication, Outreach, and Development, 2009. [Available at http://www.fda.gov/Biologics BloodVaccines/GuidanceComplianceRegula toryInformation/Guidances/Blood/ucm 071592.htm (accessed March 4, 2017).]

30. Food and Drug Administration. Guidance for industry: Assessing donor suitability and blood and blood product safety in cases of known or suspected West Nile virus infection. (June 2005) Silver Spring, MD: CBER Office of Communication, Outreach, and Develop-

ment, 2005. [Available at http://www.fda.gov/BiologicsBloodVaccines/GuidanceCompliance RegulatoryInformation/Guidances/Blood/ucm074111.htm (accessed March 4, 2017).]

31. Food and Drug Administration. Guidance for industry: Use of nucleic acid tests on pooled and individual samples from donors of whole blood and blood components (including Source Plasma and Source Leukocytes) to adequately and appropriately reduce the risk of transmission of HIV-1 and HCV. (October 2004) Silver Spring, MD: CBER Office of Communication, Outreach, and Development, 2004. [Available at http://www.fda.gov/BiologicsBloodVaccines/GuidanceCompliance RegulatoryInformation/Guidances/Blood/ucm074934.htm (accessed March 4, 2017).]

32. Food and Drug Administration. Guidance for industry: Donor screening for antibodies to HTLV-II. (August 1997) Silver Spring, MD: CBER Office of Communication, Outreach, and Development, 1997. [Available at http://www.fda.gov/BiologicsBloodVaccines/GuidanceComplianceRegulatoryInformation/Guidances/Blood/ucm170786.htm (accessed March 4, 2017).]

33. Food and Drug Administration. Memorandum to all registered blood and plasma establishments: Recommendations for the quarantine and disposition of units from prior collections from donors with repeatedly reactive screening tests for hepatitis B Virus (HBV), hepatitis C Virus (HCV) and human T-lymphotropic virus type I (HTLV-I). (July 1996) Silver Spring, MD: CBER Office of Communication, Outreach, and Development, 1996. [Available at http://www.fda.gov/downloads/BiologicsBloodVaccines/GuidanceComplianceRegulatoryInformation/Other RecommendationsforManufacturers/Memo randumtoBloodEstablishments/UCM062600.pdf (accessed March 4, 2017).]

34. Food and Drug Administration. Memorandum to all registered blood establishments: Recommendations for the management of donors and units that are initially reactive for hepatitis B surface antigen (HBsAg). (December 1987) Silver Spring, MD: CBER Office of Communication, Outreach, and Development, 1987. [Available at http://www.fda.gov/downloads/BiologicsBloodVaccines/Guid

anceComplianceRegulatoryInformation/Oth erRecommendationsforManufacturers/Mem orandumtoBloodEstablishments/UCM 063011.pdf (accessed March 4, 2017).]

35. Ooley PW, ed. Standards for blood banks and transfusion services. 30th ed. Bethesda, MD: AABB, 2016.

36. Recommendations to address residual risk of bacterial contamination of platelets. Association bulletin #12-04. Bethesda, MD: AABB, 2012.

37. Guidance on management of blood and platelet donors with positive or abnormal results on bacterial contamination tests. Association bulletin #05-02. Bethesda, MD: AABB, 2005.

38. Actions following an initial positive test for possible bacterial contamination of a platelet unit. Association bulletin #04-07. Bethesda, MD: AABB, 2004.

39. Dual enzyme immuno assay (EIA) approach for deferral and notification of anti-HTLV-I/II EIA reactive donors. Association bulletin #99-9. Bethesda, MD: AABB, 1999.

40. Food and Drug Administration. Draft guidance for industry: Amendment to "Guidance for industry: Use of serological tests to reduce the risk of transmission of *Trypanosoma cruzi* infection in whole blood and blood components intended for transfusion." (November 2016) Silver Spring, MD: CBER Office of Communication, Outreach, and Development, 2016. [Available at https://www.fda.gov/downloads/BiologicsBloodVac cines/GuidanceComplianceRegulatoryInformation/Guidances/Blood/UCM528600.pdf (accessed March 4, 2017).]

41. Food and Drug Administration. Guidance for industry: Recommendations for donor screening, deferral, and product management to reduce the risk of transfusion transmission of Zika virus. (February 2016) Silver Spring, MD: CBER Office of Communication, Outreach, and Development, 2016. [Available at http://www.fda.gov/downloads/BiologicsBloodVac cines/GuidanceComplianceRegulatoryInformation/Guidances/Blood/UCM486360.pdf (accessed March 4, 2017).]

42. Food and Drug Administration. Guidance for industry: Revised recommendations for reducing the risk of Zika virus transmission by blood and blood components. (August 2016) Silver Spring, MD: CBER Office of Communi-

cation, Outreach, and Development, 2016. [Available at http://www.fda.gov/downloads/ BiologicsBloodVaccines/GuidanceComplianceRegulatoryInformation/Guidances/ Blood/UCM518213.pdf (accessed March 4, 2017).]

43. Updated recommendations for Zika, dengue and chikungunya viruses. Association bulletin #16-07. Bethesda, MD: AABB, 2016.

44. Blajchman MA, Goldman M, Freedman JJ, Sher GD. Proceedings of a consensus conference: Prevention of post-transfusion CMV in the era of universal leukoreduction. Transfus Med Rev 2001;15:1-20.

45. Vamvakas EC. Is white blood cell reduction equivalent to antibody screening in preventing transmission of cytomegalovirus by transfusion? A review of the literature and meta-analysis. Transfus Med Rev 2005;19:181-99.

46. Bowden RA, Slichter SJ, Sayers M, et al. A comparison of filtered leukocyte-reduced and cytomegalovirus (CMV) seronegative blood products for the prevention of transfusion-associated CMV infection after marrow transplant. Blood 1995;86:3598-603.

47. Nash T, Hoffmann S, Butch S, et al. Safety of leukoreduced, cytomegalovirus (CMV)-untested components in CMV-negative allogeneic human progenitor cell transplant recipients. Transfusion 2012;52:2270-2.

48. Hall S, Danby R, Osman H, et al. Transfusion in CMV seronegative T-depleted allogeneic stem cell transplant recipients with CMV-unselected blood components results in zero CMV transmissions in the era of universal leukocyte reduction: A UK dual centre experience. Transfus Med 2015;25:418-23.

49. The ADA, HIV, and autologous blood donation. Association bulletin #98-5. Bethesda, MD: AABB, 1998.

50. Code of federal regulations. Title 21, CFR Part 1271. Washington, DC: US Government Publishing Office, 2017 (revised annually). [Available at http://www.accessdata.fda.gov/ scripts/cdrh/cfdocs/cfcfr/CFRSearch.cfm? CFRPart=1271 (accessed March 5, 2017).]

51. Food and Drug Administration. Guidance for industry: Eligibility determination for donors of human cells, tissues, and cellular and tissue-based products (HCT/Ps). (August 2007) Silver Spring, MD: CBER Office of Communication, Outreach, and Development, 2007.

[Available at http://www.fda.gov/downloads/ biologicsbloodvaccines/guidancecompliance regulatoryinformation/guidances/tissue/ ucm091345.pdf (accessed March 4, 2017).]

52. Food and Drug Administration. Guidance for industry: Use of donor screening tests to test donors of human cells, tissues and cellular and tissue-based products for infection with *Treponema pallidum* (syphilis). (September 2015) Silver Spring, MD: CBER Office of Communication, Outreach, and Development, 2015.

53. Food and Drug Administration. Guidance for industry: Use of nucleic acid tests to reduce the risk of transmission of West Nile virus from living donors of human cells, tissues, and cellular and tissue-based products (HCT/Ps). (September 2016) Silver Spring, MD: CBER Office of Communication, Outreach, and Development, 2016. [Available at http:// www.fda.gov/downloads/BiologicsBloodVac cines/GuidanceComplianceRegulatoryInfor mation/Guidances/Tissue/UCM372084.pdf (accessed March 4, 2017).]

54. Food and Drug Administration. Tissue guidances. Silver Spring, MD: CBER Office of Communication, Outreach, and Development, 2016. [Available at http://www.fda.gov/Bio logicsBloodVaccines/GuidanceCompliance RegulatoryInformation/Guidances/Tissue/ default.htm (accessed March 4, 2017).]

55. Food and Drug Administration. Testing HCT/ P donors: Specific requirements. Silver Spring, MD: CBER Office of Communication, Outreach, and Development, 2015. [Available at http://www.fda.gov/BiologicsBloodVaccines/ SafetyAvailability/TissueSafety/ucm151757. htm (accessed March 4, 2017).]

56. Anderson SA, Yang H, Gallagher LM, et al. Quantitative estimate of the risks and benefits of possible alternative blood donor deferral strategies for men who have had sex with men. Transfusion 2009;49:1102-14.

57. Zou S, Dorsey KA, Notari EP, et al. Prevalence, incidence, and residual risk of human immunodeficiency virus and hepatitis C virus infections among United States blood donors since the introduction of nucleic acid testing. Transfusion 2010;50:1495-504.

58. Stramer SL, Glynn SA, Kleinman SH, et al. Detection of HIV-1 and HCV infections among antibody-negative blood donors by nucleic

acid-amplification testing. N Engl J Med 2004; 351:760-8.

59. Dodd RY, Notari EP, Stramer SL. Current prevalence and incidence of infectious disease markers and estimated window-period risk in the American Red Cross blood donor population. Transfusion 2002;42:975-9.

60. Stramer SL, Notari EP, Krysztof DE, Dodd RY. Hepatitis B virus testing by minipool nucleic acid testing: Does it improve blood safety? Transfusion 2013;53(Suppl 3):2449-58.

61. Stramer SL, Hollinger FB, Katz LM, et al. Emerging infectious disease agents and their potential threat to transfusion safety. Transfusion 2009;49(Suppl 2):1S-235S.

62. Emerging infectious disease agents and their potential threat to transfusion safety. Bethesda, MD: AABB, 2017. [Available at http://www.aabb.org/tm/eid/Pages/default.aspx (accessed March 4, 2017).]

63. Stramer SL, Yu G, Herron R, et al. Two human immunodeficiency virus Type 2 cases in US blood donors including serologic, molecular, and genomic characterization of an epidemiologically unusual case. Transfusion 2016;56(6 Pt 2):1560-8.

64. Centers for Disease Control and Prevention. HIV surveillance report, 2014; vol. 26. Atlanta, GA: National Center for HIV/AIDS, Viral Hepatitis, STD, and TB Prevention, 2014. [Available at http://www.cdc.gov/hiv/pdf/library/reports/surveillance/cdc-hiv-surveillance-report-us.pdf (accessed March 4, 2017).]

65. HIV prevalence, unrecognized infection, and HIV testing among men who have sex with men—five U.S. cities, June 2004-April 2005. MMWR Morb Mortal Wkly Rep 2005;54:597-601.

66. Truong HM, Kellogg T, Klausner JD, et al. Increases in sexually transmitted infections and sexual risk behaviour without a concurrent increase in HIV incidence among men who have sex with men in San Francisco: A suggestion of HIV serosorting? Sex Transm Infect 2006;82:461-6.

67. Food and Drug Administraion. Guidance for industry: Revised recommendations for reducing the risk of human immunodeficiency virus transmission by blood and blood products. (December 2015) Silver Spring, MD: CBER Office of Communication, Outreach, and Development, 2015. [Available at http://www.fda.gov/downloads/BiologicsBloodVaccines/GuidanceComplianceRegulatoryInformation/Guidances/Blood/UCM446580.pdf (accessed March 4, 2017).]

68. Kleinman SH, Busch MP. Assessing the impact of HBV NAT on window period reduction and residual risk. J Clin Virol 2006;36(Suppl 1):S23-9.

69. Stramer SL. Pooled hepatitis B virus DNA testing by nucleic acid amplification: Implementation or not. Transfusion 2005;45:1242-6.

70. Linauts S, Saldanha J, Strong DM. PRISM hepatitis B surface antigen detection of hepatits B virus minipool nucleic acid testing yield samples. Transfusion 2008;48:1376-82.

71. Stramer SL, Wend U, Candotti D, et al. Nucleic acid testing to detect HBV infection in blood donors. N Engl J Med 2011;364:236-47.

72. Alter HJ. Descartes before the horse: I clone, therefore I am: The hepatitis C virus in current perspective. Ann Intern Med 1991;115:644-9.

73. Smith BD, Morgan RL, Beckett GA, et al. Centers for Disease Control and Prevention. Recommendations for the identification of chronic hepatitis C virus infection among persons born during 1945-1965. MMWR Recomm Rep 2012;61(No. RR-4):1-32.

74. Page-Shafer K, Pappalardo BL, Tobler LH, et al. Testing strategy to identify cases of acute hepatitis C virus (HCV) infection and to project HCV incidence rates. J Clin Microbiol 2008; 46:499-506.

75. Guidelines for counseling persons infected with human T-lymphotropic virus type I (HTLV-I) and type II (HTLV-II). Centers for Disease Control and Prevention and the U.S.P.H.S. Working Group. Ann Intern Med 1993;118:448-54.

76. Vrielink H, Zaaijer HL, Reesink HW. The clinical relevance of HTLV type I and II in transfusion medicine. Transfus Med Rev 1997;11:173-9.

77. Petrik J, Lozano M, Seed CR, et al. Hepatitis E. Vox Sang 2016;110:93-130.

78. Hewitt PE, Ijaz S, Brailsford SR, et al. Hepatitis E virus in blood components: A prevalence and transmission study in southeast England. Lancet 2014;384:1766-73.

79. Stramer SL, Moritz ED, Foster GA, et al. Hepatitis E virus: Seroprevalence and frequency of viral RNA detection among US blood donors. Transfusion 2016;56:481-8.

80. Orton S. Syphilis and blood donors: What we know, what we do not know, and what we need to know. Transfus Med Rev 2001;15:282-92.

81. Katz LM. A test that won't die: The serologic test for syphilis. Transfusion 2009;49:617-19.

82. Zou S, Notari EP, Fang CT, et al. Current value of serologic test for syphilis as a surrogate marker for blood-borne viral infections among blood donors in the United States. Transfusion 2009;49:655-61.

83. Food and Drug Administration. Fatalities reported to FDA following blood collection and transfusion: Annual summary for fiscal year 2015. Silver Spring, MD: CBER Office of Communication, Outreach, and Development, 2015 [Available at https://www.fda.gov/downloads/BiologicsBloodVaccines/SafetyAvailability/ReportaProblem/TransfusionDonationFatalities/UCM518148.pdf (accessed March 4, 2017).]

84. Food and Drug Administration. Draft guidance for industry: Bacterial risk control strategies for blood collection establishments and transfusion services to enhance the safety and availability of platelets for transfusion. (March 2016) Silver Spring, MD: CBER Office of Communication, Outreach, and Development, 2016. [Available at http://www.fda.gov/downloads/BiologicsBloodVaccines/GuidanceComplianceRegulatoryInformation/Guidances/Blood/UCM425952.pdf (accessed March 4, 2017).]

85. Eder AF, Kennedy JM, Dy BA, et al. Limiting and detecting bacterial contamination of apheresis platelets: Inlet-line diversion and increased culture volume improve component safety. Transfusion 2009;49:1554-63.

86. Ramirez-Arcos SM, Goldman M, Blajchman MA. Bacterial infection: Bacterial contamination, testing and post-transfusion complications. In: Hillyer CD, Silberstein LE, Ness PM, et al, eds. Blood banking and transfusion medicine: Basic principles and practice. 2nd ed. Philadelphia: Churchill Livingstone, 2007:639-51.

87. Suggested options for transfusion services and blood collectors to facilitate implementation of BB/TS Interim Standard 5.1.5.1.1. Association bulletin #10-05. Bethesda , MD: AABB; 2010.

88. Benjamin RJ, Klein L, Dy BA, et al. Bacterial contamination of whole-blood-derived platelets: The introduction of sample diversion and prestorage pooling with culture testing in the American Red Cross. Transfusion 2008;48:2348-55.

89. Jacobs MR, Smith D, Heaton WA, et al for the PGD Study Group. Detection of bacterial contamination in prestorage culture-negative apheresis platelets on day of issue with the Pan Genera Detection test. Transfusion 2011;51:2573-82.

90. Biggerstaff BJ, Petersen LR. Estimated risk of West Nile virus transmission through blood transfusion in the US. Transfusion 2003;43:1007-17.

91. Pealer LN, Marfin AA, Petersen LR, et al. Transmission of West Nile virus through blood transfusion in the United States in 2002. N Engl J Med 2003;349:1236-45.

92. Zou S, Foster GA, Dodd RY, et al. West Nile fever characteristics among viremic persons identified through blood donor screening. J Infect Dis 2010;202:1354.

93. Dodd RY, Foster GA, Stramer SL. Keeping blood transfusion safe from West Nile virus: American Red Cross experience, 2003-2012. Transfus Med Rev 2015;29:153-61.

94. Groves JA, Shafi H, Nomura JH, et al. A probable case of West Nile virus transfusion transmission. Transfusion 2017;57:850-6.

95. Petersen LR, Jamieson DJ, Powers AM, Honein MA. Zika virus. N Engl J Med 2016;374:1552-63.

96. Rasmussen SA, Jamieson DJ, Honein MA, Petersen LR. Zika virus and birth defects—Reviewing the evidence for causality. N Engl J Med 2016;374:1981-7.

97. Brasil P, Pereira JP, Gabaglia C, et al. Zika virus infection in pregnant women in Rio de Janeiro. N Engl J Med 2016;375:2321-34.

98. França GV, Schuler-Faccini L, Oliveira WK, et al. Congenital Zika virus syndrome in Brazil: A case series of the first 1501 livebirths with complete investigation. Lancet 2016;388:891-7.

99. Johansson MA, Mier YT-RL, Reefhuis J, et al. Zika and the risk of microcephaly. N Engl J Med 2016;375:1-4.

100. Garcez PP, Loiola EC, da Costa M, et al. Zika virus impairs growth in human neurospheres and brain organoids. Science 2016;352:816-18.

101. Cao-Lameau V, Blake A, Mons S, et al. Guillain-Barré syndrome outbreak associated with Zika virus infection in French Polynesia: A case-control study. Lancet 2016;387:1531-9.

102. Gallain P, Cabié A, Richard P, et al. Zika virus in asymptomatic blood donors in Martinique. Blood 2017;129:263-6.

103. Musso D, Nhan T, Robin E, et al. Potential for Zika virus transmission through blood transfusion demonstrated during an outbreak in French Polynesia, November 2013 to February 2014. Euro Surveill 2014;19:20761.

104. Kuehnert MJ, Basavaraju SV, Moseley RR, et al. Screening of blood donations for Zika virus infection—Puerto Rico, April 3–June 11, 2016. MMWR Morb Mortal Wkly Rep 2016;65:627-8.

105. Benjamin RJ. Zika virus in the blood supply. Blood 2017;129:144-5.

106. Barjas-Castro ML, Angerami RN, Cunha MS, et al. Probable transfusion-transmitted Zika virus in Brazil. Transfusion 2016;56:1684-8.

107. Motta IJF, Spencer BR, Cordeiro da Silva SG, et al. Evidence for transmission of Zika virus by platelet transfusion. N Engl J Med 2016;375:1101-3.

108. Davidson A, Slavinski S, Komoto K, et al. Suspected female-to-male sexual transmission of Zika virus—New York City, 2016. MMWR Morb Mortal Wkly Rep 2016;65:716-17.

109. Lessler JT, Ott C, Carcelen A, et al. Times to key events in Zika virus infection and implications for blood donation: A systematic review. Bull World Health Organ 2016;94:841-9.

110. Lustig Y, Mendelson E, Puran N, et al. Detection of Zika virus RNA in whole blood of imported Zika virus disease cases up to 2 months after symptom onset, Israel, December 2015 to April 2016. Euro Surveill 2016;21:7-11.

111. Bingham AM, Cone M, Mock V, et al. Comparison of test results for Zika virus RNA in urine, serum, and saliva specimens from persons with travel-associated Zika virus disease - Florida, 2016. MMWR Morb Mortal Wkly Rep 2016;65:475-8.

112. Centers for Disease Control and Prevention. Interim guidance for Zika virus testing of urine – United States, 2016. MMWR Morb Mortal Wkly Rep 2016;65:474.

113. Atkinson B, Hearn P, Afrough B, et al. Detection of Zika virus in semen. Emerg Infect Dis 2016;22:940.

114. Mansuy JM, Pasquier C, Daudin M, et al. Zika virus in semen of a patient returning from a non-epidemic area. Lancet Infect Dis 2016; 16:894-5.

115. Gaskell KM, Houlihan C, Nastouli E, Checkley AM. Persistent Zika virus detection in semen in a traveler returning to the United Kingdom from Brazil, 2016. Emerg Infect Dis 2017;23: 137-9.

116. Paz-Bailey G, Rosenberg ES, Doyle K, et al. Persistence of Zika virus in body fluids – preliminary report. N Engl J Med 2017 Feb 14; doi: 10.1056/NEJMoa1613108. (Epub ahead of print.)

117. Centers for Disease Control and Prevention. Zika virus: Case counts in the US. Atlanta, GA: CDC, 2017. [Available at http://www.cdc.gov/zika/geo/united-states.html (accessed February 2, 2017).]

118. Swaminathan S, Schlaberg R, Lewis J, et al. Fatal Zika virus infection with secondary nonsexual transmission. N Engl J Med 2016;375:19-21.

119. Stone M, Lanteri MC, Bakkour S, et al. Relative analytical sensitivity of donor nucleic acid amplification technology screening and diagnostic real-time polymerase chain reaction assays for detection of Zika virus RNA. Transfusion 2017;57:734-47.

120. Galel SA, Williamson PC, Busch MP, et al. First Zika-positive donations in the continental United States. Transfusion 2017;57:762-9.

121. Williamson PC, Linnen JM, Kessler DA, et al. First cases of Zika virus-infected US blood donors outside states with areas of active transmission. Transfusion 2017;57:770-8.

122. Aubry M, Richard V, Green J, et al. Inactivation of Zika virus in plasma with amotosalen and ultraviolet A illumination. Transfusion 2016; 56:33-40.

123. Laughhunn A, Santa Maria F, Broult J, et al. Amustaline (S-303) treatment inactivates high levels of Zika virus in red blood cell components. Transfusion 2017;57:779-89.

124. Blümel J, Musso D, Teitz S, et al. Inactivation and removal of Zika virus during manufacture of plasma derived medicinal products. Transfusion 2017;57:790-6.

125. Kühnel D, Müller S, Pichotta A, et al. Inactivation of Zika virus by solvent/detergent treatment of human plasma and other plasma-derived products and pasteurization of human serum albumin. Transfusion 2017; 57:802-10.

126. Anez G, Rios M. Dengue in the United States of America: A worsening scenario? Biomed Res Int 2013;2013:678645.

127. Tomashek KM, Margolis HS. Dengue: A potential transfusion-transmitted disease. Transfusion 2011;51:1654.

128. Stramer SL, Linnen JM, Carrick JM, et al. Dengue viremia in blood donors identified by RNA and detection of dengue transfusion transmission during the 2007 dengue outbreak in Puerto Rico. Transfusion 2012;52:1657-66.

129. Matos D, Tomashek KM, Perez-Padilla J, et al. Probable and possible transfusion-transmitted dengue associated with NS1-antigen negative but RNA-confirmed-positive red blood cells. Transfusion 2016;56:215-22.

130. Sabino E, Loureiro P, Lopes M, et al. Transfusion-transmission of dengue virus and associated clinical symptomatology during the 2012 epidemic in Brazil. J Infect Dis 2016; 213:694-702.

131. Chiu C, Bres V, Yu G, et al. Genomic assays for identification of chikungunya virus in blood donors, Puerto Rico, 2014. Emerg Infect Dis 2015;21:1409-13.

132. Brouard C, Bernillon P, Quatresous I, et al. Estimated risk of chikungunya viremic blood donation during an epidemic on Reunion Island in the Indian Ocean, 2005-2007. Transfusion 2008;48:1333-41.

133. Simmons G, Bres V, Lu K, et al. High incidence of chikungunya virus and frequency of viremic blood donations during epidemic, Puerto Rico, USA, 2014. Emerg Infect Dis 2016;22:1221-8.

134. Otani MM, Vinelli E, Kirchhoff LV, et al. WHO comparative evaluation of serologic assays for Chagas disease. Transfusion 2009;49:1076-82.

135. Food and Drug Administration. Blood Products Advisory Committee, 94th Meeting, Gaithersburg, MD, April 1, 2009. Silver Spring, MD: CBER Office of Communication, Outreach, and Development, 2009. [Available at http://www.fda.gov/downloads/Advisory Committees/CommitteesMeetingMaterials/ BloodVaccinesandOtherBiologics/BloodProd uctsAdvisoryCommittee/UCM155628.pdf (accessed March 4, 2017).]

136. Benjamin RJ, Stramer SL, Leiby DA, et al. *Trypanosoma cruzi* infection in North America and Spain: Evidence in support of transfusion transmission. Transfusion 2012;52:1913-21.

137. Kessler DA, Shi PA, Avecilla ST, Shaz BH. Results of lookback for Chagas disease since the inception of donor screening at New York Blood Center. Transfusion 2013;53:1083-7.

138. Blumental S, Lambermont M, Heijmans C, et al. First documented transmission of *Trypanosoma cruzi* infection through blood transfusion in a child with sickle-cell disease in Belgium. PLoS Negl Trop Dis 2015;9:e0003986.

139. Babesiosis. Association bulletin #14-05. Bethesda, MD: AABB, 2014.

140. Herwaldt BL, Linden JV, Bosserman E, et al. Transfusion-associated babesiosis in the United States: A description of cases. Ann Intern Med 2011;155:509-19.

141. Fang DC, McCullough J. Transfusion-transmitted *Babesia microti*. Transfus Med Rev 2016:30:132-8.

142. Tonnetti L, Eder AF, Dy B, et al. Transfusion-transmitted *Babesia microti* identified through hemovigilance. Transfusion 2009;49:2557-63.

143. Moritz ED, Winton CS, Tonnetti L, et al. Screening for *Babesia microti* in the U.S. blood supply. N Engl J Med 2016;375:2236-45.

144. Mali S, Steele S, Slutsker L, Arguin PM. Malaria surveillance—United States, 2007. MMWR Surveill Summ 2009;58(SS-2):1-16.

145. Mali S, Tan KR, Arguin PM. Malaria surveillance—United States, 2009. MMWR Morb Mortal Wkly Rep 2011;60:1-15.

146. Food and Drug Administration. Guidance for industry: Recommendations for donor questioning, deferral, reentry and product management to reduce the risk of transfusion-transmitted malaria. (August 2013) Silver Spring, MD: CBER Office of Communication, Outreach and Development, 2013. [Available at http://www.fda.gov/downloads/Biologics BloodVaccines/GuidanceComplianceRegula toryInformation/Guidances/Blood/UCM 080784.pdf (accessed March 4, 2017).]

147. Spencer B, Steele W, Custer B, et al. Risk for malaria in United States donors deferred for travel to malaria-endemic areas. Transfusion 2009;49:2335-45.

148. O'Brien SF, Delage G, Seed CR, et al. The epidemiology of imported malaria and transfusion policy in nonendemic countries. Transfus Med Rev 2015;29:162-71.

149. Allain JP, Owusu-Ofori AK, Assennato SM. Effect of *Plasmodium* inactivation in whole blood on the incidence of blood transfusion-transmitted malaria in endemic regions: The African Investigation of the Mirasol System (AIMS) randomised controlled trial. Lancet 2016;387:1753-61.

150. Food and Drug Administration. Guidance for industry: Revised preventive measures to reduce the possible risk of transmission of Creutzfeldt-Jakob disease (CJD) and variant Creutzfeldt-Jakob disease (vCJD) by blood and blood products. (May 2010, updated January 2016) Silver Spring, MD: CBER Office of Communication, Outreach, and Development, 2016. [Available at http://www.fda.gov/ucm/ groups/fdagov-public/@fdagov-bio-gen/doc uments/document/ucm307137.pdf (accessed March 4, 2017).]

151. Snyder EL, Stramer SL, Benjamin RJ. The safety of the US blood supply – time to raise the bar. N Engl J Med 2015;372:1882-5.

152. Webert KE, Cserti CM, Hannon J, et al. Proceedings of a consensus conference: Pathogen inactivation—making decisions about new technologies. Transfus Med Rev 2008;22:1-34.

153. Klein HG, Anderson D, Bernardi MJ, et al. Pathogen inactivation: Making decisions about new technologies. Report of a consensus conference. Transfusion 2007;47:2338-47.

154. Seghatchian J, Hervig T, Putter JS. Effect of pathogen inactivation on the storage lesion in red cells and platelet concentrates. Transfus Apher Sci 2011;45:75.

155. Food and Drug Administration. Guidance for industry: Recommendations for assessment of blood donor eligibility, donor deferral and blood product management in response to Ebola virus. (January 2017) Silver Spring, MD: CBER Office of Communication, Outreach, and Development, 2017. [Available at https:// www.fda.gov/downloads/BiologicsBloodVac cines/GuidanceComplianceRegulatoryInfor mation/Guidances/Blood/UCM475072.pdf (accessed March 4, 2017).]

Chapter 8

Molecular Biology and Immunology in Transfusion Medicine

• ● •

James D. Gorham, MD, PhD

THIS CHAPTER REVIEWS fundamental principles and approaches for
analyzing nucleic acids and proteins,
particularly antibodies, and introduces basic
concepts in humoral (antibody-mediated)
immunity.

In the practice of transfusion medicine,
analyses of nucleic acids and antibodies are
extensively employed to 1) detect infectious
pathogens in donated components; 2) predict
the phenotypic expression of antigens on the
surface of cells (red cells, platelets, and neutrophils); 3) detect and identify red cell and platelet antibodies; 4) determine HLA type; and
5) perform relationship testing. Although the
last is somewhat outside transfusion practice,
it is a component of AABB's standards and
accreditation programs.

Entire textbooks explain molecular biology and immunology. This chapter focuses on
topics immediately relevant to the practice of
transfusion testing. Moreover, within immunology, the focus is humoral immunity (medi-

ated by antibodies), which is more relevant to
the practice of transfusion medicine than is
cellular immunity. Finally, specific assay protocols are not provided, but the scientific principles underlying the molecular biological and
immunological assays used in transfusion
medicine are presented.

ANALYSIS OF DNA

The practical application of nucleic acid analysis in transfusion medicine lies in two principal areas: 1) the detection of infectious pathogens and 2) the genotyping of blood donors
and recipients. The human genome is made
up of DNA, organized into chromosomes,
which are present in the cell nucleus. Whereas
most cells in the human body are nucleated,
circulating red cells and platelets are anucle-
ate, and thus lack DNA. The genotype of an individual is his or her genetic makeup, encoded
in the DNA; in practical transfusion medicine,
the term "genotype" is commonly used to refer

James D. Gorham, MD, PhD, Professor of Pathology; Director, Division of Laboratory Medicine; and Medical
Director of the Blood Bank and Transfusion Medicine Services, University of Virginia Health System, Charlot-
tesville, Virginia
The author has disclosed no conflicts of interest.

to the specific allele present at a single gene locus. Bacteria, fungi, protozoa, and many viruses also utilize DNA to encode their genomes. Some viral pathogens use RNA instead. Either DNA or RNA encodes all known genetic material relevant to transfusion medicine, with the notable exception of prions, which appear to lack nucleic acids.

Basic Chemistry and Structure of Nucleic Acids

A brief overview of this topic is presented here, while more details are available elsewhere.[1] DNA is a nucleic acid polymer containing chains of nucleotides. Nucleotides are composed of three moieties: 1) a pentose sugar (five carbon atoms); 2) a phosphate group linked to carbon 5 (C5); and 3) a base group attached to carbon 1 (C1) [Fig 8-1 (A)]. There are four different nucleotides in DNA: adenine (A), guanine (G), cytosine (C), and thymine (T), which differ from one another in the chemical

structure of the C1 base group. Polymers of DNA consist of repeats of covalently bound sugars and phosphates that form the outside backbone of the double helical strand of DNA. DNA strands are described as having a "5' end" and a "3' end," terms that refer to the end with a free phosphate attached to C5, and the opposite end with a free hydroxyl group attached to carbon 3 (C3), respectively [Fig 8-1 (B)].

The human genome consists of double-stranded DNA (dsDNA). The bases within one strand of DNA form noncovalent hydrogen bonds with complementary bases on the other strand. Specifically, T always pairs with A, using two hydrogen bonds, and G always pairs with C, using three hydrogen bonds. When two strands have complementary sequences, they can "hybridize" via hydrogen bonding between complementary base pairs to form a dsDNA molecule [Fig 8-1 (C)]. The two complementary strands align such that the 5' and 3' ends have opposite orientations and form a

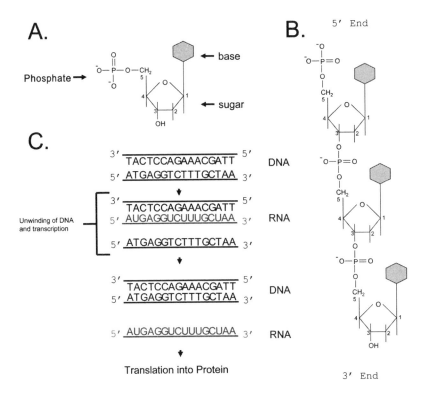

FIGURE 8-1. Chemical structure of nucleic acids and DNA.

double helix in which the phosphodiester backbone is on the outside of the helix and the hydrogen-bond-paired bases are on the inside. DNA molecules vary from each other based on the sequence of nucleotides, determined by the bases incorporated into the polymer.

When genes are expressed, the DNA encoding a given gene is used as a template to produce RNA, which is then exported from the nucleus to the cytoplasm and used as a guide to produce proteins, the workhorses of most cellular activity. The structure of RNA is similar to that of DNA, with some differences: 1) ribonucleotides have an additional hydroxyl group on carbon 2; 2) uracil (U) is used in place of thymine (T); and 3) RNA is typically single-stranded.

Several classes of RNA exist in human cells; the type that comes to be used as a blueprint for protein synthesis is termed "messenger RNA" (mRNA). When a gene is expressed, it is used as a template to generate a copy of itself in mRNA form, a process termed "transcription." The transcription machinery unwinds the DNA double helix, synthesizes a new mRNA strand of complementary sequence, and re-anneals the DNA in its wake [Fig 8-1 (C)]. Thus, the mRNA represents a copy of the gene sequence present in the DNA. mRNA is always synthesized in the "5′ to 3′ direction," and thus for a given gene, only one of the two DNA strands is transcribed into mRNA. After synthesis in the nucleus, mRNA is processed and exported to the cytoplasm, where ribosomes use it as a template to synthesize a new protein molecule, a process called "translation."

Isolation of Nucleic Acid

The first step in most DNA and RNA analyses is the isolation of nucleic acids. Because essentially all nucleated cells of an individual contain identical genomic DNA (gDNA), gDNA can be isolated from any readily obtainable cellular source, such as peripheral blood leukocytes or buccal swabs (epithelial cells). In contrast, mRNAs differ between cell types, because their differential expression patterns are important in defining the phenotypes of these

cells. The implication of this is that for mRNA analysis, the choice of source cells is critical. Kits are readily available from multiple manufacturers for the simple and rapid isolation of high-quality cellular DNA or mRNA, or of viral nucleic acids from plasma.

The Polymerase Chain Reaction

Nucleic acid detection and analysis were revolutionized by the invention of the polymerase chain reaction (PCR) in the 1980s. PCR was the first amplification-based technique for generating nucleic acid fragments for direct analysis.[2] A PCR requires: 1) a DNA sample to be analyzed (the "target" or "template"); 2) gene-specific primers of around 20 nucleotides in length; 3) a thermostable DNA polymerase enzyme that recognizes primer bound to target DNA and sequentially adds the complementary nucleotide building blocks to extend the length of the primed DNA strand; 4) the four nucleotides (ATCG); and 5) the proper buffer. PCR involves repeat cycles of heating/cooling ("thermocycling"), allowing exponential DNA amplification of the fragment of interest, carried out in a thermocycler that rapidly changes temperature with accuracy and precision. A single cycle involves 1) heating to denature the template dsDNA to allow strand separation, 2) cooling to allow annealing of primer to complementary regions on the template DNA, and 3) extension and synthesis of DNA on the primer strand. Typically, 20 to 40 cycles are performed in total, depending on the abundance of the template and the required sensitivity of the assay.

Figure 8-2 shows an example, beginning with a single copy of a dsDNA template. The dsDNA is denatured by heating to near boiling (~95 C), disrupting the hydrogen bonds between complementary bases, thereby separating the two strands. The temperature is then lowered to allow gene-specific primers in the reaction mix to anneal to their complementary targets. One primer is designed to anneal "upstream" (aka "just 5′") to the region of interest, whereas the other is designed to anneal "downstream" (aka "just 3′") to this region. The temperature is then raised to 72 C, the

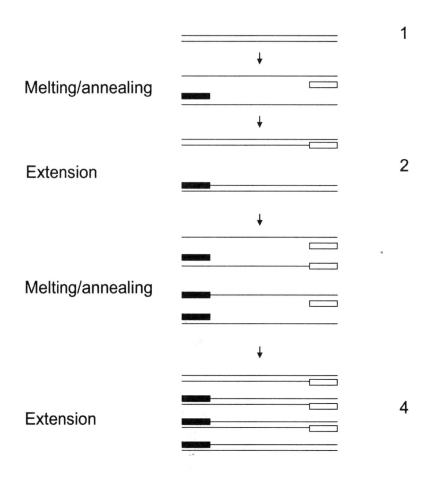

FIGURE 8-2. Overview of the polymerase chain reaction.

temperature at which the thermostable polymerase functions optimally, and the primers are extended along the length of the DNA through incorporation of complementary nucleotides. Thus, at the end of extension, there are two copies of the DNA. The process of denaturing, annealing, and extension then repeats itself. Each subsequent cycle yields a doubling in DNA copy number. PCR results in an exponential expansion of a selected DNA "amplicon," defined as the sequence bounded by the two chosen primers.

PCR Considerations

Although PCR is a robust method of detecting nucleic acids, technical considerations can affect PCR and other amplification-based techniques.

Specimen Processing and Template Degradation

DNA is stable and can usually withstand variations in storage temperature and handling before being processed for genomic analysis. Exceptions include samples in which the target DNA is present in low quantity, such as fetal typing from maternal plasma and viral testing. By contrast, RNA is far less stable, as it is susceptible both to spontaneous autodegradation and to catalytic degradation mediated by the abundant thermostable RNAse enzymes found in many biologic specimens.

Inhibitors

Because PCR amplification depends on the enzymatic activity of DNA polymerase, PCR can be inhibited by substances that negatively affect the activity. Heparin can inhibit PCR, and hemoglobin or lactoferrin released from erythrocytes or leukocytes also inhibits.[3] Most analytic systems minimize risk of interference by an inhibitor, but deviations from established protocols may introduce unintended inhibitory substances. To detect the presence of inhibitors, controls include amplifying ubiquitous target sequences (conserved regions of gDNA) and/or spiking the specimen with a positive control.

Primer Design

Although inferior performance of primers is typically not a concern for commercially available tests, understanding primer design is important in assay troubleshooting and in developing PCR-based assays for new targets. Although the ideal primer hybridizes to a target found in only one location in the entire genome, given the complexity of gDNA, primer annealing to unintended targets can occur, resulting in both the potential to amplify unintended targets and the ongoing consumption of primers. In addition, primers can anneal to each other to form a short amplicon, in a so-called primer-dimer formation.[4]

Contamination

One of the greatest strengths of PCR is its ability to amplify very small amounts of genetic material. In theory, single-copy sensitivity can be achieved. In practice, 10 copies of target DNA are about the lower limit of detection, depending on the sensitivity of the assay readout. The sensitivity makes PCR susceptible to false-positive results, due to contamination either from other specimens being analyzed or, more commonly, from amplicons generated in previous PCR runs. Beginning with just 10 molecules of DNA, 30 rounds of PCR amplification yields >10^{10} amplicons. Thus, as little as 0.0000001% of a previous reaction inadvertently introduced into a pipette or picked up from a laboratory surface or from the thermocycler can lead to a false-positive result in a subsequent reaction.

To minimize contamination, PCR laboratories routinely process samples in one geographic direction. DNA extraction is located away from testing, and PCR reactions are assembled in one room (or in a positive pressure hood) and amplified in a second room; any downstream analysis is performed in a third room. There should be no retrograde flow, and no materials or instruments used in the amplification or analysis (post-PCR) rooms should ever make their way into the DNA extraction and PCR setup (pre-PCR) room. Pipette filter tips are routinely used to minimize carryover contamination and sample aerosols.

Another effective method to avoid contamination is the addition of deoxyuridine triphosphate (dUTP) before PCR amplification. Polymerases incorporate dUTP in place of deoxythymidine triphosphate (dTTP). The enzyme uracil-DNA glycosylase (UNG) is also added to specifically cleave DNA containing uracil[5]; thus, UNG in PCR reactions destroys contaminating amplicons from previous amplifications but not native DNA in the specimen. The initial denaturation step inactivates the heat-labile UNG.

Finally, it is standard practice to include a water control, for which water rather than a DNA sample is used as the input sample. The water control (no-DNA control) reaction should yield no detectable signal above background. Signal in the water control indicates contamination of a reagent or instrument and invalidates the test run.

Reverse Transcriptase PCR

Messenger RNA is unsuitable as a template for PCR. When analysis of mRNA is desired, an additional step is employed to generate a single-stranded complementary DNA (cDNA), using mRNA as the template. The enzyme reverse transcriptase (RT) synthesizes cDNA from an RNA template (in the 5′ to 3′ direction), requiring the annealing of a primer to initiate transcription. The cDNA is then a suitable substrate for PCR.

Transcription-Mediated Amplification and Sequence-Based Amplification

There are additional non-PCR amplification techniques; among these, transcription-mediated amplification (TMA) and nucleic acid sequence-based amplification (NASBA) are further described (Fig 8-3).[6,7]

TMA plays a large role in nucleic acid testing (NAT) for human immunodeficiency virus (HIV), hepatitis C virus (HCV), and West Nile virus, for which viral RNA is the target. The reaction contains two primers, RT, DNA polymerase, RNAse H, and a sequence-specific RNA polymerase called T7 polymerase. A sequence-specific downstream primer hybridizes to the 3′ end of the target RNA, and RT synthesizes a cDNA copy (Fig 8-3, step 1). Primer 1 contains a sequence at its 3′ end that hybridizes to the target RNA, and a specific sequence at its 5′ end, that serves as a promoter for the T7 polymerase. The RNA template is degraded either by RT itself (TMA assay) or by RNAse H (NASBA assay) (step 2). A second primer (primer 2) then binds to the newly syn-thesized cDNA (step 3) and utilizes DNA polymerase to synthesize a dsDNA molecule (step 4). This molecule now has a T7 promoter at one end (from primer 1), and thus T7 polymerase drives transcription of new RNA (step 5). The numerous RNA transcripts synthesized from a single DNA template can reenter the amplification cycle, with primer 2 initiating reverse transcription, followed by RNA degradation and subsequent synthesis of DNA using primer 1 and DNA polymerase. This leads to additional amplification, with ongoing cycles of transcription and template synthesis. One advantage of NASBA over PCR is that repeat nucleic acid denaturation is unnecessary; amplification of RNA is isothermal and thus does not require a thermocycler.

Detection of Amplification Products

Initially, amplicons were detected through separation by gel electrophoresis followed by visualization of fragment length using a fluorescent DNA intercalating agent such as ethidium bromide. Because gel electrophoresis is

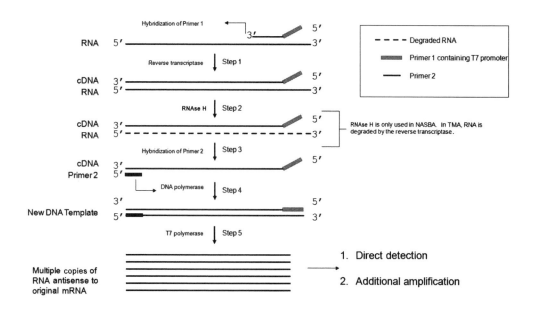

FIGURE 8-3. Overview of transcription-mediated amplification and nucleic acid sequence-based amplification. RNA = ribonucleic acid; cDNA = complementary deoxyribonucleic acid; mRNA = messenger RNA; RNAse = ribonuclease.

time-consuming and not readily automated, more advanced techniques for detecting amplicons have become routine in the clinical laboratory.

Real-Time PCR

Real-time PCR employs one or more "probes" that fluoresce only when the correct amplicon is present. A probe is a short oligomer of DNA that hybridizes to a specific cDNA sequence located within the amplicon. For real-time PCR approaches, the thermocycler used also incorporates a built-in fluorescence spectrophotometer, allowing for the detection of amplification products with each cycle. Real-time PCR is highly sensitive and quantitative and (through the use of multiple reporter dyes with distinct fluorescence spectra) permits the detection of multiple targets in a single reaction tube (multiplex amplification). In addition, because detection allows analysis without opening the reaction tube, the risk of laboratory contamination with amplicons (and subsequent false-positive results) is greatly minimized.

Several approaches can be used to detect fluorescence resulting from amplicon production. The TaqMan system (Applied Biosystems, Foster City, CA) employs a probe built with a fluorescent chemical tag (a "fluorochrome") at one end and a fluorescence quencher tag at the other [Fig 8-4 (A)]. Tethered to the probe, the two tags are close enough that the quencher effectively blocks the fluorescent signal. During amplicon synthesis, DNA polymerase, moving along the template strand, encounters the hybridized probe. DNA polymerase also has a nuclease activity, which causes probe degradation. The fluorochrome is now liberated from the probe and, no longer in proximity to the quencher, begins to fluoresce. Because fluorochrome liberation occurs only when 1) the probe hybridizes to its target and 2) DNA polymerase degrades the bound probe, fluorescence generation is a highly specific function of amplicon generation.

A second approach uses a molecular "beacon" that, like the TaqMan probe, has a fluorochrome tag at one end and a quencher tag at the other. The beacon probe is built such that the target sequence is flanked by complementary sequences. Unbound probe forms a hairpin loop, thus closely juxtaposing the fluorochrome with the quencher. As the amplicon is generated, the beacon hybridizes to its target, and the hairpin loop unfolds; the quencher is now sufficiently distant from the quencher that fluorescence is generated [Fig 8-4 (B)].

A third approach uses two probes, each of which has a distinct tag tethered to it. Fluorescence does not occur unless the two tags are near to one other. If the amplicon is present, the probes anneal so that the two tags are in close proximity, and fluorescence ensues [Fig 8-4 (C)].

A fourth method (not shown) uses a dye called SYBR green (Thermo Fisher Scientific, Waltham, MA), which fluoresces only when bound to dsDNA. Unlike the above approaches, SYBR green is not sequence-specific but detects all dsDNA in the reaction tube. It is thus less specific than approaches that use sequence-specific probes and is more prone to false-positive results. Fortunately, authentic amplicons typically can be distinguished from aberrant products by making use of a "melting curve" analysis, which assesses the temperature profile at which the amplicon denatures ("melts"). Because the melting curve is a function of amplicon size and of GC content, and the size and sequence of the correct amplicon is known, the melting curve is useful to confirm the identity of the amplicon.

These fluorescent-probe techniques are applicable not only to real-time PCR but also to other amplification technologies, such as TMA (above).

DNA Arrays

Evaluation at the DNA level of differences in the genes encoding protein blood groups is becoming much more commonly employed in the practice of transfusion medicine.[8] The vast majority of blood group antigens are the result of small differences in membrane proteins, often a single amino acid residue, that are

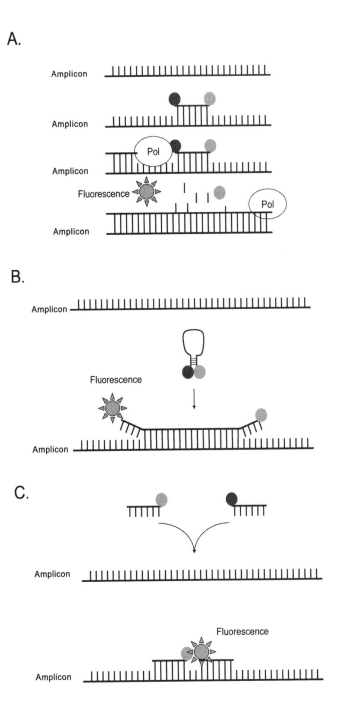

FIGURE 8-4. Methods of detection by sequence-specific probes during real-time polymerase chain reaction. Pol = polymerase enzyme.

encoded by single nucleotide polymorphisms (SNPs) at the level of gDNA.

Methods for detecting blood group SNPs primarily use PCR amplification followed by analysis by DNA-array technologies. After the region of interest in the blood group genes is amplified by PCR, specific products are detected by primers (or probes) designed such that hybridization and signal output depends on the presence of one allele but not the other. Multiplex PCR and DNA-array systems can determine the genotypes of blood group antigens in individual specimens[9-11] and offer high throughput and automated readout.

Genotyping of red cell antigens can be more efficient than traditional serologic typing. In the case of the multitransfused patient, where it is not possible to distinguish the patient's own red cells from transfused red cells, genotyping the patient's DNA can be the only reliable way to predict the patient's red cell phenotype. Genotyping is also useful in patients with sickle cell disease and other diseases in which frequent transfusion is expected and blood group matching to prevent alloimmunization is a component of care.[12]

Occasionally, however, genotype may not correlate with phenotype. Genotyping typically focuses on known polymorphisms but does not provide information on the entire sequence of the gene or on its regulatory regions. Therefore, genotyping might not predict phenotype when, for example, new (hitherto unknown) polymorphisms in the coding region alter protein structure, or new polymorphisms appear in regions that regulate expression (such as the gene promoter) but do not affect the coding sequence per se.

ANALYSIS OF PROTEIN

Much laboratory testing in transfusion medicine involves the detection and identification of antibodies in patients' plasma. In the following sections, the principles of the more common laboratory assays used to detect antibodies are described. Less routinely used technologies that are nevertheless important to understand are also presented.

Fluid-Phase Assays (Agglutination-Based Methods)

Depending on antibody isotype, immunoglobulins (Igs) contain two (IgG) to 10 (IgM) antigen-binding sites per molecule. Each antibody can bind more than one target molecule, allowing antibodies to crosslink antigens present in multiple copies on red cells. A standard serologic method for detecting antibody-antigen interactions, agglutination, is used extensively in transfusion medicine.

The antigen copy number and density vary depending on the blood group. Agglutination is used for serologic crossmatching (donor red cells incubated with recipient plasma or serum), screening for unexpected antibodies (reagent red cells of known blood group antigen composition incubated with recipient plasma or serum), and blood group antigen phenotyping of the donor or recipient (test red cells incubated with monoclonal antibodies or reagent-quality antisera of known specificity).

Agglutination can be detected by several methods. With manual tube testing, agglutination is visually detected by the adhesion of red cells to one another in the postcentrifuge pellet. Agglutination in microtiter plates is visualized by the spread pattern of red cells in individual wells. Gel-based testing is used widely; after agglutination is allowed to take place, the reaction mixture is centrifuged through a gel matrix, typically composed of dextran-acrylamide. Unagglutinated red cells pass through the gel, while the larger, agglutinated complexes are retained at the top of, or within, the matrix. Advantages of gel-based testing over tube testing include standardization of reaction strength, sensitivity, and streamlined throughput, because of both the use of automated platforms and the opportunity to eliminate some wash steps.[13]

Although agglutination reaction tests are sensitive and easy to perform, the formation of agglutinates depends on the proper stoichiometric ratio of antibody to antigen. The "zone of equivalence" refers to the ratio of antigen to antibody that permits ready agglutination. Each arm of the antibody binds to a different particle, and a network (lattice) of linked particles results in agglutination [Fig 8-5 (B)]. A false-negative result is generated if the stoichiometric ratio is outside the zone of equivalence at either extreme. A prozone effect can occur with unusually high antibody concentration, diminishing the likelihood of an antibody binding to two separate particles or red cells [Fig 8-5 (A)]. Although unusual in classical red cell serology, prozone has been observed when titers of red cell antibodies are very high, and can cause discrepant reverse ABO typing.[14] Diluting the serum being tested, or using diluents containing EDTA, decreases the likelihood of prozone.[15] False-negative agglutination reactions can also be the result of a postzone effect, which occurs when there is excess antigen [Fig 8-5 (C)] and each antibody binds to multiple epitopes on the same particle, thereby preventing crosslinking and agglutination.

Solid-Phase Assays

In solid-phase assays, a specific antigen or antibody is immobilized on a solid matrix, typically made of plastic. A solution containing the protein of interest is placed into a well; the polystyrene (or other plastic employed) directly absorbs protein from solution and irreversibly binds protein to the plastic. The well is washed, the analyte is added and incubated with the protein-coated solid phase, and its adherence is measured. Several combinations of adherence and detection approaches have been described.

Solid-Phase Assays for Phenotyping Red Cells

Antibodies specific for a known blood group antigen are coated onto round-bottom microtiter plates [Fig 8-6 (A)]. Red cells to be analyzed are added to the plate wells, allowed to

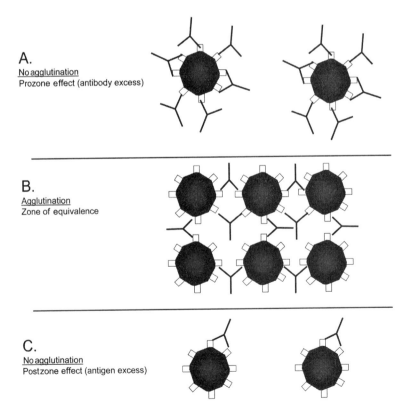

A.
No agglutination
Prozone effect (antibody excess)

B.
Agglutination
Zone of equivalence

C.
No agglutination
Postzone effect (antigen excess)

FIGURE 8-5. Effects of relative concentrations of antigen and antibody on the outcome of agglutination reactions.

adhere, and then the plate is centrifuged. If no binding occurs (negative reaction), the red cells cluster together as a "button" at the well bottom. In contrast, specific binding results in dispersion of the red cells over the surface of the entire well (positive reaction), which indicates the presence of the antigen on the red cells.

Solid-Phase Assays for Detecting Antibodies to Red Cell Antigens

Antigen-coated particles, typically red cells (or red cell fragments), are coated onto microtiter plate wells [Fig 8-6 (B)]. Patient serum is then added, followed by incubation and washing. If the patient serum contains antigen-specific antibodies, they will bind to the red cells. Indicator red cells (coated with antihuman IgG) are then added. A positive reaction is demonstrated by diffuse adherence of the indicator red cells to the well, whereas a negative reaction is demonstrated by clustering of indicator cells in a button.

Solid-Phase Assays for Platelet Testing

Using the approaches described above, solid-phase red cell adherence (SPRCA) technology has been adapted to detect antigens on platelets, such as HPA-1a, as well as to detect antibodies against platelet antigens.[16]

Enzyme-Linked Immunosorbent Assay (ELISA)

The ELISA (aka "enzyme immunoassay") can detect either antibodies or antigens. To generate a signal, a secondary antibody is used that is tethered to an enzyme, which modifies an added enzyme-specific substrate to generate either color (chromogenic reaction) or photons (chemiluminescent reaction). The use of secondary antibodies and enzymatic signal generation renders ELISAs capable of robust signal amplification; ELISAs are therefore much more sensitive than fluid-phase agglutination or SPRCA assays.

ELISAs typically use purified or recombinant antigens or antibodies, depending on the analyte to be detected. However, intact red cells can be used to screen for red cell antibodies, and this is referred to as the "enzyme-linked antiglobulin test."[17]

Detection of Antibodies by the Indirect ELISA. To detect antibodies against a specific antigen, the antigen is coated onto microtiter

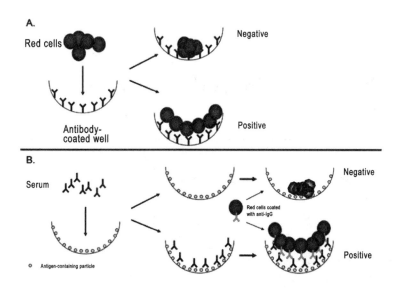

FIGURE 8-6. Schematic representation of (A) phenotyping red cells and (B) detecting antibodies by solid-phase assay.

plate wells [Fig 8-7 (A)]. The test sample is then added, incubated, and washed. Antigen-specific antibodies bound to the antigen-coated well are then detected by incubating with an antibody (eg, anti-IgG) that serves as a reporter, as it is engineered to be tethered to an enzyme such as alkaline phosphatase or horseradish peroxidase. After further washing, enzyme substrate is added and enzymatically converted to a detectable color. A spectrophotometer is used to measure light absorbance at the wavelength specific for that enzyme/substrate. Color intensity is positively related to the amount of antibody bound to the antigen. Quantification is possible through use of a standard curve. Sometimes samples need to be diluted to ensure that they yield absorbance

values in the linear range of the assay. Detection of antigens carried on multipass transmembrane proteins can be difficult in ELISA, because epitopes may not retain antigenic conformation when deposited onto a solid surface such as a microtiter well.

Detection of Antigens by Sandwich ELISA. The sandwich ELISA is used to detect and quantify a specific soluble antigen. For this assay, two different antibodies [typically monoclonal antibodies (MoAbs)] are used, each of which binds separate epitopes on the same target antigen without cross-interference. Microtiter plate wells are first coated with one MoAb (the "capture" antibody) [Fig 8-7 (B)]. The sample is then added, and antigen in solution binds to the capture antibody. Next, the

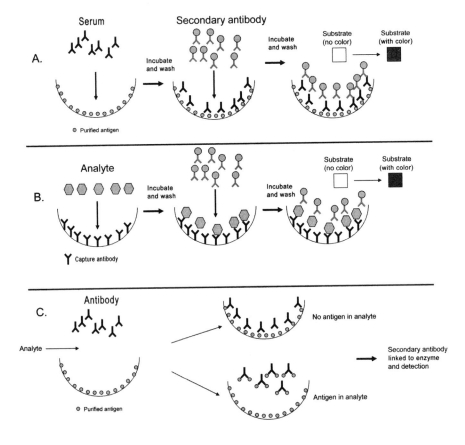

FIGURE 8-7. Schematic representation of (A) indirect enzyme-linked immunosorbent assay (ELISA), (B) sandwich ELISA, and (C) competitive ELISA.

plate is washed and incubated with a second MoAb linked to a reporter enzyme. Because it is specific for the target antigen, the reporter antibody binds to the well only if antigen is already bound via the capture antibody. After additional washing, enzyme substrate is added, and it is converted to a detectable color if antibody with enzyme has been bound.

Detection of Antigens by Competitive ELISA. Competitive ELISA begins similarly to indirect ELISA, using wells in which target antigen is already bound. The test sample is preincubated with solution-phase antibody, and this mixture is added to the well [Fig 8-7 (C)]. If no antigen is in the specimen, then reagent antibodies bind unimpeded to the solid-phase antigen. If antigen is present in the specimen, the antigen binds to reagent antibodies, preventing them from binding to the solid-phase antigen. As the amount of soluble antigen in the specimen increases, the amount of reagent antibody free to bind to the solid-phase antigen decreases. Thus, the signal is *inversely* related to the amount of soluble antigen in the specimen.

Competitive ELISA is also used for antibody detection. In this case, the test sample is added to an antigen-coated well along with a labeled antigen-specific reagent antibody. Patient antibody and labeled reagent antibody compete with each other for antigen-binding sites in the well. Again, a higher signal is generated if the antibody level in the sample is low or absent. Although more difficult to optimize than sandwich ELISAs, competitive ELISAs do not require two separate antibodies against different epitopes on the target antigen.

Technical Problems with ELISAs. ELISAs are usually straightforward and robust. False-negative signals can result from enzymatic inhibitors in the sample, and false-positive signals, from nonspecific enzymatic activity; however, the use of proper controls and thorough washing typically prevents these problems. Falsely low signals can occur if the amount of antigen exceeds the amount of antibody present, a phenomenon termed the "hook effect." Similar to the prozone effect (see "Fluid-Phase Assays" section above), excess antigen can cause the signal to decrease

in some sandwich ELISAs in which the antigen and detection antibody are added simultaneously. The hook effect can be readily overcome by diluting the antigen. Finally, patients exposed to mice or to mouse-based biologic drugs may develop human antimouse antibodies (HAMAs) that crosslink the capture antibody and/or detection antibody in sandwich ELISAs, resulting in very high signals.

Protein Assay Technologies Encountered Less Commonly in Transfusion Medicine

A number of other technological approaches can be used in the analysis of proteins. For a variety of reasons, these approaches have not been adopted widely in blood banking and transfusion medicine, with notable exceptions as indicated.

Protein Microarrays

Microarray technology dramatically increases the number of substrates that can be simultaneously assayed by solid-phase methods. When numerous different proteins are placed (spotted) on a small chip, a single specimen can be assayed for binding activity to multiple analytes simultaneously. For example, a microarray chip spotted with different blood group antigens can be used to assess a single patient specimen for several alloantibodies simultaneously. Like ELISA, protein microarrays require that the structural conformation required for antibody recognition be maintained. The practical application of protein microarrays to blood bank serology has yet to be realized.

Western Blotting

While highly sensitive, ELISA is prone to false-positive results if the antigen used to coat the well is not pure (eg, cell lysates of viruses grown in tissue culture), leading to cross-reactivity with other components in the antigen preparation. In Western blot (WB) assays, the antigen mixture is first separated by high-resolution protein electrophoresis, using polyacrylamide gels. The separated proteins are then transferred to a membrane to serve as the solid phase for probing with an antibody-containing patient sample. Using molecular weight size markers in an adjacent lane, one can determine the molecular weight of the antigens recognized by the antibodies. Alternatively, antigens can be separated on the basis of other physical properties, such as charge.

Because of the low likelihood of a cross-reactive antigen sharing the same physical characteristics as the intended analyte, WB provides more specificity than ELISA. Thus, WB is used to confirm positive serologic screening assays to detect infectious agents, such as HIV or HCV.

Flow Cytometry

Flow cytometry revolutionized the analysis of cell populations. The basic principle is that fluorescent-tag-labeled antibodies against cell-surface molecules are incubated with a target population of cells; these "stained" cells are then passed through a flow cytometer. As they travel, cells are exposed to lasers that excite the fluorescent tags, causing emission of photons of very specific wavelengths that can be detected by sensors in the flow cytometer. Fluorescence is assessed on a cell-by-cell basis, allowing for the visualization and quantification of minor populations of cells within a complex mixture.[18]

Suspension Array Technology

Suspension array technology (SAT) combines the specificity of solid-state antibody/antigen interaction (ELISA) with the sensitivity and high throughput of optical detection by flow cytometry.[19] Through selection of fluorescent dyes during the manufacturing process, populations of microspheres (beads) are generated with distinct fluorescent properties and used as solid supports for the initial binding of specific receptors (capture antigens or antibodies). By pairing beads of specific fluorescent optical properties with specific receptors, it is possible to prepare arrays of microspheres capable of detecting multiple analytes at the same time.

For sample analysis, a suspension of beads covalently tethered with receptors is first incubated with the solution of interest (eg, plasma) to bind the target analyte (antigen or antibody). Next, the bead-receptor-analyte suspension is incubated with a secondary MoAb. The secondary (reporter) MoAb is labeled with its own fluorochrome, rather than with an enzyme (as done in ELISA). Detection is rendered by sending bead suspensions through a flow cytometer, which detects individual beads (as opposed to individual cells). Software in the flow cytometer can recognize the specific capture antibody on each individual bead based on the unique fluorescent signature of the bead, and can determine the quantity of analyte bound based on the fluorescent intensity of the secondary MoAb. Multiple specific analytes can be measured simultaneously. The system allows for high throughput using very small quantities of sample.

An example of SAT applicable to transfusion medicine is the use of the Luminex system (Luminex, Austin, TX) in the detection and identification of HLA-specific alloantibodies for screening platelet donors and for workup of platelet refractoriness.[20] This system is also used for blood group genotyping.

BASIC IMMUNOLOGY

The process by which the immune system generates antibodies against foreign antigens (yet maintains tolerance to self-antigens) is complicated and elegant, with multiple cellular players and intricate regulation. Of necessity, this section is limited to antibody structure, function, and role in transfusion complications.

Antibody Structure

At its simplest, an antibody is a tetramer comprising two identical heavy chains and two identical light chains (Fig 8-8). Each heavy chain and light chain contains a variable region, which is the part of the molecule that varies between antibodies and binds antigen, and a constant region. Two light-chain fami-

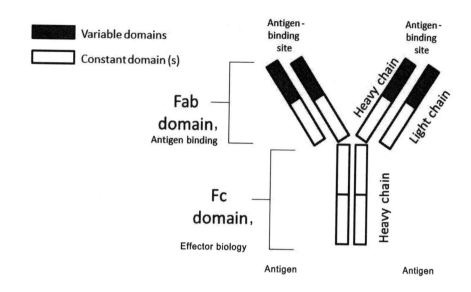

FIGURE 8-8. General structure of a monomeric immunoglobulin.

lies (kappa and lambda) are found in humans. A given antibody has either two kappa light chains or two lambda light chains.

Igs treated with the enzyme papain can be digested into two functional fragments. The "Fab" fragment consists of the heavy- and light-chain variable regions, the light-chain constant regions, and one heavy-chain constant region domain. The Fab fragment binds antigen but does not activate effector mechanisms. In contrast, the Fc fragment, consisting only of heavy-chain constant regions, activates effector mechanisms, allowing destruction of the antibody target. Fc constant regions differ between antibody molecules based on antibody isotype and subclass.

There are five different antibody isotypes (IgM, IgG, IgE, IgA, IgD), determined by the constant region of the heavy chain. Antibodies of different isotypes differ both in the number of antigen-binding sites per molecule and in the potency of their effector functions [Fig 8-9 (A)]. The "affinity" of an antibody for its antigen reflects the binding ability of a single binding site, where the "avidity" refers to the total binding strength conferred by the combined effects of multiple binding sites. Thus, al-

though the individual binding sites of IgM are of relatively low affinity, IgM demonstrates high antigen avidity because it has 10 antigen-binding sites. In IgM, the five Ig molecules are held together by an additional protein (the J chain) and by extensive disulfide binding. Treatment with dithiothreitol (DTT) can destroy IgM binding because it cleaves (reduces) disulfide bonds; DTT treatment is used in the clinical laboratory to distinguish IgM antibodies from IgG antibodies. IgM potently activates complement by changing its three-dimensional structure after antigen binding. In general, IgM (and some IgG) can cause hemolysis during transfusion reactions and in autoimmune hemolytic anemia. Importantly, unlike IgG, IgM does not cross the placenta and is therefore not involved in hemolytic disease of the fetus and newborn.

Whereas IgM is expressed early in the antigen-specific immune response, IgG antibodies are important in mature humoral immune effector functions, and are divided into four subclasses: IgG1, IgG2, IgG3, and IgG4. Each subclass has a different constant region and a different capacity to either activate complement and/or interact with Fc receptors on

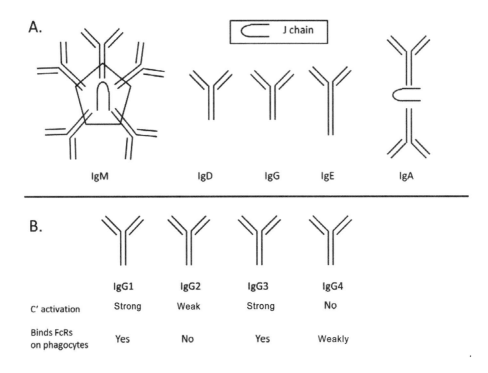

FIGURE 8-9. Immune globulin (Ig) isotypes (A), IgG subclasses, and their relative activation of complement and binding to Fc-gamma receptors (FcγRs) (B).

phagocytes [Fig 8-9 (B)]. IgG1 and IgG3 are the most potent, whereas IgG2 only weakly activates complement, and IgG4 largely lacks effector activity. Consistent with these observations, patients with only IgG4 subclass red cell antibodies typically do not exhibit hemolysis. In contrast, IgG1, IgG2, and IgG3 red cell antibodies can all induce hemolysis.

IgA is the primary antibody isotype secreted at mucosal surfaces; therefore, it is largely responsible for neutralizing pathogens encountered in the gastrointestinal, genitourinary, and respiratory tracts. Although IgA exists in either monomeric or dimeric forms (Fig 8-9 shows a dimer), in serum it is often monomeric. IgA is further divided into IgA1 and IgA2 subclasses (not shown). Dimeric IgA is composed of monomers connected by the J chain (the same J chain found in IgM). Only rarely is Ig-mediated hemolysis due to IgA. Antiglobulin (Coombs) reagents do not detect IgA, and

the potential presence of IgA red cell antibodies should be considered when analyzing a patient with both hemolysis and a negative direct antiglobulin test result.

IgE antibodies bind to Fc receptors on mast cells, inducing histamine release upon antigen encounter, and are the predominant cause of allergic and anaphylactic responses (Type I hypersensitivity). IgD primarily remains membrane bound on the B-cell surface, with only minimal levels in serum, but its functions remain unclear.

Antibody Receptors (FcγRs) in Target Clearance

The Fc regions of antigen-bound IgGs are recognized by the gamma family of Fc receptors (FcγRs) found on the surface of cells. At least four FcγRs have been described, each with different properties that can have opposite functions. For example, FcγR2a and FcγR3 promote phagocytosis of targets. Because of the relatively low affinity of these receptors, monomeric IgG does not engage FcγR2a or FcγR3; these receptors are engaged only when an antigenic target is bound by multiple IgGs simultaneously. In contrast, FcγR2b is an inhibitory receptor that prevents phagocytosis. FcγR1 has an unusually high affinity for IgG, and binds monomeric IgG, such that FcγR1 binds IgG whether or not it is complexed with a target; the function of this activity is currently unclear.

FcγR biology is complex, as 1) a given IgG-bound cell or particle may simultaneously activate multiple (potentially antagonistic) receptors, and 2) each IgG subclass (IgG1, IgG2, IgG3, IgG4) has a different affinity for the various FcγRs [Fig 8-9 (B)]. A mixture of IgGs may bind a particle or cell bearing a foreign antigen. The net effect on phagocytosis depends on the relative binding of different IgG subclasses and their interactions with different FcγRs. Thus, direct binding of Fc domains to FcγRs promotes red cell clearance in many but not all cases.

Complement in Target Cell Opsonization and Destruction

Fc regions of IgG antibodies can also activate complement. The complement system consists of a cascade of proteases that, once activated, amplifies the initial signal, leading to the production of a large number of effector molecules. Although there are several pathways to complement activation, this discussion focuses on the "classical pathway" initiated by Fc regions.

IgM is highly efficient in activating complement. However, to avoid indiscriminant activation, IgM must undergo a conformational shift, which occurs only after binding antigen, thereby exposing complement-binding sites in the heavy-chain constant region. This interaction is so potent that, in theory, a single antigen-bound IgM is sufficient to lyse a target.

In contrast, complement activation by IgG does not involve a conformational change.

Rather, complement activation requires clustered binding to the same target by multiple IgG molecules. This ensures against indiscriminate complement activation by unbound circulating IgG.

Once activated, the complement system initiates at least two distinct mechanisms of target destruction. The first involves decoration of the target by complement components labeling it for destruction; this process is known as "opsonization." Early in activation, a portion of one complement component (termed "C3") covalently attaches (by thioester bonds) to the surface of the antigen. Multiple copies of C3b can be recognized by specific receptors on phagocytic cells. Upon encountering a C3b-coated molecule, a phagocyte ingests and destroys it. However, C3b can also rapidly degrade to C3dg, which is not recognized by phagocytes, thus bypassing phagocytosis.

In the second mechanism, activation of C3 promotes the assembly of the membrane attack complex (MAC). The MAC consists of complement proteins (C5b-C9) arranged into a structure resembling a hollow tube that is inserted into the membrane of the target cell. This creates a channel between the inside of a target cell and its external environment, typically resulting in osmotic lysis of the target.

Outcomes of Complement Activation

The effector mechanisms induced by antibody binding have different effects on bacteria, viruses, particles, and various human tissues. In general, once an IgG antibody binds to a red cell, the target cell may undergo FcγR-mediated phagocytosis (Fig 8-10). If the antibody initiates the complement cascade, C3b deposition on the red cell surface contributes to opsonization, leading to phagocytosis mediated by the C3b receptors CR1 and CRIg. Finally, if complement activation is complete, MAC insertion causes red cell lysis.

The relative contribution of each pathway varies based on the relative amounts of antibody isotype and subclass, and on the properties of the antigen (eg, antigen density or linkage to cytoskeleton). The sections below describe what is known about these processes with regard to red cell destruction and the clinical manifestations of hemolysis.

Extravascular Hemolysis

Extravascular hemolysis refers to the consumption of antibody- and/or C3b-bound red cells by phagocytes in the reticuloendothelial system (RES), found predominantly in the spleen and liver. The term "extravascular" is used because the red cells are destroyed outside of their normal compartment, the intravascular space. This process is also commonly referred to as a "delayed hemolytic transfusion reaction" (DHTR) because it typically occurs days after transfusion. In contrast, "intravascular" hemolysis (see below) occurs rapidly during or following transfusion and is associated with an "acute hemolytic transfusion reaction" (AHTR). DHTRs demonstrate delayed kinetics both because the manifestations of extravascular hemolysis are more mild and because the antibodies implicated are often absent or of low titer initially, requiring some time to develop and increase in titer before the onset of significant red cell destruction.

Extravascular hemolysis is markedly different from intravascular hemolysis, in which red cell contents are directly released into the circulating blood. The term "hemolysis" in this context can cause confusion for health-care providers not accustomed to transfusion medicine terminology; hemolysis is often thought of as just described—the rupture of red cells within the circulation. In contrast, in extravascular hemolysis, the red cells are destroyed by phagocytes, typically within the lysosomes. This is a very important distinction because phagocytes in the RES consume a substantial number of senescent, autologous red cells each day in the normal process of red cell turnover. Thus, consumption of red cells by this pathway follows a process that evolved specifically to break down and recycle red cell contents (hemoglobin and iron) in a manner that avoids tissue damage.

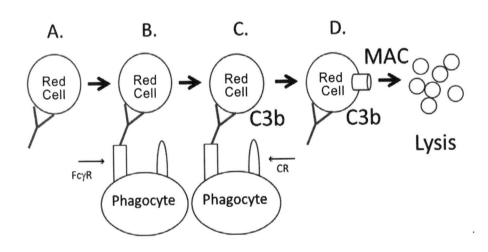

FIGURE 8-10. Mechanisms of red cell destruction by antibody binding. Upon binding (A), an immune globulin G (IgG) represents a ligand for Fc-gamma receptors (FcγRs) on phagocytes (B). If the red cell avoids FcγR-mediated phagocytosis, opsonization may be increased by activation of complement with deposition of C3b (C). If the combined opsonization of FcγR binding and C3b is not sufficient to mediate clearance, completion of the complement cascade may lead to insertion of the membrane attack complex (MAC) into the red cell surface, resulting in lysis (D). These processes likely occur simultaneously, with the outcome representing the aggregate effect of competing pathways.
CR = complement receptor.

This does not mean, however, that extravascular removal of antibody-coated red cells is biologically equivalent to clearance of normal, senescent red cells. On the contrary, DHTRs can cause substantial morbidity (and occasional mortality).

It is not clear why some red cell antibodies preferentially promote opsonization and phagocytosis instead of osmotic lysis by the MAC. The antibody type and the topology and copy number of the target antigen on the red cells are important. In addition, although complement may be activated, the aggregate opsonization of red cells by C3b and antibody may result in phagocytosis before MAC-induced lysis occurs. Consistent with these explanations, extravascular hemolysis is typically induced by IgG red cell antibodies, whereas intravascular hemolysis is typically induced by IgM red cell antibodies. IgM is much more efficient at activating complement and promoting MAC formation.

Intravascular Hemolysis

In some cases of incompatible transfusion, the MAC rapidly assembles and lyses the red cells before C3b and/or IgG opsonization can induce phagocytosis. Because these red cells lyse while still circulating, this process is termed "intravascular hemolysis." In addition, because antibody-mediated intravascular hemolysis occurs at a brisker pace than extravascular hemolysis (or, at least, is more quickly noticed because of dramatic signs and symptoms), this hemolytic transfusion reaction is called "acute."

As discussed, AHTRs are typically caused by IgM antibodies, which efficiently activate complement, leading to rapid formation of the MAC. Although an IgM-specific Fc receptor has been described (FcγR), it is predominantly expressed on nonphagocytic lymphocytes[21] and is unlikely to promote phagocytosis of IgM-coated red cells. Complement activation by IgM red cell antibodies can result in opsonization by C3b, leading to some receptor-mediated phagocytosis. Overall, however, IgM antibodies predominantly induce intravascular hemolysis.

Intravascular hemolysis, unlike extravascular hemolysis, does not occur at any appreciable level under normal conditions. The release of red cell contents directly into the circulation can be highly toxic, with free hemoglobin inducing perhaps the greatest insult. Although much free hemoglobin is scavenged by the circulating molecule haptoglobin, this system is easily overwhelmed. AHTRs often result in tea-colored urine (hemoglobinuria) and can induce renal dysfunction. Moreover, the signs and symptoms of AHTRs can be dramatic and include disseminated intravascular coagulation, shock, and death. This type of reaction most often occurs as a result of a clerical error with ABO-incompatible transfusion, and current practices have evolved multiple redundant checkpoints to prevent AHTRs from ABO incompatibility.

Nonhemolytic Red Cell Antibodies

Given the redundant pathways leading to the destruction of antibody-coated red cells, it makes sense that transfusions of crossmatch-incompatible red cells can produce hemolysis. Curiously, however, most red cell antibodies are actually not hemolytic. For some blood group antigens, hemolysis is only very rarely observed following incompatible transfusion (eg, JMH, Chido, Rodgers antigens). Moreover, approximately 1% of healthy blood donors have positive direct antiglobulin test results (indicating that IgG autoantibodies are bound to their own red cells), yet there is no evidence of hemolysis. For antigens known to be frequently responsible for antibody-mediated hemolysis (in the Rh, Kell, Kidd, Duffy, and Ss systems), hemolysis is variable. Indeed, in patients mistakenly transfused with ABO-incompatible Red Blood Cell (RBC) units, clinically significant hemolysis occurs in only 50% of cases even for this robustly hemolytic antigen/antibody combination.

Several explanations may account for the lack of hemolysis during incompatible transfusions. For antigens that are essentially never involved in hemolysis, the antigen cell surface density or topography may prevent hemolysis.

For antigens that are variably involved in hemolysis, the antibody response (titer, affinity, isotype, or IgG subclass) may play roles. Distinct antibodies of the same antigenic specificity may have different capacities for activating complement. This is the rationale for including the anti-C3 component in the antiglobulin (Coombs) reagent: it provides information on whether an antibody can activate (fix) complement.

IgG blood group antibodies are typically polyclonal responses, and a number of early studies demonstrated that clinically significant red cell IgG responses are primarily IgG1 and IgG3 isotypes, with IgG2 and IgG4 isotypes much less frequently observed[22-24]; indeed, some clinically insignificant blood group antibodies (eg, anti-Chido) show a converse relationship, exhibiting a higher frequency of IgG4.[22] In this regard, it is notable that one antihuman globulin MoAb in common use in pretransfusion testing fails to detect IgG4 isotypes as well as some IgG3 allelic variants present in specific populations.[25] The studies establishing that clinically significant antibodes are often IgG1 and IgG3, and clinically insignificant antibodies are IgG2 and IgG4, are now decades old. Utilizing new exquisitely specific reagents could potentially establish, for each blood group antigen, the relationship between IgG isotype and clinical significance.

A number of different genetic polymorphisms and/or deficiencies may also regulate hemolysis vs red cell survival on a patient-by-patient basis, including perturbations in complement, complement-regulatory proteins, and allelic polymorphisms in FcγRs. Thus, in some cases, regulation of hemolysis may be independent of the nature of the antibody.

It is fair to state that there is only a rudimentary understanding of the underlying basis for the development and manifestation of immune red cell destruction.[26] From a practical standpoint, crossmatch-incompatible RBC units may be issued for transfusion if the offending entity is in the category of a "clinically insignificant antibody," especially if the antigen is of very high frequency and antigen-negative blood is difficult or impossible to obtain. The transfusion service must be prepared to address appropriate concerns from healthcare providers managing these patients. Although an antibody deemed "clinically significant" may not actually produce hemolysis in all patients, there is no practical method of predicting hemolysis in a given recipient. Thus, transfusion with a unit that is antigen matched to the patient for common clinically significant blood group antigens should be considered, and RBC units that are crossmatch-incompatible should not be issued for clinically significant antibodies except as a lifesaving intervention. If compatible RBC units are unavailable, it might be determined that hemolysis occurring over several days (in the case of a DHTR) is less dangerous than the consequences of the patient's severe anemia. In such cases, close and frequent communication between managing physicians and the blood bank is required.

Summary of Efferent Immunity

In aggregate, when an antibody binds a red cell, multiple pathways are activated that can lead to cell destruction. Complement activation promotes phagocytosis through the opsonizing properties of C3b and through direct red cell lysis via assembly of the MAC. The presence of IgG Fc domains promotes red cell phagocytosis by binding FcγRs on the phagocyte surface. The relative contributions of these different pathways vary depending on the nature of the target antigen and the properties of the cognate antibodies. The activation of immune pathways, and the toxicity associated with red cell hemolysis, can lead to negative clinical consequences far beyond simple loss of efficacy of the transfused red cells. Indeed, substantial toxicity can occur, leading to morbidity and, in some cases, mortality. The reader is referred to a more in-depth reference[27] if additional mechanistic details on immunobiology and the immune response are desired.

KEY POINTS

1. Hybridization-based methods can be used to detect genes, gene products, and polymorphisms. However, hybridization methods are less sensitive than amplification-based methods.
2. Amplification-based nucleic acid detection methods (PCR, TMA, NASBA) are highly sensitive but susceptible to false-positive or false-negative results caused by contamination (eg, amplicons) or inhibitors, respectively.
3. Analysis of protein expression detects the actual gene product(s), whereas nucleic acid testing predicts protein expression.
4. Protein analysis is less sensitive than NAT because no amplification is involved, but it is also less susceptible to contamination and inhibition.
5. Methods of detecting protein suffer from non-amplification-based artifacts (HAMA, prozone effects, hook effects) that can lead to erroneous results.
6. Different methods of detecting antigens and antibodies can result in variability in test performance.
7. IgMs and IgGs cause destruction of red cells by multiple mechanisms, based largely on the antigen recognized and the antibody structure.
8. IgG antibodies that cause red cell destruction induce extravascular hemolysis by promoting phagocyte consumption of red cells (through Fc receptors and/or complement-based opsonization). Such destruction typically presents as a delayed hemolytic transfusion reaction.
9. IgM antibodies (and in some rare cases IgG) that cause red cell destruction typically induce intravascular hemolysis through complement activation, resulting in insertion of the membrane attack complex. Such destruction typically presents as an acute hemolytic transfusion reaction.
10. Not all antibodies to red cell antigens result in destruction of red cells. Incompatibility is best avoided whenever possible, but if compatible blood is unavailable, incompatible RBC units can be used when the antibodies are known to be clinically insignificant. Transfusion of incompatible blood should be considered on a-case-by-case basis and with extensive communication with the clinicians requesting the blood components.

REFERENCES

1. Alberts B, Johnson A, Lewis J, et al. Molecular biology of the cell. 6th ed. New York: Garland Science, 2014.
2. Mullis KB, Faloona FA. Specific synthesis of DNA in vitro via a polymerase-catalyzed chain reaction. Methods Enzymol 1987;155:335-50.
3. Al-Soud WA, Radstrom P. Purification and characterization of PCR-inhibitory components in blood cells. J Clin Microbiol 2001;39:485-93.
4. Rychlik W. Selection of primers for polymerase chain reaction. Mol Biotechnol 1995;3:129-34.
5. Pang J, Modlin J, Yolken R. Use of modified nucleotides and uracil-DNA glycosylase (UNG) for the control of contamination in the PCR-based amplification of RNA. Mol Cell Probes 1992;6:251-6.
6. Compton J. Nucleic acid sequence-based amplification. Nature 1991;350:91-2.
7. Kwoh DY, Davis GR, Whitfield KM, et al. Transcription-based amplification system and detection of amplified human immunodeficiency virus type 1 with a bead-based sandwich hybridization format. Proc Natl Acad Sci U S A 1989;86:1173-7.
8. Elkins MB, Davenport RD, O'Malley BA, Bluth MH. Molecular pathology in transfusion medicine. Clin Lab Med 2013;33:805-16.
9. Denomme GA, Van Oene M. High-throughput multiplex single-nucleotide polymorphism

analysis for red cell and platelet Ag genotypes. Transfusion 2005;45:660-6.

10. Bugert P, McBride S, Smith G, et al. Microarray-based genotyping for blood groups: Comparison of gene array and 5′-nuclease assay techniques with human platelet Ag as a model. Transfusion 2005;45:654-9.

11. Hashmi G, Shariff T, Seul M, et al. A flexible array format for large-scale, rapid blood group DNA typing. Transfusion 2005;45:680-8.

12. Chou ST, Westhoff CM. The role of molecular immunohematology in sickle cell disease. Transfus Apher Sci 2011;44:73-9.

13. Harmening DM, Walker PS. Alternative technologies and automation in routine blood bank testing. In: Harmening DM, ed. Modern blood banking and transfusion practices. 5th ed. Philadelphia: FA Davis, 2005:293-302.

14. Judd WJ, Steiner EA, O'Donnell DB, Oberman HA. Discrepancies in reverse ABO typing due to prozone. How safe is the immediate-spin crossmatch? Transfusion 1988;28:334-8.

15. Salama A, Mueller-Eckhardt C. Elimination of the prozone effect in the antiglobulin reaction by a simple modification. Vox Sang 1982;42:157-9.

16. Procter JL, Vigue F, Alegre E, et al. Rapid screening of platelet donors for PIA1 (HPA-1a) alloAg using a solid-phase microplate immunoassay. Immunohematology 1998;14:141-5.

17. Leikola J, Perkins HA. Enzyme-linked antiglobulin test: An accurate and simple method to quantify red cell Abs. Transfusion 1980;20:138-44.

18. Arndt PA, Garratty G. A critical review of published methods for analysis of red cell antigen-antibody reactions by flow cytometry, and approaches for resolving problems with red cell agglutination. Transfus Med Rev 2010;24:172-94.

19. Nolan JP, Sklar LA. Suspension array technology: Evolution of the flat-array paradigm. Trends Biotechnol 2002;20:9-12.

20. Kopko PM, Warner P, Kresie L, Pancoska C. Methods for the selection of platelet products for alloimmune-refractory patients. Transfusion 2015;55:235-44.

21. Wang H, Coligan JE, Morse HC 3rd. Emerging functions of natural IgM and its Fc receptor FCMR in immune homeostasis. Front Immunol 2016;7:99.

22. Devey ME, Voak D. A critical study of the IgG subclasses of Rh anti-D antibodies formed in pregnancy and in immunized volunteers. Immunology 1974;27:1073-9.

23. Szymanski IO, Huff SR, Delsignore R. An autoanalyzer test to determine immunoglobulin class and IgG subclass of blood group antibodies. Transfusion 1982;22:90-5.

24. Michaelsen TE, Kornstad L. IgG subclass distribution of anti-Rh, anti-Kell, and anti-Duffy antibodies measured by sensitive haemagglutinition assays. Clin Exp Immunol 1987;67:637-45.

25. Howie HL, Delaney M, Wang X, et al. Serological blind spots for variants of human IgG3 and IgG4 by a commonly used anti-immunoglobulin reagent. Transfusion 2016;56:2953-62.

26. Flegel WA. Pathogenesis and mechanisms of antibody-mediated hemolysis. Transfusion 2015;55(Suppl 2):S47-58.

27. Murphy K, Weaver C. Janeway's immunobiology. 9th ed. New York: Garland Science, 2016.

Chapter 9

Blood Group Genetics

• ● •

Christine Lomas-Francis, MSc, FIBMS

THE SCIENCE OF genetics is the study of heredity—that is, the mechanisms by which particular characteristics are passed from parents to offspring. This chapter describes the genetics of blood groups. The term "blood group" can be applied to any detectable, variable characteristic of a component of the blood, including platelet and white blood cell (WBC) groups, serum groups, red cell enzymes, and hemoglobin variants. In this chapter, the term "blood group" applies primarily to antigens on the surface of the red cell membrane that are defined serologically by an antibody. Platelet and WBC blood groups are discussed in Chapter 15.

That blood groups are inherited characteristics was first shown by von Dungern and Hirszfeld in 1910, ten years after Landsteiner's discovery of the ABO blood group. Blood groups became an ideal tool for geneticists because they could be identified by specific antibodies in simple hemagglutination tests and, once identified, their inheritance could easily be followed in family studies. Red cell antigens were (and still are) valuable as **markers** (detectable characteristics to recognize a gene's presence) in genetic and anthropologic studies as well as in relationship testing.

The detection of inherited differences on the red cells from different people is the basis of safe blood transfusion. Therefore, an understanding of the principles of human genetics (including the patterns of inheritance and the language or terminology in use) is an important aspect of immunohematology and transfusion medicine. This chapter outlines the fundamental principles of genetics as they apply to blood group antigens and relates them to examples relevant to transfusion medicine. This requires the use of numerous genetic terms; each term, when first used or when fully described, will be in **bold** text and usually is closely followed by a definition.

Technical advances in genetics and molecular biology have ushered in the age of molecular genetics, when genes are routinely sequenced and inheritance and disease are studied at the nucleic acid level.[1,2] These advances have provided an understanding of the regulatory elements and genes that control the expression of blood groups so that the presence or absence of blood groups can be predicted through DNA-based analysis[3] with the potential to revolutionize transfusion medicine and patient care. Knowledge of the fundamental principles of classical genetics aids

9

Christine Lomas-Francis, MSc, FIBMS, Technical Director, Laboratory of Immunohematology and Genomics, New York Blood Center, Long Island City, New York
The author has disclosed no conflicts of interest.

understanding of the molecular aspects of individual blood groups.

BASIC PRINCIPLES OF GENETICS

Gregor Mendel established the basic techniques of genetic analysis when, in 1865, he published his classic breeding experiments with pea plants. Mendel's observations led him to conclude that there is a "factor" or unit of inheritance, now known as a gene, that is passed from one generation to another according to two simple rules: the principles of independent segregation and independent assortment. (See "Inheritance of Genetic Traits" section below.)

Cytology studies toward the end of the 19th century showed that each living cell has a characteristic set of chromosomes in the nucleus. In the early part of the 20th century it was realized that chromosomes carry genes. Biochemical studies showed that the chromosomal material is primarily made up of nucleic acids and associated proteins.[1,2]

Many excellent texts offer greater insight into classical genetics.[4] The fundamental principles of genetics outlined in this chapter are intended to serve as a review of inheritance and expression of blood group antigens.

Genes (Alleles) and Chromosomes

A **gene** is a segment of deoxyribonucleic acid (DNA) that encodes a particular protein. A gene is the basic unit of inheritance of any **trait** (defined as a genetically determined characteristic or condition), including blood group antigens, that is passed from parents to offspring. Genes are arranged on chromosomes, with each gene occupying a specific location known as the **gene locus**. A locus may be occupied by one of several alternative forms of the gene called **alleles**. For example, the gene that encodes the protein carrying the Jk^a antigen is an alternative form (allele) of the one that encodes the Jk^b antigen. The terms "gene" and "allele" can be used interchangeably. Based on internationally accepted gene and allele terminology, the written gene or allele name is italicized—for example, *RHD* for the gene encoding the RhD protein. The name usually is not italicized when the word "gene" or "allele" follows the name: for example, "RHD gene," or "RHD allele." The International Society of Blood Transfusion (ISBT) Working Party on Red Cell Immunogenetics and Blood Group Terminology[5,6] provides allele terminology for use in transfusion medicine. For alleles encoding polymorphic common antigens, the name is based on the ISBT antigen name: eg, *FY*01* or *JK*02* refer to the alleles encoding the Fy^a and Jk^b antigens, respectively. Alternatively, where letters are commonly used, symbols such as *FY*A* or *JK*B* are acceptable.

Chromosomes are the gene-carrying structures that are visible during nuclear division in the nucleus of the cell; they contain the genetic material (DNA) necessary to maintain the life of the cell and the organism. A human somatic cell contains 46 chromosomes that make up 23 pairs; each pair has one paternally and one maternally derived chromosome. In males and females, 22 of the pairs are **homologous chromosomes** (a pair of chromosomes in which males and females carry equivalent genes) and are referred to as the **autosomes** (any chromosome that is not a sex chromosome). The remaining pair is nonhomologous and consists of the **sex chromosomes** that determine an individual's gender. The sex-determining chromosomes of the male are X and Y, whereas females have two X chromosomes. The **karyotype** represents the chromosome complement of a person; this is written as "46,XY" and "46,XX" for a normal male and female, respectively. The hereditary information carried by the chromosomes is passed from a parent cell to a daughter cell during somatic cell division and from parents to offspring (children) by the gametes during reproduction.

Chromosomes are best studied during cell division (mitosis; see "Mitosis" section below), when they become discrete structures in the nucleus and can be visualized by various microscopic techniques. All chromosomes have some common morphologic features but differ in other characteristics, including size, location of the centromere, and staining properties. Each chromosome has two sections, or arms, that are joined at a central constriction called the **centromere** (Figs 9-1 and 9-2). Chromosomes are distinguished by their length and the position of the centromere. These characteristics serve as the basis for numbering the autosomes 1 through 22 such that chromosome 1 is the largest and chromosome 22 is the smallest. An internationally recognized terminology is used to describe chromosomes. The chromosomal arms are of different length, although the difference between the arms of chromosome 1 is not obvious (Fig 9-2). The "p" (or petite) arm is the shorter and, in diagrams, is at the top of the chromosome. The longer arm is termed the "q" arm. Thus, the short arm of chromosome 1 is referred to as "1p," and the long arm of chromosome 4 is "4q." The terminal portion of a chromosome is referred to as "ter"; "pter" and "qter" indicate the terminus of the short (p) and long (q) arms, respectively.

Staining techniques provide a more detailed means to distinguish individual chromosomes. Selected dyes do not stain chromosomes uniformly and, depending on the dye used, different banding patterns are obtained so that each human chromosome has a unique banding pattern. As shown in Fig 9-2, Giemsa staining reveals a specific pattern of dark (G) and light (reverse or R) bands. Quina-

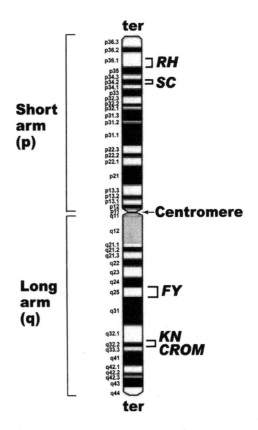

FIGURE 9-2. The morphology and banding pattern of a Giemsa-stained human chromosome 1. The locations of the genes controlling the expression of antigens for the Rh *(RH)*, Scianna *(SC)*, Duffy *(FY)*, Knops *(KN)*, and Cromer *(CROM)* blood group systems are shown.

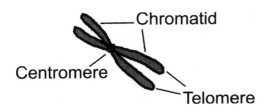

FIGURE 9-1. Diagram of a metaphase chromosome. At the metaphase stage of the cell cycle, the chromosomes have condensed and become visible by light microscopy. As shown in the diagram above, metaphase chromosomes have replicated in preparation for cell division so that each chromosome consists of two sister chromatids connected by the centromere. The telomere is the end or terminal part of a chromosome.

crine, used to stain chromosomal preparations for fluorescence microscopy, results in fluorescent bands equivalent to the dark G bands seen in light microscopy. The G bands are heterochromatin (condensed DNA) and the lighter bands are euchromatin, which is involved in the transcription of DNA to mRNA. The bands are numbered from the centromere outward. Using chromosome 1 as an example, the region closest to the centromere on the short or long arm is numbered 1p1 or 1q1, respectively. With greater resolution, there is further distinction into subbands (eg, 1p11 and 1p12) that, in turn, can be subdivided (eg, 1p11.1 and 1p11.2). Genes can be individually mapped to a specific band location (Fig 9-2), and the chromosomal location of the genes encoding the 36 red cell systems[5-9] are listed in Table 9-1.

Cell Division

As a cell divides, the chromosomes replicate and each daughter cell receives a full complement of genetic material. In somatic cells, this occurs through mitosis; in reproductive cells a similar process called "meiosis" takes place. A feature common to both types of cell division is that, before the start of the process, each chromosome replicates to form two identical daughter **chromatids** attached to each other through the centromere (Fig 9-1).

Mitosis

Somatic cells divide for growth and repair by **mitosis** (Fig 9-3). Through this process, a single cell gives rise to two daughter cells with identical sets of chromosomes. The daughter cells, like the parent cell, are **diploid (2N)**; that is, they contain 46 chromosomes in 23 pairs and have all the genetic information of the parent cell.

Meiosis

Meiosis occurs only in germ cells that are intended to become gametes (sperm and egg cells). Somatic cells are diploid (2N), whereas gametes are **haploid** [having half the chromosomal complement of somatic cells (1N)]. **Meiosis** is a process of cell division and replication that leads to the formation of haploid gametes. During meiosis, diploid cells undergo DNA replication, followed by two cycles of cell division to produce four haploid gametes. (See Fig 9-4.) Because sperm and egg cells fuse at fertilization, the gametes must be haploid. If each gamete carried a diploid (2N) set of 46 chromosomes, the resulting zygote would have 92 chromosomes, which would be incompatible with life.

Meiosis ensures genetic diversity through two mechanisms: independent assortment and crossing over. Through independent assortment, each daughter cell randomly receives either maternally or paternally derived homologous chromosomes. The chromosomal crossing over involves exchange of genetic material between homologous chromosome pairs. Such shuffling of genetic material ensures diversity and produces genetically unique gametes that fuse to produce a unique zygote.

X Chromosome Inactivation (Lyonization)

Females have two copies of X-borne genes in their somatic cells, while males have only one copy of X-borne genes. Because most X-borne genes do not have a homolog on the Y chromosome, there is a potential imbalance in the dosage of X-borne genes between males and females. This difference is compensated for by **X chromosome inactivation** (also called lyonization), a process through which most of the genes on one of the two X chromosomes in each female somatic cell are inactivated at a very early stage of embryonic development.[19] It is a matter of chance whether the maternal or paternal X chromosome is inactivated in any one cell, but once inactivation has occurred, all descendants of that cell will have the same inactive X chromosome. Some X-borne genes escape inactivation; the first gene found to escape inactivation was *XG*, the gene encoding the antigens of the Xg blood group system. Like *XG*, most of the genes that escape inactivation are located on the extreme tip of the short arm of the X chromosome, but several are clustered in regions on the short and long arms of the chromosome.[20(pp359-370),21]

The XK gene, which encodes the Kx blood group system, is the only other X-borne gene known to encode red cell antigens. Changes or deletions in *XK* result in McLeod phenotype red cells that lack Kx antigen and have reduced expression of Kell antigens.[22,23] The XK gene, unlike *XG*, is subject to X chromosome inactivation, with the result that a female who is a **carrier** (a person who carries one gene for a recessive trait and one normal gene) of a gene that is responsible for the McLeod phenotype can have a dual population of Kx– (McLeod phenotype) and Kx+ (non-McLeod) red cells. Flow cytometry, using selected Kell antibodies,

TABLE 9-1.　Blood Group Systems

ISBT System Name (Number)	Gene Name ISBT (HGNC)*	Chromosome Location	Gene Product and Component Name [CD number]	Associated Blood Group Antigens [Null phenotype]
ABO (001)	*ABO* (*ABO*)	9q34.2	Glycosyltransferase, carbohydrate	A; B; A,B; A1 [Group O]
MNS (002)	*MNS* (*GYPA* *GYPB* *GYPE*)	4q31.21	Glycophorin A (GPA) [CD235a] Glycophorin B (GPB) [CD235b]	M, N, S, s, U, He, Mi^a, Vw, and 41 more [En(a–); U–; M^kM^k]
P1PK (003)	*P1* (*A4GALT*)	22q13.2	Galactosyltransferase, carbohydrate	P1, P^k, NOR
Rh (004)	*RH* (*RHD* *RHCE*)	1p36.11	RhD [CD240D] RhCE [CD240CE]	D, G, Tar C, E, c, e, V, Rh17, and 45 more [Rh_{null}]
Lutheran (005)	*LU* (*LU*)	19q13.32	Lutheran glycoprotein, B-cell adhesion molecule [CD239]	Lu^a, Lu^b, Lu3, Lu4, Au^a, Au^b, and 18 more [Recessive Lu(a–b–)]
Kell (006)	*KEL* (*KEL*)	7q34	Kell glycoprotein [CD238]	K, k, Kp^a, Kp^b, Ku, Js^a, Js^b, and 29 more [K_0 or K_{null}]
Lewis (007)	*LE* (*FUT3*)	19p13.3	Fucosyltransferase, carbohydrate (adsorbed from plasma)	Le^a, Le^b, Le^{ab}, Le^{bh}, ALe^b, BLe^b [Le(a–b–)]
Duffy (008)	*FY* (*ACKR1, previously DARC*)	1q23.2	Duffy glycoprotein [CD234]	Fy^a, Fy^b, Fy3, Fy5, Fy6 [Fy(a–b–)]
Kidd (009)	*JK (SLC14A1)*	18q12.3	Human urea transporter (HUT), Kidd glycoprotein	Jk^a, Jk^b, Jk3 [Jk(a–b–)]
Diego (010)	*DI* (*SLC4A1*)	17q21.31	Band 3, anion exchanger 1 [CD233]	Di^a, Di^b, Wr^a, Wr^b, Wd^a, Rb^a, and 16 more
Yt (011)	*YT* (*ACHE*)	7q22.1	Acetylcholinesterase	Yt^a, Yt^b
Xg (012)	*XG* (*MIC2*)	Xp22.33 Yp11.2	Xg^a glycoprotein CD99 (*MIC2* product)	Xg^a CD99
Scianna (013)	*SC* (*ERMAP*)	1p34.2	Erythroid membrane-associated protein (ERMAP)	Sc1, Sc2, Sc3, Rd, and 3 more [Sc:–1,–2,–3]

(Continued)

TABLE 9-1. Blood Group Systems (Continued)

ISBT System Name (Number)	Gene Name ISBT (HGNC)*	Chromosome Location	Gene Product and Component Name [CD number]	Associated Blood Group Antigens [Null phenotype]
Dombrock (014)	DO (ART4)	12p12.3	Do glycoprotein, ART 4 [CD297]	Do^a, Do^b, Gy^a, Hy, Jo^a, and 5 more [Gy(a–)]
Colton (015)	CO (AQP1)	7p14.3	Aquaporin 1 (AQP1)	Co^a, Co^b, Co3, Co4 [Co(a–b–)]
Landsteiner-Wiener (016)	LW (ICAM4)	19p13.2	LW glycoprotein, intracellular adhesion molecule 4 (ICAM4) [CD242]	LW^a, LW^{ab}, LW^b [LW(a–b–)]
Chido/Rodgers (017)	CH/RG (C4A, C4B)	6p21.32	Complement component: C4A, C4B	Ch1, Ch2, Rg1, and 6 more [Ch–Rg–]
H (018)	H (FUT1)	19q13.33	Fucosyltransferase, carbohydrate [CD173]	H [Bombay (O_h)]
Kx (019)	XK (XK)	Xp21.1	XK glycoprotein	Kx [McLeod phenotype]
Gerbich (020)	GE (GYPC)	2q14.3	Glycophorin C (GPC) [CD236] Glycophorin D (GPD)	Ge2, Ge3, Ge4, and 8 more [Leach phenotype]
Cromer (021)	CROM (CD55)	1q32.2	DAF [CD55]	Cr^a, Tc^a, Tc^b, Tc^c, Dr^a, Es^a, IFC, and 12 more [Inab phenotype]
Knops (022)	KN (CR1)	1q32.2	CR1 [CD35]	Kn^a, Kn^b, McC^a, Sl^a, Yk^a, and 4 more
Indian (023)	IN (CD44)	11p13	Hermes antigen [CD44]	In^a, In^b, and 3 more
Ok (024)	OK (BSG)	19p13.3	Neurothelin, basigin [CD147]	Ok^a, OKGV, OKGM
Raph (025)	RAPH (CD151)	11p15.5	CD151	MER2 [Raph–]
JMH (026)	JMH (SEMA7A)	15q24.1	Semaphorin 7A [CD108]	JMH and 5 more [JMH–]
I (027)	GCNT2 (IGNT)	6p24.2	Glucosaminyltransferase, carbohydrate	I [I– or i adult]
Globoside (028)	GLOB (B3GALNT1)	3q26.1	Transferase, carbohydrate (Gb_4, globoside)	P [P–]
Gill (029)	GIL (AQP3)	9p13.3	Aquaporin 3 (AQP3)	GIL [GIL–]

TABLE 9-1. Blood Group Systems (Continued)

ISBT System Name (Number)	Gene Name ISBT (HGNC)*	Chromosome Location	Gene Product and Component Name [CD number]	Associated Blood Group Antigens [Null phenotype]
Rh-associated glycoprotein (030)	*RHAG*	6p21.3	Rh-associated glycoprotein [CD241]	Duclos, Ol[a], DSLK[†], RHAG4 [Rh$_{null}$ (regulator type)][5]
FORS[10] (031)	*FORS (GBGT1)*	9q34.2	Globoside 3-α-N-acetylgalactosaminyl-transferase 1, Forssman glycolipid	FORS1
JR[11,12] (032)	*JR (ABCG2)*	4q22.1	Jr glycoprotein, ATP-binding cassette, subfamily G, member 2 (ABCG2) [CD338]	Jr[a] [Jr(a–)]
Lan[13] (033)	*LAN (ABCB6)*	2q36	Lan glycoprotein, ATP-binding cassette, subfamily B, member 6 (ABCB6)	Lan [Lan–]
Vel[14-16] (034)	*VEL (SMIM1)*	1p36	Small integral membrane protein 1 (SMIM1)	Vel [Vel–]
CD59[17] (035)	*CD59*	11p13.33	CD59	CD59.1 [CD59:–1]
Augustine[18] (036)	*ENT1 (SLC29A1)*	6p21.1	Equilibrative nucleoside transporter 1 (ENT1)	AUG1, At[a] (AUG2) [AUG:–1,–2]

*If the genetic information is obtained by blood group typing, the gene name is the italicized form of the of the blood group system ISBT name. For example, *SLC14A1* (HGNC terminology) would be written as *JK*A* and *JK*B* or *JK*01/02* (ISBT terminology).

†Provisionally numbered by the ISBT because of limited genetic evidence.

ISBT = International Society of Blood Transfusion; HGNC = Human Gene Nomenclature Committee; ATP = adenosine triphosphate.

shows the weakening of Kell antigens on red cells of the McLeod phenotype and demonstrates two red cell populations in carrier females. This mixed-cell population reflects the randomness of whether the maternal or paternal X chromosome is inactivated in any single somatic cell lineage.

Genotype and Phenotype

The **genotype** of a person is the complement of genes inherited from his or her parents; the term is frequently also used to refer to the set of alleles at a single gene locus. The **phenotype** is the observable expression of the genes inherited by a person and reflects the biologic activity of the gene(s). Thus, the presence or absence of antigens on the red cells, as determined by serologic testing, represents the phenotype. The presence or absence of antigens on the red cells predicted by DNA-based testing represents the genotype. Sometimes the genotype can be predicted from the

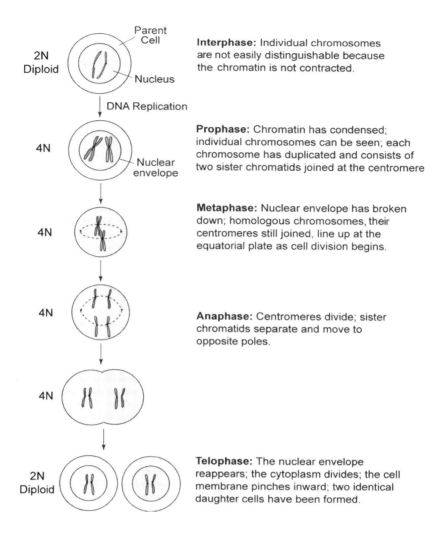

FIGURE 9-3. Diagram showing mitosis.

phenotype; for example, when a person's red cells are reactive with anti-Jk^a and anti-Jk^b, which is a Jk(a+b+) phenotype, a *JK*A/JK*B* genotype can be inferred. Frequently, the phenotype provides only a partial indication of the genotype; for example, red cells that are group B reflect the presence of a B gene, but the genotype may be *ABO*B/B* or *ABO*B/O*. For decades, family studies were often the only way to determine a person's genotype, but now that most antigens and phenotypes can be defined at the DNA level, family studies to determine genotype can be mostly replaced by DNA analysis. (See "Blood Group Genomics" section below.)

Alleles

A gene at a given locus on a chromosome may exist in more than one form; that is, it may be allelic. Each person has two alleles for a trait, one that is maternally derived and another that is paternally derived. At the simplest level, and for the purpose of explaining the concept, the ABO gene locus can be considered to have three alleles: *A*, *B*, and *O* (although genotyping has revealed many variant alleles). With three alleles, there are six possible genotypes (*A/A*, *A/O*, *A/B*, *B/B*, *B/O*, and *O/O*). Depending on the parental contribution, a person could inherit any combination of two of the alleles and

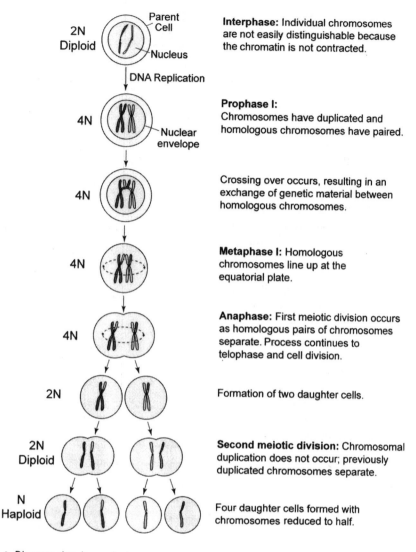

Interphase: Individual chromosomes are not easily distinguishable because the chromatin is not contracted.

DNA Replication

Prophase I: Chromosomes have duplicated and homologous chromosomes have paired.

Crossing over occurs, resulting in an exchange of genetic material between homologous chromosomes.

Metaphase I: Homologous chromosomes line up at the equatorial plate.

Anaphase: First meiotic division occurs as homologous pairs of chromosomes separate. Process continues to telophase and cell division.

Formation of two daughter cells.

Second meiotic division: Chromosomal duplication does not occur; previously duplicated chromosomes separate.

Four daughter cells formed with chromosomes reduced to half.

2N Diploid — Parent Cell — Nucleus — Nuclear envelope — 4N — 2N — N Haploid

FIGURE 9-4. Diagram showing meiosis.

express the corresponding antigens on their red cells. For example, inheritance of *A/A* and *A/O* would result in group A red cells, *A/B* would result in group AB red cells, *B/B* and *B/O* would result in group B red cells, and *O/O* would result in group O red cells.

When identical alleles for a given locus are present on both chromosomes, the person is said to be **homozygous** for the particular allele. A person who is **hemizygous** for an allele has only a single copy of an allele instead of the customary two copies; an example is the deletion of one *RHD* in a D+ phenotype. When different (ie, not identical) alleles are present at a particular locus, the person is said to be **heterozygous**. For example, a person who is homozygous at the *KEL* locus for the allele (*KEL*02*) encoding the k antigen will have K–k+ red cells. A person who is heterozygous for *KEL*01* and *KEL*02* (*KEL*01/02* genotype), would have red cells that are K+k+.

Antigens that are encoded by alleles at the same locus are said to be **antithetical** (meaning "opposite"); thus, K and k are a pair of antithetical antigens. It is incorrect to refer to red cells that are, for example, K–k+ or Kp(a–b+) as being homozygous for the k or Kp^b antigen; rather, it should be said that the cells have a double dose of the antigen and that they are from a person who is homozygous for the allele. Genes are allelic whereas antigens are antithetical.

The quantity of antigen expressed (antigen density) is influenced by whether a person is heterozygous or homozygous for an allele; the antigen density is generally greater when a person is homozygous. In some blood group systems, this difference in antigen density is manifested by antibodies giving stronger reactions with cells that have a double dose of the antigen. Red cells with the Jk(a+b−) phenotype, encoded by a *JK*A/A* genotype, have a double dose of the Jk^a antigen and often are more strongly reactive with anti-Jk^a than those that are Jk(a+b+) and have a single dose of the antigen. Similarly, M+N− red cells tend to be more strongly reactive with anti-M than are M+N+ red cells. Antibodies that are weakly reactive may not be detected if they are tested with red cells expressing a single dose of the antigen. This observable difference in strength of reaction, based on homozygosity or heterozygosity for an allele, is termed "the **dosage effect**."

Polymorphism

For blood group genetics, **polymorphism** refers to the occurrence in the population of genomes with allelic variation (two or more alleles at one locus) producing different phenotypes, each with appreciable (>1%) frequency. Some blood group systems (Rh and MNS, for example) are highly polymorphic and have many more alleles at a given locus than other systems such as Duffy and Colton.[5] An allele that is polymorphic in one population is not necessarily polymorphic in all populations; for example, the FY allele associated with silencing of Fy^b in red cells (*FY*02N.01*) is polymorphic in populations of African ethnicity, with a prevalence of >70%, but this allele is not found in other populations. A gene polymorphism may represent an evolutionary advantage for a population, and a polymorphic population is likely to adapt to evolutionary

change more rapidly than if the population had genetic uniformity. It is not yet understood what, if any, evolutionary advantages were derived from the extensive polymorphism displayed by red cell antigens, but many publications associate resistance to, or susceptibility for, a particular disease with a particular blood type.[24]

The difference between two alleles is the result of a permanent change in the DNA. An event that leads to the production of an altered gene and a new allele or polymorphism that did not exist in the biologic parents is referred to as a **mutation**. The mutation rate of expressed genes resulting *in a new phenotype* has been estimated to be <10^{-5} (<1 in 100,000) in humans, and a mutation has to occur in the germ cells (gametes) to be inherited.

A mutation can occur spontaneously or be brought about by agents such as radiation (eg, ultraviolet rays or x-rays) or chemicals. A mutation may occur within a gene or in the intergenic regions. It may be **silent**—that is, have no effect on the encoded protein—or it may alter the gene product and potentially cause an observable effect in the phenotype. In the context of an allele that encodes a protein that carries red cell antigens, any genetically induced change must be recognized by a specific antibody before an allele can be said to encode a new antigen.

Numerous genetic events that generate red cell antigens and phenotypes have been identified. The event can occur at the level of the chromosome (eg, deletion or translocation of part of a chromosome), the gene (eg, deletion, conversion, or rearrangement), the exon (eg, deletion or duplication), or the nucleotide (eg, deletion, substitution, or insertion). The mechanism that has given rise to most diversity in the human genome is single nucleotide polymorphism (SNP)—that is, a single nucleotide change in the DNA.[25-27] Accordingly, the majority of polymorphic blood group antigens are the result of SNPs.[3,28,29] DNA analysis to predict the red cell phenotype is discussed in more detail in the section on "Blood Group Genomics."

INHERITANCE OF GENETIC TRAITS

A genetic trait is the observed expression of one or more genes. The inheritance of a trait (and red cell antigens) is determined by whether the gene responsible is located on an autosome or on the X chromosome (sex-linked) and whether the trait is dominant or recessive.

Pedigrees

A family study follows the inheritance of a genetic characteristic—for example, an allele encoding the expression of a red cell antigen—as it is transmitted through a kinship. A diagram that depicts the relationship of family members and shows which family members express (are **affected**), or do not express, the trait under study is termed a **pedigree**. A review of a pedigree should reveal the pattern or type of inheritance for the trait, or antigen, of interest. The person who first caused the family to be investigated is considered the index case and is often referred to as the **proband** or **propositus/proposita** (male singular form or gender unknown/female singular form); propositi is the plural form regardless of gender. Details of the conventions and the symbols used for the construction of pedigrees are provided in Figs 9-5 and 9-6.

Autosomal Dominant Inheritance

An antigen (or any trait) that is inherited in an **autosomal dominant** manner is always expressed when the relevant allele is present, regardless of whether a person is homozygous or heterozygous for the allele. The antigen appears in every generation and occurs with equal frequency in both males and females. A person who carries an autosomal dominant trait transmits it, on average, to half of his or her children. The pedigree in Fig 9-7 demonstrates autosomal dominant inheritance and shows that the B allele is dominant over *O*.

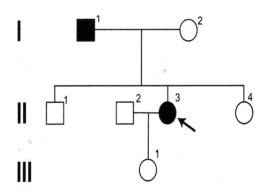

FIGURE 9-5. An example of a pedigree. Males are denoted by squares and females by circles, and each different generation in a pedigree is identified by Roman numerals. Persons in each generation are identified by Arabic numbers; the numbering is sequential from left to right, with the eldest child for each family unit being placed on the left of any series of siblings. Closed symbols represent family members affected by the trait, whereas open symbols are unaffected members.

Autosomal Codominant Inheritance

Blood group antigens that appear to be autosomal dominant may be encoded by alleles that are inherited in a **codominant** manner—that is, when two different alleles are present (the heterozygous condition), the products of both alleles are expressed. Thus, when red cells have the S+s+ phenotype, the presence of one allele encoding S and another allele encoding s [or an *S/s* (*GYPB*S/s*) genotype] can be inferred.

Autosomal Recessive Inheritance

A trait with autosomal recessive inheritance is expressed only in a person who is homozygous for the allele and has inherited the recessive allele from both parents. When a person inherits a single copy of a recessive allele in combination with a silent or deleted (null) allele—that is, a nonfunctioning allele or one that encodes a product that cannot be detected—the recessive trait is expressed and the person appears to be homozygous. It is difficult or impossible to distinguish such a combination from

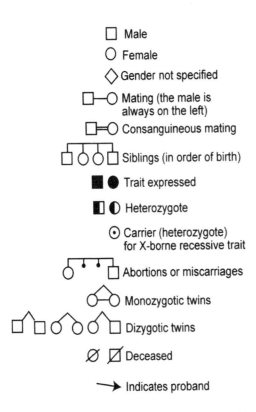

FIGURE 9-6. Symbols, and their significance, used in the construction of pedigrees.

homozygosity for the recessive allele through serologic testing, but DNA-based testing can usually make this distinction.

A mating between two heterozygous carriers results in one chance in four that the children will be homozygous for the trait. The parents of a child who is homozygous for a recessive trait must be obligate carriers of the trait. If the frequency of the recessive allele is low, the condition is rare and usually found only among **siblings** (brothers and sisters) of the person and not in other relatives. The condition is not found in preceding or successive generations unless **consanguineous** mating (ie, between blood relatives) occurs. When a recessive allele is rare, the parents of an affected person are most likely consanguineous because a rare allele is more likely to occur in blood relatives than in unrelated persons in a random population. When a recessive trait is one that is common, consanguinity is not a prerequisite for homozygosity; for example, the O allele of the ABO system, although recessive, is not rare, and persons who are homozygous for O are easily found in the random population.

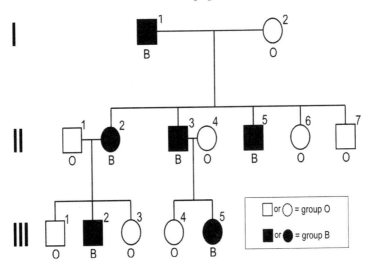

FIGURE 9-7. Autosomal dominant inheritance of the ABO alleles. Based on the ABO groups of his children, I-1 would be expected to have a *B/O* rather than a *B/B* genotype (showing that the B allele is dominant over *O*) because two of his children (II-6 and II-7) are group O and must have inherited an O allele from their father (I-1) in addition to the O allele inherited from their mother (I-2). Similarly, II-2 and II-3 are *B/O*, based on the ABO type of their children, showing the dominance of *B* over *O*.

In blood group genetics, a recessive trait or condition almost always means that red cells express a null phenotype [eg, the Lu(a–b–) or Rh$_{null}$ or O phenotypes] because of homozygosity for a **silent** or **amorphic gene** that either results in no product or encodes a defective product. The family in Fig 9-8 demonstrates the inheritance of a recessive silent LU gene, which in the homozygous state results in the Lu(a–b–) phenotype. The proband, II-3, who was multitransfused, was identified because of the presence of anti-Lu3 (an antibody to a high-prevalence Lutheran antigen) in his plasma. Because his Lu(a–b–) phenotype is the result of recessive inheritance, any potential donors in the family can be found by testing his siblings. About 25%, or one in four of the offspring of the mating between I-1 and I-2, is expected to have the Lu(a–b–) phenotype; in this case, only the proband has Lu(a–b–) red cells.

Sex-Linked Inheritance

A **sex-linked** trait is one that is encoded by a gene located on the X or Y chromosome. The Y chromosome carries few functional genes, and discussion of sex-linked inheritance generally is synonymous with inheritance of X-borne genes. In females (who have two X chromosomes) the inheritance of X-borne genes, like the inheritance of genes carried on the autosomes, can be dominant or recessive. Males, in contrast, have one X chromosome (always maternally derived) and one Y chromosome (always paternally derived) and are hemizygous for genes on the X or Y chromosome because only one chromosome (and thus one copy of a gene) is present. Most X-borne genes do not have a **homolog** (a similar sequence of DNA) on the Y chromosome. As a consequence, inheritance of an X-borne dominant trait is the same in males and females. However, an X-borne trait that is recessive in females is

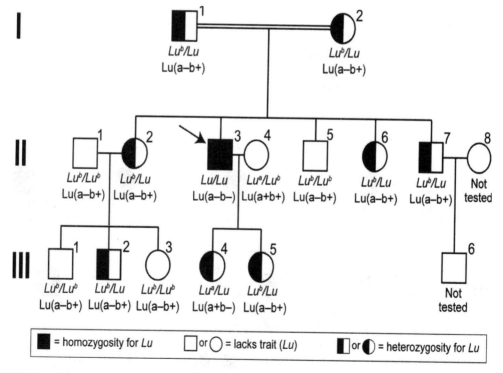

FIGURE 9-8. Autosomal recessive inheritance. The offspring of II-3, the Lu(a–b–) proband, and II-4, his Lu(a+b+) wife, demonstrate that *Lu* (depicting a Lutheran null allele, or *LU*02N*) is recessive to *Lu^a* (*LU*A*) and *Lu^b* (*LU*B*) and that the presence of the silenced Lutheran allele is masked by the product of *Lu^a* (*LU*A*) or *Lu^b* (*LU*B*) at the phenotype level.

expressed by all males who carry the gene for the trait. The most striking feature of both dominant and recessive X-linked inheritance is that there is no male-to-male transmission; that is, the trait is never transmitted from father to son.

Sex-Linked Dominant Inheritance

A trait encoded by an X-borne allele that has **sex-linked dominant** inheritance is expressed by hemizygous males and by both heterozygous and homozygous females. A male passes his single X chromosome to all of his daughters and all daughters will express the condition or trait. When a female is heterozygous for an allele that encodes a dominant trait, each of her children, whether male or female, has a 50% chance of inheriting the trait. When a female is homozygous for an X-borne allele with dominant inheritance, the encoded trait is expressed by all her children.

The Xg^a antigen (Xg blood group system) is encoded by an allele on the X chromosome and is inherited in a sex-linked dominant manner. The first indication that the Xg^a antigen is X-borne came from the observation that the prevalence of the Xg(a–) and Xg(a+) phenotypes differed noticeably between males and females; the Xg^a antigen has a prevalence of 89% in females and only 66% in males.[5]

Figure 9-9 shows the inheritance of the Xg^a antigen in a three-generation family. In generation I, the father (I-1) is Xg(a+) and has transmitted Xg^a to all his daughters but to none of his sons. His eldest daughter (II-2), for example, must be heterozygous for Xg^a/Xg; she received the allele encoding the Xg^a antigen from her Xg(a+) father and a silent allele, Xg, from her Xg(a–) mother. II-2 has transmitted Xg^a to half her children, regardless of whether they are sons or daughters.

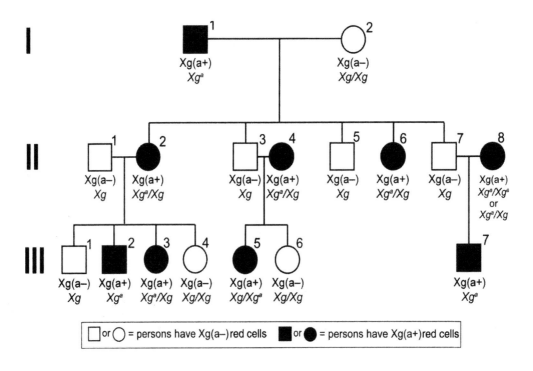

FIGURE 9-9. Sex-linked dominant inheritance. The Xg^a antigen is encoded by an allele on the tip of the short arm of the X chromosome. This family demonstrates the sex-linked dominant inheritance of the Xg^a antigen.

Sex-Linked Recessive Inheritance

A trait encoded by an **X-borne recessive** allele is carried, but not expressed, by a heterozygous female. A male inherits the trait from his mother, who is usually a carrier (or could be homozygous for the trait if she is the offspring of a male who expresses the trait and a carrier female). An affected male transmits the trait to all of his daughters, who in turn transmit the trait to approximately half of their sons. Therefore, the prevalence of the expression of an X-borne recessive trait is much higher in males than in females. A carrier female who mates with a male lacking the trait transmits the trait to one-half of her daughters (who will also be carriers) and to one-half of her sons (who will be affected). If mating is between an affected male and a female who lacks the trait, all of the sons will lack the trait and all of the daughters will be carriers. If an X-borne recessive trait is rare in the population, the trait is expressed almost exclusively in males.

The XK gene encodes the Kx protein and demonstrates X-borne recessive inheritance. Mutations in *XK* result in red cells with the McLeod phenotype; such red cells lack Kx and have reduced expression of Kell antigens (McLeod syndrome). McLeod syndrome is associated with late-onset clinical or subclinical myopathy, neurodegeneration, and central nervous system manifestations, as well as with acanthocytosis and, frequently, compensated hemolytic anemia. More than 30 different *XK* gene mutations associated with a McLeod phenotype have been found. Different *XK* mutations appear to have different clinical effects and may account for the variability in the prognosis.[30] Sequencing of *XK* to determine the specific type of mutation in individuals with McLeod phenotypes has clinical prognostic value. McLeod syndrome is an X-linked recessive condition and, as demonstrated by the family in Fig 9-10, is found only in males.

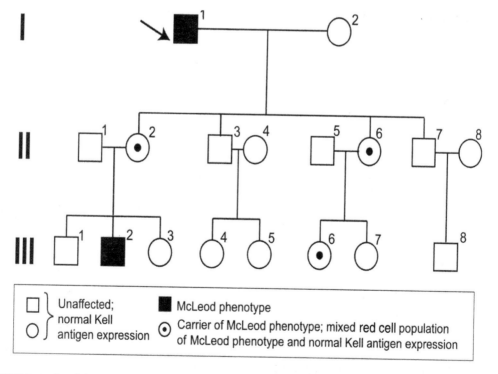

FIGURE 9-10. Sex-linked recessive inheritance. This family demonstrates that a sex-linked trait that is recessive in females will be expressed by any male who inherits the trait. Homozygosity for such a trait is required for it to be expressed in females. The trait skips one generation and is carried through females.

The Principles of Independent Segregation and Independent Assortment

The passing of a trait from one generation to the next follows certain patterns or principles. The principle of **independent segregation** refers to the separation of homologous chromosomes and their random distribution to the gametes during meiosis. Only one member of an allelic pair is passed on to the next generation, and each gamete has an equal probability of receiving either member of a parental homologous allelic pair; these chromosomes are randomly united at fertilization and thus segregate independently from one generation to the next. The family in Fig 9-11 demonstrates the independent segregation of the ABO alleles on chromosome 9.

The principle of **independent assortment** states that alleles determining various traits are inherited independently from each other. In other words, the inheritance of one allele (eg, a B allele, on chromosome 9, encoding B antigens) does not influence the inheritance of another allele (eg, an M allele, on chromosome 4, encoding M antigens). This is demonstrated by the family in Fig 9-11.

Linkage and Crossing Over

Linkage is the physical association between two genes that are located on the same chromosome and are inherited together. Examples include *RHD* and *RHCE* encoding the antigens of the Rh system, which are both on chromosome 1 and represent linked loci that do not assort independently.

Crossing over is the exchange of genetic material between homologous chromosome pairs (Fig 9-4). In this process, a segment from one chromatid (and any associated genes) changes places with the corresponding part of the other chromatid (and its associated genes); the segments are rejoined, and some genes will have switched chromosomes. Thus, crossing over is a means to shuffle genetic material. Because crossing over can result in new gene combinations on the chromosomes involved, it is also referred to as **recombination**, and the

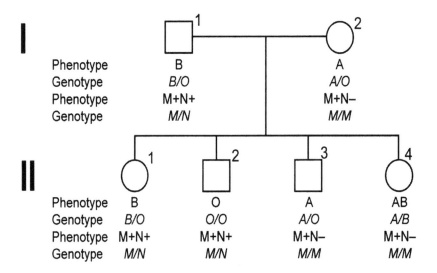

FIGURE 9-11. Independent segregation and independent assortment are illustrated by the inheritance of blood group alleles in one family. Parental ABO alleles were randomly transmitted (independent segregation), and each child has inherited a different combination. The family also illustrates that the alleles encoding antigens of the ABO and MNS blood group systems are inherited independently from each other.

rearranged chromosomes can be referred to as **recombinants**. Crossing over and recombination, using chromosome 1 as an example, are explained in Fig 9-12.

Two gene loci carried by the same chromosome that are not closely linked are referred to as being **syntenic**. For example, the loci for *RH* and *FY*, both located on chromosome 1, are syntenic because the distance between them (*RH* on the short arm and *FY* on the long arm) is great enough for them to undergo crossing over and to assort independently.

The frequency of crossing over involving two genes on the same chromosome is a measure of the distance [measured in centimorgans (cM)] between them; the greater the distance between two loci, the greater the probability that crossing over (and recombination) will occur. In contrast, genes located very close together (linked) tend to be transmitted together with no recombination. The degree of crossing over between two genes can be calculated by analyzing pedigrees of families informative for the genes of interest and observing the extent of recombination. The traditional method of linkage analysis requires the use of lod (logarithm of the odds) scores.[31] Linkage analysis was the basis through which chromosomes were mapped and the relative position and distance between genes established. Linkage between Lutheran (*LU*) and ABH secretion (*SE* or *FUT2*) was the first recognized example

of autosomal linkage in humans and is explained in Fig 9-13.

Although crossing over occurs readily between distant genes, rare examples of recombination have been documented for genes that are very closely linked or adjacent on a chromosome. Such genes include those encoding the MN (*GYPA*) and Ss (*GYPB*) antigens on chromosome 4 and are reviewed by Daniels.[20(pp96-142)]

Linkage Disequilibrium

Genes at closely linked loci tend to be inherited together and constitute a **haplotype** (a combination of alleles at two or more closely linked loci on the same chromosome). The alleles encoding the MNS antigens are inherited as four haplotypes: *MS*, *Ms*, *NS*, or *Ns* (in the ISBT allele terminology these haplotypes would be written as *GYPA*M-GYPB*S*, *GYPA*M-GYPB*s*, *GYPA*N-GYPB*S*, or *GYPA*N-GYPB*s*, respectively). Because linked genes do not assort independently, the antigens encoded by each of these haplotypes have a different prevalence in the population than would be expected by random assortment. If *M* and *S* were not linked, the expected prevalence for M+ and S+ in the population would be 17% (from frequency calculations), whereas the actual or observed prevalence (obtained from testing and analyzing families) of the *MS* haplotype is 24%.[20(pp96-142)] This constitutes **linkage disequilibrium**, which is the tendency

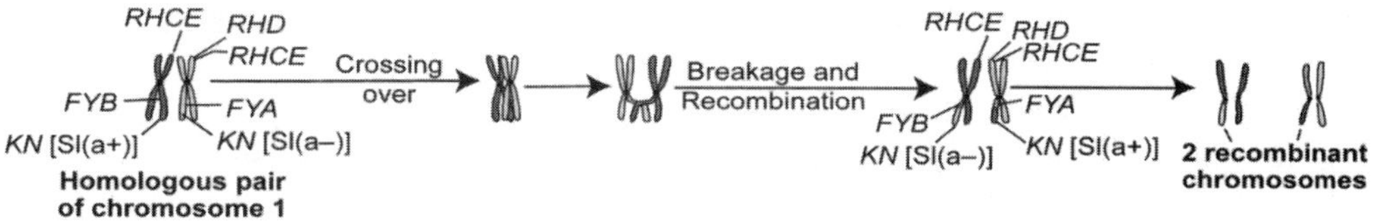

FIGURE 9-12. Crossing over and recombination. In the diagram, chromosome 1 is used as an example. The very closely linked RH genes, *RHD* and *RHCE,* are located near the tip of the short arm of chromosome 1. The loci for *FY* and *KN* are on the long arm of the chromosome and are not linked. During meiosis, crossing over occurs between this homologous chromosome pair, and portions of chromosome break and become rejoined to the partner chromosome. Crossing over of the long arm of chromosome 1 results in recombination between the loci for *FY* and *KN* such that the gene encoding Fy[b] antigen is now traveling with a gene that encodes the Sl(a−) phenotype of the Knops system.

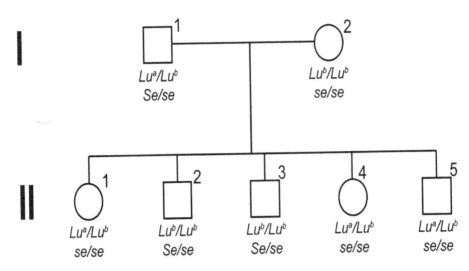

FIGURE 9-13. Linkage between *LU* and *SE* (*FUT2*). I-2 is homozygous for *Lu^b* (*LU**B) and *se* and must transmit these alleles to all her offspring. I-1 is doubly heterozygous [*Lu^a/Lu^b* (*LU***A/B*) and *Se/se*]. He has transmitted *Lu^b* (*LU**B) with *Se*, and *Lu^a* (*LU**A) with *se*, showing linkage between *LU* and *Se* (*FUT2*). Several such informative families would need to be analyzed to statistically confirm linkage.

of specific combinations of alleles at two or more linked loci to be inherited together more frequently than would be expected by chance.

Gene Interaction and Position Effect

Alleles that are carried on the same chromosome are referred to as being in *cis* position, whereas those on opposite chromosomes of a homologous pair are in *trans* position. Alleles that are in *cis* and linked are always inherited together on the same chromosome, whereas genes in *trans* segregate independently.

Historically, the Rh blood group system was used to explain the meaning of *cis* and *trans*. For example, the *DCe/DcE* genotype was described as having C and e alleles in *cis* in the *DCe* haplotype, with c and E alleles in *cis* in the partner *DcE* haplotype, whereas *C* and *E* and also *c* and *e* are in opposing haplotypes and are in *trans*. In this alignment, *C* and *e*, for example, are always inherited together, but *C* and *E* are not. The preceding explanation, which implies that one gene encodes C and c antigens while another linked gene encodes E and e antigens, was based on the Fisher-Race theory of three genes at the *RH* locus. In contrast, genomic analysis indicates that only one gene (*RHCE*), with four alleles (*RHCE**Ce, *RHCE**cE, *RHCE**ce, and *RHCE**CE), encodes one protein that carries the CcEe antigens. Thus, for Rh, *DCe* is an example of a haplotype, and the RHD allele is in *cis* to the RHCE*Ce allele.

The expression of red cell antigens may be modified or affected by gene or protein interactions that manifest primarily as reduced antigen expression. One example in which the haplotype on one chromosome affects the expression of the haplotype on the paired chromosome is commonly referred to as the **position effect** and can be observed with Rh antigen expression. When a *Ce* haplotype (note the absence of *RHD*) is in *trans* to a D antigen-encoding haplotype, the expression of D is dramatically reduced and a weak D phenotype can result. When the same D-encoding haplotype is inherited with either *ce* or *cE*, D antigen is normally expressed. The cause of this reduced antigen expression is not known, but it may involve differences in gene expression levels or altered assembly of proteins in the membrane. In the presence of the Kell system antigen Kp^a, expression of other Kell system antigens encoded by the same allele is suppressed to varying degrees (*cis*-modifier effect). This is best observed in persons who have a silenced K_0 (a Kell$_{null}$ gene) in *trans*. The amino acid change that results in the expression of Kp^a adversely affects trafficking of the Kell glycoprotein to the red cell surface, so that the quantity of Kp^a-carrying Kell glycoprotein that reaches the red cell surface is greatly reduced.

Suppressor or modifier genes affect the expression of another gene, or genes. For example, *KLF1*, located on chromosome 19p13.3-p13.12, encodes erythroid Krüppel-like factor, which is a transcription factor essential for terminal differentiation of red cells. Singleton et al[32] first discovered that heterozygosity for nucleotide changes in *KLF1* is responsible for the dominant Lu(a–b–) phenotype,[5] which is also known as the In(Lu) phenotype. This heterozygosity is characterized by reduced expression of antigens in the Lutheran system (Lu$_{mod}$) and for P1, In^b, and AnWj antigens.

In kind, the transcription factor GATA-1, encoded by the X-borne GATA-1 gene, is essential for erythroid and megakaryocyte differentiation. Changes in this gene were associated with the X-linked type of Lu$_{mod}$ that initially presented as a Lu(a–b–) phenotype.[33] Serologic differentiation of these Lu$_{mod}$ phenotypes from the true Lu(a–b–) (Lu$_{null}$) phenotype can be challenging, yet has clinical value. Now that the genetic basis of these phenotypes is understood, sequencing of the relevant genes can be used to make the distinction.

In the past, independent, unidentified modifier or regulator genes were postulated to be the basis of several null or variant phenotypes when a silent or inactive (nonfunctioning) gene was not evident. For example, the regulator type (as opposed to the amorph type) of Rh$_{null}$ was shown through family studies to result from a gene not at the *RH* locus. This phenotype is now known to result from various silencing changes in *RHAG*, a gene located on chromosome 6 (and thus independent of *RH*). *RHAG* encodes the Rh-associated glycoprotein RhAG, which is required in the red cell membrane for Rh antigen expression. Similarly, genomic analysis indicates that the modifying gene that causes the Rh$_{mod}$ phenotype is a mutated *RHAG*.[5]

Several red cell antigens require the interaction of the products of two or more independent genes for their expression. The high-prevalence antigen Wr^b of the Diego blood group system requires GPA (or more precisely, amino acids 75 to 99 of GPA), which carries MN antigens, to be present in the red cell membrane for Wr^b expression. The Wr^a/Wr^b polymorphism is encoded by *DI* and carried on band 3, whereas GPA is the product of *GYPA*, a gene that is independent of *DI*. An absence of RhD and RhCE protein (Rh$_{null}$) results in red cells that lack LW antigens and lack or have reduced expression of U and S or s antigens, again demonstrating the interaction in the membrane of the products of two or more independent blood group genes.

The sequential interaction of genes at several loci is required for the expression of ABO, H, Lewis, and I antigens on red cells and in secretions. These antigens are carbohydrate determinants carried on glycoproteins or glycolipids, and the genetics of these antigens is more complex than that of protein-based antigens. The carbohydrate antigens are carried on oligosaccharide chains that are assembled by the stepwise addition of monosaccharides. ABO genes and the genes encoding the other carbohydrate-based antigens do not encode membrane proteins but do encode an enzyme, a glycosyltransferase, that catalyzes the sequential transfer of the appropriate immunodominant monosaccharide. Each monosaccharide structure is transferred by a separate glycosyltransferase, such that two genes are required for a disaccharide, three for a trisaccharide, and so on. An inactivating change at one locus can prevent or modify the expression of the other gene products. The product encoded by the H gene is the biosynthetic precursor for A and B antigen production; if the H gene is silenced, A or B antigens cannot be produced. A mutated A or B allele may result in a glycosyltransferase that is inactive or that causes more or less antigen to be expressed. Details on the biosynthesis of the ABO, H, Lewis, and I antigens may be found in Chapter 10.

POPULATION GENETICS

Population genetics is the study of the distribution patterns of genes and of the factors that maintain or change gene (or allele) frequencies. A basic understanding of population genetics, probability, and the application of simple algebraic calculations is important for relationship (identity) testing. In transfusion medicine, the knowledge can be applied to clinical situations such as predicting the likelihood of finding compatible blood for a patient who has made antibody(ies) to red cell antigens. It may be helpful to define three commonly used words so that their appropriate use is understood. **Frequency** is used to describe prevalence at the genetic level—that is, the occurrence of an allele (gene) in a population. **Prevalence** is used to describe the occurrence of a permanent inherited characteristic at the phenotypic level—for example, a blood group—in any given population. **Incidence** is used when describing the rate of occurrence in a population of a condition that changes over time, such as a disease.

Phenotype Prevalence

The prevalence of a blood group antigen or phenotype is determined by testing red cells from a large random sample of people of the same race or ethnicity with a specific antibody and calculating the percentage of positive and negative reactions. The larger the cohort being tested, the more statistically significant is the result. The sum of the percentages for the prevalence of the phenotypes should equal 100%. For example, in the Duffy blood group system, the prevalence in a random population of African ethnicity for the Fy(a+b–), Fy(a–b+), Fy(a+b+), and Fy(a–b–) phenotypes is 9%, 22%, 1%, and 68%, respectively; together, these percentages total 100%. If the red cells from 1000 donors of European ethnicity are tested with anti-c, and 800 of the samples are positive and 200 are negative for the Rh antigen c, the prevalence of the c+ phenotype is 80% and that of the c– phenotype is 20%. Thus, in this donor population, approximately 20% of ABO-compatible units of blood, or 1 in 5, should be compatible with serum from a patient who has made anti-c.

Calculations for Antigen-Negative Phenotypes

When blood is provided for a patient with antibodies directed at one or more red cell antigens, a simple calculation can be used to estimate the number of units that need to be tested to find the desired antigen combination. To calculate the prevalence of the combined antigen-negative phenotype, the prevalence of each of the individual antigens are multiplied together because the antigens are inherited independently of each other. An exception occurs when the antigens are encoded by alleles that are closely linked and are inherited as haplotypes (M, N, S, s) or reside on the same carrier protein (C, c, E, e). If a patient with antibodies to K, S, and Jk^a antigens requires 3 units of blood, for example, the prevalence of the antigen-negative phenotype and the number of units that need to be tested to find it can be calculated as follows:

- The prevalence of: K– donors = 91%; S– donors = 48%; Jk(a–) donors = 23%.
- The percentage of donors negative for each antigen is expressed as a decimal and multiplied: 0.91(K–) × 0.48(S–) × 0.23[Jk(a–)] = 0.10.
- 0.10 expressed as a % = 0.10 × 100% = 10%.
- 10% expressed as occurrence = 10/100 = 1/10.
- Thus, approximately 1 in 10 ABO-compatible Red Blood Cell (RBC) units are expected to be K– S– Jk(a–).
- The patient in question requires 3 units, so on average, 30 units would need to be tested.

The prevalence of a particular antigen (or phenotype) can vary with race,[5] and the prevalence for a combined antigen-negative phenotype calculation should be selected on the basis of the predominant race found in the donor population.

Allele (Gene) Frequency

The allele frequency is the proportion of one allele relative to all alleles at a particular gene locus in a given population at a given time. This frequency can be calculated from the prevalence of each phenotype observed in a population. The sum of allele frequencies at any given locus must equal 100% (or 1 in an algebraic calculation) in the population sample tested. The genotype frequency is the number of individuals with a given genotype divided by the total number of individuals sampled in a population.

The Hardy-Weinberg Equilibrium

Gene frequencies tend to remain constant from generation to generation in any relatively large population unless they are influenced by factors such as selection, mutation, migration, or nonrandom mating, any of which would have to be rampant to have a discernible effect. According to the principles proposed by the British mathematician Hardy and the German physician Weinberg, gene frequencies reach equilibrium. This equilibrium can be expressed in algebraic terms by the Hardy-Weinberg formula or equation:

$$p^2 + 2pq + q^2 = 1$$

If two alleles, classically referred to as A and a, have gene frequencies of p and q, the homozygotes and heterozygotes are present in the population in the following proportions:

$$AA = p^2; Aa = 2pq; aa = q^2$$

In such a two-allele system, if the gene frequency for one allele, say p, is known, q can be calculated by $p + q = 1$.

The Hardy-Weinberg equation permits the estimation of genotype frequencies from the phenotype prevalence in a sampled population and, reciprocally, allows the determination of genotype frequency and phenotype prevalence from the gene frequency. The equation has a number of applications in blood group genetics, and its use is demon-

strated below. In a population of European ethnicity, the frequencies of the two alleles encoding K (*KEL*01*) or k (*KEL*02*) can be determined as follows:

Frequency of the KEL*01 allele = p
    Frequency of the KEL*02 allele = q

Frequency of the *KEL*01* genotype = p^2
    Frequency of the *KEL*01/02* genotype = 2pq
    Frequency of the *KEL*02/02* genotype = q^2

The K antigen is expressed on the red cells of 9% of people of European ethnicity; therefore:

$p^2 + 2pq$ = the frequency of people who carry *KEL*01* and are K+

Thus, $p^2 + 2pq = 0.09$

$q^2 = 1 - (p^2 + 2pq)$ = the frequency of people who carry *KEL*02/02* and are K–

$q^2 = 1 - 0.09$

$q^2 = \sqrt{0.91}$

$q = 0.91$

$q = 0.95$ = the frequency of *KEL*02*

Because the sum of the frequencies of both alleles must equal 1.00:

$p + q = 1$

$p = 1 - q$

$p = 1 - 0.95$

$p = 0.05$ = the frequency of *KEL*01*

Having calculated the allele frequencies for *KEL*01* and *KEL*02*, it is possible to calculate the percentage of k+ (both K+k+ and K–k+) and K+ (both K+k– and K+k+) people:

Prevalence of k+   = $2pq + q^2$
         = $2(0.05 \times 0.95) + (0.95)^2$
         = 0.9975×100
         = a calculated prevalence of 99.75% (the observed prevalence of the k+ phenotype is 99.8%)

Prevalence of K+
$$= 2pq + p^2$$
$$= 2(0.05 \times 0.95) + (0.05)^2 = 0.0975$$
$$= 0.0975 \times 100 = \text{a calculated prevalence for K+ of 9.75\% (the observed prevalence of the K+ phenotype is 9\%)}$$

The Hardy-Weinberg equation also can be applied to calculate the frequencies of the three possible genotypes $KEL*01/01$, $KEL*01/02$, and $KEL*02/02$ from the gene frequencies $KEL*01$ (p) = 0.05 and $KEL*02$ (q) = 0.95:

$$p^2 + 2pq + q^2 = 1$$

Frequency of $KEL*01/01 = p^2 = 0.0025$

Frequency of $KEL*01/02 = 2pq = 0.095$

Frequency of $KEL*02/02 = q^2 = 0.9025$

If antibodies are available to test for the products of the alleles of interest (in this example, anti-K and anti-k), the allele frequencies also can be obtained by direct counting as demonstrated in Table 9-2. The allele frequencies obtained by direct testing are the **observed frequencies** for the population being sampled, whereas those obtained by gene frequency calculations (above) are the **expected frequencies**. The various calculations above,

when applied to a two-allele situation, are relatively simple; the calculations for three or more alleles are much more complex and beyond the scope of this chapter.

For a given population, if the prevalence of one genetic trait, such as a red cell antigen, is known, the Hardy-Weinberg equation can be applied to calculate allele and genotype frequencies. The Hardy-Weinberg equilibrium principle is valid when the population is sufficiently large that chance alone cannot alter an allele frequency and when the mating is random. A selective advantage or disadvantage of a particular trait and other influencing factors, such as mutation or migration in or out of the population, are assumed to be absent when the Hardy-Weinberg equilibrium principle is applied. When all of these conditions are met, the gene pool is in equilibrium and allele frequencies do not change from one generation to the next. If the conditions are not met, changes in allele frequencies may occur over a few generations and may explain many of the differences in allele frequencies between populations.

RELATIONSHIP TESTING

Polymorphisms are inherited characteristics or genetic markers that can distinguish between people. The blood groups with the

TABLE 9-2. Allele Frequencies of K $(KEL*01)$ and k $(KEL*02)$ Calculated Using Direct Counting (assuming the absence of null alleles)

Phenotype	No. of Persons	No. of Kk Alleles	K ($KEL*01$)	k ($KEL*02$)
K+k−	2	4	4	0
K+k+	88	176	88	88
K−k+	910	1820	0	1820
Totals	1000	2000	92	1908
Allele frequency			0.046	0.954

A random sample of 1000 people tested for K and k antigens has a total of 2000 alleles at the *KEL* locus because each person inherits two alleles, one from each parent. Therefore, the two persons with a K+k− phenotype (each with two alleles) contribute a total of four alleles. To this are added 88 K ($KEL*01$) alleles from the K+k+ group, for a total of 92 K ($KEL*01$) alleles or an allele frequency of 0.046 (92 ÷ 2000). The frequency of the k ($KEL*02$) allele is 0.954 (1908 ÷ 2000).

greatest number of alleles (greatest polymorphism) have the highest power of discrimination and are the most useful for determining relationships. Blood is a rich source of inherited characteristics that can be detected, including red cell, HLA, and platelet antigens. Red cell and HLA antigens are easily identifiable, are polymorphic, and follow Mendelian laws of inheritance. The greater the polymorphism of a system, the less chance there is of finding two people who are identical. The extensive polymorphism of the HLA system alone allows the exclusion of >90% of falsely accused men in cases of disputed paternity.

Serologic methods of identity testing have been surpassed and replaced by DNA-based assays[34] (referred to as DNA fingerprinting, DNA profiling, or DNA typing) that were pioneered by Jeffreys and colleagues.[35,36] Tandemly repeated sequences of DNA of varying lengths occur predominantly in the noncoding genomic DNA, and they are classified into groups depending on the size of the repeat region. The extensive variation of these tandemly repeated sequences between individuals makes it unlikely for the same number of repeats to be shared by two individuals, even if these individuals are related. Minisatellite [also referred to as variable number of tandem repeats (VNTR)] loci have tandem repeat units of 9 to 80 base pairs, whereas microsatellite [also referred to as short tandem repeat (STR)] loci consist of two to five base-pair tandem repeats.[37] Microsatellites and minisatellites are reviewed by Bennett.[38]

Assays for VNTR and STR sequences involve the electrophoretic separation of DNA fragments according to size. DNA profiling involves amplification of selected, informative VNTR and STR loci using locus-specific oligonucleotide primers, with the subsequent measurement of the size of the polymerase chain reaction (PCR) products. Hundreds of STR loci have been mapped throughout the human genome, and many have been applied to identity testing. Analysis of different STR loci (usually at least 12) is used to generate a person's DNA profile that is virtually guaranteed to be unique to that person (or to two identical twins). DNA fingerprinting is a powerful tool

not only for identity testing and population genetics but also for monitoring chimerism after marrow transplantation.[39,40] STR analysis also has been used to monitor patients for graft-vs-host disease after organ transplantation, particularly after a liver transplant.[41]

In a case of disputed paternity, if an alleged father cannot be excluded from paternity, the probability of his paternity can be calculated. The calculation compares the probability that the alleged father transmitted the paternal obligatory genes with the probability that any other randomly selected man from the same racial or ethnic group transmitted the genes. The result is expressed as a likelihood ratio (paternity index) or as a percentage. AABB has developed standards and guidance documents for laboratories that perform relationship testing.[42]

BLOOD GROUP GENE MAPPING

Gene mapping is the process through which a gene locus is assigned to a location on a chromosome. The initial mapping of blood group genes was accomplished by testing many families for selected red cell antigens. Pedigrees were analyzed for evidence of recombination between the genes of interest to rule out or establish linkage of a blood group with another marker having a known chromosomal location.

The gene encoding the antigens of the Duffy blood group system was the first to be assigned to a chromosome, by showing that the gene is linked to an inherited deformity of chromosome 1. More recently, recombinant DNA methods were used to establish the physical locations of genes, and today, with sequencing of the human genome, determining the location of a gene involves a computer database sequence search. The Human Genome Project (http://web.ornl.gov/sci/techresources/Human_Genome/index.shtml) has resulted in construction of a physical gene map indicating the position of gene loci, and the distance between loci is expressed by the number of base pairs of DNA.

Currently, 36 blood group systems are recognized by the ISBT.[6] The genes for all of them have been cloned and assigned to their respective chromosomes. (See Table 9-1.) Details on procedures for gene mapping are beyond the scope of this chapter, but reviews are available.[8]

CHIMERISM

The observation that a sample gives mixed-field agglutination is not an unusual one in transfusion medicine. Often this is the result of artificially induced chimerism through the transfusion of donor red cells or a stem cell transplant. On rare occasions, the observation of mixed-field agglutination identifies a true **chimera**, that is, a person with a dual population of cells derived from more than one zygote. Indeed, the first example of a human chimera was a female blood donor discovered through mixed-field agglutination during antigen typing. Most human chimeras can be classified as either twin chimeras or tetragametic (dispermic) chimeras. Chimerism is not a hereditary condition.[43]

Twin chimerism occurs through the formation of placental blood vessel anastomoses, which results in the mixing of blood between two fetuses. This vascular bridge allows hematopoietic stem cells to migrate to the marrow of the opposite twin. Each twin may have two distinct populations of cells (red cells and leukocytes), that of his or her true genetic type and that of the twin. The percentage of the two cell lines in each twin tends to vary; the major cell line is not necessarily the autologous cell line, and the proportions of the two cell lines may change throughout life. Chimeric twins have immune tolerance; they do not make antibody against the A or B antigens that are absent from their own red cells but are present on the cells of the engrafted twin. This tolerance extends beyond red cells to negative mixed-lymphocyte cultures and the mutual acceptance of skin grafts.

In twin chimeras, the dual cell population is strictly confined to blood cells. Tetragametic or dispermic chimeras present chimerism in all tissues and are more frequently identified because of infertility than because of mixed populations of red cells. The mechanism(s) leading to the development of tetragametic chimeras are unknown, but they arise through the fertilization of two maternal nuclei by two sperm followed by fusion of the two zygotes and development into one person containing two cell lineages.

More commonly, chimeras occur through medical intervention and arise from the transfer of actively dividing cells, such as through hematopoietic cell transplantation.[43] However, chimerism may be more prevalent than once thought, based on the discovery of people with dual red cell populations when performing DNA analysis to predict red cell phenotypes, and chimerism has been the cause of disputed maternity.[44,45]

BLOOD GROUP TERMINOLOGY

Antigens were originally named using an alphabetical (eg, A/B, C/c) notation, or they were named after the proband whose red cells carried the antigen or who made the first known antibody (eg, Duclos). A symbol with a superscript letter (eg, Lu^a, Lu^b; Jk^a, Jk^b) was used, and a numerical terminology (eg, Fy3, Jk3, Rh32) was introduced. In blood group systems, antigens are named using more than one scheme (eg, the Kell blood group system: K, k, Js^a, Js^b, K11, K17, TOU).

In 1980, the ISBT established its Working Party on Terminology for Red Cell Surface Antigens. The working party was charged to develop a uniform nomenclature that would be "both eye and machine readable" and "in keeping with the genetic basis of blood groups." **A blood group system** consists of one or more antigens under the control of a single gene locus or of two or more homologous genes. Thus, each blood group system is genetically independent from every other blood group system and represents a single gene or a cluster of two or three homologous genes.

The failure of an antibody to be reactive with red cells of a particular null phenotype is not sufficient for assignment of the corresponding antigen to a system. Some null phenotypes are the result of inhibitor or modifying genes that may suppress the expression of antigens from more than one system [eg, the Rh$_{null}$ phenotype lacks not only Rh antigens but also LW system antigens, Fy5 antigen (Duffy system), and sometimes U (MNS system) antigen]. Similarly, a blood group antigen must be shown to be inherited through family studies, or the expression of the antigen must be demonstrated to be associated with a variation in the nucleotide sequence of the gene controlling the system, to be assigned antigen status by the ISBT terminology working party. A blood group antigen must be defined serologically by an antibody; a polymorphism that is detectable only by DNA analysis and for which there is no corresponding antibody cannot be called a blood group antigen.

The working party established a terminology consisting of uppercase letters and Arabic numerals to represent blood group systems and antigens.[6,46] Each system can be identified by a set of numbers (eg, ABO system = 001; Rh system = 004). Similarly, each antigen in the system is assigned a number (eg, A antigen = 001; B antigen = 002; D antigen = 001). Thus, 001001 identifies the A antigen and 004001 identifies the D antigen. Alternatively, the sinistral zeros may be omitted so that the A antigen becomes 1.1 and the D antigen becomes 4.1. Each system also has an alphabetical abbreviation (Table 9-1 gives the italicized gene names analogous to the system names); thus KEL is the ISBT symbol for the Kell system, the Rh ISBT system symbol is RH, and an alternative name for the D antigen is RH1. This alphanumeric terminology, which was designed primarily for computer use, is not ideal for

everyday communication. To achieve uniformity, a recommended list of user-friendly alternative names was compiled.[47]

The ISBT working party meets periodically to assign names and numbers to newly discovered antigens. The working party is also charged to develop, maintain, and monitor a terminology for blood group genes and their alleles; this is reflected by its recent change of name to Red Cell Immunogenetics and Blood Group Terminology working party.[6] The terminology takes into account the guidelines for human gene nomenclature published by the Human Genome Organization (HUGO), which is responsible for naming genes based on the International System for Human Gene Nomenclature.[48] For antigen terminology criteria; tables listing the systems, antigens, and phenotypes; and information regarding the current status of gene and allele terminology, see ISBT Red Cell Immunogenetics and Blood Group Terminology web resources.[6] An example of ISBT terminology as it applies to alleles, genotypes, phenotypes, and antigens is shown in Table 9-3.

BLOOD GROUP GENOMICS

As discussed in earlier sections of this chapter, the antigens expressed on red cells are the products of genes and can be detected directly by hemagglutination techniques (as long as relevant antisera are available). Their detection is an important aspect of the practice of transfusion medicine because an antigen can,

TABLE 9-3. Example of Allele, Genotype, Phenotype, and Antigen Terminology

Duffy System	Traditional	ISBT Terminology
Allele	None[†]	*FY*01* or *FY*A*, *FY*02* or *FY*B*, *FY*01N* or *FY*02N*
Genotype/haplotype	None[†]	*FY*A/FY*B* or *FY*01/FY*02*
Phenotype	Fy(a+b+)	FY:1,2
Antigen	Fy^a, Fy^b	FY1, FY2 *or* 008001, 008002 or 8.1, 8.2

[†]Historical terminology used the italicized form of the antigen for the allele, genotype, and haplotype (eg, *Fy^a*, *Fy^b*). The historical terminology is still used in some areas of this chapter for simplicity of the discussion.
ISBT = International Society of Blood Transfusion; N denotes "null"; *FY*01N* or *FY*02N* indicates that the null mutation is on an *FY*A* or *FY*B* background, and *FY*AN* or *FY*BN* are not used.

if it is introduced into the circulation of an individual who lacks that antigen, elicit an immune response.

It is the antibody from such an immune response that causes problems in clinical practice, such as patient/donor blood transfusion incompatibility or maternal-fetal incompatibility, and it is the reason why antigen-negative blood is required for safe transfusion in these patients. Hemagglutination is simple, quick, and relatively inexpensive. When carried out correctly, it has a specificity and sensitivity that is appropriate for most testing. However, hemagglutination has limitations; for example, it is difficult and often impossible to obtain an accurate phenotype for a recently transfused patient or to type red cells that are coated with IgG, and some typing reagents are in short supply or not available. Because the genes encoding the 36 known blood group systems have been cloned and sequenced and the genetic bases of most blood group antigens and phenotypes are known, DNA-based methods (genotyping) are increasingly being used as an indirect method to predict a blood group phenotype. This approach has introduced blood group genomics, often referred to as "molecular immunohematology," into the practice of transfusion medicine. Prediction of a blood group antigen by testing DNA is simple and reliable for the majority of antigens because most result from SNPs that are inherited in a straightforward Mendelian manner. For example, the antithetical antigens S and s arise from GYPB alleles that differ by one nucleotide—143T for S and 143C for s—and the resulting proteins differ by one amino acid, methionine at residue 48 for S and threonine for s (designated c.143T>C p.Met48Thr). As a result, assay design and interpretation are fairly straightforward for the prediction of most phenotypes.

However, detailed serologic and genetic studies, including whole genome sequencing, have shown that there are far more alleles than phenotypes, and this is especially relevant clinically for ABO and Rh. More than 380 different alleles encoding the glycosyltransferases responsible for the four ABO types have been identified, and a single nucleotide change in an A or B allele can result in an inactive transferase and a group O phenotype. (See Chapter 10.) Testing for the common Rh antigens D, C/c, and E/e is uncomplicated for most populations, but antigen expression is more complex in some ethnic groups. There are >490 RHD alleles encoding weak D or partial D phenotypes, and >150 RHCE alleles encoding altered, or novel, hybrid Rh proteins, some of which result in weakened antigen expression. (See Chapter 11.) RH genotyping, particularly in minority populations, requires sampling of multiple regions of the gene(s) and algorithms for interpretation.

The basis of DNA assays is the amplification of a target gene sequence through PCR, followed by manual, semi-automated, or automated downstream analysis. (See also Chapter 8.) Commonly used methods are sequence-specific primer PCR (SSP-PCR) and allele-specific PCR (AS-PCR). For manual methods, gel electrophoresis is used to separate the PCR products for fragment size determination. As an alternative, the assay may include digestion of the PCR products with a restriction fragment length polymorphism (RFLP), followed by electrophoresis and visualization of the fragments. Semi-automated approaches include real-time PCR using fluorescent probes with quantitative and qualitative automated readout. Manual methods are labor-intensive, and each assay is performed separately on each sample. Automated DNA arrays allow for higher throughput with a larger number of target alleles in the PCR reaction, which makes possible the determination of numerous antigens in a single assay. Most available platforms are based on fluorescent bead technology or mass spectrometry. Routine ABO and RhD testing is not currently available on automated platforms because the expression of these antigens is complex, and further development is required.

Specialty referral laboratories use methods that are similar to those used for high-resolution HLA typing, that is, gene-specific amplification of coding exons followed by sequencing, or gene-specific complementary DNA amplification and sequencing. These methods are used to investigate new alleles and resolve serologic and genotyping discrepancies. The application of these methods has been reviewed by several groups.[48-51]

Clinical Application of the Prediction of Blood Groups by DNA Analysis

A major use of DNA-based assays is to predict the red cell phenotype of a fetus or of a patient who has been transfused, or when red cells are coated with IgG. Additional applications include the resolution of discrepancies in the ABO and Rh systems and identification of the genetic basis of unusual serologic results. DNA analysis also affords the capability of distinguishing alloantibodies from autoantibodies. This section gives an overview of some of the major applications of DNA-based analysis that are currently employed in patient and donor testing. These and additional clinical applications are summarized in Table 9-4.

DNA-Based Assays to Predict the Red Cell Phenotype: Recently Transfused Patients

In patients receiving chronic or massive transfusions, the presence of donor red cells makes typing by hemagglutination inaccurate. Time-consuming and cumbersome cell separation methods that are often unsuccessful in isolating the patient's reticulocytes for typing can be avoided when DNA typing is used. PCR-based assays primarily use DNA extracted from WBCs isolated from a sample of peripheral blood. Interference from donor-derived DNA is avoided by targeting and amplifying a region of the gene that is common to all alleles so that the minute quantity of donor DNA is not detected. This approach makes possible reliable blood group determination with DNA prepared from a blood sample collected after transfusion. DNA isolated from a buccal swab or urine sediment is also suitable for testing. In transfusion-dependent patients who produce alloantibodies, an extended antigen profile is important to determine additional blood group antigens to which the patient can become sensitized.

In the past, when a patient with autoimmune hemolytic anemia was transfused before the patient's red cell phenotype for minor antigens was established, time- and resource-consuming differential allogeneic adsorptions were required to determine the presence or absence of alloantibodies underlying the autoantibody. Establishing the patient's most probable phenotype through DNA-based assays makes it possible to match the antigen profile of the adsorbing red cells to that of the patient, thereby reducing the number of cell types required for adsorption. This approach also allows matching of the antigen profile of the donor to that of the patient for the most clinically significant, common antigens (eg, Rh, Jk^a, Jk^b; S, s) when transfusion is required. Matching avoids the use of "least incompatible" blood for transfusion and allows transfusion of units that are "antigen-matched for clinically significant blood group antigens" to prevent delayed transfusion reactions and circumvent additional alloimmunization.

DNA-Based Assays to Predict the Red Cell Phenotype: When Red Cells Are Coated with IgG

In patients with or without autoimmune hemolytic anemia, the presence of immunoglobulin bound to the red cells [positive result on direct antiglobulin testing (DAT)] often makes antigen typing results by serologic methods invalid. Certain methods, such as treatment of the red cells with chloroquine diphosphate or EDTA-glycine acid (EGA), may be employed to remove the red-cell-bound IgG. These methods are not always successful; the antigen of interest may be denatured by the treatment (eg, EGA destroys antigens of the Kell blood group system), and direct agglutinating antibodies for the antigen of interest may not be available. DNA testing allows determination of an extended antigen profile to select antigen-negative RBC units for transfusion.

TABLE 9-4. Applications of DNA-Based Assays for Patient and Donor Testing

To predict a patient's red cell phenotype:

- After a recent transfusion.
  - Aid in antibody identification and RBC unit selection.
  - Select RBCs for adsorption.

- When antibody typing reagent is not available (eg, anti-Do^a, -Do^b, -Js^a, -V, -VS).

- Distinguish an alloantibody from an autoantibody (eg, anti-e, anti-Kp^b).

- Help identify alloantibody when a patient's type is antigen-positive and a variant phenotype is possible (eg, anti-D in a D-positive patient, anti-e in an e-positive patient).

- When the patient's red cells are coated with immunoglobulin (DAT+).
  - When direct-agglutinating antibodies are not available.
  - When the antigen is sensitive to the IgG removal treatment (eg, antigens in the Kell system are denatured by EDTA-glycine-acid elution).
  - When testing requires the indirect antiglobulin test and IgG removal techniques are not effective at removing cell-bound immunoglobulin.
  - When antisera are weakly reactive and reaction is difficult to interpret (eg, anti-Do^a, anti-Do^b, anti-Fy^b).

- After allogeneic stem cell transplantation.
  - If an antibody problem arises, test stored DNA samples (or buccal swab) from the patient and the donor(s) to guide selection of units for transfusion.

- To detect weakly expressed antigens (eg, Fy^b with the Fy^X phenotype).

- Identify genetic basis of unusual serologic results, especially Rh variants.

- Resolve discrepancies, eg, A, B, and Rh.

- Aid in the resolution of complex serologic investigations, especially those involving high-prevalence antigens when reagents are not available.

- Identify if a fetus is or is not at risk for hemolytic disease of the fetus and newborn.
  - Predict if the partner of a prospective mother with anti-D is homozygous or heterozygous for *RHD*.

To predict a donor's red cell phenotype:

- Screen for antigen-negative donors.

- When antibody is weak or not available (eg, anti-Do^a, -Do^b; -Js^a, -Js^b; -V/VS).

- Mass screening to increase antigen-negative inventory.

- Find donors whose red cells lack a high-prevalence antigen.

- Resolve blood group A, B, and Rh discrepancies.

- Detect genes that encode weak antigens.

- Type donors for reagent red cells for antibody screening cells and antibody identification panels (eg, Do^a, Do^b, Js^a, V, VS).

- Determine zygosity of donors on antibody detection/identification reagent panels, especially D, S, Fy^a, and Fy^b.

RBCs = Red Blood Cells; DAT = direct antiglobulin test.

DNA-Based Assays to Distinguish Alloantibody from Autoantibody

When an antibody specificity is found in a patient whose red cells express the corresponding antigen, it is essential to know whether the antibody is an allo- or autoantibody, and a DNA-based investigation is helpful for transfusion management. If DNA typing predicts the red cells to be antigen positive, further investigation by high-resolution gene sequencing should be considered because the sample may have a novel amino acid change in the protein carrying the blood group antigen. These novel amino acid changes result in new epitopes and altered (weakened or partial) expression of the conventional antigen.

This is especially relevant in patients with sickle cell disease (SCD) or thalassemia who require long-term transfusion support and are at risk of alloimmunization that is often complicated by the presence of autoantibodies. In patients of African ancestry who have SCD, partial expression of common Rh antigens (D, C, c, and e) is prevalent. Such patients frequently present with a combination of anti-D, -C, and -e, and yet their red cells type serologically as D+, C+, and e+. Although such patients may make alloantibodies to these antigens, autoantibody production with Rh-related specificity is prevalent, and distinguishing between the two is critical for safe transfusion practice to avoid hemolytic transfusion reactions (and conserve rare blood).[52,53] Delayed hemolytic transfusion reaction, in particular, places patients with SCD at risk for life-threatening anemia, pain crisis, acute chest syndrome, and/or acute renal failure. Patients may also experience hyperhemolysis, in which hemoglobin levels drop below pretransfusion levels as a result of bystander hemolysis of the patients' own antigen-negative red cells. RH genotyping has revealed that many of these patients have variant RHD and/or RHCE alleles that encode amino acid changes in Rh proteins, resulting in altered or partial antigens. For details on RHD and RHCE alleles that encode partial antigens, refer to Chapter 11.

Reports of autoantibodies to Jk^a and Jk^b are not uncommon. With the discovery of variant JK alleles that encode partial Jk^a and Jk^b antigens, it is probable that some previously identified autoantibodies were alloantibodies. (See Chapter 12.) DNA analysis for JK variants is helpful to clarify the situation. As in some other blood group systems, Kidd system genetic diversity is higher in populations of African ancestry.

DNA-Based Testing in Prenatal Practice

DNA-based testing has affected prenatal practice in the areas that are discussed below. Hemagglutination, including antibody titers, gives only an indirect indication of the risk and severity of hemolytic disease of the fetus and newborn (HDFN). Antigen prediction by DNA-based assays can be used to identify the fetus who is not at risk of HDFN (ie, who is predicted to be antigen-negative) so that the mother need not be aggressively monitored. Testing of fetal DNA should be considered when a mother's serum contains an IgG alloantibody that has been associated with HDFN and the father's status for the corresponding antigen is heterozygous or indeterminable, or he is not available for testing.

DNA-Based Testing to Identify a Fetus at Risk for Anemia of the Neonate

The first application of DNA-based assays for the prediction of blood group phenotype occurred in the prenatal setting and was reported by Bennett et al,[54] who tested fetal DNA for the presence of *RHD*. Because of the clinical significance of anti-D, *RHD* is probably the most frequent target gene, but DNA-based assays can be used to predict the antigen type of the fetus for any antigen if the genetic basis is known. When the implicated IgG antibody in the maternal circulation is not anti-D, it is prudent, when possible, to also test the fetal DNA for *RHD* to preempt unnecessary requests for D– blood for intrauterine transfusion; this is particularly relevant to avoid the use of rare r'r' or r"r" blood when anti-c or anti-e is the implicated antibody.

PCR analyses for the prediction of fetal D phenotype are based on detecting the presence or absence of specific portions of *RHD*. In populations of European ancestry, the genetic basis of the D– phenotype is usually associated with deletion of the entire *RHD*, but several other molecular bases have been described. In populations of Asian ancestry, 15% to 30% of D– people have an intact but inactive *RHD*, while others with red cells that are nonreactive with anti-D have the D_{el} phenotype. Approximately a quarter of D– people of African ethnicity have an *RHD* pseudogene (*RHDΨ*), which does not encode the D antigen, and many others have a hybrid *RHD-CE-D* gene (eg, the r'^{s} phenotype). Predicting the D type by DNA analysis requires probing for multiple nucleotide changes. The choice of assays depends on the patient's ethnicity and the degree of discrimination desired. Establishing the fetal *KEL* genotype is also of great clinical value in determining whether a fetus is at risk for severe anemia, because the strength of the mother's K antibody often does not correlate with the severity of the infant's anemia. The same is true for anti-Ge3.[55]

Amniocytes, harvested from amniotic fluid, are the most common source of fetal DNA. Chorionic villus sampling and cordocentesis are not favored because of their more invasive nature and associated risk to the fetus. A noninvasive sample source is the cell-free fetal DNA that is present in maternal plasma as early as 5 weeks of gestation; the amount of DNA increases with gestational age, and reliable results in DNA-based assays are obtained starting at about 15 weeks of gestation (sometimes earlier, depending on the gene of interest).[56,57] These assays are particularly successful for D typing because the D– phenotype in the majority of samples is due to the absence of the RHD gene.

Testing for the presence or absence of a gene is less demanding than testing for a single gene polymorphism or SNP to predict, for example, the K/k antigen status. Cell-free fetal DNA from the maternal plasma is routinely tested in Europe for the presence of a fetal RHD gene to eliminate the unnecessary administration of antepartum Rh Immune Globulin (RhIG) to the approximately 40% of D– women who are carrying a D– fetus.

DNA-Based Testing for D in Pregnant Women

Serologic typing for D cannot easily distinguish women whose red cells lack some epitopes of D (partial D) and are at risk for D immunization, from those with a weak D phenotype who are not at risk for D immunization. Red cells with partial D type as D+, some by direct tests and others by indirect tests. These women might benefit from receiving RhIG prophylaxis if they deliver a D+ fetus. *RHD* genotyping can distinguish weak D from partial D to guide RhIG prophylaxis and blood transfusion recommendations.[58]

DNA-Based Testing of Paternal Samples

The father's red cells should be tested for the antigen corresponding to the antibody in the maternal plasma. If the red cells are negative, the fetus is not at risk. If the father is positive for the antigen, zygosity testing can determine whether the father is homozygous or heterozygous for the gene encoding the antigen. This is particularly relevant when there is no allelic antigen or no antisera to detect the allelic product.

Zygosity testing of paternal samples is most often performed when testing for possible HDFN due to anti-D or anti-K. If the paternal red cells are K+ and the mother has anti-K, they can be tested serologically for expression of the allelic k antigen. However, many centers do not have a licensed reagent available, and genetic counselors often request DNA testing. If the paternal red cells are K–, the maternal anti-K is most likely the result of immunization through transfusion.

For maternal anti-D, DNA testing of *RHD* zygosity is the only method to determine the paternal gene copy number. Several different genetic events cause a D– phenotype, and multiple assays must be conducted to accurately determine *RHD* zygosity, especially in non-European ethnic groups. If the father is *RHD* homozygous, all of his children will be

D+, and any pregnancy in his partner needs to be monitored. If the father is heterozygous, the fetus has a 50% chance of being at risk. The D type of the fetus should be determined to prevent unnecessary testing so the mother need not be aggressively monitored or receive immune-modulating agents.

DNA-Based Testing for Antigen-Negative Blood Donors

DNA-based typing to predict donor antigen profiles in the search for antigen-negative units is now a standard procedure for blood centers, especially when suitable antibodies are not available. Because red cell typing for Dombrock antigens is notoriously difficult, one of the most frequent approaches is to type for Do^a and Do^b. Many other antibody specificities are unavailable for mass donor screening. These specificities include anti-Hy, -Jo^a, -Js^a, -Js^b, -C^W, -V, and -VS. Even specificities considered to be common, such as anti-S and anti-Fy^b, are not always readily available.

DNA arrays can be used to screen for multiple minor antigens in a single assay format and have the potential to be used for mass screening of donors. A platform licensed by the Food and Drug Administration (FDA) is now available. The results can be used for the labeling of donor units for extended antigen profiles. This practice not only increases the antigen-negative inventory by expanding combinations of the minor antigens and some high-prevalence antigens, but also allows provision of donor components that are DNA matched to the patient's type. Licensed DNA methods that predict ABO and RhD are not available for the labeling of donor units.

DNA-Based Testing to Confirm D Type of Donors

Donor centers must test donors for weak D to avoid labeling a product as D– that might result in anti-D in response to transfused RBCs. Some donor red cells with very weak D expression (weak D type 2, and especially those with the D$_{el}$ phenotype) are not typed as D+ using current methods and are labeled as D–. The prevalence of weak D red cells not detected by serologic reagents is approximately 0.1% (but may vary depending on the test method and population). Although the clinical significance has not been established, donor red cells with weak D expression have been associated with alloimmunization. *RHD* genotyping would improve donor testing by confirming D– phenotypes,[59] but a high-throughput and cost-effective platform is not yet available.

Discrepancies Between Serologic (Phenotype) and DNA (Genotype) Testing

Differences between serologic and DNA testing results do occur and should be investigated. Often, these discrepancies lead to interesting discoveries such as the presence of a novel allele or genetic variant, particularly when people of diverse ethnicities are tested. Causes of discrepancies include recent transfusions, stem cell transplantation, and natural chimerism. Stem cell transplantation and natural chimerism also may cause differences between the results of testing DNA from somatic cells and results of testing DNA extracted from peripheral WBCs. Thus, when using DNA testing, it is important to obtain an accurate medical history. Many genetic events can cause apparent discrepant results between hemagglutination and DNA test results. Weak antigen expression may not be detected by hemagglutination, and the genotype may not always predict the phenotype.[3,5,29] (See Table 9-5.)

Silenced or Nonexpressed Genes

DNA testing interrogates a single SNP or a few SNPs associated with antigen expression and cannot sample every nucleotide in the gene. Although a gene may be detected by DNA testing, there are times when the gene product is not expressed on the red cells, because of a mutation that silences the gene or reduces expression levels, and is not detected by routine hemagglutination testing. Such changes result in discrepancies in the typing of patients and donors. Homozygosity (or compound heterozygosity) for a silenced gene results in a null

TABLE 9-5. Examples of Some Molecular Events Where Analysis of Gene and Phenotype May Not Agree

Molecular Event	Mechanism	Observed Blood Group Phenotype
Alternative splicing	Nt change in splice site: partial/complete skipping of exon	S–s–; Gy(a–)
	Deletion of nt(s)	Dr(a–)
Premature stop codon	Deletion of nt(s) → frameshift	Fy(a–b–); D–; c–E–; Rh_{null}; Gy(a–); GE:–2,–3,–4; K_0; McLeod
	Insertion of nt(s) → frameshift	D–; Co(a–b–)
	Nt change	Fy(a–b–); r′; Gy(a–); K_0; McLeod
Amino acid change	Missense nucleotide change	D–; Rh_{null}; K_0; McLeod
Reduced amount of protein	Missense nucleotide change	Fy^X; Co(a–b–)
Hybrid genes	Crossing over	GP.Vw; GP.Hil; GP.TSEN
	Gene conversion	GP.Mur; GP.Hop; D– –; R_0^{Har}
Interacting protein	Absence of RhAG	Rh_{null}
	Absence of Kx	Weak expression of Kell antigens
	Absence of aas 75 to 99 of GPA	Wr(b–)
	Absence of protein 4.1	Weak expression of Ge antigens
Modifying gene	*In(Jk)*	Jk(a–b–)

Nt = nucleotide; aas = amino acids.

phenotype, and most null phenotypes have more than one genetic basis.[5]

With donor typing, the presence of a grossly normal gene whose product is not expressed on the red cell surface results in the donor being falsely typed as antigen-positive. Although this situation means loss of an antigen-negative donor, it does not jeopardize the safety of blood transfusion. However, if a grossly normal gene is detected in a patient but the gene is not expressed, the patient remains at risk for the corresponding antibody if he or she receives a transfusion of antigen-positive blood.

To avoid misinterpretation, routine assays must include appropriate tests to detect a change that silences gene expression if prevalent in the population tested. Silenced alleles can be specific to a particular ethnic group. For example, in the Duffy blood group system, a single nucleotide change (–67T>C) within the promoter region (GATA box) of *FY* prevents transcription of *FY*A* and/or *FY*B* in red cells but not in other tissues. Although silencing of *FY*A* is rare, silencing of *FY*B* is frequent in persons of African ethnicity where homozygosity for the –67T>C change in *FY*B* results in the Fy(a–b–) phenotype, which has a prevalence of 60% or higher. To ensure accuracy, testing for the GATA box mutation must be included in typing for Duffy in persons of African ethnicity.

When the assay is used to predict the presence or absence of D antigen, particularly in populations of African ancestry, it is essential to include a test for the complete but inactive *RHD* pseudogene (*RHDψ*), which has a 37-bp sequence duplication. If the assay tests for *GYPB*S* (S antigen), additional testing should be performed to detect a C>T change at nucleotide 230 in *GYP*B* exon 5 or a change in intron 5 (+5g>t); both changes prevent expression of S antigen when testing persons of African ancestry.

Other common causes of discrepancies include the presence in the sample of an altered FY*B allele that encodes an amino acid change causing an Fy^X phenotype with greatly reduced expression of Fy^b antigen. The red cells type as Fy(b–) with most serologic reagents. The prevalence of the allele encoding the Fy^X phenotype in people of European ancestry is as high as 2%, and the allele has been found in persons of African ancestry also. Silencing mutations associated with the loss of Kidd antigen expression occur more often in people of Asian ancestry, whereas nucleotide changes encoding amino acid changes that weaken Kidd expression occur in people of African ethnicity.

The routine detection of some blood group polymorphisms by DNA analysis is not practical at this time. This includes situations where 1) a large number of alleles encode one phenotype (eg, ABO, Rh, and null phenotypes in many blood group systems), 2) a phenotype results from alleles with a large deletion (eg, GE:–2,3 and GE:–2,–3,–4), or 3) a phenotype results from hybrid alleles (eg, in the Rh and MNS systems). In addition, not all alleles in all ethnic populations are known.

Summary

Blood group genomics has become an essential component of the practice of transfusion medicine.[60] Genomics has provided a greater understanding of genetic blood group variants, including the complexity of Rh variants, such as those that encode the Hr–hr^S– and hr^B–Hr^B– phenotypes[61,62] and the associated partial Rh antigens that are a daily challenge for the management of patients with SCD.[52,53] RH genotyping expands and extends matching for Rh in this patient population. High-throughput platforms provide a means to test relatively large numbers of donors, thereby opening up the possibility of changing the way antigen-negative blood is provided to patients to prevent immunization or to eliminate transfusion reactions for those who are already immunized.

KEY POINTS

1. Genetics is the study of heredity; that is, the mechanisms by which a particular characteristic, such as a blood group, is passed from parents to offspring.
2. A gene is a segment of DNA and is the basic unit of inheritance; it occupies a specific location on a chromosome (the gene locus). Alleles are alternative forms of a gene at the same gene locus (eg, alleles *JK*A* and *JK*B* encode the Jk^a and Jk^b antigens, respectively).
3. A human somatic (body) cell is diploid, containing 46 chromosomes in 23 pairs: 22 pairs are alike (homologous) in males and females and are termed autosomes. The remaining pair are the sex chromosomes: X and Y for males, or two X chromosomes for females.
4. Somatic cells divide for growth and repair by mitosis. Mitosis replicates the chromosomes and produces two identical nuclei in preparation for cell division. The new cells are diploid, like the parent cell, and have all the genetic information of the parent cell.
5. Meiosis is the process by which germ cells divide to become gametes (sperm and egg cells); diploid cells undergo DNA replication and two divisions to form four gametes, each of which is haploid, having half the chromosomal complement of the parent somatic cell.
6. The term "genotype" traditionally refers to the complement of genes inherited by each person from his or her parents; the term is also used to refer to the set of alleles at a single gene locus. Whereas the genotype of a person is his or her genetic constitution, the phenotype is the observable expression of the genes and reflects the biologic activity of the gene(s). Thus,

the presence or absence of antigens on the red cells, as determined by serologic testing, represents the phenotype.

7. When identical alleles for a given locus are present on both chromosomes, a person is homozygous for the particular allele, whereas when nonidentical alleles are present at a particular locus, the person is heterozygous. Antigens encoded by alleles at the same locus are said to be antithetical. Thus, genes are allelic but not antithetical, whereas antigens are antithetical but not allelic.

8. The expression of blood group antigens on the red cell may be modified or affected by gene interaction. Homozygosity (or compound heterozygosity) for a silenced gene results in a null phenotype, and most null phenotypes have more than one genetic basis.

9. A blood group system consists of one or more antigens under the control of a single gene locus (eg, *KEL* encodes the Kell blood group antigens) or of two or more homologous genes (eg, *RHD* and *RHCE* encode the Rh blood group antigens). Thus, each blood group system is genetically independent. Currently 36 blood group systems are recognized.

10. The genes encoding the 36 blood group systems have been sequenced, and the genetic bases of most antigens and phenotypes are known, so that DNA-based methods (genotyping) can be used to predict a blood group phenotype.

11. DNA-based assays (blood group genotyping) have major applications in patient and donor testing. They can be used to predict the red cell phenotype of a fetus or of a patient who was transfused, or when red cells are coated with IgG; they can be used to resolve ABO and Rh discrepancies and to identify the molecular basis of unusual serologic results. DNA analysis aids in distinguishing alloantibodies from autoantibodies and is being applied to high-throughput screening of donors.

REFERENCES

1. Brown TA. Introduction to genetics: A molecular approach. London, UK: Garland Science, 2011.

2. Clark DP, Russell LD. Molecular biology: Made simple and fun. St. Louis, MO: Cache River Press, 2010.

3. Reid ME, Denomme GA. DNA-based methods in the immunohematology reference laboratory. Transfus Apher Sci 2011;44:65-72.

4. Nussbaum RL, McInnes RR, Willard HF. Thompson & Thompson genetics in medicine. 8th ed. Philadelphia: Elsevier/Saunders, 2016.

5. Reid ME, Lomas-Francis C, Olsson ML. The blood group antigen factsbook. 3rd ed. San Diego, CA: Academic Press, 2012.

6. International Society of Blood Transfusion. Red Cell Immunogenetics and Blood Group Terminology (working group). Blood group terminology. Amsterdam, the Netherlands: ISBT, 2017. [Available at http://www.isbt web.org/working-parties/red-cell-immunoge netics-and-blood-group-terminology/ (accessed March 20, 2017).]

7. An international system for human cytogenetic nomenclature (1978) ISCN (1978). Report of the Standing Committee on Human Cytogenetic Nomenclature. Cytogenet Cell Genet 1978;21:309-404.

8. Lewis M, Zelinski T. Linkage relationships and gene mapping of human blood group loci. In: Cartron J-P, Rouger P, eds. Molecular basis of major human blood group antigens. New York: Plenum Press, 1995:445-75.

9. Lögdberg L, Reid ME, Zelinski T. Human blood group genes 2010: Chromosomal locations and cloning strategies revisited. Transfus Med Rev 2011;25:36-46.

10. Svensson L, Hult AK, Stamps R, et al. Forssman expression on human erythrocytes: Biochemical and genetic evidence of a new histo-blood group system. Blood 2013;121:1459-68.

11. Zelinski T, Coghlan G, Liu XQ, et al. ABCG2 null alleles define the Jr(a–) blood group phenotype. Nat Genet 2012;44:131-2.

12. Saison C, Helias V, Ballif BA, et al. Null alleles of ABCG2 encoding the breast cancer resistance protein define the new blood group system Junior. Nat Genet 2012;44:174-7.

13. Helias V, Saison C, Ballif BA, et al. ABCB6 is dispensable for erythropoiesis and specifies the

new blood group system Langereis. Nat Genet 2012;44:170-3.

14. Storry JR, Jöud M, Christophersen MK, et al. Homozygosity for a null allele of SMIM1 defines the Vel-negative blood group phenotype. Nat Genet 2013;45:537-41.

15. Cvejic A, Haer-Wigman L, Stephens JC, et al. SMIM1 underlies the Vel blood group and influences red cell traits. Nat Genet 2013;45:542-5.

16. Ballif BA, Helias V, Peyrard T, et al. Disruption of SMIM1 causes the Vel– blood type. EMBO Mol Med 2013;5:751-61.

17. Anliker, M, von Zabern I, Höchsmann B, et al. A new blood group antigen is defined by anti-CD59, detected in a CD59 deficient patient. Transfusion 2014;54:1817-22.

18. Daniels G, Ballif BA, Helias V, et al. Lack of the nucleoside transporter ENT1 results in the Augustine-null blood type and ectopic mineralization. Blood 2015;125:3651-4.

19. Lyon MF. X-chromosome inactivation. Curr Biol 1999;9:R235-R237.

20. Daniels G. Human blood groups. 3rd ed. Oxford, UK: Blackwell Science, 2013.

21. Clemson CM, Hall LL, Byron M, et al. The X chromosome is organized into a gene-rich outer rim and an internal core containing silenced nongenic sequences. Proc Natl Acad Sci U S A 2006;103:7688-93.

22. Redman CM, Reid ME. The McLeod syndrome: An example of the value of integrating clinical and molecular studies. Transfusion 2002;42:284-6.

23. Russo DCW, Lee S, Reid ME, Redman CM. Point mutations causing the McLeod phenotype. Transfusion 2002;42:287-93.

24. Garratty G. Blood groups and disease: A historical perspective. Transfus Med Rev 2000;14:291-301.

25. Thorisson GA, Stein LD. The SNP consortium website: Past, present and future. Nucleic Acids Res 2003;31:124-7.

26. Blumenfeld OO, Patnaik SK. Allelic genes of blood group antigens: A source of human mutations and cSNPs documented in the Blood Group Antigen Gene Mutation Database. Hum Mutat 2004;23:8-16.

27. US Department of Energy and National Institutes of Health. Human Genome Project. Washington, DC: US Department of Energy Genome Programs, Office of Biological and Environmental Research, 2010. [Available at http://web.ornl.gov/sci/techresources/Hu man_Genome/index.shtml (accessed March 20, 2017).]

28. Reid ME. Molecular basis for blood groups and function of carrier proteins. In: Silberstein LE, ed. Molecular and functional aspects of blood group antigens. Arlington, VA: AABB, 1995:75-125.

29. Storry JR, Olsson ML. Genetic basis of blood group diversity. Br J Haematol 2004;126:759-71.

30. Danek A, Bader B. Neuroakanthozytose-Syndrome. München, Germany: Ludwig-Maximilians Universitat München, 2013. [Available at http://www.klinikum.uni-muenchen.de/Klinik-und-Poliklinik-fuer-Neurologie/de/Klinik/Neurologische_Po liklinik/Kogni tive_Neurologie/Forschung/Ak anthozyten/index.html (accessed March 20, 2017).]

31. Race RR, Sanger R. Blood groups in man. 6th ed. Oxford, UK: Blackwell, 1975.

32. Singleton BK, Burton NM, Green C, et al. Mutations in EKLF/KLF1 form the molecular basis of the rare blood group In(Lu) phenotype. Blood 2008;112:2081-8.

33. Singleton BK, Roxby D, Stirling J, et al. A novel GATA-1 mutation (Ter414Arg) in a family with the rare X-linked blood group Lu(a–b–) phenotype (abstract). Blood 2009;114:783.

34. Pena SDJ, Chakraborty R. Paternity testing in the DNA era. Trends Genet 1994;10:204-9.

35. Jeffreys AJ, Wilson V, Thein SL. Hypervariable 'minisatellite' regions in human DNA. Nature 1985;314:67-73.

36. Jeffreys AJ, Wilson V, Thein SL. Individual-specific 'fingerprints' of human DNA. Nature 1985;316:76-9.

37. Butler JM, Reeder DJ. Short tandem repeat DNA internet database. NIST standard reference database SRD 130. Gaithersburg, MD: National Institute of Standards and Technology, 2017. [Available at http://www.cstl. nist.gov/div831/strbase/index.htm (accessed March 20, 2017).]

38. Bennett P. Demystified . . . microsatellites. Mol Pathol 2000;53:177-83.

39. Khan F, Agarwal A, Agrawal S. Significance of chimerism in hematopoietic stem cell transplantation: New variations on an old theme. Bone Marrow Transplant 2004;34:1-12.

40. Thiede C, Bornhauser M, Ehninger G. Evaluation of STR informativity for chimerism testing—comparative analysis of 27 STR

systems in 203 matched related donor recipient pairs. Leukemia 2004;18:248-54.

41. Domiati-Saad R, Klintmalm GB, Netto G, et al. Acute graft versus host disease after liver transplantation: Patterns of lymphocyte chimerism. Am J Transplant 2005;5:2968-73.

42. Maha GC, ed. Standards for relationship testing laboratories. 13th ed. Bethesda, MD: AABB, 2018.

43. Bluth MH, Reid ME, Manny N. Chimerism in the immunohematology laboratory in the molecular biology era. Transfus Med Rev 2007; 21:134-46.

44. Wagner FF, Frohmajer A, Flegel WA. RHD positive haplotypes in D negative Europeans. BMC Genet 2001;2:10.

45. Cho D, Lee JS, Yazer MH, et al. Chimerism and mosaicism are important causes of ABO phenotype and genotype discrepancies. Immunohematology 2006;22:183-7.

46. Daniels GL, Anstee DJ, Cartron J-P, et al. Blood group terminology 1995. ISBT Working Party on Terminology for Red Cell Surface Antigens. Vox Sang 1995;69:265-79.

47. Garratty G, Dzik WH, Issitt PD, et al. Terminology for blood group antigens and genes: Historical origins and guidelines in the new millennium. Transfusion 2000;40:477-89.

48. HGNC searches. Cambridge, UK: HUGO Gene Nomenclature Committee, 2016. [Available at http://www.genenames.org/ (accessed June 21, 2016).]

49. Avent ND. Large scale blood group genotyping. Transfus Clin Biol 2007;14:10-15.

50. Monteiro F, Tavares G, Ferreira M, et al. Technologies involved in molecular blood group genotyping. ISBT Science Series 2011;6:1-6.

51. Gassner C, Meyer S, Frey BM, et al. Matrix-assisted laser desorption/ionization, time of flight mass spectrometry-based blood group genotyping – the alternative approach. Transfus Med Rev 2013;27:2-9.

52. Chou ST, Westhoff CM. The role of molecular immunohematology in sickle cell disease. Transfus Apher Sci 2011;44:73-9.

53. Noizatt-Pirenne F, Tournamille C. Relevance of RH variants in transfusion of sickle cell patients. Transfus Clin Biol 2011;18:527-35.

54. Bennett PR, Le Van Kim C, Colin Y, et al. Prenatal determination of fetal RhD type by DNA amplification. N Engl J Med 1993;329:607-10.

55. Pate LL, Myers J, Palma J, et al. Anti-Ge3 causes late-onset hemolytic disease of the newborn: The fourth case in three Hispanic families. Transfusion 2013;53:2152-7.

56. Daniels G, Finning K, Martin P, Soothill P. Fetal blood group genotyping from DNA from maternal plasma; an important advance in the management and prevention of haemolytic disease of the fetus and newborn. Vox Sang 2004;87:225-32.

57. Clausen FB, Christiansen M, Steffensen R, et al. Report of the first nationally implemented clinical routine screening for fetal RHD in D– pregnant women to ascertain the requirement for antenatal RhD prophylaxis. Transfusion 2012;52:752-8.

58. Sandler S, Flegel W, Westhoff CM, et al. It's time to phase in RHD genotyping for patients with a serologic weak D phenotype. Transfusion 2015;55:680-9.

59. Wagner FF. RHD PCR of D-negative blood donors. Transfus Med Hemother 2013;40:172-81.

60. Hillyer C, Shaz B, Winkler A, Reid ME. Integrating molecular technologies for red blood cell typing and compatibility testing into blood centers and transfusion services. Transfus Med Rev 2008;22:117-32.

61. Pham B-N, Peyrard T, Tourret S, et al. Anti-HrB and anti-hrB revisited. Transfusion 2009;49:2400-5.

62. Reid ME, Hipsky CH, Velliquette RW, et al. Molecular background of RH in Bastiaan, the RH:-31,-34 index case, and two novel RHD alleles. Immunohematology 2012;28:97-103.

Chapter 10

ABO and Other Carbohydrate Blood Group Systems

• ● •

Julia S. Westman, PhD, and Martin L. Olsson, MD, PhD

THE 18 BLOOD group antigens in the ABO, P1PK, Lewis, H, I, Globoside, and FORS blood group systems are defined by immunodominant carbohydrate epitopes on glycoproteins and glycolipids. The synthesis of these antigens requires the action of a series of enzymes known as glycosyltransferases [Fig 10-1 (A)]. These enzymes reside mainly in the Golgi apparatus and are responsible for adding specific sugars, in a specific sequence and steric or anomeric linkage (α-linked or β-linked), to growing oligosaccharide chains on glycolipids and/or glycoproteins.[1,2] Most, but not all, blood group antigens are located at the ends of these chains. Because of their wide tissue distribution, the carbohydrate-based systems are often referred to as histo-blood groups.[3]

Previously, the dogma was that a glycosyltransferase typically uses a specific donor molecule and a specific acceptor molecule, but many examples of broader, more "promiscuous" use of acceptor substrates have come to light, including those involving carbohydrate-based blood groups. Transcriptional regulation together with the specificity of these enzymes for both their nucleotide sugar donor substrates [eg, uridine diphosphate (UDP)-galactose] and acceptor substrates (eg, type 1 chain vs type 2 chain) are responsible for the tissue-specific distribution of many blood group antigens.[4,5] Studies have shown that these blood groups have roles in development, cell adhesion, malignancy, and infectious disease, although many of the exact mechanisms underlying these roles remain unknown.[4,6,7]

THE ABO SYSTEM

The ABO system was originally described by Karl Landsteiner in 1900 and remains the most important blood group system in transfusion medicine.[7] In blood, ABO antigens are found in substantial amounts on red cells and platelets. In individuals who have the secretor phenotype, antigens are present in body fluids as well. ABO antigens are also expressed on many other tissues, including those of the endothelium,

Julia S. Westman, PhD, postdoctoral scientist, Division of Hematology and Transfusion Medicine, Department of Laboratory Medicine, Lund University, Lund, Sweden; and Martin L. Olsson, MD, PhD, Professor of Transfusion Medicine, Division of Hematology and Transfusion Medicine, Department of Laboratory Medicine, Lund University, Lund, Sweden, and Medical Director, Nordic Reference Laboratory for Genetic Blood Group Typing, LabMedicine, Region Skåne, Sweden
The authors have disclosed no conflicts of interest.

10

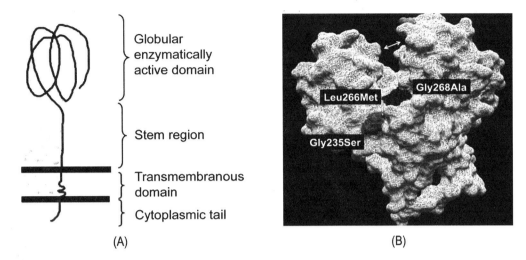

(A)   (B)

FIGURE 10-1. Model of a glycosyltransferase anchored in the Golgi membrane (A), and three-dimensional surface model of the human ABO glycosyltransferase (B). The arrow at the top shows the catalytic cleft, and the dark surfaces highlighted with black labels correspond to the amino acid positions that determine A vs B specificity.

kidney, heart, bowel, pancreas, and lung.[5] This is the reason these antigens constitute a barrier against ABO-incompatible organ transplantation.[8]

Transfusion of ABO-incompatible blood can be associated with acute intravascular hemolysis and renal failure, and can be fatal.[9,10] Similarly, transplanted ABO-incompatible solid organs can undergo hyperacute humoral rejection if the patient has not been pretreated to remove naturally occurring anti-A and/or anti-B from plasma. Because of the serious clinical consequences associated with ABO incompatibilities, ABO typing and ABO compatibility testing remain the foundation of safe pretransfusion testing and a crucial part of a pretransplantation workup.

The ABO system contains four major ABO phenotypes: A, B, O, and AB. The four phenotypes are determined by the presence or absence of two antigens (A and B) on red cells. (See Table 10-1.) The ABO system is also characterized by the presence or absence of naturally occurring antibodies, termed isohemagglutinins, directed against the missing A and B antigens. As shown in Table 10-1, an inverse

relationship exists between the presence of A and/or B antigens on red cells and the presence of anti-A, anti-B, or both, in sera, a phenomenon often referred to as Landsteiner's rule. For example, group O individuals, who lack A and B antigens on red cells, possess both anti-A and anti-B. It is believed that the immunizing sources for such naturally occurring antibodies are gut and environmental bacteria, such as the *Enterobacteriaceae*, which have been shown to possess ABO-like structures on their lipopolysaccharide coats.[11,12]

Biochemistry

The A and B antigens are defined by three sugar terminal epitopes on glycolipids and glycoproteins.[7] As shown in Fig 10-2, the H antigen is characterized by a terminal α1,2 fucose, which is the immediate and required biosynthetic precursor for expression of either the A or B antigen. The presence of this fucose is required for the A and B glycosyltransferases to be able to use the oligosaccharide chain as its acceptor substrate. In group A individuals, an *N*-acetylgalactosamine is added in an α1,3 linkage to the subterminal galactose of the H

TABLE 10-1. Routine ABO Grouping

Reaction of Red Cells with Antisera (Red Cell Grouping)		Reaction of Serum/Plasma with Reagent Red Cells (Serum Grouping)			Interpre-tation	Prevalence (%) in US Population	
Anti-A	Anti-B	A₁ Cells	B Cells	O Cells	ABO Group	European Ethnicity	African Ethnicity
0	0	+	+	0	0	45	49
+	0	0	+	0	A	40	27
0	+	+	0	0	B	11	20
+	+	0	0	0	AB	4	4
0	0	+	+	+	Bombay*	Rare	Rare

*H-negative phenotype (see section on H antigen).
+ = agglutination; 0 = no agglutination.

antigen to form A antigen. In group B individuals, an α1,3 galactose is added to the same subterminal galactose to form B antigen. In group AB individuals, both A and B structures are synthesized. In group O individuals, neither A nor B antigens are synthesized, as a result of alterations in the ABO genes.[7,13] Consequently, group O individuals express only H antigen. A and B antigens are also absent in the very rare Bombay phenotype because of the absence of the H-antigen precursor. (See "The H system" below.)

As terminal epitopes, the A and B antigens can be displayed on a number of oligosaccharide scaffolds that differ in their size, composition, linkages, and tissue distribution. On red cells, ABH antigens are mainly present as the N-linked portions of glycoproteins but also, to a lesser degree, as the O-linked part of glycoproteins and as glycosphingolipids (Fig 10-3). ABH antigens are subclassified by the carbohydrate sequence immediately next to the ABH-defining sugars. In humans, ABH is expressed predominantly on four different oligosaccharide peripheral core structures. (See Table 10-2.) On human red cells, the majority of endogenous ABH antigen synthesized is present on type 2 chain structures. In addition, ABH-active type 1 chain structures can be adsorbed onto the red cell, especially in secretor individuals.[14]

The ability to synthesize and use different carbohydrate chains is genetically determined. In addition to the four main ABO groups mentioned (as phenotypes) above, subgroups of the A and B phenotypes can be identified based on the quantity of A or B antigen expression and which types of carbohydrate chains contain the A or B antigen. (See "ABO Subgroups" section.) For example, the A phenotype can be subdivided into a number of subgroups, with A₁ and A₂ being the most common and second most common A subgroup, respectively. The A₁ phenotype, compared to A₂, has approximately five times the number of A antigens on red cells as a result of a more active A transferase.[13] There are also antigenic differences between the two. For instance, the A₁ transferase is more prone to make type 3 (repetitive A) and type 4 (globo-A) A antigens than the A₂ transferase.[15,16] As an example, ABH antigens on type 1 chain substrates can be recognized by antibodies directed against both ABH and Le^b antigens.[13,17] (See "The Lewis System".)

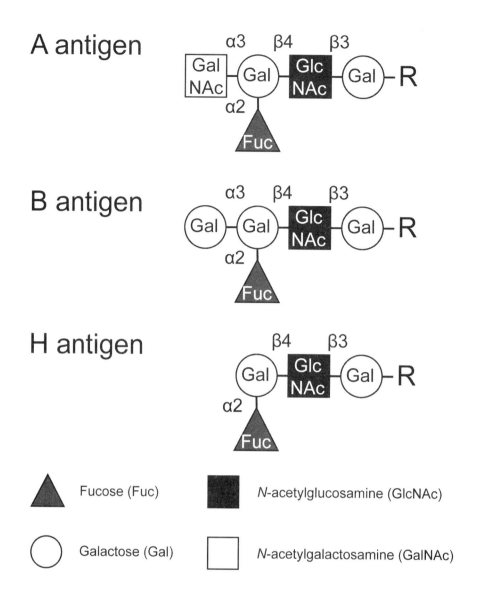

FIGURE 10-2. Schematic representation of the ABH antigens. Standard symbols for glycan annotation are used. Type 2 ABH antigens, the most common type on red cells, are shown. (See also Table 10-2.) R = upstream carbohydrate sequence.

ABO in Development and Aging

ABO antigens can be detected on red cells of embryos as early as 5 to 6 weeks of gestation.[17] The quantity of ABO antigens on umbilical cord red cells is less than that of adults, as the result of the immaturity of type 2 chain precursors on cord red cells.[18] (See section on the I blood group system below.) With increasing age, precursor chains become increasingly branched, thereby allowing more A and B antigen to be expressed.[19] Adult levels of ABO expression are generally present by age 2 to 4 years.[17,18]

Anti-A and anti-B are not present at birth or, if present, they are of maternal origin. Endogenous synthesis of anti-A and anti-B can

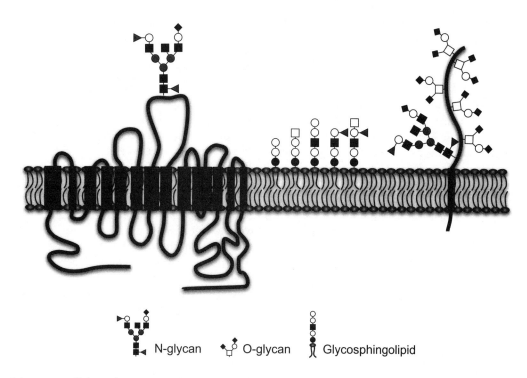

N-glycan   O-glycan   Glycosphingolipid

FIGURE 10-3. Schematic representation of the red cell membrane with selected carbohydrate-carrying blood group molecules representing different kinds of glycans.

TABLE 10-2. The Most Important Peripheral Core Chain Variants of A Antigen in Humans

Antigen	Oligosaccharide Sequence*
A epitope	GalNAcα1-3(Fucα1-2)Galβ1-R
A type 1	GalNAcα1-3(Fucα1-2)<u>Galβ**1-3**GlcNAc</u>β1-3-R
A type 2†	GalNAcα1-3(Fucα1-2)<u>Galβ**1-4**GlcNAc</u>β1-3-R
A type 3 (repetitive A)	GalNAcα1-3(Fucα1-2)Galβ**1-3**GalNAcα1-3(Fucα1-2)Galβ**1-4**GlcNAcβ1-3-R
A type 4 (globo-A)	GalNAcα1-3(Fucα1-2)Galβ**1-3**<u>GalNAcβ1-3Galα</u>1-4Galβ1-4Glc-Cer

*Underlined sequences denote the critical differences between type 1, 2, and 4 chains. Linkages and anomery (α- or β-linked) of the galactose in these A antigen variants are shown in bold. Bracketed sequences denote the repetitive sequence characteristic of type 3 chain A antigen. Note: There is also an alternative type 3 chain that is denoted the O-linked mucin type, which has the characteristic Galβ**1-3**GalNAc binding but not the repetitive A sequence.
†By far the predominant type on human red cells.
Cer = ceramide; Fuc = fucose; Gal = galactose; GalNAc = *N*-acetylgalactosamine; Glc = glucose; GlcNAc = *N*-acetylglucosamine; R = upstream carbohydrate sequence.

develop as early as age 3 to 6 months, with nearly all children displaying the appropriate isohemagglutinins in their sera at 1 year of age.[17,20] Titers of anti-A and anti-B continue to increase during early childhood and achieve adult levels within 5 to 10 years.

Among healthy adults, ABO titers can naturally vary from 4 to 2048 or higher.[17,20,21] High-titer ABO antibodies can be present in group O multiparous women and in patients taking certain bacteria-based nutritional supplements.[7,12,17] Although early reports indicated a fall in isohemagglutinin titers in the elderly, subsequent studies have disputed these findings.[20] In industrialized countries, isohemagglutinin titers have generally decreased, and some studies suggest that increasing consumption of processed foods is a factor.[21]

Genetics

The ABO gene is located on chromosome 9q34 and consists of seven coding exons spread over ~19 kb.[7] The largest portion of the open reading frame is located in exons 6 and 7. The gene is transcriptionally regulated by several mechanisms, including promoter methylation, antisense RNA, tissue-specific transcription-factor-binding motifs, and a minisatellite enhancer region 4 kb upstream of exon 1.[7] In addition, recent studies have shown the importance of an erythro-specific GATA-binding motif in intron 1[22] and the possibility that micro-RNAs may be involved by binding to the 3' end of the sequence.[23] ABO expression is also regulated by the FUT(1) H gene, which is responsible for the synthesis of H antigen, the precursor of A and B antigens. The FUT(1) H gene is in turn tightly regulated in a tissue-specific manner through transcription factors and promoters. In the total absence of H, no A or B antigen can be expressed regardless of *ABO* genotype. This results in the Bombay or O_h phenotype.[7,13]

Following the purification of A glycosyltransferase from lung tissue[24] and the subsequent cloning of the ABO gene,[25] a series of studies has identified the molecular basis for A, B, O, *cis*-AB, and weak ABO subgroups.[7,13,26] Although hundreds of ABO alleles have been found and characterized, the vast majority of individuals have alleles giving rise to A_1, A_2, B, or O expression. The A^1 and B consensus alleles [written as *ABO*A1.01* and *ABO*B.01*, respectively, in the blood group allele terminology developed by the International Society of Blood Transfusion (ISBT)] are codominantly expressed, and their coding regions differ by only seven nucleotides, of which four alter amino acids in the resulting glycosyltransferases.[7,25,26] Three amino acid substitutions (A vs B; p.Gly235Ser, p.Leu266Met, and p.Gly268Ala) are important in determining whether the glycosyltransferase uses UDP-*N*-acetylgalactosamine or UDP-galactose donor substrate to synthesize A or B antigens, respectively [Fig 10-1 (B)].[7,13] The rare *cis*-AB phenotype results from a chimeric enzyme with a mix of A- and B-specific amino acids at or nearby those amino acid positions.[26] A plethora of mutations associated with weak A and B subgroups has been described. As an example, group A_2 (the second most common A subgroup after A_1) is commonly the product of a nucleotide deletion and frameshift, resulting in an enzyme with an additional 21 amino acids at the C-terminus of the molecule.[7,26] Most of the weak A or B subgroups described below and in Table 10-3 depend on single nonsynonymous changes compared to *A* or *B* consensus, resulting in the substitution of a conserved amino acid that is important for the activity, specificity, or localization of the enzyme.

An O allele encodes a gene product without enzymatic function or no protein at all. The blood group O phenotype, therefore, is an autosomal recessive trait representing inheritance of two nonfunctional ABO genes. Overall, close to 100 O alleles have been identified.[7,26] The two most common O alleles are *ABO*O.01.01* (formerly known as O^1 or *O01*) and *ABO*O.01.02* (known as $O^{1variant}$ or *O02*). They contain the same nucleotide deletion, 261delG, which leads to a frameshift and premature truncation of the protein that lacks the enzymatically active domain. A principally different but infrequent O allele is *ABO*O.02* (originally described as O^2 but later also called *O03*), a group of nondeletional O alleles that contains a nonsynonymous polymorphism

TABLE 10-3. Serologic Reactions Observed in Selected A and B Subgroups

Red Cell Phenotype	Red Cell Reactions with Antisera or Lectins				Serum Reactions with Reagent Red Cells			Saliva (Secretors)
	Anti-A*	Anti-B	Anti-A,B	Anti-H	A_1 Cells	B Cells	O Cells	
A_1	4+	0	4+	0	0	4+	0	A, H
A_2	4+	0	4+	2+	0/2+†	4+	0	A, H
A_3	3+mf‡	0	3+mf‡	3+	0/2+†	4+	0	A, H
A_x	0/±	0	1-2+	4+	0/2+†	4+	0	H
A_{el}	0	0	0	4+	0/2+†	4+	0	H
A_m	0/±	0	0/±	4+	0	4+	0	A, H
B	0	4+	4+	0	4+	0	0	B, H
B_3	0	3+mf‡	3+mf‡	4+	4+	0	0	B, H
B_{weak}	0	±/2+	±/2+	4+	4+	0	0	H
B_{el}	0	0	0	4+	4+	0	0	H
B_m	0	0/±	0/±	4+	4+	0	0	B, H

*Positive adsorption/elution test with anti-A.

†The occurrence of anti-A1 is variable in these phenotypes.

‡This reaction can be read as 2+ or 3+ mixed field but typically looks like one or a few large agglutinates among a large number of free cells.

1+ to 4+ = agglutination of increasing strength; ± = weak agglutination; mf = mixed-field agglutination; 0 = no agglutination.

(c.802G>A) encoding the amino acid 268 (p.Gly268Arg), which is otherwise a critical residue for donor substrate binding. These alleles were found to be involved in cases of suspected A subgroups.[27,28] A subsequent study found that alleles with this alteration were responsible for 25% of all serologic ABO typing discrepancies caused by reverse-grouping problems in healthy donors, despite the frequency of this type of O allele being 1% to 2% in people of European ethnicity.[29] It was speculated that the weak anti-A observed in plasma could reflect weak residual glycosyltransferase activity. However, a later study was unable to demonstrate A antigen or enzyme activity in group O donors with the ABO*O.02 allele but confirmed that the anti-A titers appear to be lower.[30] The clinical significance, if any, is unclear, and the units are labeled group O.

ABO Subgroups

ABO subgroups are phenotypes that differ in the amount of A and B antigen carried on red cells and present in secretions (for those individuals who have the "secretor" phenotype). Clinically, the two most common subgroups encountered are A_1 and A_2. A_1 represents the majority of group A donors (~80% among people of European ethnicity) and is characterized by approximately five times more A antigen epitopes per red cell compared to A_2, which is the second most common subgroup (20%). It is difficult to estimate the absolute number of A antigen sites per red cell. Some investigators have suggested approximately 1 million for A_1 and 220,000 for A_2,[31] but others have suggested two to three times as many.[32] Both A_1 and A_2 are strongly agglutinated by reagent anti-A in routine direct testing. A_1 can be distinguished from A_2 by the lectin *Dolichos biflorus,* which agglutinates A_1 red cells but is diluted to a level that should not agglutinate A_2 red cells. Because the A_2 phenotype reflects the inefficient conversion of H to A antigen, A_2 red cells have increased reactivity with anti-H lectin *Ulex europaeus.* Enzyme studies comparing A_1 and A_2 glycosyltransferase activity show that the A_1 enzyme is five to ten times more active than the A_2 enzyme, resulting in quantitative and qualitative differences in A antigen expression.[7,13] The latter includes the synthesis of unusual type 3 and type 4 chain A antigen on A_1 red cells that are either not present or expressed at much lower levels on A_2 cells or weaker A subgroups.[13,15,16]

In addition to A_2, several weaker A subgroups have been described (eg, A_3, A_x, A_m, and A_{el}). Similarly, multiple weak B subgroups have been described (eg, B_3, B_x, B_m, and B_{el}). The weak A and B subgroups are infrequently encountered and are usually recognized by apparent discrepancies between red cell (forward) and serum or plasma (reverse) grouping. Most weak A and B subgroups were originally described before the advent of monoclonal typing reagents, and the hemagglutination patterns reported were based on reactivity with human polyclonal anti-A, anti-B, and anti-A,B reagents. Weak A subgroups are frequently nonreactive with human polyclonal anti-A (see Table 10-3) and can show variable reactivity with human polyclonal anti-A1 and anti-A,B and murine monoclonal antibodies (not shown).[13,15,26] The degree of reactivity with commercial murine monoclonal reagents is clone dependent, and clones may be used together in monoclonal blends as an anti-A,B reagent to allow for the agglutination of A_x red cells. This is a requirement of the European in-vitro diagnostic directive (IVDD), although it is not required in the United States. Because of the reciprocal relationship between H and synthesis of A and B antigens, most weak A and B subgroups have H expression similar to group O cells.[7] In clinical practice, it is seldom necessary to identify a patient's specific A or B subgroup except where identifying a group A_2 kidney donor allows for transplantation of the kidney to a group O recipient. To avoid unnecessary use of group O red cell units, however, it can be worthwhile to define the ABO blood group carefully in chronically transfused patients. Great care should be exercised to understand the underlying reason for any ABO discrepancy in a blood donor. For instance, a chimera must be differentiated from an A_3 subgroup, even if both may exhibit a mixed-field agglutination pattern.

When performed, serological classification of weak A subgroups is typically based on the following:

1. Degree of red cell agglutination by monoclonal (and possibly polyclonal) anti-A and anti-A1 (in the case of the latter, *Dolichos biflorus* lectin can also be used).
2. Degree of red cell agglutination by human polyclonal and some monoclonal anti-A,B.
3. Degree of H antigen expression (reactivity with monoclonal anti-H and/or *Ulex europaeus* lectin).
4. Presence or absence of anti-A_1 in serum (Method 2-9).
5. Presence of A and H in saliva (an analysis now seldom performed).
6. Adsorption and elution studies with polyclonal anti-A.
7. Family (pedigree) studies.

In the case of suspected weak B subgroups, the investigation is similar to the above, but anti-B replaces anti-A (and anti-A1). Presence of B and H can be investigated in saliva.

Currently, many reference laboratories also use genetic typing of the ABO gene as a complement to establish the underlying reason for an ABO discrepancy.[33] Sanger sequencing of the ABO gene or next-generation sequencing may be used. In addition, some ABO subgroups exhibit characteristic patterns when tested by flow cytometry with selected monoclonal ABO reagents.[34] This method is very useful for differentiating a low-grade chimera from a weak subgroup, or the inherited A_3 subgroup from a mixed-field pattern after transfusion.

B(A), A(B), and cisAB Phenotypes

The B(A) phenotype is an autosomal dominant phenotype characterized by weak A expression on group B red cells.[17,35] Serologically, red cells from B(A)-phenotype individuals are strongly reactive with anti-B and weakly reactive with certain monoclonal anti-A (<2+), and they may possess a strong anti-A that is reactive with both A_1 and A_2 red cells in their sera. B(A) red cells can show varying reactivity with monoclonal anti-A reagents. Testing the sample with a panel of polyclonal and monoclonal anti-A may resolve the discrepancy; however, genetic testing is the most accurate. Absence of the B-characteristic c.703G>A polymorphism (p.Gly235Ser) in a B allele will make it a B(A) allele, but also other genetic alterations in B alleles will result in this phenotype.[26] The basis of the phenotype is that the B-like glycosyltransferase in these individuals has an increased capacity to use UDP-*N*-acetylgalactosamine in addition to UDP-galactose, resulting in detectable A antigen synthesis.

An A(B) phenotype has also been described, using monoclonal anti-B. The A(B) phenotype was associated with elevated H antigen and plasma H-transferase activity.[17] It has been hypothesized that the increased H precursor on these cells may permit the synthesis of some B antigen by the A glycosyltransferase.

The cisAB phenotype can occur when an individual has inherited an ABO gene encoding an ABO glycosyltransferase that can use both A- and B-specific nucleotide sugars in a more equal way than in the B(A) or A(B) phenotypes.[36] If a cisAB allele is inherited together *in trans* with an O allele, an unusual phenotype with weak expression of A and B is observed (eg, A_2B_3). Anti-B is often present in serum. There are different variants of cisAB, but the most common one (*ABO*cisAB.01*) is relatively prevalent in some parts of East Asia, and consequently in individuals with ancestry from these regions. In this variant, an A^1 allele exhibits the presence of a B-specific polymorphism, c.803G>C (p.Gly268Ala), which alters the enzyme's specificity for donor substrate.

Acquired B Phenotype

The acquired B phenotype phenomenon is a transient serologic discrepancy in group A individuals that causes red cell grouping discrepancies.[37] Acquired B should be suspected when a patient or donor who has historically typed as group A newly presents with weak B expression on forward red cell typing. Serologically, the acquired B phenotype shows strong agglutination with anti-A, typically shows weak agglutination (2+ or less) with certain monoclonal and most polyclonal anti-B, and contains a strong anti-B in serum. Despite reactivity of the patient's red cells with anti-B, the patient's serum is not reactive with autologous red cells.

Acquired B is the result of deacetylation of the A antigen *N*-acetylgalactosamine, yielding a B-like galactosamine sugar.[38,39] In patients' samples, acquired B is often present in the setting of infection by gastrointestinal bacteria. Many enteric bacteria possess a deacetylase enzyme capable of converting A antigen to a B-like analog.[39] Identification of the acquired B phenotype can also be influenced by reagent pH and specific monoclonal anti-B typing reagents.[37] In the past, anti-B reagents containing the ES-4 clone were associated with an increased detection of acquired B.

To resolve a patient's true red cell type and confirm the presence of acquired B, red cells should be retyped using a different monoclonal anti-B or acidified (pH 6.0) human anti-B. Acidified human anti-B does not react with acquired B antigen. ABO genotyping can also be useful. Monoclonal anti-B reagents that recognize acquired B should not be used in clinical practice.

ABO Antibodies

Anti-A and Anti-B

Immunoglobulin M (IgM) is the predominant isotype found in group A and group B individuals, although small quantities of IgG antibody can be detected. In group O serum, IgG is a major isotype of anti-A and anti-B. As a consequence, the incidence of ABO hemolytic disease of the fetus and newborn (ABO HDFN) is higher among the offspring of group O mothers than of mothers with other blood types, because IgG can cross the placenta but IgM cannot. However, ABO HDFN is less of a clinical problem than RhD-related HDFN.

Both IgM and IgG anti-A and anti-B preferentially agglutinate red cells at room temperature (20 to 24 C) or cooler, and both can efficiently activate complement at 37 C. The complement-mediated lytic capability of these antibodies becomes apparent if serum testing includes an incubation phase at 37 C. Hemolysis caused by ABO antibodies should be suspected when either the supernatant serum is pink to red or the cell button is smaller or absent. Hemolysis must be interpreted as a positive result. The use of plasma for testing or the use of reagent red cells suspended in solutions that contain EDTA prevents complement activation and hemolysis.

Anti-A,B

Sera from group O individuals contain an antibody known as "anti-A,B" because it is reactive with both A and B red cells. Such anti-A and anti-B reactivity cannot be separated by differential adsorption, suggesting that the antibody recognizes a common epitope shared by the A and B antigens.[7,40] This is the reason that ISBT has acknowledged A,B as the third antigen of the ABO system. Saliva containing secreted A or B substance can inhibit the activity of anti-A,B against both A and B red cells.

Anti-A1

Anti-A1 is present as an alloantibody in the serum of 1% to 8% of A_2 individuals and 22% to 35% of A_2B individuals and is sometimes present in the sera of individuals with other weak A subgroups. Group O serum contains a mixture of anti-A and anti-A1.[39] Because of the presence of the antibody, ISBT has recognized the A1 antigen as the fourth antigen in the ABO system. Anti-A1 can cause ABO discrepancies during routine testing and lead to incompatible crossmatches with A_1 and A_1B red cells. Anti-A1 is usually of IgM isotype, reacting best at room temperature or below, and is usually considered clinically insignificant. Anti-A1 is

considered clinically significant if reactivity is observed at 37 C.[39] Group A_2 patients with an anti-A1 that is reactive at 37 C should be transfused with group A_2 or O red cells; group A_2B patients should receive group A_2, A_2B, B, or O red cells.

Routine Testing for ABO

Donor blood samples are routinely typed for ABO at the time of donation and on receipt of red cell units by the hospital transfusion service (confirmatory typing). The latter is not always practiced outside the US. Recipient samples are typed before transfusion. ABO grouping requires both antigen typing of red cells for A and B antigen (red cell grouping or forward type) and screening of serum or plasma for the presence of anti-A and anti-B isohemagglutinins (serum/plasma grouping or reverse type). Both red cell and serum/plasma grouping are required for donors and patients because each grouping serves as a control for the other. Reverse or serum grouping is not required in two circumstances: 1) for confirmation testing of labeled, previously typed donor red cells and 2) in infants younger than 4 months of age. As previously discussed, isoagglutinins are not present at birth and develop only after 3 to 6 months of age.

Commercially available anti-A and anti-B for red cell typing are extremely potent and agglutinate most antigen-positive red cells directly, even without centrifugation. Most monoclonal typing reagents have been formulated to detect many weak ABO subgroups. (See manufacturers' inserts for specific reagent characteristics.) Additional reagents (anti-A1 and anti-A,B) and special techniques to detect weak ABO subgroups are not necessary for routine testing but are helpful for resolving ABO typing discrepancies.

In contrast to commercial ABO typing reagents, human anti-A and anti-B in the sera of patients and donors can be relatively weak, requiring incubation and centrifugation. Tests for serum grouping, therefore, should be performed using a method that adequately detects human anti-A and anti-B. Several methods are available for determining ABO group, including slide, tube, microplate, and column agglutination techniques.

ABO Discrepancies

Table 10-1 shows the results and interpretations of routine red cell and serum tests for ABO. A discrepancy exists when the results of red cell tests do not agree with those of serum tests, usually because of unexpected negative or positive results in either the forward or reverse typing. (See Table 10-3.) ABO discrepancies may arise from intrinsic problems with either red cells or serum or from technical errors in performing the test. (See Table 10-4 and section on resolving ABO discrepancies.)

When a discrepancy is encountered, the discrepant results must be recorded, but interpretation of the ABO group must be delayed until the discrepancy has been resolved. If the specimen is from a donor unit, the unit must be quarantined and cannot be released for transfusion. When an ABO discrepancy is identified in a patient, it may be necessary to transfuse group O red cells pending an investigation. It is important to obtain a sufficient pretransfusion blood sample from the patient to complete any additional studies that may be required.

Red Cell Testing Problems

ABO testing of red cells may give unexpected results for several reasons, including the following:

1. Weak ABO expression that results from inheritance of a weak ABO subgroup. Some patients with leukemia and other malignancies can also show weakened ABO expression.[13,41]
2. Mixed-field agglutination with circulating red cells of more than one ABO group following out-of-group red cell transfusion or hematopoietic progenitor cell (HPC) transplantation (eg, group O to group A). Mixed-field agglutination is also present in some ABO subgroups (eg, A_3), blood group chi-

merism in fraternal twins, and very rare cases of mosaicism arising from dispermy.

3. Neutralization of anti-A and anti-B typing reagents by high concentrations of A or B blood group substance in serum, resulting in unexpected negative reactions with serum- or plasma-suspended red cells.
4. Spontaneous agglutination or autoagglutination of serum- or plasma-suspended red cells caused by heavy coating of red cells by potent autoagglutinins.
5. Nonspecific aggregation of serum- or plasma-suspended red cells caused by abnormal concentrations of serum proteins or infused macromolecular solutions.
6. False-positive reactions caused by a pH-dependent autoantibody, a reagent-dependent antibody (eg, EDTA or paraben), or rouleaux.
7. Anomalous red cell grouping resulting from acquired B, B(A), cisAB, or A(B) phenotypes.
8. Polyagglutination (eg, T activation) resulting from inherited or acquired abnormalities of the red cell membrane, with exposure of "cryptic autoantigens."[39] Because all human sera contain naturally occurring antibodies to such cryptic antigens, those abnormal red cells are agglutinated also by ABO-compatible human sera. Monoclonal anti-A and anti-B reagents do not detect polyagglutination.

Problems with Serum or Plasma Testing

Problems may arise during ABO testing of serum or plasma, including the following:

1. Small fibrin clots in plasma or incompletely clotted serum that can be mistaken for red cell agglutinates.
2. Lack of detectable isoagglutinins in infants younger than 4 to 6 months. Children do not develop isoagglutinins until 3 to 6 months of age. ABO antibodies present at birth are passively acquired from the mother.

TABLE 10-4. Possible Causes of ABO Typing Discrepancies

Category	Causes
Weak/missing red cell reactivity	ABO subgroup
	Leukemia/malignancy
	Transfusion
	Pregnancy
	Intrauterine fetal transfusion
	Transplantation
	Excessive soluble blood group substance
Extra red cell reactivity	Autoagglutinins/excess protein coating red cells
	Unwashed red cells: plasma proteins
	Unwashed red cells: antibody in patient's serum to reagent constituent
	Transplantation
	Acquired B antigen or other polyagglutinable conditions
	cisAB or B(A) phenomenon
	Out-of-group transfusion
Mixed-field red cell reactivity	ABO subgroup
	Recent transfusion
	Transplantation
	Fetomaternal hemorrhage
	Twin or dispermic (tetragametic) chimerism
Weak/missing serum reactivity	Age related (<4-6 months old or elderly)
	ABO subgroup
	Hypogammaglobulinemia
	Transplantation
	Excessive anti-A or anti-B (prozone effect)
	Hemodilution, eg, by excessive infusion of IV fluids
Extra serum reactivity	Cold autoantibody
	Cold-reactive alloantibody
	Serum antibody to reagent constituent
	Excess serum protein
	Transfusion of plasma components
	Transplantation
	Infusion of intravenous immune globulin

3. Unexpected absence of ABO agglutinins caused by a weak A or B subgroup. (See Table 10-3.)

4. Unexpected absence of anti-B in children receiving long-term parenteral and enteral nutrition who are in a sterile environment and free of bacteria.[42]

5. Unexpected absence of anti-A agglutinins in patients receiving equine-derived immunoglobulins.[43]

6. ABO-incompatible HPC transplantation with induction of tolerance. For example, a group A patient receiving a group O marrow transplant will have circulating group O-like red cells but will produce only anti-B in serum.[44] (Refer to Chapter 27 for more information on ABO-mismatched transplantation.)

7. Severe hypogammaglobulinemia secondary to inherited immunodeficiency or disease therapy. Hypogammaglobulinemia with dilution of isoagglutinins can also occur after several courses of plasma exchange with albumin replacement.

8. Cold alloantibodies (eg, anti-M) or autoantibodies (eg, anti-I) that are reactive with corresponding antigen-positive reverse-grouping cells.

9. Antibodies directed against constituents in the diluents used to preserve reagent A_1 and B red cells.[39]

10. Nonspecific aggregation or agglutination caused by high-molecular-weight plasma expanders, rouleaux, high serum-protein concentrations, or altered serum-protein ratios.

11. Recent transfusion of out-of-group plasma-containing components (eg, a group A patient transfused with platelets from a group O donor, causing unexpected passively acquired anti-A in the patient's plasma).

12. Recent infusion of intravenous immunoglobulin, which can contain ABO isoagglutinins.

Technical Errors

Technical problems with a sample or during testing can also lead to problems in ABO grouping, including:

1. Specimen mix up.
2. Too heavy or too light red cell suspensions.
3. Failure to add reagents.
4. Missed observation of hemolysis.
5. Failure to follow the manufacturer's instructions.
6. Under- or overcentrifugation of tests.
7. Incorrect interpretation or recording of test results.

Resolving ABO Discrepancies

The first step in resolving an apparent serologic testing discrepancy should be to repeat the test with the same sample to exclude the possibility of a technical error during testing. Additional studies may include testing a new sample to avoid mix-up; testing washed red cells; testing for unexpected red cell alloantibodies; and reviewing the patient's medical record for conditions, medications, or recent transfusions that may have contributed to the conflicting test results (Method 2-4). Samples with apparent weak or missing ABO antigens and/or antibodies may require tests using methods that enhance antigen-antibody binding, including incubating red cells at 4 C (Method 2-5), using enzyme-treated red cells (Method 2-6), and conducting adsorption and elution studies (Method 2-7) and molecular testing when warranted. In some instances, it may be useful to test for the secretion of ABH antigens in saliva (Method 2-8). Patients with suspected B(A), acquired B, or A(B) phenotypes should be retested using different monoclonal and human polyclonal reagents.

ABO discrepancies caused by unexpected serum reactions are not uncommon. Commonly encountered causes of serum-grouping discrepancies include cold autoantibodies, rouleaux, cold-reacting alloantibodies (eg, anti-M), and weak A subgroups with an anti-A1. In addition, the presence of certain nondeletional O alleles (*ABO*O.02*) is a common reason for lower anti-A titers in group O individuals, as discussed above.[29,45] To resolve an ABO discrepancy caused by an anti-A1 in a group A individual, red cells should be tested with *Dolichos biflorus* lectin, which agglutinates group A_1 but not A_2 and weaker A subgroups. The presence of an anti-A1 should be confirmed by testing serum against A_1, A_2, and O red cells (Method 2-9). Reverse-grouping problems resulting from either a cold alloantibody (Method 2-10) or autoantibody can be identified with a room-temperature antibody detection test and an autologous control at room temperature. Techniques to identify ABO antibodies in the presence of cold autoantibodies include testing at 37 C without centrifugation (Method 2-11) and cold autoadsorption (Method 4-5). Serum or plasma properties can induce rouleaux formation that resembles agglutination with A_1 and B red cells. Saline replacement or saline dilution (Method 3-7) can be used to distinguish rouleaux from agglutination and identify ABO antibodies.

Cold autoantibodies can cause autoagglutination of red cells and unexpected reactions during red cell typing. Red cells heavily coated with autoantibodies can spontaneously agglutinate and cause false-positive reactions in tests with anti-A and anti-B. Usually, false-positive reactions caused by cold autoantibodies can be eliminated by washing red cells with warm saline (Method 2-17). Autoagglutination caused by IgM can also be inhibited or dispersed by incubating red cells in the presence of either dithiothreitol or 2-aminoethylisothiouronium bromide (Method 3-16). These reagents reduce the disulfide bonds on IgM molecules, decreasing their polyvalency and ability to directly agglutinate red cells.

THE H SYSTEM

H antigen is expressed on all red cells except the rare Bombay phenotype. Because H antigen serves as the precursor to both A and B antigens, the amount of H antigen on red cells depends on an individual's ABO type. H antigen is highly expressed on group O red cells because group O individuals lack a functional ABO gene. In group A and B individuals, the amount of H antigen is considerably less because H is converted to the A and B antigens, respectively. The amount of H antigen on red cells, based on agglutination with the anti-H lectin *Ulex europaeus*, is represented thus: $O>A_2>B>A_2B>A_1>A_1B$. H antigen is present on HPCs, red cells, megakaryocytes, and other tissues.[5,46,47] H antigen has been implicated in cell adhesion, normal hematopoietic differentiation, and several malignancies.[6,7,48]

Biochemistry and Genetics

H antigen is defined by the terminal disaccharide fucose(α1,2)galactose. Two different fucosyltransferase (Fuc-T) enzymes are capable of synthesizing H antigen: α2Fuc-T1 (encoded by *FUT1*, also known as the H gene) and α2Fuc-T2 (encoded by *FUT2*, the secretor gene). The *FUT1* enzyme preferentially fucosylates type 2 chain oligosaccharides on red cell glycoproteins and glycolipids to form H type 2. In contrast, the *FUT2*-encoded enzyme prefers the type 1 chain precursors needed to form H type 1 and Le^b antigens in secretions (Fig 10-4).[13] Secretion of type 1 chain ABH antigens in saliva and other fluids requires a functional FUT2 (secretor) gene. *FUT2* is not expressed in red cells but is expressed in salivary glands, gastrointestinal tissues, and genitourinary tissues.[4,13] Type 1 chain ABH antigens present on red cells are passively adsorbed from circulating glycolipid antigens present in plasma.[39] (See "The Lewis System.") Several inactivating and weakening mutations have been described in both the FUT1 and FUT2 genes.[26] Many of the mutations are geographically and ethnically distributed. For instance, approximately 20% of people of European descent are nonsecretors, and this is mainly the result of homozygosity for the common FUT2*01N.02 allele with c.428G>A, which leads to a premature stop codon (p.Trp143Stop) and a nonfunctional enzyme.

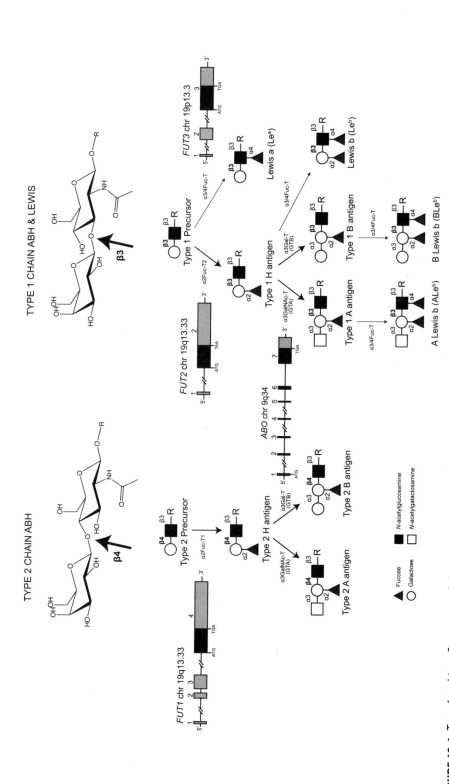

FIGURE 10-4. Type 1 and type 2 precursor chains are shown in the two figures at the top, and the difference (β3 vs β4 linkage) is highlighted with arrows. The genes and enzymes involved in the elongation of precursor to type 1 ABH and Lewis antigens, as well as type 2 ABH antigens, are shown in the lower section of the figure.
Fuc-T = fucosyltransferase; Gal-T = galactosyltransferase; GalNAc-T = *N*-acetylgalactosaminyltransferase; R = upstream carbohydrate sequence.

Null Phenotypes

Bombay (O_h) Phenotype

Originally described in Bombay, India, the O_h or Bombay phenotype is a rare, autosomal recessive phenotype characterized by the absence of H, A, and B antigens on red cells and in secretions. Genetically, O_h individuals are homozygous (or compound heterozygous) for nonfunctional FUT1 and FUT2 genes, resulting in a complete absence of H type 1 and H type 2 chains, and consequently also loss of A and B independent of *ABO* genotype. The original Bombay phenotype is actually the result of a missense mutation (c.725T>G, p.Leu242Arg) in *FUT1* while the entire FUT2 gene is deleted. O_h red cells type as H negative with anti-H lectin *Ulex europaeus*, monoclonal anti-H, and human polyclonal anti-H from other O_h individuals. Because these individuals lack a functional FUT2 (secretor) gene necessary for Le^b synthesis, O_h individuals also type as Le(b–). (See "The Lewis System.") Genotyping studies have described a wide range of inactivating mutations in both the FUT1 and FUT2 genes in O_h individuals.[13,26] The O_h phenotype is also present in leukocyte adhesion deficiency type 2 disease (LAD2) because of a mutation in the GDP-fucose transporter gene.[49]

Because they lack all ABH antigens, O_h individuals possess natural isoagglutinins to A, B, and H. (See Table 10-1.) In routine ABO typing, these individuals initially type as group O. The O_h phenotype becomes apparent during antibody detection tests with group O red cells, which are rich in H antigen. The anti-H present in O_h individuals strongly agglutinates all group O red cells and sometimes demonstrates in-vitro hemolysis. The O_h phenotype can be confirmed by demonstrating an absence of H antigen on red cells and the presence of a strong anti-H in serum that is reactive with group O red cells but not with O_h red cells from other individuals.

Para-Bombay Phenotype

Individuals with the para-Bombay phenotype can be secretors whose red cells are apparently deficient of H antigen.[7,13] Genetically, these individuals are homozygous for a nonfunctional FUT1 gene, but they have inherited at least one functional FUT2 (secretor) gene. The red cells from these H-deficient secretors lack serologically detectable H antigen but can carry small amounts of H, A, and/or B antigen because, unlike persons with classic Bombay phenotype, para-Bombay persons express type 1 chain ABH antigens in their secretions and plasma (Method 2-8).[39] Type 1 chain A and/or B antigens in plasma are then passively adsorbed onto red cells, resulting in weak A or B antigen expression. Red cells from para-Bombay individuals are designated "A_h," "B_h," and "AB_h." Para-Bombay can also occur in group O individuals, as evidenced by trace type 1 chain H on their red cells and in their secretions.

In laboratory testing, red cells from para-Bombay individuals may (or may not) have weak reactions with anti-A and anti-B reagents. In some cases, A and B antigens may be detected only after adsorption and elution. A_h and B_h para-Bombay red cells are nonreactive with anti-H lectin, monoclonal anti-H, and human anti-H from O_h individuals. The sera of para-Bombay individuals contain anti-H, anti-HI, or both and, depending on their ABO type, anti-A and anti-B.[17,39] The anti-H is typically weaker and less clinically significant in para-Bombay than Bombay individuals.

The para-Bombay phenotype can also occur in nonsecretors (ie, without a functional FUT2 gene). In these rare cases, both FUT1 alleles carry mutations that diminish, but do not abolish, the enzyme activity. Therefore, these individuals express small amounts of H type 2 antigen on red cells but lack H type 1 in secretions (and on red cells). If A or B alleles are inherited at the *ABO* locus, the phenotypes can be described as A_h and B_h, respectively.

Anti-H

Alloanti-H (Bombay and Para-Bombay)

The anti-H found in Bombay (O_h) individuals is clinically significant and associated with acute hemolytic transfusion reactions. These antibodies are predominantly of IgM isotype and exhibit a broad thermal range (4 to 37 C) with all red cells except O_h red cells. As with anti-A and anti-B, alloanti-H is capable of activating complement and causing red cell hemolysis intravascularly. The anti-H found in para-Bombay individuals may show lower titers and be less prone to cause direct lysis in vitro but can still be significant.

Autoanti-H and Autoanti-HI

Autoantibodies to H and HI antigens can be encountered in healthy individuals. When present, these autoantibodies are most common in A_1 individuals, who have low levels of H antigen on their red cells. Autoanti-H and autoanti-HI are usually of IgM isotype and are reactive at room temperature.

Transfusion Practice

Alloanti-H is highly clinically significant and is capable of fixing complement and causing hemolytic transfusion reactions. As a result, patients with alloanti-H caused by the Bombay phenotype must be transfused with H-negative (O_h) red cells. The same is true for para-Bombay patients, but in an acute situation, evaluation of the clinical significance in the individual para-Bombay case may be worthwhile.

In contrast, autoantibodies against H and HI are generally clinically insignificant. In most patients, transfused group-specific or group O red cells should have normal in-vivo survival. Occasionally, autoanti-HI can result in decreased red cell survival and hemolytic transfusion reactions after transfusion of group O red cells.[17,39] Hemolysis may follow transfusion of group O red cells to a group A_1, B, or A_1B patient with an unusually potent high-titer anti-HI that is reactive at 37 C.[39] In such patients, transfusion of group-specific (A_1, B, or AB) red cells is advised.

THE LEWIS SYSTEM

The Lewis blood group system consists of two main antigens, Le^a (LE1) and Le^b (LE2), and three common phenotypes, Le(a+b–), Le(a–b+), and Le(a–b–). Four additional Lewis

antigens represent composite reactivity between Le^a, Le^b, and ABH antigens: Le^{ab} (LE3), Le^{bH} (LE4), ALe^b (LE5), and BLe^b (LE6).[26,49] In addition to being present on red cells, Lewis antigens are widely expressed on platelets, endothelial cells, and kidney tissue, as well as on genitourinary and gastrointestinal epithelium.

Lewis antigens are not synthesized by the erythroid cells but are passively adsorbed onto red cell membranes from a pool of soluble Lewis glycolipid present in plasma.[49] The gastrointestinal tract, which is rich in Lewis-active glycolipid and glycoprotein, is thought to be the primary source of Lewis glycolipid in plasma. Because Lewis antigens are passively adsorbed onto red cell membranes, they can be eluted from red cells after transfusion or by increases in plasma volume and increased circulating lipoproteins, which also adsorb Lewis glycolipid. For example, Lewis antigen is often decreased on red cells during pregnancy, with some women transiently typing as Le(a–b–), which is attributed to an increase in circulating plasma volume and a fourfold increase in lipoprotein.[39] The levels of Lewis antigens also decrease on stored red cells, and therefore Lewis phenotyping should be performed sooner than later to avoid false-negative results. Le^b expression and immunoreactivity are also influenced by ABH type as a result of the synthesis of hybrid structures with both Lewis and ABH activity (Fig 10-4).[5,13,47]

Biochemistry and Synthesis

Lewis antigen synthesis depends on the interaction of fucosyltransferases encoded by two distinct genes (Fig 10-4): *FUT3* (the Lewis gene) and *FUT2* (the secretor gene).[49,50] Unlike the enzyme encoded by *FUT1*, which prefers type 2 chain substrates, the enzymes encoded by *FUT2* and *FUT3* preferentially fucosylate type 1 chain substrates. The FUT2 gene therefore controls addition of a terminal $\alpha1,2$ fucose to type 1 chain precursors to form H type 1 antigen. *FUT3*, the Lewis gene, encodes an $\alpha1,3/4$ fucosyltransferase that transfers a fucose, in an $\alpha1,4$ linkage, to the penultimate *N*-acetylglucosamine of the type 1 chain precursor (also known as "Lewis c") to form Le^a

antigen. The Lewis enzyme can also add a second fucose to H type 1 antigen to form Le^b antigen. Le^b cannot be formed from Le^a because the presence of a subterminal fucose on Le^a sterically inhibits binding by the secretor enzyme.[4]

In individuals with both Lewis and secretor enzymes, type 1 chain H is favored over Le^a synthesis. As a result, most of the Lewis antigen synthesized is Le^b [Le(a–b+) phenotype]. In group A$_1$ and B individuals, Le^b and type 1 chain H can be further modified by ABO glycosyltransferases to form LE5 and LE6, the A type 1 and B type 1 antigens, respectively.[5,50] In group A$_1$ individuals, the majority of Lewis antigen in plasma is actually ALe^b.[51]

Genetics and Lewis Phenotypes

The three Lewis phenotypes commonly encountered represent the presence or absence of Lewis and secretor enzymes. (See Table 10-5.) Le(a+b–) individuals have inherited at least one functional FUT3 gene (also denoted *Le*) but are homozygous for nonfunctional FUT2 alleles (denoted *se/se*). As a result, such individuals synthesize and secrete Le^a antigen but lack Le^b and type 1 chain ABH antigens as well as LE5 and LE6. The Le(a–b+) phenotype re-

flects inheritance of both functional FUT3 (Le) and FUT2 (Se) alleles, leading to the synthesis of Le^a, Le^b, and type 1 chain ABH. Because most type 1 chain precursor is converted to Le^b in those individuals, they appear to type as Le(a–). An Le(a+b+) phenotype is transiently observed in infants because secretor activity increases with developmental age. An Le(a+b+) phenotype is also commonly present in individuals of Asian ethnicity (eg, 16% of Japanese individuals) as a result of inheritance of a weak secretor gene (*FUT2*01W.02*, previously *Se^w*).[26] In the absence of a functional FUT3 gene (*le/le*), neither Le^a nor Le^b can be synthesized, leading to the Le(a–b–), or Lewis null, phenotype. Type 1 chain ABH antigens may still be synthesized and secreted in individuals who have inherited at least one functional FUT2 allele (Method 2-8). The Le(a–b–) phenotype is significantly more common in persons of African ethnicity. Although rare, an Le(a–b–) phenotype is also present in individuals with LAD2 due to defects in fucose transport.[49]

Several inactivating mutations have been identified in both the FUT3 (Lewis) and FUT2 (secretor) genes.[26] Many of the mutations are geographically and ethnically distributed, with

TABLE 10-5. Adult Phenotypes and Prevalence Rates in the Lewis System

Red Cell Reactions			Prevalence (%)		Genotype*		
Anti-Le^a	Anti-Le^b	Phenotype	European Ethnicity	African Ethnicity	Lewis	Secretor	Saliva†
+	0	Le(a+b–)	22	23	*Le*	*se/se*	Le^a
0	+	Le(a–b+)	72	55	*Le*	*Se*	Le^a, Le^b, ABH
0	0	Le(a–b–)	6	22	*le/le* *le/le*	*se/se* *Se*	Type 1 precursor Type 1 ABH
+	+	Le(a+b+)‡	Rare	Rare	*Le*	*Se^w*	Le^a, Le^b, ABH

*Probable genotype at the Lewis (*FUT3*) and Secretor (*FUT2*) loci.
†Type 1 chain antigens present in saliva and other secretions.
‡Le(a+b+) is present in 16% of Japanese individuals and is also transiently observed in infants.
Le = at least one FUT3 gene encoding functional Lewis enzyme (represents the genotypes *Le/Le* or *Le/le*); *le/le* = homozygous for FUT3 gene encoding an inactive enzyme; *Se* = At least one FUT2 gene encoding active secretor enzyme (represents the genotypes *Se/Se* or *Se/se*); *se/se* = homozygous for FUT2 gene encoding an inactive enzyme; *Se^w* = FUT2 gene encoding a weak secretor enzyme.

many populations displaying a few predominant alleles.

Lewis Expression in Children

Table 10-5 shows the distribution of Lewis types in adults. In contrast, most newborns type as Le(a–b–). Approximately 50% of newborns subsequently type as Le(a+) after ficin or papain treatment. The prevalence of Le^b antigen, however, is low in newborns compared to adults because of developmental delays in secretor (*FUT2*) activity. An Le(a+b+) phenotype can be transiently present in children as the level of secretor activity approaches adult levels. A valid Lewis phenotype is not developed until age 5 or 6.[17]

Lewis Antibodies

Antibodies against Lewis antigens are generally of IgM isotype and occur naturally. Clinically, Lewis antibodies are most often encountered in the sera of Le(a–b–) individuals and may contain a mixture of anti-Le^a, anti-Le^b, and anti-Le^{ab}, an antibody capable of recognizing both Le(a+) and Le(b+) red cells. Because small amounts of Le^a are synthesized in the Le(a–b+) phenotype, Le(a–b+) individuals do not make anti-Le^a. Anti-Le^b is present infrequently in the Le(a+b–) phenotype. Lewis antibodies, accompanied by a transient Le(a–b–) phenotype, may be present during pregnancy. Finally, anti-Le^b can demonstrate ABO specificity (anti-Le^{bH}, anti-ALe^b, and anti-BLe^b) and is preferentially reactive with Le(b+) red cells of a specific ABO group.[39,47] Anti-Le^{bH}, the most common specificity, is more strongly reactive with Le(b+) group O and A$_2$ red cells than with group A$_1$ and B red cells, which have low H antigen levels. Anti-Le^{bL} is strongly reactive with all Le(b+) red cells, regardless of ABO group.

Most examples of Lewis antibodies are saline agglutinins that are reactive at room temperature. Unlike ABO, the agglutination is relatively fragile and easily dispersed, requiring gentle resuspension after centrifugation. Agglutination is sometimes observed after 37 C incubation, but the reaction is typically weaker than that at room temperature. On occasion, Lewis antibodies can be detected in the anti-human globulin (AHG) phase. Such detection may reflect either IgG or bound complement (if polyspecific AHG reagent is used). Lewis antibodies can sometimes cause hemolysis in vitro, especially when fresh serum and enzyme-treated red cells are used.

Transfusion Practice

In general, Lewis antibodies are not considered clinically significant. Red cells that are compatible in tests at 37 C, regardless of Lewis phenotype, are expected to have normal in-vivo survival. It is not necessary to transfuse antigen-negative red cells in most patients. Unlike ABO antigens, Lewis antigens are extrinsic glycolipid antigens that are readily eluted and shed from transfused red cells within a few days of transfusion.[49] Furthermore, Lewis antigens in transfused plasma can neutralize Lewis antibodies in the recipient. For these reasons, hemolysis in vivo is very rare following transfusion of either Le(a+) or Le(b+) red cells, but exceptions occur.[52]

Lewis antibodies are not a cause of HDFN.[17] Lewis antibodies are predominantly of IgM isotype and do not cross the placenta. In addition, Lewis antigens are poorly expressed on neonatal red cells, with many newborns typing as Le(a–b–).

THE I BLOOD GROUP SYSTEM AND Ii COLLECTION

The I and i antigens are ubiquitous, structurally related antigens present on all cell membranes. The minimum epitope common to both i and I is a repeating lactosamine (Galβ1-4GlcNAc) or type 2 chain precursor. The minimum i antigen epitope is a linear, nonbranched structure containing at least two successive lactosamine motifs.[18] The I antigen is a polyvalent, branched glycan derived from the i antigen (Fig 10-5). Both i and I serve as substrates and scaffolds for the synthesis of ABH, Lewis X [Galβ1-4(Fucα1-3)GlcNAc], and other type 2 chain antigens.[4,5,18] On red cells, i and I antigens are present on *N*-linked glycoproteins and glycosphingolipids. The I antigen belongs to the I system, whereas the i anti-

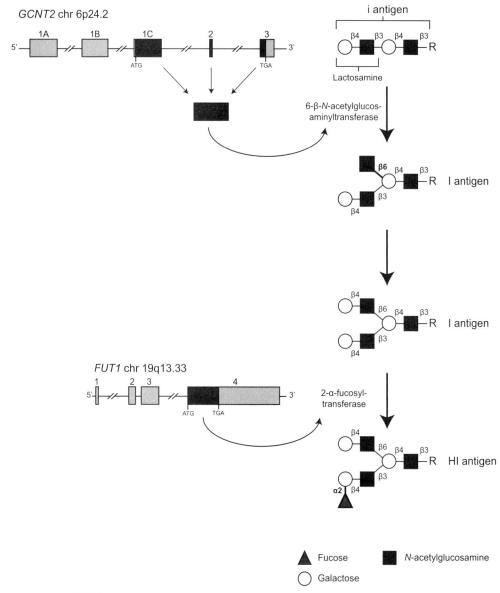

FIGURE 10-5. *GCNT2* and its erythroid transcript that gives rise to the enzyme synthesizing the I antigen from i antigen on red cells. Further elongation by *FUT1*-encoded fucosyltransferase results in the HI antigen. The linkages created by each enzyme are highlighted in bold. ATG and TGA represent the start and stop codons of the gene, respectively.
R = upstream carbohydrate sequence.

gen represents the sole member of the Ii collection.

Phenotypes

Two phenotypes are recognized according to the presence or absence of I antigen: I and i (I–).

The i phenotype is characteristic of neonatal red cells, whereas I+ is the common phenotype in adults. With increasing age, there is a gradual increase in I antigen accompanied by a reciprocal decrease in i antigen as glycan chains are branched; most children develop an adult I+ phenotype by age 2.[18] An increase in i antigen can occur in people with chronic hemolytic disorders and is a sign of stressed erythropoiesis.[53]

Two genetic disorders are associated with an increase in i antigen.[18] The i_{adult} phenotype (I–i+) is an autosomal recessive phenotype caused by mutations in *GCNT2* (previously known as the I or IGnT gene). In populations of Asian ancestry, the i_{adult} phenotype can be associated with congenital cataracts. Increased i antigen levels are also present in people with congenital dyserythropoietic anemia type II (also known as hereditary erythroblastic multinuclearity with positive acidified serum lysis test).

Genetics

The GCNT2 gene encodes a β1-6 *N*-acetylglucosaminyltransferase that converts the linear i antigen into the branched I antigen.[18,26] The gene resides on chromosome 6p24 and contains five exons, including three tissue-specific, alternative exons (exons 1A, 1B, and 1C). As a result, three different mRNA transcripts are synthesized, depending on which exon 1 is used.

In the i_{adult} phenotype without cataracts, there are mutations in exon 1C, which is specific for I antigen synthesis in red cells. Consequently, I antigen is missing on red cells but is still synthesized in other tissues that use either exon 1A or exon 1B. In the i_{adult} phenotype with cataracts, there is a loss of I antigen synthesis in all tissues, caused by either gene deletion or mutations in exons 2 and 3.

Antibodies

Anti-I

Anti-I is common in the serum of healthy individuals. Anti-I is usually of IgM isotype and is strongly reactive at 4 C with titers of <64. Samples with higher titers may also be detectable at room temperature. Anti-I is identified by strong reactions with adult red cells and the autocontrol but weak or no agglutination with cord red cells. (See Table 10-6.) Anti-I can be enhanced by 4 C incubation, the presence of albumin, or use of enzyme-treated red cells. An alloanti-I can be seen in the i_{adult} phenotype.

Some examples of anti-I can demonstrate complex reactivity and are more strongly reactive with red cells of specific ABO, P_1, or Lewis phenotypes. Many of those antibodies appear to recognize branched oligosaccharides that have been further modified to express additional blood group antigens. Anti-HI is commonly present in the serum of A_1 individuals. Anti-HI is more strongly reactive with group O and group A_2 red cells, which are rich in H antigen, than with group A_1 red cells. Anti-HI is suspected when serum from a group A individual directly agglutinates all group O red cells but is compatible with most group A donor blood tested. Other examples of complex reactivity include anti-IA, -IP1, -IBH, and -ILe^{bH}.[39]

TABLE 10-6. Comparative Typical Serologic Behavior of I/i Blood Group Antibodies with Saline Red Cell Suspensions

Temperature	Cell Type	Anti-I	Anti-i
4 C	I adult	4+	0-1+
	i cord	0-2+	3+
	i adult	0-1+	4+
22 C	I adult	2+	0
	i cord	0	2-3+
	i adult	0	3+

Anti-i

Autoanti-i is a relatively uncommon cold agglutinin in sera from healthy individuals. Like
anti-I, anti-i is primarily of IgM isotype but is
weakly reactive at 4 to 10 C. Anti-i is most
strongly reactive with cord and i_{adult} red cells
and more weakly reactive with I+ adult red
cells (Table 10-6). Patients with infectious
mononucleosis often have transient but potent anti-i. As with anti-I, complex reactivity
can sometimes occur (eg, anti-iH).

Cold Agglutinin Syndrome

Autoanti-I and autoanti-i are pathologically
significant in cold agglutinin syndrome (CAS)
and mixed-type autoimmune hemolytic anemia. In those disorders, autoanti-I (or anti-i)
behaves as a complement-binding antibody
with a high titer and wide thermal range. Primary CAS occurs with lymphoproliferative disorders (eg, Waldenström macroglobulinemia,
lymphoma, and chronic lymphocytic leukemia). A potent autoanti-I can also occur in the
setting of infection. *Mycoplasma pneumoniae*
infections are a common cause of autoanti-I
and can be accompanied by a transient, typically intravascular hemolysis. [See Chapter 14
for additional information on CAS (aka cold
agglutinin disease, or CAD).]

The specificity of the autoantibody in CAS
may not be apparent when undiluted samples
are tested. Titration and thermal amplitude
studies may be required to discern the specificity of the autoantibodies and their potential
clinical significance. Table 10-6 illustrates the
serologic behavior of anti-I and anti-i at 4 C
and 22 C. (See Chapter 14 and Method 4-7 for
additional information regarding titration and
thermal amplitude studies.)

Transfusion Practice

Autoanti-I can interfere with ABO typing, antibody screening, and compatibility testing. In
laboratory testing, these antibodies can also
be reactive in the AHG phase of testing, particularly when polyspecific AHG is used. Such reactions rarely indicate antibody activity at 37 C
but are the consequence of antibody binding, followed by complement binding, at
low temperatures. Typically, avoiding room-
temperature testing and using anti-IgG-
specific AHG prevents detection of nuisance
cold autoantibodies. For stronger antibody
samples, autoantibody can be removed from
serum by cold autoadsorption techniques.
(See Method 4-5.) Cold-autoadsorbed serum
can also be used for ABO testing.

**P1PK AND GLOBOSIDE BLOOD
GROUP SYSTEMS AND THE
GLOB COLLECTION**

The first antigen of (what was previously
known as) the P blood group system was discovered by Landsteiner and Levine in 1927 in a
series of experiments that also led to the discovery of M and N antigens. Because this was
actually what is now called the P1 antigen [and
the P antigen belongs to another system,
Globoside (symbol: GLOB)], it was decided in
2010 to change the name of this system to
P1PK. Several related glycosphingolipid antigens belong to the P1PK system (P1, P^k, NOR),
the GLOB system (P, PX2), or the GLOB collection (LKE).[26,54] P^k, P, PX2, and LKE are high-
prevalence antigens expressed on nearly all individuals' red cells except in rare null phenotypes, which lack P, PX2, and LKE (P^k phenotype), or P, P^k, and LKE antigens (p phenotype).
(See Table 10-7.) On the other hand, PX2 is
particularly strongly expressed on red cells of p
phenotype.[55] Red cells are particularly rich in P
antigen (also known as globoside), which
makes up nearly 6% of total red cell lipid. P^k
and P antigens are also widely expressed in
plasma and on nonerythroid cells, including
lymphocytes, platelets, and kidney, lung,
heart, endothelium, placenta, and synovium
cells.[56] In contrast, P1 antigen seems to be
mainly expressed on red cells.[56]

Phenotypes

More than 99.9% of donors have the P_1 (P1+) or
P_2 (P1–) phenotypes. (See Table 10-7.) Both
phenotypes express P^k and P antigens and differ only in the expression of the P1 antigen.
Three rare, autosomal recessive phenotypes

TABLE 10-7. Phenotypes and Prevalence in the P1PK and GLOB Group Systems

Red Cell Reactions with Antisera						Prevalence (%)		
Anti-P1	Anti-P	Anti-P^k	Anti-PP1P^k	Antibodies in Serum	Pheno-type	European Ethnicity	African Ethnicity	Asian Ethnicity
+	+	0/+	+	None	P_1	79	94	20
0	+	0/±	+	Anti-P1*	P_2	21	6	80
0	0[†]	0	0	Anti-PP1$P^{k‡}$	p	Rare	Rare	Rare
+	0	+	+	Anti-P, -PX2	P_1^k	Rare	Rare	Rare
0	0	+	+	Anti-P, -P1, -PX2	P_2^k	Rare	Rare	Rare

*An anti-P1 is detected in approximately 25% of P_2 individuals.
†Usually negative. Some examples of anti-P may be weakly positive as a result of cross-reactivity of anti-P with PX2 on p red cells.
‡Formerly known as anti-Tj^a.

have been identified (p, P_1^k, P_2^k), as well as some rare weak variants.[57,58] Analogous to the ABO system, the rare p and P^k phenotypes are associated with the presence of naturally occurring antibodies against the missing antigens (anti-P1, anti-P, and anti-P^k).

Biochemistry

The synthesis of the P^k, P, and P1 antigens proceeds through the stepwise addition of sugars to lactosylceramide, a ceramide dihexose (CDH) (Fig 10-6 and Table 10-8). The first step in this process is the synthesis of the P^k antigen, the precursor of all globo-series glycosphingolipids. To make the P^k antigen, $\alpha1,4$-galactosyltransferase (which is encoded by *A4GALT*) adds a terminal galactose, in an $\alpha1,4$ linkage, to CDH. The P^k antigen can then serve as a substrate for $\beta1,3$-*N*-acetylgalactosaminyltransferase (encoded by *B3GALNT1*), which adds a $\beta1,3$-linked *N*-acetylgalactosamine to the terminal galactose of P^k (Gb_3) to form P antigen (Gb_4). In some cells, including red cells, the P antigen is further elongated to form additional, globo-family antigens, such as Luke (LKE), type 4 chain ABH antigens (globo-H, -A, and -B), and NOR. NOR, a rare polyagglutinable red cell phenotype, is the re-sult of unusual globo-family antigens characterized by the addition of an $\alpha1-4$ galactose to the terminus of P and related long-chain globoglycolipids (Table 10-8).[59]

Unlike P^k and P antigens, the P1 antigen is not a globo-series glycosphingolipid but is a member of the neolacto family (type 2 chain glycosphingolipids). In P_1 individuals, *A4GALT* adds an $\alpha1-4$ galactose to the terminus of paragloboside. The P1 antigen is not thought to be expressed on red cell glycoproteins.[60] The weak P-like activity on p red cells is conferred by x_2 (renamed PX2 in 2010), a related type 2 chain glycolipid. Recent studies have shown that *B3GALNT1* is capable of synthesizing PX2 and that this is lacking on P^k phenotype red cells.[55]

Genetics

Several inactivating mutations have been identified in both *A4GALT* and *B3GALNT1*.[26,61] The p phenotype is the consequence of mutations in the protein-coding sequence of *A4GALT* but can also be the result of deletions in noncoding upstream exons.[62] In the absence of *A4GALT*-encoded activity, there is a loss of all globo-family and P1 antigens. These individuals have a compensatory increase in type

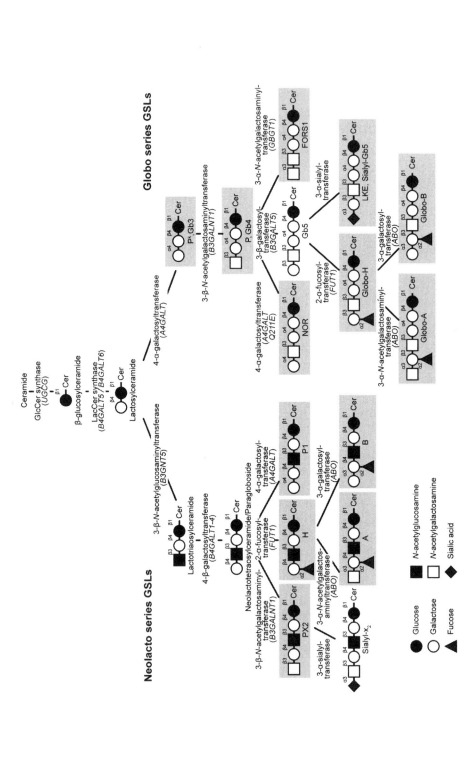

FIGURE 10-6. Synthetic pathways of glycosphingolipids in the neolacto and globo series. Structures acknowledged as blood group antigens are highlighted with a grey box. Glycosyltransferases synthesizing all glycosphingolipids depicted are included, as are the underlying genes (italicized and in brackets), if known. The ABH antigens are presented on type 2 chains in the neolacto series and as type 4 chains in the globo series. GlcCer = glucosylceramide; GSLs = glycosphingolipids; LacCer = lactosylceramide.

TABLE 10-8. Structures of Blood-Group-Carrying Molecules in the P1PK, GLOB, and FORS Systems, and Related Glycosphingolipids

Family*	Name	Oligosaccharide Structure
	CDH	Galβ1-4Glcβ1-1Cer
Globo (Gb)	Gb$_3$, P^k	Galα1-4Galβ1-4Glcβ1-1Cer
	Gb$_4$, P	GalNAcβ1-3Galα1-4Galβ1-4Glcβ1-1Cer
	Gb$_5$	Galβ1-3GalNAcβ1-3Galα1-4Galβ1-4Glcβ1-1Cer
	NOR1	Galα1-4GalNAcβ1-3Galα1-4Galβ1-4Glcβ1-1Cer
	FORS1	GalNAcα1-3GalNAcβ1-3Galα1-4Galβ1-4Glcβ1-1Cer
	Globo-H	Fucα1-2Galβ1-3GalNAcβ1-3Galα1-4Galβ1-4Glcβ1-1Cer
	LKE	NeuAcα2-3Galβ1-3GalNAcβ1-3Galα1-4Galβ1-4Glcβ1-1Cer
	NOR2	Galα1-4GalNAcβ1-3Galα1-4GalNAcβ1-3Galα1-4Galβ1-4Glcβ1-1Cer
Neolacto (nLc)	Lc$_3$	GlcNAcβ1-3Galβ1-4Glcβ1-1Cer
	nLc$_4$, PG	Galβ1-4GlcNAcβ1-3Galβ1-4Glcβ1-1Cer
	P1	Galα1-4Galβ1-4GlcNAcβ1-3Galβ1-4Glcβ1-1Cer
	SPG	NeuAcα2-3Galβ1-4GlcNAcβ1-3Galβ1-4Glcβ1-1Cer
	PX2 (x$_2$)	GalNAcβ1-3Galβ1-4GlcNAcβ1-3Galβ1-4Glcβ1-1Cer
	Sialyl-x$_2$	NeuAcα2-3GalNAcβ1-3Galβ1-4GlcNAcβ1-3Galβ1-4Glcβ1-1Cer

*Glycosphingolipid family. Note: Neolacto are type 2 chain glycosphingolipids.
CDH = ceramide dihexose or lactosylceramide; Cer = ceramide; Gal = galactose; GalNAc = *N*-acetylgalactosamine; Glc = glucose, GlcNAc = *N*-acetylglucosamine; NeuAc = *N*-acetylneuraminic acid (sialic acid); PG = paragloboside; SPG = sialylparagloboside.

2 chain glycolipid synthesis, as evidenced by increased paragloboside, sialoparagloboside, and PX2.[55] Mutations in *B3GALNT1* give rise to the P^k phenotype, which is characterized by a loss of P, LKE, and PX2 antigens and by increased P^k expression. The mechanism underlying the P$_1$ vs P$_2$ phenotype is still under investigation, but polymorphisms have been identified in a novel exon in *A4GALT* as well as in the surrounding intron sequences.[57,63] Interestingly, individuals with weak P1 expression are heterozygous for P^{1}P^2 alleles.[57]

P1PK and GLOB System Antibodies

Anti-P1

Anti-P1 is present in the sera of one-quarter to two-thirds of P$_2$ donors.[39] Anti-P1 is a naturally occurring antibody of IgM isotype and is often detected as a weak, room-temperature agglutinin. In rare cases, anti-P1 is reactive at 37 C or shows in-vitro hemolysis. Because anti-P1 is nearly always IgM, anti-P1 does not cross the placenta and has not been reported to cause HDFN. Anti-P1 has only rarely been reported to cause in-vivo hemolysis. Anti-P1 titers are often elevated in patients with hydatid cyst disease or fascioliasis (liver fluke) and in bird handlers. It is believed that P1-like substance in bird excrement can stimulate anti-P1 levels. Some people with anti-P1 also have I blood group specificity (anti-IP1).[39]

P1 expression varies in strength among individuals according to genotype[57] and has been reported to decrease during in-vitro storage.[39] As a consequence, anti-P1 may not be reactive with all P1+ red cells tested. Anti-P1 can be enhanced by incubation at low temperatures (eg, 4 C) or by testing serum against enzyme-treated red cells. Anti-P1 reactivity can be inhibited in the presence of hydatid cyst fluid or P1 substance derived from pigeon eggs. Inhibiting P1 activity may be helpful when testing sera containing multiple antibodies.

Alloanti-PP1P^k and Alloanti-P

Anti-PP1P^k (historically known as anti-Tj^a) is a separable mixture of anti-P, anti-P1, and anti-P^k in the sera of p individuals. Alloanti-P is present in the sera of P$_1^k$ and P$_2^k$ individuals (see Table 10-7), occurs naturally, and is predominantly of IgM isotype or a mixture of IgM and IgG. The antibodies are potent hemolysins and are associated with hemolytic transfusion reactions and, occasionally, HDFN. There is an association between anti-PP1P^k (in the p phenotype) or anti-P (in the P$_1^k$/P$_2^k$ phenotypes) and early, recurrent spontaneous abortions. The placenta, which is of fetal origin, is rich in P^k and P antigen and is a target for maternal cytotoxic IgG antibodies.[64]

Autoanti-P (Donath-Landsteiner)

An autoantibody with P specificity is present in patients with paroxysmal cold hemoglobinuria (PCH), a clinical syndrome that most commonly occurs in children following viral infection. In PCH, autoanti-P is an IgG biphasic hemolysin capable of binding red cells at colder temperatures, which is followed by intravascular hemolysis at body temperature. This characteristic can be demonstrated in vitro in the Donath-Landsteiner test. (See Chapter 14 and Method 4-11.)

Transfusion Practice

Alloanti-PP1P^k and alloanti-P are clinically significant antibodies associated with acute hemolytic transfusion reactions and spontaneous abortion. Rare individuals of p and P^k phenotypes should be provided with antigen-negative, crossmatch-compatible red cells for transfusion. Because P^k individuals have both anti-P and anti-PX2 in their sera, the provision of red cell units of p phenotype should be

avoided even if they are P negative. The p phenotype exhibits the highest expression of PX2 of all phenotypes.[55]

In general, anti-P1 is a clinically insignificant, room-temperature agglutinin. Patients with anti-P1, which is reactive only at room temperature or below, can be safely transfused with P1+ red cells, which results in normal red cell survival. It is not necessary to provide antigen-negative units to these patients. Very rarely, anti-P1 can cause decreased red cell survival and hemolytic transfusion reactions.

Anti-P1 that is capable of fixing complement at 37 C and is strongly reactive in the AHG phase of testing is considered potentially clinically significant. In such rare instances, units selected for transfusion should be nonreactive at 37 C and in an indirect antiglobulin test with either polyspecific AHG or anti-C3.[39]

THE FORS BLOOD GROUP SYSTEM

The latest addition to the carbohydrate blood group systems came in 2012, when the FORS system was acknowledged by ISBT. This system harbors a single low-prevalence antigen, FORS1, a glycosphingolipid synthesized by addition of N-acetylgalactosamine in an $\alpha 1,3$ linkage to the P antigen (Fig 10-6). Because this antigen bears a certain resemblance to the A antigen, which terminates with the same $\alpha 1,3$-linked sugar residue, some polyclonal anti-A reagents may react with FORS1-positive red cells of group O. Thus, the FORS1-positive phenotype was originally reported in 1987 as a new ABO subgroup, A$_{pae}$, found in three English families.[65] These red cells reacted weakly with some anti-A but were strongly positive with *Helix pomatia* lectin and negative with *Dolichos biflorus*. When *ABO* genotyping showed homozygosity for common O alleles, it was revealed that the reactive antigen was not A but FORS1.[66] The responsible gene is *GBGT1*, which encodes Forssman synthase, a glycosyltransferase able to create this specific linkage in many mammals. This gene had previously been considered a pseudogene in humans but was shown to be reactivated by c.887G>A (p.Arg296Gln) in FORS1-positive individuals.[66] Interestingly, most people have naturally occurring anti-FORS1 in plasma. These antibodies may cause hemolysis in vitro, but their clinical relevance is not yet known. A summary of more information about this new blood group system was recently published.[67]

ACKNOWLEDGMENT

The current authors thank the previous authors of this chapter, in particular Dr. Laura Cooling, for their contributions.

KEY POINTS

1. The antigens of the ABO, H, Lewis, I, P1PK, GLOB and FORS blood group systems are defined by carbohydrate epitopes on glycoproteins and glycosphingolipids. They are synthesized by a group of Golgi-residing enzymes called glycosyltransferases and are considered histo-blood-group antigens because of their broad tissue distribution.

2. The ABO system contains four major ABO phenotypes: A, B, O, and AB. The four phenotypes result from the combination of ABO alleles inherited, and are determined by the presence or absence of A and B glycosyltransferase, which synthesize A and B antigens, respectively, on red cells. An inverse reciprocal relationship exists between the presence of A and B antigens on red cells and the presence of anti-A, anti-B, or both, in sera.

3. ABO grouping requires both antigen typing of red cells for A and B antigen (red cell grouping or forward type) and typing of serum or plasma for the presence of anti-A and anti-B isoagglutinins (serum grouping or reverse type). ABO discrepancies occur when forward and reverse typing do not agree, and can be resolved with additional testing with methods to enhance missing reactivity or eliminate spurious reactivity, and if available, the use of ABO and FUT1/FUT2 gene sequencing.

4. H antigen is ubiquitously expressed on all red cells, except in the rare Bombay (O_h) phenotype, in which both H-synthesizing fucosyltransferases encoded by the FUT1 and FUT2 genes are inactive or absent.

5. H antigen is the precursor to both A and B antigens; thus, the amount of H antigen on red cells depends on the person's ABO group. H antigen is highly expressed on group O red cells because group O persons lack a functional ABO gene. In group A_1 and B persons, the amount of H antigen is considerably less because H is converted to the A and B antigens, respectively.

6. Lewis antigens are not synthesized by red cells but are passively adsorbed onto red cell membranes from soluble Lewis glycolipids present in plasma.

7. The three common Lewis phenotypes indicate the presence or absence of functional glycosyltransferases encoded by the FUT3 (Lewis) and FUT2 (secretor) genes.

8. With increasing age, there is a gradual increase in I antigen accompanied by a reciprocal decrease in i antigen. Most children develop an adult I+ phenotype by age 2.

9. Autoanti-I and autoanti-i are pathogenetically significant in cold agglutinin syndrome and mixed-type autoimmune hemolytic anemia.

10. More than 99.9% of donors have the P_1 (P1+) or P_2 (P1–) phenotypes. Both phenotypes synthesize P^k and P antigens and differ mainly in the expression of the P1 antigen. Other rare phenotypes (P_1^k, P_2^k, and p) exist, in which naturally occurring antibodies against P^k and P can give rise to hemolytic transfusion reactions and recurrent spontaneous abortions.

11. FORS is a newly recognized blood group system. The frequency of its FORS1 antigen is very low in all populations tested, but most people have naturally occurring anti-FORS1 in their plasma.

REFERENCES

1. Paulson JC, Colley KJ. Glycosyltransferases: Structure, localization, and control of cell type-specific glycosylation. J Biol Chem 1989; 264:17615-18.

2. Hansen SF, Bettler E, Rinnan A, et al. Exploring genomes for glycosyltransferases. Mol Biosyst 2010;6:1773-81.

3. Clausen H, Hakomori S. ABH and related histo-blood group antigens; immunochemical differences in carrier isotypes and their distribution. Vox Sang 1989;56:1-20.

4. Lowe JB, Marth JD. A genetic approach to mammalian glycan function. Ann Rev Biochem 2003;72:643-91.

5. Marionneau S, Cailleau-Thomas A, Rocher J, et al. ABH and Lewis histo-blood group antigens, a model for the meaning of oligosaccharide diversity in the face of a changing world. Biochimie 2001;83:565-73.

6. Anstee DJ. The relationship between blood groups and disease. Blood 2010;115:4635-43.

7. Storry JR, Olsson ML. The ABO blood group system revisited: A review and update. Immunohematology 2009;25:48-59.

8. Rydberg L. ABO-incompatibility in solid organ transplantation. Transfus Med 2001;11:325-42.

9. Sazama K. Reports of 355 transfusion-associated deaths: 1976 through 1985. Transfusion 1990;30:583-90.

10. Linden JV, Wagner K, Voytovich AE, Sheehan J. Transfusion errors in New York state: An analysis of 10 years' experience. Transfusion 2000; 40:1207-13.

11. Springer GF. Blood-group and Forssman antigenic determinants shared between microbes and mammalian cells. Prog Allergy 1971;15:9-77.

12. Daniel-Johnson J, Leitman S, Klein H, et al. Probiotic-associated high-titer anti-B in a group A platelet donor as a cause of severe hemolytic transfusion reactions. Transfusion 2009;49:1845-9.

13. Daniels G. Human blood groups. 3rd ed. Oxford: Wiley-Blackwell, 2013.

14. Henry S, Oriol R, Samuelsson B. Lewis histo-blood group system and associated secretory phenotypes. Vox Sang 1995;69:166-82.

15. Clausen H, Levery SB, Nudelman E, et al. Repetitive A epitope (type 3 chain A) defined by blood group A1-specific monoclonal antibody TH-1: Chemical basis of qualitative A1 and A2 distinction. Proc Natl Acad Sci U S A 1985;82: 1199-203.

16. Svensson L, Rydberg L, de Mattos LC, Henry SM. Blood group A(1) and A(2) revisited: An immunochemical analysis. Vox Sang 2009; 96:56-61.

17. Klein HG, Anstee DJ. ABO, H, LE, P1PK, GLOB, I and FORS blood group systems. In: Mollison's blood transfusion in clinical medicine. 12th ed. Oxford: Wiley-Blackwell, 2014:118-66.

18. Cooling L. Polylactosamines, there's more than meets the "Ii": A review of the I system. Immunohematology 2010;26:133-55.

19. Twu YC, Hsieh CY, Lin M, et al. Phosphorylation status of transcription factor C/EBP alpha determines cell-surface poly-LacNAc branching (I antigen) formation in erythropoiesis and granulopoiesis. Blood 2010;115:2491-9.

20. Auf der Maur C, Hodel M, Nydegger UE, Rieben R. Age dependency of ABO histo-blood group antibodies: Reexamination of an old dogma. Transfusion 1993;33:915-18.

21. Mazda T, Yabe R, NaThalang O, et al. Differences in ABO antibody levels among blood donors: A comparison between past and present Japanese, Laotian, and Thai populations. Immunohematology 2007;23:38-41.

22. Sano R, Nakajima T, Takahashi K, et al. Expression of ABO blood-group genes is dependent upon an erythroid cell-specific regulatory element that is deleted in persons with the B(m) phenotype. Blood 2012;119:5301-10.

23. Kronstein-Wiedemann R, Nowakowska P, Milanov P, et al. miRNA regulation of blood group ABO genes (abstract). Blood 2015;126:158.

24. Clausen H, White T, Takio K, et al. Isolation to homogeneity and partial characterization of a histo-blood group A defined Fuc-alpha1-2Gal alpha1-3-N-acetylgalactosaminyltransferase from human lung tissue. J Biol Chem 1990;265: 1139-45.

25. Yamamoto F, Clausen H, White T, et al. Molecular genetic basis of the histo-blood group ABO system. Nature 1990;345:229-33.

26. Reid ME, Lomas-Francis C, Olsson ML. The blood group antigen factsbook. 3rd ed. London: Academic Press, 2012.

27. Hosseini-Maaf B, Irshaid NM, Hellberg Å, et al. New and unusual O alleles at the ABO locus are implicated in unexpected blood group phenotypes. Transfusion 2005;45:70-81.

28. Seltsam A, Das Gupta C, Wagner FF, Blasczyk R. Nondeletional ABO*O alleles express weak blood group A phenotypes. Transfusion 2005; 45:359-65.

29. Wagner FF, Blasczyk R, Seltsam A. Nondeletional ABO*O alleles frequently cause blood donor typing problems. Transfusion 2005;45: 1331-4.

30. Yazer MH, Hult AK, Hellberg Å, et al. Investigation into A antigen expression on O2 heterozygous group O-labeled red blood cell units. Transfusion 2008;48:1650-7.

31. Cartron JP. [Quantitative and thermodynamic study of weak A erythrocyte phenotypes]. Rev Fr Transfus Immunohematol 1976;19:35-54.

32. Berneman ZN, Van Bockstaele DR, Uyttenbroeck WM, et al. Flow-cytometric analysis of erythrocytic blood group A antigen density profile. Vox Sang 1991;61:265-74.

33. Hosseini-Maaf B, Hellberg Å, Chester MA, Olsson ML. An extensive PCR-ASP strategy for clinical ABO blood group genotyping that avoids potential errors caused by null, subgroup and hybrid alleles. Transfusion 2007;47: 2110-25.

34. Hult AK, Olsson ML. Many genetically defined ABO subgroups exhibit characteristic flow cytometric patterns. Transfusion 2010;50:308-23.

35. Beck ML, Yates AD, Hardman J, Kowalski MA. Identification of a subset of group B donors reactive with monoclonal anti-A reagent. Am J Clin Pathol 1989;92:625-9.

36. Yazer MH, Olsson ML, Palcic MM. The cis-AB blood group phenotype: Fundamental lessons in glycobiology. Transfus Med Rev 2006;20: 207-17.

37. Garratty G, Arndt P, Co A, et al. Fatal hemolytic transfusion reaction resulting from ABO mistyping of a patient with acquired B antigen detectable only by some monoclonal anti-B reagents. Transfusion 1996;36:351-7.

38. Okubo Y, Seno T, Tanaka M, et al. Conversion of group A red cells by deacetylation to ones that react with monoclonal antibodies specific for the acquired B phenotype. Transfusion 1994;34:456-7.

39. Issitt PD, Anstee DJ. Applied blood group serology. 3rd ed. Miami, FL: Montgomery Scientific Publications, 1998.

40. Obukhova P, Korchagina E, Henry S, Bovin N. Natural anti-A and anti-B of the ABO system: Allo- and autoantibodies have different epitope specificity. Transfusion 2012;52:860-9.

41. Olsson ML, Irshaid NM, Hosseini-Maaf B, et al. Genomic analysis of clinical samples with serologic ABO blood grouping discrepancies: Identification of 15 novel A and B subgroup alleles. Blood 2001;98:1585-93.

42. Cooling LW, Sitwala K, Dake LR, et al. ABO typing discrepancies in children requiring long-term nutritional support: It is the gut after all! (abstract) Transfusion 2007;47(Suppl 1):10A.

43. Shastry S, Bhat SS, Singh K. A rare case of missing antibody due to anti-snake venom. Transfusion 2009;49:2777-8.

44. Hult AK, Dykes JH, Storry JR, Olsson ML. A and B antigen levels acquired by group O donor-derived erythrocytes following ABO-non-identical transfusion or minor ABO-incompatible haematopoietic stem cell transplantation. Transfus Med 2017;27:181-91.

45. Yazer MH, Hosseini-Maaf B, Olsson ML. Blood grouping discrepancies between ABO genotype and phenotype caused by O alleles. Curr Opin Hematol 2008;15:618-24.

46. Molne J, Bjorquist P, Andersson K, et al. Blood group ABO antigen expression in human embryonic stem cells and in differentiated hepatocyte- and cardiomyocyte-like cells. Transplantation 2008;86:1407-13.

47. Larson G, Svensson L, Hynsjö L, et al. Typing for the human Lewis blood group system by quantitative fluorescence-activated flow cytometry: Large differences in antigen presentation on erythrocytes between A(1), A(2), B, O phenotypes. Vox Sang 1999;77:227-36.

48. Hosoi E, Hirose M, Hamano S. Expression levels of H-type alpha(1,2)-fucosyltransferase gene and histo-blood group ABO gene corresponding to hematopoietic cell differentiation. Transfusion 2003;43:65-71.

49. Combs MR. Lewis blood group system review. Immunohematology 2009;25:112-18.

50. Cooling L. Carbohydrate blood group antigens and collections. In: Petrides M, Stack G, Cooling L, Maes L, eds. Practical guide to transfusion medicine. 2nd ed. Bethesda, MD: AABB Press, 2007:59-91.

51. Lindstrom K, Breimer ME, Jovall PA, et al. Non-acid glycosphingolipid expression in plasma of an A1 Le(a-b+) secretor human individual: Identification of an ALeb heptaglycosylceramide as major blood group component. J Biochem 1992;111:337-45.

52. Höglund P, Rosengren-Lindquist R, Wikman AT. A severe haemolytic transfusion reaction

caused by anti-Le(a) active at 37 degrees C. Blood Transfus 2013;11:456-9.

53. Navenot JM, Muller JY, Blanchard D. Expression of blood group i antigen and fetal hemoglobin in paroxysmal nocturnal hemoglobinuria. Transfusion 1997;37:291-7.

54. Storry JR, Castilho L, Chen Q, et al. International Society of Blood Transfusion Working Party on Red Cell Immunogenetics and Terminology: Report of the Seoul and London meetings. ISBT Sci Ser 2016;11:118-22.

55. Westman JS, Benktander J, Storry JR, et al. Identification of the molecular and genetic basis of PX2, a glycosphingolipid blood group antigen lacking on globoside-deficient erythrocytes. J Biol Chem 2015;290:18505-18.

56. Cooling L, Downs T. Immunohematology. In: McPherson RA, Pincus MR, eds. Henry's clinical diagnosis and management by laboratory methods. 22nd ed. Philadelphia: Saunders, 2007:618-68.

57. Thuresson B, Westman JS, Olsson ML. Identification of a novel *A4GALT* exon reveals the genetic basis of the P1/P2 histo-blood groups. Blood 2011;117:678-87.

58. Cooling L, Dake LR, Haverty D, et al. A hemolytic anti-LKE associated with a rare LKE-negative, "weak P" red blood cell phenotype: Alloanti-LKE and alloanti-P recognize galactosylgloboside and monosialo-galactosylgloboside (LKE) antigens. Transfusion 2015;55:115-28.

59. Duk M, Singh S, Reinhold VN, et al. Structures of unique globoside elongation products present in erythrocytes with a rare NOR phenotype. Glycobiology 2007;17:304-12.

60. Yang Z, Bergström J, Karlsson KA. Glycoproteins with Gal alpha 4Gal are absent from human erythrocyte membranes, indicating that glycolipids are the sole carriers of blood group P activities. J Biol Chem 1994;269:14620-4.

61. Hellberg Å, Ringressi A, Yahalom V, et al. Genetic heterogeneity at the glycosyltransferase loci underlying the GLOB blood group system and collection. Br J Haematol 2004;125:528-36.

62. Westman JS, Hellberg Å, Peyrard T, et al. Large deletions involving the regulatory upstream regions of *A4GALT* give rise to principally novel P1PK-null alleles. Transfusion 2014;54:1831-5.

63. Lai YJ, Wu WY, Yang CM, et al. A systematic study of single-nucleotide polymorphisms in the *A4GALT* gene suggests a molecular genetic basis for the P1/P2 blood groups. Transfusion 2014;54:3222-31.

64. Lindström K, von dem Borne AE, Breimer ME, et al. Glycosphingolipid expression in spontaneously aborted fetuses and placenta from blood group p women. Evidence for placenta being the primary target for anti-Tja-antibodies. Glycoconj J 1992;9:325-9.

65. Stamps R, Sokol RJ, Leach M, et al. A new variant of blood group A. Apae. Transfusion 1987;27:315-18.

66. Svensson L, Hult AK, Stamps R, et al. Forssman expression on human erythrocytes: Biochemical and genetic evidence of a new histo-blood group system. Blood 2013;121:1459-68.

67. Hult AK, Olsson ML. The FORS awakens: A review of a blood group system reborne. Immunohematology 2017;33:64-72.

11

The Rh System

• ● •

Gregory A. Denomme, PhD, FCSMLS(D)

THE RH SYSTEM is composed of two genes, each encoding a polypeptide, that together are responsible for the expression of 54 antigens (Table 11-1). The genetic alterations underlying the expression of Rh antigens make this system one of the most complex among the 36 human blood group systems. The attention to red cell alloimmunization relative to this system stems from the D antigen, which is the most immunogenic of all minor blood group antigens. Mollison's textbook states[2]: "When a relatively large amount of D-positive red cells (200 ml or more) is transfused to D-negative subjects, within 2-5 months anti-D can be detected in the plasma of some 85% of the recipients." Although the frequency of anti-D alloimmunization among transfusion recipients varies widely,[3] the impact of alloimmunization in Rh-negative females of childbearing potential and the significant risk of harm to an Rh-positive fetus make D-antigen matching a routine practice in transfusion medicine.

A true success story in transfusion medicine therapy in the mid-1960s, the development of Rh Immune Globulin (RhIG) prophylaxis arose partly from the observation that ABO incompatibility between a mother and fetus had a partial protective effect against immunization to D.[4] The administration of immunoglobulin G (IgG) anti-D obtained from human plasma was effective in the prevention of hemolytic disease of the fetus and newborn (HDFN).[5] With the use of RhIG, alloimmunization to D in pregnancy has been reduced to about 1 in 4000 live births.[6]

HISTORICAL PERSPECTIVE

The clinical impact of the D antigen dates to 1939 when Levine and Stetson made the key observation that the serum of a pregnant woman agglutinated some 80% of ABO-compatible samples. The authors proposed that "products of the disintegrating fetus" and an adverse transfusion reaction in the mother to a blood transfusion from her husband were related to the hemagglutinin found in her serum.[7] Initially, the D antigen was confused with LW because of the development of an antiserum raised against Rhesus macaque monkey red cells. A good historical account of confusion of the D antigen with the LW system has been described by Rosenfield.[8]

"Rh positive" and "Rh negative" refer to the D antigen status of red cells. The D and

Gregory A. Denomme, PhD, FCSMLS(D), Senior Director of Immunohematology and Innovation, Diagnostic Laboratories, and Senior Investigator, Blood Research Institute, BloodCenter of Wisconsin, Milwaukee, Wisconsin

The author has disclosed a financial relationship with Grifols.

TABLE 11-1. Rh Antigens by Common Name, ISBT Terminology, and Prevalence

| Antigen | ISBT Terminology | | Prevalence | Comment |
	Number	Symbol		
D	004.001	RH1	Common	85%/92% Whites/Blacks
C	004.002	RH2	Common	68%/27% Whites/Blacks
E	004.003	RH3	Common	29%/22% Whites/Blacks
c	004.004	RH4	High	80%/96% Whites/Blacks
e	004.005	RH5	98%	
ce or f	004.006	RH6	Common	65%/92% Whites/Blacks
Ce or rh_i	004.007	RH7	Common	68%/27% Whites/Blacks
C^W	004.008	RH8	2%	Whites
C^X	004.009	RH9	~2%	Finns
V	004.010	RH10	30%	Blacks
E^W	004.011	RH11	Low	
G	004.012	RH12*	Common	84%/92% Whites/Blacks
...	...	RH13-RH16	...	Obsolete
Hr_0	004.017	RH17[†]	High	
Hr	004.018	RH18[‡]	High	
hr^S	004.019	RH19[§]	High	98% Blacks
VS	004.020	RH20	Common	32% Blacks
C^G	004.021	RH21	Common	68% Whites
CE	004.022	RH22	Low	<1%
D^W	004.023	RH23[◊]	Low	on DVa
...	...	RH24/RH25	...	Obsolete
c-like	004.026	RH26	High	
cE	004.027	RH27	Common	28%/22% Whites/Blacks
hr^H	004.028	RH28	Low	
total Rh	004.029	RH29[¶]	High	100% except Rh_{null}
Go^a	004.030	RH30[◊]	Low	
hr^B	004.031	RH31[§]	High	
Rh32	004.032	RH32[#]	Low	1% Blacks on DBT
Ro^{Har}, DHAR	004.033	RH33	Low	<1% Germans
Hr^B	004.034	RH34**	High	
Rh35	004.035	RH35	Low	
Be^a	004.036	RH36	Low	

TABLE 11-1. Rh Antigens by Common Name, ISBT Terminology, and Prevalence (Continued)

Antigen	ISBT Terminology Number	ISBT Terminology Symbol	Prevalence	Comment
Evans	004.037	RH37	Low	on D/CE hybrids
...	...	RH38	...	Obsolete
C-like	004.039	RH39	High	
Tar	004.040	RH40	Low	on DVII
Ce-like	004.041	RH41	High	70% Whites
Ce^S	004.042	RH42	Low	2% Blacks
Crawford	004.043	RH43	Low	0.1% Blacks
Nou	004.044	RH44	High	
Riv	004.045	RH45	Low	
Sec	004.046	RH46	High	
Dav	004.047	RH47	High	
JAL	004.048	RH48	Low	
STEM	004.049	RH49[††]	Low	6% Blacks
FPTT	004.050	RH50	Low	on DFR, R_0^{Har}
MAR	004.051	RH51	High	
BARC	004.052	RH52[◊]	Low	on DVI
JAHK	004.053	RH53	Low	
DAK	004.054	RH54[◊]	Low	$DIII^a$, DOL, R^N
LORC	004.055	RH55	Low	
CENR	004.056	RH56	Low	
CEST	004.057	RH57	High	Antithetical to JAL
CELO	004.058	RH58	High	Antithetical to RH43
CEAG	004.059	RH59	High	
PARG	004.060	RH60	Low	
CEVF	004.061	RH61	Low	

*Present on red cells expressing C or D antigen.
†Antibody made by individuals with D-deletion phenotypes D−−, Dc−, and DC^w−.
‡Antibody made by individuals with altered e and/or D phenotypes prevalent in groups of African ethnicity.
§Absent from red cells with DcE/DcE (R_2R_2) phenotype or variant e found in groups of African ethnicity.
◊Low-prevalence antigen associated with the partial D indicated.
¶Antibody made by individuals with Rh_{null} red cells.
#Low-prevalence antigen expressed by red cells with R^N or the partial DBT antigen.[1]
**Antibody made by individuals with altered C, E, and/or D phenotypes prevalent in groups of African ethnicity.
††Associated with 65% of hr^S− Hr− and 30% of hr^B−Hr^B− red cells.

ABO antigens are the principal antigens matched for transfusion. Along with the D antigen, four Rh antigens—antithetical C/c and E/e, named by Fisher using the next available letters of the alphabet—are responsible for the majority of clinically significant Rh antibodies.

Rh proteins, unlike most membrane proteins, are neither glycosylated nor phosphorylated.[9,10] The use of immunoprecipitation followed by sodium dodecylsulfate polyacrylamide gel electrophoresis led to the discovery that Rh proteins have a molecular weight of 30,000 to 32,000 kDa.[11,12] N-terminal amino acid sequencing of Rh was accomplished in the late 1980s.[13] The findings led to the cloning of the RHCE gene in 1990[14] and of the RHD gene in 1992.[15,16] The genetic basis of four different RHCE alleles was identified in 1994.[17]

TERMINOLOGY

Early Rh nomenclature reflects the differences in opinion concerning the number of genes that encode DCE antigens. The Fisher-Race terminology was based on the premise that three closely linked genes, C/c, E/e, and D, were responsible. In contrast, the Wiener nomenclature (Rh-Hr) was based on the belief that a single gene encoded several blood group factors. However, the Rh system is composed of two genes, as proposed by Tippett.[18]

The Fisher-Race CDE terminology is often preferred for written communication, but a modified version of Wiener's nomenclature makes it possible to identify the Rh antigens present on one chromosome using a single term, that is, using a haplotype (Table 11-2). In the modified Wiener's nomenclature, "R" indicates that D is present, and a number or letter indicates the C/c and E/e antigens: R1 for Ce, R2 for cE, R0 for ce, and Rz for CE. The lowercase "r" indicates haplotypes lacking D, with the C/c and E/e antigens indicated using symbols: r' for Ce, r" for cE, and r^y for CE (Table 11-2).

The International Society of Blood Transfusion (ISBT) Working Party on Red Cell Immunogenetics and Blood Group Terminology adopted six-digit numbers to indicate red cell antigens. The first three numbers represent the system, and the remaining three digits refer to the antigenic specificity; the Rh system was assigned number 004. The Rh system has recorded 61 antigens, with 7 antigens deemed obsolete. In 2008, the ISBT committee recog-

TABLE 11-2. Prevalence of the Principal Rh Haplotypes

Fisher-Race Haplotype	Modified Wiener Haplotype	Prevalence (%)		
		White	Black	Asian
Rh positive				
DCe	R1	42	17	70
DcE	R2	14	11	21
Dce	R0	4	44	3
DCE	Rz	<0.01	<0.01	1
Rh negative				
ce	r	37	26	3
Ce	r'	2	2	2
cE	r"	1	<0.01	<0.01
CE	r^y	<0.01	<0.01	<0.01

nized antigens of the Rh-associated glycopro-tein (RHAG) as the 30th blood group system.

RH LOCUS

Chromosomal Structure

The two genes responsible for the expression of Rh antigens, *RHD* and *RHCE*, are closely linked near the 3′ end of chromosome 1p36.11. *RHD* and *RHCE* are oriented in a tail-to-tail arrangement: telomere – 5′-*RHD*-3′ – 3′-*RHCE*-5′ – centromere, with a blood-group-irrelevant gene, *TMEM50A*, overlapping the 3′ end of *RHCE*, and another gene, *RSRP1*, com-pletely overlapping *RHD* but in the opposite orientation [Fig 11-1 (A)]. *RHD* likely arose from *RHCE* in a duplication event.[19] Each gene has 10 exons, and overall the two genes share 97% sequence identity in the coding region.

Nucleotide changes are common for both genes and are thought to be facilitated by their inverted orientation.[20] The inverted orienta-tion promotes hairpin loop formation and subsequent genetic exchange via template conversion; one gene acts as a donor template during replication but remains unchanged in the process. The donated region can be one nucleotide or span several base pairs, single exons, or multiple exons.

Gene Products (Rh Proteins)

RHD encodes the D antigen, and *RHCE* en-codes the CcEe antigens in four combinations (ce, cE, Ce, or CE). Both genes encode 417 ami-no acids. The two polypeptides encoded by *RHD* vs *RHCE* differ by 32 to 35 amino acids, depending on whether RhD is compared to RhC or Rhc. The last decade has witnessed the development of an abundance of information on the genetic diversity of the *RH* locus, and antigen variants identified by DNA-based test-ing have far exceeded the number identified by serology. More than 500 RHD and 150 RHCE alleles have been documented. A direc-tory of RHD alleles is maintained by the Rhe-susBase database,[21] and RHCE and RHD alleles are listed on the National Center for Biotechnology Information human blood

group mutation website,[22] and on the ISBT website, where the Working Party on Red Cell Immunogenetics and Blood Group Termin-ology maintains, names, and catalogs new alleles.[23]

Most D-negative (Rh-negative) pheno-types are the result of complete deletion of the RHD gene, likely through a non-sister chroma-tid exchange involving regions termed the "Rhesus boxes" that flank *RHD* [Fig 11-1 (B)].[20] The *RHD*-deleted or *RHD*-inactive haplotype provides the immunologic rationale for why the transfusion of D-positive blood to a D-negative individual often results in produc-tion of anti-D. The immunogenicity of a pro-tein correlates with the degree of foreignness to the host. The large number of amino acid differences between RhD and RhCE explains why exposure can result in a robust immune response.

RHCE is found in all but rare D– – individ-uals (the dashes represent missing antigens) and encodes both C/c and E/e antigens on a single protein. C and c antigens differ by four amino acids (p.Trp16Cys, p.Leu60Ile, p.Asn68Ser, p.Ser103Pro), but only the serine to proline at position 103 is predicted to be ex-tracellular. The E and e antigens differ by one amino acid: a proline or alanine at position 226 (p.Pro226Ala), located on the fourth extra-cellular loop of the protein.

The five principal antigens are responsi-ble for the majority of Rh incompatibilities, al-though the Rh system as a whole is more com-plex (Table 11-1). New antigens may result from single nucleotide polymorphisms (SNPs) or major gene rearrangements. For example, the genetic exchanges between *RHD* and *RHCE* can create hybrid proteins that express an RhD protein with a portion of RhCE, or vice versa.

RHD GENOTYPE

Inheritance studies of the five principal Rh an-tigens have been used to determine Rh haplo-types (Table 11-3) and to predict *RHD* zygosity. However, some haplotypes inferred from the antigens present on red cells are equally common in certain ethnic groups. Therefore,

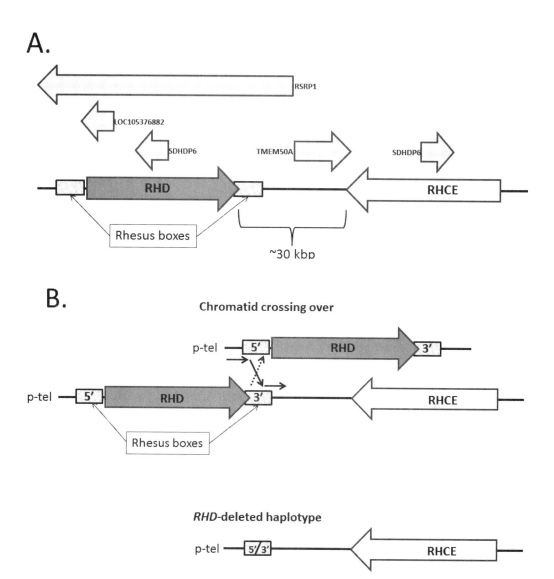

FIGURE 11-1. The *RH* locus. (A) Organization of *RHD* and *RHCE* in the short arm (p) region of chromosome 1p36.11. The two genes are each approximately 55,000 base pairs (bp) in size and are separated by approximately 30,000 bp (~30 kpb). *RHD* is flanked by two long homologous regions (Rhesus boxes) of approximately 9000 bp. The orientation of the *RH* locus is: p-telomere (p-tel) – *RHD* – *RHCE*. Other genes are in the region but are irrelevant to the expression of RH. (B) The origin of the *RHD*-deleted haplotype. During meiosis, a chromatid crossing-over misalignment occurs between the upstream Rhesus box (5′) of one chromatid and downstream Rhesus box (3′) of another (upper figure). An *RHD*-deleted haplotype (lower figure) results from the resolution of the chromatid exchange (solid arrows), with the formation of a hybrid Rhesus box (5′/3′). The alternate haplotype, two *RHD* in tandem (hatch arrow), has not been observed.

TABLE 11-3. Results of Tests with Five Principal Rh Antisera with Phenotype and Predicted RH Genotype

Anti-D	Anti-C	Anti-E	Anti-c	Anti-e	Phenotype	Predicted Genotype*	Alternative Genotype
			Antisera				

Anti-D	Anti-C	Anti-E	Anti-c	Anti-e	Phenotype	Predicted Genotype*	Alternative Genotype
					Rh positive†		
+	+	0	+	+	D, C, c, e	*R1 r*	*R1 R0*
						DCe/ce	*DCe/Dce*
							R0 r'
							Dce/Ce
+	+	0	0	+	D, C, e	*R1 R1*	*R1 r'*
						DCe/DCe	*DCe/Ce*
+	+	+	+	+	D, C, c, E, e	*R1 R2*	*R1 r''*
						DCe/DcE	*DCe/cE*
							R2 r'
							DcE/Ce
							Rz r
							DCE/ce
							R0 Rz
							Dce/DCE
+	0	0	+	+	D, c, e	*R0 r*	*R0 R0*
						Dce/ce	*Dce/Dce*
+	0	+	+	+	D, c, E, e	*R2 r*	*R2 R0*
						DcE/ce	*DcE/Dce*
							R0 r''
							Dce/cE
+	0	+	+	0	D, c, E	*R2 R2*	*R2 r''*
						DcE/DcE	*DcE/cE*
+	+	+	0	+	D, C, E, e	*R1 Rz*	*Rz r'*
						DCe/DCE	*DCE/Ce*
+	+	+	+	0	D, C, c, E	*R2 Rz*	*Rz r''*
						DcE/DCE	*DCE/cE*
+	+	+	0	0	D, C, E	*Rz Rz*	*Rz rʸ*
						DCE/DCE	*DCE/CE*

(Continued)

TABLE 11-3. Results of Tests with Five Principal Rh Antisera with Phenotype and Predicted RH Genotype (Continued)

Antisera						Predicted	Alternative
Anti-D	Anti-C	Anti-E	Anti-c	Anti-e	Phenotype	Genotype*	Genotype
Rh negative‡							
0	0	0	+	+	c, e	*r r*	
						ce/ce	
0	+	0	+	+	C, c, e	*r' r*	
						Ce/ce	
0	0	+	+	+	c, E, e	*r'' r*	
						cE/ce	
0	+	+	+	+	C, c, E, e	*r' r''*	
						Ce/cE	

*Each genotype is shown in both Wiener and Fisher-Race nomenclature.

†Rare genotypes (*R0 r^y*, *R1 r^y*, and *R2 r^y*) not shown (prevalence of <0.01%).

‡Rare genotypes (*rr^y*, *r'r^y*, *r''r^y*, and *r^{y}r^y*) not shown (prevalence of <0.01%).

the combination of some haplotypes makes the prediction of *RHD* zygosity uncertain (eg, the frequencies of R0R0 vs R0r are nearly identical in persons of African ethnicity). Moreover, the use of inferred haplotype frequencies in multiethnic societies makes prediction of *RHD* zygosity uncertain. Serologic testing to determine the strength of D antigen expression also cannot confirm whether red cells are homozygous (*RHD/RHD*) or hemizygous (*RHD/–*). The strength of anti-D hemagglutination cannot reliably show a difference between a single or a double dose of the D antigen. In addition, the Rh haplotype can influence the level of D antigen expression. Less D antigen is expressed when the C antigen is expressed—a phenomenon called the "Ceppellini effect."[24] Red cells from a DCe/Ce (R1r') individual express significantly fewer D antigen sites than red cells from a DCe/ce (R1r) individual. For this reason, it is important to choose red cells with the same Rh phenotype when performing serial anti-D titers in the antenatal setting because significantly different titers can be obtained if the red cells differ in their underlying zygosity.

RHD zygosity (see below) can be determined by DNA-based testing that relies on *RHD* deletion as the mechanism for hemizygosity. However, many different nonfunctional *RHD* have been reported.[25]

ANTIGENS

Manufactured licensed reagents are available to detect the expression of the principal Rh antigens—D, C, c, E, and e (Table 11-3). D antigen phenotyping is routinely performed on donors and patients. Testing for the common CcEe antigens is performed primarily during antibody investigations or to provide antigen-matched blood for certain chronic transfusion recipients, such as patients with sickle cell disease (SCD) and thalassemia, to minimize alloimmunization.

D Antigen

The D antigen is composed of numerous epitopes (designated by "epD") that were originally defined by antibodies from D-positive people who made anti-D. Subsequent studies with monoclonal antibodies defined 30 or more epitopes assigned to the designations "epD1" to "epD9."[26] Each epitope has additional subdivisions (eg, epD6.1). D epitopes are highly conformational and consist of more than simple linear amino acid residues. The use of monoclonal antibodies to assign a D variant to a specific partial type may not be reliable.[27]

D-Positive (Rh-Positive) Phenotypes

Most individuals with a D-positive red cell phenotype express a conventional RhD protein. However, >500 RHD alleles have been reported that encode amino acid changes. These alleles can cause numerous variations in the expression of D antigen, and red cells with some form of altered D expression are encountered in routine transfusion practice. An estimated 1% of individuals of European ethnicity carry RHD alleles that encode altered D antigens, and the incidence in individuals of African ethnicity is higher. Altered D is organized into four groups: weak D, partial D (including category D), D_{el}, and nonfunctional *RHD*.[28-31]

Weak D Types. Traditionally, the weak D phenotype was defined as red cells with a reduced amount of D antigen that required an indirect antiglobulin test (IAT) for detection (formerly called "D^u"). However, the number of samples identified as having weak D expression depends on the typing reagent and method used, which have changed over the years. Wagner and Flegel proposed a system to classify altered D red cells on the basis of their nucleotide substitutions (reviewed in Flegel and Denomme[32]). Weak D types are the result of an SNP that encodes amino acid changes predicted to be located within the intracellular or transmembrane region of the protein, rather than on the exofacial domain of the RhD protein. (See Fig 11-2.) Generally, intracellular amino acid changes are thought to affect the insertion of the polypeptide into the membrane and thus result in a reduced number of D-antigen sites on the red cells. Not included in the definition is whether a person with a weak D type can or cannot make alloanti-D.

Uniquely different SNPs cause weak D types 1 to 135.[21] The most common is weak D type 1, which has a valine-to-glycine amino acid substitution at position 270 (p.Val270Gly).

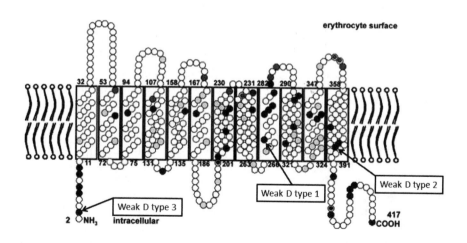

FIGURE 11-2. Structural models of weak D and partial D. The locations of amino acid changes are shown as solid circles in the plasma membrane or on the interior. Weak D types 1, 2, and 3 (shown by the arrows) are found in approximately 90% of people of European ethnicity with weak D phenotypes. Partial D types are encoded by single amino acid changes that are generally present on the exterior (erythrocyte surface) of the cell. Adapted from Flegel.[33]

Types 1, 2, and 3 represent approximately 90% of the weak D types in persons of European ethnicity.[29] Weak D types can be further weakened when C is present in *trans* to a weak D type; for example, r′ in *trans* with weak D type 2 (R2r′).

Partial D Types. Red cells with "category D" have historically been classified using monoclonal antibodies to evaluate D epitope expression. The red cells of these D individuals type as D positive, but these individuals can make anti-D when exposed to the conventional D antigen. The term "category D" is no longer used because these phenotypes are included with partial D types. The majority of partial D phenotypes are caused by hybrid genes in which portions of *RHD* are replaced by corresponding portions of *RHCE*. The novel sequences of the hybrid protein resulting from regions of RhD joined to RhCE can result in the loss of D epitopes and also generate new antigens. For example, DVI red cells carry the BARC antigen. A few partial D phenotypes are the result of multiple nucleotide changes. Some partial D types are detected using direct tests, and others only by the IAT. In contrast to weak D types, partial changes are predicted to be located on the exterior membrane surface,[34] or alternatively, can be internal but alter extracellular epitopes.

D$_{el}$ Types. Red cells that express extremely low levels of D antigen that cannot be detected by routine serologic methods (including IAT) are designated as "D-elution" or D$_{el}$ types. These red cells have D antigens that can be detected by adsorption/elution studies only. D$_{el}$ cells are found in 10% to 30% of D-negative people of Asian ethnicity and result from several different *RHD* mutations. D$_{el}$ cells are much less common in individuals of European ethnicity (0.027%) and carry different nucleotide substitutions than those in individuals of Asian ethnicity.[30,31]

Nonfunctional RHD Alleles. RHD genes that do not encode a full-length polypeptide are nonfunctional and have been given the ISBT allele designation *RHD*01N* (with "N" indicating "null") to indicate that they are not expressed.[23]

D Epitopes on Rhce. Expression of D epitopes by the protein product of the RHCE gene, in the absence of *RHD*, further complicates serologic determination of D status. Several Rhce proteins have D-specific amino acids and epitopes that are reactive with some monoclonal anti-D. These are more often found in a specific population. Examples include DHAR (Rhce'Har'), which is found in individuals of European ethnicity, and Crawford (*ceCF*), found in individuals of African ethnicity. These two examples are notable because the red cells show strong reactivity with some monoclonal reagents but are nonreactive with others, and are thus a source of D typing discrepancies (Table 11-4). Less dramatic are changes in the Rhce polypeptide that mimic a D epitope. They are encoded by alleles designated by the amino acid changes as "*ceRT*" and "*ceSL*."[35,36] The red cells are weakly reactive with some, but not all, monoclonal anti-D. Most important, individuals with DHAR and Crawford lack the expression of a conventional RhD and can be sensitized to D.[37,38]

Elevated D. Several rare deletion phenotypes, designated as "D––," "Dc–," and "DC^w–," have an enhanced expression of D antigen and no or weak or altered C/c and E/e antigens.[39] These variants are the converse of partial D and result from the replacement of portions of *RHCE* by *RHD*. The additional *RHD* sequences in *RHCE* result in the additional expression of (hybrid) D antigen along with a normal *RHD* often *in trans*, which explains the enhanced D expression and reduced or missing C/c and E/e antigens.

D-Negative (Rh-Negative) Phenotype

The D-negative phenotype is most common in people of European ethnicity (15%-17%), is less common in people of African ethnicity (approximately 8% in African-Americans), and is rare in people of Asian ethnicity (<0.1%).[40] The D-negative phenotype has arisen multiple times in human history, as evidenced by the different nonfunctional alleles responsible for the lack of D expression in various ethnic groups.

TABLE 11-4. Reactivity of FDA-Licensed Anti-D Reagents with Some D Variant Red Cells

Reagent	IgM Monoclonal	IgG	DVI IS/AHG*	DBT IS/AHG*	DHAR (Whites) IS/AHG*	Crawford (Blacks) IS/AHG*	ceRT	ceSL
Gammaclone	GAMA401	F8D8 monoclonal	Neg/Pos	Pos	Pos	Pos/Neg†		
Immucor Series 4	MS201	MS26 monoclonal	Neg/Pos	Pos	Pos	Neg/Neg	Weakly pos	Neg
Immucor Series 5	Th28	MS26 monoclonal	Neg/Pos	Pos	Pos	Neg/Neg	Weakly pos	Weakly pos
Ortho BioClone	MAD2	Polyclonal	Neg/Pos	Neg/Pos	Neg/Neg	Neg/Neg		
Ortho Gel (ID-MTS)	MS201		Neg	Pos	Pos	Neg	Weakly pos	Neg
Biotest RH1	BS226		Neg		Pos	Neg		
Biotest RH1 Blend	BS221	BS232 H4111B7	Neg/Pos		Pos†	Neg		
Alba Bioscience alpha	LDM1		Neg		Pos	Neg		
Alba Bioscience beta	LDM3		Neg		Pos	Neg		
Alba Bioscience delta	LDM1 ESD1-M		Neg		Pos	Neg		
ALBAclone blend	LDM3	ESD1	Neg/Pos		Pos	Pos/Neg†		
Polyclonal			Neg/Pos	Neg/Pos	Neg/Neg	Neg/Neg	Weakly pos‡	Neg

*Result following slash denotes anti-D test result by the indirect antiglobulin test (IAT).

†Test result is positive in the direct agglutination phase and will be negative in the IAT phase.

‡Enzyme-treated cells.

FDA = Food and Drug Administration; IgM = immunoglobulin M; IS = immediate spin; AHG = antihuman globulin; pos = positive; neg = negative.

In most people of European ethnicity, the D-negative phenotype results from a deletion of the entire RHD gene.[41] There are exceptions, however, and red cell samples with uncommon haplotypes [r′ (Ce) or r″ (cE)] are more likely to carry a weak D or nonfunctional *RHD*. In other ethnic groups, D-negative phenotypes are primarily caused by inactivating changes in *RHD*. In D-negative individuals of African ethnicity, a nonfunctional allele is prevalent, which contains a 37-bp insertion and results in a premature stop codon rendering the gene nonfunctional. It has been designated *RHDΨ*.[25] D-negative phenotypes in people of Asian ethnicity result from mutations in *RHD* that are most often associated with a Ce (r′) haplotype, although 10% to 30% of people of Asian ethnicity who type as D-negative are actually D_{el}.[30]

Testing for D

Monoclonal antibody production technology introduced in the 1980s freed manufacturers from reliance on human source material to manufacture anti-D reagents. These antibodies are specific for a single D epitope and do not detect all D-positive red cells. By the 1990s it became apparent that monoclonal antibodies could be used in a "blended" fashion to avoid deeming a pregnant woman or transfusion recipient D positive if she or he expressed the category DVI variant. It had been known for many years that category DVI types could make anti-D and cause significant HDFN.[31] Reagents for D phenotyping were selected to circumvent this problem. The immediate spin (IS) phase uses an IgM monoclonal anti-D that fails to react with red cells with partial DVI. This antibody is blended with a monoclonal or polyclonal IgG that requires an antiglobulin test (IAT) for the detection of D. In this way, typing partial DVI as D positive could be avoided in pregnancy and transfusion by performing only the IS phase of testing. Cord blood is tested in both the IS phase and the IAT phase to assign a D-positive status to all D variants.

Since their development, "blended" anti-D reagents from various manufacturers have used different monoclonal anti-D. Most Food and Drug Administration (FDA)-approved anti-D reagents combine a monoclonal IgM, which causes direct agglutination at room temperature, with a monoclonal or polyclonal IgG that is reactive by IAT, for the determination of weak expression of D. Anti-D for column agglutination testing contains only a monoclonal IgM. FDA-licensed reagents contain unique IgM clones, and these may exhibit different reactivity with red cells that have certain weak D, partial D, or D-like epitopes, including DHAR and Crawford (Table 11-4).

Typing Donors for D

The goal of D typing of donors, including the identification of units with weak D or partial D types, is to prevent anti-D immunization of transfusion recipients. The AABB *Standards for Blood Banks and Transfusion Services* (*Standards*) requires donor blood to be tested using a method that is designed to detect weak expression of D. There is no requirement that the typing be done using an IAT, and automated systems use enzymes to enhance detection of weak D. If the test results are positive, the unit is labeled "Rh positive."[42(p31)] Most weak or partial D-antigen units are detected, but infrequently some very weak D red cells or unusual partial D types are not detected; D_{el} red cells will be nonreactive with anti-D. Red cells with weak D antigen are less immunogenic than normal D-positive red cells, but even D_{el} donor units may stimulate anti-D.[43-47] Once shipped to an institution, a unit labeled "Rh negative" must be confirmed D negative by testing an integrally attached segment before transfusion, but testing by IAT is not required. Units labeled "Rh positive" do not require a confirmatory test.[42(p35)]

Typing Patients for D

When the D type of a patient is determined, a weak D test is not necessary except to assess the red cells of a newborn to determine maternal risk for D immunization. Today, monoclonal IgM reagents type many samples as D positive by IS that would have previously been detected only by IAT.

DVI is the most common partial D found in people of European ethnicity, and anti-D produced by women with partial DVI has resulted in fatal hemolytic disease.[48] Current FDA-licensed monoclonal IgM reagents are selected to be nonreactive with red cells with partial DVI in direct tests (Table 11-4). Therefore, performing only the direct test on red cells from female children and women of childbearing potential avoids the risk of sensitization by classifying women with DVI as D negative for transfusion and RhIG prophylaxis. However, the results of positive rosetting tests (to detect fetomaternal hemorrhage) must be carefully evaluated; maternal weak D types that are reactive only in the IAT phase have a false-positive rosette test result.

D Typing Discrepancies

D typing discrepancies should always be investigated and resolved. (See "Resolving D Typing Discrepancies.") D-negative blood is an appropriate option for female patients needing immediate transfusion, but a thorough clerical and serologic investigation should be performed. *RHD* genotyping is also useful to resolve D typing discrepancies.[49] (See "Clinical Considerations.")

Because donor centers use test methods to detect weak D phenotypes, and generally hospitals do not, a donor who is correctly classified as D positive may be classified as Rh negative as a transfusion recipient. This discrepancy should not be considered problematic but, rather, should be communicated to the patient and health-care staff and be noted in the patient's medical record.

Clinical Considerations

The long history of transfusing recipients who have weak D phenotype cells with D-positive red blood cells (RBCs) has suggested that some weak D phenotypes are unlikely to make anti-D. In 2015, a work group evaluated the scientific literature on anti-D alloimmunization among individuals whose red cells have a weak D phenotype and concluded that weak D types

1, 2, and 3 can be safely treated as D positive in pregnancy.[50] The recommendations have been adopted by AABB, the College of American Pathologists, the American College of Obstetricians and Gynecologists, and the Armed Services Blood Program. *RHD* genotyping can be performed with reasonable cost recovery that is in line with the costs associated with unnecessary administration of RhIG.[51] Thus, implementing the committee recommendation can help to avoid exposing pregnant women to RhIG unnecessarily. Other weak D types such as 11 and 15 have been reported to make anti-D,[1] and information on risk for alloanti-D for other weak D types is not yet available.

Unfortunately, licensed anti-D reagents cannot distinguish individuals with partial D from those expressing a normal D antigen. Many partial D red cells such as DIIIa or DAR, two of the most common partial D types in people of African ethnicity, type strongly D positive in the IS phase and, in the absence of *RHD* genotyping, are recognized as a D variant only after the patients produce anti-D.

Policies regarding D typing procedures and selection of blood components for transfusion should be based on the patient population, risk of immunization to D, and supply of D-negative blood. Policies should address procedures when an unexpected D phenotype is encountered. While it is important to prevent D immunization in females of childbearing potential to avoid HDFN, for other patients the complications of anti-D are less serious, and the decision to transfuse D-positive or D-negative blood should take into consideration the D-negative blood supply.[52]

As previously stated, not all D-negative patients make anti-D when they are exposed to D-positive red cells. The incidence in D-negative hospitalized patients given D-positive blood components is variable but approximates 30%.[3,53] AABB *Standards* requires that transfusion services have policies that address the administration of D-positive red cells to D-negative patients and the use of RhIG, which is a human blood product that is not entirely without risk.[42(pp37,46)]

G Antigen

The G antigen is found on red cells possessing C or D and maps to the shared exon 2 and the 103Ser residue on RhD, RhCe, and RhCE. Antibodies to G appear as anti-D plus anti-C that cannot be separated. However, the antibody can be adsorbed by either D–C+ or D+C– red cells. The presence of anti-G can explain why a D-negative person who was transfused with D– (C+) blood, or a D-negative woman who delivered a D– (C+) child, can subsequently appear to have made anti-D. Anti-D, -C, and -G can usually be distinguished by adsorption and elution studies.[54] The analyses are not often necessary in the pretransfusion setting. However, it is important to provide RhIG prophylaxis to pregnant women who have anti-G only and are at risk for anti-D.

C/c and E/e Antigens

The RHCE alleles encode the principal C/c and E/e antigens. More than 150 different RHCE alleles are known, and many are associated with altered or weak expression of the principal antigens and, in some cases, loss of high-prevalence antigens.[23] Partial C and many partial e antigens are well recognized, with the majority reported among individuals of African ethnicity.

Altered or Variant C and e Antigens

Nucleotide changes in *RHCE* result in quantitative and qualitative changes in C/c or E/e antigen expression; altered or partial C and e antigens are encountered most frequently. In persons of European ethnicity, altered C is associated with amino acid changes on the first extracellular loop of RhCe and the expression of C^W (Gln41Arg) or C^X (Ala36Thr) antigens. In people of African ethnicity, altered or partial C is associated with changes that result in the expression of the novel antigens JAHK (p.Ser122Leu) and JAL (p.Arg114Trp), but partial C expression most often results from the inheritance of an *RHD*DIIIa-CE(4-7)-D* hybrid, and less often of an *RHD-CE(4-7)-D* hybrid.[39] These two hybrids are located in the RHD gene but do not encode D antigen; rather, they encode C antigen on a hybrid background that differs from the normal background (Fig 11-3). The gene has an incidence of approximately 20% in people of African ethnicity. It is inherited with an RHCE allele designated as "*RHCE*ce^S*" that encodes partial e antigen and a V–VS+ phenotype.[55] The expressed product of the hybrid *RHD*DIIIa-CE(4-7)-D* linked to *RHCE*ce^S* is referred to as the "(C)ce^S" or "r'^S" haplotype. Red cells with the r'^S haplotype type as strongly C positive with monoclonal reagents, and the presence of the partial C is undetected. Anti-C is not uncommon among people of African ethnicity receiving C+ blood.

Transfusion recipients who express partial e antigens frequently appear to make antibodies with e-like specificity. The red cells may lack the high-prevalence hr^B or hr^S antigens.[56-58] Partial e expression is associated with several RHCE*ce alleles.[58] These alleles are found primarily in people of African ethnicity; some examples are shown in Fig 11-3. Red cells designated as hr^B– or hr^S– by serologic testing may not be compatible with anti-hr^B or -hr^S produced by patients with the same apparent partial antigen.[59,60]

An additional complication is that altered *RHCE*ce* is often inherited with a partial *RHD* (eg, DIII, DAU, or DAR).[61] As discussed above, patients with partial D red cells are at risk of producing anti-D.

CE, Ce, cE, and ce Compound Antigens

Compound antigens define epitopes that depend on conformational changes resulting from amino acids associated with both C/c and E/e. These antigens were referred to previously as "*cis* products" to indicate that the antigens were expressed from the same haplotype, that is, on a single Rhce polypeptide protein. These antigens are shown in Table 11-5 and include ce (f), Ce (rh_i), CE (Rh22), and cE (Rh27).

Clinical Considerations

It has long been recognized that alloimmunization represents a significant problem in

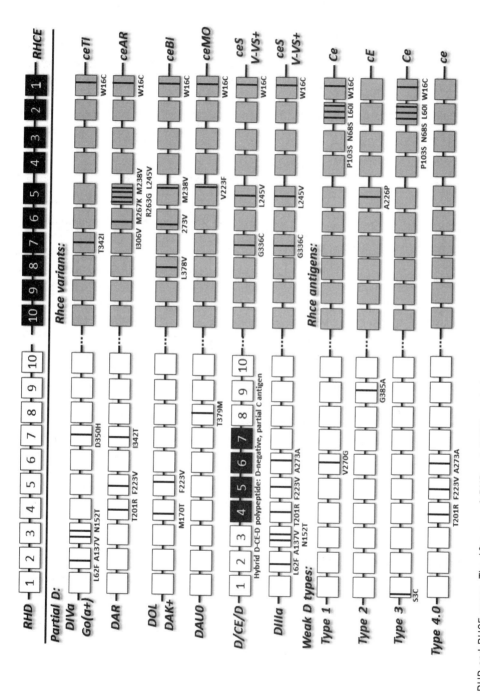

FIGURE 11-3. RHD and RHCE genes. The 10 exons of *RHD* and *RHCE* are depicted as white and gray boxes, respectively. Also shown are examples of *RHD* encoding partial D and weak D types, and of RHCE alleles with nucleotide polymorphisms often found in *cis* with the RHD alleles shown. The expression of the RHCE alleles with nucleotide polymorphisms can result in alloimmunization to conventional Rh proteins, which complicates transfusions in patients with sickle cell disease.

TABLE 11-5. Compound Rh Antigens on Rh Proteins

Compound Antigen Designation	Rh Protein	Present on Red Cells with These Haplotypes
ce or f	Rhce	Dce (R0) or ce (r)
Ce or rh$_i$, Rh7	RhCe	DCe (R1) or Ce (r')
cE or Rh27	RhcE	DcE (R2) or cE (r'')
CE or Rh22	RhCE	DCE (Rz) or CE (r^y)

patients with SCD because 25% to 30% or more of those who are chronically transfused develop red cell antibodies in the absence of minor blood group antigen matching.[62] To address the problem, many treatment programs determine the pretransfusion red cell phenotype in patients with SCD and transfuse RBCs that are C, E, and K antigen matched (ie, antigen negative if the patient lacks the antigen), because these antigens are considered to be the most immunogenic. In addition, some programs attempt to supply RBCs from donors of African ethnicity whenever that is possible. Antigen-matching reduces alloimmunization significantly, although there is not complete consensus on antigen-matching for all patients with SCD.[63,64]

Despite matching for D, C/c, and E/e, some patients become sensitized because they express Rh variants.[65] It is not possible to predict who will become alloimmunized, and prophylactic antigen-matching of blood for these patients is not feasible because of the low prevalence of antigen-negative blood.

RH GENOTYPING

RH genotyping is a powerful adjunct to serologic testing for the typing of transfused patients, *RHD* zygosity determination, fetal *RHD* typing, confirmation of D status, and identifi-

cation of antigen-matched blood for patients with SCD.

Typing Transfused Patients

In patients receiving chronic or massive transfusions, the presence of donor red cells in the peripheral blood makes red cell phenotyping by agglutination inaccurate. Genotyping overcomes this limitation because blood grouping can be determined with DNA prepared from a blood sample, even if the sample was collected after transfusion.[66]

RHD Zygosity Testing

RHD zygosity can be determined by two approaches: assaying *RHD* dosage or confirming the presence of a hybrid Rhesus box.[20,67] In prenatal practice, paternal *RHD* zygosity testing is important to predict fetal D status when the mother has anti-D. The management of HDFN can vary depending on whether the father is homozygous or hemizygous *RHD* positive. Care must be taken in the interpretation of testing results using either approach. For *RHD* dosage, at least two target exons must be tested to accurately determine zygosity, and nucleotide polymorphisms in hybrid Rhesus boxes can confound the analysis, especially in ethnic minorities.[67,68] The presence of the nonfunctional *RHDΨ* pseudogene should be included in zygosity analysis as a routine practice because it is common among persons of African ethnicity.[25]

Fetal *RHD* Typing

To determine the D antigen status of a fetus, fetal DNA can be isolated from cells obtained by amniocentesis or chorionic villus sampling. An alternative, noninvasive approach is to test the maternal plasma, which contains cell-free, fetal-derived DNA beyond 5 weeks' gestation.[69,70] In the future, determination of fetal *RHD* status using this noninvasive procedure could become routine in clinical practice to eliminate the unnecessary administration of antepartum RhIG to women who are carrying a D-negative fetus.[70]

Confirming D Status

RHD genotyping is useful to distinguish partial D from weak D or to resolve serologic D typing discrepancies. Although patients with an uncertain D status can be treated as D negative for transfusion and RhIG administration, this approach may be unsatisfactory for females of childbearing potential who face unnecessary RhIG injections, and it puts a strain on the limited D-negative blood supply. *RHD* genotyping in pregnancy allows informed decisions to be made on the administration of antenatal RhIG. (See "D Typing Discrepancies" and "Clinical Considerations" in the "Testing for D" section above.)

For donors, D typing discrepancies must be resolved because errors in determining D status may be reportable to the FDA and result in the recall of blood components. D-negative, first-time donors are screened for *RHD* to detect red cells with very weak D in some centers.[71,72]

RH Genotyping for Patients with SCD

Currently, extensive RH genotyping is time consuming and is used primarily for patients with complex Rh antibody reactivity and to find compatible donors in the American Rare Donor Program for patients with antibodies to high-prevalence Rh antigens.[57] The future availability of high-throughput RH genotyping platforms enables donors to be identified by genotyping. However, RH genotype-matching for patients with SCD who have rare Rh variant types may not be possible for chronic prophylactic transfusions.[73] Patients with SCD who cannot be supported with crossmatch-compatible transfusions may be candidates for stem cell transplantation.[74]

RH$_{NULL}$ SYNDROME AND RHAG BLOOD GROUP SYSTEM

Erythrocytes express a third Rh protein, RhAG, which shares 38% of its identity with RhD/RhCE, has the same topology in the membrane, and is encoded by a single gene on chromosome 6. RhAG associates with the Rh blood group proteins in the membrane to form an Rh-core complex. Four red cell antigens resulting from single amino acid substitutions form the RHAG blood group system: Duclos is RHAG1, Ol^a is RHAG2, and DSLK is RHAG3 and RHAG4.[75]

Red cells lacking all Rh antigens are designated as "Rh$_{null}$." Although uncommon, the phenotype most often results from nucleotide changes in *RHAG* known as a "regulator" type Rh$_{null}$, indicating that the RhAG protein plays a critical role in trafficking RhCE and RhD to the membrane. Less often, Rh$_{null}$ individuals have *RHCE* nucleotide changes along with the common deletion of *RHD*, and these individuals are called "amorph."

Rh$_{null}$ red cells are stomatocytic and associated with mild anemia, suggesting that the Rh proteins have an important structural role in the erythrocyte membrane. The Rh complex is associated with the membrane skeleton through CD47 protein 4.2, ankyrin band 3, Duffy, and glycophorin B and C interactions.[76,77]

RH ANTIBODIES

Most Rh antibodies are IgG but may have an IgM component. Typically, Rh antibodies do not activate complement, although rare exceptions have been reported. As a result, in a transfusion reaction involving Rh antibodies, hemolysis is primarily extravascular rather than intravascular.

Rh antibodies have the potential to cause clinically significant HDFN. Anti-c may cause severe HDFN, but anti-C, -E, and -e often do not cause HDFN, and when they do, it is usually mild. For antibody investigations, Rh antibodies are enhanced by enzyme treatment of red cells, and most are optimally reactive at 37 C.

Concomitant Rh Antibodies

Some Rh antibodies are often found together. For example, a DCe/DCe (R1R1) patient with anti-E most certainly has been exposed to the c antigen as well. Anti-c may be present in addition to anti-E, but the anti-c may be weak and undetectable at the time of testing. When seemingly compatible E-negative blood is transfused, it is most likely to be c-positive and may elicit an immediate or delayed transfusion reaction. Therefore, some experts advocate for avoiding the transfusion of c-positive blood in this situation. In contrast, testing for anti-E in serum containing anti-c is not warranted because the patient has probably been exposed to c without being exposed to E. In addition, the vast majority of c-negative donor blood is E negative. (See Table 11-3.)

Antibodies to High-Prevalence Rh Antigens

Alloantibodies to high-prevalence Rh antigens include anti-Rh29, made by some Rh_{null} individuals who lack Rh antigens, and others (anti-hr^S, -hr^B, -Hr^B, and -Hr) that are most often encountered in transfused patients with SCD.

TECHNICAL CONSIDERATIONS FOR RH TYPING

High-Protein Reagents and Controls

Some Rh reagents for use in slide, rapid tube, or microplate tests contain high concentrations of protein (20% to 24%) and other macromolecular additives. These reagents are prepared from pools of human sera and give reliable results; however, high protein levels and macromolecular additives may cause false-positive reactions. (See "Causes of False-Positive and False-Negative Rh Typing Results" below.) These reagents must be used according to the manufacturers' instructions and with the appropriate controls. False-positive results could cause a D-negative patient to receive D-positive blood and become immunized. If red cells exhibit aggregation in the control test, the results of the test are not valid.

Low-Protein Reagents and Controls

Most Rh antisera in routine use are low-protein reagents formulated predominantly with IgM monoclonal antibodies. Spontaneous agglutination causing a false-positive result can occur, although this happens much less frequently than with high-protein reagents. A negative result from a test that was performed concurrently with a similar reagent serves as a control. For example, for ABO and Rh typing, the absence of agglutination by anti-A or anti-B serves as a negative control for spontaneous hemagglutination. For red cells that show agglutination with all reagents (eg, group AB or D+), a control performed as described by the reagent manufacturer is required (with the exception of donor retyping).

In most cases, a suitable control is a suspension of the patient's red cells with autologous serum or 6% to 10% albumin. Indirect antiglobulin testing is not valid for red cells with a positive direct antiglobulin test (DAT) result unless a method is used to remove the IgG antibody. Antigen-positive and -negative controls should be tested, and the positive control cells should have a single dose of the antigen or be known to demonstrate weak reactivity.

Rh Testing Considerations in HDFN

Red cells from an infant with HDFN are coated with immunoglobulin, and a low-protein reagent is usually necessary to test these cells. Occasionally, red cells with a strongly positive DAT result may be so heavily coated that they are not agglutinated by a reagent with the same specificity as the bound antibody. This "blocking" phenomenon probably results from steric hindrance, or the epitope targeted by the monoclonal antiserum is occupied by maternal anti-D, causing a false-negative result. Heat elution of the antibody performed at 45 C permits red cell typing, but elution must be performed with appropriate controls to control for antigen denaturation. Detection of the antibody in an eluate confirms the presence of the antigen on the red cells, and *RHD* genotyping can be used for confirmation of D typing.

Causes of False-Positive and False-Negative Rh Typing Results

False-positive typing results can be caused by any of the following:

1. Immunoglobulin-coating of the cells as a result of warm or cold autoagglutinins. The red cells should be washed several times and retested with low-protein reagents by direct methods. If an IAT is required, IgG coating on the red cells can be removed by treating the cells with glycine/EDTA (Method 2-21) or chloroquine (Method 2-20) and retesting.
2. Induction of rouleaux by serum factors that can be eliminated by thoroughly washing the red cells and retesting.
3. Use of the wrong reagent.
4. Contamination with reagent from another vial.
5. Nonspecific aggregation of the red cells due to some component of the reagent other than the antibody (ie, a preservative, antibiotic, or dye).
6. Testing of polyagglutinable red cells agglutinated with reagents that contain human serum.

False-negative typing results can be caused by any of the following:

1. Failure to add the reagent. It is good practice to add typing reagent to all test tubes or wells before adding the red cells.
2. Use of the wrong reagent.
3. A red cell suspension that is too heavy for a tube test or too weak for a slide test.
4. Failure to detect a weak D reaction with direct testing (immediate centrifugation).
5. Nonreactivity of a reagent with a weak or partial form of the antigen.
6. Aggressive resuspension of the red cell button, dispensing the agglutination.
7. Contamination, improper storage, or outdating of the reagent.

8. Red cells with a strongly positive DAT result and antigen sites blocked because of a large amount of bound antibody (most common in severe HDFN caused by anti-D).

Resolving D Typing Discrepancies

To investigate D typing discrepancies, errors in sample identification or of a clerical nature should be eliminated by obtaining and testing a new sample. Beyond clerical errors, multiple variables contribute to D typing discrepancies. These variables include the use of different methods (ie, slide, tube, microplate, gel, and automated analyzers using enzyme-treated red cells), the phase of testing (direct or IAT), different IgM clones in manufacturers' reagents, and the large number of RHD gene variations that affect the level of expression and epitopes of the D antigen.

It is important to know the characteristics of the D typing reagent used and to always consult and follow the manufacturer's instructions during D typing. The FDA has drafted recommendations that require manufacturers to specify the reactivity of their reagents with partial DIV, DV, and DVI red cells.[78]

The IgM anti-D in all of the tube reagents currently licensed by the FDA is reactive by direct testing (initial spin) with DIV and DV red cells but has been selected to be nonreactive with partial DVI red cells in direct testing. Limited studies have been performed to characterize the reactivity of anti-D reagents with other partial D and weak D red cells. These studies have shown that the anti-D reagents cannot reliably predict whether a D variant is a weak or partial D antigen.[79,80] Table 11-4 shows the reactivity of important D variant red cells that have predictable patterns among the different anti-D reagents. In general, females of childbearing potential with partial D should be considered to be D-positive when they are blood donors, but D-negative when they are transfusion recipients.

KEY POINTS

1. The Rh system is highly immunogenic, complex, and polymorphic. More than 50 Rh antigens have been characterized, although the five principal antigens—D, C, c, E, and e—are responsible for the majority of clinically significant antibodies.
2. "Rh positive" and "Rh negative" refer to the presence or absence, respectively, of the D antigen.
3. Contemporary Rh terminology distinguishes between antigens (such as D and C), genes (such as *RHD* and *RHCE*), alleles (such as *RHCE*ce* and *RHCE*Ce*), and proteins (such as RhD and Rhce).
4. Most D-negative (Rh negative) phenotypes result from complete deletion of the RHD gene. Exposure of D-negative individuals to RhD can result in the development of anti-D.
5. *RHCE* encodes both C/c and E/e antigens on a single protein. C and c differ by four amino acids, whereas E and e differ by one amino acid.
6. Routine donor and patient Rh typing procedures test only for D. Testing for other common Rh antigens is used to resolve or confirm antibody identification and, for many SCD transfusion programs or for other patients receiving chronic transfusions, to match patients and donors for D, C, and E.
7. Weak D phenotypes are defined as having a reduced amount of D antigen and may require an IAT for detection. Weak D usually results from amino acid changes that impair the insertion of the protein in the membrane. Many different mutations cause weak expression of D.
8. *RHD* genotyping can identify those pregnant females and blood transfusion recipients with a serologic weak D phenotype who can be managed safely as D positive.
9. Most anti-D reagents approved by the FDA combine a monoclonal IgM (that is reactive at room temperature for routine testing) and a monoclonal or polyclonal IgG (that is reactive by IAT for the determination of weak D). The exception is anti-D for column agglutination testing, which contains only IgM. These reagents may show different reactivity with red cells that have weak D, partial D, or D-like epitopes.
10. When determining the D type of a patient, an IAT for weak expression of D is not necessary except when testing the red cells of an infant born to a mother at risk of D immunization. D-negative donors must be tested by a method that detects weak D.
11. Most Rh antibodies are IgG, although some may have an IgM component. With rare exceptions, Rh antibodies do not activate complement and, thus, cause primarily extravascular rather than intravascular hemolysis. Antibodies almost always result from red cell immunization through pregnancy or transfusion.

REFERENCES

1. Flegel WA. Homing in on D antigen immunogenicity. Transfusion 2005;45:466-8.
2. Klein HG, Anstee DJ. The Rh blood group system (including LW and RHAG). In: Mollison's blood transfusion in clinical medicine. 12th ed. Hoboken, NJ: Wiley-Blackwell, 2014:167-213.
3. Selleng K, Jenichen G, Denker K, et al. Emergency transfusion of patients with unknown blood type with blood group O Rhesus D positive red blood cell concentrates: A prospective, single-centre, observational study. Lancet Haematol 2017;4:e218-24.
4. Mollison PL, Hughes-Jones NC, Lindsay M, Wessely J. Suppression of primary RH immunization by passively-administered antibody: Experiments in volunteers. Vox Sang 1969;16:421-39.
5. Freda V, Gorman J, Pollack W. Rh factor: Prevention of isoimmunization and clinical trials in mothers. Science 1966;151:828-30.

6. Zwingerman R, Jain V, Hannon J, et al. Alloimmune red blood cell antibodies: Prevalence and pathogenicity in a Canadian prenatal population. J Obstet Gynaecol Can 2015;37:784-90.

7. Levine P, Stetson RE. An unusual case of intragroup agglutination. JAMA 1939;113:126-7.

8. Rosenfield R. Who discovered Rh? A personal glimpse of the Levine-Wiener argument. Transfusion 1989;29:355-7.

9. Green FA. Phospholipid requirement for Rh antigenic activity. J Biol Chem 1968;243:5519.

10. Gahmberg CG. Molecular characterization of the human red cell Rho(D) antigen. EMBO J 1983;2:223-7.

11. Bloy C, Blanchard D, Lambin P, et al. Human monoclonal antibody against Rh(D) antigen: Partial characterization of the Rh(D) polypeptide from human erythrocytes. Blood 1987;69:1491-7.

12. Moore S, Woodrow CF, McClelland DB. Isolation of membrane components associated with human red cell antigens Rh(D), (c), (E) and Fy. Nature 1982;295:529-31.

13. Saboori AM, Smith BL, Agre P. Polymorphism in the Mr 32,000 Rh protein purified from Rh(D)-positive and -negative erythrocytes. Proc Natl Acad Sci U S A 1988;85:4042-5.

14. Cherif-Zahar B, Bloy C, Le Van Kim C, et al. Molecular cloning and protein structure of a human blood group Rh polypeptide. Proc Natl Acad Sci U S A 1990;87: 6243-7.

15. Le Van Kim C, Mouro I, Cherif-Zahar B, et al. Molecular cloning and primary structure of the human blood group RhD polypeptide. Proc Natl Acad Sci U S A 1992;89:10925-9.

16. Arce MA, Thompson ES, Wagner S, et al. Molecular cloning of RhD cDNA derived from a gene present in RhD-positive, but not RhD-negative individuals. Blood 1993;82:651-5.

17. Simsek S, de Jong CAM, Cuijpers HTM, et al. Sequence analysis of cDNA derived from reticulocyte mRNAs coding for Rh polypeptides and demonstration of E/e and C/c polymorphism. Vox Sang 1994;67:203-9.

18. Tippett P. A speculative model for the Rh blood groups. Ann Hum Genet 1986;50(Pt 3):241-7.

19. Wagner FF, Flegel WA. RHCE represents the ancestral RH position, while RHD is the duplicated gene. Blood 2002;99:2272-3.

20. Wagner FF, Flegel WA. RHD gene deletion occurred in the Rhesus box. Blood 2000;95:3662-8.

21. Wagner FF, Flegel WA. The human RhesusBase. Version 2.0. [Available at http://www.rhesusbase.info (accessed March 26, 2017).]

22. Blumenfeld OO, Patnaik SK. Allelic genes of blood group antigens: A source of human mutations and cSNPs documented in the Blood Group Antigen Gene Mutation Database. Hum Mutat 2004;23:8-16. [See also https://www.ncbi.nlm.nih.gov/gv/mhc/xslcgi.cgi?cmd=bgmut/home (accessed March 26, 2017).]

23. International Society of Blood Transfusion Working Group on Red Cell Immunogenetics and Blood Group Terminology. Blood group terminology: Blood group allele tables. Amsterdam: ISBT, 2017. [Available at http://www.isbtweb.org/working-parties/red-cell-immunogenetics-and-blood-group-terminology/ (accessed March 26, 2017).]

24. Ceppellini R, Dunn LC, Turri M. An interaction between alleles at the RH locus in man which weakens the reactivity of the Rh(0) Factor (D). Proc Natl Acad Sci U S A 1955;41:283-8.

25. Singleton BK, Green CA, Avent ND, et al. The presence of an RHD pseudogene containing a 37 base pair duplication and a nonsense mutation in Africans with the Rh D-negative blood group phenotype. Blood 2000;95:12-18.

26. Scott ML, Voak D, Liu W, et al. Epitopes on Rh proteins. Vox Sang 2000;78(Suppl 2):117-20.

27. Denomme GA, Dake LR, Vilensky D, et al. Rh discrepancies caused by variable reactivity of partial and weak D types with different serologic techniques. Transfusion 2008;48:473-8.

28. Ye L, Wang P, Gao H, et al. Partial D phenotypes and genotypes in the Chinese population. Transfusion 2012;52:241-6.

29. Wagner FF, Gassner C, Muller TH, et al. Molecular basis of weak D phenotypes. Blood 1999;93:385-93.

30. Shao CP, Maas JH, Su YQ, et al. Molecular background of Rh D-positive, D-negative, D(el) and weak D phenotypes in Chinese. Vox Sang 2002;83:156-61.

31. Lacey PA, Caskey CR, Werner DJ, Moulds JJ. Fatal hemolytic disease of a newborn due to anti-D in an Rh-positive Du variant mother. Transfusion 1983;23:91-4.

32. Flegel WA, Denomme GA. Allo- and autoanti-D in weak D types and in partial D. Transfusion 2012;52:2067-9.

33. Flegel WA. Molecular genetics of RH and its clinical application. Transfus Clin Biol 2006;13:4-12.

34. Wagner FF, Frohmajer A, Ladewig B, et al. Weak D alleles express distinct phenotypes. Blood 2000;95:2699-708.

35. Wagner FF, Ladewig B, Flegel WA. The RHCE allele ceRT: D epitope 6 expression does not require D-specific amino acids. Transfusion 2003;43:1248-54.

36. Chen Q, Hustinx H, Flegel WA. The RHCE allele ceSL: The second example for D antigen expression without D-specific amino acids. Transfusion 2006;46:766-72.

37. Beckers EA, Porcelijn L, Ligthart P, et al. The Ro[HAR] antigenic complex is associated with a limited number of D epitopes and alloanti-D production: A study of three unrelated persons and their families. Transfusion 1996;36:104-8.

38. Westhoff CM. Review: The Rh blood group D antigen: Dominant, diverse, and difficult. Immunohematol 2005;21:155-63.

39. Daniels G. Human blood groups. 2nd ed. Cambridge, MA: Blackwell Science, 2002.

40. Race RR, Sanger R. Blood groups in man. 6th ed. Oxford: Blackwell, 1975.

41. Colin Y, Cherif-Zahar B, Le Van Kim C, et al. Genetic basis of the RhD-positive and RhD-negative blood group polymorphism as determined by Southern analysis. Blood 1991;78: 2747-52.

42. Ooley PW, ed. Standards for blood banks and transfusion services. 30th ed. Bethesda, MD: AABB, 2016.

43. Schmidt PJ, Morrison EC, Shohl J. The antigenicity of the Rh₀ (D[u]) blood factor. Blood 1962;20:196-202.

44. Wagner T, Kormoczi GF, Buchta C, et al. Anti-D immunization by D[EL] red blood cells. Transfusion 2005;45:520-6.

45. Yasuda H, Ohto H, Sakuma S, Ishikawa Y. Secondary anti-D immunization by D[el] red blood cells. Transfusion 2005;45:1581-4.

46. Flegel WA, Khull SR, Wagner FF. Primary anti-D immunization by weak D type 2 RBCs. Transfusion 2000;40:428-34.

47. Mota M, Fonseca NL, Rodrigues A, et al. Anti-D alloimmunization by weak D type 1 red blood cells with a very low antigen density. Vox Sang 2005;88:130-5.

48. Lacey PA, Caskey CR, Werner DJ, Moulds JJ. Fatal hemolytic disease of a newborn due to anti-D in an Rh-positive D[u] variant mother. Transfusion 1983;23:91-4.

49. Flegel WA, Denomme GA, Yazer MH. On the complexity of D antigen typing: A handy decision tree in the age of molecular blood group diagnostics. J Obstet Gynaecol Can 2007;29: 746-52.

50. Sandler SG, Flegel WA, Westhoff CM, et al. It's time to phase in RHD genotyping for patients with a serologic weak D phenotype. College of American Pathologists Transfusion Medicine Resource Committee Work Group. Transfusion 2015;55:680-9.

51. Kacker S, Vassallo R, Keller MA, et al. Financial implications of RHD genotyping of pregnant women with a serologic weak D phenotype. Transfusion 2015;55:2095-103.

52. Schonewille H, van de Watering LM, Brand A. Additional red blood cell alloantibodies after blood transfusions in a nonhematologic alloimmunized patient cohort: Is it time to take precautionary measures? Transfusion 2006;46: 630-5.

53. Frohn C, Dumbgen L, Brand J-M, et al. Probability of anti-D development in D– patients receiving D+ RBCs. Transfusion 2003;43:893-8.

54. Issitt PD, Anstee DJ. Applied blood group serology. 4th ed. Durham, NC: Montgomery Scientific Publications, 1998.

55. Daniels GL, Faas BH, Green CA, et al. The VS and V blood group polymorphisms in Africans: A serologic and molecular analysis. Transfusion 1998;38:951-8.

56. Reid ME, Storry JR, Issitt PD, et al. Rh haplotypes that make e but not hr[B] usually make VS. Vox Sang 1997;72:41-4.

57. Vege S, Westhoff CM. Molecular characterization of GYPB and RH in donors in the American Rare Donor Program. Immunohematol 2006;22:143-7.

58. Noizat-Pirenne F, Lee K, Pennec PY, et al. Rare RHCE phenotypes in black individuals of Afro-Caribbean origin: Identification and transfusion safety. Blood 2002;100:4223-31.

59. Pham BN, Peyrard T, Tourret S, et al. Anti-HrB and anti-hrb revisited. Transfusion 2009;49: 2400-5.

60. Pham BN, Peyrard T, Juszczak G, et al. Analysis of RhCE variants among 806 individuals in France: Considerations for transfusion safety, with emphasis on patients with sickle cell disease. Transfusion. 2011;51:1249-60.

61. Westhoff CM, Vege S, Halter-Hipsky C, et al. DIIIa and DIII Type 5 are encoded by the same allele and are associated with altered RHCE*ce alleles: Clinical implications. Transfusion 2010;50:1303-11.

62. Vichinsky EP, Earles A, Johnson RA, et al. Alloimmunization in sickle cell anemia and trans-

fusion of racially unmatched blood. N Engl J Med 1990;322:1617-21.

63. Ness PM. To match or not to match: The question for chronically transfused patients with sickle cell anemia. Transfusion 1994;34:558-60.

64. Vichinsky EP, Luban NL, Wright E, et al. Prospective RBC phenotype matching in a stroke prevention trial in sickle cell anemia: A multicenter transfusion trial. Transfusion 2001;41: 1086-92.

65. Chou ST, Jackson T, Vege S, et al. High prevalence of red blood cell alloimmunization in sickle cell disease despite transfusion from Rh-matched minority donors. Blood 2013;122: 1062-71.

66. Reid ME, Rios M, Powell VI, et al. DNA from blood samples can be used to genotype patients who have recently received a transfusion. Transfusion 2000;40:48-53.

67. Pirelli KJ, Pietz BC, Johnson ST, et al. Molecular determination of RHD zygosity: Predicting risk of hemolytic disease of the fetus and newborn related to anti-D. Prenat Diagn 2010;12-13: 1207-12.

68. Matheson KA, Denomme GA. Novel 3′ rhesus box sequences confound RHD zygosity assignment. Transfusion 2002;42:645-50.

69. Lo YM, Corbetta N, Chamberlain PF, et al. Presence of fetal DNA in maternal plasma and serum. Lancet 1997;350:485-7.

70. Van der Schoot CE, Soussan AA, Koelewijn J, et al. Non-invasive antenatal RHD typing. Transfus Clin Biol 2006;13:53-7.

71. Gassner C, Doescher A, Drnovsek TD, et al. Presence of RHD in serologically D–, C/E+ individuals: A European multicenter study. Transfusion 2005;45:527-38.

72. Polin H, Danzer M, Hofer K, et al. Effective molecular RHD typing strategy for blood donations. Transfusion 2007;47:1350-5.

73. Chou St, Westhoff CM. The role of molecular immunohematology in sickle cell disease. Transfus Apher Sci 2011;44:73-9.

74. Fasano RM, Monaco A, Meier ER, et al. RH genotyping in a sickle cell disease patient contributing to hematopoietic stem cell transplantation donor selection and management. Blood 2010;116:2836-8.

75. Tilley L, Green C, Poole J, et al. A new blood group system, RHAG: Three antigens resulting from amino acid substitutions in the Rh-associated glycoprotein. Vox Sang 2010;98: 151-9.

76. Dahl KN, Parthasarathy R, Westhoff CM, et al. Protein 4.2 is critical to CD47-membrane skeleton attachment in human red cells. Blood 2004;103:1131-6.

77. Nicolas V, Le Van Kim C, Gane P, et al. RhRhAG/ankyrin-R, a new interaction site between the membrane bilayer and the red cell skeleton, is impaired by Rh(null)-associated mutation. J Biol Chem 2003;278:25526-33.

78. Food and Drug Administration. Draft guidance: Recommended methods for blood grouping reagents evaluation. (March 1992) Silver Spring, MD: CBER Office of Communication, Outreach, and Development, 1992. [Available at https://www.fda.gov/downloads/BiologicsBloodVaccines/GuidanceComplianceRegulatoryInformation/Guidances/Blood/UCM080926.pdf (accessed March 30, 2017).]

79. Judd WJ, Moulds M, Schlanser G. Reactivity of FDA-approved anti-D reagents with partial D red blood cells. Immunohematol 2005;21:146-8.

80. Denomme GA, Dake LR, Vilensky D, et al. Rh discrepancies caused by variable reactivity of partial and weak D types with different serologic techniques. Transfusion 2008;48:473-8.

Chapter 12

Other Blood Group Systems and Antigens

• ● •

Jill R. Storry, PhD, FIBMS

THE INTERNATIONAL SOCIETY of Blood Transfusion (ISBT) currently recognizes 352 antigen specificities, of which 314 belong to one of 36 blood group systems.[1,2] Each system represents either a single gene or two or three closely linked homologous genes. The ABO and Rh systems are the best known and clinically most important systems and are described in detail in Chapters 10 and 11. The antigens of the H, Lewis, I, P1PK, and Globoside systems are carbohydrate structures that are biochemically closely related to ABO antigens and are discussed in Chapter 10. The remaining systems are described in this chapter; some, generally the most important in transfusion medicine, are described in some detail, others in a few lines. They are listed in ISBT order, as in Table 12-1.

In addition to the 36 systems, some groups of antigens that are serologically, biochemically, or genetically related but not eligible to join a system are classified together as collections (200 series). Other antigens that are not eligible to join a system or collection are of either low or high prevalence in most major populations and make up the 700 and 901 series, respectively.[1] These are discussed at the end of the chapter.

The full ISBT classification can be found on the ISBT website (http://www.isbtweb.org/working-parties/red-cell-immunogenetics-and-blood-group-terminology/), and Appendix 6 lists all antigens assigned to systems. Many more references to blood group systems and antigens than can be provided here are available in various textbooks and reviews.[3-5]

The most important aspect of blood group antigens in transfusion medicine is whether their corresponding antibodies are hemolytic and therefore have the potential to cause hemolytic transfusion reactions (HTRs) and hemolytic disease of the fetus and newborn (HDFN). A guide to the potential clinical significance of blood group antibodies is provided in Table 12-1.

THE MNS SYSTEM

MNS is a highly complex blood group system consisting of 49 antigens. As with the Rh system, much of its complexity arises from

Jill R. Storry, PhD, FIBMS, Associate Professor, Division of Hematology and Transfusion Medicine, Department of Laboratory Medicine, Lund University, and Technical Director, Immunohematology, Clinical Immunology and Transfusion Medicine, Office of Medical Services, Lund, Sweden
The author has disclosed no conflicts of interest.

TABLE 12-1. Clinical Significance of Antibodies to Blood Group Antigens

ISBT No.	System Name or Symbol	No. of Antigens	Hemolytic Transfusion Reaction (HTR), Acute (AHTR) or Delayed (DHTR)	Hemolytic Disease of the Fetus and Newborn (HDFN)
001	ABO	4	See Chapters 10 and 22.	See Chapters 10 and 23.
002	MNS	49	Rare examples of anti-M and -N active at 37 C cause AHTRs and DHTRs; anti-S, -s, -U, and some other antibodies may cause AHTRs and DHTRs.	Anti-S, -s, -U, and some other antibodies cause severe HDFN; anti-M rarely causes severe HDFN.
003	P1PK	3	Only very rare examples active at 37 C cause AHTRs and DHTRs.	No.
004	Rh	54	Rh antibodies can cause severe AHTRs and DHTRs. (See Chapters 11 and 22.)	Anti-D can cause severe HDFN. (See Chapter 23.)
005	Lutheran	24	Anti-Lu^a and -Lu^b have caused mild DHTRs; anti-Lu8 has caused AHTRs.	No.
006	Kell	36	Kell antibodies can cause severe AHTRs and DHTRs.	Anti-K can cause severe HDFN.
007	Lewis	6	Anti-Le^a and -Le^b are not generally considered to be clinically significant.	No.
008	Duffy	5	Anti-Fy^a, -Fy^b, and -Fy3 cause AHTRs and DHTRs; anti-Fy5 causes DHTRs.	Anti-Fy^a and -Fy^b cause HDFN.
009	Kidd	3	Anti-Jk^a is a common cause of DHTRs; anti-Jk^a and -Jk3 also cause AHTRs.	No. Anti-Jk^a does not usually cause HDFN.
010	Diego	22	One anti-Di^a caused a DHTR, but there is little evidence; anti-Di^b has rarely caused mild DHTRs; and anti-Wr^a causes HTRs.	Anti-Di^a, -Di^b, and -Wr^a, plus some others, have caused severe HDFN.
011	Yt	2	Anti-Yt^a has very rarely caused HTRs.	No.
012	Xg	2	No.	No.
013	Scianna	7	No.	No.
014	Dombrock	10	Anti-Do^a and -Do^b cause AHTRs and DHTRs.	No.

	System		HTR	HDFN
015	Colton	4	Anti-Co^a causes AHTRs and DHTRs; anti-Co^b and -Co3 have caused mild HTRs.	Anti-Co^a has caused severe HDFN, and anti-Co3 has caused mild HDFN.
016	LW	3	No.	No.
017	Ch/Rg	9	No.	No.
018	H	1	Anti-H in Bombay phenotype can cause severe intravascular HTRs; anti-H in para-Bombay is not usually clinically significant. (See Chapter 10.)	Anti-H in Bombay phenotype has the potential to cause severe HDFN.
019	Kx	1	Anti-Kx and -Km in McLeod syndrome has caused severe HTRs.	Antibodies found only in males.
020	Gerbich	11	Anti-Ge3 has caused mild to moderate HTRs.	Three examples have been reported of anti-Ge3 causing HDFN.
021	Cromer	19	No.	No.
022	Knops	9	No.	No.
023	Indian	5	There is one example of anti-In^b causing an HTR. Anti-AnWj has caused severe HTRs.	No.
024	Ok	3	Anti-Ok^a is very rare and no cases of HTR have been reported.	No.
025	Raph	1	No.	No.
026	JMH	6	One example has been reported of anti-JMH causing AHTR.	No.
027	I	1	Anti-I in adult i phenotype has caused increased destruction of I+ red cells.	No.
028	Globoside	1	Globoside has caused intravascular HTRs.	No, but anti-PP1P^k is associated with a high rate of spontaneous abortion.
029	Gill	1	No.	No.
030	RHAG	4	No.	RHAG4 has caused one case of HDFN.

(Continued)

TABLE 12-1. Clinical Significance of Antibodies to Blood Group Antigens (Continued)

ISBT No.	System Name or Symbol	No. of Antigens	Hemolytic Transfusion Reaction (HTR), Acute (AHTR) or Delayed (DHTR)	Hemolytic Disease of the Fetus and Newborn (HDFN)
031	FORS	1	No.	No.
032	JR	1	Mild DHTRs and one case of AHTR have been reported to be caused by anti-Jr[a].	Two examples of severe HDFN due to anti-Jr[a] have been reported.
033	LAN	1	Mild to severe HTR due to anti-Lan has been reported.	Anti-Lan is generally not a cause of HDFN, although cases of mild HDFN have been reported.
034	Vel	1	Severe AHTR and mild to severe DHTR due to anti-Vel have been reported.	Anti-Vel is generally not a cause of HDFN, although cases of severe HDFN have been reported.
035	CD59	1	One example of anti-CD59 has been reported but was not associated with reduced red cell survival.	No data.
036	AUG	2	Mild to severe DHTR has been reported.	None to mild.

ISBT = International Society of Blood Transfusion.

recombination between closely linked homologous genes.

The MNS Glycoproteins and the Glycophorin A Gene Family

The antigens of the MNS system are located on one or both of two glycoproteins: glycophorin A (GPA, CD235A) and glycophorin B (GPB, CD235B). Each crosses the membrane once and has an external N-terminal domain and a C-terminal cytosolic domain. The extracellular domains of both molecules have many sialic-acid-rich O-glycans; GPA is N-glycosylated at asparagine-45 (position 26 in the mature protein), whereas GPB is not N-glycosylated. The long cytosolic tail of GPA interacts with the cytoskeleton. GPA is abundant, with about 10^6 copies per red cell, whereas GPB has only about 200,000 copies per cell. GPA forms an association in the membrane with band 3 (Diego blood group system), and both GPA and GPB appear to be part of the band 3/Rh ankyrin macrocomplex (Fig 12-1).[6]

GYPA and *GYPB*, the genes encoding GPA and GPB, are located on chromosome 4q31.21 and include seven and five exons, respectively. A region of intron 3 of *GYPB* is homologous to exon 3 of *GYPA* but is not expressed because of a defective splice site (Fig 12-2).[7] Exon 1 of each gene encodes a 19-amino-acid signal peptide that is not present in the mature protein. A third gene in this GPA gene family, *GYPE*, probably produces a third glycoprotein, glycophorin E, but this plays little or no part in MNS antigen expression and is not detectable by routine methods.

GPA is restricted to blood cells of erythroid origin and is often used as an erythroid marker. Both GPA and GPB are exploited by the malaria parasite *Plasmodium falciparum* as receptors for binding to red cells and may be critical to the invasion process.[8] A GPA-like molecule has been detected on renal endothelium.

M (MNS1), N (MNS2), S (MNS3), AND s (MNS4)

M and N (as detected by most anti-N reagents) are antithetical antigens and polymorphic in all populations tested (Table 12-2). M and N are located at the N-terminus of GPA. M-active GPA has serine and glycine at the first and fifth positions of the mature protein (positions 20 and 25); N-active GPA has leucine and glutamic acid at those positions. The amino-terminal 26 amino acids of GPB mature protein are usually identical to those of the N form of GPA. Thus, in almost all people of European ethnicity and most people of other ethnicities, GPB expresses 'N.' However, because GPB is much less abundant than GPA, most anti-N reagents do not detect the 'N' antigen on GPB.

S and s are another pair of polymorphic antithetical antigens of the MNS system, carried on GPB. Family studies show tight linkage between *M/N* and *S/s*.

The N-terminal region of GPA is cleaved from intact red cells by trypsin, whereas that of GPB is not. Consequently, M and N antigens on GPA are trypsin sensitive, and S, s, and 'N' on GPB are trypsin resistant. In contrast, with α-chymotrypsin treatment of red cells, M and N activity is only partially reduced, whereas S, s, and 'N' expression is completely destroyed. M, N, S, s, and 'N' are all destroyed by treatment of the red cells with papain, ficin, bromelin, or pronase, although this effect with S and s may be variable.

S–s–U– Phenotype

The red cells of about 2% of Americans of African ancestry and a higher proportion of Africans are S–s– and lack the high-prevalence antigen U (MNS5). The S–s–U– phenotype often results from homozygosity for a deletion of the coding region of *GYPB*, but other, more complex molecular phenomena involving hybrid genes may also give rise to an S–s– phenotype with expression of a variant U antigen. U is generally resistant to denaturation by proteases—papain, ficin, trypsin, α-chymotrypsin—although anti-U is not reactive with papain-treated red cells in rare cases.

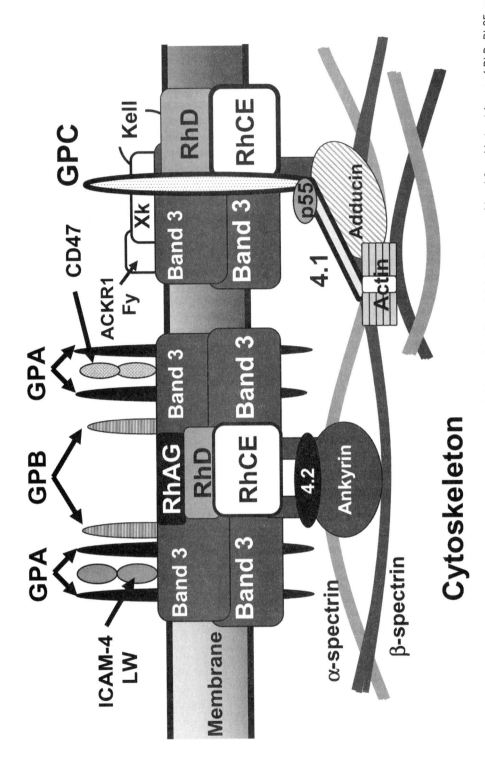

FIGURE 12-1. Model of two proposed membrane complexes containing band 3 and Rh proteins: 1) containing tetramers of band 3 and heterotrimers of RhD, RhCE, and RhAG, and linked to the spectrin matrix of the cytoskeleton through band 3, protein 4.2, and ankyrin; and 2) containing band 3, RhD, and RhCE, and linked to the spectrin/actin junction through glycophorin C (GPC), p55, and protein 4.1, and through band 3 and adducin.

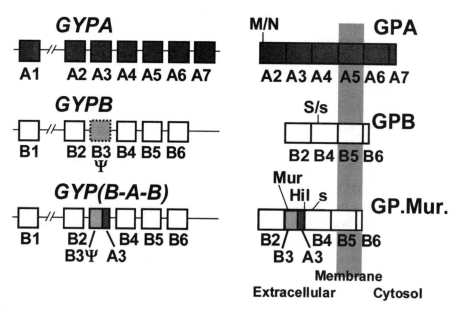

FIGURE 12-2. *GYPA, GYPB,* and the hybrid *GYP(B–A–B)* gene responsible for GP. Mur, and a representation of the proteins they encode, showing the regions of proteins encoded by the various exons.
ψ = pseudoexon not represented in the mRNA or the encoded protein.

M, N, S, s, and U Antibodies and Their Clinical Significance

Anti-M is a relatively common antibody, whereas anti-N is quite rare. Most anti-M and -N are not active at 37 C, are not clinically sig-

TABLE 12-2. Prevalence of Some Phenotypes of the MNS System

Phenotype	Prevalence (%)	
	Whites	US Blacks
M+ N−	30	25
M+ N+	49	49
M− N+	21	26
S+ s−	10	6
S+ s+	42	24
S− s+	48	68
S− s−	0	2

nificant, and can generally be ignored in transfusion practice. If room-temperature incubation is eliminated from compatibility testing and screening for antibodies, these antibodies are not detected. When M or N antibodies active at 37 C are encountered, antigen-negative red cells or those that are compatible by an indirect antiglobulin test (IAT) should be provided. Very occasionally, anti-M and -N have been implicated as the cause of acute and delayed HTRs, and anti-M has very rarely been responsible for severe HDFN.[9] A few cases of warm autoimmune hemolytic anemia (AIHA) caused by autoanti-N have been described, one of which had a fatal outcome. Autoanti-M responsible for warm AIHA has not been reported.

Anti-S and -s are usually IgG antibodies that are active at 37 C. They have been implicated in HTRs and have caused severe and fatal HDFN. Autoanti-S has caused AIHA. If immunized, individuals with S–s–U– red cells may produce anti-U. Anti-U has been responsible for severe and fatal HTRs and HDFN. Autoanti-U has been implicated in AIHA.

Other MNS Antigens and Antibodies

The other MNS antigens are either of high or low prevalence in most populations. The similarity of sequence between certain regions of *GYPA* and *GYPB* may occasionally lead to *GYPA* pairing with *GYPB* during meiosis. If recombination then occurs, either by crossing over or by gene conversion, a hybrid gene can be formed consisting partly of *GYPA* and partly of *GYPB*. A large variety of these rare hybrid genes exists, and they give rise to low-prevalence antigens and, in the homozygous state, to phenotypes that lack high-prevalence antigens.[7] Red cells of some of the phenotypes resulting from hybrid genes react with an antibody called "anti-Mi[a]." Thought for many years to be a cross-reactive epitope on several hybrids, the Mi[a] antigen has been shown to be a discrete antigen. The best-known example of the Mi(a+) phenotype is created by the hybrid gene that is responsible for the GP.Mur (previously Mi.III) phenotype. The hybrid gene is mostly *GYPB*, but a small region of *GYPB* encompassing the 3′ end of the pseudoexon and the 5′ end of the adjacent intron has been replaced by the equivalent region from *GYPA*. This means that the defective splice site in *GYPB* is now replaced by the functional splice site from *GYPA*, and the new, composite exon is expressed in the messenger RNA (mRNA) and represented in the protein.[10] This provides an unusual amino acid sequence that is immunogenic and represents the antigen Mur (and the Mi[a] antigen). The amino acid sequence that results from the junction of exons B3 and A3 gives rise to Hil and MINY (Fig 12-2).

Mur antigen is rare in people of European and African ethnicity but has a prevalence of about 7% in people of Chinese ethnicity and 10% in people of Thai ethnicity. Anti-Mur has the potential to cause severe HTRs and HDFN. In Hong Kong and Taiwan, anti-Mur is the most common blood group antibody after anti-A and -B. In Southeast Asia, it is important that red cells for antibody detection include a Mur+ sample.[11]

Antibodies to regions of GPA with the generic name En[a] that may be made by very rare individuals who lack all or part of GPA have caused severe HTRs and HDFN.

THE LUTHERAN SYSTEM

Lutheran is a polymorphic system consisting of 24 antigens, the majority of which are highly prevalent in all populations tested. There are four antithetical pairs—Lu[a]/Lu[b], Lu6/Lu9, Lu8/Lu14, and Au[a]/Au[b]—of which Lu[a], Lu9, and Lu14 are of low prevalence.[12] Au[a] and Au[b] have a prevalence of around 80% and 50%, respectively, in people of European ethnicity. Of most relevance in transfusion medicine, Lu[a] (LU1) has a prevalence of about 8% in people of European or African ethnicity but is rare elsewhere; its antithetical antigen, Lu[b] (LU2), is common everywhere.

Lutheran antigens are destroyed by treatment of the red cells with trypsin or α-chymotrypsin, whereas papain and ficin have little effect. Most Lutheran antibodies are not reactive with red cells treated with the sulfhydryl reagents 2-aminoethylisothiouronium bromide (AET) or dithiothreitol (DTT), which reduce the disulfide bonds of the immunoglobulin superfamily (IgSF) domains (Method 3-18).

The Lutheran antigens are located on a pair of glycoproteins that differ by the length of their cytoplasmic domains as a result of alternative RNA splicing. They are encoded by *BCAM* located on chromosome 19q13.2. The proteins span the membrane once and have five extracellular IgSF domains. The isoform with the longer cytoplasmic domain interacts with spectrin of the membrane skeleton. The location of the Lutheran antigens on the IgSF domains is shown in Fig 12-3. The Lutheran glycoproteins are adhesion molecules that bind isoforms of laminin that contain α-5 chains. Laminin is a glycoprotein of the extracellular matrix, and Lutheran-laminin interactions may play a role in the migration of mature erythroid cells from the marrow to the peripheral blood at the latest stages of erythropoiesis. Upregulation of Lutheran glycoproteins on red cells of patients with sickle cell disease could play a part in adhesion of these cells to the vascular endothelium and the resultant crises of vascular occlusion.[13]

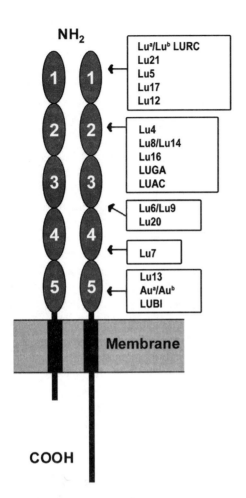

FIGURE 12-3. Diagram of the two isoforms of the Lutheran glycoprotein, showing the five extracellular immunoglobulin superfamily domains and the location of the Lutheran antigens on these domains, the single membrane-spanning domain, and the cytoplasmic domains.

The extremely rare Lu_{null} phenotype arises from homozygosity for inactive LU gene.[14] The red cells lack any expression of Lutheran antigens, and individuals with this phenotype may produce anti-Lu3, which is reactive with all red cells except those from other Lu(a–b–) individuals. Heterozygosity for inactivating mutations in the erythroid transcription factor gene *KLF1* is responsible for In(Lu), a phe-

notype with extremely weak expression of Lutheran antigens that are detectable only by adsorption/elution techniques. Mutations in *KLF1* also affect other blood group genes and cause weakened expression of several other antigens, including P1, In[b], and AnWj.[15] The In(Lu) phenotype has a prevalence of around 0.03%. In one family, hemizygosity for a mutation in the X-linked gene for the major erythroid transcription factor GATA-1 resulted in a Lu(a–b–) phenotype with an X-linked mode of inheritance.[16]

Lutheran antibodies are most often IgG and demonstrate reactivity best by IAT but have generally been implicated only in mild delayed HTRs and have not caused severe HDFN. Anti-Lu[a] may be "naturally occurring" or immune, and it is often IgM but may also be IgG and IgA. These antibodies are usually reactive by direct agglutination of Lu(a+) red cells but often also reactive by an IAT and may show a "mixed-field"-like agglutination that is characteristic of this and other antibodies to Lutheran antigens.

THE KELL AND KX SYSTEMS

The antigen often referred to as "Kell," but correctly named "K" or "KEL1," is the original antigen of the Kell system and the first blood group antigen to be identified following the discovery of the antiglobulin test in 1946. Its antithetical antigen, k or KEL2, was identified 3 years later. The Kell system now consists of 36 antigens numbered from KEL1 to KEL39, of which three are obsolete.[17] The Kell system includes seven pairs (K/k, Js[a]/Js[b], K11/K17, K14/K24, VLAN/VONG, KYO/KYOR, and KHUL/KEAL) and one triplet (Kp[a]/Kp[b]/Kp[c]) of Kell antithetical antigens. Initially, most antigens joined the Kell system through genetic associations observed in family studies. These associations have now been confirmed by DNA sequencing of the KEL gene.

The Kell Glycoprotein and the KEL Gene

The Kell antigens are located on a red cell membrane glycoprotein (CD238) with four

(KEL1 isoform) or five (KEL2 isoform) N-glycans but no O-glycosylation. Kell is a type II membrane glycoprotein; it spans the membrane once and has a short N-terminal domain in the cytosol and a large C-terminal domain outside the membrane (Fig 12-4).[18] The extracellular domain has 15 cysteine residues and is extensively folded by disulfide bonding, although crystallographic studies are required to determine the molecule's three-dimensional structure. Kell system antigens depend on the conformation of the glycoprotein and are sensitive to disulfide-bond-reducing agents, such as DTT and AET.

The Kell glycoprotein is linked through a single disulfide bond to the Xk protein (Fig 12-4), an integral membrane protein that expresses the Kx blood group antigen (XK1). Absence of Xk protein from the red cell results in reduced expression of the Kell glycoprotein and weakened Kell antigens (McLeod phenotype, see below).

The KEL gene is located on chromosome 7q33. It is organized into 19 exons: Exon 1 encodes the probable translation-initiating methionine; exon 2, the cytosolic domain; exon 3, the membrane-spanning domain; and exons 4 through 19, the large extracellular domain.

Kell Antigens

K has a prevalence of about 9% in people of European ethnicity and about 2% in people of African ethnicity (Table 12-3). It is rare in East Asia. The k antigen is highly prevalent in all populations. K and k result from a single nucleotide polymorphism (SNP) in exon 6, which encodes Met193 in K and Thr193 in k.

Kp^a (KEL3) is found in about 2% of people of European ethnicity and is not present in people of African or Japanese ethnicity (Table 12-3); Kp^b (KEL4) has high prevalence in all populations. Kp^c (KEL21), an antigen with very low prevalence, is the product of another allele at the same locus as *Kp^a* and *Kp^b*, and the

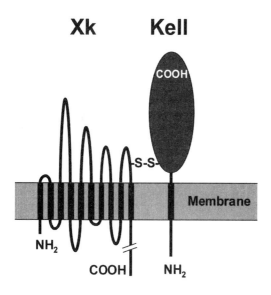

FIGURE 12-4. Diagram of the Kell and Xk proteins linked by a single disulfide bond. The Xk protein has cytoplasmic N- and C-terminal domains and 10 membrane-spanning domains. The Kell glycoprotein has a large, folded, extracellular, C-terminal domain and an intracellular N-terminal domain.

TABLE 12-3. Prevalence of Some Kell Phenotypes

Phenotype	Prevalence (%)	
	Whites	US Blacks
K– k+	91.0	98
K+ k+	8.8	2
K+ k–	0.2	Rare
Kp(a–b+)	97.7	100
Kp(a+b+)	2.3	Rare
Kp(a+b–)	Rare	0
Js(a–b+)	100.0	80
Js(a+b+)	Rare	19
Js(a+b–)	0	1

K, Kp^a, and Js^a are extremely rare in populations of Asian ancestry.

antigen results from different single nucleotide substitutions within codon 281. The mutation associated with Kpª expression reduces the quantity of Kell glycoprotein in the red cell membranes, giving rise to a slight reduction in expression of Kell antigens in *Kpª/Kpª* homozygotes but a more obvious weakening of Kell antigens in individuals who are heterozygous for *Kpª* and the null allele *K⁰*.

Jsª (KEL6) is almost completely confined to people of African ethnicity. The prevalence of Jsª in African Americans is about 20% (Table 12-3). Jsᵇ (KEL7) is highly prevalent in all populations, and Js(a+b–) has not been found in persons of non-African ethnicity.

The remaining five antithetical antigen pairs (K11/K17, K14/K24, VLAN/VONG, KYO/KYOR, KHUL/KEAL); the low-prevalence antigens Ulª and K23; and the high-prevalence antigens K12, K13, K18, K19, K22, TOU, RAZ, KALT, KTIM, KUCI, KANT, KASH, KELP, and KETI all result from single amino acid substitutions in the Kell glycoprotein.

Kell antigens are resistant to papain, ficin, trypsin, and α-chymotrypsin but are destroyed by a mixture of trypsin and α-chymotrypsin. They are also destroyed by DTT and AET (see above) and by EDTA-glycine.

Clinical Significance of Antibodies to Kell Blood Group Antigens

Kell antibodies are usually IgG, predominantly IgG1. They should be considered potentially clinically significant from the perspective of causing severe HDFN and HTRs. Patients with Kell antibodies should be transfused with antigen-negative blood whenever possible.

Anti-K is the most common immune red cell antibody outside the ABO and Rh systems; one-third of all non-Rh red cell immune antibodies investigated are anti-K. An antiglobulin test is usually the method of choice for detecting anti-K, although occasional samples may agglutinate red cells directly. Most anti-K appears to be induced by blood transfusion. Because anti-K can cause severe HDFN, it is usual practice in some countries for girls and women of childbearing potential to receive only K– red cells. Antibodies to K, k, Kpª, Kpᵇ,

Jsª, Jsᵇ, Ku, Ulª, K11, K19, K22, and KEAL are all reported to have caused severe HDFN and many have been implicated in acute or delayed HTRs.

The pathogenesis of HDFN caused by anti-K differs from that resulting from anti-D. Anti-K HDFN is associated with lower concentrations of amniotic fluid bilirubin than anti-D HDFN of comparable severity. Postnatal hyperbilirubinemia is not prominent in infants with anemia caused by anti-K. There is also reduced reticulocytosis and erythroblastosis in HDFN caused by anti-K compared with anti-D. These symptoms suggest that anti-K HDFN is associated with a lower degree of hemolysis and that fetal anemia in anti-K HDFN results predominantly from a suppression of erythropoiesis.[19] The Kell glycoprotein appears on erythroid progenitors at a much earlier stage of erythropoiesis than do Rh antigens. Consequently, anti-K probably facilitates phagocytosis of K+ erythroid progenitors at an early stage of development by macrophages in the fetal liver, before the erythroid cells produce hemoglobin.

Antibodies mimicking Kell specificities have been responsible for severe AIHA. Presence of the autoantibody is often associated with apparent depression of all Kell antigens. Although most examples of anti-K are stimulated by pregnancy or transfusion, a few cases of apparently non-red-cell immune anti-K have been described. In some cases, the antibodies were found in untransfused, healthy, male blood donors; in others, microbial infection was implicated as an immunizing agent.

Null (K₀) and Mod Phenotypes

Like most blood group systems, Kell has a null phenotype (K₀), in which none of the Kell antigens are expressed and the Kell glycoprotein cannot be detected in the membrane. Immunized K₀ individuals may produce anti-Ku (anti-KEL5), an antibody that is reactive with all cells except those of the K₀ phenotype. Homozygosity for a variety of nonsense, missense, and splice-site mutations have been associated with K₀ phenotype.[20]

K_{mod} red cells have only very weak expression of Kell antigens, and individuals with this phenotype are homozygous (or doubly heterozygous) for missense mutations, resulting in single-amino-acid substitutions within the Kell glycoprotein. Some K_{mod} individuals make an antibody that resembles anti-Ku but differs in being nonreactive with K_{mod} red cells. Other phenotypes in which Kell antigens have substantially depressed expression result from Kp^a/K_0 heterozygosity (see above), absence of Xk protein (see below), and absence of the Gerbich antigens Ge2 and Ge3, which are located on the glycophorins C and D (GPC, GPD). The reason for this phenotypic association between Kell and Gerbich is not well defined, although there is biochemical evidence to show that Kell glycoprotein, Xk, GPC, and GPD are all located within the 4.1R membrane protein complex (Fig 12-1).[21,22]

Functional Aspects

The Kell protein has structural and sequence homology with a family of zinc-dependent endopeptidases that process a variety of peptide hormones. Although the physiologic function of the Kell glycoprotein is not known, it is enzymatically active and can cleave the biologically inactive peptide big-endothelin-3 to create the biologically active vasoconstrictor endothelin-3. Consequently, Kell might play a role in regulating vascular tone, but there is no direct evidence for this.[23] No obvious pathogenesis is associated with the K_0 phenotype.

In addition to erythroid cells, Kell antigens may be present on myeloid progenitor cells, and Kell glycoprotein has been detected in testis and lymphoid tissues, and with Xk protein in skeletal muscle.

Kx Antigen (XK1), McLeod Syndrome, and McLeod Phenotype

Kx is the only antigen of the Kx blood group system. It is located on a polytopic protein that spans the red cell membrane 10 times and is linked to the Kell glycoprotein by a single disulfide bond (Fig 12-4). Xk protein is encoded by the XK gene on chromosome Xp21.1.

McLeod syndrome is a very rare X-linked condition that develops almost exclusively in males and is associated with acanthocytosis and a variety of late-onset muscular, neurologic, and psychiatric symptoms. It results from hemizygosity for inactivating mutations and deletions of the XK gene.[24] McLeod syndrome is associated with the McLeod phenotype, in which Kell antigens are expressed weakly and Km (KEL20) as well as Kx are absent. When transfused, people with the McLeod phenotype without chronic granulomatous disease (CGD) produce anti-Km only, which is compatible with both McLeod and K_0 phenotype red cells. The function of the Xk-Kell complex is not known, but Xk has structural resemblance to a family of neurotransmitter transporters.

Deletion of part of the X chromosome that includes *XK* may also include *CYBB*, absence of which is responsible for X-linked CGD. When transfused, CGD patients with McLeod syndrome usually produce anti-Kx plus anti-Km, making it almost impossible to find compatible donors. It is recommended that transfusion of males with CGD and McLeod syndrome be avoided where possible.

THE DUFFY SYSTEM

The Duffy system includes five antigens that reside on a glycoprotein also known as the atypical chemokine receptor 1 (ACKR1, previously known as DARC). The ACKR1 gene consists of two exons, with exon 1 encoding only the first seven amino acids of the Duffy glycoprotein.[25] *ACKR1* is on chromosome 1q21-q22.

Fy^a (FY1) and Fy^b (FY2)

The antigens Fy^a and Fy^b differ by a single amino acid change in the N-terminus of the Duffy glycoprotein (Gly42 and Asp42, respectively; see Fig 12-5). They are polymorphic in people of European ethnicity, giving rise to three phenotypes: Fy(a+b–), Fy(a+b+), and Fy(a–b+) (Table 12-4). In Asia, Fy^a is a high-prevalence antigen, and the phenotype Fy(a–b+) is rarely encountered. In individuals of African descent, the Fy(a–b–) phenotype is most com-

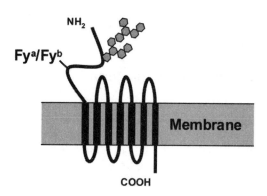

FIGURE 12-5. Diagram of the Duffy glycoprotein (previously DARC but renamed ACKR1), with a glycosylated external N-terminal domain, seven membrane-spanning domains, and a cytoplasmic C-terminus. The position of the Fy^a/Fy^b polymorphism is shown.

mon, caused by homozygosity for a silenced FY*B allele (*FY*02N.01*). Fy^a and Fy^b are very sensitive to most proteolytic enzymes, including bromelin, α-chymotrypsin, ficin, papain, and pronase, but are not destroyed by trypsin.

The FY*02N.01 allele in people of African ethnicity encodes the Fy^b antigen but is silenced by a mutation in the promoter region, –67T>C.[26] This mutation disrupts the binding site for the erythroid-specific GATA-1 transcription factor and prevents expression of the gene in erythroid tissue. Duffy glycoprotein is present on many cells throughout the body; thus, Fy(a–b–) people of African ethnicity lack Duffy on their red cells only. This explains why they do not make anti-Fy^b and only very rarely make anti-Fy3 or anti-Fy5. (See below.) The GATA-1 binding-site mutation in people of African ethnicity has been found only in Duffy genes encoding Fy^b; however, the same mutation has been detected in FY*A alleles in people of Papua New Guinea and Brazil.

A weak form of Fy^b antigen known as Fy^x occurs. The allele, *FY*02W.01*, encodes an amino acid substitution, Arg89Cys, in the cytosolic domain of the glycoprotein. Fy^b antigen may be undetected in some samples of anti-Fy^b, although the antigen can be detected by adsorption/elution.

Fy3, Fy4, Fy5, and Fy6

Very rare people of non-African ethnicity with Fy(a–b–) red cells are homozygous for inactivating mutations in *ACKR1*. These individuals make no Duffy glycoprotein at all and were identified through the presence in their sera of anti-Fy3, an antibody that is reactive with all red cells except those of the Fy(a–b–) phenotype. Fy6, like Fy^a and Fy^b, is sensitive to protease treatment, whereas Fy3 and Fy5 are resistant. Fy5 is absent not only from cells of the Fy(a–b–) phenotype but also from cells of the Rh$_{null}$ phenotype. The Duffy glycoprotein may belong to the junctional membrane protein complex, which also contains Rh proteins (Fig 12-1).[27] Anti-Fy5 has been found only in multitransfused individuals of African ethnicity. Anti-Fy6 is defined by monoclonal antibodies only, and reacts with all red cells except Fy(a–b–) cells. It reacts with an epitope on the N-terminus of the Duffy glycoprotein regardless of Fy^a/Fy^b phenotype. Anti-Fy4 is obsolete.

TABLE 12-4. Duffy Phenotypes and Genotypes in Selected Populations

	Genotype		Frequency (%)		
Phenotype	Whites or Asians	US Blacks	Whites	US Blacks	Japanese
Fy(a+b–)	*Fy^a/Fy^a*	*Fy^a/Fy^a* or *Fy^a/Fy*	20	10	81
Fy(a+b+)	*Fy^a/Fy^b*	*Fy^a/Fy^b*	48	3	15
Fy(a–b+)	*Fy^b/Fy^b*	*Fy^b/Fy^b* or *Fy^b/Fy*	32	20	4
Fy(a–b–)	*Fy/Fy*	*Fy/Fy*	0	67	0

Duffy Antibodies and Their Clinical Significance

Anti-Fy^a is a relatively common antibody; anti-Fy^b is about 20 times less common. IgG1 usually predominates, and naturally occurring examples are very rare. Anti-Fy^a and anti-Fy^b may cause acute or delayed HTRs. Although generally mild, some have proven fatal. These antibodies have also been responsible for mild to severe HDFN. Anti-Fy3 has been responsible for acute and delayed HTRs, and anti-Fy5 for delayed HTRs.

Functional Aspects of the Duffy Glycoprotein

The Duffy glycoprotein is a red cell receptor for a variety of chemokines, including interleukin-8, monocyte chemotactic protein-1, and melanoma growth stimulatory activity.[28] It traverses the membrane seven times, with a 63-amino-acid extracellular N-terminal domain that contains two potential N-glycosylation sites and a cytoplasmic C-terminal domain (Fig 12-5). This arrangement is characteristic of the G-protein-coupled superfamily of receptors that includes chemokine receptors.

The function of ACKR1 on red cells is not known. It has been suggested that it might act as a clearance receptor for inflammatory mediators and that red cells function as a "sink," or as scavengers, for the removal of unwanted chemokines. If so, this function must be of limited importance because Duffy is absent on the red cells of most individuals of African ethnicity. It has been suggested that ACKR1 on red cells reduces angiogenesis and, consequently, the progression of prostate cancer by clearing angiogenic chemokines from the tumor microenvironment. This potential effect of erythroid ACKR1 could provide an explanation for the substantially higher levels of prostate cancer in men of African ethnicity compared with those of European ethnicity.[29]

ACKR1 is present in many organs, where it is expressed on endothelial cells lining postcapillary venules. Duffy glycoprotein on vascular endothelium may be involved in the inhibition of cancer-cell metastasis and induc-tion of cellular senescence.[30] ACKR1 may also facilitate movement of chemokines across the endothelium.

The Duffy Glycoprotein and Malaria

The Duffy glycoprotein is a receptor for merozoites of *Plasmodium vivax*, the parasite responsible for a form of malaria that is widely distributed in Africa and Asia but is less severe than malaria resulting from *P. falciparum* infection. Red cells with the Fy(a–b–) phenotype are resistant to invasion by *P. vivax* merozoites. Consequently, the FY*02N.01 allele confers a selective advantage in geographic areas where *P. vivax* is endemic; this advantage probably balances out any potential disadvantage resulting from the absence of the chemokine receptor on red cells.

THE KIDD SYSTEM

The Kidd system consists of three antigens located on a glycoprotein with 10 membrane-spanning domains, cytoplasmic N- and C-termini, and one extracellular N-glycosylation site (Fig 12-6).[22,31] The Kidd gene (*SLC14A1*) is located on chromosome 18q11-q12 and contains 11 exons, of which 4 through 11 encode the mature protein.

Jk^a (JK1) and Jk^b (JK2)

Jk^a and Jk^b are the products of antithetical alleles and represent Asp280 and Asn280 in the fourth external loop of the Kidd glycoprotein (Fig 12-6). They have similar prevalence in populations of European and Asian ethnicity, but Jk^a is more common than Jk^b in people of African ethnicity (Table 12-5). The antigens are resistant to proteolytic enzymes, such as papain and ficin.

Jk(a–b–) and Jk3

The null phenotype, Jk(a–b–) Jk:–3, usually results from homozygosity for a silent gene at the *JK* locus. Although very rare in most populations, the null phenotype is relatively common in people of Polynesian ethnicity, with a prevalence of around 1 in 400 but as high as

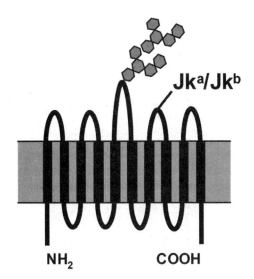

Jkᵃ/Jkᵇ

NH₂   COOH

FIGURE 12-6. Diagram of the Kidd glycoprotein, a urea transporter, with cytoplasmic N- and C-terminal domains, 10 membrane-spanning domains, and an N-glycan on the third extracellular loop. The position of the Jkᵃ/Jkᵇ polymorphism is shown on the fourth external loop.

1.4% in those of Niuean ancestry. The Polynesian null allele (*JK*02N.01*) contains a splice site mutation in intron 5 that results in the absence of the protein from the membrane. In people of Finnish ancestry, where Jk(a–b–) is less rare than in other populations of European ethnicity, the allele responsible (*JK*02N.06*) encodes a Ser291Pro substitution. Immunized individuals with the Jk(a–b–) phenotype may produce anti-Jk3. An extremely rare form of Jk(a–b–) phenotype found in people of Japanese ethnicity results from heterozygosity for a

TABLE 12-5. Kidd Phenotypes in Three Populations

Phenotype	Prevalence (%)		
	Whites	US Blacks	Asians
Jk(a+b–)	26	52	23
Jk(a+b+)	50	40	50
Jk(a–b+)	24	8	27

dominant inhibitor gene, named *In(Jk)* in analogy with the *In(Lu)* dominant inhibitor of Lutheran and other antigens. Very weak expression of Jkᵃ and/or Jkᵇ can be detected on In(Jk) red cells by adsorption/elution tests.

Kidd Antibodies and Their Clinical Significance

Anti-Jkᵃ and -Jkᵇ are usually IgG1 and IgG3, but some are partly IgG2, IgG4, or IgM. About 50% of anti-Jkᵃ and -Jkᵇ bind complement and are often found in antibody mixtures.

Kidd antibodies are often difficult to detect. Some agglutinate antigen-positive cells directly, but the reactions are usually weak. Generally, an antiglobulin test is required, and use of enzyme-treated cells may be necessary to detect weaker antibodies.

Kidd antibodies may cause severe acute HTRs. They are also a very common cause of delayed HTRs, probably because they may not be detected in pretransfusion testing due to their tendency to drop to low or undetectable levels in plasma. Anti-Jk3 can also cause acute or delayed HTRs. Despite their hemolytic potential, Kidd antibodies only very rarely cause severe HDFN. Kidd antibodies have been implicated in acute renal transplant rejection, suggesting that Kidd antigens can behave as histocompatibility antigens.[31]

The Kidd Glycoprotein in Urea Transportation

The Kidd antigens are located on the red cell urea transporter, SLC14A1 (also known as HUT11 or UT-B1). When red cells approach the renal medulla, which contains a high concentration of urea, the urea transporter permits rapid uptake of urea and prevents the cells from shrinking in the hypertonic environment. As the red cells leave the renal medulla, urea is transported rapidly out of the cells, preventing the cells from swelling and carrying urea away from the kidney. SLC14A1 has been detected on endothelial cells of the vasa recta, the vascular supply of the renal medulla, but it is not present in renal tubules.

Normal red cells are rapidly lysed by 2M urea because urea transported into the cells makes them hypertonic and they burst as a result of the osmotic influx of water. Because of the absence of the urea transporter, Jk(a–b–) cells are not hemolyzed by 2M urea, and this can be used as a method for screening for Jk(a–b–) donors.[32]

The Jk(a–b–) phenotype is not associated with any clinical defect, although two unrelated Jk(a–b–) individuals had a mild urine-concentrating defect.[33]

THE DIEGO SYSTEM

Band 3, the Red Cell Anion Exchanger

The 22 antigens of the Diego system are located on band 3, the common name for the red cell anion exchanger or solute carrier family 4 A1 (*SLC4A1*). Band 3 is a major red cell membrane glycoprotein with ~10^6 copies per red cell. Band 3 has a transmembrane domain that traverses the membrane 14 times, with an N-glycan on the fourth extracellular loop. Band 3 also has a long cytoplasmic N-terminal domain that interacts with the membrane skeleton proteins ankyrin, 4.1R, and protein 4.2 and functions as a binding site for hemoglobin (Figs 12-1 and 12-7). The short cytoplasmic C-terminal domain binds carbonic anhydrase II.

Band 3 in red cells has at least two major functions: the rapid exchange of HCO_3^- and Cl^- ions, which are important in CO_2 transport, and attachment of the red cell membrane to the cytoskeleton.[27] Tetramers of band 3 form the core of the band 3/Rh ankyrin macrocomplex of red cell membrane proteins, which could function as a gas channel for O_2 and CO_2. Band 3 is also a component of the junctional complex that links the red cell membrane to the membrane skeleton via GPC and protein 4.1 (Fig 12-1). *SLC4A1* encodes band 3. It is located on chromosome 17q21.31 and consists of 20 exons.

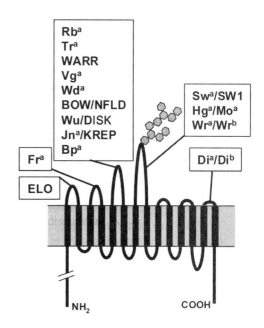

FIGURE 12-7. Diagram of band 3, the Diego glycoprotein and anion exchanger, with cytoplasmic N- and C-terminal domains, 14 membrane-spanning domains, and an N-glycan on the fourth extracellular loop (although the precise conformation is still controversial). The locations of 22 antigens of the Diego system on the extracellular loops are shown.

Di^a (DI1) and Di^b (DI2); Anti-Di^a and -Di^b

Di^a, the original Diego antigen, is very rare in people of European or African ethnicity but has a prevalence of 5% in people of Chinese or Japanese ethnicity and an even higher prevalence in the indigenous peoples of North and South America, reaching 54% in the Kainganges Indians of Brazil. Di^b is a high-prevalence antigen in almost all populations. Di^a and Di^b represent an amino acid substitution in the seventh extracellular loop of band 3: Leu854 and Pro854, respectively.

Anti-Di^a and -Di^b are usually IgG1 plus IgG3 and typically require an antiglobulin test for detection, although a few directly agglutinating samples have been found. Anti-Di^a occasionally binds complement and lyses untreated red cells. Anti-Di^a, which is present in ~3.6% of multitransfused patients in Brazil, can cause severe HDFN. Anti-Di^b has, very rarely, been responsible for serious HDFN. Generally, neither anti-Di^a nor anti-Di^b cause HTRs; one example of anti-Di^a causing a delayed reaction has been reported, and anti-Di^b rarely causes mild delayed reactions.[17]

Wr^a (DI3) and Wr^b (DI4); Anti-Wr^a and -Wr^b

The low-prevalence antigen Wr^a and its antithetical antigen of extremely high prevalence, Wr^b, represent an amino acid substitution in the fourth loop of band 3: Lys658 and Glu658, respectively. Wr^b expression, however, also depends on the presence of GPA. Despite the presence of Glu658 on band 3, Wr^b is not expressed in the rare phenotypes associated with a complete absence of the MN glycoprotein GPA or of the part of GPA that is close to insertion into the red cell membrane. This provides strong evidence for an interaction between band 3 and GPA within the red cell membrane.

Anti-Wr^a is a relatively common antibody, usually detected by an antiglobulin test but sometimes by direct agglutination of red cells. Wr^a antibodies are mostly IgG1 but sometimes IgM or IgM plus IgG. Anti-Wr^a has been responsible for severe HDFN and HTRs. Alloanti-Wr^b is rare and little is known about its clinical significance, but autoanti-Wr^b is a relatively common autoantibody and may be implicated in AIHA.

Other Diego Antigens

Over the years, many antigens of very low prevalence have been shown to represent amino acid substitutions in band 3 and have joined the Diego system: Wd^a, Rb^a, WARR, ELO, Wu, Bp^a, Mo^a, Hg^a, Vg^a, Sw^a, BOW, NFLD, Jn^a, KREP, Tr^a, Fr^a, and SW1. Anti-DISK detects a high-prevalence antigen that is antithetical to Wu and has caused severe HDFN. Anti-ELO and anti-BOW have also caused severe HDFN.

Antigens of the Diego system are not destroyed by proteolytic enzymes, such as papain, ficin, or trypsin; however, the antigens carried on the third extracellular loop (Rb^a, Tr^a, WARR, Vg^a, Wd^a, BOW, NFLD, Wu,

DISK, Jn^a, KREP, and Bp^a) are sensitive to α-chymotrypsin.

THE YT SYSTEM

Yt^a (YT1; His353) and Yt^b (YT2; Asn353) are antithetical antigens on acetylcholinesterase, an enzyme that is important in neurotransmission but of unknown function on red cells. Yt^b has a prevalence of about 8% in people of European ethnicity but is more common in people from the eastern Mediterranean; Yt^a has relatively high prevalence in all populations. Yt^a is not affected by trypsin but is destroyed by α-chymotrypsin treatment of the red cells; papain and ficin may also destroy the antigen, but this ability appears to depend on the anti-Yt^a used. Yt^a and Yt^b are sensitive to the disulfide-bond-reducing agents AET and DTT.

Yt antibodies are usually IgG and require an IAT for detection. They are not generally considered to be clinically significant, although anti-Yt^a may cause accelerated destruction of Yt(a+) transfused red cells and has been implicated in acute and delayed HTRs.[34]

THE XG SYSTEM

The two antigens of the XG blood group system, Xg^a (XG1) and CD99 (XG2), are encoded by homologous genes. The XG gene lies partly within the X chromosome pseudoautosomal region (Xp22.32), a section at the tip of the short arm that pairs with the Y chromosome. *XG* is one of few genes not inactivated by lyonization.[35] The CD99 gene is homologous to *XG* and is located on both X and Y chromosomes (Yp11), with pairing occurring at meiosis. Xg^a is polymorphic and has a prevalence of about 66% in males and 89% in females. Both CD99 and Xg^a expression appear to be controlled by a common regulator gene, *XGR*. Although Xg^a antibodies occasionally agglutinate red cells directly, they are generally IgG and are reactive by an IAT. They are not reactive with red cells treated with proteolytic enzymes. Anti-Xg^a is not clinically significant. CD99 antibodies in common use are mostly monoclonal and of mouse origin; a few human alloanti-CD99 occur, although little is known about their characteristics.

THE SCIANNA SYSTEM

The Scianna system consists of seven antigens on erythrocyte membrane-associated protein (ERMAP), a member of the IgSF that has one IgSF domain.[36] Sc1 (Gly57) and Sc2 (Arg57) are antithetical antigens of high and low prevalence, respectively. Rd (SC4) is of low prevalence; Sc3, STAR, SCER, and SCAN are of high prevalence. Anti-Sc3 is produced by individuals with the very rare Scianna-null phenotype.

While antibodies to Scianna antigens have not been implicated in an HTR, mild to severe HDFN has been reported; however, evidence is limited because of the scarcity of the antibodies. Although directly agglutinating SC1 antibodies are known, Scianna antibodies are generally reactive by an IAT. Treatment of red cells by proteolytic enzymes has little effect, but disulfide-bond-reducing agents (AET and DTT) substantially reduce reactivity.

THE DOMBROCK SYSTEM

The Dombrock system consists of 10 antigens: the polymorphic antithetical antigens Do[a] (DO1; Asn265) and Do[b] (DO2; Asp265) and the high-prevalence antigens Gy[a], Hy, Jo[a], DOYA, DOMR, DOLG, DOLC, and DODE.[37] Do[a] and Do[b] have a prevalence of 66% and 82%, respectively, in populations of European ethnicity (Table 12-6). The prevalence of Do[a] is somewhat lower in populations of African ethnicity and substantially lower in people of East Asian ethnicity. Anti-Gy[a] is the antibody that is characteristically produced by immunized individuals with the Dombrock-null [Gy(a–)] phenotype that results from various inactivating mutations. Two uncommon phenotypes are present in individuals of African ethnicity: Hy– Jo(a–) (Gly108Val) and Hy+[w] Jo(a–) (Thr117Ile). These are usually associated with weak expression of Do[b] and Do[a], respectively (Table 12-6). The Dombrock glycoprotein (ART4; CD297) is an adenosine diphosphate ribosyltransferase encoded by *ART4* located on chromosome 12p13-p12, although its function on red cells is not known.

Dombrock antigens are resistant to papain and ficin treatment of red cells but are sensitive to trypsin, α-chymotrypsin, and pronase. They are also sensitive to the disulfide-bond-reducing agents AET and DTT.

Dombrock antibodies are usually IgG and reactive by an IAT. They are rare and are often of poor quality, with very weak reactivity.

TABLE 12-6. Phenotypes of the Dombrock System and Their Approximate Prevalence

Phenotype	Do[a]	Do[b]	Gy[a]	Hy	Jo[a]	Prevalence (%) Whites	Prevalence (%) US Blacks
Do(a+b–)	+	–	+	+	+	18	11
Do(a+b+)	+	+	+	+	+	49	44
Do(a–b+)	–	+	+	+	+	33	45
Gy(a–)	–	–	–	–	–	Rare	0
Hy–	–	+[w]	+[w]	–	–	0	Rare
Jo(a–)	+[w]	–/+[w]	+	+[w]	–	0	Rare
DOYA–	–	–	+[w]	+[w]	+[w]	Rare	Rare
DOMR–	–	+	–	+[w]	+[w]	Rare	Rare
DOLG–	+	–	+[w]	+	+	Rare	Rare

+[w] = weakened expression of antigen.

Screening for Dombrock-compatible donors, therefore, is best performed by molecular genotyping.

Anti-Do^a and -Do^b have been responsible for acute and delayed HTRs. There is little information regarding the clinical significance of other Dombrock antibodies. No Dombrock antibody has caused HDFN.

THE COLTON SYSTEM

Co^a (CO1; Ala45) is a high-prevalence antigen; Co^b (CO2; Val45), its antithetical antigen, has a prevalence of about 8% in people of European ethnicity but is less common in other ethnic groups.[38] Anti-Co3 is reactive with all red cells except those of the extremely rare Co(a–b–) phenotype that results from various inactivating mutations. Co4 (Gln47) is a high-prevalence antigen whose presence is required for the expression of Co^a because of the proximity of the polymorphism.[39] The Colton antigens

are located on the red cell's water transporter, aquaporin-1, encoded by *AQP1* on chromosome 7p14 (Fig 12-8). Colton antibodies are usually IgG and reactive by an IAT, although agglutinating IgM anti-Co^a has been found. Colton antibodies have been implicated in severe HDFN and HTRs. Colton antigens are resistant to proteolytic enzymes.

THE LANDSTEINER-WIENER SYSTEM

LW^a (LW5) and LW^b (LW7; Gln100Arg) are antithetical antigens of high and low prevalence, respectively.[40] Anti-LW^{ab} is reactive with all red cells except those of the extremely rare LW-null phenotype and Rh$_{null}$ cells, which are also LW(a–b–). LW antigens are expressed more strongly on D+ than D– red cells and more strongly on umbilical cord red cells than on those of adults. LW antigens are unaffected by treatment of the red cells with papain, ficin,

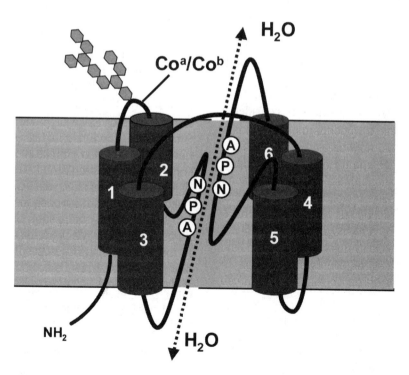

FIGURE 12-8. A model of aquaporin-1, showing the six membrane-spanning domains as cylinders. The first extracellular loop is glycosylated and contains the Co^a/Co^b polymorphism. The third extracellular loop and first intracellular loop contain alanine (A)-proline (P)-asparagine (N) motifs and form a channel in the membrane through which water molecules pass.

trypsin, or α-chymotrypsin but are destroyed by pronase. Disulfide-bond-reducing agents (AET and DTT) either destroy or greatly reduce LW^a or LW^{ab} (LW6) on red cells.

The LW glycoprotein is intercellular adhesion molecule-4 (ICAM-4), an IgSF adhesion molecule encoded by *ICAM4* on chromosome 19p13.2. ICAM-4 binds integrins on macrophages and erythroblasts, and it is probably involved in the stabilization of erythroblastic islands in the marrow during the later stages of erythropoiesis.[39] ICAM-4 is also part of the band 3/Rh ankyrin macrocomplex (Fig 12-1) of red cell surface antigens and might maintain close contact between the red cell surface and the vascular endothelium. Upregulation of ICAM-4 on red cells of patients with sickle cell disease has been implicated in the adhesion of these cells to the vascular endothelium and the resultant crises of vascular occlusion.[41]

Most LW antibodies are reactive by an IAT. They are not generally considered to be clinically significant and have not been implicated in HTRs or HDFN. Acquired and often temporary LW-negative phenotypes sometimes occur with production of anti-LW^a or anti-LW^{ab}, a phenomenon that is usually associated with pregnancy or hematologic malignancy. The transient antibodies behave like alloantibodies but, strictly speaking, should be considered autoantibodies.

THE CHIDO/RODGERS SYSTEM

The nine antigens of the Chido/Rodgers system, while considered blood group antigens, are not produced by erythroid cells. They are located on a fragment of the fourth component of complement (C4d) that attaches to the red cells from the plasma. Ch1 to Ch6, Rg1, and Rg2 each have a prevalence >90%; WH has a prevalence of about 15%. A complex relationship exists between the nine determinants and SNPs in *C4A* and *C4B*, the genes encoding the C4α chains. The expression of Chido/Rodgers on red cells is destroyed by treatment of the cells with proteolytic enzymes, such as papain or ficin.

No Chido/Rodgers antibodies are known to have caused HTRs or HDFN, and antigen-

negative blood is not required for transfusion. However, rare cases of anaphylactic reactions caused by these antibodies have been described. Chido/Rodgers antibodies are generally IgG. Detection of these antibodies with native red cells usually requires an IAT, but they directly agglutinate red cells coated artificially with C4d. Binding of Chido/Rodgers antibodies to red cells is readily inhibited by plasma from Ch/Rg+ individuals; this is a useful aid to identification of these antibodies (Method 3-17).

THE GERBICH SYSTEM

The Gerbich system consists of six highly prevalent antigens—Ge2, Ge3, Ge4, GEPL, GEAT, and GETI—and five antigens with very low prevalence: Wb, Ls^a, An^a, Dh^a, and GEIS. These antigens are located on GPC, GPD, or both. These two glycoproteins are produced by the same gene, *GYPC*, located on chromosome 2q14-q21, by initiation of translation at two different sites on the mRNA. GPD lacks the N-terminal 21 amino acids of GPC. GPC and GPD are part of the junctional complex of membrane proteins.[42] Their C-terminal cytoplasmic domains interact with the membrane skeleton through 4.1R, p55, and adducin and serve as an important link between the membrane and its skeleton.

GPC is exploited as a receptor by some strains of the malaria parasite *P. falciparum*. There are three types of "Gerbich-negative" phenotypes (Table 12-7). Ge:–2,–3,–4 is the true null in which both GPC and GPD are absent from the red cells, and the cells are elliptocytic. In the other phenotypes,

TABLE 12-7. Phenotypes Lacking High-Prevalence Gerbich Antigens and the Antibodies That May Be Produced

Phenotype	Antibodies
Ge:–2,3,4 (Yus type)	Anti-Ge2
Ge:–2,–3,4 (Ge type)	Anti-Ge2 or -Ge3
Ge:–2,–3,–4 (Leach type)	Anti-Ge2, -Ge3, or -Ge4

Ge:–2,3,4 and Ge:–2,–3,4, GPD is absent and an abnormal form of GPC is present. Ge2, Ge3, and Ge4 are destroyed by trypsin treatment of red cells. Whereas Ge2 and Ge4 are also sensitive to papain-treatment, Ge3 is resistant. Consequently, papain-treated red cells can be used for distinguishing anti-Ge2 from anti-Ge3 in the absence of the very rare Ge:–2,3,4 phenotype red cells.

Gerbich antibodies may be IgM and directly agglutinating, but most are IgG and require an IAT for detection. Anti-Ge2 is not generally considered to be clinically significant, but anti-Ge3 has caused mild to moderate HTRs. Anti-Ge3 has caused HDFN that tends to manifest 2 to 4 weeks after birth, and with severe neonatal anemia associated with suppression of erythropoiesis. Some autoantibodies with specificities resembling anti-Ge2 or -Ge3 have been responsible for AIHA.

THE CROMER SYSTEM

The 19 Cromer antigens are located on the complement-regulatory glycoprotein called decay-accelerating factor (DAF or CD55).[43] They include the antithetical antigens Tc^a/Tc^b/Tc^c, and WES^a/WES^b. Tc^a and WES^b have high prevalence, and Tc^b, Tc^c, and WES^a, have low prevalence, although both Tc^b and WES^a are present in approximately 0.5% of people of African ethnicity, and WES^a is present in 0.6% of people of Finnish ancestry. The other antigens have high prevalence: Cr^a, Dr^a, Es, IFC, UMC, GUTI, SERF, ZENA, CROV, CRAM, CROZ, CRUE, CRAG, and CROK.

Anti-IFC is the antibody made by individuals with the very rare Cromer-null phenotype (Inab phenotype), and it is reactive with all red cells other than those of the Inab phenotype. Cromer antigens are readily destroyed by α-chymotrypsin treatment of red cells but not by papain, ficin, or trypsin treatment. The disulfide-bond-reducing agents AET and DTT reduce antigen expression only slightly.

CD55 helps protect the red cells from lysis resulting from autologous complement by inhibiting the action of C3-convertases. Inab-phenotype red cells do not undergo undue hemolysis, however, because of the activity of another complement-regulatory glycoprotein, CD59. Because CD55 and CD59 are both linked to the red cell membrane by a glycosyl-phosphatidylinositol (GPI) anchor, pathologic levels of hemolysis occur in paroxysmal nocturnal hemoglobinuria, which is associated with a clonal defect in GPI biosynthesis and the absence of both CD55 and CD59 in affected red cells. CD55 has recently been identified as a receptor for *P. falciparum.*[44]

Cromer antibodies are not usually considered to be clinically significant because there is little evidence that any of them has caused an HTR, and the evidence from functional cellular assays is equivocal. No Cromer antibodies have been implicated in HDFN, and they are probably sequestered by high levels of CD55 in the placenta. Cromer antibodies are usually IgG and require an IAT for detection. They may be inhibited by serum or concentrated urine from antigen-positive individuals.

THE KNOPS SYSTEM

The nine antigens of the Knops system are located on the complement-regulatory glycoprotein called complement receptor 1 (CR1 or CD35).[45] All are polymorphic, although Kn^a, McC^a, Sl1, Sl3, and Yk^a have relatively high prevalence (Table 12-8).

The Helgeson phenotype, an apparent null phenotype, indicates very low levels of red cell CR1 and very weak expression of Knops antigens. Knops antigens are generally resistant to papain and ficin, although this may depend on the antibodies used, and are destroyed by trypsin or α-chymotrypsin treatment. They are also destroyed, or at least weakened, by AET and DTT.

CR1 is a receptor for *P. falciparum* and appears to be involved in the rosetting of red cells that is associated with severe malaria. The McC^b and Sl2 alleles, present almost exclusively in individuals of African ethnicity, may confer a degree of protection from the parasite. This might explain the very strong difference in the prevalence of some antigens, especially Sl1, McC^b, Sl2, and KCAM, among populations

TABLE 12-8. Approximate Prevalence of Knops Antigens in Two Populations

Antigen		Prevalence (%)	
		Whites	US Blacks
Kn^a	KN1	99	100
Kn^b	KN2	6	0
McC^a	KN3	98	94
Sl1 (Sl^a)	KN4	98	60
Yk^a	KN5	92	98
McC^b	KN6	0	45
Sl2	KN7	0	80
Sl3	KN8	100	100
KCAM	KN9	98	20

of European and African ethnicity (Table 12-8).

Knops antibodies are not clinically significant and can be ignored when selecting blood for transfusion. They are usually difficult to work with, often making it difficult to distinguish antigen-negative cells from those with weak expression. Recombinant CR1 reagents are becoming available for use as inhibiting reagents to help in detection of these antibodies. They are generally IgG and reactive only by an IAT.

THE INDIAN SYSTEM

The low-prevalence antigen In^a and its antithetical antigen In^b plus three other high-prevalence antigens (INFI, INJA, and INRA) are located on CD44, the predominant cell surface receptor for the glycosaminoglycan hyaluronan, a component of the extracellular matrix.[46] AnWj (901009), an antigen with very high prevalence, may also be located on or associated with CD44, but the evidence is incomplete. Indian antigens have reduced expression on red cells with the In(Lu) phenotype, and AnWj is virtually undetectable on In(Lu) cells. In^a and In^b are sensitive to treatment of red cells with proteolytic enzymes—papain, ficin, trypsin, α-chymotrypsin—and are also destroyed by

the disulfide-bond-reducing agents AET and DTT. AnWj, however, is resistant to all these enzymes but shows variable outcomes with reducing agents.

Anti-In^a and -In^b often agglutinate red cells directly, but the reaction is usually enhanced by an IAT. Indian antibodies are not generally considered to be clinically significant, although there is one report of anti-In^b causing an HTR. Anti-AnWj, however, has caused severe HTRs, and In(Lu) red cells should be selected for transfusion.

THE OK SYSTEM

Ok^a, OKGV, and OKVM have very high prevalence and are located on the IgSF molecule CD147, or basigin, which has two IgSF domains. Ok^a is resistant to proteolytic enzymes and disulfide-bond-reducing agents. Very few alloanti-Ok^a antibodies and a single example each of anti-OKGV and -OKVM are known; all are reactive by an IAT.[47] In-vivo survival tests and cellular functional assays with one anti-Ok^a have suggested that it could be clinically significant, but no clinical information exists. Basigin is another important receptor for *P. falciparum* invasion.[48]

THE RAPH SYSTEM

MER2 (RAPH1), which is located on the tetraspanin CD151, was initially defined by mouse monoclonal antibodies that recognized a quantitative polymorphism, and about 8% of the population has undetectable levels of MER2 on their mature red cells. Alloanti-MER2 was found in three Israeli Jews originating from India who had a RAPH-null phenotype resulting from a single nucleotide deletion that led to a premature stop codon. These three individuals were CD151-deficient and had end-stage renal failure, sensorineural deafness, and pretibial epidermolysis bullosa, suggesting that CD151 is essential for the proper assembly of basement membranes in kidney, inner ear, and skin.[49,50] MER2-negative individuals with anti-MER2 but only single amino acid substitutions in CD151 do not have these symptoms.

MER2 antigen is resistant to treatment of red cells with papain but is destroyed by trypsin, α-chymotrypsin, and pronase and by AET and DTT. MER2 antibodies react in an IAT. There is no evidence that anti-MER2 is clinically significant.

THE JOHN MILTON HAGEN SYSTEM

This system consists of six antigens with very high prevalence—JMH, JMHK, JMHL, JMHG, JMHM, and JMHQ—on the semaphorin glycoprotein CD108 (Sema7A). Anti-JMH is typically produced by individuals with an acquired loss of CD108. This most often occurs in elderly patients and is associated with a weakly positive direct antiglobulin test (DAT) result. The absence of the other JMH antigens results from different missense mutations in *SEMA7A*.[51] JMH antigens are destroyed by proteolytic enzymes and disulfide-bond-reducing agents. They are not detected on cord red cells. Sema7A has also been shown to be a receptor for *P. falciparum*.[8]

JMH antibodies are usually reactive in an IAT. They are not generally considered to be clinically significant, although one example was implicated in an acute HTR.

THE GILL SYSTEM

GIL antibodies detect a very high-prevalence antigen, GIL, located on aquaporin 3 (AQP3), a member of the aquaporin superfamily of water and glycerol channels (like the Colton blood group system).[52] AQP3 enhances the permeability of the red cell membrane by glycerol and water.

GIL antigen is resistant to proteolytic enzymes and disulfide-bond-reducing agents. GIL antibodies are reactive by an IAT. Anti-GIL has not been implicated in HTRs or HDFN, although monocyte monolayer assays have suggested a potential to cause accelerated destruction of GIL+ red cells.

THE RHAG SYSTEM

The four antigens of the RHAG system are located on the Rh-associated glycoprotein (RhAG), which is described in more detail in Chapter 11.[53] RhAG is closely associated with the Rh protein in the membrane as part of the band 3/Rh ankyrin macrocomplex (Fig 12-1). Ol^a is very rare, and homozygosity for the allele encoding Ol^a is associated with an Rh$_{mod}$ phenotype. Duclos and DSLK have high prevalence, and absence of these antigens is associated with an aberrant U (MNS5) antigen. RHAG4 is a low-prevalence antigen whose antibody was associated with a single case of severe HDFN.

THE FORS SYSTEM

FORS is a new blood group system consisting of a single antigen, Forssman glycosphingolipid antigen (FORS1). The presence of FORS1 on human erythrocytes is unusual and was shown to be the result of an enzyme-activating amino acid substitution arising from a missense mutation in the human Forssman synthase gene *GBGT1*. FORS1 was demonstrated biochemically on the red cells of two blood donors from different families with the A$_{pae}$ phenotype.[54] (See Chapter 10.) A$_{pae}$ had been previously thought to constitute a subgroup of A in the ABO system but has now been shown to be based on the presence of FORS1 antigen on red cells. Forssman synthase adds a terminal 3-α-*N*-acetylgalactosamine to its globoside acceptor. FORS1 is not usually present on the red cells of primates but is highly expressed on the red cells and uroepithelia of lower mammals, such as dogs and sheep. As with other carbohydrate blood group antigens, naturally occurring antibodies to FORS1 are present in all human sera, with the exception of rare FORS1+ individuals, and have the potential to cause a positive crossmatch.

THE JR SYSTEM

The high-prevalence antigen Jr^a is currently the only antigen in the JR blood group system, following the independent findings of two groups demonstrating that the Jr(a–) pheno-type was the result of inactivating nucleotide changes in *ABCG2*.[55,56] The gene encodes ABCG2, a multipass membrane-protein family member of the adenosine triphosphate (ATP)-binding cassette transporters that is broadly distributed throughout the body. Jr[a] has long been associated with drug resistance in cancer and resistance to xenobiotics, and it might be important for porphyrin homeostasis.[57]

The Jr(a–) phenotype is present predomi-nantly in people of Japanese ancestry. Jr[a] anti-gen is resistant to proteolytic enzymes and disulfide-bond-reducing agents. Anti-Jr[a] is re-active by an IAT and has caused HTRs. It is not usually implicated in HDFN, although two fa-tal cases have been reported.

THE LAN SYSTEM

Lan, another high-prevalence antigen, was also elevated to become a new blood group system following the discovery that it was car-ried on ABCB6, another ATP-binding cassette transporter molecule on the erythrocyte mem-brane.[58] Unlike Jr[a], Lan is not associated with any single geographic or ethnic group, and this is mirrored by the diversity of mutant alleles in the Lan– individuals studied. ABCB6 is associ-ated with porphyrin transport and was thought to have an important role in heme synthesis; however, the existence of ABCB6-deleted individuals indicates that there may be compensation by other transporters in the ab-sence of ABCB6.

Lan antigen is expressed variably on red cells in different individuals but is resistant to proteolytic enzymes and disulfide-bond-reducing agents. Anti-Lan is reactive by an IAT and has been implicated in HTRs but not gen-erally in HDFN.

THE VEL SYSTEM

Vel is a high-prevalence blood group antigen that has been shown to depend on the pres-ence of small integral protein 1 (SMIM1), a protein of unknown function newly discovered on the erythrocyte surface.[59-61] Absence of Vel antigen in the vast majority of individuals, re-gardless of ethnic background, is caused by a 17-base-pair deletion in *SMIM1*, which results in the absence of the protein at the cell membrane.

Vel antigen expression is generally weak on cord red cells and differs substantially from one individual to another. Patterns of expres-sion are a consequence both of zygosity for the 17-bp deletion and of polymorphism in the transcription regulatory region in intron 2. Se-rologic expression is not affected by protease treatment, although sensitivity to reducing agents such as 0.2-M DTT is variable. Anti-Vel are often a mixture of IgG and IgM, readily ac-tivate complement, and have been implicated in mild to severe HTRs, although HDFN is rare.

THE CD59 SYSTEM

An antibody to a high-prevalence antigen de-tected in the plasma of a transfused CD59-deficient child was shown to be specific for CD59.[62] The antibody was readily inhibited with soluble protein. Sequence analysis of samples from the family revealed that the par-ents (first-degree cousins) were heterozygous and the child homozygous for a silencing mu-tation in *CD59*. The antibody was IgG, and al-though the child's red cells had been weakly DAT-positive following transfusion, incompat-ible blood was well tolerated. Thus, CD59 has been ratified as a blood group system and the antigen to which the antibody was directed was named CD59.1.[2]

THE AUGUSTINE SYSTEM

The erythrocyte protein called equilibrative nucleoside transporter 1 (ENT1) was identified as the carrier of the At[a] antigen. Daniels and colleagues showed that the At(a–) phenotype in individuals of African origin is defined by an amino acid polymorphism on the ENT1 pro-tein, and that the At(a–) members of a rare family affected by bone malformation lacked the protein because of an inactivating muta-tion in the ENT1 gene.[63] Based on the evi-dence, the blood group system Augustine (symbol: AUG) was created. The antigen de-fined by the antibody produced by the null phenotype was named AUG1, and the antigen defined by the amino acid Glu391 (At^a) was named AUG2.

Anti-At^a is reactive by the IAT, and while it may cause decreased red cell survival of antigen-positive cells, it has been implicated in a case of mild HDFN only.

ANTIGENS THAT DO NOT YET BELONG TO A BLOOD GROUP SYSTEM

Blood Group Collections

Although many antigens are categorized to one of the 36 known blood group systems, others remain as yet uncharacterized. These are mostly antigens with either very high or very low prevalence. Some of them are included in blood group collections that contain two or more antigens that are related serologically, biochemically, or genetically but do not fit the criteria for system status.[1]

The Cost collection contains Cs^a and Cs^b, antithetical antigens with relatively high and low prevalence, respectively. These antigens are serologically related to those of the Knops system but do not appear to be located on CR1. Cost antibodies are not clinically significant.

Er^a and Er^b are antithetical antigens with very high and low prevalence, respectively. Anti-Er3 is produced by individuals with Er(a–b–) red cells. There is no evidence that Er antibodies are clinically significant.

Carbohydrate antigens of the Ii and GLOB collections are described in Chapter 10.

Carbohydrate antigens associated with MNS antigens that are not encoded by *GYPA* or *GYPB* are included in the collection called MNS CHO. These antigens have been shown to result from altered glycosylation of the *O*-linked sugars on GPA and GPB.

High-Prevalence Antigens (901 Series)

The 901 series of the ISBT classification contains six antigens (Table 12-9): five have a prevalence well in excess of 99%, whereas Sd^a has a prevalence of about 91%. All are inherited, though none is eligible to join a system. All six antigens are resistant to papain, trypsin, α-chymotrypsin, and AET treatment of the red cells, and all except AnWj and Sd^a are well-expressed on cord cells.

AnWj is a high prevalence antigen that serves as the receptor for *Haemophilus influenza* on red cells. Alloanti-AnWj has been reported in few individuals and may cause severe HTR, although no cases are known of HDFN. Autoanti-AnWj is more common and is associated with a transiently AnWj– phenotype. The antigen may be carried on CD44. AnWj is absent on cord red cells and is severely depressed in red cells of the In(Lu) phenotype.

Little is known about the Emm antigen. Seven examples of anti-Emm have been described, and of those, six have occurred as naturally occurring antibodies, all in

TABLE 12-9. Antigens of the ISBT 901 Series (High Prevalence)

Antigen	Number	Clinical Significance
Emm	901008	No evidence of clinical significance
AnWj	901009	Severe AHTRs
Sd^a	901011	No evidence of clinical significance
PEL	901014	No evidence of clinical significance
ABTI	901015	No evidence of clinical significance
MAM	901016	Severe HDFN

ISBT = International Society of Blood Transfusion; AHTR = acute hemolytic transfusion reaction; HDFN = hemolytic disease of the fetus and newborn.

nontransfused males. The clinical significance is unknown.

Sd^a is a carbohydrate antigen on red cells synthesized by an enzyme, $\alpha(1,4)N$-acetylgalactosaminyltransferase. The strength of Sd^a on red cells is highly variable, and Sd^a is not detected on cord red cells. Agglutination of Sd(a+) red cells has a characteristic mixed-field appearance of agglutinates and free red cells; when viewed microscopically, the agglutinates are refractile. Anti-Sd^a is inhibited by urine from Sd(a+) individuals (Method 3-19) and by guinea pig urine.

The PEL– phenotype has been found in only two families, and only two examples of anti-PEL have been described. A related antibody, anti-MTP, was nonreactive with PEL– red cells, but anti-PEL was weakly reactive with red cells of the antibody makers.

The high-prevalence antigen ABTI is serologically related to Vel. However, it has been excluded from SMIM1 by sequencing analysis and thus has returned to the 901 series. Like Vel, ABTI expression differs substantially, and it is generally expressed only weakly on cord red cells. ABTI is resistant to treatment of red cells with proteolytic enzymes or disulfide-bond-reducing agents. Anti-ABTI has not caused HDFN, and clinical data are limited.

MAM is the sixth antigen belonging to this series and one for which there is good evidence that the antibodies are clinically important. Severe HDFN and, in one case, neonatal thrombocytopenia have been reported to be caused by anti-MAM.

Low-Prevalence Antigens (700 Series)

Seventeen antigens of very low prevalence in all of the populations tested constitute the 700 series of the ISBT classification: By, Chr^a, Bi, Bx^a, To^a, Pt^a, Re^a, Je^a, Li^a, Milne, RASM, JFV, Kg, JONES, HJK, HOFM, and REIT. All are inherited and do not fit any criteria for joining or forming a system.

Antibodies to low-prevalence antigens do not present transfusion problems because compatible blood is readily available; however, these antibodies remain undetected if a serologic crossmatch is not employed. Antibodies to JFV, Kg, JONES, HJK, and REIT have all caused HDFN.

HLA Antigens on Red Cells

"Bg" is the name given to HLA Class I antigens expressed on mature red cells. Bg^a represents HLA-B7; Bg^b, HLA-B17 (B57 or B58); and Bg^c, HLA-A28 (A68 or A69, which cross-reacts with HLA-A2). Many individuals, however, do not express Bg antigens on their red cells, despite having the corresponding HLA antigens on their lymphocytes.

There are a few reports of Bg antibodies causing HTRs.[64] These antibodies are sometimes present as contaminants in reagents. HLA antigens on red cells are not destroyed by papain, ficin, pronase, trypsin, α-chymotrypsin, AET, or DTT. They can be stripped from red cells with chloroquine (Method 2-20) or acid glycine/EDTA (Method 2-21).

ERYTHROID PHENOTYPES CAUSED BY MUTATIONS IN TRANSCRIPTION FACTOR GENES

Mutations in genes encoding erythroid transcription factors are emerging as important modifiers of blood group antigen expression. As described in the Lutheran system section above, heterozygosity for different mutations in *KLF1* has been identified in individuals with the In(Lu) phenotype. In these individuals, expression of antigens carried on CD44 (In^a/In^b) and the AnWj and P1 antigens is weak.[15] However, *KLF1* mutations have also been shown to affect other genes, notably the β-globin gene, resulting in the hereditary persistence of fetal hemoglobin syndrome.[65] Affected individuals have elevated hemoglobin F levels, some >30%, and demonstrate an In(Lu) phenotype. Furthermore, discrete mutations in *KLF1* appear to give rise to different phenotypes; for example, the change of Glu325Lys does not result in the In(Lu) phenotype but is associated with severe congenital dyserythropoietic anemia. These red cells demonstrate weakened expression of the antigens in the Colton (AQP1), Cromer (DAF), and Landsteiner-Wiener (ICAM-4) blood group systems.[66]

Although mentioned above in the Lutheran system section, it is worth repeating that a mutation in *GATA-1* resulted in the X-linked Lu(a–b–) phenotype in one family.[16] It is likely that additional mutations in these and other erythroid-specific transcription factors will be identified as the causes of altered blood group antigen expression.

KEY POINTS

1. Of 352 recognized antigen specificities, 314 belong to 1 of 36 blood group systems representing either a single gene or two or three closely linked homologous genes. Some groups of antigens that are not eligible to join a system are classified together as collections. Antigens not classified in a system or collection have either low or high prevalence and make up the 700 and 901 series, respectively.

2. M and N are antithetical, polymorphic antigens. M, N, S, s, and 'N' are all destroyed by treatment of the red cells with papain, ficin, bromelin, or pronase, although this effect with S and s is variable. M and N, but not S, s, or 'N', are destroyed by trypsin treatment.

3. Anti-M is relatively common, while anti-N is quite rare. Most anti-M and -N are not clinically significant. When M or N antibodies active at 37 C are encountered, antigen-negative or -compatible red cells should be provided. Anti-S, -s, and -U are generally IgG antibodies that are active at 37 C. They have been implicated in HTRs and severe and fatal HDFN.

4. The antigen often referred to as "Kell" is correctly named "K" or "KEL1"; its antithetical antigen is k or KEL2.

5. Because Kell antibodies can cause severe HDFN and HTRs, patients with Kell antibodies should be transfused with antigen-negative blood whenever possible. Anti-K is the most common immune red cell antibody not in the ABO and Rh systems.

6. The Duffy polymorphism consists of two antigens, Fy^a and Fy^b, and three phenotypes, Fy(a+b–), Fy(a+b+), and Fy(a–b+). Fy^a and Fy^b are very sensitive to most proteolytic enzymes. In people of African ethnicity, a silent allele, *FY*02N.01*, is often present. These individuals do not express Fy^b on their red cells but are not at risk for anti-Fy^b because expression in tissues is not silenced. Individuals who are homozygous for *FY*02N.01* have the red cell phenotype Fy(a–b–).

7. Anti-Fy^a (common) and anti-Fy^b (rare) are generally detected by an IAT and may cause acute or delayed HTRs that are usually mild, although some have been fatal.

8. The polymorphic antigens Jk^a and Jk^b in the Kidd system are resistant to proteolytic enzymes, such as papain and ficin.

9. Anti-Jk^a and -Jk^b are not common, are generally present in antibody mixtures, and are often difficult to detect. An IAT is usually required, and use of enzyme-treated cells may be necessary to detect weaker antibodies. Kidd antibodies may cause severe acute HTRs and are a common cause of delayed HTRs.

10. The 22 antigens of the Diego system are located on band 3, the red cell anion exchanger. Anti-Di^a and -Wr^a can cause severe HDFN. Anti-Wr^a can also cause HTRs.

REFERENCES

1. Daniels GL, Fletcher A, Garratty G, et al. Blood group terminology 2004: From the International Society of Blood Transfusion committee on terminology for red cell surface antigens. Vox Sang 2004;87:304-16.

2. Storry JR, Castilho L, Chen Q, et al. International Society of Blood Transfusion Working Party on Red Cell Immunogenetics and Terminology: Report of the Seoul and London meetings. ISBT Sci Ser 2016;11:118-22.

3. Poole J, Daniels G. Blood group antibodies and their significance in transfusion medicine. Transfus Med Rev 2007;21:58-71.

4. Reid ME, Lomas-Francis C, Olsson ML. The blood group antigen factsbook. 3rd ed. London: Academic Press, 2012.

5. Daniels G. Human blood groups. 3rd ed. Oxford: Wiley-Blackwell, 2013.

6. Lux SE 4th. Anatomy of the red cell membrane skeleton: Unanswered questions. Blood 2016; 127:187-99.

7. Blumenfeld OO, Huang CH. Molecular genetics of the glycophorin gene family, the antigens for MNSs blood groups: Multiple gene rearrangements and modulation of splice site usage result in extensive diversification. Hum Mutat 1995;6:199-209.

8. Satchwell TJ. Erythrocyte invasion receptors for *Plasmodium falciparum*: New and old. Transfus Med 2016;26:77-88.

9. Wikman A, Edner A, Gryfelt G, et al. Fetal hemolytic anemia and intrauterine death caused by anti-M immunization. Transfusion 2007; 47:911-17.

10. Huang CH, Blumenfeld OO. Molecular genetics of human erythrocyte MiIII and MiVI glycophorins: Use of a pseudoexon in construction of two delta-alpha-delta hybrid genes resulting in antigenic diversification. J Biol Chem 1991;266:7248-55.

11. Heathcote DJ, Carroll TE, Flower RL. Sixty years of antibodies to MNS system hybrid glycophorins: What have we learned? Transfus Med Rev 2011;25:111-24.

12. Crew VK, Green C, Daniels G. Molecular bases of the antigens of the Lutheran blood group system. Transfusion 2003;43:1729-37.

13. Eyler CE, Telen MJ. The Lutheran glycoprotein: A multifunctional adhesion receptor. Transfusion 2006;46:668-77.

14. Karamatic Crew V, Mallinson G, Green C, et al. Different inactivating mutations in the LU genes of three individuals with the Lutheran-null phenotype. Transfusion 2007;47:492-8.

15. Singleton BK, Burton NM, Green C, et al. Mutations in EKLF/KLF1 form the molecular basis of the rare blood group In(Lu) phenotype. Blood 2008;112:2081-8.

16. Singleton BK, Roxby DJ, Stirling JW, et al. A novel GATA1 mutation (Stop414Arg) in a family with the rare X-linked blood group Lu(a-b-) phenotype and mild macrothrombocytic thrombocytopenia. Br J Haematol 2013;161: 139-42.

17. Westhoff CM, Reid ME. Review: The Kell, Duffy, and Kidd blood group systems. Immunohematology 2004;20:37-49.

18. Lee S, Zambas ED, Marsh WL, Redman CM. Molecular cloning and primary structure of Kell blood group protein. Proc Natl Acad Sci U S A 1991;88:6353-7.

19. Daniels G, Hadley A, Green CA. Causes of fetal anemia in hemolytic disease due to anti-K. Transfusion 2003;43:115-16.

20. Denomme GA. Kell and Kx blood group systems. Immunohematology 2015;31:14-19.

21. Salomao M, Zhang X, Yang Y, et al. Protein 4.1R-dependent multiprotein complex: New insights into the structural organization of the red blood cell membrane. Proc Natl Acad Sci U S A 2008;105:8026-31.

22. Azouzi S, Collec E, Mohandas N, et al. The human Kell blood group binds the erythroid 4.1R protein: New insights into the 4.1R-dependent red cell membrane complex. Br J Haematol 2015;171:862-71.

23. Lee S, Debnath AK, Redman CM. Active amino acids of the Kell blood group protein and model of the ectodomain based on the structure of neutral endopeptidase 24.11. Blood 2003;102: 3028-34.

24. Danek A, Rubio JP, Rampoldi L, et al. McLeod neuroacanthocytosis: Genotype and phenotype. Ann Neurol 2001;50:755-64.

25. Meny GM. The Duffy blood group system: A review. Immunohematology 2010;26:51-6.

26. Tournamille C, Colin Y, Cartron JP, Le Van Kim C. Disruption of a GATA motif in the Duffy gene promoter abolishes erythroid gene expression in Duffy-negative individuals. Nat Genet 1995;10:224-8.

27. Mohandas N, Gallagher PG. Red cell membrane: Past, present, and future. Blood 2008; 112:3939-48.

28. Horuk R, Chitnis CE, Darbonne WC, et al. A receptor for the malarial parasite *Plasmodium vivax*: The erythrocyte chemokine receptor. Science 1993;261:1182-4.

29. Shen H, Schuster R, Stringer KF, et al. The Duffy antigen/receptor for chemokines (DARC) regulates prostate tumor growth. FASEB J 2006;20:59-64.

30. Xu L, Ashkenazi A, Chaudhuri A. Duffy antigen/receptor for chemokines (DARC) attenuates angiogenesis by causing senescence in endothelial cells. Angiogenesis 2007;10:307-18.

31. Holt S, Donaldson H, Hazlehurst G, et al. Acute transplant rejection induced by blood transfusion reaction to the Kidd blood group system. Nephrol Dial Transplant 2004;19:2403-6.

32. Heaton DC, McLoughlin K. Jk(a-b-) red blood cells resist urea lysis. Transfusion 1982;22:70-1.

33. Sands JM, Gargus JJ, Frohlich O, et al. Urinary concentrating ability in patients with Jk(a-b-) blood type who lack carrier-mediated urea transport. J Am Soc Nephrol 1992;2:1689-96.

34. Byrne KM, Byrne PC. Review: Other blood group systems—Diego, Yt, Xg, Scianna, Dombrock, Colton, Landsteiner-Wiener, and Indian. Immunohematology 2004;20:50-8.

35. Johnson NC. XG: The forgotten blood group system. Immunohematology 2011;27:68-71.

36. Velliquette RW. Review: The Scianna blood group system. Immunohematology 2005;21:70-6.

37. Reid ME. Complexities of the Dombrock blood group system revealed. Transfusion 2005;45:92S-9S.

38. Halverson GR, Peyrard T. A review of the Colton blood group system. Immunohematology 2010;26:22-6.

39. Daniels G. Functions of red cell surface proteins. Vox Sang 2007;93:331-40.

40. Grandstaff Moulds MK. The LW blood group system: A review. Immunohematology 2011;27:136-42.

41. Zennadi R, Moeller BJ, Whalen EJ, et al. Epinephrine-induced activation of LW-mediated sickle cell adhesion and vaso-occlusion in vivo. Blood 2007;110:2708-17.

42. Walker PS, Reid ME. The Gerbich blood group system: A review. Immunohematology 2010;26:60-5.

43. Storry JR, Reid ME, Yazer MH. The Cromer blood group system: A review. Immunohematology 2010;26:109-18.

44. Egan ES, Jiang RH, Moechtar MA, et al. Malaria. A forward genetic screen identifies erythrocyte CD55 as essential for *Plasmodium falciparum* invasion. Science 2015;348:711-14.

45. Moulds JM. The Knops blood-group system: A review. Immunohematology 2010;26:2-7.

46. Xu Q. The Indian blood group system. Immunohematology 2011;27:89-93.

47. Smart EA, Storry JR. The OK blood group system: A review. Immunohematology 2010;26:124-6.

48. Crosnier C, Bustamante LY, Bartholdson SJ, et al. Basigin is a receptor essential for erythrocyte invasion by *Plasmodium falciparum*. Nature 2011;480:534-7.

49. Karamatic Crew V, Burton N, Kagan A, et al. CD151, the first member of the tetraspanin (TM4) superfamily detected on erythrocytes, is essential for the correct assembly of human basement membranes in kidney and skin. Blood 2004;104:2217-23.

50. Hayes M. Raph blood group system. Immunohematology 2014;30:6-10.

51. Seltsam A, Strigens S, Levene C, et al. The molecular diversity of Sema7A, the semaphorin that carries the JMH blood group antigens. Transfusion 2007;47:133-46.

52. Roudier N, Ripoche P, Gane P, et al. AQP3 deficiency in humans and the molecular basis of a novel blood group system, GIL. J Biol Chem 2002;277:45854-9.

53. Chou ST, Westhoff CM. The Rh and RhAG blood group systems. Immunohematology 2010;26:178-86.

54. Svensson L, Hult AK, Stamps R, et al. Forssman expression on human erythrocytes: Biochemical and genetic evidence of a new histo-blood group system. Blood 2013;121:1459-68.

55. Saison C, Helias V, Ballif BA, et al. Null alleles of ABCG2 encoding the breast cancer resistance protein define the new blood group system Junior. Nat Genet 2012;44:174-7.

56. Zelinski T, Coghlan G, Liu XQ, Reid ME. ABCG2 null alleles define the Jr(a-) blood group phenotype. Nat Genet 2012;44:131-2.

57. Robey RW, To KK, Polgar O, et al. ABCG2: A perspective. Adv Drug Deliv Rev 2009;61:3-13.

58. Helias V, Saison C, Ballif BA, et al. ABCB6 is dispensable for erythropoiesis and specifies the new blood group system Langereis. Nat Genet 2012;44:170-3.

59. Storry JR, Joud M, Christophersen MK, et al. Homozygosity for a null allele of SMIM1 defines the Vel-negative blood group phenotype. Nat Genet 2013;45:537-41.

60. Ballif BA, Helias V, Peyrard T, et al. Disruption of SMIM1 causes the Vel- blood type. EMBO Mol Med 2013;5:751-61.

61. Cvejic A, Haer-Wigman L, Stephens JC, et al. SMIM1 underlies the Vel blood group and influences red blood cell traits. Nat Genet 2013;45:542-5.

62. Anliker M, von Zabern I, Hochsmann B, et al. A new blood group antigen is defined by anti-CD59, detected in a CD59-deficient patient. Transfusion 2014;54:1817-22.

63. Daniels G, Ballif BA, Helias V, et al. Lack of the nucleoside transporter ENT1 results in the Augustine-null blood type and ectopic mineralization. Blood 2015;125:3651-4.

64. Nance ST. Do HLA antibodies cause hemolytic transfusion reactions or decreased RBC survival? Transfusion 2003;43:687-90.

65. Borg J, Papadopoulos P, Georgitsi M, et al. Haploinsufficiency for the erythroid transcription factor KLF1 causes hereditary persistence of fetal hemoglobin. Nat Genet 2010;42:801-5.

66. Arnaud L, Saison C, Helias V, et al. A dominant mutation in the gene encoding the erythroid transcription factor KLF1 causes a congenital dyserythropoietic anemia. Am J Hum Genet 2010;87:721-7.

Chapter 13

Identification of Antibodies to Red Cell Antigens

• • •

Janis R. Hamilton, MS, MT(ASCP)SBB, and
Debra J. Bailey, MT(ASCP)SBB

13

NATURALLY OCCURRING ANTI-A and anti-B are the only red cell antibodies that are commonly found in human serum or plasma. All other antibodies are called "unexpected red cell antibodies." This chapter discusses methods for identifying unexpected red cell antibodies once pretransfusion testing (see Chapter 17) indicates an unexpected antibody is present.

There are two types of unexpected red cell antibodies: alloantibodies and autoantibodies. When an individual produces an antibody to an antigen that he or she lacks, the antibody is called an alloantibody. When an individual produces an antibody to an antigen that she or he possesses, the antibody is called an autoantibody. Therefore, by definition, alloantibodies react only with allogeneic red cells that express the corresponding antigens—not with the antibody producer's red cells. Conversely, autoantibodies are reactive with the red cells of the antibody producer. In fact, autoantibodies usually are reactive with most reagent red cells as well as with autologous red cells.

Immunization to red cell antigens may result from pregnancy, transfusion, transplantation, needle sharing, or injections of immunogenic material. The incidence of alloimmunization is extremely variable depending on the patient population being studied. In chronically transfused patient populations, such as those with sickle cell anemia or thalassemia, as many as 14% to 50% of individuals are reported to be alloimmunized.[1-3]

In some instances, no specific immunizing event can be identified. "Naturally occurring" antibodies have presumably resulted from exposure to environmental, bacterial, or viral antigens that are similar to blood group antigens. Antibodies detected in serologic tests may also be passively acquired from injected immunoglobulin, donor plasma, passenger lymphocytes in transplanted organs, or hematopoietic progenitor cells (HPCs).

After an antibody has been detected, its type (auto and/or allo) and specificity should be determined and its clinical significance assessed. A clinically significant red cell antibody

Janis R. Hamilton, MS, MT(ASCP)SBB, Manager, and Debra J. Bailey, MT(ASCP)SBB, Lead Technologist, Reference Laboratory, American Red Cross Blood Services, Detroit, Michigan
J. Hamilton has disclosed financial relationships with Grifols and Immucor, Inc. D. Bailey has disclosed no conflicts of interest.

is defined as an antibody that is frequently associated with hemolytic disease of the fetus and newborn (HDFN), hemolytic transfusion reactions, or a notable decrease in transfused red cell survival. Determining the specificity of the antibody is the most commonly used way of predicting its possible clinical significance. Yet, the degree of clinical significance varies among antibodies with the same specificity; some cause destruction of incompatible red cells within hours or even minutes, whereas others decrease red cell survival by only a few days, and still others do not shorten red cell survival discernibly. Some antibodies are known to cause HDFN, whereas others may cause a positive direct antiglobulin test (DAT) result in the fetus without clinical evidence of HDFN.

BASIC CONCEPTS IN RED CELL ANTIGEN EXPRESSION

Antibody identification is dependent on the reactivity of the serum or plasma with red cells of known antigen expression. A basic understanding of variables in antigen expression is critical to interpreting reactivity in identification studies.

Zygosity and Dosage

The reaction strength of some antibodies may vary because of dosage, meaning that antibodies are more strongly reactive (or only reactive) with red cells that possess a "double-dose" expression of the antigen. Double-dose antigen expression occurs when an individual is homozygous for the gene that encodes the antigen. Red cells from individuals who are heterozygous for the gene may express fewer antigens and, therefore, may be weakly reactive or nonreactive with a weak example of the corresponding antibody. Alloantibodies vary in their tendency to demonstrate dosage. Many antibodies to antigens in the Rh, Duffy, MNS, and Kidd blood groups demonstrate dosage.

Variation in Adults and Neonates

Some antigens (eg, I, P1, Le^a, and Sd^a) show variable expression on red cells from different adults. The antigenic differences can be demonstrated serologically; however, the variability from one antigen-positive adult to another is unrelated to zygosity. Some antigens are expressed differently on cord/neonate red cells compared to adult red cells of the same individual. Antigen expression on cord/neonate red cells may be absent, weaker, or stronger as compared to adult red cells. (Table 13-1 provides some examples.)

Changes with Storage

Blood group antibodies may be more weakly reactive with stored red cells than with fresh red cells. Some antigens (eg, Fy^a, Fy^b, M, P1, Kn^a, McC^a, and Bg) deteriorate more rapidly than others during storage, and the rate varies among red cells from different individuals.[4] Because red cells from donors are often fresher than commercial reagent red cells, some antibodies have stronger reactions with donor red cells than with reagent red cells. Similarly, storage of red cells in a freezer may cause antigens to deteriorate, thus producing misleading antibody identification results.

The pH or other characteristics of the storage medium can affect the rate of antigen deterioration.[4,5] For example, Fy^a and Fy^b antigens may weaken when the red cells are stored in a medium with low pH and low ionic strength. Thus, certain antibodies may demonstrate differences in reactivity with red cells

TABLE 13-1. Antigen Expression on Cord Red Cells*

Expression	Antigens
Negative	Le^a, Le^b, Sd^a, Ch, Rg, and AnWj
Weak	I, H, P1, Lu^a, Lu^b, Yt^a, Vel, Bg, KN and DO antigens, Yk^a, Cs^a, and Fy3
Strong	i, LW^a, and LW^b

*Modified with permission from Reid et al.[28]

from different manufacturers if the suspending media are different.

The age and nature of the specimen must be considered when red cells are typed. Antigens on red cells from clotted samples tend to deteriorate more quickly than antigens on red cells from donor units that are collected in citrate anticoagulants, such as acid-citrate-dextrose or citrate-phosphate-dextrose. Red cells in donor units collected in approved anticoagulants retain their antigens throughout the standard shelf life of the blood component. Samples with EDTA up to 14 days old are suitable for antigen typing.[6] However, the manufacturer's instructions should always be consulted when commercial typing reagents are used.

INITIAL ANTIBODY IDENTIFICATION CONSIDERATIONS

Specimen Requirements

Serum and plasma are interchangeable for antibody testing unless complement is required for antibody detection. In such rare cases, only serum provides complement. Throughout this chapter, serum can be considered to be interchangeable with plasma unless the text indicates otherwise. The use of serum or plasma may also be dictated by the test method employed.

Depending on the test methods used, a 5-mL to 10-mL aliquot of whole blood usually contains enough serum or plasma for identifying simple antibody specificities; more whole blood may be required for complex studies. When autologous red cells are tested, the use of samples anticoagulated with EDTA avoids problems associated with the in-vitro uptake of complement components by red cells, which may occur when clotted samples are used.

Reagents and Test Methods

Antibody Detection Red Cells

Group O red cells suitable for pretransfusion antibody screening are commercially available and most frequently offered as sets of either two or three samples of reagent single-donor red cells. All reagent red cell sets licensed by the US Food and Drug Administration (FDA) for this purpose must contain red cell samples that collectively express the following antigens: D, C, E, c, e, M, N, S, s, P1, Le^a, Le^b, K, k, Fy^a, Fy^b, Jk^a, and Jk^b. Three-red-cell-sample antibody-detection sets usually offer red cells from presumed homozygous donors with double-dose expression for the following common antigens: D, C, E, c, e, k, M, N, S, s, Fy^a, Fy^b, Jk^a, and Jk^b. As mentioned above, antibodies in the Rh, MNS, Duffy, and Kidd systems most commonly demonstrate dosage. Each laboratory should decide whether to use two or three reagent single-donor red cell samples for antibody detection testing. When antibody detection is automated, the instrument platform may dictate the reagent red cell configuration. In the United States, pooled red cells for antibody detection are obtained from two different donors and may be used only when testing donor samples. Reagent red cells should be refrigerated when not in use and should not be used for antibody detection after their expiration date.

Antibody Identification Red Cell Panels

Identification of antibodies to red cell antigens detected in pretransfusion antibody screening requires testing the serum/plasma against a panel of red cell samples (typically 8-14) with known antigenic composition. Usually, the red cell samples are obtained from commercial suppliers, but institutions may assemble their own panels using red cells from local sources. Except in special circumstances, panel cells are group O, thereby allowing serum/plasma of any ABO group to be tested.

Each reagent red cell sample in the panel is from a different donor. The reagent red cells are selected so a distinctive pattern of positive and negative reactions will result when the reactivity of all the panel cells is considered. To be functional, a reagent red cell panel must make it possible to identify with confidence those clinically significant alloantibodies that are most commonly encountered, such as anti-D, -E, -K, and -Fy^a. The phenotypes of the reagent red cells should be distributed so that single common alloantibody specificities can be clearly identified and most others can be excluded. Ideally, patterns of reactivity for most examples of single alloantibodies should not overlap with any other (eg, all of the K+ red cells should not be the only ones that are also E+). Reagent red cells with double-dose antigen expression are included to detect common antibodies that frequently show dosage. Commercial panels are accompanied by an antigen extended-profile sheet that lists the phenotypes of the red cells. It is essential to use the correct panel sheet when interpreting results because the combination of red cell samples is different for each lot of reagent. Commercial reagent red cells for tube testing are diluted to a 2% to 5% suspension in a preservative solution that can be used directly from the bottle. Washing the red cells before use is usually unnecessary unless the preservative solution is suspected of interfering with antibody identification.

Panel cells beyond their expiration date should not be used as the sole resource for antibody identification. Most laboratories use in-date reagent red cells for initial antibody identification and, if necessary, use expired reagent red cells to exclude or confirm uncommon specificities. Any laboratory that uses expired reagent red cells should establish a policy and validate any procedures associated with this practice.[7(p22)]

Test Methods

All techniques for antibody detection and identification in general use today are based on the principle of hemagglutination (tube or column agglutination systems) or red cell adherence (solid phase). AABB *Standards for Blood Banks and Transfusion Services* requires that "methods of testing shall be those that demonstrate clinically significant antibodies" and "include incubation at 37 C preceding an antiglobulin test."[8(p36)] All methods meet this standard, but each method offers different advantages. Tube testing offers flexibility to test at different phases and the option to use a va-

riety of enhancement media (and thus obtain varying degrees of sensitivity). It also requires little specialized equipment. Column agglutination and solid-phase technology offer stable and possibly less subjective endpoints, workflow standardization, and the ability to be incorporated into semiautomated or automated systems. They provide a sensitive detection system for most blood-group antibodies. Column agglutination, solid-phase methods, and very sensitive tube tests have also been shown to enhance serologic reactivity that may not be clinically significant in the selection of units for transfusion, including the reactivity of warm autoantibodies. The different methods offer laboratories choice in selecting a primary antibody detection and identification method that, with its sensitivity, specificity, automation capabilities (if desired), and cost, is suitable for the patient population served, the laboratory size, and its staff expertise/experience.

Published studies have compared the various methods for detection of wanted and unwanted red cell alloantibodies as well as the potential effect of using red cell membranes vs intact red cells.[9-13] Laboratories should be familiar with the unique reactivity characteristics of their selected method. They frequently will choose to have one or more additional methods available and develop testing algorithms that involve the different methods to aid in the investigation and resolution of results that are not easily apparent with their primary method.

Enhancement Media

Although the test method may consist solely of serum or plasma and red cells (either reagent red cells as provided by the manufacturer or saline-suspended red cells), as in Method 3-2, most serologists use some type of enhancement medium when tube methods are used to decrease incubation time and increase sensitivity. Several different enhancement media are available, including low-ionic-strength saline (LISS), polyethylene glycol (PEG), and 22% bovine albumin. Additional enhancement techniques may be used for complex studies. Some enhancement techniques are discussed in more detail later in this chapter. Specifics regarding the mechanism of action for 22% bovine albumin, LISS, and PEG can be found in the methods describing their use (Methods 3-3, 3-4, and 3-5). Non-tube methods typically prescribe the use of an enhancement medium for the same reasons they are used in tube methods.

Antiglobulin Reagents

Most antibody detection and identification studies include an indirect antiglobulin test (IAT) phase. Either antihuman globulin (AHG) specific only for human immunoglobulin G (IgG) or a polyspecific reagent that contains anti-IgG and anticomplement may be used. A polyspecific reagent may detect—or may detect more readily—antibodies that bind complement, because a single IgG molecule can deposit multiple complement molecules. Therefore, presence of a low-level IgG antibody may be visualized by its complement activation. To detect complement binding, serum rather than plasma must be used: the anticoagulant in plasma binds calcium, making it unavailable for complement activation. Complement binding may be advantageous in some rare instances, such as the detection of certain JK system antibodies. Because of the sensitivity of current test methods, most serologists prefer IgG-specific AHG reagents for routine use. This avoids unwanted reactivity resulting from in-vitro complement binding by cold-reactive antibodies.[14]

   Antiglobulin reagents may be derived from monoclonal or polyclonal source material. Polyclonal reagents, by nature, contain antibodies from many B-cell clones, and collectively their reactivity is directed at many epitopes of the target antigen. Monoclonal reagents have selective reactivity with only specific epitopes. Reagents made from different clones may have subtle reactivity differences: some monoclonally based reagents are blended to cover a wider range of epitope specificities. The anticomplement reagents licensed in the United States are monoclonal. Anti-IgG can be either polyclonal or monoclonal. US-licensed monoclonal anti-IgG does not detect

antibodies of IgG4 subclass. This has little clinical significance, as red cell antibodies of pure IgG4 subclass are rare, and they are not associated with increased red cell destruction because monocytes do not have receptors for the Fc portion of IgG4 molecules. A recent report has described lack of reactivity of this monoclonal anti-IgG also with several IgG3 isoallotypes (genetic variations within an IgG subclass).[15] These reactivity patterns could lead to missing a clinically significant IgG3 red cell antibody if it is predominantly of an isoallotype not detected by the reagent. Differences in anti-IgG reactivity can also be a source of variation in detection of antibody reactivity between laboratories testing the same sample.

BASIC ANTIBODY IDENTIFICATION

Patient History

Before antibody identification testing begins, the patient's medical history should be considered, if such information can be obtained. Multiple aspects of the patient's medical history may influence antibody identification test selection as well as interpretation.

Prior Red Cell Exposure

Exposure to foreign red cells through blood transfusion or pregnancy is the usual cause of red cell immunization. It is uncommon for patients who have never been transfused or pregnant to produce clinically significant alloantibodies, although naturally occurring antibodies may be present. Women are more likely to have alloantibodies than men because of exposure to foreign (ie, fetal) red cells during pregnancy. Infants <6 months usually do not produce alloantibodies, but newborns may have passive antibody of maternal origin.

   If the patient has been transfused, it is critical to know when the most recent transfusion was given. If the patient was transfused during the past 3 months, primary immunization to red cell antigens may be a risk, and the presence of circulating donor red cells affects testing. Mixed-field results caused by the donor red cells in antigen typing tests interfere with interpretation of an autologous phenotype. Autologous adsorption techniques would not be used because alloantibodies could be adsorbed onto transfused donor red cells.

Diagnosis and Disease

Certain diseases have been associated with red cell antibodies; depending on the methods used, such antibodies may be detectable in antibody detection and identification tests. Cold agglutinin syndrome, Raynaud phenomenon, and infections with *Mycoplasma pneumoniae* are often associated with anti-I. Infectious mononucleosis is sometimes associated with anti-i. Patients with paroxysmal cold hemoglobinuria, which is associated with syphilis in adults and viral infections in children, may demonstrate autoantibodies with anti-P specificity by the Donath-Landsteiner test. Warm autoantibodies often accompany diagnoses such as warm autoimmune hemolytic anemia, systemic lupus erythematosus, multiple myeloma, chronic lymphocytic leukemia, or lymphoma. Patients who have received solid-organ or HPC transplants may demonstrate passive antibodies that originate from donor passenger lymphocytes.

Medications and Biologic Therapies

Certain drugs are known to cause antibody identification problems. (See Chapter 14 for a discussion of drug-related mechanisms and drugs that are associated with serologic problems.) Administration of intravenous immune globulin (IVIG) and Rh Immune Globulin (RhIG) can interfere with antibody screening tests. Some lots of IVIG have been reported to contain unexpected antibodies, including anti-A and anti-B. Intravenous RhIG, which is sometimes used to treat immune thrombocytopenia, could explain the presence of anti-D in an Rh-positive patient.

Monoclonal antibodies developed as immunotherapeutic agents may also interfere with serologic results. Anti-CD38 treatment for multiple myeloma and other B-cell malignancies [daratumumab (Darzalex; Janssen Bio-

tech, Horsham, PA)] causes positive reactions in serologic tests employing the antiglobulin phase when infused IgG anti-CD38 binds to the small amount of CD38 present on all normal red cells.[16,17] Anti-CD38 can also, although less often, be the cause of a weakly positive DAT. Development of other novel immunotherapies might cause similar serologic interferences depending on their target antigen. Communication from the health-care team identifying patients being treated with a monoclonal immunotherapy can streamline pretransfusion testing.

Elements of Basic Antibody Identification

Autologous Control and DAT

The autologous control (autocontrol), in which serum or plasma and autologous red cells are tested under the same conditions as testing against reagent red cells, is an important part of antibody identification and should be performed when the test method allows. The autocontrol is not the same as or equivalent to a DAT (Method 3-14). Incubation and the presence of enhancement reagents may cause reactivity in the autocontrol that is an in-vitro phenomenon only. If the autocontrol is positive in the antiglobulin phase, a DAT should be performed. If the DAT result is negative, antibodies to an enhancement medium constituent or autoantibodies that are reactive only in the enhancement medium should be considered. Warm autoantibodies and cold autoantibodies, such as anti-I, -IH, or -Pr, may be reactive in an IAT when certain enhancement media are used; therefore, testing should be repeated in another medium. If the DAT result is positive, it must be interpreted with careful attention to the transfusion history. Autoantibodies or drugs could explain a positive DAT result; however, if the patient has an alloantibody and was recently transfused with blood that expressed the corresponding antigen, the positive DAT may be caused by coating of the donor red cells with alloantibody. This situation is associated with a clinically significant delayed transfusion reaction. More information about interpreting a positive DAT can be found in Chapter 14.

Initial Identification Panel

For initial antibody identification, it is common to use a complete commercial reagent red cell panel in the same methods and test phases as in the antibody detection test or crossmatch. The gel-column and solid-phase methods involve a single reading of the test at the IAT phase. Tube-testing protocols have greater flexibility for reading at different test phases (eg, immediate spin, room temperature, 37 C, and IAT), but many serologists also use a single IAT reading because this test detects the overwhelming majority of clinically significant alloantibodies.

Some serologists using tube methods may choose to include an immediate centrifugation reading, a room-temperature incubation that is read before an enhancement medium is added, or both during initial antibody identification. Such an approach may enhance the detection of certain antibodies (eg, anti-M, -N, -P1, -I, -Le^a, or -Le^b) and may help explain reactions detected in other phases. These steps are frequently omitted in initial antibody identification studies because most antibodies that are reactive only at lower temperatures have little or no clinical significance.

Readings for direct agglutination taken after 37 C incubation in tube testing are influenced by the enhancement media used. Tests employing PEG enhancement cannot be centrifuged and read because the reagent causes nonspecific aggregation of all red cells. LISS, albumin, and saline (no enhancement) tests do not have this restriction. A 37 C reading can detect some antibodies (eg, potent anti-D, -E, or -K) that may cause direct agglutination of red cells. Other antibodies (eg, anti-Le^a or -Jk^a) may occasionally be detected by the lysis of antigen-positive red cells during the 37 C incubation if serum is tested. Omitting centrifugation and the reading at 37 C should lessen the detection of unwanted positive reactions caused by clinically insignificant autoantibodies and alloantibodies. However, in some instances, potentially clinically significant antibodies are detected only by their 37 C reactivity. In 87,480 samples, 103 examples of such antibodies were identified (63 anti-E; 27 -K; 5 -Jk^a; 4 -D; 3 -cE; and 1 -C).[18] If the 37 C reading is desired in a specific antibody study, an alternative strategy is to set up duplicate tests. One test is read after the 37 C incubation, and the other test is read only at the IAT phase.

Abbreviated Identification Panel

If a patient has antibodies that were identified previously, the known antibodies should be considered when selecting reagent red cells to test. For example, if the patient has known anti-e, it will not be helpful to test the patient's serum with a complete commercial reagent red cell panel in which 9 of 10 red cell samples are e-positive. Testing a selected panel of e-negative red cells is a better approach to find any newly formed antibodies. It is not necessary to test e-positive red cells to reconfirm the previously identified anti-e because e-negative donor units will be selected for transfusion regardless of the reactivity.

If the patient's red cell phenotype is known, reagent red cells may be selected to detect only those alloantibodies that the patient would potentially form. For example, if the patient's Rh phenotype is C–E+c+e–, red cells selected to exclude anti-E and anti-c should not be necessary or can be limited to a single selected cell sample because the patient is not expected to form alloantibodies to these antigens. Exceptions include patients with weak or altered (partial) Rh antigens, which are usually found in populations of African descent and patients whose Rh phenotype was predicted by DNA testing rather than serology and who could be carrying a silenced or altered allele. This approach can minimize the amount of testing required.

Autologous Red Cell Phenotype

Determining the phenotype of an individual's autologous red cells by serology or genotyping is an important part of antibody identification because the antibody maker's red cells are expected to lack antigens to which they make alloantibodies. This information can guide the antibody identification process.

Obtaining an autologous red cell phenotype may not always be simple. Recent transfusions or immunoglobulins coating the patient's red cells make obtaining a valid phenotype difficult. Misleading results may occur unless techniques are used to circumvent these issues.[19] Many of these special phenotyping techniques, such as separation of autologous cells or removal of bound immunoglobulin, can be found later in this chapter under "Selected Procedures." Red cell genotyping is now commonly performed to obtain phenotype information. This approach avoids interference from circulating donor red cells or Ig-coated patient red cells. Molecular testing relies on the extraction of DNA from white cells. Because of nearly universal leukocyte reduction, the short life span of white cells in vivo, and, importantly, the assay design, the presence of transfused white cells from donors, if present, is not a limiting factor in determining the patient's red cell genotype. There are situations, however, where the genotype of a person may not predict the red cell phenotype. Mutations that inactivate gene expression or rare new alleles may not be identified by the specific assay performed. In addition, the genotype obtained from DNA isolated from leukocytes and hematopoietic cells may differ from that of other tissues in people with a history of transplantation.[20]

Interpretation of Results

Antibody detection results are interpreted as positive or negative according to the presence or absence of reactivity (ie, agglutination, hemolysis in serum tests, or red cell effacement in solid-phase tests). Interpretation of antibody identification results can be a very complex process combining technique, knowledge, and intuitive skills. Identification panels generally include both positive and negative results, sometimes at different phases of testing; each positive result should ultimately be explained. The following sections describe a systematic process for antibody identification interpretation.

General Assessment of Positive and Negative Reactions

Both positive and negative reactions are equally important in antibody identification, and they may be initially assessed to provide a general idea of the specificity(ies) present in the sample. (See Method 1-9 for grading agglutination in hemagglutination assays.) The phase and strength of positive reactions may be compared to the antigen patterns of the panel red cells to help suggest specificity. Negative reactions support the specificity suggested by the positive reactions. A single common alloantibody usually produces a clear pattern with antigen-positive and antigen-negative reagent red cells. In Table 13-2, if a sample is reactive only with red cell samples 3 and 5 of the reagent red cell panel, anti-E is very likely present. Both reactive red cells express the antigen, and all cells lacking the antigen are nonreactive. This general assessment is only the first part of the interpretation process. The rest of the process as described below must be completed even when a specificity looks apparent at this stage. Exclusion of antibodies must be performed to ensure proper identification of all antibodies potentially present.

Antibody Exclusion and Initial Specificity Assessment

A widely used first approach to the interpretation of panel results is to exclude specificities on the basis of nonreactivity of the patient's sample with red cells that express the antigen. Such a system is sometimes referred to as a "cross-out," "rule-out," or "exclusion" method. Once all panel results have been recorded, the antigen profile on the antigen worksheet of the first nonreactive red cell is examined. If an antigen is *present* on the red cell and the patient sample *was not reactive* with it, the presence of the corresponding antibody may tentatively be excluded. Many technologists actually cross out such antigens from the list at the top of the antigen profile sheet to facilitate the process. After all of the antigens for that red cell sample have been crossed out, the same process is performed with the other nonreactive red

TABLE 13-2.   Example of a Reagent Red Cell Panel for Antibody Identification

Cell	Rh								MNS				Kell				P1	Lewis		Duffy		Kidd		Others	Cell	Results
	D	C	E	c	e	f	Cʷ	V	M	N	S	s	K	k	Kpᵃ	Jsᵃ	P1	Leᵃ	Leᵇ	Fyᵃ	Fyᵇ	Jkᵃ	Jkᵇ			37 C AHG
1	+	+	0	0	+	0	0	0	+	0	0	+	0	+	0	0	+	0	+	+	+	0	+	Bg(a+)	1	
2	+	+	0	0	+	0	+	0	+	+	+	0	0	+	0	0	+	0	0	0	0	+	0		2	
3	+	0	+	+	0	0	0	0	0	+	0	+	0	+	0	0	0	+	0	0	+	+	+		3	
4	0	+	0	+	+	0	0	0	+	0	+	+	0	+	0	0	+	0	+	+	0	+	0		4	
5	0	0	+	+	+	+	0	0	0	+	+	+	0	+	0	0	+	0	+	0	+	0	+		5	
6	0	0	0	+	+	+	0	0	+	0	+	0	+	+	0	0	+	0	+	+	0	0	+		6	
7	0	0	0	+	+	+	0	0	+	+	+	+	0	+	0	0	+	0	+	0	+	+	0		7	
8	+	0	0	+	+	+	0	+	0	+	0	0	0	0	0	0	+	0	0	0	0	0	+		8	
9	0	0	0	+	+	+	0	0	+	+	+	+	+	0	0	0	0	+	0	+	0	+	+		9	
10	0	0	0	+	+	+	0	0	+	0	0	+	+	+	+	0	+	0	0	0	+	+	+	Yt(b+)	10	
11	+	+	0	0	+	0	0	0	+	+	0	+	0	+	0	0	+	0	+	0	+	0	+		11	
AC																									AC	

+ indicates presence of antigen; 0 indicates absence of antigen; AC = autocontrol; AHG = antihuman globulin.

cells; additional specificities are then excluded. In most cases, this process leaves a group of antibodies that have not been excluded.

Exclusion of clinically significant alloantibodies should involve, at a minimum, those to the following antigens: D, C, E, c, e, K, Fy^a, Fy^b, Jk^a, Jk^b, S, and s. Antibodies to Le^a, Le^b, M, N, P1, and other antigens specific to certain patient populations may also be added to this list. Laboratories should have a policy for their antibody exclusion. The policy should list alloantibodies requiring exclusion as well as, based on their chosen test method and available resources, whether the exclusion is to be performed using single- or double-dose antigen-positive red cells. Ideally, antibody exclusion is performed on a nonreactive double-dose antigen-positive red cell sample. As antibody investigations become more complex, double-dose exclusion may become more difficult. The laboratory policy should also include any exceptions to the exclusion criteria.

The ethnicity of the donor serving as a panel cell source affects antibody exclusions. Panel red cells may appear to be double dose based on phenotype. Yet, for blood group systems having a very common silencing allele, the panel cells may carry only a single dose of the antithetical antigen. Most common is the Fy(a+b–) phenotype on the red cells of a donor of African ancestry. Because of the high frequency of the FY*02N.01 allele with silenced Fy^b red cell expression in this population, these Fy(a+b–) cells often have only one dose of Fy^a antigen. If the Fy(a+b–) sample is also D+C–E–, V+, or Js(a+), the donor is likely of African ancestry. Exclusion of anti-Fy^a on such a panel red cell would probably represent only a single-dose exclusion.

The red cells that are reactive are then evaluated. If there is an antigen pattern that matches the test reactivity exactly, this most likely identifies the specificity of the antibody. Additional testing may be needed to eliminate remaining specificities that were not excluded and confirm the suspected specificity. This process of selecting red cells for exclusion and confirmation is described in the next section. When additional testing is not needed after the initial identification panel because an initial

specificity can be assigned and all other specificities can be excluded, the probability of an accurate identification can be directly assessed. (See below.)

Selected Red Cells for Exclusion and Confirmation

Selected red cells, chosen for the specific antigens they carry or lack, are used to confirm or rule out the presence of antibodies. For example, if a pattern of reactive red cells fits anti-Jk^a exactly, but anti-K and anti-S were not excluded, the serum should be tested with selected red cells. Ideally, red cells with the following phenotypes should be chosen: Jk(a–), K+, S–; Jk(a–), K–, S+; and Jk(a+), K–, S–. The reaction pattern with these red cells should both confirm the presence of anti-Jk^a and include or exclude anti-K and anti-S. Whenever possible, selected red cells should have a strong expression of the antigen being tested (ie, from presumed homozygous donors or red cells with double-dose expression). Such red cells help ensure that nonreactivity with the selected red cell sample indicates the absence of the antibody and not that the antibody was too weak to be reactive with a selected red cell that had a weak expression of the antigen. It must be remembered that confirmation of double-dose expression of an antigen can only be accomplished by demonstrating homozygosity of the corresponding allele through genotyping. As explained above, ethnicity influences the apparent zygosity of the FY*A allele. Testing at this stage of the investigation can also reveal errors in the presumptive identification when the expected positive and negative results in confirmatory testing are not obtained.

Probability of Accurate Identification

Accurate identification of antibody specificity greatly depends on the antibody having a sufficient titer (ie, quantity of circulating antibody) to provide reliably positive reactions. Secondly, antigen strength on test cells must be adequate to provide a consistent target antigen. It is difficult to know exactly when both of these criteria are met. Test protocols are designed to enhance clinically significant reactivity, and good laboratory practices attempt to minimize antigen deterioration. Assuming these two variables are controlled to the greatest degree possible, it is still necessary to ensure that an observed pattern of reactions is not the result of chance alone. Conclusive antibody identification requires the sample to be tested against a sufficient number of reagent red cell samples that lack—and express—the antigen that corresponds with the antibody's apparent specificity. A standard approach (which is based on Fisher's exact method) has been to require that three antigen-positive red cell samples are reactive and that three antigen-negative red cell samples are not reactive for each specificity identified.[21] When that approach is not possible, a more liberal approach (which is derived from calculations by Harris and Hochman[22]) allows the minimum requirement for a probability (p) value of ≤0.05 to be met with two reactive and three nonreactive red cell samples or with one reactive and seven nonreactive red cell samples (or the reciprocal of either combination). In some cases, the use of two reactive and two nonreactive red cell samples is also an acceptable approach for antibody confirmation.[7,23] Additional details on calculating probability may be found in the suggested readings list at the end of this chapter.

Consistency of Antibody Identified with Autologous Red Cell Phenotype

The patient's autologous red cell phenotype is used to support the presumptive antibody identification: the red cells should lack the corresponding antigen. The phenotype as determined by serology or genotyping may also indicate the need for further investigation. For example, if an individual appears to have anti-Fy[a], his or her red cells should type Fy(a–). However, if the autologous red cells type as Fy(a+) (and have a negative DAT), the identification of an anti-Fy[a] is in conflict with the phenotype, and additional testing should be performed. A serologically derived antigen-positive typing should be reconfirmed by testing with more than one antibody source when

possible. If genotyping predicted the antigen-positive status, this discrepancy may indicate that the patient's red cells do not actually express the antigen because of a gene-silencing mutation not targeted by the assay. Alternatively, the patient might have an altered or partial antigen because of an additional gene polymorphism. It is important to remember that the antibody in the sample could be, in fact, an alloantibody.

COMPLEX ANTIBODY IDENTIFICATION

Not all antibody identifications are straightforward. The interpretation process described above does not always lead directly to an answer, and additional testing and/or consultation with an immunohematology reference laboratory (IRL) may be required. The autologous control that is tested with initial antibody identification studies provides a starting point for complex antibody problem resolution. If the test method does not allow for testing of an autocontrol, the DAT result can be used to plan additional testing. Figure 13-1 shows some approaches to identifying antibodies in a variety of situations when the autocontrol is negative, and Fig 13-2 shows some approaches to identifying antibodies when the autocontrol is positive. Common types of antibody investigations mentioned in Figs 13-1 and 13-2 as well as others are further described below.

Multiple Antibodies

When a sample contains two or more alloantibodies, it may be difficult to interpret the results of testing performed with a single panel of reagent red cells. The presence of multiple antibodies may be suggested by a variety of test results, such as the following:

1. *The observed pattern of reactive and nonreactive red cells does not fit a single antibody.* When the exclusion approach fails to indicate a specific pattern, it is helpful to determine whether the pattern matches two combined specificities. For example, if the

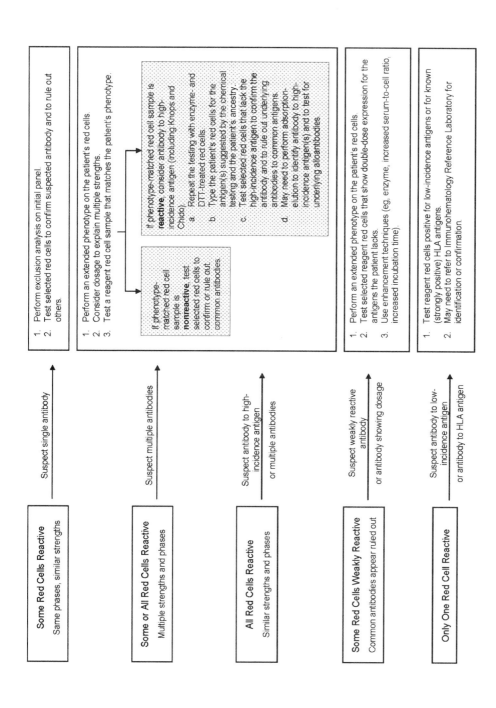

FIGURE 13-1. Antibody identification with negative autocontrol.
DTT = dithiothreitol.

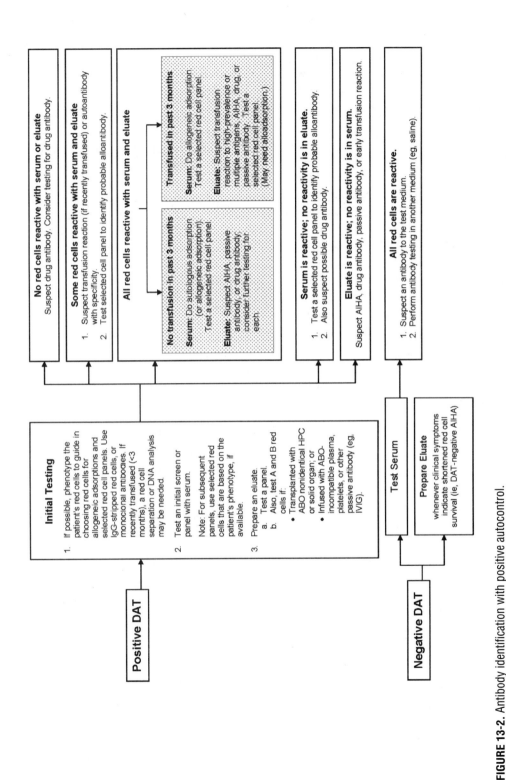

Positive DAT

Initial Testing

1. If possible, phenotype the patient's red cells to guide in choosing red cells for allogeneic adsorptions and selected red cell panels. Use IgG-stripped red cells, or monoclonal antibodies. If recently transfused (<3 months), a red cell separation or DNA analysis may be needed.

2. Test an initial screen or panel with serum.

   Note: For subsequent panels, use selected red cells that are based on the patient's phenotype, if available.

3. Prepare an eluate.
   a. Test a panel.
   b. Also, test A and B red cells if:
      • Transplanted with ABO nonidentical HPC or solid organ, or
      • Infused with ABO-incompatible plasma, platelets, or other passive antibody (eg, IVIG).

No red cells reactive with serum or eluate
Suspect drug antibody. Consider testing for drug antibody.

Some red cells reactive with serum and eluate

1. Suspect transfusion reaction (if recently transfused) or autoantibody with specificity.
2. Test selected cell panel to identify probable alloantibody.

All red cells reactive with serum and eluate

No transfusion in past 3 months

Serum: Do autologous adsorption (or allogeneic adsorption). Test a selected red cell panel

Eluate: Suspect AIHA, passive antibody, or drug antibody; consider further testing for each.

Transfused in past 3 months

Serum: Do allogeneic adsorption. Test a selected red cell panel

Eluate: Suspect transfusion reaction to high-prevalence or multiple antigens, AIHA, drug, or passive antibody. Test a selected red cell panel. (May need alloadsorption.)

Serum is reactive; no reactivity is in eluate.

1. Test a selected red cell panel to identify probable alloantibody.
2. Also suspect possible drug antibody.

Eluate is reactive; no reactivity is in serum.
Suspect AIHA, drug antibody, passive antibody, or early transfusion reaction.

Test Serum

All red cells are reactive.

1. Suspect an antibody to the test medium.
2. Perform antibody testing in another medium (eg, saline).

Prepare Eluate
whenever clinical symptoms indicate shortened red cell survival (ie, DAT-negative AIHA)

Negative DAT

FIGURE 13-2. Antibody identification with positive autocontrol.

HPC = hematopoietic progenitor cell; IVIG = intravenous immune globulin; DAT = direct antiglobulin test; A1HA = autoimmune hemolytic anemia.

reactive red cells on the panel in Table 13-2 are numbers 3, 5, 6, 9, and 10, none of the specificities remaining after crossing out fits a pattern exactly. However, if both E and K are considered together, a pattern is discerned, with reagent cells 3 and 5 showing reactivity because of anti-E, and reagent cells 6, 9, and 10 because of anti-K. If the reaction pattern does not fit two combined specificities, the possibility that more than two antibodies are present must be considered. The more antibodies a sample contains, the more complex identification and exclusion become, but the basic process remains the same.

2. *Reactivity occurs at different test phases.* When tube tests are performed and reactivity occurs at several phases, each phase should be analyzed separately. The pattern at room temperature may indicate a different specificity from the pattern at the IAT phase. It is also helpful to look for variations in the strength of the reactions at each phase of testing. Table 13-3 provides information about the characteristic reactivity of many antibodies.

3. *Unexpected reactions occur when attempts are made to confirm the specificity of a suspected single antibody.* If a sample suspected to contain anti-e is reactive with some e-negative red cells, another antibody may be present or the suspected antibody may not be anti-e at all. Testing a panel of selected e-negative red cells may help identify an additional specificity.

4. *A phenotypically similar red cell is nonreactive.* When all or nearly all panel red cells are reactive, the easiest way to recognize multiple antibodies is to test a phenotypically similar red cell. A phenotypically similar red cell is one that lacks the same common antigens as the patient's red cells. Lack of reactivity with this type of red cell indicates that the alloantibodies are directed at common antigens lacking from the test red cell. A selected red cell panel

can then be tested to identify or exclude the common antibodies to the red cell antigens that the patient lacks. (See the discussion on selected red cells earlier in this chapter.)

Reactivity without Apparent Specificity

Zygosity (ie, copy number), variation in antigen expression, and other factors may contribute to difficulty in interpreting results of antibody identification tests. If the reactivity of the serum is very weak and/or the pattern of reactivity and the cross-out process have excluded all likely specificities, alternative approaches should be used. Some helpful techniques and considerations include the following.

Alternate Test Method

Depending on the method originally used, it may be necessary either to enhance antibody reactivity by using a more sensitive method (eg, PEG, enzymes, increased incubation time, or increased serum-to-cell ratio; see Methods 3-5 and 3-8 through 3-13) or to decrease the sensitivity of the method to avoid the detection of unwanted and clinically insignificant reactivity. Methods to inactivate certain antigens on the reagent red cells may also be helpful. Enzyme treatment renders red cells negative for such antigens as Fy^a and Fy^b. (See Table 13-3.) Observation of the effect a reagent red cell treatment has on the unknown serum reactivity can provide clues about its possible specificity. Adsorption or elution methods to separate antibodies (Methods 3-20, 4-1, and 4-2) may also be useful because selective adsorption can isolate unknown reactivity, and elution of unknown reactivity from adsorbing red cells can concentrate the antibody.

Optimal Phase or Temperature for Antibody Was Not Tested

If weak or questionable positive results are obtained at the IAT phase, it may be helpful to perform tube tests with readings at immediate spin, room temperature, or 37 C if these phases were not included in the original

TABLE 13-3. Serologic Reactivity of Some Common Blood Group Antibodies

Antibody	Immuno-globulin Class	Reactivity				Papain/ Ficin	DTT (200 mM)	Associated with	
		4 C	22 C	37 C	AHG			HDFN	HTR
Anti-M	IgG > IgM	Most	Most		Rare	Sensitive	Resistant	Rare	Rare
Anti-N	IgM > IgG	Most	Most		Rare	Sensitive	Resistant	No	Rare
Anti-S	IgG > IgM		Most		Most	Variable	Resistant	Yes	Yes
Anti-s	IgG > IgM				Most	Variable	Resistant	Yes	Yes
Anti-U	IgG				Most	Resistant	Resistant	Yes	Yes
Anti-P1	IgM (IgG rare)	Most	Most			Resistant	Resistant	No	Rare
Anti-D	IgG > IgM (IgA rare)		Some	Some	Most	Resistant	Resistant	Yes	Yes
Anti-C	IgG > IgM		Some	Some	Most	Resistant	Resistant	Yes	Yes
Anti-E	IgG > IgM		Some	Some	Most	Resistant	Resistant	Yes	Yes
Anti-c	IgG > IgM		Some	Some	Most	Resistant	Resistant	Yes	Yes
Anti-e	IgG > IgM		Some	Some	Most	Resistant	Resistant	Yes	Yes
Anti-Lu^a	IgM > IgG		Most		Most	Resistant or weakened	Variable	No	Mild
Anti-Lu^b	IgG > IgM		Some		Most	Resistant or weakened	Variable	No	Mild
Anti-K	IgG > IgM		Some		Most	Resistant	Sensitive	Yes	Yes
Anti-k	IgG > IgM				Most	Resistant	Sensitive	Yes	Yes
Anti-Kp^a	IgG				Most	Resistant	Sensitive	Yes	Yes
Anti-Kp^b	IgG > IgM				Most	Resistant	Sensitive	Yes	Yes
Anti-Js^a	IgG > IgM				Most	Resistant	Sensitive	Yes	Yes
Anti-Js^b	IgG				Most	Resistant	Sensitive	Yes	Yes
Anti-Le^a	IgM > IgG	Most	Most	Most	Most	Resistant	Resistant	No	Rare
Anti-Le^b	IgM > IgG	Most	Most	Most	Most	Resistant	Resistant	No	No
Anti-Fy^a	IgG > IgM				Most	Sensitive	Resistant	Yes	Yes
Anti-Fy^b	IgG > IgM				Most	Sensitive	Resistant	Yes	Yes
Anti-Jk^a	IgG > IgM				Most	Resistant	Resistant	Rare	Yes
Anti-Jk^b	IgG > IgM				Most	Resistant	Resistant	Rare	Yes
Anti-Di^a	IgG				Most	Resistant	Resistant	Yes	Rare

(Continued)

TABLE 13-3. Serologic Reactivity of Some Common Blood Group Antibodies (Continued)

Antibody	Immuno-globulin Class	Reactivity				Papain/ Ficin	DTT (200 mM)	Associated with	
		4 C	22 C	37 C	AHG			HDFN	HTR
Anti-Di^b	IgG				Most	Resistant	Resistant	Yes	Rare
Anti-Yt^a	IgG				Most	Variable	Sensitive or weakened	No	Yes
Anti-Yt^b	IgG				Most	Variable	Sensitive or weakened	No	No
Anti-Xg^a	IgG > IgM		Some		Most	Sensitive	Resistant	No	No
Anti-Sc1	IgG				Most	Resistant	Variable	No	No
Anti-Sc2	IgG				Most	Resistant	Variable	No	No
Anti-Do^a	IgG				Most	Resistant	Variable	No	Yes
Anti-Do^b	IgG				Most	Resistant	Variable	No	Yes
Anti-Co^a	IgG > IgM				Most	Resistant	Resistant	Yes	Yes
Anti-Co^b	IgG				Most	Resistant	Resistant	Yes	Yes

AHG = antihuman globulin; DTT = dithiothreitol; HDFN = hemolytic disease of the fetus and newborn; HTR = hemolytic transfusion reaction; Ig = immunoglobulin.

testing. This may allow an antibody that optimally reacts as a direct agglutinin at 37 C or below to be more clearly visualized.

Potential Phenotype Exclusions

When serum reactivity has no apparent specificity, a useful approach is to type the patient's red cells by serology or genotyping for common red cell antigens, and eliminate from initial consideration specificities that correspond to antigens on the patient's autologous red cells. This combined with other techniques allows the investigation to be focused on specificities more likely to be present. Phenotyping may not be possible if the patient has been transfused recently or has had a positive DAT result.

Presence of Antigens in Common

Instead of excluding antibodies to antigens on nonreactive red cells, close observation may identify antigens that the reactive red cells have in common. For example, if all of the red cells reactive at room temperature are P1+ but the anti-P1 pattern is not complete, the antibody could be anti-P1 that is not reactive with red cells with a weaker expression of the antigen. (Such red cells are occasionally designated on the panel sheet as "+w.") In this case, it might be helpful to use a method that enhances anti-P1, such as testing at low temperature.

If all of the reactive red cells are Jk(b+) but not all Jk(b+) red cells are reactive, the reactive red cells might be Jk(a–b+) with a double-dose expression of the antigen. In this case, enhancement techniques such as enzymes or PEG might help demonstrate reactivity with all of the Jk(b+) red cells. Typing the patient's red cells to confirm that they lack the corresponding antigen is also helpful.

If strongly positive results are obtained, the exclusion method should be used with nonreactive cells to eliminate specificities from initial consideration. The strongly reactive reagent cells may be examined for any antigen in common.

Finally, the presence of some antigens in common may suppress the expression of other antigens. This suppression can cause weak antibodies to be missed or certain red cells to be unexpectedly nonreactive when a suspected antibody fails to show reactivity with all antigen-positive red cells. For example, In(Lu) is known to suppress the expression of Lutheran antigens, P1, In^b, and AnWj. Similarly, Kp^a is known to weaken the expression of Kell antigens. (See Chapter 12 for a more detailed discussion.)

Inherent Variability

Nebulous reaction patterns that do not appear to fit any particular specificity are characteristic of certain antibodies, such as anti-Bg^a, -Kn^a, -McC^a, -Sl^a, -Yk^a, and -Cs^a, and -JMH. Antigens corresponding to these antibodies vary markedly in their expression on red cells from different individuals. For example, the expression of Knops blood group antigens shows marked differences between individuals as a result of variations in the CR1 copy numbers on the red cells.[24]

Unlisted Antigens

A sample may react with an antigen that is not routinely listed on the antigen profile supplied by the reagent manufacturer—Do^a, Do^b, and Yt^b are some examples. Even though serum studies yield clearly reactive and nonreactive test results, such antibodies may not be recognized. In these circumstances, it is useful to review additional phenotype information supplied with the reagent panel or consult the manufacturer. If only one cell is unexpectedly reactive, this reaction is most likely caused by an antibody to a low-prevalence antigen. These antibodies are discussed in more detail later in this chapter.

ABO Type of Red Cells Tested

The sample may be reactive with many or all of the group O reagent red cells but not with red cells of the same ABO group as the autologous red cells. Such a reaction pattern occurs most frequently with anti-H, anti-IH, or anti-Le^{bH}. Group O and A$_2$ red cells have more H antigen than A$_1$ and A$_1$B red cells, which express very little H. (See Chapter 10 for more information.) Thus, sera containing anti-H or anti-IH are strongly reactive with group O reagent red cells, whereas autologous A$_1$ or A$_1$B red cells or donor red cells used for crossmatching may be weakly reactive or nonreactive. Anti-Le^{bH} is strongly reactive with group O, Le(b+) red cells but weakly reactive or nonreactive with Le(b+) red cells from A$_1$ or A$_1$B individuals.

Unexpected Reagent Red Cell Problems

Rarely, a pattern of reactive and nonreactive red cells cannot be interpreted because the typing result for a reagent red cell is incorrect or the reagent red cell has a positive DAT result. If the red cell sample is from a commercial source, the manufacturer should be notified immediately of the discrepancy.

Warm Autoantibodies

The presence of warm-reactive autoantibodies in a patient's sera creates a special challenge because the antibody is reactive with virtually all red cells tested. The majority of warm autoantibodies are IgG; IgM warm autoantibodies are unusual, but they have caused severe (often fatal) autoimmune hemolytic anemia.[25] If a patient with warm autoantibodies requires a transfusion, it is important to detect any underlying clinically significant alloantibodies. Solid-phase and gel-column methods frequently greatly enhance warm autoantibodies. PEG, enzymes, and to a lesser extent, LISS also may enhance these autoantibodies. It is often helpful to omit the enhancement media when testing sera that contain warm autoantibodies. If such tests are nonreactive, common alloantibody specificities can be excluded and the same procedure can be used for compatibility testing without the need for adsorptions. If such tests remain reactive, adsorptions are typically required to rule out underlying alloantibodies. For more information, see Chapter 14 and Methods 3-20 and 4-8 through 4-10.

Cold Autoantibodies

Cold autoantibodies may be clinically benign or pathologic. In either case, potent cold autoantibodies that are reactive with all red cells at room temperature or below, including the patient's own, can create special problems—especially if the reactivity persists at temperatures above room temperature and into the IAT phase of antibody identification. Such situations make it difficult to detect and identify potential clinically significant alloantibodies that are being masked by the cold autoantibody reactivity. The detection of cold autoantibodies can be dependent on the test method used. Gel-column tests can give a mixed-field appearance even though only one cell population is present. Solid-phase tests are designed to minimize their detection. There are different approaches to testing sera with potent cold autoagglutinins. Once the presence of a cold autoantibody has been confirmed, the goal in most situations is to circumvent or remove the interfering cold autoagglutinin reactivity in order to detect underlying and potentially clinically significant antibodies. Procedures to accomplish this include the following:

1. Omitting the room-temperature and/or immediate-spin phase of testing if one was performed.
2. The use of anti-IgG rather than polyspecific AHG reagent for the IAT phase of antibody identification.
3. Cold auto- or allogeneic adsorption of the patient's serum or plasma to remove autoantibodies but not alloantibodies (Method 4-5 and 3-20).
4. Prewarming techniques in which reagent red cells and patient serum or plasma are prewarmed to 37 C separately before they are combined (Method 3-6).
5. Adsorption with rabbit erythrocytes or rabbit erythrocyte stroma.[26,27]

The use of the last two procedures listed is controversial for the purposes of circumventing cold autoantibodies. Notes and limitations of the procedures can be found within their respective method description or references.

In some situations, the goal of testing is not to circumvent the cold autoantibody but rather define its serologic characteristics (eg, specificity, thermal amplitude, titer). This may be requested and useful if the patient's clinical situation is suggestive of a pathologic cold autoagglutinin. See Chapter 14 for a more detailed discussion.

Delayed Serologic/Hemolytic Transfusion Reactions

Delayed transfusion reactions are defined by the development of a new alloantibody in a patient following transfusion that results in laboratory evidence (serologic) or laboratory and clinical evidence (hemolytic) of the destruction of incompatible transfused red cells that were compatible at the time of infusion. If a patient has been transfused in the last 3 months and the autocontrol is positive in the IAT phase, there may be antibody-coated donor red cells in the patient's circulation, resulting in a positive DAT that can show mixed-field reactivity. An elution should be performed, especially when tests on plasma or serum are inconclusive. For example, a recently transfused patient may have a positive autocontrol and show weak reactivity with most but not all Fy(a+) red cells. It may be possible to confirm anti-Fy^a specificity in an eluate because more antibody is often bound to donor red cells, and importantly, the preparation of an eluate concentrates the antibody. It is rare for transfused red cells to make the autocontrol positive at a phase other than IAT, but this can occur, especially with a newly developing or cold-reacting alloantibody. If the DAT result does have a mixed-field appearance and the plasma or serum is reactive with all cells tested, a transfusion reaction caused by an alloantibody to a high-prevalence antigen should be considered (Fig 13-2).

Antibodies to High-Prevalence Antigens

If all reagent red cells are reactive in the same test phase and with uniform strength but the autocontrol is nonreactive, an alloantibody to a high-prevalence antigen should be considered. Antibodies to high-prevalence antigens can be identified by testing selected red cells of rare phenotypes and by typing the patient's autologous red cells with antisera to high-prevalence antigens. Knowing the ethnic or ancestral origin of the antibody producer can be helpful when selecting additional tests to perform (Table 13-4).[28] Chemically modified and/or enzyme-modified red cells (eg, DTT-treated or ficin-treated red cells) can give characteristic reactivity patterns that help limit possible specificities (Table 13-5). Testing rare red cells that lack all antigens in a blood group system [eg, K_0, Rh_{null}, or Lu(a–b–) cells] can localize the reactivity to that blood group system if nonreactive.

If red cells negative for a particular high-prevalence antigen are not available, red cells that are positive for the lower prevalence antithetical antigen can sometimes be helpful. For example, if a sample contains anti-Co[a], weaker reactions may be observed with Co(a+b+) red cells than with Co(a+b–) red cells because of a dosage effect.

Antibodies to high-prevalence antigens may be accompanied by antibodies to common antigens, which can make identification much more difficult. In such cases, it may be necessary to determine the patient's phenotype for common antigens, choose a phenotypically similar red cell sample (ie, one that lacks the same common antigens as the patient's red cells) that is incompatible with the patient's serum, and adsorb the antibody to the high-prevalence antigen onto that red cell sample. This approach leaves antibodies to common red cell antigens in the adsorbed plasma or serum, where they can be identified with a routine selected red cell panel. Because the identification of antibodies to high-prevalence antigens is complicated, it may be necessary to refer such specimens to a reference laboratory.

Ancestry of Antibody Maker

Antibodies such as anti-U, -McC[a], -Sl[a], -Js[b], -Hy, -Jo[a], -Tc[a], -Cr[a], and -At[a] should be considered if the sample is from an individual of African origin because the antigen-negative phenotypes occur almost exclusively in persons of African ancestry. Individuals with anti-Kp[b] are almost always of European ancestry. Anti-Di[b] is usually found among populations of Asian, South American Indian, and Native American ancestry. Other examples are found in Table 13-4.

Serologic Clues

Knowing the serologic characteristics of particular antibodies to high-prevalence antigens may help with identification.

1. Reactivity in tests at room temperature suggests anti-H, -I, -IH, -P, -PP1P[k] (-Tj[a]), -En[a], -LW (some), -Ge (some), -Sd[a], or -Vel.
2. Lysis of reagent red cells during testing with fresh serum is characteristic of anti-Vel, -P, -PP1P[k] (-Tj[a]), -Jk3, and some examples of anti-H and -I. Serum instead of plasma must be used in tests to see lysis.
3. Reduced or absent reactivity with enzyme-treated red cells occurs with anti-Ch, -Rg, -En[a], -In[b], -JMH, -Ge2, and some examples of anti-Yt[a].
4. Weak nebulous reactions in the IAT phase are often associated with anti-Kn[a], -McC[a], -Yk[a], and -Cs[a]. Knops system antigens are labile during storage: Antibodies may be more reactive with donor red cells and fresher reagent red cells.
5. Complement-binding autoantibodies, such as anti-I and -IH, or alloantibodies, such as anti-PP1P[k] and -Vel, may give stronger results when a polyspecific AHG reagent is used.

TABLE 13-4. High-Prevalence Antigens Absent in Certain Populations*

Phenotype	Population
AnWj–	Transient in any population>Israeli Arabs (inherited type)
At(a–)	Blacks
Cr(a–)	Blacks
Di(b–)	South Americans>Native Americans>Japanese
Fy(a–b–)	Blacks>Arabs/Jews>Mediterraneans>Whites
Ge:-2,-3 (Gerbich phenotype)	Papua New Guineans>Melanesians>Whites>any
Ge:-2,3 (Yus phenotype)	Mexicans>Israelis>Mediterraneans>any
Ge:-2,-3,-4 (Leach phenotype)	Any
Gy(a–)	Eastern Europeans (Romany)>Japanese
hr^B–	Blacks
hr^s–	Blacks
Hy–	Blacks
In(b–)	Indians>Iranians>Arabs
Jk(a–b–)	Polynesians>Finns>Japanese>any
Jo(a–)	Blacks
Jr(a–)	Japanese>Asians>Europeans>Bedouin Arabs>any
Js(b–)	Blacks
k–	Whites>any
Kn(a–)	Whites>Blacks>any
Kp(b–)	Whites>Japanese
Lan–	Whites>Japanese>Blacks>any
Lu(a–b–)	Any
LW(a–b–)	Transient in any>inherited type in Canadians
LW(a–)	Balts
O$_h$ (Bombay)	Indians>Japanese>any
Ok(a–)	Japanese
P–	Japanese>Finns>Israelis>any
PP1P^k–	Swedes>Amish>Israelis>Japanese>any
Sl(a–)	Blacks>Whites>any
Tc(a–b+c–)	Blacks
U– and S–s–U+^{var}	Blacks
Vel–	Swedes>any
WES(b–)	Finns>Blacks>any
Yk(a–)	Whites>Blacks>any
Yt(a–)	Arabs>Jews>any

*Adapted with permission from Reid et al.[28]

TABLE 13-5. Alterations of Antigens by Various Agents*

Agent	Antigens Usually Denatured or Altered[†]
Proteolytic enzymes[‡]	M, N, S, Fy[a], Fy[b], Yt[a], Ch, Rg, Pr, Tn, Mg, Mi[a]/Vw, Cl[a], Je[a], Ny[a], JMH, Xg[a], some Ge, and In[b]
Dithiothreitol (DTT) or 2-aminoethylisothiouronium bromide (AET)	Yt[a]; JMH; Kn[a]; McC[a]; Yk[a]; LW[a]; LW[b]; all Kell, Lutheran, Dombrock, Cromer, and Indian blood group antigens

*Appropriate controls should be used with modified red cells.
[†]Some antigens listed may be weakened rather than completely denatured.
[‡]Different proteolytic enzymes may have different effects on certain antigens.

Antibody to High-Prevalence Antigen vs Warm Autoantibody

When a patient produces an antibody to a high-prevalence antigen after transfusion, the patient's posttransfusion red cell sample may have a positive DAT, and both serum or plasma and the eluate may be reactive with all reagent red cells tested. Because this pattern of reactivity is identical to that of many warm-reacting autoantibodies that appear after transfusion, the two scenarios can be very difficult to differentiate. A posttransfusion DAT that is significantly weaker than the serum or plasma reactivity would be more characteristic of an alloantibody to a high-prevalence antigen than a warm autoantibody, because only the transfused cells are coated with the alloantibody. The DAT in a posttransfusion sample containing a new alloantibody to a high-prevalence antigen would be expected to give a mixed-field appearance (ie, some red cells agglutinated among many unagglutinated red cells) again because only the transfused red cells would be coated with antibody. In practice, however, weak sensitization and mixed-field agglutination can be difficult to differentiate. If a pretransfusion specimen is not available, it may be helpful to perform a red cell genotype or to use red cell separation procedures to isolate autologous red cells for testing. Performing a DAT on autologous red cells, testing the posttransfusion sample or the eluate with DAT-negative autologous red cells, or both may help distinguish an autoantibody

from an alloantibody. If a DAT result from autologous red cells is negative, the reactivity is consistent with an alloantibody. If the posttransfusion serum or plasma is reactive with DAT-negative autologous red cells, the reactivity is consistent with an autoantibody. (See Chapter 14 and Fig 13-2.)

Antibodies to Low-Prevalence Antigens

If a sample is reactive only with a single donor or reagent red cell sample after alloantibody exclusions are complete, an antibody to a low-prevalence antigen should be suspected. To identify such an antibody, a panel of reagent red cells that express low-prevalence antigens can be tested with the serum. Alternatively, the one reactive red cell sample can be tested with known antibodies to low-prevalence antigens. Unfortunately, sera that contain antibodies to low-prevalence antigens often contain multiple antibodies to low-prevalence antigens. Although low-prevalence antigens are rare by definition, naturally occurring antibodies that recognize some of them are much less rare. Many antibodies to low-prevalence antigens are reactive only at temperatures below 37 C and therefore have doubtful clinical significance. To confirm the suspected specificities, one may need the expertise and resources of a reference laboratory. Some IRLs, however, do not attempt to identify antibodies to low-prevalence antigens because many of these antibodies are not clinically meaningful, and compatible units are readily available.

If an antibody to a low-prevalence antigen is suspected and all common alloantibody specificities have been excluded, transfusion should not be delayed if identification studies are performed. Because antisera to type donor units for low-prevalence antigens are rarely available, it is usually necessary to rely on the crossmatch to avoid transfusion of antigen-positive units. When the serum is reactive with only one donor unit or reagent red cell sample, the most likely cause is an antibody to a low-prevalence antigen; however, some other possible explanations are that the red cells may be ABO incompatible, have a positive DAT result, or are polyagglutinable (ie, red cells that have crypt antigens exposed and react with all normal adult serum).

Antibodies to Low-Prevalence Antigens in Pregnancy

An antibody to a low-prevalence antigen may also be suspected when a maternal antibody screen is nonreactive but her ABO-compatible newborn has a positive DAT and/or unexplained decrease in red cell survival. A positive result when testing the mother's serum or plasma, or an eluate from the infant's DAT+ red cells, against the father's red cells can implicate an antibody to a low-prevalence antigen as the probable cause, even if the specificity is unknown. This testing can be performed only if the mother's sample is ABO compatible with the father's red cells or if the eluate from the infant's red cells does not contain anti-A or -B that would react with his red cells, or if the ABO antibodies are removed from the serum or eluate by adsorption.

Drug-Dependent Antibodies

Certain drugs induce the formation of antibodies in some patients. These drug antibodies may cause positive antibody detection/identification tests typically at the IAT phase and/or a positive DAT. Actual immune hemolytic anemia caused by drugs is a rare event, with an estimated incidence of about one in a million.[29] Prompt correlation between clinical course, drug history, and serologic findings gives opportunity for timely recognition of the event and provision of potentially lifesaving information to the patient's clinician. When antibodies to a drug or drug/red cell membrane complexes are detected in routine serology, additional and sometimes complex testing may be needed to rule out the presence of alloantibodies and exclude the possibility of a transfusion reaction (delayed or serologic) occurring in the patient. Testing for drug-dependent antibodies and information on drug-induced immune hemolytic anemia may be found in Chapter 14.

Antibodies to Reagent Components

Antibodies to a variety of drugs and chemicals in testing reagents can cause positive results in antibody detection and identification tests. The offending component may be found in the suspending media of the reagent red cells or maybe a constituent of the antibody enhancement medium that is added to the test system. Most of these anomalous reactions are in-vitro phenomena and have no clinical significance in transfusion therapy, other than causing laboratory problems that delay transfusions. A systematic comparison of the sample's reactivity with cells or enhancement media sourced from different manufacturers, with washed red cells vs cells in original diluent, or with red cells from commercial sources vs donor blood may identify the offending component. For a more complete discussion, see the suggested reading by Garratty at the end of this chapter as well as listed references.[30-32]

Rouleaux

Rouleaux is one of the most commonly encountered anomalous serologic reactions. Rouleaux are aggregates of red cells that can be mistaken for agglutination upon macroscopic examination. They can occur in any test that contains patient plasma and reagent red cells at the time of reading. If viewed microscopically, rouleaux red cell aggregates will often look like a stack of coins. Rouleaux formation is an in-vitro phenomenon that is produced by abnormal patient serum protein concentrations. It may be difficult to detect antibodies by direct agglutination in a test serum that contains rouleaux-producing proteins. Rouleaux itself is not observed in the IAT phase of testing because the washing steps remove the majority of implicated plasma proteins. Patient plasma samples exhibiting rouleaux are, however, prone to incomplete washing at the IAT and potentially false-negative results. Fortunately, such false-negative results caused by incomplete washing should easily be recognized by the failed Coomb's control cell step of the IAT. The saline replacement technique can be used to detect direct-agglutinating antibodies in the presence of rouleaux and confirm the suspected reactivity to be rouleaux if it is dispersed by the procedure (Method 3-7).

Other Anomalous Serologic Reactions

Antibodies that react only with red cells freshly washed in saline, red cells that are aged (in vitro or in vivo), and red cells that have been stored in some plastic containers, among others, have also been described. These types of anomalous reactions are less frequently encountered but are entertained as possibilities after close scrutiny of unexplained reactivity. Additional information can be found in the suggested reading by Garratty.

SELECTED PROCEDURES

Although the same method used for antibody detection tests is routinely used for basic antibody identification, alternative techniques and methods may be needed to resolve complex antibody identification problems. Some of the procedures described in this section are used routinely by many laboratories; others are used selectively and may apply only in special circumstances. It is important to remember that no single method is optimal for detecting all antibodies. When routine methods fail to indicate specificity, or the presence of an antibody is suspected but cannot be confirmed, the use of other enhancement techniques or procedures may be helpful. Techniques involving enzyme treatment of red

cells, testing at lower temperatures, or testing with various enhancement media should include an autocontrol to ensure proper interpretation of results.

Obtaining Autologous Red Cell Phenotype

It may be difficult to determine the patient's phenotype if the individual was transfused in the past 3 months. A pretransfusion specimen, if available, should be used to determine the phenotype. If a pretransfusion sample is not available, the patient's newly formed autologous red cells can be separated from the transfused red cells and then typed (Method 2-22). Separation of young red cells by centrifugation is based on the difference in the densities of new and mature red cells. Separation is most successful when ≥3 days have elapsed since the last transfusion, which will provide time for new autologous red cell production. New autologous red cells must be isolated from the sample while it is fresh. The technique is ineffective and can often result in false-positive typing if the sample is too old (>24 hours) or the patient is not producing new red cells.

Sickle cells are quite dense, making centrifugation an ineffective technique for separating the autologous red cells from the transfused donor red cells in a patient with sickle cell disease. Autologous sickle cells may be separated from donor red cells using washes with hypotonic saline (Method 2-23). Sickle cells containing hemoglobin SS are resistant to lysis by hypotonic saline, whereas donor red cells containing hemoglobin AA are lysed.

Cold and warm autoantibodies may also complicate antigen typing because of the immunoglobulins coating the patient's red cells. It may be possible to remove cold autoantibodies with warm (37 C) saline washes (Method 2-17). If the cold autoantibodies are very potent, it may be necessary to treat the red cells with 0.01 M dithiothreitol (DTT) to dissociate IgM molecules that cause spontaneous agglutination (Method 2-18). When red cells are coated with IgG autoantibodies, it is not possible to perform antigen typing with reagents that require an IAT (eg, Fy^a, Fy^b)

without first removing the bound IgG. However, it is often possible to type antibody-coated red cells with direct-agglutinating antisera, such as IgM monoclonal reagents. With rare exceptions, most direct-agglutinating monoclonal reagents give valid phenotyping results despite a positive DAT result.[33] Common techniques for removing IgG antibodies, when needed, include gentle heat elution (Method 2-19), treatment with chloroquine diphosphate (Method 2-20), and treatment with acid glycine/EDTA (Method 2-21).

LISS and PEG

LISS and PEG techniques are used to enhance reactivity and reduce incubation time compared to testing in the absence of an enhancement medium. LISS may be used to suspend test red cells for use in tube or column agglutination tests or as an additive medium for tube or solid-phase tests. Commercially prepared LISS additives or PEG additives may contain additional enhancing agents. Care should be taken to closely follow the instructions in the manufacturer's product insert to ensure that the appropriate proportion of serum to LISS or PEG is achieved. Generic LISS and PEG procedures, as well as the principles and special considerations for each technique, can be found in Methods 3-4 and 3-5. Because LISS and PEG enhance autoantibodies, their use may complicate alloantibody identification in samples that also contain autoantibodies.[34,35]

Temperature Reduction

Some antibodies (eg, anti-M, -N, -P1, -Le^a, -Le^b, and -A1) react better at room temperature or below, and their specificity may be apparent only at a temperature <22 C. An autocontrol is especially important for tests at low temperatures because many sera also contain autoanti-I or other cold-reactive autoantibodies.

Increased Serum-to-Cell Ratio

Increasing the volume of serum incubated with a standard volume of red cells may enhance the reactivity of antibodies that are present in low concentrations. One acceptable procedure involves mixing 4 volumes (drops) of serum or plasma with 1 volume of a 2% to 5% saline suspension of red cells and incubating the mixture for 60 minutes at 37 C. Periodic mixing during the incubation promotes contact between the red cells and the antibodies. It is helpful to remove the serum before washing the cells for an IAT because the standard three to four washes may be insufficient to remove all of the unbound immunoglobulin if increased amounts of serum or plasma are used. More than four washes are not recommended because bound antibody molecules may dissociate. Increasing the serum-to-red-cell ratio is not appropriate for tests using LISS or commercial PEG, which may contain LISS. Tests performed in a low-ionic-strength medium require specific proportions of serum or plasma and additive.

Increased Incubation Time

For some antibodies, the routine incubation period (typically 10 to 15 minutes minimum for some enhancement media, and 30 minutes for tests with no enhancement media) may not be sufficient to achieve maximum antibody binding; therefore, the reactions may be negative or weak, particularly in saline or albumin media. Extending the incubation time to between 30 and 60 minutes for albumin or saline tests often improves the reactivity and helps clarify the pattern of reactions. Extended incubation may be contraindicated when LISS or PEG is used. If the incubation period exceeds the recommended times for these methods, the reactivity may be diminished or lost. Care must be taken to use all reagents according to the manufacturers' directions.

Alteration in pH

Altering the pH of the test system can change the reactivity of certain antibodies, enhancing the reactivity of some and decreasing that of others.

Some examples of anti-M are enhanced when the pH of the test system is lowered to 6.5.[36] If anti-M is suspected because the only reactive red cells are M+N–, a definitive pattern (ie, reactivity with M+N+ red cells also) may be seen if the serum is acidified. The addition of 1 volume of 0.1 N HCl to 9 volumes of serum or plasma lowers the pH to approximately 6.5. The acidified serum should be tested with known M-negative red cells to control for nonspecific agglutination.

Lowering the pH, however, significantly decreases the reactivity of other antibodies.[37] If unbuffered saline with a pH <6.0 is used to prepare red cell suspensions or for washing in an IAT, antibodies in the Rh, Duffy, Kidd, and MNS blood groups may lose reactivity. Phosphate-buffered saline (Method 1-8) can be used to control the pH and enhance the detection of antibodies that are poorly reactive at a lower pH.[38]

Enzyme Modification/Destruction of Blood Group Antigens on Red Cells

Ficin and papain are the most frequently used enzymes for complex antibody identification. They destroy or weaken antigens, such as M, N, S, Fy[a], Fy[b], JMH, Ch, Rg, and Xg[a] (Table 13-5). Antibodies to these antigens are nonreactive with treated red cells. Conversely, ficin- and papain-treated red cells show persistent or enhanced reactivity with other antibodies (eg, Rh, P1PK, I, Kidd, and Lewis system antibodies). For this reason, enzyme techniques may be used to separate mixtures of antibodies. For example, if a serum sample contains anti-Fy[a] and anti-Jk[a], many of the red cell samples on the initial panel would be reactive. If a panel of enzyme-treated red cells were tested, the anti-Jk[a] reactivity would persist, whereas the anti-Fy[a] reactivity would no longer be detected because its target antigen was destroyed by the enzyme treatment. Procedures for the preparation and use of proteolytic enzymes are given in Methods 3-8 to 3-13.

Additional enzymes that are commonly used in advanced IRLs include trypsin, α-chymotrypsin, and pronase. Depending on the enzyme and method used, other antigens may be altered or destroyed. Antigens that are inactivated by one proteolytic enzyme may not be inactivated by other enzymes. Trypsin treatment has been used to remove CD38 from red cells, thereby avoiding the interference of anti-CD38 immunotherapy.[39] The clinical significance of antibodies that are reactive only with enzyme-treated cells is questionable; such "enzyme-only" antibodies may not have clinical significance.[40]

Chemical Modification/Destruction of Blood Group Antigens on Red Cells

Certain blood group antigens can be destroyed or weakened by chemical treatment of the cells (Table 13-5). Modified red cells can be useful for both confirming the presence of suspected antibodies and detecting additional antibodies. The use of modified red cells can be especially helpful if a sample contains an antibody to a high-prevalence antigen because antigen-negative red cells are rare. Sulfhydryl reagents such as 2-aminoethylisothiouronium bromide (AET), 2-mercapto-ethanol (2-ME), or DTT cleave disulfide bonds that are responsible for the conformation of certain blood group antigens and therefore can be used to weaken or destroy antigens in the Kell system and some other antigens (Method 3-18).[41-42] DTT treatment will also destroy CD38 on red cells and has commonly been used to mitigate the interference of anti-CD38 immunotherapy on serology testing.[16,17] ZZAP reagent, which contains both a proteolytic enzyme and DTT, denatures antigens that are sensitive to DTT (eg, all Kell system antigens) as well as antigens that are sensitive to enzymes (Method 4-8).[43] Glycine-HCl/EDTA treatment of red cells destroys Bg and Kell system antigens as well as the Er[a] antigen (Methods 2-21 and 4-2).[44] Chloroquine diphosphate can be used to weaken the expression of Class I HLA antigens (Bg antigens) on red cells.[45] Chloroquine treatment also weakens some other antigens, including Rh antigens (Method 2-20).

Inhibition Techniques

Soluble forms of some blood group antigens exist in body fluids, such as saliva, urine, and plasma. These substances are also present in other natural sources, or they can be prepared synthetically. Soluble substance can be used to inhibit the reactivity of the corresponding antibody that could mask the presence of underlying nonneutralizable antibodies. Also, inhibition of the reactivity by a soluble substance can help with the identification of the specificity of the antibody. For example, if a suspected anti-P1 does not produce a definitive pattern of agglutination, the loss of reactivity after the addition of soluble P1 substance strongly suggests that the specificity is anti-P1 if a parallel dilution control with saline remains reactive. Inhibition results can be interpreted only when the test is nonreactive and the dilution control that substitutes an equal volume of saline for the soluble substance is reactive.

The most commonly used substances for inhibition include the following:

1. *Lewis substances.* Le^a substances, Le^b substances, or both are present in the saliva of individuals who possess the Lewis gene (*FUT3*). Le^a substance is present in the saliva of Le(a+b–) individuals, and both Le^a and Le^b substances are present in the saliva of Le(a–b+) individuals (Method 2-8). Commercially prepared Lewis substance is available.
2. *P1 substance.* Soluble P1 substance is present in hydatid cyst fluid and the ovalbumin of pigeon eggs. Commercially prepared P1 substance is available.
3. *Sd^a substance.* Soluble Sd^a blood group-substance is present in various body fluids, but urine has the highest concentration of Sd^a.[46] To confirm the presence of anti-Sd^a in a serum sample, urine from a known Sd(a+) individual (or a pool of urine specimens) can be used to inhibit the antibody reactivity (Method 3-19).
4. *Chido and Rodgers substances.* Ch and Rg antigens are epitopes on the fourth component of human complement (C4).[47,48] Most normal red cells have a trace amount of C4 on their surface. Anti-Ch and anti-Rg are reactive with this C4 in an IAT. A useful test to identify anti-Ch and anti-Rg is inhibition of the antibodies with plasma from Ch+,

Rg+ individuals (Method 3-17). Although not an inhibition technique, soluble Ch and Rg substance in plasma can also be used to coat red cells in vitro with excess C4d. Such coated red cells will directly agglutinate anti-Ch and -Rg, allowing for their rapid identification.[49]

Denaturation of Immunoglobulins

Sulfhydryl reagents, such as DTT and 2-ME, can also be used to cleave the disulfide bonds that join the monomeric subunits of the IgM pentamer. Intact 19S IgM molecules are cleaved into 7S Ig subunits, which have altered serologic reactivity.[50] The interchain bonds of 7S Ig monomers are relatively resistant to such cleavage.

Uses of sulfhydryl reagents to denature immunoglobulins include the following:

1. Determining the Ig class of an antibody (Method 3-16). In a pregnant woman's sample, IgG antibody indicates the potential for HDFN.
2. Identifying antibodies in a mixture of IgM and IgG antibodies, particularly when an agglutinating IgM antibody masks the presence of IgG antibodies.
3. Determining the relative amounts of IgG and IgM components of a given specificity (eg, anti-A or -B).
4. Dispersing red cell agglutinates caused by IgM autoantibodies (Method 2-18).
5. Removing IgG antibodies from red cells using a mixture of DTT and proteolytic enzyme (ZZAP reagent) (Method 4-8).

Adsorption

Antibody can be removed from a serum sample by adsorption onto red cells that express the corresponding antigen. After the antibody attaches to the membrane-bound antigens, the antibody remains attached to the red cells when serum/plasma and cells are separated. It may be possible to harvest the bound antibody by elution or examine the adsorbed serum or plasma for antibody(ies) remaining after the adsorption process.

Adsorption techniques are useful for the following purposes:

1. Separating multiple antibodies present in a single serum.
2. Removing autoantibody to permit the detection or identification of underlying alloantibodies. (See Chapter 14 for more information.)
3. Removing unwanted antibody (often anti-A, anti-B, or both) from serum that contains an antibody suitable for reagent use.
4. Confirming the presence of specific antigens on red cells by their ability to remove antibody of corresponding specificity from previously characterized serum.
5. Confirming the specificity of an antibody by showing that it can be adsorbed onto red cells of only a particular blood group phenotype.

Adsorption serves different purposes in different situations; no single procedure is satisfactory for all purposes (Methods 4-5, 4-8, 4-9, and 4-10). A basic procedure for antibody adsorption can be found in Method 3-20. The usual serum/plasma-to-cell ratio is 1 volume of serum or plasma to an equal volume of washed, packed red cells. To enhance antibody removal, a larger volume of red cells increases the proportion of antigen. The incubation temperature should be that at which the antibody is optimally reactive. Pretreating red cells with a proteolytic enzyme may enhance antibody uptake and reduce the number of adsorptions required to remove an antibody completely. Because enzymes destroy some antigens, antibodies directed against those antigens are not removed by enzyme-treated red cells. To ensure that an adsorption process is complete (ie, that no unadsorbed antibody remains), it is essential to confirm that the adsorbed serum is nonreactive with a sample of the adsorbing red cells that was not used for adsorption. Adsorption requires a substantial volume of red cells, and vials of reagent red

cells are usually not sufficient. Blood samples from donor units are the most convenient sources.

When separating mixtures of antibodies, the selection of red cells of the appropriate phenotype is extremely important. If one or more antibodies have been previously identified, red cells that express the corresponding antigens can be used to remove the known antibodies. For example, if a person who types K+k–, Fy(a–b+) has produced anti-k, it may be necessary to adsorb the anti-k onto K–k+, Fy(a–b+) red cells to remove the anti-k. Then, the adsorbed sample can be tested with common K–k+, Fy(a+b–) red cells to detect or exclude anti-Fy^a.

Elution

Elution dissociates antibodies from sensitized red cells. Bound antibody may be released by changing the thermodynamics of antigen-antibody reactions, neutralizing or reversing forces of attraction that hold antigen-antibody complexes together, or disturbing the structure of the antigen-antibody binding site. The usual objective is to recover bound antibody in a usable form.

Selected elution procedures are given in Methods 4-1 through 4-4. No single method is best for all situations. Heat or freeze-thaw elution techniques are usually restricted to the investigation of HDFN caused by ABO incompatibility because these elution procedures rarely work well for other antibodies. Acid or organic solvent methods are used for eluting warm-reactive auto- and alloantibodies. Commercial kits are available for performing elution. (See Chapter 14, Table 14-2 for a list of elution methods and their uses, advantages, and disadvantages.)

Elution techniques are useful for the following:

1. Investigation of a positive DAT result (Chapter 14).
2. Concentration and purification of antibodies, detection of weakly expressed antigens, and identification of multiple antibody specificities. Such studies are used in con-

junction with an appropriate adsorption technique, as described below and in Method 2-7.

3. Preparation of antibody-free red cells for autologous adsorption studies. (Methods 4-5 and 4-8).

Technical factors that influence the outcome of elution procedures include the following:

1. *Incomplete washing.* Sensitized red cells should be thoroughly washed before an elution to prevent contamination of the eluate with unbound residual antibody. Six washes with saline are usually adequate, but more washes may be needed if the serum contains a high-titer antibody. (The considerations in Item 3 below should be kept in mind.) To confirm the efficacy of the washing process, supernatant fluid from the final wash should be tested for antibody activity and found to be nonreactive.

2. *Binding of protein to glass surfaces.* If an eluate is prepared in the test tube that was used during the sensitization or washing phases, antibody that nonspecifically binds to the test tube surface may dissociate during the elution. Similar binding can also occur from a whole blood sample when a patient has a positive DAT result and has free antibody in the serum. To avoid such contamination, red cells used to prepare an eluate should be transferred to a clean test tube before washing and then to another clean tube before the elution procedure is initiated.

3. *Dissociation of antibody before elution.* IgM antibodies, such as anti-A or anti-M, or low-affinity IgG, may spontaneously dissociate from the red cells during the wash phase. To minimize the loss of bound antibody, cold (4 C) saline or wash solution provided by the manufacturer should be used for washing.

4. *Incorrect technique.* Such factors as incomplete removal of organic solvents or failure to correct the tonicity or pH of an eluate may cause the reagent red cells used to test the eluate to hemolyze or appear "sticky." The presence of stromal debris may interfere with the reading of test results. Careful technique and strict adherence to procedures should eliminate such problems.

5. *Instability of eluates.* Dilute protein solutions, such as those obtained by elution into saline, are unstable. Eluates should be tested as soon as possible after preparation. Alternatively, bovine albumin may be added to a final concentration of 6% w/v, and the preparation may be frozen during storage. Eluates can also be prepared in antibody-free plasma, 6% albumin, or a similar protein medium. When commercial elution kits are used, the manufacturer's instructions for preparation and storage should be followed.

Combined Adsorption-Elution

Combined adsorption-elution tests can be used to separate a mixture of antibodies in a single-serum sample, detect weakly expressed antigens on red cells, or help identify weakly reactive antibodies. The process consists of first incubating serum with selected red cells and then eluting antibody from the adsorbing red cells.

Care must be taken when selecting the adsorbing cells to separate a mixture of antibodies. The cells should express only one of the antigens corresponding to an antibody in the mixture so that the eluate from the cells will contain only that antibody. Both the eluate and adsorbed serum can be used for further testing. Unmodified red cells are generally used for adsorptions when subsequent elutions are being prepared.

Titration

The titer of an antibody is usually determined by testing serial twofold dilutions of the serum with selected red cells. Results are expressed as the reciprocal of the highest serum dilution that shows macroscopic agglutination. Titration values can provide information about the relative amount of antibody present in a sample or the relative strength of antigen expression on red cells.

Titration studies are useful for the following purposes:

1. *Prenatal studies.* When the antibody has a specificity that is known to cause HDFN, or the antibody's clinical significance is unknown, the results of titration studies may contribute to the decision about performing additional procedures (eg, Doppler sonography or amniocentesis). (See Chapter 23 and Method 5-3.)

2. *Antibody identification.* Some antibodies that agglutinate virtually all reagent red cells may give an indication of specificity by demonstrating reactivity of different strengths with different red cell samples in titration studies. For example, potent undiluted autoanti-I may be reactive with both adult and umbilical cord blood red cells, but titration studies may reveal reactivity with adult I+ red cells at a higher dilution than with cord blood I+^{w} red cells. The reactivity of most antibodies weakens progressively with serial dilutions (ie, a 2+ reaction becomes 1+ in the next dilution), and weak antibodies (<1+) may lose their reactivity when diluted. Yet, some antibodies that have weak reactions when they are undiluted continue to react at dilutions as high as 1 in 2048. Such antibodies include anti-Ch, -Rg, -Cs^a, -Yk^a, -Kn^a, -McC^a, and -JMH. Titration studies may be performed on a sample showing unexplained weak IAT reactions to determine whether the reactivity is consistent with the antibodies in this group; however, not all examples of these antibodies demonstrate such high-titer, low-avidity characteristics. Thus, the serologic characteristics may suggest certain specificities, but failure to do so does not

eliminate these possibilities. The antibodies listed above are not expected to cause shortened red cell survival, although there are examples of other antibodies (eg, anti-Lu^b, -Hy, and -Yt^a) that may mimic these serologic characteristics and cause shortened red cell survival. Anti-CD38 may also show high-titered reactivity and is generally nonreactive with Lu(a–b–) cells.[39,51] If administration of this therapy to the patient is not disclosed to laboratory staff, the investigation may conclude the sample contains an antibody to a high-prevalence Lutheran system antigen. Details about titration are given in Method 3-15.

3. *Separating multiple antibodies.* Titration results may suggest that one antibody is reactive at higher dilutions than another antibody. That information can allow the serum to be diluted before it is tested with a red cell panel, which effectively removes one antibody and allows the other to be identified. For example, if a serum contains anti-Jk^a that is reactive to a titer of 2 and anti-c that is reactive to a titer of 16, it may be possible to eliminate the anti-Jk^a reactivity by diluting the serum to a titer of 8.

Other Methods

Methods other than traditional tube, gel, or solid-phase techniques may be used for antibody identification. Some methods are especially useful for testing small volumes of samples or reagents. Such methods include testing in capillary tubes, microplates, or enzyme-linked immunosorbent assays. Other methods that are useful in laboratories with specialized equipment include immunofluorescence, flow cytometry, and immunoblotting.

CONSIDERATIONS FOLLOWING ANTIBODY IDENTIFICATION

Unexpected red cell antibodies are revealed in antibody detection tests and characterized through antibody identification testing. Information obtained from this process is then used to help determine the potential clinical significance of the unexpected antibody for the purpose of providing an effective transfusion of red cell components or to identify the need for further monitoring for HDFN.

Significance of Identified Antibodies

The phases in which an antibody is identified and its specificity are the two primary means used to predict an unexpected antibody's potential clinical significance. Antibodies that are reactive at 37 C, in an IAT, or both are potentially clinically significant. Antibodies that are reactive at room temperature and below are usually not clinically significant; however, there are many exceptions. For example, anti-Vel, -P, and -PP1P^k (-Tj^a) may be reactive only at cold temperatures, yet may cause red cell destruction in vivo. Anti-Ch, anti-Rg, and many of the Knops and Cost antibodies have little or no clinical significance despite their reactivity in an IAT. Reported experience with examples of antibodies with the same specificity can be used in assessing the clinical significance.

Table 13-3 summarizes the expected reactivity and clinical significance of commonly encountered alloantibodies. For some antibodies, little or no data exist, and the decision about clinical significance must be based on the premise that clinically significant antibodies are those that are active at 37 C, in an IAT, or both.

Certain laboratory tests have been used to predict the clinical significance of antibodies. The monocyte monolayer assay, which quantifies phagocytosis, adherence of antibody-coated red cells, or both, can be used to predict the in-vivo clinical significance of some antibodies.[52,53] The test for antibody-dependent cellular cytotoxicity, which measures lysis of antibody-coated red cells, and the chemiluminescence assay, which measures the respiratory release of oxygen radicals after phagocytosis of antibody-coated red cells, have been helpful in predicting in-vivo antibody significance—particularly for predicting the severity of HDFN. For cold-reactive

antibodies, in-vitro thermal amplitude studies may be able to predict the likelihood of in-vivo hemolysis.[54]

In-vivo tests may also be used to evaluate the significance of an antibody. The most common technique is a red cell survival study in which radiolabeled, antigen-positive red cells (usually labeled with ^51Cr) are infused into the patient. After a specified period has elapsed, a sample of blood from the patient is tested for radioactivity. With this technique, it is possible to measure the survival of ≤1 mL of infused cells. Another in-vivo technique, flow cytometry, can also be used to measure the survival of infused red cells, but a larger aliquot of red cells (about 10 mL) is usually required. Interpretation of in-vivo survival test results is complicated by the fact that small aliquots of incompatible red cells may have a faster rate of destruction than an entire transfused unit of Red Blood Cells (RBCs). Comparison with documented cases in the literature and consultation with a reference laboratory should provide guidance about previous examples of similar specificities.

Subsequent Antibody Identification in Patients with a Known History of Antibodies

Once a clinically significant antibody has been identified, the patient must receive red cells negative for the corresponding antigen if at all possible, so it is rarely necessary to routinely repeat the identification of known antibodies in subsequent pretransfusion testing. AABB *Standards* states that in patients with previously identified antibodies, testing methods should be used that identify *additional* clinically significant antibodies.[8(p36)] Each laboratory should define policies and methods for the detection of additional antibodies in these patients.

Selection of Donor Units for Patients Whose Serum Contains Antibodies

Antigen-Negative Blood

RBC units selected for transfusion to a patient with potentially clinically significant antibodies should be negative for the corresponding antigen(s). Even if the antibodies are no longer detectable, all subsequent RBC transfusions to that patient should lack the antigen to prevent a secondary immune response. The transfusion service must maintain records of all patients in whom clinically significant antibodies have been previously identified, and an IAT crossmatch procedure is required if the sample contains—or has previously contained—a clinically significant antibody.[8(p76)] Exceptions to these practices should be made only in extreme clinical emergencies under the direction of a physician.

A potent example of the antibody should be used to identify antigen-negative RBC units. Often, the antibody is a commercial antiserum, but to save expensive or rare reagents, units can be tested first (often referred to as screened) for compatibility with the patient's serum. Then, the absence of the antigen in compatible units can be confirmed with commercial reagents. If the antibody is unusual and commercial antiserum is not available, a stored sample from the sensitized patient may be used to select units for transfusion at a later time, especially if the patient's later samples lose reactivity. If any patient serum or plasma is used as a typing reagent, referred to as a single-source antibody, the antibody reactivity should be well characterized and retain reactivity after storage. Appropriate negative and weak-positive controls (eg, from heterozygous donors) should be used at the time of the testing. The following criteria, established by the FDA for licensing some reagents, should be used as guidelines for human-source reagents used in lieu of commercial reagents[55]:

1. Anti-K, -k, -Jk^a, -Fy^a, and -C^w: dilution of 1:8 must produce at least a 1+ reaction.
2. Anti-S, -s, -P1, -M, -I, -c (saline), -e (saline), and -A1: dilution of 1:4 must produce at least a 1+ reaction.
3. Most other specificities: undiluted reagent must produce at least a 2+ reaction.

When selecting units for patients with clinically significant antibodies, some serologists recommend typing the units with antibodies from two different sources, but others consider this step unnecessary—especially when potent commercial reagents are available and an IAT crossmatch will be performed. Different lots of antibody from the same manufacturer and even different reagents from different manufacturers may have been prepared from the same source material because manufacturers often acquire these resources from the same entity.

If a donor unit is tested for selected antigens and labeled by the blood center, the use of licensed (commercial) reagents, if available, is required. If no licensed reagent is available, the unit must be labeled with appropriate wording (eg, "Tested and found negative for XX antigen using unlicensed typing reagents").[56] Except for results of ABO and D typing, there is no requirement that the hospital repeat testing of donor minor antigen typing if the results are on the label or on an attached tag.[8(p35)] Minor antigen typing results on packing slips or not physically attached to the donor unit should be confirmed by the hospital, if possible, when the unit is intended for transfusion to a patient with the corresponding alloantibody.

Crossmatch for Compatibility

For certain antibodies, typing the donor units may not be necessary, and the patient's serum can be used to select serologically compatible RBC units. This is especially true for antibodies that characteristically are reactive below 37 C (eg, anti-M, -N, -P1, -Le^a, -Le^b, and -A1) and that do not ordinarily produce a secondary immune response following the transfusion of antigen-positive RBC units.

Phenotype-Matched Blood

Sometimes it may be best practice to provide phenotypically matched, antigen-negative RBC units as a prophylactic measure. For example, when a patient of the R$_1$R$_1$ phenotype produces anti-E, some serologists suggest that RBC units should be negative for both the E and c antigens. This recommendation is based on the assumption that the stimulus to produce anti-E may also have stimulated anti-c or anti-cE that remains undetected by routine tests.[57] Similarly, for an R_2R_2 patient with demonstrable anti-C, the use of e-negative donor blood may be considered.

It may be prudent to select RBC units that are phenotypically matched with the patient for clinically significant antigens when a patient has potent warm autoantibody or is receiving monoclonal antibody therapy and compatibility cannot be demonstrated by routine testing. This is also true when an antibody has not been specifically demonstrated but decreased survival of transfused cells is observed.

For patients needing chronic transfusion therapy for sickle cell disease or thalassemia, limited antigen matching, specifically for Rh antigens (generally C and E) and K is becoming common practice to prevent or mitigate alloimmunization. Transfusion of phenotypically matched RBC units, however, does not prevent formation of all new alloantibodies.

When Uncommon or Rare Blood Is Needed

Rare blood includes units that are negative for high-prevalence antigens (<1:1000 units) or are negative for a combination of many common antigens (<1:100). When a patient has multiple antibodies, it is helpful to determine the prevalence of compatible donors. To calculate this prevalence, one must multiply the prevalence of donors who are negative for one antigen by the prevalence of donors who are negative for each of the other antigens. For example, if a serum contains anti-c, anti-Fy^a, and anti-S, and if the prevalence of antigen-negative individuals is 18% (c–), 34% [Fy(a–)], and 45% (S–), then the prevalence of compatible units is 0.18 × 0.34 × 0.45 = 0.028, or 2.8%. If the patient is group O, the prevalence of group O donors (45%) is factored into the calculation as follows: 0.028 × 0.45 = 0.013, or 1.3%.

If any of these antibodies is present alone, finding compatible blood is not very difficult, but the combination requires a large number of units in order to find one compatible unit. The calculation above uses the prevalence in populations of European descent, and prevalence may be different in populations of non-European descent. In calculating the probability of compatible donors, one should use the antigen prevalence that corresponds with the racial composition of the donor population, if available.

When units of rare or uncommon phenotypes are needed, the local IRL should be contacted. Local IRLs that reside within or are associated with blood centers typically have an inventory (fresh and/or frozen) of RBC units of uncommon phenotypes and sometimes rare phenotypes. When the local IRL does not have RBCs of the necessary phenotype, they typically have a mechanism for searching for the required units. (See IRL section below.)

If the clinical situation allows, autologous RBC transfusions should be considered for patients with rare phenotypes who are expected to need blood in the future. Additionally, family members are another potential source of rare blood donors. The absence of high-prevalence antigens is usually associated with the inheritance of the same rare recessive blood group gene from each heterozygous parent. Children from the same parents have one chance in four of inheriting the same two rare genetic mutations, making siblings much more likely than the general population to have the rare blood type. In most cases, blood from the patient's parents, children, and half of the patient's siblings express only one rare gene. If transfusion is essential and there is no alternative to transfusing incompatible blood, these heterozygous (single-dose) donors may be preferable to random donors. For infants with HDFN resulting from multiple antibodies or an antibody to a high-prevalence antigen, the mother (if she is ABO compatible) is often the logical donor.

IMMUNOHEMATOLOGY REFERENCE LABORATORIES

IRLs typically have the skilled staff, procedures, and, most importantly, resources (such as frozen aliquots of fully phenotyped rare red cells lacking high-prevalence antigens) to investigate and resolve many or most complex antibody problems. IRLs can also provide consultation and information to laboratories about unfamiliar or infrequently encountered complex antibody problems. Additionally, IRLs often help facilities procure units of specific phenotypes when such units cannot be found in a routine transfusion service. Many IRLs also have access to the American Rare Donor Program (ARDP), which provides a network for finding RBC units with rare phenotypes throughout the United States and also has connection to similar programs worldwide (See Method 3-21).

KEY POINTS

1. A clinically significant red cell antibody is an antibody that is frequently associated with HDFN, hemolytic transfusion reactions, or a notable decrease in the survival of transfused red cells.

2. It is important to consider the patient's medical history (transfusions, pregnancies, transplantations, diagnoses, drugs and biologic therapies/immunotherapies) before starting antibody identification testing.

3. Biologic therapies are expanding beyond IVIG and RhIG. Monoclonal antibodies developed as immunotherapeutic agents [eg, daratumumab (anti-CD38)] may also interfere with serologic results. Novel therapies may impact serologic testing in the future.

4. The autologous control, in which serum and autologous red cells are tested under the same conditions as the serum and reagent red cells, is an important part of antibody identification. The autologous control is not the same as a DAT.

5. An antibody may be tentatively excluded or ruled out if an antigen is present on a reagent cell and the patient's serum or plasma is not reactive with it.

6. The phenotype of the patient's autologous red cells is an important part of antibody identification. When an antibody has been tentatively identified, the corresponding antigen is expected to be absent from the autologous red cells, although exceptions can occur. Discrepancies between autologous phenotype and antibody specificity may indicate alloantibody in a patient having a variant or partial antigen.

7. Genotyping is an accepted method for obtaining red cell phenotype information. DNA-based methods are also used to resolve conflicting results in antibody identification or in serologic- vs genotyping-based phenotype discrepancies.

8. Common clinically significant alloantibodies that should be considered in the process of exclusion during antibody identification testing are, at a minimum, anti-D, -C, -E, -c, -e, -K, -Fy^a, -Fy^b, -Jk^a, -Jk^b, -S, and -s.

9. Based on probability, the use of two reactive and two nonreactive red cell samples is the very minimum acceptable for antibody confirmation.

10. The use of DTT or 2-ME to determine the immunoglobulin class of plasma/serum reactivity is useful in the prenatal setting, where detection of IgG antibody would indicate the ability of the antibody to cross the placenta and the potential for HDFN.

11. Elution dissociates antibodies from sensitized red cells. Bound antibody may be released by changing the thermodynamics of an antigen-antibody reaction, neutralizing or reversing forces of attraction that hold antigen-antibody complexes together, or disturbing the structures of the antigen-antibody binding site.

12. RBC units selected for transfusion to a patient with a potentially clinically significant antibody should be negative for the corresponding antigen(s). Even if the antibody is no longer detectable, all subsequent RBC transfusions to the patient should lack the antigen to prevent a secondary immune response.

REFERENCES

1. Tremi A, King K. Red blood cell alloimmunization: Lessons from sickle cell disease. Transfusion 2013;53:692-5.
2. Chou ST, Jackson T, Vege S, et al. High prevalence of red blood cell alloimmunization in sickle cell disease despite transfusion from Rh-matched minority donors. Blood 2013;122:1062-71.
3. Spanos T, Karageorga M, Ladis V, et al. Red cell alloantibodies in patients with thalassemia. Vox Sang 1990;58:50-5.
4. Issitt PD, Anstee DJ. Applied blood group serology. 4th ed. Durham, NC: Montgomery Scientific Publications, 1998.
5. Malyska H, Kleeman JE, Masouredis SP, Victoria EJ. Effects on blood group antigens from storage at low ionic strength in the presence of neomycin. Vox Sang 1983;44:375-84.
6. Westhoff CM, Sipherd BD, Toalson LD. Red cell antigen stability in K3EDTA. Immunohematol 1993;9:109-11.
7. Kaherl KJ, ed. Standards for immunohematology reference laboratories. 9th ed. Bethesda, MD: AABB, 2015.
8. Ooley PW, ed. Standards for blood banks and transfusion services. 30th ed. Bethesda, MD: AABB, 2016.
9. Casina TS. In search of the holy grail: Comparison of antibody screening methods. Immunohematology 2006;22:196-202.
10. Winters JL, Richa EM, Bryant SC, et al. Polyethylene glycol antiglobulin tube versus gel microcolumn: Influence on the incidence of delayed hemolytic transfusion reactions and delayed serologic transfusion reactions. Transfusion 2010;50;1444-52.
11. Bunker ML, Thomas CL Geyer SJ. Optimizing pretransfusion antibody detection and identification: A parallel, blinded comparison of tube PEG, solid-phase, and automated methods. Transfusion 2001;41:621-6.
12. Pisacka M, Kralova M, Sklenarova M. Solid-phase-membrane only antibodies—reactive only in Capture-R Ready but nonreactive by Capture-R Select and in other techniques (abstract). Transfusion 2011;51(Suppl 3):175A.
13. Lang N, Sulfridge DM, Hulina J, et al. Solid phase reactive only antibodies (abstract). Transfusion 2011;51(Suppl 3):172A.
14. Howard JE, Winn LC, Gottlieb CE, et al. Clinical significance of anti-complement component of antiglobulin antisera. Transfusion 1982;22:269-72.
15. Howie HL, Delaney M, Wang X. Serological blind spots for variants of human IgG3 and IgG4 by a commonly used anti-immunoglobulin reagent. Transfusion 2016;56:2953-62.
16. Oostendorp M, Lammerts van Bueren JJ, Doshi P, et al. When blood transfusion medicine becomes complicated due to interference by monoclonal antibody therapy. Transfusion 2015;55:1555-62.
17. Chapuy CL, Nicholson RT, Aguad MD, et al. Resolving the daratumumab interference with blood compatibility testing. Transfusion 2015;55:1545-54.
18. Judd WJ, Steiner EA, Oberman HA, Nance S. Can the reading for serologic reactivity following 37 degrees C incubation be omitted? Transfusion 1992;32:304-8.
19. Reid ME, Øyen R, Storry J, et al. Interpretation of RBC typing in multi-transfused patients can be unreliable (abstract). Transfusion 2000;40(Suppl):123.
20. Lomas-Francis C, DePalma H. 2007 Rock Øyen Symposium. DNA-based assays for patient testing: Their application, interpretation, and correlation of results. Immunohematology 2008;24:180-90.
21. Fisher RA. Statistical methods and scientific inference. 2nd ed. Edinburgh, Scotland: Oliver and Boyd, 1959.
22. Harris RE, Hochman HG. Revised p values in testing blood group antibodies: Fisher's exact test revisited. Transfusion 1986;26:494-9.
23. Kanter MH, Poole G, Garratty G. Misinterpretation and misapplication of p values in antibody identification: The lack of value of a p value. Transfusion 1997;37:816-22.
24. Moulds JM, Zimmerman PA, Doumbo OK, et al. Molecular identification of Knops blood group polymorphisms found in long homologous region D of complement receptor 1. Blood 2001;97:2879-85.
25. Arndt PA, Leger RM, Garratty G. Serologic findings in autoimmune hemolytic anemia associated with immunoglobulin M warm autoantibodies. Transfusion 2009;49:235-42.
26. Waligora SK, Edwards JM. Use of rabbit red cells for adsorption of cold autoagglutinins. Transfusion 1983;23:328-30.

27. Yuan S, Fang A, Davis R, et al. Immunoglobulin M red blood cell alloantibodies are frequently adsorbed by rabbit erythrocyte stroma. Transfusion 2010;50:1139-43.

28. Reid ME, Lomas-Francis C, Olsson M. The blood group antigens factsbook. 3rd ed. London: Elsevier Academic Press, 2012.

29. Arndt PA, Garratty G. The changing spectrum of drug-induced immune hemolytic anemia. Semin Hematol 2005;42:137-44.

30. Judd WJ, Steiner EA, Cochran RK. Paraben-associated autoanti-Jka antibodies: Three examples detected using commercially prepared low-ionic strength saline containing parabens. Transfusion 1982;22:31-5.

31. Judd WJ, Storry JR, Annesley TD, et al. The first example of a paraben-dependent antibody to an Rh protein. Transfusion 2001;41:371-4.

32. Dube VE, Zoes C, Adesman P. Caprylate-dependent auto-anti-e. Vox Sang 1977;33:359-63.

33. Rodberg K, Tsuneta R, Garratty G. Discrepant Rh phenotyping results when testing IgG-sensitized RBCs with monoclonal Rh reagents (abstract). Transfusion 1995;35(Suppl):67.

34. Reisner R, Butler G, Bundy K, Moore SB. Comparison of the polyethylene glycol antiglobulin test and the use of enzymes in antibody detection and identification. Transfusion 1996;36:487-9.

35. Issitt PD, Combs MR, Bumgarner DJ, et al. Studies of antibodies in the sera of patients who have made red cell autoantibodies. Transfusion 1996;36:481-6.

36. Beattie KM, Zuelzer WW. The frequency and properties of pH-dependent anti-M. Transfusion 1965;5:322-6.

37. Bruce M, Watt AH, Hare W, et al. A serious source of error in antiglobulin testing. Transfusion 1986;26:177-81.

38. Rolih S, Thomas R, Fisher F, Talbot J. Antibody detection errors due to acidic or unbuffered saline. Immunohematol 1993;9:15-18.

39. Velliquette RW, Shakarian G, Jhang J, et al. Daratumumab-derived anti-CD38 can be easily mistaken for clinically significant antibodies to Lutheran antigens or to Knops antigens (abstract). Transfusion 2015;55(3S):26A.

40. Issitt PD, Combs MR, Bredehoeft SJ, et al. Lack of clinical significance of "enzyme-only" red cell alloantibodies. Transfusion 1993;33:284-93.

41. Advani H, Zamor J, Judd WJ, et al. Inactivation of Kell blood group antigens by 2-aminoethyli-sothiouronium bromide. Br J Haematol 1982;51:107-15.

42. Branch DR, Muensch HA, Sy Siok Hian AL, Petz LD. Disulfide bonds are a requirement for Kell and Cartwright (Yta) blood group antigen integrity. Br J Haematol 1983;54:573-8.

43. Branch DR, Petz LD. A new reagent (ZZAP) having multiple applications in immunohematology. Am J Clin Pathol 1982;78:161-7.

44. Liew YW, Uchikawa M. Loss of Era antigen in very low pH buffers. Transfusion 1987;27:442-3.

45. Swanson JL, Sastamoinen R. Chloroquine stripping of HLA A,B antigens from red cells. Transfusion 1985;25:439-40.

46. Morton JA, Pickles MM, Terry AM. The Sda blood group antigen in tissues and body fluids. Vox Sang 1970;19:472-82.

47. O'Neill GJ, Yang SY, Tegoli J, et al. Chido and Rodgers blood groups are distinct antigenic components of human complement C4. Nature 1978;273:668-70.

48. Tilley CA, Romans DG, Crookston MC. Localization of Chido and Rodgers determinants to the C4d fragment of human C4 (abstract). Transfusion 1978;18:622.

49. Judd WJ, Kraemer K, Moulds JJ. The rapid identification of Chido and Rodgers antibodies using C4d-coated red blood cells. Transfusion 1981;21:189-92.

50. Freedman J, Masters CA, Newlands M, Mollison PL. Optimal conditions for use of sulphydryl compounds in dissociating red cell antibodies. Vox Sang 1976;30:231-9.

51. Aye T, Arndt PA, Leger RM, et al. Myeloma patients receiving daratumumab (anti-CD38) can appear to have an antibody with Lutheran-related specificity (abstract). Transfusion 2015;55(3S):28A.

52. Nance SJ, Arndt P, Garratty, G. Predicting the clinical significance of red cell alloantibodies using a monocyte monolayer assay. Transfusion 1987;27:449-52.

53. Arndt PA, Garratty G. A retrospective analysis of the value of monocyte monolayer assay results for predicting the clinical significance of blood group alloantibodies. Transfusion 2004;44:1273-81.

54. Petz LD, Garratty G. Immune hemolytic anemias. 2nd ed. Philadelphia: Churchill Livingstone, 2004.

55. Code of federal regulations. Title 21, CFR Parts 660.25 and 660.26. Washington, DC: US

Government Publishing Office, 2016 (revised annually).

56. Food and Drug Administration. 7342.001: Inspection of licensed and unlicensed blood banks, brokers, reference laboratories, and contractors. Compliance Program guidance manual. Silver Spring, MD: CBER Office of Compliance and Biologics Quality, 2010:50-3. [Available at http://www.fda.gov/downloads/BiologicsBloodVaccines/GuidanceComplianceRegulatoryInformation/ComplianceActivities/Enforcement/CompliancePrograms/UCM337001.pdf (accessed April 16, 2017).]

57. Shirey RS, Edwards RE, Ness PM. The risk of alloimmunization to c (Rh4) in R1R1 patients who present with anti-E. Transfusion 1994;34:756-8.

SUGGESTED READINGS

Daniels G. Human blood groups. 3rd ed. Hoboken, NJ: Wiley-Blackwell, 2013.

Daniels G, Poole J, de Silva M, et al. The clinical significance of blood group antibodies. Transfus Med 2002;12:287-95.

Engelfriet CP, Overbeeke MA, Dooren MC, et al. Bioassays to determine the clinical significance of red cell antibodies based on Fc receptor-induced destruction of red cells sensitized with IgG. Transfusion 1994;34: 617-26.

Garratty G. In-vitro reactions with red blood cells that are not due to blood group antibodies: A review. Immunohematology 1998;14:1-11.

Harmening DM. Modern blood banking and transfusion practices. 6th ed. Philadelphia: FA Davis, 2012.

Issitt PD, Anstee DJ. Applied blood group serology. 4th ed. Durham, NC: Montgomery Scientific Publications, 1998.

Judd WJ, Johnson S, Storry J. Judd's methods in immunohematology. 3rd ed. Bethesda, MD: AABB Press, 2008.

Kaherl, KJ, ed. Standards for immunohematology reference laboratories. 9th ed. Bethesda, MD: AABB, 2015.

Kanter MH. Statistical analysis. In: Busch MP, Brecher ME, eds. Research design and analysis. Bethesda, MD: AABB, 1998:63-104.

Klein HG, Anstee DJ. Mollison's blood transfusion in clinical medicine. 12th ed. Oxford, UK: Wiley-Blackwell, 2014.

Lomas-Francis C, DePalma H. 2007 Rock Øyen Symposium. DNA-based assays for patient testing: Their application, interpretation, and correlation of results. Immunohematology 2008;24:180-90.

Menitove JE. The Hardy-Weinberger principle: Selection of compatible blood based on mathematic principles. In: Fridey JL, Kasprisin CA, Chambers LA, Rudmann SV, eds. Numbers for blood bankers. Bethesda, MD: AABB, 1995:1-11.

Ooley PW, ed. Standards for blood banks and transfusion services. 30th ed. Bethesda, MD: AABB, 2016.

Reid ME, Lomas-Francis C, Olsson M. The blood group antigen factsbook. 3rd ed. London: Elsevier Academic Press, 2012.

Rolih S. A review: Antibodies with high-titer, low-avidity characteristics. Immunohematology 1990;6:59-67.

Rudmann SV, ed. Serologic problem-solving: A systematic approach for improved practice. Bethesda, MD: AABB Press, 2005.

Weisbach V, Kohnhauser T, Zimmermann R, et al. Comparison of the performance of microtube column systems and solid-phase systems and the tube low-ionic-strength solution additive indirect antiglobulin test in the detection of red cell alloantibodies. Transfus Med 2006;16:276-84.

Westhoff C. 2007 Rock Øyen Symposium. Potential of blood group genotyping for transfusion medicine practice. Immunohematology 2008;24:190-5.

Chapter 14

The Positive Direct Antiglobulin Test and Immune-Mediated Hemolysis

• • •

Regina M. Leger, MSQA, MT(ASCP)SBB, CMQ/OE(ASQ), and
P. Dayand Borge Jr, MD, PhD

14

HEMOLYTIC ANEMIA IS the short-ening of red cell survival. The normal life span of red cells is approximately 110 to 120 days. In healthy individuals, 1% of red cells are removed by the reticuloendothelial system each day, but this is matched by red cell production in the marrow. Normal marrow can increase red cell production to compensate for blood loss. Thus, in the absence of bleeding, an increased reticulocyte count is an indirect measure of hemolysis. If the marrow is able to adequately compensate, a reduced red cell survival may not result in anemia.

Immune-mediated hemolysis, the subject of this chapter, is only one cause of hemolytic anemia, and many causes of hemolysis are unrelated to immune reactions. Immune hemolytic anemia is the result of an immune response. The diagnosis of hemolytic anemia rests on clinical findings and laboratory data, such as hemoglobin or hematocrit values; reticulocyte count; red cell morphology; and bilirubin, haptoglobin, and lactate dehydrogenase (LDH) levels.

In some cases, the destruction of red cells takes place in the intravascular space with the release of free hemoglobin into the plasma. The red cells are ruptured following activation of the classical complement cascade. The characteristic features of this rare type of hemolysis are hemoglobinemia and, when the plasma hemoglobin level exceeds the renal threshold, hemoglobinuria. Conversely and more commonly, extravascular hemolysis results when macrophages in the spleen and liver phagocytose red cells completely or partially (producing spherocytes) or destroy red cells by cytotoxic events, resulting in an increase in serum bilirubin. This distinction is a simplification, however, because hemoglobin can also be released into the plasma following extravascular destruction if hemolysis is brisk.

Regina M. Leger, MSQA, MT(ASCP)SBB, CMQ/OE(ASQ), Lead Technologist, Special Immunohematology Laboratory, American Red Cross Blood Services, Southern California Region, Pomona, California; and P. Dayand Borge Jr, MD, PhD, Chief Medical Officer, East Division, American Red Cross Blood Services, Penn-Jersey Region, Philadelphia, Pennsylvania

The authors have disclosed no conflicts of interest.

The serologic investigations carried out in the blood bank help determine whether the hemolysis has an immune basis and, if so, what type of immune hemolytic anemia is present. This is important because the treatment for each type is different but generally involves some type of immunomodulatory therapy. Although there is no evidence-based algorithm for therapy, treatment options can include corticosteroids, intravenous immunoglobulin (IVIG), splenectomy, rituximab, and other more potent immunosuppressive medications.[1] As more patient outcome data with different treatment modalities become available, the determination of what is considered first-line therapy will change. For example, although rituximab is considered to be first-line therapy for cold agglutinin disease (CAD), eculizumab, an antibody that mitigates complement-mediated hemolysis, may be more effective in patients with acute, brisk hemolysis.[2]

The direct antiglobulin test (DAT) is a simple test used to determine if red cells have been coated in vivo with immunoglobulin (Ig), complement, or both. The DAT is used primarily for the investigation of hemolytic transfusion reactions (HTRs), hemolytic disease of the fetus and newborn (HDFN), autoimmune hemolytic anemia (AIHA), and drug-induced immune hemolytic anemia (DIIHA). A positive DAT result may or may not be associated with immune-mediated hemolysis. As shown in Table 14-1, there are many causes of a positive DAT result.

THE DAT

The DAT should be performed on every patient in whom the presence of hemolysis has been established to distinguish immune from nonimmune hemolytic anemia. The DAT should also be performed when a positive autocontrol is found in antibody identification studies (see Chapter 13), but there is no benefit to performing a DAT (or autocontrol) as part of routine pretransfusion testing. The DAT should not be performed as a screening test for hemolytic anemia. The predictive value of a positive DAT result is 83% in a patient with hemolytic anemia, but only 1.4% in a patient without hemolytic anemia.[3]

Small amounts of IgG and complement that are lower than the detection limit of routine testing techniques appear to be present on all red cells. Using sensitive testing techniques, 5 to 90 IgG molecules/red cell[4] and 5 to 40 C3d molecules/red cell[5] have been detected in healthy individuals. Depending on the technique and reagents used, the DAT can detect 100 to 500 molecules of IgG/red cell and 400 to 1100 molecules of C3d/red cell. Positive DAT results are reported in 1:1000 to 1:14,000 blood donors and 1% to 15% of hospital patients.[6]

TABLE 14-1. Some Causes of a Positive DAT Result

● Autoantibodies to intrinsic red cell antigens
● Hemolytic transfusion reactions
● Hemolytic disease of the fetus and newborn
● Drug-induced antibodies
● Passively acquired alloantibodies (eg, from donor plasma, derivatives, or immunoglobulin)
● Nonspecifically adsorbed proteins (eg, hypergammaglobulinemia, high-dose intravenous immune globulin, or modification of red cell membrane by some drugs)
● Complement activation due to bacterial infection, autoantibodies, or alloantibodies
● Antibodies produced by passenger lymphocytes (eg, in transplanted organs or hematopoietic components)

DAT = direct antiglobulin test.

These large differences in incidence are probably related to the different DAT techniques used.

Most blood donors with a positive DAT result appear to be perfectly healthy, and most patients with positive DAT results have no obvious signs of hemolytic anemia. However, a careful evaluation may show evidence of increased red cell destruction. Studies suggest that a positive DAT result in a healthy blood donor may be a marker of risk of future development of malignancy.[7,8]

A positive DAT result in a patient with hemolytic anemia indicates that the most likely diagnosis is one of the immune hemolytic anemias. However, the DAT result can be positive, coincidentally, in patients with hemolytic anemia that is not immune mediated. Conversely, some patients with immune hemolytic anemia have a negative DAT result. (See "DAT-Negative AIHA" section below.)

The DAT can also be positive for IgG or complement without a clear correlation with anemia in patients with sickle cell disease, beta-thalassemia, renal disease, multiple myeloma, autoimmune disorders, AIDS, or other diseases associated with elevated serum globulin or blood urea nitrogen levels.[9-11] The interpretation of a positive DAT result should take into consideration the patient's history, clinical data, and results of other laboratory tests.

Initial transfusion reaction investigations include a DAT on a posttransfusion specimen. In the presence of immune-mediated hemolysis, the DAT result may be positive if sensitized red cells have not been destroyed, or negative if hemolysis and rapid clearance have occurred. Preparation and testing of an eluate from DAT-positive posttransfusion-reaction red cells is indicated. Even if the DAT result is only weakly positive or negative, testing of an eluate may be informative. If the DAT result is positive on the postreaction specimen, a DAT should also be performed on the pretransfusion specimen for comparison and appropriate interpretation.

The Principles of the DAT

The DAT is based on the test developed by Coombs, Mourant, and Race[12] for the detection of antibodies attached to red cells that do not produce direct agglutination. This test, an indirect antiglobulin test, was initially used to demonstrate antibody in serum, but it was later applied to demonstrate the in-vivo coating of red cells with antibody or complement components (the DAT).

Most of the antiglobulin reactivity is directed at the heavy chains (eg, Fc portion of the sensitizing antibody) or the complement component, thus bridging the gap between adjacent red cells to produce visible agglutination. The strength of the observed agglutination is usually proportional to the amount of bound protein.

The DAT is performed by testing freshly washed red cells directly with antiglobulin reagents containing anti-IgG and anti-C3d. In the United States, only polyspecific anti-IgG,-C3d and monospecific anti-IgG, anti-C3d, and anti-C3b,-C3d reagents are currently licensed. The red cells need to be washed to remove free plasma globulins and complement; otherwise, the antiglobulin reagent can be neutralized, leading to a false-negative result. The saline used for washing the red cells should be at room temperature; washing red cells with warm (eg, 37 C) saline can result in the loss of red-cell-bound, low-affinity IgG. The red cells should be tested immediately after washing to prevent false-negative results caused by the elution of IgG. Performing a DAT using a column agglutination test (eg, gel test) does not require washing of the red cells before testing because plasma proteins do not neutralize detection of red-cell-bound reactivity. This may represent a positive bias for detection of red-cell-bound low-affinity IgG.

Although any red cells may be tested, EDTA-anticoagulated blood samples are preferred. The EDTA prevents in-vitro fixation of complement by chelating the calcium that is needed for C1 activation. If red cells from a clotted blood sample have a positive DAT result due to complement, the results should be confirmed on red cells from freshly collected blood kept at 37 C or an EDTA-anticoagulated specimen if these results are to be used for diagnostic purposes.

The DAT can be initially performed with a polyspecific antihuman globulin (AHG) reagent that is capable of detecting both IgG and C3d. (See Method 3-14.) If the results are positive, tests with monospecific reagents (anti-IgG and anticomplement separately) need to be performed to appropriately characterize the immune process involved and determine the diagnosis. Because polyspecific reagents are usually blended, and testing conditions for optimally detecting IgG and C3d on red cells may differ, some laboratories perform the DAT initially with anti-IgG and anti-C3d reagents separately. If the polyspecific reagent is polyclonal, proteins other than IgG or C3d (eg, IgM, IgA, or other complement components) can occasionally be detected; however, specific reagents to distinguish these other proteins by serologic techniques are not readily available. If umbilical cord blood samples are to be tested, it is appropriate to use anti-IgG only, because HDFN results from fetal red cell sensitization with maternally derived IgG antibody, and complement activation rarely occurs.[6]

It is important to follow the reagent manufacturer's instructions and recognize any product limitations. False-negative or weaker results can be obtained if the washed red cells are allowed to sit before they are tested with anti-IgG or if the reading of the results is delayed. Some anticomplement reagents, in contrast, demonstrate stronger reactivity if centrifugation is delayed for a short time after the reagent has been added. When the DAT result is positive with both anti-IgG and anti-C3, the red cells should be tested with an inert control reagent (eg, 6% albumin or saline). Lack of agglutination of the red cells in the control reagent provides some assurance that the test results are accurately interpreted. If the control is reactive, the DAT result is invalid. [See sections below on warm AIHA (WAIHA) and CAD.] Reactivity with this control reagent can indicate spontaneous agglutination caused by heavy coating of IgG or rare warm-reactive IgM, or it can indicate IgM cold autoagglu-tinins that were not dissociated during routine washing.

Evaluation of a Positive DAT Result

A positive DAT result alone is not diagnostic of hemolytic anemia. Understanding the significance of this positive result requires knowledge of the patient's diagnosis; recent drug, pregnancy, transfusion, and hematopoietic transplantation history; and the presence of acquired or unexplained hemolytic anemia. Dialogue with the attending physician is important. Clinical considerations together with laboratory data should dictate the extent to which a positive DAT result is evaluated.

Patient History

The following situations may warrant further investigation of a positive DAT result.

1. *Evidence of in-vivo hemolysis (ie, red cell destruction).* If a patient with anemia who has a positive DAT result shows evidence of hemolysis, testing to evaluate a possible immune etiology is appropriate. Reticulocytosis; spherocytes observed on the peripheral blood film; hemoglobinemia; hemoglobinuria; decreased serum haptoglobin; and elevated levels of serum unconjugated (indirect) bilirubin or LDH, especially LDH1, may be associated with increased red cell destruction. These factors are indicative of hemolytic anemia but not specifically immune hemolytic anemia. *If there is no evidence of hemolytic anemia, no further studies are necessary* unless the patient requires a red cell transfusion and the serum contains incompletely identified antibodies to red cell antigens. Testing an eluate may be helpful for antibody identification. (See "Elution" section below and Chapter 13.)

2. *Recent transfusion.* When a patient has recently been transfused, a positive DAT result may be the first indication of a developing immune response. The developing

antibody sensitizes the transfused red cells that have the corresponding antigen, and the DAT result becomes positive. The antibody may not be present in sufficient quantity to be detected in the serum. Antibody may appear as early as 7 to 10 days after transfusion in a primary immunization or as early as 1 to 2 days in a secondary response.[6,13] These alloantibodies could shorten the survival of red cells that have already been transfused or are administered in subsequent transfusions. A mixed-field appearance in the posttransfusion DAT result (ie, agglutination of donor red cells and no agglutination of the patient's red cells) may or may not be observed.

3. *Administration of drugs associated with immune-mediated hemolysis.* Many drugs have been reported to cause a positive DAT result and/or immune-mediated hemolysis, but this occurrence is not common.[14] (See "Drug-Induced Immune Hemolytic Anemia" section below.)

4. *History of hematopoietic progenitor cell or organ transplantation.* Passenger lymphocytes of donor origin produce antibodies directed against ABO or other blood group antigens on the recipient's red cells, causing a positive DAT result.[6]

5. *Administration of IVIG or intravenous (IV) anti-D.* IVIG may contain ABO antibodies, anti-D, or sometimes, other antibodies.[15] IV anti-D used to treat immune thrombocytopenia (previously known as "immune thrombocytopenic purpura") causes Rh-positive patients to develop a positive DAT result. IV anti-D may also contain other antibodies, including ABO antibodies.[16]

6. *Administration of therapeutic monoclonal antibodies that may react with target antigen on red cells.* For example, anti-CD38 administered to treat myeloma causes reactivity with all red cells because of the presence of low amounts of CD38 on red cells.[17-18]

The DAT may or may not be positive. A complete history (eg, diagnosis, medications) is important in these cases.

Serologic Investigation

Three investigative approaches are helpful in the evaluation of a positive DAT result:

1. Test the DAT-positive red cells with anti-IgG and anti-C3d reagents to characterize the type of protein(s) coating the red cells. This will help to classify an immune-mediated hemolytic anemia.

2. Test the serum/plasma to detect and identify clinically significant antibodies to red cell antigens. Additional tests that are useful in classifying the immune hemolytic anemias and procedures for detecting alloantibodies in the presence of autoantibodies are described later in this chapter.

3. Test an eluate prepared from the DAT-positive red cells with reagent red cells to determine whether the coating protein has red cell antibody specificity. When the only coating protein is complement, the eluate is likely to be nonreactive. However, an eluate from the patient's red cells coated only with complement should be tested if there is clinical evidence of antibody-mediated hemolysis, for example, after transfusion. The eluate preparation can concentrate small amounts of IgG that may not be detectable in routine testing of the patient's plasma.

Results of these tests combined with the patient's history and clinical data should assist in classification of the problem involved.

Elution

Elution can be informative in the following situations:

• Clinical signs and symptoms of immune hemolysis are present.

- Serum test results are negative or inconclusive for a patient who has been recently transfused.
- HDFN is suspected but no alloantibodies were detected in the maternal plasma.

Performing an elution routinely on the red cells of all patients who have a positive DAT result is not recommended. The majority of pretransfusion patients with a positive DAT result have a nonreactive eluate that is often associated with an elevated serum globulin level.[9-11]

Elution frees antibody from sensitized red cells and recovers antibody in a usable form. Multiple elution methods have been described and reviewed.[19] Many laboratories use commercial acid elution kits, primarily for ease of use and decreased exposure to potentially harmful chemicals; these kits are suitable to recover antibody in most cases. False-positive eluate results associated with high-titer antibodies have been reported when the low-ionic wash solution supplied with the commercial acid eluates was used.[20] Because no single elution method is ideal in all situations, an alternative elution method (eg, an organic solvent) may be used in some high-complexity reference laboratories when a nonreactive acid eluate result is not in agreement with clinical data.[21]

Table 14-2 lists the uses of some common elution methods. Typically, eluates are tested only at the antiglobulin phase. If an IgM antibody is being investigated or suspected, however, centrifugation and reading after the 37 C incubation should be performed. Technical considerations for elution are discussed in Chapter 13.

In cases of HTR or HDFN, specific antibody (or antibodies) is usually detected in the eluate that may or may not be detectable in the serum. For transfusion reactions, newly developed antibodies that are initially detectable only in the eluate are usually detectable in the serum after about 14 to 21 days.[22] If the eluate is nonreactive and a non-group-O patient has received plasma containing anti-A or anti-B (as a result of the transfusion of group O platelets, for example) and the recipient appears to have immune hemolysis, the eluate should be tested against A_1 and/or B cells. It may be appropriate to test the eluate against red cells from recently transfused donor units, which could have caused immunization to a rare antigen. For cases of HDFN when no maternal antibody has been detected and paternal red cells are ABO incompatible with maternal plasma, testing an eluate prepared from the infant's red cells with the paternal red cells may detect a maternally derived antibody to a low-prevalence antigen.

TABLE 14-2. Antibody Elution Methods

Method	Use	Comments
Lui freeze-thaw	ABO HDFN	Quick, small volume of red cells needed, poor recovery of other antibodies
Heat (56 C)	ABO HDFN, IgM agglutinating antibodies	Easy, poor recovery of IgG allo- and autoantibodies
Acid elution kits (commercial)	Warm auto- and alloantibodies	Easy, possible false-positive eluate results when high-titer antibody is present[20]
Chemical/organic solvent	Warm auto- and alloantibodies	Chemical hazards; eg, flammability, toxicity, or carcinogenicity

HDFN = hemolytic disease of the fetus and newborn; IgM = immunoglobulin M.

When the eluate reacts with all cells tested, autoantibody is the most likely explanation, especially if the patient has not been transfused recently. However, if the patient has been recently transfused, an antibody to a high-prevalence antigen should be considered. When no unexpected antibodies are present in the serum and the patient has not been transfused recently, no further serologic testing of an autoantibody detected only in the eluate is necessary.

The patient's complete history, including the presence of potential passive antibodies, needs to be reviewed when the serologic test results are evaluated. If both the serum and eluate are nonreactive, there is evidence of immune hemolysis, and the patient has received a drug reported to have caused immune-mediated hemolysis, testing to demonstrate drug-related antibodies should be considered. (See "Laboratory Investigation of Drug-Induced Immune Hemolysis" section below.)

AUTOIMMUNE HEMOLYTIC ANEMIA

Immune hemolytic anemias can be classified in various ways. One classification system is shown in Table 14-3. The AIHAs are subdivided into the major types: WAIHA, CAD, mixed- or combined-type AIHA, and paroxysmal cold hemoglobinuria (PCH). Other classification

TABLE 14-3. Classification of Immune Hemolytic Anemias

Autoimmune hemolytic anemia (AIHA)
● Warm AIHA
● Cold agglutinin disease
● Mixed-type AIHA
● Paroxysmal cold hemoglobinuria
Alloimmune hemolytic anemia
● Hemolytic transfusion reaction
● Hemolytic disease of the fetus and newborn
Drug-induced immune hemolytic anemia

schemes consider PCH as one of the cold-reactive AIHAs. Not all cases fit neatly into these categories. Table 14-4 shows the typical serologic characteristics of the AIHAs. Drugs (discussed in the "Drug-Induced Immune Hemolytic Anemia" section below) may also induce immune hemolysis; the effects of drug-induced *auto*antibodies are serologically indistinguishable from WAIHA.

Warm Autoimmune Hemolytic Anemia

The majority of AIHA cases are caused by warm-reactive autoantibodies that are optimally reactive with red cells at 37 C. The autoantibody is usually IgG, but it can be IgM or IgA.

Serologic Characteristics

The DAT result may be positive because of IgG plus complement (67% of cases), IgG without complement (20%), or complement without IgG (13%).[6] Performing an elution at initial diagnosis and/or during pretransfusion testing is useful to demonstrate that the IgG coating the patient's red cells is autoantibody.

Typically in WAIHA, the eluate is reactive with virtually all red cells tested, and reactivity is enhanced in tests against enzyme-treated red cells, with polyethylene glycol (PEG) enhancement, or in column agglutination and solid-phase tests. The eluate usually has no serologic activity if the only protein coating the red cells is complement.

If the autoantibody has been adsorbed by the patient's red cells in vivo, the serum may not contain detectable free antibody. The serum contains free antibody when the amount of autoantibody exceeds the available binding sites on the patient's red cells; thus, serum autoantibody reactivity is "left over," that is, what was not adsorbed by the patient's red cells in vivo. The DAT result in such cases is usually strongly positive.

Autoantibody in the serum typically is reactive against all cells by an IAT. Approximately 60% of patients with WAIHA have serum antibodies that react with untreated saline-

TABLE 14-4. Typical Serologic Findings in AIHA

	WAIHA	CAD	Mixed-Type AIHA	PCH
DAT (routine)	IgG IgG + C3 C3	C3 only	IgG + C3 C3	C3 only
Ig type	IgG	IgM	IgG, IgM	IgG
Eluate	IgG antibody	Nonreactive	IgG antibody	Nonreactive
Serum	By IAT, 35% agglutinate untreated red cells at 20 C	IgM agglutinating antibody, titer ≥1000 (60%) at 4 C, reactive at 30 C	IgG IAT-reactive antibody plus IgM agglutinating antibody reactive at 30 C	Negative routine IAT result, IgG biphasic hemolysin in Donath-Landsteiner test
Specificity	Broadly reactive, multiple specificities reported	Usually anti-I	Usually unclear	Anti-P

AIHA = autoimmune hemolytic anemia; WAIHA = warm AIHA; CAD = cold agglutinin disease; PCH = paroxysmal cold hemoglobinuria; DAT = direct antiglobulin test; IgG = immunoglobulin G; IgM = immunoglobulin M; IAT = indirect antiglobulin test.

suspended red cells. When tested with PEG, enzyme-treated red cells, column agglutination, or solid-phase methods, >90% of these sera can be shown to contain autoantibody. Agglutination at room temperature is present in about one-third of patients with WAIHA, but these cold agglutinins have normal titers at 4 C and are nonreactive at 30 C and 37 C. Thus, these cold agglutinins are nonpathogenic and the patient does not have CAD in addition to WAIHA.[6]

An unusual subcategory of WAIHA is associated with IgM agglutinins in the plasma that are reactive at 37 C.[6,23] This type of WAIHA is characterized by severe hemolysis, and the prognosis for these patients can be poor. The red cells are typically spontaneously agglutinated in the DAT; that is, the washed red cells are reactive with all reagents tested, including a control, such as 6% albumin or saline. (See "Serologic Problems" section below.) Complement is usually detected on the red cells; IgG or IgM may or may not be detected. IgM agglutinins are often detected in an eluate (eg, acid) when it is inspected for agglutination after the 37 C incubation and before the antiglobulin test is conducted. Some serum IgM warm au-

toagglutinins may be difficult to detect; some are enhanced in the presence of albumin or at low pH. Optimal reactivity of the agglutinin sometimes occurs between 20 C and 30 C rather than at 37 C. These antibodies have low titers at 4 C, usually <64, which easily differentiates this IgM warm antibody from those in CAD. To prevent misinterpretation of titration results, titrations at different temperatures (eg, 37 C, 30 C, room temperature, and 4 C) need to be carried out with separate sets of tubes to avoid carryover agglutination.[6,23] Testing for the presence of a warm hemolysin can sometimes define the AIHA as consistent with a warm IgM AIHA.[23]

Serologic Problems

Warm autoantibodies can cause technical difficulties during red cell testing. Spontaneous agglutination can occur if the red cells are heavily coated with IgG and the reagent contains a potentiator, such as albumin. This has been observed when high-protein Rh typing sera are used. If the control reagent provided by the manufacturer for these antisera is reactive, the typing is invalid. IgG can less commonly cause spontaneous agglutination in lower-protein reagents (eg, monoclonal typing sera); this reactivity is often weaker or more fragile than true agglutination and may not be detected by a 6% albumin control.[24] Spontaneous agglutination caused by red cells heavily coated with IgG is less frequently observed.

Warm-reactive IgM agglutinins can also cause spontaneous agglutination, resulting in ABO and Rh typing problems and/or reactivity with the negative control reagent for the DAT.[23] In these cases, treatment with dithiothreitol (DTT) or 2-mercaptoethanol (2-ME) (Method 2-18) to disrupt the IgM agglutinin is required to accurately interpret typing and DAT results. When the spontaneous agglutination is disrupted, the control reagent is nonreactive.

When the DAT result is positive due to IgG, antiglobulin-reactive typing reagents cannot be used unless the red-cell-bound IgG is first removed. (See Methods 2-20 and 2-21.) An alternative is to use low-protein antisera (eg, monoclonal reagents) that do not require an antiglobulin test. (Refer to the manufacturer's instructions for the detection of spontaneous agglutination.) It is helpful to know which of the common red cell antigens are lacking on the patient's red cells to predict which clinically significant alloantibodies the patient may have produced or may produce in the future. Antigens absent from autologous cells could well be the target of present or future alloantibodies. The patient's phenotype for the common antigens can be determined serologically or predicted using DNA-based methods.

The presence of autoantibody in the serum increases the complexity of the serologic evaluation and the time needed to complete pretransfusion testing. If a patient who has warm-reactive autoantibodies in the serum needs a transfusion, it is important to determine whether alloantibodies are also present. Some alloantibodies may make their presence known by reacting more strongly or at different phases than the autoantibody, but quite often, routine testing may not suggest the existence of masked alloantibodies.[25,26]

Methods to detect alloantibodies in the presence of warm-reactive autoantibodies are used to attempt to remove, reduce, or circumvent the autoantibody. Antibody detection methods that use PEG, enzymes, column agglutination, or solid-phase red cell adherence usually enhance autoantibodies. Antibody detection tests using low-ionic-strength saline (LISS) or saline tube methods may not detect autoantibodies but they do detect most clinically significant alloantibodies. Other procedures involve adsorption; two widely used adsorption approaches are discussed below.

Adsorption with Autologous Red Cells

In a patient who has not been transfused recently, adsorption with autologous red cells (autologous adsorption; see Method 4-8) is the best way to detect alloantibodies in the presence of warm-reactive autoantibodies. Only autoantibodies are removed, and alloantibodies, if present, remain in the serum.

Autologous adsorption typically requires some initial preparation of the patient's red cells. At 37 C, in-vivo adsorption has occurred, and all antigen sites on the patient's own red cells may be blocked. A gentle heat elution at 56 C for 3 to 5 minutes can dissociate some of the bound IgG. This can be followed by treatment of the autologous red cells with proteolytic enzymes to increase their capacity to adsorb autoantibody. (Treatment with proteolytic enzyme alone does not remove IgG coating the red cells.) Treatment of the red cells with ZZAP, a mixture of papain or ficin and DTT, accomplishes both of these actions in one step. It is proposed that the sulfhydryl component makes the IgG molecules more susceptible to the protease and dissociates the antibody molecules from the cell.[27] Multiple sequential autologous adsorptions with new aliquots of red cells may be necessary if the serum contains high levels of autoantibody. Once autoantibody has been removed, the adsorbed serum is tested for alloantibody reactivity.

Autologous adsorption is not recommended for patients who have been transfused within the last 3 months because a blood sample may contain some transfused red cells that might adsorb alloantibody. Red cells normally survive for about 110 to 120 days. In patients with AIHA, autologous and transfused red cells can be expected to have shortened survival. However, determining how long transfused red cells remain in circulation in patients who need repeated transfusions is not feasible. It has been demonstrated that very small amounts (<10%) of antigen-positive red cells are capable of removing alloantibody reactivity in in-vitro studies.[28] Therefore, it is recommended to wait for 3 months after transfusion before performing autologous adsorptions.

Adsorption with Allogeneic Red Cells

The use of allogeneic red cells for adsorption (allogeneic adsorption) may be helpful when the patient has been recently transfused or insufficient autologous red cells are available. The goal is to remove autoantibody and leave the alloantibody in the adsorbed serum. The adsorbing red cells must not have the antigens against which the alloantibodies are reactive. Because alloantibody specificity is unknown, red cells of different phenotypes are usually used to adsorb several aliquots of the patient's serum.

Given the number of potential alloantibodies, the task of selecting the red cells may appear formidable. However, red cell selection is based only on those few antigens for which alloantibodies of clinical significance are likely to be present. These include the common Rh antigens (D, C, E, c, and e), K, Fy^a and Fy^b, Jk^a and Jk^b, and S and s. Red cell selection is made easier by the fact that some of these antigens can be destroyed by appropriate pretreatment (eg, with enzymes or ZZAP) before use in adsorption procedures. (See Chapter 13, Table 13-5.) Antibodies to high-prevalence antigens cannot be excluded by allogeneic adsorptions because the adsorbing red cells are expected to express the antigen and adsorb the alloantibody along with autoantibody.

When the patient's phenotype is not known, group O red cell samples of three different Rh phenotypes (R_1R_1, R_2R_2, and rr) should be selected. (See Method 4-9.) One sample should lack Jk^a, and another, Jk^b. As shown in Table 14-5, ZZAP or enzyme pretreatment of the adsorbing red cells reduces the phenotype requirements. Untreated red cells may be used, but the adsorbing red cells must

TABLE 14-5. Selection of Red Cells for Allogeneic Adsorption

Step 1. Select red cells for each Rh phenotype.

R_1R_1
R_2R_2
rr

Step 2. On the basis of the red cell treatment or lack of treatment (below), at least one of the Rh-phenotyped cells should be negative for the antigens listed below.

ZZAP-Treated Red Cells	Enzyme-Treated Red Cells	Untreated Red Cells
Jk(a–)	Jk(a–)	Jk(a–)
Jk(b–)	Jk(b–)	Jk(b–)
	K–	K–
		Fy(a–)
		Fy(b–)
		S–
		s–

include at least one sample that is negative for the S, s, Fy^a, Fy^b, and K antigens in addition to the Rh and Kidd requirements stated above.

If the patient's phenotype is known or can be determined, adsorption with a single sample of red cells may be possible. Red cells can be selected that match the patient's phenotype or at least match the Rh and Kidd phenotypes if ZZAP treatment is used. For example, if a patient's phenotype is E– K– S– Fy(a–) Jk(a–), untreated adsorbing red cells need to lack all five antigens, but enzyme-treated red cells only need to be E– K– Jk(a–), and ZZAP-treated red cells only need to be E– Jk(a–). Adsorption using untreated red cells in the presence of PEG (Method 4-10) or LISS[29,30] are modifications that have been used to decrease the incubation time for adsorptions and increase efficiency.

Testing of Adsorbed Serum

In some cases, each aliquot of serum may need to be adsorbed two or three times to remove the autoantibody. The fully adsorbed aliquots are then tested against reagent red cells known to either lack or carry common antigens of the Rh, MNS, Kell, Duffy, and Kidd blood group systems (eg, antibody detection cells). If an adsorbed aliquot is reactive, the aliquot should be tested to identify the antibody. Adsorbing several aliquots with different red cell samples provides a battery of potentially informative specimens. For example, if the aliquot adsorbed with Jk(a–) red cells subsequently is reactive only with Jk(a+) red cells, the presence of alloanti-Jk^a can be inferred confidently.

Sometimes, autoantibody is not removed by three sequential adsorptions. Additional adsorptions can be performed, but the performance of multiple adsorptions has the potential to dilute the serum. If the adsorbing cells do not appear to remove the antibody, the autoantibody may have an unusual specificity that is not reactive with the red cells used for adsorption. For example, autoantibodies with Kell, LW, or En^{a}FS specificity are not removed by ZZAP-treated red cells. (See Table 14-5 for a list of antigens altered by various agents.) The

possibility that the sample contains an auto- or alloantibody to a high-prevalence antigen should always be considered when adsorption fails to remove the reactivity.

Autoantibodies sometimes have patterns of reactivity that suggest the presence of alloantibody. For example, the serum of a D– patient may have apparent anti-C reactivity. The anti-C reactivity may reflect warm-reactive autoantibody even if the patient's red cells lack C. The apparent alloanti-C would, in this case, be adsorbed by C– red cells, both autologous and allogeneic. This is unlike the behavior of a true alloanti-C, which would be adsorbed only by C+ red cells. In one study, the serum adsorbed with autologous red cells often retained autoantibodies that mimicked alloantibodies in addition to the true alloantibody(ies) present, whereas serum adsorbed with allogeneic red cells most often contained only alloantibodies.[31] This reflects an inefficiency of autologous adsorption that is primarily caused by limited volumes of autologous red cells available for removing all of the autoantibody reactivity from the serum.

Specificity of Autoantibody

In many cases of WAIHA, no autoantibody specificity is apparent. The patient's serum reacts with all of the red cell samples tested. If testing is performed with cells of rare Rh phenotypes, such as D–– or Rh$_{null}$, some autoantibodies are weakly reactive or are nonreactive, and the autoantibody appears to have broad specificity in the Rh system. Apparent specificity for simple Rh antigens (D, C, E, c, and e) is occasionally seen, especially in saline or LISS indirect antiglobulin tests. A "relative" specificity based on stronger reactivity with cells of certain phenotypes may also be seen; relative specificity may also be apparent after adsorption. Autoantibody specificities can be clearer in the serum than in the eluate.

Apart from Rh specificity, warm autoantibodies with many other specificities have been reported (eg, specificities in the LW, Kell, Kidd, Duffy, and Diego systems).[32,33] Patients with autoantibodies of Kell, Rh, LW, Ge, Sc, Lu, and Lan specificities may have transiently depressed expression of the respective antigen, and the DAT result may be negative or very weakly positive.[33] In these cases, the autoantibody may initially appear to be alloantibody. Proof that it is truly autoantibody is demonstration that after the antibody and hemolytic anemia subside, the antigen strength returns to normal, and stored serum containing antibody is reactive with the patient's red cells.

Tests against red cells of a rare phenotype and by special techniques to determine autoantibody specificity have limited clinical or practical application. If the autoantibody reacts with all red cells except those of a rare Rh phenotype (eg, Rh_{null}), compatible donor blood is unlikely to be available. Such blood, if available, should be reserved for alloimmunized patients of that uncommon phenotype.

Selection of Blood for Transfusion

The most important consideration is to exclude the presence of potentially clinically significant alloantibodies *before* selecting RBC units for transfusion. There are multiple reports in the literature demonstrating that patients who have warm autoantibodies in their sera have a higher rate of alloimmunization (eg, 12% to 40%, with a mean of 32%).[25,34-37] Although these patients present a serologic challenge, they deserve the same protection from HTRs as any other patient. Autoantibodies that react with all reagent red cells, even weakly, are capable of masking alloantibody reactivity (ie, reactivity of red cells with both alloantibody and autoantibody may not be any stronger than with autoantibody alone).[25,26]

It is the exclusion of newly formed alloantibodies that is of concern. Because of the presence of autoantibodies, all crossmatches are incompatible. This is unlike the case of clinically significant alloantibodies without autoantibodies, where a compatible crossmatch with antigen-negative red cells is possible. Monitoring for evidence of red cell destruction caused by *alloantibodies* is difficult in patients who already have AIHA; these patients' own red cells and transfused red cells have shortened survival.

If no alloantibodies are detected in adsorbed serum, random units of the appropriate ABO group and Rh type may be selected for transfusion. If clinically significant alloantibodies are present, the transfused cells should lack the corresponding antigen(s). For patients facing long-term transfusion support, it is prudent to obtain an extended phenotype or predicted phenotype by genotyping. Consideration can then be given to transfusion with donor units that are antigen matched for clinically significant blood group antigens to avoid additional alloimmunization and potentially decrease the number of adsorptions required and the complexity of pretransfusion workup.

If the autoantibody has clear-cut specificity for a single antigen (eg, anti-e) and active hemolysis is ongoing, blood lacking that antigen should be selected. There is evidence that such red cells survive longer than the patient's own red cells.[6] If the autoantibody shows broader reactivity—reacting with all cells but showing some relative specificity (eg, preferentially reacting with e+ red cells), whether to transfuse blood lacking the corresponding antigen is debatable. In the absence of hemolysis or evidence of compromised survival of transfused cells, autoantibody specificity is not important. However, donor units that are negative for the antigen may be chosen because this is a simple way to circumvent the autoantibody and detect potential alloantibodies.

It may be undesirable to expose the patient to Rh antigens absent from autologous cells, especially D and especially in females of childbearing potential, merely to improve serologic compatibility testing results with the autoantibody. (For example, when a D– patient has autoanti-e, available e– units are likely to be D+; D–e– units are extremely rare.) Referral of the sample for molecular investigation to determine the risk for allo- or autoantibody production will aid in decision-making in these complex cases and potentially improve patient care.

Some laboratories use the adsorbed serum to screen and select nonreactive units (units that are antigen-negative for clinically significant alloantibodies, if detected) for transfusion. Other laboratories do not perform a crossmatch with the adsorbed serum because all units will be incompatible in vivo due to the autoantibody. Issuing a unit that is serologically compatible with adsorbed serum may provide some assurance that the correct unit has been selected and avoid incompatibility because of additional antibodies (eg, anti-Wr[a]), but this practice can also provide a false sense of security about the safety of the transfusion for these patients.

A transfusion management protocol using prophylactic antigen-matched units for patients with warm autoantibodies, where feasible, in combination with streamlined adsorption procedures has been described.[38] The same antigens for the commonly occurring, clinically significant antibodies (D, C, E, c, e, K, Fy[a], Fy[b], Jk[a], Jk[b], S, and s) are taken into account, as discussed in the previous section on adsorptions. The ability to implement such a protocol depends on the ability of the transfusion service, and more often the blood supplier, to maintain an adequate inventory of phenotyped units to meet the antigen-matching needs. In recent years, molecular technologies have been applied to red cell genotyping for patients with warm autoantibodies to determine which common alloantibodies the patient can make. DNA tests are attractive for determining the predicted phenotype of patients with a positive DAT (IgG) result because IgG is not always successfully removed and some red cell antigens are sensitive to IgG removal treatment.[39,40] Recent transfusions do not interfere with molecular testing. It must be remembered that genotyping may not accurately predict the phenotype if uncommon or rare silencing mutations are present or the patient has received a stem cell transplant.

Some experts propose that an electronic crossmatch can be safely used for patients with autoantibodies when the presence of common, clinically significant alloantibodies has been excluded.[41,42] This approach circumvents the need to issue units that are labeled "incompatible"; however, as discussed above, this practice can also lead to a false sense of security.

Although resolving serologic problems for these patients is important, delaying transfu-sion in the hope of finding serologically compatible blood may, in some cases, cause greater danger to the patient. Only clinical judgment can resolve this dilemma; therefore, having a dialogue with the patient's physician is important.

Transfusion of Patients with Warm-Reactive Autoantibodies

Patients with warm-reactive autoantibodies may have no apparent hemolysis or may have life-threatening anemia. Patients with little or no evidence of significant hemolysis tolerate transfusion quite well. The risk of transfusion is somewhat increased in these patients because of the difficulties with pretransfusion testing. The duration of survival of the transfused red cells is about the same as that of the patient's own red cells.

In patients with active hemolysis, transfusion may increase hemolysis, and the transfused red cells may be destroyed more rapidly than the patient's own red cells. This is related to the increased red cell mass available from the transfusion and the kinetics of red cell destruction.[6] Destruction of transfused cells may increase hemoglobinemia and hemoglobinuria. Disseminated intravascular coagulation can develop in patients with severe posttransfusion hemolysis.

The transfusion of patients with AIHA is a clinical decision that should be based on the balance between the risks and clinical need. Transfusion should not be withheld solely because of serologic incompatibility. The volume transfused should usually be the smallest amount required to maintain adequate oxygen delivery and not necessarily the amount required to reach an arbitrary hemoglobin level.[6] The patient should be carefully monitored throughout the transfusion.

DAT-Negative AIHA

Clinical and hematologic evidence of WAIHA is present in some patients whose DAT result is negative. The most common causes of AIHA associated with a negative DAT result are red-cell-bound IgG below the detection threshold of the antiglobulin test, red-cell-bound IgM and IgA that are not detectable by routine AHG reagents, and low-affinity IgG that is washed off the red cells during the washing phase for the DAT.[6,43]

Nonroutine tests can be applied in these situations. Unfortunately, these assays require standardization and many have a low predictive value. One of the easier tests is for low-affinity antibodies. Washing with ice-cold (eg, 4 C) saline or LISS may help retain antibody on the cells; a control (eg, 6% albumin) is necessary to confirm that cold autoagglutinins are not causing the positive results.[6,43] Methods that have been used to detect lower levels of red-cell-bound IgG include the complement fixation antibody consumption assay, the enzyme-linked antiglobulin test, radiolabeled anti-IgG, flow cytometry, solid-phase testing, the direct PEG test, the direct Polybrene test, column agglutination, and concentrated eluates.[43]

Anti-IgG, anti-C3d, and the combined anti-C3b,-C3d reagents are the only licensed products available in the United States for use with human red cells. AHG reagents that react with IgA or IgM are available commercially but probably have not been standardized for use with red cells in agglutination tests. They must be used cautiously, and their hemagglutination reactivity must be carefully standardized by the user.[6] Outside the United States, AHG reagents for the detection of IgM and IgA in tube tests or column agglutination tests may be available.

Cold Agglutinin Disease

CAD, which is less common than WAIHA, is the hemolytic anemia that is most commonly associated with autoantibodies that react preferentially in the cold. CAD occurs as an acute or chronic condition. The acute form is often secondary to *Mycoplasma pneumoniae* infection. The chronic form is often seen in elderly patients and is sometimes associated with lymphoma, chronic lymphocytic leukemia, or Waldenström macroglobulinemia. Acrocyanosis and hemoglobinuria may occur in cold weather; thus, patients should be advised to avoid cold. CAD is often characterized by agglutination, at room temperature, of red cells in an EDTA specimen, sometimes to the degree that the red cells appear to be clotted.

Serologic Characteristics

Complement is the only protein detected on red cells in almost all cases of CAD. If the red cells have been collected properly and washed at 37 C, there will be no immunoglobulin on the cells and no reactivity in the eluate. If other proteins are detected, a negative control for the DAT (eg, 6% albumin or saline) should be tested to ensure that the cold autoagglutinin is not causing a false-positive result. The cold-reactive autoagglutinin is usually IgM, which binds to red cells in the lower temperature of the peripheral circulation and causes complement components to attach to the red cells. As the red cells circulate to warmer areas, the IgM dissociates but the complement remains.

IgM cold-reactive autoagglutinins associated with immune hemolysis usually react at 30 C, and 60% have a titer of ≥1000 when tested at 4 C.[6] If 22% to 30% bovine albumin is included in the test system, pathologic cold agglutinins will react at 30 C or 37 C.[6] On occasion, pathologic cold agglutinins have a lower titer (ie, <1000), but they have a high thermal amplitude (ie, reactive at 30 C with or without the addition of albumin). The thermal amplitude of the antibody has greater significance than the titer. Hemolytic activity against untreated red cells can sometimes be demonstrated at 20 C to 25 C. Except in rare cases with Pr specificity, enzyme-treated red cells are hemolyzed in the presence of adequate complement.

To determine the true thermal amplitude or titer of the cold autoagglutinin, the specimen is collected and maintained strictly at 37 C until the serum and red cells are separated to avoid in-vitro autoadsorption. Alternatively, plasma can be used from an EDTA-anticoagulated specimen that has been warmed for 10 to 15 minutes at 37 C (with repeated mixing) and then separated from the cells, ideally at 37 C. This process should release autoadsorbed antibody back into the plasma.

In chronic CAD, the IgM autoagglutinin is usually a monoclonal protein with kappa light chains. In the acute form induced by *Mycoplasma* or viral infections, the antibody is polyclonal IgM with normal kappa and lambda light-chain distribution. Rare examples of IgA and IgG cold-reactive autoagglutinins have also been described.[6]

Serologic Problems

Problems with ABO and Rh typing and other tests are not uncommon. Often, it is only necessary to maintain the blood sample at 37 C immediately after collection and to wash the red cells with warm (37 C) saline before testing. Alternatively, an EDTA sample can be warmed to 37 C for about 10 minutes, after which the red cells are washed with warm saline. It is helpful to perform a parallel control test with 6% bovine albumin to determine whether autoagglutination persists. If the control test result is nonreactive, the results obtained with anti-A and anti-B are usually valid. If autoagglutination still occurs, it may be necessary to treat the red cells with sulfhydryl reagents. Because cold-reactive autoagglutinins are almost always IgM and sulfhydryl reagents denature IgM molecules, reagents (such as 2-ME or DTT) can be used to abolish autoagglutination. (See Method 2-18.) The red cells can also be treated with ZZAP reagent, as in the preparation for adsorptions. (See Method 4-8.)

When the serum agglutinates group O reagent red cells, ABO serum tests are invalid. Repeating the tests using prewarmed serum and group A_1, B, and O red cells and allowing the red cells to "settle" after incubation at 37 C for 1 hour (instead of centrifuging the sample) often resolves any discrepancy. (See Method 2-11.) By eliminating the centrifugation step, interference by cold-reactive autoantibodies might be avoided. Weak anti-A and/or -B in some patients' sera may not react at 37 C. Alternatively, adsorbed serum (either autoadsorbed or adsorbed with allogeneic group O red cells) can be used. Serum adsorbed with rabbit erythrocyte stroma should not be used for ABO serum tests because anti-B and anti-A1 may be removed.[44,45]

Detection of Alloantibodies in the Presence of Cold-Reactive Autoantibodies

Cold-reactive autoagglutinins rarely mask clinically significant alloantibodies if serum tests are conducted at 37 C and IgG-specific reagents are used for the antiglobulin phase. The use of potentiators (eg, albumin or PEG) is not recommended because they may increase the reactivity of the autoantibodies. In rare instances, it may be necessary to perform autologous adsorption at 4 C. (See Method 4-5.) Achieving the complete removal of potent cold-reactive autoagglutinins is very time consuming and usually unnecessary. Sufficient removal of cold autoagglutinins may be facilitated by treating the patient's cells with enzymes or ZZAP before adsorption. One or two cold autologous adsorptions should remove enough autoantibody to make it possible to detect alloantibodies at 37 C that were otherwise masked by the cold-reactive autoantibody. As an alternative, the allogeneic adsorption process used for WAIHA can be performed at 4 C. Rabbit erythrocyte stroma, which removes autoanti-I and -IH from sera, should be used with caution because this method can remove clinically significant alloantibodies—notably anti-D, -E, and -Vel, and IgM antibodies regardless of blood group specificity.[46,47]

Specificity of Autoantibody

The autoantibody specificity in CAD is most often anti-I but is usually of academic interest only. Anti-i is found less commonly, and it is usually associated with infectious mononucleosis. On rare occasions, other specificities are seen.

Autoantibody specificity is not diagnostic for CAD. Autoanti-I may be seen in healthy individuals as well as in patients with CAD. The nonpathologic forms of autoanti-i, however, rarely react at titers above 64 at 4 C and are usually nonreactive with I– (cord i and adult i) red cells at room temperature. In contrast, the autoanti-I of CAD may react quite strongly with I– red cells in tests at room temperature, and equal or even stronger reactions occur with I+ red cells. Autoanti-i reacts in the opposite manner, demonstrating stronger reactions with I– red cells than with red cells that are I+. Anti-I^T, originally thought to recognize a transition state of i to I (explaining the designation "I^T"), reacts strongly with cord red cells, weakly with normal adult I red cells, and most weakly with the rare adult i red cells. In rare cases, the cold agglutinin specificity may be anti-Pr, which reacts equally well with untreated red cells of I or i phenotypes but does not react with enzyme-treated red cells. Procedures to determine the titer and specificity of cold-reactive autoantibodies are given in Methods 4-6 and 4-7. Typical reactivity patterns of cold autoantibodies are shown in the table in Method 4-6.

Mixed-Type AIHA

Although about one-third of patients with WAIHA have nonpathologic IgM antibodies that agglutinate at room temperature, another group of patients with WAIHA have cold agglutinins that react at or above 30 C. This latter group is referred to as having "mixed" or "combined warm and cold" AIHA and can be subdivided into patients with high-titer, high-thermal-amplitude IgM cold antibodies (the rare WAIHA plus classic CAD) and patients with normal-titer (<64 at 4 C), high-thermal-amplitude cold antibodies.[48-50] Patients with mixed-type AIHA often present with hemolysis and complex serum reactivity in all phases of testing.

Serologic Characteristics

In mixed-type AIHA, both IgG and C3 are usually detectable on patients' red cells; however, C3, IgG, or IgA alone may be detectable on the red cells.[6] An eluate contains a warm-reactive IgG autoantibody. Both warm-reactive IgG autoantibodies and cold-reactive, agglutinating IgM autoantibodies are present in the serum. These autoantibodies usually result in reactivity at all phases of testing and with virtually all cells tested. The IgM agglutinating autoanti-

body reacts at 30 C or above. If adsorptions are performed to detect alloantibodies, it may be necessary to perform them at both 37 C and 4 C.

Specificity of Autoantibodies

The unusual cold-reactive IgM agglutinating autoantibody can have specificities that are typical of CAD (ie, anti-I or -i) but often has no apparent specificity.[48,49] The warm-reactive IgG autoantibody often appears to be serologically indistinguishable from autoantibodies encountered in typical WAIHA.

Transfusion of Patients with Mixed-Type AIHA

If blood transfusions are necessary, the considerations for the exclusion of alloantibodies and the selection of blood for transfusion are identical to those described for patients with acute hemolysis caused by WAIHA and CAD. (See above.)

Paroxysmal Cold Hemoglobinuria

PCH is the rarest form of DAT-positive AIHA. Historically, PCH was associated with syphilis, but this association is now unusual.[51] More commonly, PCH presents as an acute transient condition that is secondary to a viral infection, particularly in young children. In such cases, the biphasic hemolysin may be only transiently detectable. PCH can also occur as an idiopathic chronic disease in older people.

Serologic Characteristics

PCH is caused by a cold-reactive IgG complement-binding antibody. As with IgM cold-reactive autoagglutinins, reactivity occurs with red cells in colder areas of the body (usually the extremities) and causes C3 to bind irreversibly to red cells. The antibody then dissociates from the red cells as the blood circulates to warmer parts of the body. Red cells washed in a routine manner for the DAT are usually coated only with complement, but IgG may be detectable on cells that have been washed with cold saline and tested with cold anti-IgG reagent.[6] Keeping the test system close to its optimal binding temperature allows the cold-reactive IgG autoantibody to remain attached to its antigen. Because complement components are usually the only globulins present on circulating red cells, eluates prepared from the red cells of patients with PCH are almost always nonreactive.

The IgG autoantibody in PCH is classically described as a biphasic hemolysin because binding to red cells occurs at low temperatures, but hemolysis does not occur until the complement-coated red cells are warmed to 37 C. This is the basis of the diagnostic test for the disease, the Donath-Landsteiner test. (See Method 4-11.) The autoantibody may agglutinate normal red cells at 4 C but rarely to titers >64. Because the antibody rarely reacts above 4 C, pretransfusion antibody detection tests are usually nonreactive, and the serum is usually compatible with random donor cells by routine crossmatch procedures.

Specificity of Autoantibody

The autoantibody of PCH has most frequently been shown to have P specificity. The autoantibody reacts with all red cells by the Donath-Landsteiner test (including the patient's own red cells), except those of the very rare p or P^k phenotypes.

Transfusion of Patients with PCH

Transfusion is rarely necessary for adult patients with PCH, unless their hemolysis is severe. In young children, the thermal amplitude of the antibody tends to be much wider than in adults and hemolysis is often more brisk, so transfusion may be required as a lifesaving measure. Although there is some evidence that p red cells survive longer than P+ (P1+ or P1–) red cells, the prevalence of p blood is approximately 1 in 200,000, and the urgent need for transfusion usually precludes attempts to obtain this rare blood. Transfusion of donor blood should not be withheld from patients with PCH whose need is urgent. Transfusion of red cells that are negative for the P antigen should be considered only for those patients who do not respond adequately to randomly selected units of donor blood.[6]

DRUG-INDUCED IMMUNE HEMOLYTIC ANEMIA

Drugs rarely cause immune hemolytic anemia; the estimated incidence is 1 in 1 million people.[52] Many drugs have been implicated in hemolytic anemia over the years, as can be seen in the list provided in Appendix 14-1 and reviewed elsewhere.[14]

Drugs sometimes induce the formation of antibodies against the drug, red cell membrane components, or an antigen formed by the drug and the red cell membrane. These antibodies may cause a positive DAT result, immune red cell destruction, or both.[14,52] In some instances, a positive DAT result can be caused by nonimmunologic protein adsorption (NIPA) onto the red cell, which is caused by the drug.[14]

Theoretical Mechanisms of Drug-Induced Antibodies

Numerous theories have been suggested to explain how drugs induce immune responses and what relation such responses may have to the positive DAT result and immune-mediated cell destruction observed in some patients.[6] For many years, drug-associated positive DAT results were classified by four mechanisms: drug adsorption (penicillin-type), immune complex formation, autoantibody production, and NIPA. This classification has been useful serologically, but many aspects lack definitive proof. In addition, some drugs demonstrate serologic reactivity that appears to involve more than one mechanism. A more comprehensive approach, termed a "unifying hypothesis," is shown in Fig 14-1. One or more populations of antibodies may be present. In addition, NIPA, which is independent of antibody production, appears to play a role in drug-induced immune hemolytic anemia.[14]

Serologic Classification

Drug-induced antibodies can be classified into two groups: drug dependent (those that require the presence of the drug in the test system to be detected) and drug independent (those that do not require the in-vitro addition

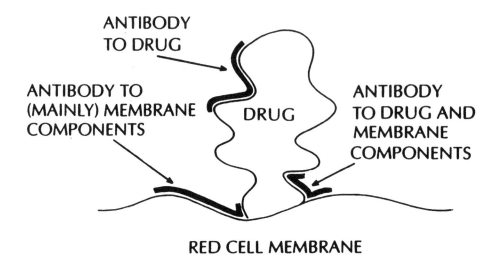

FIGURE 14-1. Proposed unifying theory of drug-induced antibody reactions (based on a cartoon by Habibi as cited by Garratty[32]). The thicker lines represent antigen-binding sites for the Fab region of the drug-induced antibody. Drugs (haptens) bind loosely or firmly to cell membranes, and antibodies may be made to 1) the drug [producing in-vitro reactions typical of a drug adsorption (penicillin-type) reaction]; 2) membrane components or mainly membrane components (producing in-vitro reactions typical of autoantibody); or 3) part-drug, part-membrane components (producing an in-vitro reaction typical of the so-called immune complex mechanism).[32(p55)]

of the drug for detection).[6] Drug-dependent antibodies are subdivided into those that react with drug-treated red cells (eg, antibodies to penicillin and some cephalosporins) and those that react with untreated red cells in the presence of a solution of the drug (eg, antibodies to quinine and ceftriaxone). Drug-independent antibodies (eg, autoantibodies induced by methyldopa and fludarabine) have serologic reactivity that is independent of the drug despite the fact that the drug originally induced the immune response. Because the drug does not need to be added to the test system, drug-independent antibodies behave like autoantibodies that are serologically indistinguishable from idiopathic warm auto-antibodies.

If a patient is suspected of having DIIHA, then the suspected drug should be stopped. Laboratory testing to detect drug-dependent antibodies can be performed, but DIIHA caused by drug-independent antibodies or NIPA can be suggested only by showing a tem-poral association of the drug administration and hemolysis.

The historical details of penicillin- and methyldopa-induced antibodies are not described in this chapter but have been extensively reviewed elsewhere.[6,52] DIIHA caused by high-dose intravenous penicillin therapy is no longer seen, and methyldopa, the prototype for drug-independent antibodies, is not used as frequently as in the past. Currently, the drugs most commonly associated with DIIHA are piperacillin, ceftriaxone, and cefotetan; there has also been a small increase in DIIHA caused by drugs in the platinum family.[14]

Drug-Dependent Antibodies That Are Reactive with Drug-Treated Red Cells

Some drugs (eg, penicillin, ampicillin, and many cephalosporins) covalently bind to red cells, thus making it possible to coat red cells in the laboratory with the drug. Antibodies directed to these drugs will react with the drug-treated red cells but not with untreated red cells (ie, no reaction unless the patient also has alloantibodies to red cell antigens present on these cells).

Penicillin and the cephalosporins are beta-lactam antibiotics. It was thought for some time that antibodies to any drug in the penicillin and cephalosporin families could be detected by testing red cells with drug-treated cells using methods previously described for penicillin and cephalothin. It is now known that this is not the case. Synthetic penicillins and newer cephalosporins cannot be assumed to have the same red-cell-binding characteristics as penicillin and cephalothin (a first-generation cephalosporin). Cefotetan (a second-generation cephalosporin) binds very well to red cells, and antibodies caused by cefotetan typically react to very high titers with cefotetan-treated red cells. However, ceftriaxone (a third-generation cephalosporin) does not bind well to red cells; therefore, antibodies to ceftriaxone cannot be tested by this method.[53] Piperacillin, a semisynthetic penicillin, binds to red cells at high pH. However, a large percentage of plasma from healthy blood donors and patients reacts with piperacillin-treated red cells, so this method is not recommended for testing for piperacillin antibodies.[53] For drug antibodies detected using drug-treated red cells, the following are expected:

- The DAT result is usually positive for IgG, but complement may also be present.
- The serum contains an antibody that reacts with the drug-treated red cells but not the untreated red cells.
- Antibody eluted from the patient's red cells reacts with drug-treated red cells but not untreated red cells.

Hemolysis develops gradually but may be life threatening if the etiology is unrecognized and drug administration is continued. The patient may or may not have been previously exposed to the drug and, in the case of cefotetan, even only a single dose given prophylactically can result in severe hemolysis. Normal plasma has been shown to react with some drug-treated red cells (eg, red cells treated with cefotetan, piperacillin, or oxaliplatin),[53] suggesting

prior exposure to these drugs through environmental routes.

Drug-Dependent Antibodies That Are Reactive with Untreated Red Cells in the Presence of Drug

Antibodies to many drugs that have been reported to cause immune hemolytic anemia are detected by testing untreated red cells in the presence of the drug. Piperacillin and some of the second- and third-generation cephalosporins react by this method; anti-ceftriaxone has been detected only by testing red cells in the presence of drug.[53] The following observations are characteristic:

- Complement may be the only protein easily detected on the red cells, but IgG may be present.
- The serum antibody can be IgM, IgG, or IgM with IgG.
- A drug (or metabolite) must be present in vitro for the antibody in the patient's serum to be detected. Antibodies may cause hemolysis, agglutination, and/or sensitization of red cells in the presence of the drug.
- The patient need only take a small amount of the drug (eg, a single dose).
- Acute intravascular hemolysis with hemoglobinemia and hemoglobinuria is the usual presentation. Renal failure is quite common.
- Once antibody has been formed, severe hemolytic episodes may recur after exposure to very small quantities of the drug.

On occasion, it appears that a patient's serum contains an "autoantibody" in addition to a drug antibody reacting in the presence of the drug. Rather than a true autoantibody, it is believed that this reactivity results from the presence of circulating drug or drug-plus-antibody complexes.[53] In these cases, an eluate is usually nonreactive when the drug is not present in the system. However, in some cases involving piperacillin, the eluate reacts while the patient is still taking the drug. A sample collected several days after the drug has been discontinued will be nonreactive. A true warm autoantibody is expected to be reactive in an eluate prepared from the patient's red cells, and autoantibody in the serum persists. Consequently, DIIHA caused by piperacillin can be misdiagnosed as WAIHA, especially if the eluate reacts. Differentiation of warm-reactive autoantibody from DIIHA is important for clinical management.[53]

Drug-Independent Antibodies: Autoantibody Production

Some drugs induce autoantibodies that appear serologically indistinguishable from those of WAIHA. Red cells are coated with IgG, and the eluate as well as the serum react with virtually all cells tested in the absence of the drug. The antibody has no direct or indirect in-vitro interaction with the drug. The prototype drug for such cases is methyldopa, which is now used much less frequently than in the past. Currently, fludarabine, used to treat chronic lymphocytic leukemia, is the most commonly used drug that produces drug-independent antibodies and AIHA.[52]

Nonimmunologic Protein Adsorption

The positive DAT result associated with some drugs is caused by modification of the red cell membrane by the drug and is independent of antibody production. Hemolytic anemia associated with this mechanism is rare.

Cephalosporins (primarily cephalothin) are the drugs with which positive DAT results and NIPA were originally associated. In vitro, red cells coated with cephalothin in pH 9.8 buffer and incubated with normal plasma adsorb albumin, IgA, IgG, IgM, C3, and other proteins in a nonimmunologic manner. For this reason, the indirect antiglobulin test result with virtually all plasma will be positive. Other drugs that cause NIPA and a positive DAT result include diglycoaldehyde, cisplatin, oxaliplatin, and beta-lactamase inhibitors (clavulanic acid, sulbactam, and tazobactam).[14]

NIPA should be suspected when a patient's plasma/serum and most normal plasma/sera are reactive in an indirect antiglobulin test with drug-treated red cells but the

eluate from the patient's red cells is nonreactive with the drug-treated cells.

Laboratory Investigation of Drug-Induced Immune Hemolysis

The drug-related problems that are most commonly encountered in the blood bank are those associated with a positive DAT result and a nonreactive eluate. Recent red cell transfusions and/or dramatic hemolysis may result in a weak DAT result by the time hemolysis is suspected. When other, more common causes of immune-mediated hemolysis have been excluded *and* a temporal relationship exists between the administration of a drug and the hemolytic anemia, a drug antibody investigation should be pursued.

The patient's serum should be tested for unexpected antibodies by routine procedures. If the serum does not react with untreated red cells, the tests should be repeated with the drug(s) suspected of causing the problem.[53] Some drug formulations contain inert ingredients (eg, pill or capsule forms), and other drugs are combinations of two drugs (eg, piperacillin plus tazobactam). Although it would seem logical to test the patient's serum with the actual drug that the patient received, inert ingredients or drug combinations can make preparation of drug-treated red cells difficult or make the results confusing. It is preferable to test serum using pure drug formulations as well as separate components of combination drugs.

If the drug has already been reported to cause hemolytic anemia, testing methods may be described in the case reports. Far more drug antibodies are detected by testing serum in the presence of drug; therefore, when a previous report of antibodies to a drug is not available, an initial screening test can be performed with a solution of the drug at a concentration of approximately 1 mg/mL in phosphate-buffered saline.[53] (See Method 4-13.) Serum, rather than plasma, is the preferred specimen for testing for hemolysis to be observed; this also allows for the addition of fresh normal serum (as a source of complement) to the test system. The addition of the fresh complement increases the sensitivity of the test for the detection of in-vitro hemolysis resulting from complement activation.

If these tests are not informative, attempts can be made to coat normal red cells with the drug.[53] The patient's serum and an eluate from the patient's red cells can be tested against the drug-treated red cells. (See Method 4-12.) This is the method of choice when cephalosporins (except for ceftriaxone) are thought to be implicated. Results that are definitive for a drug-induced positive DAT result are reactivity of the eluate with drug-treated red cells and absence of reactivity with untreated red cells.

Drug-treated red cells should always be tested with saline and normal serum (or plasma) as negative controls. This approach ensures that the observed reactivity with the patient's serum/plasma is appropriately interpreted. Antibodies reactive with red cells treated with some drugs (eg, beta-lactams and platinums) have been detected in the plasma from blood donors and patients without hemolytic anemia and are thought to be caused by environmental exposure. Therefore, misinterpretation of reactivity in a patient's serum is possible.[53]

Whenever possible, a positive control should be tested with drug-treated red cells. Negative results of a patient's serum and eluate without a positive control can only be interpreted as showing that antibodies to that drug were not detected. The drug may or may not be bound to the test red cells.

If the drug in question is known to cause NIPA, the patient's serum and the controls (negative and positive) should also be tested at a dilution of 1 in 20. Normal sera at this dilution do not usually contain enough protein for NIPA to be detected.

When a patient is receiving more than one drug that has a temporal relationship to hemolysis, the coadministered drugs should be tested. Antibodies to more than one drug have been reported in cases where chemotherapeutics have been administered multiple times.[54] In addition, an immune response may be caused by a metabolite of a drug rather than the drug itself. If the clinical picture is consistent with immune-mediated hemolysis and the above tests are noninformative, it may be helpful to test metabolites of the parent drug that are present in the serum or urine of an individual who is taking that drug.[55] Antibodies to some nonsteroidal anti-inflammatory drugs have required testing in the presence of metabolite.[56] The metabolism and half-life of the drug determines when the drug metabolite should be collected. Pharmacology information for the metabolite(s) detectable in serum or urine and previous reports for the drug under investigation should be consulted.

KEY POINTS

1. The DAT is used to determine whether red cells have been coated in vivo with immunoglobulin, complement, or both. The DAT is used primarily for the investigation of hemolytic transfusion reactions, HDFN, AIHA, and drug-induced immune hemolysis.
2. The DAT should be used to determine whether a hemolytic anemia has an immune etiology.
3. A positive DAT result may or may not be associated with hemolysis.
4. Performance of the DAT on postreaction specimens is part of the initial investigation of a transfusion reaction. The DAT result may be positive if sensitized red cells have not been destroyed, or may be negative if hemolysis and rapid clearance have occurred.
5. The DAT is performed by testing freshly washed red cells directly with antiglobulin reagents containing anti-IgG and anti-C3d. False-negative or weaker results can be obtained if the washed red cells are allowed to sit before testing with anti-IgG or if the reading is delayed.
6. When the DAT result is positive with both anti-IgG and anti-C3, the red cells should be tested with an inert control reagent (eg, 6% albumin or saline). If the control is reactive, the DAT result is invalid, possibly indicating spontaneous agglutination from heavy coating of IgG or

rare warm-reactive IgM. The invalid DAT result could also be caused by IgM cold autoagglutinins that were not dissociated during routine washing.

7. A positive DAT result alone is not diagnostic of hemolytic anemia. The interpretation of the significance of this positive result requires additional patient-specific information. Dialogue with the attending physician is important. Clinical considerations together with laboratory data should dictate the extent to which a positive DAT result is evaluated.

8. The following situations may warrant further investigation of a positive DAT:
   - Evidence of in-vivo red cell destruction.
   - Recent transfusion.
   - Administration of drugs that have previously been associated with immune-mediated hemolysis.
   - History of hematopoietic progenitor cell or organ transplantation.
   - Administration of IVIG or intravenous anti-D.
   - Administration of therapeutic monoclonal antibodies that may react with target antigen on red cells.

9. Elution frees antibody from sensitized red cells and recovers antibody in a usable form. Elution is useful in certain situations for implicating an autoantibody, detecting specific antibodies that may not be detectable in the serum, and deciding to test the patient's serum for drug-related antibodies.

10. AIHAs are subdivided into the major types: WAIHA, CAD, mixed- or combined-type AIHA, and PCH. Drugs may also induce immune hemolysis.

REFERENCES

1. Zanella A, Barcellini W. Treatment of autoimmune hemolytic anemias. Haematologica 2014;99:1547-54.
2. Shapiro R, Chin-Yee I, Lam S. Eculizumab as a bridge to immunosuppressive therapy in severe cold agglutinin disease of anti-Pr specificity. Clin Case Rep 2015;3:942-4.
3. Kaplan HS, Garratty G. Predictive value of direct antiglobulin test results. Diagnostic Med 1985;8:29-32.
4. Garratty G. The significance of IgG on the red cell surface. Transfus Med Rev 1987;1:47-57.
5. Freedman J. The significance of complement on the red cell surface. Transfus Med Rev 1987; 1:58-70.
6. Petz LD, Garratty G. Immune hemolytic anemias. 2nd ed. Philadelphia: Churchill-Livingstone, 2004.
7. Rottenberg Y, Yahalom V, Shinar E, et al. Blood donors with positive direct antiglobulin tests are at increased risk for cancer. Transfusion 2009;49:838-42.
8. Hannon JL. Management of blood donors and blood donations from individuals found to have a positive direct antiglobulin test. Transfus Med Rev 2012;26:142-52.
9. Toy PT, Chin CA, Reid ME, Burns MA. Factors associated with positive direct antiglobulin tests in pretransfusion patients: A case control study. Vox Sang 1985;49:215-20.
10. Heddle NM, Kelton JG, Turchyn KL, Ali MAM. Hypergammaglobulinemia can be associated with a positive direct antiglobulin test, a nonreactive eluate, and no evidence of hemolysis. Transfusion 1988;28:29-33.
11. Clark JA, Tanley PC, Wallas CH. Evaluation of patients with positive direct antiglobulin tests and nonreactive eluates discovered during pretransfusion testing. Immunohematology 1992;8:9-12.
12. Coombs RRA, Mourant AE, Race RR. A new test for the detection of weak and "incomplete" Rh agglutinins. Br J Exp Pathol 1945;26:255-66.
13. Heddle NM, Soutar RL, O'Hoski PL, et al. A prospective study to determine the frequency and clinical significance of alloimmunization post-transfusion. Br J Haematol 1995;91:1000-5.
14. Garratty G, Arndt PA. Drugs that have been shown to cause drug-induced immune hemolytic anemia or positive direct antiglobulin tests: Some interesting findings since 2007. Immunohematology 2014;30:66-79.

15. Desborough MJ, Miller J, Thorpe SJ, et al. Intravenous immunoglobulin-induced haemolysis: A case report and review of the literature. Transfus Med 2014;24:219-26.

16. Rushin J, Rumsey DH, Ewing CA, Sandler SG. Detection of multiple passively acquired alloantibodies following infusions of IV Rh immune globulin. Transfusion 2000;40:551-4.

17. Chapuy CI, Nicholson RT, Aguad MD, et al. Resolving the daratumumab interference with blood compatibility testing. Transfusion 2015; 55:1545-54.

18. Oostendorp M, Lammerts van Bueren JJ, Doshi P, et al. When blood transfusion medicine becomes complicated due to interference by monoclonal antibody therapy. Transfusion 2015;55:1555-62.

19. Judd WJ. Elution—dissociation of antibody from red blood cells: Theoretical and practical considerations. Transfus Med Rev 1999;13: 297-310.

20. Leger RM, Arndt PA, Ciesielski DJ, Garratty G. False-positive eluate reactivity due to the low-ionic wash solution used with commercial acid-elution kits. Transfusion 1998;38:565-72.

21. Judd WJ, Johnson ST, Storry JR. Judd's methods in immunohematology. 3rd ed. Bethesda, MD: AABB Press, 2008.

22. Judd WJ, Barnes BA, Steiner EA, et al. The evaluation of a positive direct antiglobulin test (autocontrol) in pretransfusion testing revisited. Transfusion 1986;26:220-4.

23. Arndt PA, Leger RM, Garratty G. Serologic findings in autoimmune hemolytic anemia associated with immunoglobulin M warm autoantibodies. Transfusion 2009;49:235-42.

24. Rodberg K, Tsuneta R, Garratty G. Discrepant Rh phenotyping results when testing IgG-sensitized RBCs with monoclonal Rh reagents (abstract). Transfusion 1995;35(Suppl):67S.

25. Leger RM, Garratty G. Evaluation of methods for detecting alloantibodies underlying warm autoantibodies. Transfusion 1999;39:11-16.

26. Church AT, Nance SJ, Kavitsky DM. Predicting the presence of a new alloantibody underlying a warm autoantibody (abstract). Transfusion 2000;40(Suppl):121S.

27. Branch DR, Petz LD. A new reagent (ZZAP) having multiple applications in immunohematology. Am J Clin Pathol 1982;78:161-7.

28. Laine EP, Leger RM, Arndt PA, et al. In vitro studies of the impact of transfusion on the detection of alloantibodies after autoadsorption. Transfusion 2000;40:1384-7.

29. Chiaroni J, Touinssi M, Mazet M, et al. Adsorption of autoantibodies in the presence of LISS to detect alloantibodies underlying warm autoantibodies. Transfusion 2003;43:651-5.

30. Magtoto-Jocom J, Hodam J, Leger RM, Garratty G. Adsorption to remove autoantibodies using allogeneic red cells in the presence of low ionic strength saline for detection of alloantibodies (abstract). Transfusion 2011;51(Suppl): 174A.

31. Issitt PD, Combs MR, Bumgarner DJ, et al. Studies of antibodies in the sera of patients who have made red cell autoantibodies. Transfusion 1996;36:481-6.

32. Garratty G. Target antigens for red-cell-bound autoantibodies. In: Nance SJ, ed. Clinical and basic science aspects of immunohematology. Arlington, VA: AABB, 1991:33-72.

33. Garratty G. Specificity of autoantibodies reacting optimally at 37° C. Immunohematology 1999;15:24-40.

34. Branch DR, Petz LD. Detecting alloantibodies in patients with autoantibodies (editorial). Transfusion 1999;39:6-10.

35. Young PP, Uzieblo A, Trulock E, et al. Autoantibody formation after alloimmunization: Are blood transfusions a risk factor for autoimmune hemolytic anemia? Transfusion 2004; 44:67-72.

36. Maley M, Bruce DG, Babb RG, et al. The incidence of red cell alloantibodies underlying panreactive warm autoantibodies. Immunohematology 2005;21:122-5.

37. Ahrens N, Pruss A, Kähne A, et al. Coexistence of autoantibodies and alloantibodies to red blood cells due to blood transfusion. Transfusion 2007;47:813-16.

38. Shirey RS, Boyd JS, Parwani AV, et al. Prophylactic antigen-matched donor blood for patients with warm autoantibodies: An algorithm for transfusion management. Transfusion 2002;42:1435-41.

39. Hillyer CD, Shaz BH, Winkler AM, Reid M. Integrating molecular technologies for red blood cell typing and compatibility testing into blood centers and transfusion services. Transfus Med Rev 2008;22:117-32.

40. Denomme GA. Prospects for the provision of genotyped blood for transfusion. Br J Haematol 2013;163:3-9.

41. Lee E, Redman M, Burgess G, Win N. Do patients with autoantibodies or clinically insignificant alloantibodies require an indirect

antiglobulin test crossmatch? Transfusion 2007;47:1290-5.

42. Richa EM, Stowers RE, Tauscher CD, et al. The safety of electronic crossmatch in patients with warm autoantibodies (letter). Vox Sang 2007;93:92.

43. Leger RM, Co A, Hunt P, Garratty G. Attempts to support an immune etiology in 800 patients with direct antiglobulin test-negative hemolytic anemia. Immunohematology 2010;26: 156-60.

44. Waligora SK, Edwards JM. Use of rabbit red cells for adsorption of cold autoagglutinins. Transfusion 1983;23:328-30.

45. Dzik WH, Yang R, Blank J. Rabbit erythrocyte stroma treatment of serum interferes with recognition of delayed hemolytic transfusion reaction (letter). Transfusion 1986;26:303-4.

46. Mechanic SA, Maurer JL, Igoe MJ, et al. Anti-Vel reactivity diminished by adsorption with rabbit RBC stroma. Transfusion 2002;42:1180-3.

47. Storry JR, Olsson ML, Moulds JJ. Rabbit red blood cell stroma bind immunoglobulin M antibodies regardless of blood group specificity (letter). Transfusion 2006;46:1260-1.

48. Sokol RJ, Hewitt S, Stamps BK. Autoimmune haemolysis: An 18-year study of 865 cases referred to a regional transfusion centre. Br Med J 1981;282:2023-7.

49. Shulman IA, Branch DR, Nelson JM, et al. Autoimmune hemolytic anemia with both cold and warm autoantibodies. JAMA 1985;253: 1746-8.

50. Garratty G, Arndt PA, Leger RM. Serological findings in autoimmune hemolytic anemia (AIHA) associated with both warm and cold autoantibodies (abstract). Blood 2003;102 (Suppl):563a.

51. Eder AF. Review: Acute Donath-Landsteiner hemolytic anemia. Immunohematology 2005; 21:56-62.

52. Garratty G. Immune hemolytic anemia associated with drug therapy. Blood Rev 2010;24: 143-50.

53. Leger RM, Arndt PA, Garratty G. How we investigate drug-induced immune hemolytic anemia. Immunohematology 2014;30:85-94.

54. Leger RM, Jain S, Nester TA, Kaplan H. Drug-induced immune hemolytic anemia associated with anti-carboplatin and the first example of anti-paclitaxel. Transfusion 2015;55:2949-54.

55. Salama A, Mueller-Eckhardt C, Kissel K, et al. Ex vivo antigen preparation for the serological detection of drug-dependent antibodies in immune haemolytic anaemias. Br J Haematol 1984;58:525-31.

56. Johnson ST, Fueger JT, Gottschall JL. One center's experience: The serology and drugs associated with drug-induced immune hemolytic anemia—a new paradigm. Transfusion 2007; 47:697-702.

● **APPENDIX 14-1**
Drugs Associated with Immune Hemolytic Anemia

Drug	Method of Detection			
Aceclofenac			+Drug	
Acetaminophen			+ Drug	
Acyclovir		DT		
Alemtuzumab	AA			
Aminopyrine		DT		
Amoxicillin		DT		
Amphotericin B			+ Drug	
Ampicillin		DT	+ Drug	
Antazoline			+ Drug	
Azapropazone	AA	DT		
Bendamustine	AA			
Butizide			+ Drug	
Carbimazole	AA	DT	+ Drug	
Carboplatin	AA	DT	+ Drug	NIPA
Carbromal		DT		
Cefamandole		DT		
Cefazolin		DT		
Cefixime		DT	+ Drug	
Cefotaxime		DT	+ Drug	
Cefotetan	AA	DT	+ Drug	NIPA
Cefoxitin	AA	DT	+ Drug	
Cefpirome			+ Drug	
Ceftazidime	AA	DT	+ Drug	
Ceftizoxime		DT	+ Drug	
Ceftriaxone			+ Drug	
Cefuroxime		DT		
Cephalexin		DT		
Cephalothin		DT	+ Drug	NIPA
Chloramphenicol	AA	DT		
Chlorinated hydrocarbons	AA	DT	+ Drug	

(Continued)

● **APPENDIX 14-1**
Drugs Associated with Immune Hemolytic Anemia (Continued)

Drug		Method of Detection		
Chlorpromazine	AA		+ Drug	
Chlorpropamide			+ Drug	
Cimetidine		DT	+Drug	
Ciprofloxacin			+Drug	
Cisplatin		DT	+Drug	NIPA
Cladribine	AA			
Clavulanate				NIPA
Cyanidanol	AA	DT	+ Drug	
Cyclofenil	AA		+ Drug	
Cyclosporine		DT		
Diclofenac	AA	DT	+ Drug	
Diethylstilbestrol			+ Drug	
Diglycoaldehyde				NIPA
Dipyrone		DT	+ Drug	
Erythromycin		DT		
Etodolac			+ Drug	
Fenoprofen	AA		+ Drug	
Fluconazole		DT	+ Drug	
Fludarabine	AA			
Fluorescein		DT	+ Drug	
Fluorouracil			+ Drug	
Furosemide			+ Drug	
Hydralizine		DT		
Hydrochlorothiazide		DT	+ Drug	
Hydrocortisone		DT	+ Drug	
9-Hydroxy-methyl-ellipticinium			+ Drug	
Ibuprofen			+Drug	
Imatinib mesylate		DT		
Insulin		DT		
Isoniazid		DT	+ Drug	
Levodopa	AA			

● **APPENDIX 14-1**
Drugs Associated with Immune Hemolytic Anemia (Continued)

Drug	Method of Detection		
Levofloxacin		DT	+Drug
Mefenamic acid	AA		
Mefloquine		DT	+Drug
Melphalan			+Drug
6-Mercaptopurine		DT	
Methadone		DT	
Methotrexate	AA	DT	+Drug
Methyldopa	AA		
Nabumetone			+Drug
Nafcillin		DT	
Naproxen			+Drug
Oxaliplatin		DT	+Drug	NIPA
Paclitaxel		DT	+Drug
p-Aminosalicylic acid			+Drug
Pemetrexed			+Drug
Penicillin G		DT	
Phenacetin			+Drug
Phenytoin		DT	
Piperacillin		DT	+Drug
Probenicid			+Drug
Procainamide	AA		
Propyphenazone			+Drug
Pyrazinamide		DT	+Drug
Pyrimethamine		DT	
Quinidine		DT	+Drug
Quinine			+Drug
Ranitidine		DT	+Drug
Rifabutin			+Drug
Rifampicin		DT	+Drug

(Continued)

● **APPENDIX 14-1**
Drugs Associated with Immune Hemolytic Anemia (Continued)

Drug		Method of Detection	
Sodium pentothal/thiopental			+ Drug
Stibophen			+ Drug
Streptokinase		DT	
Streptomycin	AA	DT	+ Drug
Sulbactam			NIPA
Sulfamethoxazole			+ Drug
Sulfasalazine			+ Drug
Sulfisoxazole			+Drug
Sulindac	AA	DT	+ Drug
Suprofen	AA		+ Drug
Tazobactam			NIPA
Teicoplanin	AA		+ Drug
Teniposide	AA		+ Drug
Tetracycline		DT	
Ticarcillin	AA	DT	
Tolbutamide		DT	
Tolmetin	AA		+ Drug
Triamterene		DT	+ Drug
Trimethoprim			+ Drug
Vancomycin			+ Drug
Vincristine		DT	+ Drug
Zomepirac	AA		+ Drug

AA = drug-independent autoantibody; DT = testing with drug-treated red cells; + Drug = testing in the presence of drug; NIPA = nonimmunologic protein adsorption.

Chapter 15

Platelet and Granulocyte Antigens and Antibodies

• • •

Ralph R. Vassallo, MD, FACP, and
Brian R. Curtis, PhD, D(ABMLI), MT(ASCP)SBB

THIS CHAPTER DISCUSSES antigens expressed on platelets and granulocytes and the antibodies formed by sensitized individuals. These antigens and the immune responses to them are of importance in alloimmune, autoimmune, and drug-induced immune syndromes involving platelets and granulocytes.

PLATELET ANTIGENS AND ANTIBODIES

Platelets express a variety of antigenic markers on their surface. Some of these antigens are shared with other cells, such as ABH and HLA determinants, whereas others are essentially platelet specific, such as human platelet alloantigens (HPAs).

HPA

Platelets play roles in inflammation, immune responses, cardiovascular disease, and even cancer.[1-3] However, their primary function is hemostasis. Platelets perform all these functions through multiple ligand-receptor interactions involving glycoproteins expressed on their cell surface membranes.

Platelet membrane glycoproteins are expressed in different forms as a result of single nucleotide polymorphisms (SNPs) in the genes that encode them. The amino acid changes resulting from these SNPs in turn result in glycoprotein structural and antigenic changes capable of eliciting alloantibody responses after pregnancy or transfusion. Currently, 35 different HPAs expressed on six different platelet membrane glycoproteins (GPs)—GPIIb, GPIIIa, GPIbα, GPIbβ, GPIa, and CD109—have been identified (Table 15-1).[4] These antigens are often referred to as "platelet specific," and although some are found on cells other than platelets (especially leukocytes and endothelial cells), their chief clinical importance appears to be linked to their presence on platelets.

Ralph R. Vassallo, MD, FACP, Executive Vice President/Chief Medical and Scientific Officer, Blood Systems, Inc., Scottsdale, Arizona; and Brian R. Curtis, PhD, D(ABMLI), MT(ASCP)SBB, Director, Platelet and Neutrophil Immunology Lab, BloodCenter of Wisconsin, Milwaukee, Wisconsin

R. Vassallo has disclosed a financial relationship with Fresenius Kabi and New Health Sciences, Inc. B. Curtis has disclosed a financial relationship with Gen-Probe Inc.

TABLE 15-1. Human Platelet Alloantigens

Current Nomenclature	Legacy Nomenclature	Phenotypic Frequency*	Glycoprotein	Amino Acid Change	Gene/ Nucleotide Change
HPA-1a	Zw[a], Pl[A1]	72% a/a	GPIIIa	Leu33Pro	ITGB3 176T>C
HPA-1b	Zw[b], Pl[A2]	26% a/b 2% b/b			
HPA-2a	Ko[b]	85% a/a	GPIbα	Thr145Met	GPIBA 482C>T
HPA-2b	Ko[a], Sib[a]	14% a/b 1% b/b			
HPA-3a	Bak[a], Lek[a]	37% a/a	GPIIb	Ile847Ser	ITGA2B 1T>G
HPA-3b	Bak[b]	48% a/b 15% b/b			
HPA-4a	Yuk[b], Pen[a]	>99.9% a/a	GPIIIa	Arg143Gln	ITGB3 506G>A
HPA-4b	Yuk[a], Pen[b]	<0.1% a/b <0.1% b/b			
HPA-5a	Br[b], Zav[b]	88% a/a	GPIa	Glu505Lys	ITGA2 1600G>A
HPA-5b	Br[a], Zav[a], Hc[a]	20% a/b 1% b/b			
HPA-6bw	Ca[a], Tu[a]	<1% a/b or b/b	GPIIIa	Arg489Gln	ITGB3 1544G>A
HPA-7bw	Mo[a]	<1% a/b or b/b	GPIIIa	Pro407Ala	ITGB3 1297C>G
HPA-8bw	Sr[a]	<1% a/b or b/b	GPIIIa	Arg636Cys	ITGB3 1984C>T
HPA-9bw (assoc. with HPA-3b)	Max[a]	<1% a/b or b/b	GPIIb	Val837Met	ITGA2B 2602G>A
HPA-10bw	La[a]	<1% a/b or b/b	GPIIIa	Arg62Gln	ITGB3 263G>A
HPA-11bw	Gro[a]	<1% a/b or b/b	GPIIIa	Arg633His	ITGB3 1976G>A
HPA-12bw	Iy[a]	<1% a/b or b/b	GPIbα	Gly15Glu	GPIBB 119G>A
HPA-13bw	Sit[a]	<1% a/b or b/b	GPIa	Met799Thr	ITGA2 2483C>T
HPA-14bw (assoc. with HPA-1b)	Oe[a]	<1% b/b	GPIIIa	Lys611del	ITGB3 1909-1911delAAG
HPA-15a	Gov[b]	35% a/a	CD109	Ser682Tyr	CD109 2108C>A
HPA-15b	Gov[a]	42% a/b 23% b/b			

TABLE 15-1. Human Platelet Alloantigens (Continued)

Current Nomenclature	Legacy Nomenclature	Phenotypic Frequency*	Glycoprotein	Amino Acid Change	Gene/ Nucleotide Change
HPA-16bw	Duva	<1% a/b or b/b	GPIIIa	Thr140Ile	*ITGB3* 497C>T
HPA-17bw	Va[a]	<1% a/b or b/b	GPIIIa	Thr195Met	*ITGB3* 662C>T
HPA-18bw	Cab[a]	<1% a/b or b/b	GPIa	Gln716His	*ITGA2* 2235G>T
HPA-19bw	Sta	<1% a/b or b/b	GPIIIa	Lys137Gln	*ITGB3* 487A>C
HPA-20bw	Kno	<1% a/b or b/b	GPIIb	Thr619Met	*ITGA2B* 1949C>T
HPA-21bw	Nos	<1% a/b or b/b	GPIIIa	Glu628Lys	*ITGB3* 1960G>A
HPA-22bw	Sey	<1% a/b or b/b	GPIIb	Lys164Thr	*ITGA2B* 584A>C
HPA-23bw	Hug	<1% a/b or b/b	GPIIIa	Arg622Trp	*ITGB3* 1942C>T
HPA-24bw	Cab2[a+]	<1% a/b or b/b	GPIIb	Ser472Asn	*ITGA2B* 1508G>A
HPA-25bw	Swi[a]	<1% a/b or b/b	GPIa	Thr1087Met	*ITGA2* 3347C>T
HPA-26bw	Sec[a]	<1% a/b or b/b	GPIIIa	Lys580Asn	*ITGB3* 1818G>T
HPA-27bw	Cab3[a+]	<1% a/b or b/b	GPIIb	Leu841Met	*ITGA2B* 2614C>A
HPA-28bw	War	<1% a/b or b/b	GPIIb	Val740Leu	*ITGA2B* 2311G>T
HPA-29bw	Kha[b]	<1% a/b or b/b	GPIIIa	Thr7Met	*ITGB3* 98C>T

*Phenotypic frequencies are for people of European ancestry who live in North America. Human platelet alloantigen (HPA) frequencies in other races and ethnic groups can be found in the Immuno Polymorphism Database at http://www.ebi.ac.uk/ipd/hpa/freqs_1.html.

Twelve antigens are clustered into six important biallelic groups (HPA-1, HPA-2, HPA-3, HPA-4, HPA-5, and HPA-15). The nomenclature for HPAs consists of numbering the antigens in their order of discovery, with the higher-frequency antigens designated "a" and the lower-frequency antigens designated "b."[5] HPAs for which antibodies against only one of the two antithetical (non-wild-type) antigens have been detected are labeled with a "w" for "workshop," such as HPA-6bw.

Platelet Alloantigens on GPIIb/IIIa

HPA-1a is the platelet alloantigen that was discovered first and is most familiar.[6] Originally named "Zw^a" and more commonly referred to as "Pl^{A1}," it is expressed on GPIIIa, the β-subunit of the integrin GPIIb/IIIa (α_{2b}/β_3) complex.

Integrins are a broadly distributed family of adhesion molecules consisting of an α and a β chain held together by divalent cations in a heterodimeric complex.[7] Integrins are essential for platelet adhesion and aggregation because they serve as receptors for ligands, such as fibrinogen, collagen, fibronectin, von Willebrand factor (vWF), and other extracellular matrix proteins.

Postactivation binding of fibrinogen by GPIIb/IIIa results in platelet aggregation, which forms the "platelet plug" to stop bleeding. GPIIb/IIIa's hemostatic importance is demonstrated by the serious bleeding in patients with Glanzmann thrombasthenia, a rare disorder that is caused by congenital absence or dysfunction of the GPIIb/IIIa genes *ITGA2B* and/or *ITGB3*.[8] Patients with Glanzmann thrombasthenia who are exposed to normal platelets by transfusion or pregnancy can make isoantibodies against GPIIb/IIIa.

GPIIb/IIIa is the most abundantly expressed (approximately 80,000 molecules/platelet) glycoprotein complex on the platelet membrane, making it highly immunogenic. Antibodies against HPA-1a account for the vast majority (>80%) of the HPA-specific platelet antibodies detected in the sera of alloimmunized people of European ancestry. HPA-1a antibodies are produced by the 2% of individuals with the platelet type HPA-1b/1b.

Twenty-two of the 35 HPAs are carried by GPIIb (7) and GPIIIa (15). Like HPA-1a/1b, the HPA-4a/4b antigens are also expressed on GPIIIa and have been implicated in fetal and neonatal alloimmune thrombocytopenia (FNAIT), posttransfusion purpura (PTP), and platelet transfusion refractoriness. The low-frequency HPA-4b antigen is more common in populations of Japanese and Chinese ancestry.

The HPA-3a/3b antigens are expressed on GPIIb, but despite the high rate of incompatibility for both antigens in the general population, detection of HPA-3 antibodies is uncommon. Some HPA-3 antibodies are difficult to detect in monoclonal antigen capture assays, such as the modified antigen capture enzyme-linked immunosorbent assay (MACE) and monoclonal antibody-specific immobilization of platelet antigens (MAIPA), in which GPIIb is extracted from platelets with detergents that can denature the antigenic epitopes recognized by various HPA-3 antibodies.[9,10]

In addition to HPA-1b, -3b, and -4b, 19 other low-frequency platelet antigens are expressed on either GPIIb or GPIIIa (Table 15-1). These antigens were all discovered in cases of FNAIT by specific antibodies in maternal sera reactive solely with paternal GPIIb/IIIa. The vast majority of these antigens are private antigens restricted to the single families in which they were discovered. HPA-6bw and HPA-21bw are exceptions, having antigen frequencies of 1% and 2%, respectively, in people of Japanese ancestry, and HPA-9bw has been implicated in several cases of FNAIT.[11-14]

Platelet Alloantigens on GPIb/V/IX

The GPIb/V/IX complex forms the vWF receptor on platelets, and platelets express approximately 12,500 copies of this seven-unit complex. Following vascular injury, binding of the GPIb/V/IX complex to vWF facilitates platelet adhesion to vascular subendothelium and initiates signaling events within adherent platelets that lead to platelet activation, aggregation, and hemostasis. GPIb is composed of two α (GPIbα) and two β (GPIbβ) subunits (25,000 surface copies) that form noncovalent associations with two GPIX and one GPV. GPIbα carries HPA-2a/2b, and GPIbβ carries HPA-12bw. Antibodies against HPA-2a, -2b, and -12bw have all been implicated in FNAIT.

Deficiency of the entire GPIb/V/IX complex can occur from mutations in the encoding genes *GPIBA*, *GPIBB*, or *GP9*, and is the cause of Bernard Soulier syndrome (BSS). BSS is a disorder characterized by prolonged bleeding time, thrombocytopenia, and the presence of "giant platelets," and affects approximately one person per million.[8,15] BSS patients whose platelets are devoid of GPIb/V/IX can produce isoantibodies when they are exposed to the protein complex on normal platelets through transfusions or pregnancy.

Platelet Alloantigens on GPIa/IIa

The integrin GPIa/IIa, also known as integrin $\alpha_2\beta_1$, is a major collagen receptor on platelets. The GPIa protein carries the HPA-5a/5b antigens. Antibodies against HPA-5 antigens are the second most frequently detected, after anti-HPA-1a, in patients with FNAIT and are also frequently detected in patients with PTP and transfusion refractoriness. About 3000 to 5000 molecules of the GPIa/IIa heterodimeric complex are expressed on platelets.[16] HPA-13bw, -18bw, and -25bw are low-frequency antigens that are also expressed on GPIa and have all been implicated in FNAIT. Interestingly, the HPA-13bw polymorphism has been reported to cause functional defects that reduce platelet responses to collagen-induced aggregation and spreading on collagen-coated surfaces.[5]

Platelet Alloantigens on CD109

CD109 is a glycosylphosphatidylinositol (GPI)-linked protein and a member of the α_2-macroglobulin/complement superfamily. Its function is still not completely understood, but CD109 has been reported to bind to and negatively regulate the signaling of transforming growth factor beta. CD109 is also expressed on activated T lymphocytes, CD34+ hematopoietic cells, and endothelial cells, and it carries the HPA-15 antigens.

Platelets express an average of 2000 molecules of CD109, though interindividual copy numbers vary significantly.[17] Studies show the presence of HPA-15 antibodies in 0.22% to 4% of maternal sera in patients with suspected FNAIT, and several reports suggest that HPA-15 antibodies are more frequently detected in sera from patients with immune platelet refractoriness.[17-20]

Other Antigens on Platelets

ABO and Other Blood Groups

Most of the ABH antigen on platelets is carried on saccharides attached to the major platelet membrane glycoproteins (Table 15-2). GPIIb and platelet endothelial cell adhesion molecule 1 (PECAM-1/CD31) carry the largest amounts of A and B antigens.[21] Platelet A and B antigen levels are quite variable from individual to individual, with 5% to 10% of non-group-O individuals expressing extremely high levels of A1 or B on their platelets.[21,22] These "high expressers" have highly active glycosyltransferases, which are much more efficient at attaching A or B antigens.[21]

Interestingly, although individuals with the subgroup A_2 red cell phenotype express

TABLE 15-2. Other Platelet Antigens

Antigen	Phenotypic Frequency	Glycoprotein (GP)*	Amino Acid Change†	Encoding Gene	Nucleotide Change‡
ABO	Same as for red cells	GPIIb, IIIa, IV, Ia/IIa, GPIb/V/IX, CD31	Multiple	ABO	Multiple
HLA-A, -B, and -C	Same as for leukocytes	Class I HLA	Multiple	MHC	Multiple
GPIV	90%-97% (African ancestry) 90%-97% (Asian ancestry) 99.9% (European ancestry)	CD36	Tyr325Thr* Pro90Ser*	CD36	1264T>G* 478C>T* Exons 1-3 del
GPVI	N/A	GPVI	N/A	GP6/N/A	N/A

*ABO saccharides are attached to platelet GPs during their glycosylation.
†Only the most common changes are shown.
‡Only the most common mutations are shown.
N/A = not applicable.

lower levels of A on their red cells than A_1 individuals, they do not express detectable A antigens on their platelets. As a result, A_2 platelets may be successfully transfused to group O patients with high-titer immunoglobulin G (IgG) anti-A or -A,B who are refractory to non-group-O platelets.[23]

Although platelets are often transfused without regard to ABO compatibility, the use of major-mismatched platelets (eg, A or B platelets into group O recipients) frequently results in lower posttransfusion recovery rates, while minor mismatches (eg, O platelets into A or B recipients) do not.[24,25] Clinical trials comparing ABO-identical to -unmatched platelets in patients with cancer who require multiple platelet transfusions have suggested that rates of refractoriness are significantly higher when unmatched components are used.[26] Although other red cell antigens (eg, Le^a, Le^b, I, i, P, P^k, and Cromer) are also present on platelets, there is no evidence that these antigens significantly reduce platelet survival in vivo.[27,28]

GPIV/CD36

Platelets, monocytes/macrophages, and nucleated erythrocytes are the only blood cells that express GPIV/CD36 (Table 15-2). GPIV belongs to the Class B scavenger receptor family and binds a number of different ligands, including low-density lipoprotein cholesterol, thrombospondin, Types I and IV collagen, and malaria-infected red cells. A number of mutations in *CD36* have been described that result in a complete lack of protein expression on both platelets and monocytes in populations of Asian and African ancestry.[29-31] CD36-deficient individuals exposed to normal platelets can produce antibodies to CD36 that have been reported to cause FNAIT, PTP, and platelet transfusion refractoriness.[30,32,33]

GPVI

GPVI is a major collagen receptor on platelets and a member of the Ig superfamily. GPVI interactions with collagen exposed on the extracellular matrix result in platelet activation and aggregation. To date, no HPAs have been identified on GPVI, but platelet autoantibodies

formed against GPVI have been reported to cause a mild form of autoimmune thrombocytopenia.[34,35] Interestingly, GPVI autoantibodies induce shedding of GPVI from platelets, resulting in reduced collagen binding and clinically significant bleeding.

HLA

HLA is present on all nucleated cells of the body. (See Chapter 16.) HLA associated with platelets is the main source of Class I HLA in whole blood.[36] Most Class I HLA on platelets is expressed as integral membrane proteins, whereas smaller amounts may be adsorbed from surrounding plasma. HLA-A and -B locus antigens are significantly represented, but there appears to be only minimal platelet expression of HLA-C.[37] With rare exceptions, Class II HLA is not present on the platelet membrane.

Transfusion-associated HLA alloimmunization appears to be influenced by the underlying disease, immunosuppressive effects of treatment regimens, and whether the blood components contain a significant amount of leukocytes. Widespread use of leukocyte-reduced blood components has considerably reduced HLA alloimmunization from transfusion. HLA antibodies also commonly develop following pregnancy and are present in the sera of >32% of women who have had four or more pregnancies.[38] HLA antibodies have also been identified in 1.4% to 3.3% of never-pregnant or -transfused women and men with no previous transfusions.[39] Sensitization to HLA antigens becomes important in platelet-transfused patients when HLA antibodies cause destruction of allogeneic platelets, contributing to transfusion refractoriness.

Alloimmune Platelet Disorders

Platelet Transfusion Refractoriness

A less-than-expected increase in platelet count occurs in about 20% to 70% of multitransfused patients with thrombocytopenia.[40] Patients treated for malignant hematopoietic disorders are particularly likely to become refractory to platelet transfusions. Responses to platelet transfusions are often determined 10 to 60 minutes after transfusion by calculating either a corrected platelet count increment (CCI) or a posttransfusion platelet recovery (PPR), both of which normalize transfusion responses for patient blood volume and platelet dose. (See Chapter 19 for more on CCIs.) Most experts would agree that a 1-hour posttransfusion CCI of <5000 to 7500/μL/m^2/10^{11} platelets transfused after two consecutive transfusions adequately defines the refractory state.

HLA sensitization is the most common immune cause of refractoriness and can be diagnosed by demonstration of significant levels of antibodies to Class I HLA in the refractory patient's serum. (See Chapter 16 for more information on detecting HLA antibodies.) Other immune causes to be considered include antibodies to HPA, ABO incompatibility, and drug-induced antibodies.

Poor platelet recovery (1-hour CCI) is usually caused by antibody-mediated destruction, severe splenic sequestration, massive bleeding, or a combination of nonimmune factors affecting platelet survival (18- to 24-hour CCI). Some of the most commonly cited nonimmune factors associated with refractoriness are listed in Table 15-3. Even when possible immune causes of refractoriness are

TABLE 15-3. Some Nonimmune Causes of Platelet Refractoriness

- Massive bleeding
- Fever
- Sepsis
- Splenomegaly (splenic sequestration)
- Disseminated intravascular coagulation
- Allogeneic transplantation and treatment regimens
- Poor storage of platelets before transfusion
- Effects of drugs (may include immune mechanisms)
- Intravenous amphotericin B
- Thrombotic thrombocytopenic purpura

identified, nonimmune factors are often simultaneously present.[41,42]

Selection of Platelets for Transfusion in Patients with Alloimmune Refractoriness

Several strategies may be considered when selecting platelets for transfusion to patients with alloimmune refractoriness. When HLA antibodies are present, a widely used approach is to supply apheresis platelets from donors whose HLA-A and -B antigens match those of the patient. A pool of 1000 to 3000 or more HLA-typed, apheresis donors is generally necessary to find sufficient HLA-identical donors to support a typical patient.[43] Alternatively, "best-mismatch" units are often required when identical units are unavailable. This is accomplished by estimating which antibodies the recipient is statistically least likely to have, in lieu of actual determination. This is accomplished through a grading of a potential HLA-matched component, including the grading of the mismatched HLA antigens, and a determination of whether these mismatched HLA antigens share any common epitopes with those of the patient, defined as being in the same cross-reactive groups (CREGs) (Table 15-4). Platelets received following an HLA-matched request are not infrequently grade B or C matches, the closest match obtainable within the constraints of time and donor availability. In one study, 43% were relatively poor grade B or C matches.[44] In alloimmune-refractory patients, the best increases in CCI occur with grade A, B1U, or B2UX matched platelets, but platelets mismatched for some antigens (eg, B44, 45) that are poorly expressed on platelets can also be successfully transfused.[41]

An alternative approach for supplying HLA-compatible transfusions is to determine the specificity of the patient's HLA antibodies and select donors whose platelets lack the corresponding antigens.[41,42,45] This antibody specificity prediction (ASP) method is at least as effective as selection by HLA matching or platelet crossmatching and is superior to random selection of platelets. Furthermore, many

TABLE 15-4. Degree of Matching for HLA-Matched Platelets

Match Grade	Description	Examples of Donor Phenotypes for a Recipient Who Is A1, 3; B8, 27
A	4-antigen match	A1, 3; B8, 27
B1U	1 antigen unknown or blank	A1, –; B8, 27
B1X	1 cross-reactive group	A1, 3; B8, 7
B2UX	1 antigen blank and 1 cross-reactive	A1, –; B8, 7
C	1 mismatched antigen present	A1, 3; B8, 35
D	2 or more mismatched antigens present	A1, 32; B8, 35
R	Random	A2, 28; B7, 35

more potential HLA-typed donors are identified by the ASP method than are available using traditional HLA-matching criteria.[45]

Pretransfusion crossmatching of the patient's serum against platelets from potential donors is an additional approach to provide effective platelet transfusions to patients with alloimmune refractoriness.[46] Each potential platelet unit is tested in the crossmatch assay with a current sample of the patient's serum. The solid-phase red cell adherence (SPRCA) test is the most widely used method.[47] Though less successful than published HLA-identical or antigen-negative success rates, crossmatching is more widely available and significantly faster than waiting for HLA test results.[46] It avoids exclusion of HLA-mismatched but compatible donors and has the added advantage of facilitating the selection of platelets when platelet-specific antibodies are present.

Platelet crossmatching, however, will not always be successful, particularly when patients are highly alloimmunized or have interfering ABO antibodies, which can make finding sufficient amounts of compatible platelets problematic. Although the incidence of platelet-specific antibodies causing patients to be refractory to most or all platelet transfusions is very small, this possibility should be investigated when most of the crossmatches are unexpectedly incompatible or when HLA-matched transfusions fail. If platelet-specific antibodies are present, donors of known plate-let antigen phenotype or family members, who may be more likely to share the patient's phenotype, should be tested. Platelet crossmatching or HPA genotyping should be considered for patients who do not respond to ABO- and HLA-compatible platelets.

HLA-selected platelets should be irradiated to prevent transfusion-associated graft-vs-host disease (GVHD).[48(p40)] Because these platelets are selected to minimize incompatible antigens, they are more likely to cause GVHD because the recipient's immune system may fail to recognize donor T lymphocytes as foreign. Irradiation prevents the lymphocyte proliferation required for GVHD.

Fetal and Neonatal Alloimmune Thrombocytopenia

FNAIT (also known as neonatal alloimmune thrombocytopenia and abbreviated as NATP or NAIT) is a syndrome involving immune destruction of fetal platelets by maternal antibody analogous to red cell destruction in hemolytic disease of the fetus and newborn. During pregnancy, a mother may become sensitized to an incompatible paternal antigen on fetal platelets. IgG specific for the platelet antigen crosses the placenta, causing immune platelet destruction and thrombocytopenia.

FNAIT is the most common cause of severe fetal/neonatal thrombocytopenia, and affected infants are at risk of major bleeding complications, especially intracranial hemorrhage. The most commonly implicated platelet antigen incompatibility in FNAIT is HPA-1a, but all HPAs identified to date have been implicated.[49] A serologic diagnosis of FNAIT may be made by: 1) testing maternal serum for platelet antibodies using assays that can differentiate platelet-specific from non-platelet-specific reactivity, and 2) performing platelet genotyping on parental DNA.[50] Demonstration of both a platelet-specific (HPA) antibody in the maternal serum and the corresponding incompatibility for the antigen in the parental platelet types confirms the diagnosis.

Treatment of acutely thrombocytopenic newborns includes the administration of intravenous immune globulin (IVIG) with or without antigen-compatible platelet transfusions that are sometimes provided by the mother as washed platelet components.[51] Once the diagnosis of FNAIT has been made in a family, subsequent fetuses are at risk. Antenatal treatment with IVIG with or without steroids has proven to be an effective means of moderating fetal thrombocytopenia and preventing intracranial hemorrhage.[52] (For a more in-depth discussion of FNAIT, see Chapter 23.)

Posttransfusion Purpura

PTP is a rare syndrome characterized by the development of dramatic, sudden, and self-limiting thrombocytopenia 5 to 10 days after a blood transfusion in patients with a previous history of HPA sensitization by pregnancy or transfusion.[53] Coincident with the thrombocytopenia is the recrudescence of a potent platelet-specific alloantibody, usually anti-HPA-1a, in the patient's serum. Other specificities have been implicated; these are almost always associated with antigens on GPIIb/IIIa. The patient's own antigen-negative platelets as well as transfused platelets are destroyed. The pathogenesis of autologous platelet destruction is not fully understood. Mounting evidence suggests the development of transient platelet autoantibodies along with the alloantibodies.[54] These panreactive autoantibodies often target the same glycoprotein that expresses the allo-targeted HPA.

Platelet antibody assays usually reveal serum antibody specificity, usually anti-HPA-1a. Genotyping documents the absence of HPA-1a or other platelet-specific antigens. IVIG is first-line therapy, successfully elevating platelet counts in days. Plasma exchange, which is less effective than the primary therapy, is employed in the 10% to 15% of IVIG failures.[53] Antigen-negative platelets transfused following the institution of treatment appear to survive somewhat better than unselected units.[55]

After recovery, future platelet transfusions should be from antigen-negative donors. Washed red cells may offer some protection against recurrence; however, there is at least one report of PTP precipitated by a frozen deglycerolized red cell transfusion.[56] Interestingly, the frequency of PTP has significantly decreased with the introduction of leukocyte-reduced blood components.[57] Although no data have been reported to explain this trend, use of leukocyte-reduced components may also be of benefit in reducing the risk of PTP.

Drug-Induced Thrombocytopenia

Thrombocytopenia caused by drug-induced platelet antibodies is a recognized complication of drug therapy. Drugs commonly implicated include quinine, sulfa drugs, vancomycin, GPIIb/IIIa antagonists, and heparin.[58,59] Both drug-dependent antibodies and non-drug-dependent antibodies may be produced. Non-drug-dependent antibodies, although stimulated by drugs, do not require the continued presence of the drug to be reactive with platelets and are serologically indistinguishable from other platelet autoantibodies.

Although several mechanisms for drug-induced antibody formation have been described, most clinically relevant drug-dependent platelet antibodies are thought to result when a drug interacts with platelet membrane glycoproteins, inducing conformational changes recognized by the humoral immune system and development of drug-dependent antibodies.[60,61] These antibodies can cause the sudden, rapid onset of thrombocytopenia that usually resolves within 3 to 4 days after drug discontinuation.

Immune responses triggered by exposure to heparin are particularly important because of both the widespread use of this anticoagulant and the devastating thrombotic complications associated with the heparin-induced thrombocytopenia (HIT) syndrome.[62] The incidence rate of HIT is unknown, but it may develop in up to 5% of patients treated with unfractionated heparin. Low-molecular-weight heparin is less likely to be associated with HIT than unfractionated heparin.

A reduction in baseline platelet count by 30% to 50% generally occurs within 5 to 14 days after primary exposure to heparin, or sooner if the patient has been exposed to heparin within the last 3 months. The platelet count is often <100,000/μL but usually recovers within 5 to 7 days upon discontinuation of heparin. More than 50% of patients with HIT develop thrombosis, which can occur in the arterial or venous system, or both.[63] Patients may develop sometimes-fatal stroke, myocardial infarction, limb or other organ ischemia, or deep venous thrombosis. It is thus of critical importance to discontinue heparin therapy when a diagnosis of HIT is suspected. Moreover, strong consideration should be given to using an alternative (nonheparin) anticoagulant (eg, a direct thrombin inhibitor) to prevent thrombosis.[63]

The mechanism of HIT involves formation of a complex between heparin and platelet factor 4 (PF4), a tetrameric protein released from platelet α granules. IgG antibodies to the complex attach secondarily to platelet FcγRIIa receptors via their Fc region, resulting in platelet activation, thrombin generation, and thrombosis.

Autoimmune or Immune Thrombocytopenic Purpura

Immune thrombocytopenia (ITP) is an immune platelet disorder in which autoantibodies are directed against platelet antigens, resulting in platelet destruction.[64] Chronic ITP, which is most common in adults, is characterized by an insidious onset and moderate thrombocytopenia that may exist for months to years before diagnosis. Females are twice as likely to be affected as males.

Spontaneous remissions are rare, and treatment is usually required to raise the platelet count. First-line therapy consists of steroids or IVIG followed by more potent immunosuppressive agents or splenectomy in nonresponders. Many other therapies have been used in patients who do not respond to splenectomy, with variable results.

Chronic autoimmune thrombocytopenia may be idiopathic or associated with other conditions, such as human immunodeficiency virus infection, malignancy, or other autoimmune diseases. Acute ITP is mainly a childhood disease characterized by the abrupt onset of severe thrombocytopenia and bleeding symptoms, often after a viral infection. The majority of cases resolve spontaneously over a 2- to 6-month period. If treatment is required, IVIG or anti-D immunoglobulin infusions given to D-positive patients are usually effective in raising platelet counts. Steroids are used less often because of their serious side effects in children. Splenectomy, if used, is reserved for children whose disease is severe and lasts >6 months; this condition is similar to chronic ITP in adults. Rituximab and various thrombopoietin receptor agonists have been used as second-line therapies for acute ITP.[65]

Studies of both sera and washed platelets from patients with ITP have identified IgG, IgM, and IgA autoantibodies that are reactive with a number of platelet surface-membrane structures that most often include GP complexes IIb/IIIa, Ia/IIa, and Ib/IX but can also include GPIV, GPV, and GPVI.[66] In the majority of cases, platelet-associated autoantibodies are reactive with two or more platelet glycoproteins.[67] There is no compelling evidence to date suggesting that a patient's profile of autoantibody specificities correlates with the severity of the disease or predicts that patient's response to therapy.

Testing for Platelet Antigens and Antibodies

Laboratory detection of platelet antibodies provides important results to aid in clinical diagnosis of an immune platelet disorder. A comprehensive workup for platelet antibodies requires the use of multiple test methods, including a glycoprotein-specific assay, a test employing intact/whole platelets, and HPA genotyping.[68] Glycoprotein-specific assays are the most sensitive and specific for identifying the HPA specificity of serum antibodies (Fig 15-1). The inclusion of assays that use intact platelet targets is critical for detection of antibodies that can be missed by glycoprotein-specific tests because the process of platelet lysis with detergent and capture of glycoprotein with a specific monoclonal antibody can disrupt HPA epitopes recognized by some antibodies. HPA genotyping by DNA methods is helpful to confirm the HPA specificity of the antibodies and for prenatal typing of a fetus in suspected cases of FNAIT. The test methods that follow are examples of the current state-of-the-art methods used by reference laboratories. For in-depth descriptions of platelet antibody and antigen testing, readers should consult recent reviews.[50,69,70]

Assays Using Intact Platelets

An assay that is widely used for the detection of platelet-specific antibodies and for platelet crossmatching is the SPRCA.[47] Intact platelets are immobilized in round-bottomed wells of a microtiter plate and are then incubated with

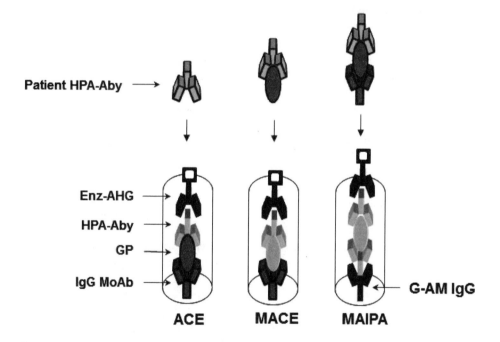

FIGURE 15-1. Enzyme-linked immunosorbent assay (ELISA) testing. Antigen-capture ELISA (ACE), which screens patient serum for glycoprotein (GP)-specific antibody, can be modified (modified-ACE, MACE) to involve preincubation of serum with target platelets, followed by washing and solubilization of the platelets in nonionic detergent. The lysate is added to microtiter plate wells for capture of platelet GP by a specific mouse immunoglobulin G (IgG) monoclonal antibody (MoAb). Platelet-specific antibodies [human platelet alloantigen (HPA)-Aby] in the patient's serum bound to the GP are detected by the addition of an enzyme-labeled goat antihuman IgG (Enz-AHG) and chromogenic substrate. The monoclonal antibody-specific immobilization of platelet antigens (MAIPA) assay is very similar to the MACE, but the patient's serum and MoAb are incubated with platelets before washing and platelet solubilization, and the HPA-Aby/GP/IgG MoAb complex is captured by goat antimouse IgG (G-AM IgG) adherent to the well bottom. There is a progressive increase in test sensitivity from ACE to MAIPA.

the patient's serum. After washing, detector red cells coated with antihuman IgG are added, and the mixture is centrifuged and examined visually. The method's main limitations are its subjective end point and failure to distinguish platelet-specific from non-platelet-specific antibodies.

Flow cytometry is commonly used for immunofluorescent detection of platelet antibodies using intact platelets.[50] Following incubation of platelets with the patient's serum, platelet-bound antibodies are detected with a fluorescent-labeled antiglobulin reagent specific for human IgG or IgM. The results can be expressed as a ratio of mean or median channel fluorescence of platelets sensitized with patient serum to that of platelets incubated with negative control serum. Platelet autoantibodies coating patient platelets can also be detected in a direct flow cytometry assay.[71]

Flow cytometry has proven to be a very sensitive method for detection of antibodies to platelets. Alloantibodies specific for labile epitopes and unreliably detected by antigen capture assays (ACAs) can be detected with intact platelets using flow cytometry.[9] Flow cytometry does not differentiate between platelet-specific (ie, platelet glycoprotein-directed/HPA) and non-platelet-specific antibodies (ie, ABO or HLA antibodies). This is a drawback when investigating FNAIT or PTP because more relevant platelet-specific antibodies can be obscured by non-platelet-specific reactivity.

Antigen Capture and Other Assays

Platelet glycoprotein ACAs are used to determine the HPA that is recognized by platelet antibodies in a patient's serum. The assays developed for this purpose include an enzyme-linked immunosorbent assay (ELISA), MACE, and MAIPA (Fig 15-1).[50,72] The assays require the use of monoclonal antibodies that recognize the target antigens of interest but do not compete with the patient's antibody. These assays capture specific platelet glycoproteins on plastic wells of a microplate after sensitization with patient's serum. The patient's bound antibody is detected with an enzyme-labeled anti-

human globulin. Because only the glycoproteins of interest are immobilized, interference by reactions from non-platelet-specific antibodies, especially anti-HLA, is eliminated. A different solid-phase assay affixes HPA antigens to microbeads that are exposed first to patient serum and then a fluorescently labeled antihuman globulin. Specific binding can be detected with the use of a Luminex mini-flow platform.[73,74]

Platelet Genotyping

Genotyping for the SNPs in the genes encoding HPA can be performed by any of the myriad molecular methods available. Allele-specific polymerase chain reaction (PCR) or restriction fragment length polymorphism analysis are two methods that have been used successfully.[67] These techniques are reliable, but they are also laborious and time consuming. Higher-throughput methods have been developed, such as real-time PCR, melting curve analysis, and allele-specific fluorescent beadchip probes.[69]

Testing for Platelet Autoantibodies

Numerous assays have been developed to detect platelet autoantibodies in patients with ITP. Although many tests are quite sensitive, particularly in detecting cell-surface, platelet-associated Igs, none has been sufficiently specific to be particularly useful in either the diagnosis or the management of ITP. The American Society of Hematology practice guidelines for ITP state that serologic testing is unnecessary, assuming that the clinical findings are compatible with the diagnosis.[64] However, platelet antibody tests may be helpful in the evaluation of patients suspected of having ITP when nonimmune causes may be present. The goal of serologic testing in ITP is to detect autoantibody bound to the patient's own platelets with or without demonstration of similar reactivity in patient plasma.

Newer assays are designed to detect immunoglobulin binding to platelet-specific epitopes found on platelet GPIIb/IIIa, GPIa/IIa, and/or GPIb/V/IX complexes. These solid-phase, GP-specific assays appear to have improved specificity in distinguishing ITP from nonimmune thrombocytopenia, but this benefit is often balanced by a decrease in sensitivity.[67,75] One commercially available test uses eluates prepared from the patient's washed platelets.[67] The eluates are tested against a panel of monoclonal-antibody-immobilized platelet glycoprotein complexes, and platelet antibodies are detected using an enzyme-linked antihuman globulin. In the indirect phase of the assay, patient plasma is tested against the same glycoprotein panel. Although autoantibodies are most often detected in the eluates, they are infrequently detected (in approximately 17% of cases) in the plasma. Patients with ITP may have antibodies that are reactive with one or several GP targets.[67]

Testing for Drug-Dependent Platelet Antibodies

Any platelet serology test used to detect platelet-bound Ig can be modified to detect drug-dependent antibodies. Each patient serum or plasma sample must be tested against normal platelets in the presence and absence of the drug. Moreover, at least one normal serum sample should be tested with and without the drug to control for nonspecific antibody binding that may occur in the drug's presence. A positive control sample known to be reactive with the drug being assayed should be tested with and without the drug to complete the evaluation. A positive result demonstrates greater reactivity against normal platelets in the presence of the drug than without and that the drug did not nonspecifically cause a positive result with normal serum controls. Flow cytometry is the most sensitive and most commonly used method to detect both IgG and IgM drug-dependent antibodies.[50,76] Limitations to detection of drug-dependent platelet antibodies include the following: 1) for many drugs, the optimal concentration for antibody detection has not been determined, and hydrophobic drugs are difficult to solubilize; 2) the presence of nondrug antibodies can mask drug-related antibodies; and 3) a patient may

be sensitized to a drug metabolite and not the native drug.

Assays for heparin-dependent antibodies include ELISA using microtiter wells coated with complexes of PF4 and heparin or heparin-like molecules (eg, polyvinyl sulfonate).[77] Optical density values above cutoff that can be inhibited by added high-dose heparin confirms the presence of heparin-dependent antibodies. Although IgG antibodies are the most clinically relevant antibodies, a few patients with HIT appear to have only IgM or IgA antibodies detectable in variants of this assay.

These assays are sensitive but not specific for the subset of antibodies that result in clinically significant platelet activation and thrombosis. The ^{14}C-serotonin release assay (SRA) is a functional assay for detection of this type of antibody.[78] Other functional tests include heparin-induced platelet aggregation and various other measures of platelet activation (adenosine triphosphate release, phosphatidyserine exposure, etc). In asymptomatic patients receiving heparin or anticipating its use, neither PF4 ELISA nor functional tests are sufficiently predictive of HIT to warrant use as screening tests.[79]

GRANULOCYTE ANTIGENS AND ANTIBODIES

Antibodies against granulocyte (neutrophil) antigens are implicated in the following clinical syndromes: neonatal alloimmune neutropenia (NAN), transfusion-related acute lung injury (TRALI), febrile transfusion reactions, primary or secondary autoimmune neutropenia (AIN), refractoriness to granulocyte transfusion, transfusion-related alloimmune neutropenia, and immune neutropenia after hematopoietic progenitor cell (HPC) transplantation. To date, nine neutrophil antigens carried on five different glycoproteins have been characterized and given human neutrophil alloantigen (HNA) designations by the Granulocyte Antigen Working Party of the International Society of Blood Transfusion (Table 15-5).[80] This nomenclature system follows a convention similar to that used for HPA nomenclature. Several of the antigens on

TABLE 15-5. Human Neutrophil Antigens

Antigen	Phenotypic Frequency*	Glycoprotein	Amino Acid Change	Encoding Gene	Nucleotide Change
HNA-1a	12% a/a	CD16b	Multiple[†]	*FCGR3B*	Multiple[†]
HNA-1b	54% a/b				
	46% b/b				
HNA-1c	5%				
HNA-2	97% CD177+	CD177	N/A	CD177	N/A
	3% CD177−				
HNA-3a	56%-59% a/a	CTL2	Arg152Gln	SLC44A2	455G>A
HNA-3b	34%-40% a/b				
	3%-6% b/b				
HNA-4a	78.6% a/a	CD11b	Arg61His	ITGAM	230G>A
HNA-4b	19.3% a/b				
	2.1% b/b				
HNA-5a	54.3% a/a	CD11a	Arg766Thr	ITGAL	2466G>C
HNA-5bw	38.6% a/b				
	7.1% b/b				

	Nucleotide Changes						Amino Acid Changes					
	141	147	227	266	277	349	36	38	65	78	82	106
HNA-1a	G	C	A	C	G	G	Arg	Leu	Asn	Ala	Asp	Val
HNA-1b/d	C	T	G	C	A	A	Ser	Leu	Ser	Ala	Asn	Ile
HNA-1c/b	C	T	G	A	A	A	Ser	Leu	Ser	Asp	Asn	Ile

*Phenotypic frequencies are for people of European ancestry who live in North America.
†HNA-1 amino acid and nucleotide changes are shown in a separate section of the table.
HNA = human neutrophil antigen; N/A = not applicable.

granulocytes are shared with other cells and are not granulocyte specific.

HNA

Antigens on FcγRIIIb

The first granulocyte-specific antigen detected was NA1, later named "HNA-1a." Five alleles of HNA-1 have now been identified, encoding three antigens: HNA-1a, HNA-1b, and HNA-1c, which are located on the protein FcγRIIIb

(CD16b).[80] Recently, another epitope on HN-1b, termed HNA-1d, was described.[81] FcγRIIIb is a GPI-linked protein receptor for the Fc region of IgG and is present only on the surfaces of neutrophils. Three alleles encode HNA-1b: one encoding HNA-1b alone, one along with HNA-1c, and another with HNA-1d.[81] Neutrophils express 100,000 to 200,000 molecules of FcγRIIIb, but there are rare individuals (approximately 0.1%) whose neutrophils express no FcγRIIIb (CD16 null) and who can produce antibodies that are reactive with FcγRIIIb when they are exposed to it through transfusion or pregnancy.[82,83] Antibodies to HNA-1a and -1b have been implicated in TRALI, NAN, and AIN, while antibodies to HNA-1c and -1d have resulted in NAN.[81,84,85]

Antigens on CD177

HNA-2 (previously known as "NB1") is not an alloantigen because HNA-2 antibodies are iso-antibodies that recognize common epitopes on CD177 protein, which is missing from the neutrophils of immunized individuals. Neutrophils from approximately 1% to 11% of people lack expression of CD177.[84-86] Originally thought to be due to messenger ribonucleic acid splicing defects, absence of CD177 is primarily caused by DNA point mutations that result in a truncated protein that cannot be expressed.[87] Interestingly, CD177 is expressed only on a neutrophil subpopulation in CD177-positive individuals.[88] The proportion of the CD177-positive neutrophil population ranges from 0% to 100%.[89]

Antibodies against HNA-2 have been implicated in NAN, TRALI, AIN, and neutropenia in marrow transplant recipients.[90-92]

Antigens on CTL2

HNA-3a and HNA-3b are carried on the choline transporter-like protein 2 (CTL2), and an SNP in the gene (*SLC44A2*) accounts for the polymorphism (Table 15-5).[93,94] CTL2 is also expressed on both T and B lymphocytes, platelets, and vascular endothelium. HNA-3a antibodies are usually agglutinins. They occasionally develop in women after pregnancy, and HNA-3a antibodies are the most frequent cause of fatal TRALI, in addition to causing febrile reactions and NAN.[95] HNA-3b antibodies are rarely detected, but several have been found during screening of the serum of multiparous blood donors.

Antigens on CD11a and CD11b

HNA-4a/4b and HNA-5a antigens are present on monocytes and lymphocytes as well as granulocytes. HNA-4a is carried on the CD11b/18 (Mac-1, CR3, $\alpha_m\beta_2$) glycoprotein.[80] CD11b/18 plays a role in neutrophil adhesion to endothelial cells and phagocytosis of C3bi opsonized microbes. There is some evidence showing that pathogenic alloantibodies against HNA-4a interfere with CD11b/18-dependent neutrophil adhesion and enhance neutrophil respiratory burst.[96] Antibodies against HNA-4a and -4b have been implicated in NAN, and autoantibodies against CD11b/18 have also been described.[97,98]

HNA-5a is carried on CD11a/18 (LFA-1, $\alpha_L\beta_2$) glycoprotein.[99] CD11a/18, like CD11b/18, plays a role in neutrophil adhesion to endothelial cells. Antibodies that are reactive with HNA-5a have been found in a chronically transfused patient with aplastic anemia and have also been reported to be associated with NAN.[100] The patient who made the original HNA-5a antibody experienced prolonged survival of an HLA-nonidentical skin graft that was associated with the HNA-5a antibody.[99]

Other Neutrophil Antigens

Neutrophils do not express ABH or other red cell group antigens, but they do express modest amounts of Class I and II HLA only upon activation.

Immune Neutrophil Disorders

Neonatal Alloimmune Neutropenia

NAN is caused by maternal antibodies against the antigens on fetal neutrophils; the most frequent specificities are those against HNA-1a, HNA-1b, and HNA-2 antigens, although HNA-1c, -1d, -3a, -4a, -4b, and -5a have caused this syndrome. NAN may also occur in the children of women who lack the FcγRIIIb protein. Neutropenia in NAN can occasionally be life-threatening because of increased susceptibility to infection.[101] Management with antibiotics, IVIG, granulocyte colony-stimulating factor, and/or plasma exchange may be helpful.

TRALI

TRALI is an acute, often life-threatening reaction characterized by respiratory distress, hypo- or hypertension, and noncardiogenic pulmonary edema that occurs within 6 hours of a blood component transfusion.[102] TRALI has been the most common cause of transfusion-related death for more than 10 years.[103] In severe TRALI, causative antibodies are most often found in the plasma of blood donors. When these antibodies are transfused, they cause activation of primed neutrophils that are sequestered in the lungs of certain patients. The activated neutrophils undergo oxidative burst, releasing toxic substances that damage pulmonary endothelium and resulting in capillary leak and pulmonary edema. HNA and Class II HLA antibodies are thought to be more pathogenic than Class I HLA antibodies.[104] (For a more in-depth discussion of TRALI, see Chapter 22.)

Autoimmune Neutropenia

AIN may occur in adults or in infants. When present in adults, it is generally persistent and may be idiopathic or secondary to autoimmune diseases, malignancies, or infections.[105] In AIN of infancy, the autoantibody has neutrophil antigen specificity (usually HNA-1a, occasionally -1b or -4a) in about 60% of patients. This condition is generally self-limiting and relatively benign, with recovery usually occurring in 7 to 24 months.[106]

Testing for Granulocyte Antibodies and Antigens

Granulocyte antibody testing is technically complex and labor intensive. The inability to maintain the integrity of granulocytes at room temperature, in refrigerated conditions, or by cryopreservation requires that cells be isolated from fresh blood on each day of testing. This demands that readily available blood donors typed for the various granulocyte antigens be available. Class I HLA antibodies that are often present in patient sera complicate detection and identification of granulocyte antibodies. For these reasons, it is critical that granulocyte antibody and antigen testing be performed by an experienced laboratory using appropriate controls.

Granulocyte Agglutination Test

This was one of the first tests developed for the detection of granulocyte antibodies. It is typically performed by overnight incubation of small volumes of isolated fresh neutrophils with the patient's serum in a microplate. The wells are viewed under an inverted phase microscope for neutrophil agglutination or aggregation.

Granulocyte Immunofluorescence Test

This test also requires fresh target cells that are incubated, usually at room temperature for 30 minutes, and washed in EDTA and phosphate-buffered saline. Neutrophil-bound antibodies are then detected with fluorescein isothiocyanate-labeled antihuman IgG or IgM using either a fluorescence microscope or a flow cytometer.[107] A combination of agglutination and immunofluorescence tests is beneficial.[94] Other methods include chemiluminescence, SPRCA, and the monoclonal antibody-specific immobilization of granulocyte antigens (MAIGA) assay, which is similar to the MAIPA assay but uses monoclonal antibodies to capture the various glycoproteins that express HNA. The MAIGA assay is used to differentiate between HLA- and HNA-specific antibodies.

Luminex-Based Antibody Identification

Microbeads coated with HNA antigens have been under development without many peer-reviewed publications available to gauge their accuracy.[108,109] Newer versions may detect all but anti-HNA-1d.

HNA Typing

As with HPA, typing for HNA is largely performed using molecular methods to detect the allelic variants that determine the antigens. Any methods used in HPA typing can be applied to HNA typing with simple modifications to the primer and probe sequences. Readers are referred to several publications on this subject.[110,111] Because the understanding of the molecular defect that results in CD177 deficiency is controversial, typing for HNA-2/ CD177 has traditionally required serologic testing on freshly isolated neutrophils using specific monoclonal antibodies. Testing may evolve as the SNPs responsible for some individuals' loss of expression are confirmed.[87]

KEY POINTS

1. Platelets express a variety of antigenic markers on their surfaces. Some of these types of antigens, such as ABH and HLA, are shared with other cells, whereas HPAs are essentially platelet specific. There are currently 35 HPAs carried on six platelet glycoproteins.
2. HLA Class I sensitization is the most common immune cause of platelet refractoriness and can be diagnosed by the demonstration of significant levels of antibodies to HLA-A and -B in patient serum. When antibodies to HLA antigens are demonstrated, widely used treatment approaches supply apheresis platelets from HLA-identical donors, those without antigens to which the recipient is sensitized, or crossmatch-compatible platelets. Presumed-compatible HLA mismatches perform least-well. HLA-selected platelets should be irradiated to prevent transfusion-associated GVHD.
3. HPA antibodies are less commonly responsible for platelet transfusion refractoriness, but in such cases, genotypically matched or crossmatch-compatible apheresis units are required.
4. Sensitization to HPA is the most common cause of FNAIT, a syndrome involving immune destruction of fetal platelets by maternal antibody. Platelet-specific antibodies are also involved in PTP, a rare syndrome characterized by severe thrombocytopenia that occurs 5 to 10 days after a blood transfusion. The most commonly implicated antibody in both conditions is anti-HPA-1a. Serologic testing using intact platelets and antigen capture assays together with HPA genotyping is used to confirm both of these diagnoses.
5. Autoantibodies directed against platelet antigens may result in ITP. Chronic ITP, which is most common in adults, is characterized by an insidious onset and moderate thrombocytopenia that may be present for months to years before diagnosis. Females are twice as likely to be affected as males. The goal of serologic testing in ITP is to detect autoantibody bound to the patient's own platelets, though testing infrequently affects management.
6. Granulocyte (neutrophil) antigens are implicated in the clinical syndromes NAN, TRALI, febrile transfusion reactions, AIN, refractoriness to granulocyte transfusion, transfusion-related alloimmune neutropenia, and immune neutropenia after HPC transplantation.
7. Granulocyte antibody testing remains low-throughput and requires both immunofluorescence and agglutination methods supplemented by MAIGA to fully evaluate patient sera for antibodies.

REFERENCES

1. Jenne CN, Kubes P. Platelets in inflammation and infection. Platelets 2015;26:286-92.
2. Mezouar S, Frère C, Darbousset R. Role of platelets in cancer and cancer-associated thrombosis: Experimental and clinical evidences. Thromb Res 2016;139:65-76.
3. Pasalic L, Wang SS, Chen VM. Platelets as biomarkers of coronary artery disease. Semin Thromb Hemost 2016;42:223-33.
4. Immuno polymorphism database. All HPA genetic information. Hinxton, UK: European Bioinformatics Institute, 2016. [Available at http://www.ebi.ac.uk/ipd/hpa/table2.html (accessed March 15, 2017).]
5. Metcalfe P, Watkins NA, Ouwehand WH, et al. Nomenclature of human platelet antigens. Vox Sang 2003;85:240-5.

6. Aster RH, Newman PJ. HPA-1a/b(PlA1/A2,Zwa/b): The odyssey of an alloantigen system. Immunohematology 2007;23:2-8.

7. Bennett JS, Berger BW, Billings PC. The structure and function of platelet integrins. J Thromb Haemost 2009;7(Suppl 1):200-5.

8. Nurden AT, Freson K, Seligsohn U. Inherited platelet disorders. Haemophilia 2012;18(Suppl 4):154-60.

9. Harrison CR, Curtis BR, McFarland JG, et al. Severe neonatal alloimmune thrombocytopenia caused by antibodies to human platelet antigen 3a (Bak^a) detectable only in whole platelet assays. Transfusion 2003;43:1398-402.

10. Socher I, Zwingel C, Santoso S, Kroll H. Heterogeneity of HPA-3 alloantibodies: Consequences for the diagnosis of alloimmune thrombocytopenic syndromes. Transfusion 2008;48:463-72.

11. Koh Y, Ishii H, Amakishi E, et al. The first two cases of neonatal alloimmune thrombocytopenia associated with the low-frequency platelet antigen HPA-21bw (Nos) in Japan. Transfusion 2012;52:1468-75.

12. Peterson JA, Pechauer SM, Gitter ML, et al. The human platelet antigen-21bw is relatively common among Asians and is a potential trigger for neonatal alloimmune thrombocytopenia. Transfusion 2012;52:915-16.

13. Peterson JA, Balthazor SM, Curtis BR, et al. Maternal alloimmunization against the rare platelet-specific antigen HPA-9b (Max^a) is an important cause of neonatal alloimmune thrombocytopenia. Transfusion 2005;45:1487-95.

14. Kaplan C, Porcelijn L, Vanlieferinghen P, et al. Anti-HPA-9bw (Max^a) fetomaternal alloimmunization, a clinically severe neonatal thrombocytopenia: Difficulties in diagnosis and therapy and report on eight families. Transfusion 2005;45:1799-803.

15. Nurden P, Nurden AT. Congenital disorders associated with platelet dysfunctions. Thromb Haemost 2008;99:253-63.

16. Corral J, Rivera J, Gonzalez-Conejero R, Vicente V. The number of platelet glycoprotein Ia molecules is associated with the genetically linked 807 C/T and HPA-5 polymorphisms. Transfusion1999;39:372-8.

17. Ertel K, Al-Tawil M, Santoso S, Kroll H. Relevance of the HPA-15 (Gov) polymorphism on CD109 in alloimmune thrombocytopenic syndromes. Transfusion 2005;45:366-73.

18. Mandelbaum M, Koren D, Eichelberger B, et al. Frequencies of maternal platelet alloantibodies and autoantibodies in suspected fetal/neonatal alloimmune thrombocytopenia, with emphasis on human platelet antigen-5 alloimmunization. Vox Sang 2005;89:39-43.

19. Berry JE, Murphy CM, Smith GA, et al. Detection of Gov system antibodies by MAIPA reveals an immunogenicity similar to the HPA-5 alloantigens. Br J Haematol 2000;110:735-42.

20. Vassallo RR. Recognition and management of antibodies to human platelet antigens in platelet transfusion-refractory patients. Immunohematology 2009;25:119-24.

21. Curtis BR, Edwards JT, Hessner MJ, et al. Blood group A and B antigens are strongly expressed on platelets of some individuals. Blood 2000;96:1574-81.

22. Ogasawara K, Ueki J, Takenaka M, Furihata K. Study on the expression of ABH antigens on platelets. Blood 1993;82:993-9.

23. Skogen B, Rossebø Hansen B, Husebekk A, et al. Minimal expression of blood group A antigen on thrombocytes from A2 individuals. Transfusion 1988;28:456-9.

24. Slichter SJ, Davis K, Enright H, et al. Factors affecting posttransfusion platelet increments, platelet refractoriness, and platelet transfusion intervals in thrombocytopenic patients. Blood 2005;105:4106-14.

25. Triulzi DJ, Assmann SF, Strauss RG, et al. The impact of platelet transfusion characteristics on post-transfusion platelet increments and clinical bleeding in patients with hypoproliferative thrombocytopenia. Blood 2012; 119:5553-62.

26. Heal JM, Rowe JM, Blumberg N. ABO and platelet transfusion revisited. Ann Hematol 1993;66:309-14.

27. Dunstan RA, Simpson MB. Heterogeneous distribution of antigens on human platelets demonstrated by fluorescence flow cytometry. Br J Haematol 1985;61:603-9.

28. Spring FA, Judson PA, Daniels GL, et al. A human cell-surface glycoprotein that carries Cromer-related blood group antigens on erythrocytes and is also expressed on leucocytes and platelets. Immunology 1987;62:307-13.

29. Ghosh A, Murugusan G, Chen K, et al. Platelet CD36 surface expression levels affect functional responses to oxidized LSL and are associated with inheritance of specific genetic polymorphisms. Blood 2011;117:6355-66.

30. Curtis BR, Ali S, Glazier AM, et al. Isoimmunization against CD36 (glycoprotein IV): Description of four cases of neonatal isoimmune thrombocytopenia and brief review of the literature. Transfusion 2002;42:1173-9.

31. Rac ME, Safranow K, Poncyljusz W. Molecular basis of human CD36 gene mutations. Mol Med 2007;13:288-96.

32. Bierling P, Godeau B, Fromont P, et al. Posttransfusion purpura-like syndrome associated with CD36 (Nak^a) isoimmunization. Transfusion 1995;35:777-82.

33. Ikeda H, Mitani T, Ohnuma M, et al. A new platelet-specific antigen, Nak^a, involved in the refractoriness of HLA-matched platelet transfusion. Vox Sang 1989;57:213-17.

34. Boylan B, Chen H, Rathore V, et al. Anti-GPVI-associated ITP: An acquired platelet disorder caused by autoantibody-mediated clearance of the GPVI/FcRγ-chain complex from the human platelet surface. Blood 2004;104:1350-5.

35. Akiyama M, Kashiwagi H, Todo K, et al. Presence of platelet-associated anti-glycoprotein (GP)VI autoantibodies and restoration of GPVI expression in patients with GPVI deficiency. J Thromb Haemost 2009;7:1373-83.

36. Bialek JW, Bodmer W, Bodmer J, Payne R. Distribution and quantity of leukocyte antigens in the formed elements of the blood. Transfusion 1966;6:193-204.

37. Saito S, Ota S, Seshimo H, et al. Platelet transfusion refractoriness caused by a mismatch in HLA-C antigens. Transfusion 2002;42:302-8.

38. Triulzi DJ, Kleinman S, Kakaiya RM, et al. The effect of previous pregnancy and transfusion on HLA alloimmunization in blood donors: Implications for a transfusion-related acute lung injury risk reduction strategy. Transfusion 2009;49:1825-35.

39. Vassallo RR, Hsu S, Einarson M, et al. A comparison of two robotic platforms to screen plateletpheresis donors for HLA antibodies as part of a transfusion-related acute lung injury mitigation strategy. Transfusion 2010;50:1766-77.

40. Kerkhoffs JL, Eikenboom JC, Van De Watering LM, et al. The clinical impact of platelet refractoriness: Correlation with bleeding and survival. Transfusion 2008;48:1959-65.

41. Vassallo RR Jr. New paradigms in the management of alloimmune refractoriness to platelet transfusions. Curr Opin Hematol 2007;14:655-63.

42. Hod E, Schwartz J. Platelet transfusion refractoriness. Br J Haematol 2008;142:348-60.

43. Bolgiano DC, Larson EB, Slichter SJ. A model to determine required pool size for HLA-typed community donor apheresis programs. Transfusion 1989;29:306-10.

44. Dahlke MB, Weiss KL. Platelet transfusion from donors mismatched for crossreactive HLA antigens. Transfusion 1984;24:299-302.

45. Petz LD, Garratty G, Calhoun L, et al. Selecting donors of platelets for refractory patients on the basis of HLA antibody specificity. Transfusion 2000;40:1446-56.

46. Vassallo RR, Fung M, Rebulla P, et al. Utility of cross-matched platelet transfusions in patients with hypoproliferative thrombocytopenia: A systematic review. Transfusion 2014;54:1180-91.

47. Rachel JM, Summers TC, Sinor LT, Plapp FV. Use of a solid phase red blood cell adherence method for pretransfusion platelet compatibility testing. Am J Clin Pathol 1988;90:63-8.

48. Ooley PW, ed. Standards for blood banks and transfusion services. 30th ed. Bethesda, MD: AABB, 2016.

49. Davoren A, Curtis BR, Aster RH, McFarland JG. Human platelet antigen-specific alloantibodies implicated in 1162 cases of neonatal alloimmune thrombocytopenia. Transfusion 2004;44:1220-5.

50. Curtis B, McFarland J. Detection and identification of platelet antibodies and antigens in the clinical laboratory. Immunohematol 2009;25:125-35.

51. Peterson JA, McFarland JG, Curtis BR, Aster RH. Neonatal alloimmune thrombocytopenia: Pathogenesis, diagnosis and management. Br J Haematol 2013;161:3-14.

52. Pacheco LD, Berkowitz RL, Moise KJ Jr, et al. Fetal and neonatal alloimmune thrombocytopenia: A management algorithm based on risk stratification. Obstet Gynecol 2011;118:1157-63.

53. McFarland JG. Posttransfusion purpura. In: Popovsky MA, ed. Transfusion reactions. 4th ed. Bethesda, MD: AABB Press, 2012:263-87.

54. Taaning E, Tonnesen F. Pan-reactive platelet antibodies in post-transfusion purpura. Vox Sang 1999;76:120-3.

55. Brecher ME, Moore SB, Letendre L. Posttransfusion purpura: The therapeutic value of Pl^{A1}-negative platelets. Transfusion 1990;30:433-5.

56. Godeau B, Fromont P, Bettaieb A, et al. [Posttransfusion purpura. An unknown cause of

acute immune thrombocytopenia. 4 new cases]. Presse Med 1990;19:1974-7.

57. Thomas D, Bolton-Maggs P, Serious Hazards of Transfusion (SHOT) Steering Group. The 2014 annual SHOT report. Manchester, UK: SHOT, 2015. [Available at http://www.shotuk.org/wp-content/uploads/summary-20141.pdf (accessed March 15, 2017).]

58. Drug-induced immune thrombocytopenia: Results of the testing for drug-dependent platelet-reactive antibodies by the BloodCenter of Wisconsin, 1995-2015. Linked from: George JN. Platelets on the web: Drug-induced thrombocytopenia. Oklahoma City, OK: OUHSC, 2015. [Available at http://www.ouhsc.edu/platelets/ditp.html (accessed March 15, 2017).]

59. Reese JA, Li X, Hauben M, et al. Identifying drugs that cause acute thrombocytopenia: An analysis using 3 distinct methods. Blood 2010;116:2127-33.

60. Aster RH, Bougie DW. Drug-induced immune thrombocytopenia. N Engl J Med 2007;357:580-7.

61. Bougie DW, Wilker PR, Aster RH. Patients with quinine-induced immune thrombocytopenia have both "drug-dependent" and "drug-specific" antibodies. Blood 2006;108:922-7.

62. Warkentin TE. Heparin-induced thrombocytopenia. Curr Opin Crit Care 2015;21:576-85.

63. Linkins LA, Dans AL, Moores LK, et al. Treatment and prevention of heparin-induced thrombocytopenia: Antithrombotic therapy and prevention of thrombosis. 9th ed. American College of Chest Physicians evidence-based clinical practice guidelines. Chest 2012;141(Suppl 2):e495S-530S.

64. Neunert C, Lim W, Crowther M, et al. The American Society of Hematology 2011 evidence-based practice guideline for immune thrombocytopenia. Blood 2011;117:4190-207.

65. Ghanima W, Godeau B, Cines DB, Bussel JB. How I treat immune thrombocytopenia: The choice between splenectomy or a medical therapy as a second-line treatment. Blood 2012;120:960-9.

66. McMillan R. Antiplatelet antibodies in chronic immune thrombocytopenia and their role in platelet destruction and defective platelet production. Hematol Oncol Clin North Am 2009;23:1163-75.

67. Davoren A, Bussel J, Curtis BR, et al. Prospective evaluation of a new platelet glycoprotein (GP)-specific assay (PakAuto) in the diagnosis of autoimmune thrombocytopenia (AITP). Am J Hematol 2005;78:193-7.

68. Wu GG, Kaplan C, Curtis BR, Pearson HA. Report on the 14th International Society of Blood Transfusion Platelet Immunology Workshop. Vox Sang 2010;99:375-81.

69. Veldhuisen B, Porcelijn L, van der Schoot CE, de Haas M. Molecular typing of human platelet and neutrophil antigens (HPA and HNA). Transfus Apher Sci 2014;50:189-99.

70. Reil A, Bux J. Geno- and phenotyping of human neutrophil antigens. Methods Mol Biol 2015;1310:193-203.

71. Christopoulos CG, Kelsey HC, Machin SJ. A flow-cytometric approach to quantitative estimation of platelet surface immunoglobulin G. Vox Sang 1993;64:106-15.

72. Kiefel V, Santoso S, Weisheit M, Mueller-Eckhardt C. Monoclonal antibody-specific immobilization of platelet antigens (MAIPA): A new tool for the identification of platelet-reactive antibodies. Blood 1987;70:1722-6.

73. Porcelijn L, Huiskes E, Comijs-van Osselen I, et al. A new bead-based human platelet antigen antibodies detection assay versus the monoclonal antigen immobilization of platelet antigens assay. Transfusion 2014;54:1486-92.

74. Cooper N, Bein G, Heidinger K, et al. A bead-based assay in the work-up of suspected platelet alloimmunization. Transfusion 2016;56:115-18.

75. McMillan R, Tani P, Millard F, et al. Platelet-associated and plasma anti-glycoprotein auto-antibodies in chronic ITP. Blood 1987;70:1040-5.

76. Curtis BR, McFarland JG, Wu GG, et al. Antibodies in sulfonamide-induced immune thrombocytopenia recognize calcium-dependent epitopes on the glycoprotein IIb/IIIa complex. Blood 1994;84:176-83.

77. McFarland J, Lochowicz A, Aster R, et al. Improving the specificity of the PF4 ELISA in diagnosing heparin-induced thrombocytopenia. Am J Hematol 2012;87:776-81.

78. Sheridan D, Carter C, Kelton JG. A diagnostic test for heparin-induced thrombocytopenia. Blood 1986;67:27-30.

79. Warkentin TE. Laboratory testing for heparin-induced thrombocytopenia. J Thromb Thrombolysis 2000;10(Suppl 1):35-45.

80. Flesch BK. Human neutrophil antigens: A nomenclature update based on new alleles and

new antigens. ISBT Sci Ser 2015;10(Suppl 1): 243-9.

81. Reil A, Sach UJ, Siahanidou T, et al. HNA-1d: A new human neutrophil antigen located on Fcγ receptor IIb associated with neonatal immune neutropenia. Transfusion 2013;53:2145-51.

82. de Haas M, Kleijer M, van Zwieten R, et al. Neutrophil Fc gamma RIIIb deficiency, nature, and clinical consequences: A study of 21 individuals from 14 families. Blood 1995;86:2403-13.

83. Stroncek DF, Skubitz KM, Plachta LB, et al. Alloimmune neonatal neutropenia due to an antibody to the neutrophil Fc-γ receptor III with maternal deficiency of CD16 antigen. Blood 1991;77:1572-80.

84. Muschter S, Bertold T. Greinacher A. Developments in the definition and clinical impact of human neutrophil antigens. Curr Opin Hematol 2011;18:452-60.

85. Moritz E, Norcia AMMI, Cardone JDB, et al. Human neutrophil alloantigens systems. An Acad Bras Cienc 2009;81:559-69.

86. Sachs UJ, Andrei-Selmer CL, Maniar A, et al. The neutrophil-specific antigen CD177 is a counter-receptor for platelet endothelial cell adhesion molecule-1 (CD31). J Biol Chem 2007;282:23603-12.

87. Li Y, Mair DC, Schuller RM, et al. Genetic mechanism of human neutrophil antigen 2 deificiency and expression variations. PLoS Genet 2015;11:e1005255.

88. Moritz E, Chiba AK, Kimura EY, et al. Molecular studies reveal that A134T, G156A and G133A SNPs in the CD177 gene are associated with atypical expression of human neutrophil antigen-2. Vox Sang 2010;98:160-6.

89. Matsuo K, Lin A, Procter JL, et al. Variations in the expression of granulocyte antigen NB1. Transfusion 2000;40:654-62.

90. Lalezari P, Murphy GB, Allen FH Jr. NB1, a new neutrophil-specific antigen involved in the pathogenesis of neonatal neutropenia. J Clin Invest 1971;50:1108-15.

91. Bux J, Becker F, Seeger W, et al. Transfusion-related acute lung injury due to HLA-A2-specific antibodies in recipient and NB1-specific antibodies in donor blood. Br J Haematol 1996;93: 707-13.

92. Stroncek DF, Shapiro RS, Filipovich AH, et al. Prolonged neutropenia resulting from antibodies to neutrophil-specific antigen NB1 following marrow transplantation. Transfusion 1993;33:158-63.

93. Curtis BR, Cox NJ, Sullivan MJ, et al. The neutrophil alloantigen HNA-3a (5b) is located on choline transporter-like protein 2 and appears to be encoded by an R>Q154 amino acid substitution. Blood 2010;115:2073-6.

94. Greinacher A, Wesche J, Hammer E, et al. Characterization of the human neutrophil alloantigen-3a. Nat Med 2010;16:45-8.

95. Reil A, Keller-Stanislawski B, Gunay S, Bux J. Specificities of leucocyte alloantibodies in transfusion-related acute lung injury and results of leucocyte antibody screening of blood donors. Vox Sang 2008;95:313-17.

96. Sachs UJ, Chavakis T, Fung L, et al. Human alloantibody anti-Mart interferes with Mac-1-dependent leukocyte adhesion. Blood 2004; 104:727-34.

97. Fung YL, Pitcher LA, Willett JE, et al. Alloimmune neonatal neutropenia linked to anti-HNA-4a. Transfus Med 2003;13:49-52.

98. Hartman KR, Wright DG. Identification of autoantibodies specific for the neutrophil adhesion glycoproteins CD11b/CD18 in patients with autoimmune neutropenia. Blood 1991; 78:1096-104.

99. Simsek S, van der Schoot CE, Daams M, et al. Molecular characterization of antigenic polymorphisms (Ond(a) and Mart(a)) of the beta 2 family recognized by human leukocyte alloantisera. Blood 1996;88:1350-8.

100. Porcelijn L, Abbink F, Terraneo L, et al. Neonatal alloimmune neutropenia due to immunoglobulin G antibodies against human neutrophil antigen-5a. Transfusion 2011;51: 574-7.

101. van den Tooren-de Groote R, Ottink M, Huiskes E. Management and outcome of 35 cases with foetal/neonatal alloimune neutropenia. Acta Paed 2014;103:e467-74.

102. Kleinman S, Caulfield T, Chan P, et al. Toward an understanding of transfusion-related acute lung injury: Statement of a consensus panel. Transfusion 2004;44:1774-89.

103. Food and Drug Administration. Fatalities reported to FDA following blood collection and transfusion: Annual summary for fiscal year 2015. Silver Spring, MD: CBER Office of Communication, Outreach, and Development, 2015. [Available at https://www.fda.gov/downloads/BiologicsBloodVaccines/SafetyAvailability/ReportaProblem/TransfusionDonationFatalities/UCM518148.pdf (accessed March 15, 2017).]

104. Toy P, Gajic O, Bacchetti P, et al. Transfusion-related acute lung injury: Incidence and risk factors. Blood 2012;119:1757-67.

105. Akhtari M, Curtis B, Waller EK. Autoimmune neutropenia in adults. Autoimmun Rev 2009; 9:62-6.

106. Audrain M, Martin J, Fromont P, et al. Autoimmune neutropenia in children: Analysis of 116 cases. Pediatr Allergy Immunol 2011;22:494-6.

107. Clay ME, Schuller RM, Bachowski GJ. Granulocyte serology: Current concepts and clinical significance. Immunohematology 2010;26:11-21.

108. Fromont P, Prie N, Simon P, et al. Granulocyte antibody screening: Evaluation of a bead-based assay in comparison with classical methods. Transfusion 2010;50:2643-8.

109. Heinzl MW, Schonbacher M, Dauber EM, et al. Detection of granulocyte-reactive antibodies: A comparison of different methods. Vox Sang 2015;108:287-93.

110. Stroncek DF, Fadeyi E, Adams S. Leukocyte antigen and antibody detection assays: Tools for assessing and preventing pulmonary transfusion reactions. Transfus Med Rev 2007;21: 273-86.

111. Bux J. Molecular genetics of granulocyte polymorphisms. Vox Sang 2000;78(Suppl 2):125-30.

Chapter 16

The HLA System

• ● •

Arthur B. Eisenbrey III, MD, PhD, and Patricia M. Kopko, MD

THE HLA SYSTEM is composed of a complex array of genes located within the human major histocompatibility complex (MHC) on the short arm of chromosome 6. Their protein products, the HLA antigens, contribute to the recognition of self and nonself, the immune responses to antigenic stimuli, and the coordination of cellular and humoral immunity.

HLA molecules play a key role in antigen presentation and the initiation of the immune response. The HLA system is generally viewed as second in importance only to the ABO antigens in influencing the survival of transplanted solid organs. In hematopoietic progenitor cell (HPC) transplantation, the HLA system is paramount with regard to graft rejection and graft-vs-host disease (GVHD). HLA antigens and antibodies are also important in complications of transfusion therapy, such as platelet refractoriness, febrile nonhemolytic transfusion reactions (FNHTRs), transfusion-related acute lung injury (TRALI), and transfusion-associated GVHD (TA-GVHD).

The biologic roles of the genes in the MHC continue to be identified (neither transfusion nor transplantation are natural events), and the tremendous polymorphism of the HLA genes is utilized outside of transplantation. Studies correlating HLA genes with disease susceptibility and disease resistance began soon after serologic techniques for HLA Class I typing were developed and have resurged with the adoption of molecular methods. The polymorphisms identified by HLA antigen typing were used in relationship assessments and forensic investigations, although they have been replaced by other loci evaluated with various molecular methods. Functional cellular responses measured in mixed lymphocyte culture (MLC) were used to select matched donor-recipient pairs for hematopoietic stem cell/HPC transplantation until replaced by DNA-based typing methods for HLA antigens and alleles. Understanding the relationships between the polymorphisms of the HLA genes and antigen presentation by the HLA molecules has permitted the analysis of peptide-binding restriction parameters needed for effective vaccine development. The MHC and HLA genetic polymorphisms have been used by anthropologists and population geneticists as accurate tools for population studies. Because of the complexity of the MHC

16

Arthur B. Eisenbrey III, MD, PhD, Associate Professor of Pathology, University of Toledo College of Medicine, Toledo, Ohio, and Assistant Professor of Pathology, Wayne State University School of Medicine, Detroit, Michigan; and Patricia M. Kopko, MD, Professor of Pathology, University of California San Diego Medical Center, San Diego, California

P. Kopko has disclosed a financial relationship with Cerus. A. Eisenbrey has disclosed no conflicts of interest.

and the extent of polymorphism in the HLA genes, a complex nomenclature was developed (and continues to evolve) to define unique allele sequences based on the relationship of each allele's protein sequence to the serologic specificity of the corresponding antigen.[1,2]

BIOCHEMISTRY, TISSUE DISTRIBUTION, AND STRUCTURE

Characteristics of Class I and Class II Antigens

Class I antigens (HLA-A, -B, and -C) have a molecular weight of approximately 57,000 Daltons and consist of two protein chains: a glycoprotein heavy chain (45,000 Daltons) encoded on the short arm of chromosome 6 and, as a light chain, the β_2-microglobulin molecule (12,000 Daltons) encoded by a gene on chromosome 15. The heavy chain penetrates the cell membrane, whereas β_2-microglobulin does not. Rather, β_2-microglobulin associates (noncovalently) with the heavy chain through the latter's nonvariable (α3) domain. (See Fig 16-1.) The external portion of the heavy chain consists of three amino acid domains (α1, α2, and α3), of which the outermost domains, α1 and α2, contain the majority of polymorphic regions conferring serologic HLA antigen specificity.

The "classical" HLA Class I molecules (HLA-A, -B, and -C) are present on platelets and most nucleated cells in the body, with some exceptions that include neurons, corneal epithelial cells, trophoblasts, and germinal cells. Only vestigial amounts remain on mature red cells, with certain allotypes better expressed than others. These Class I types were independently recognized as red cell antigens by serologists and designated as "Bennett-Goodspeed" (Bg) antigens. The specificities called "Bg^a," "Bg^b," and "Bg^c" are actually HLA-B7, HLA-B17 (B57 or B58), and HLA-A28 (A68 or A69), respectively. Platelets express primarily HLA-A and HLA-B antigens. HLA-C antigens are present at very low levels, and Class II antigens are generally not present on platelets.

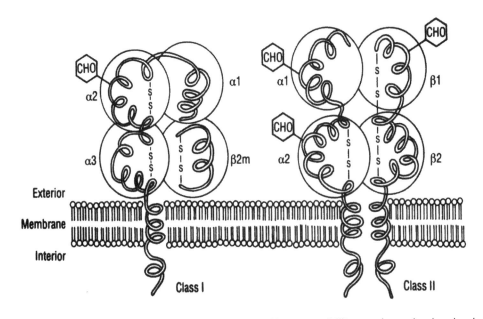

FIGURE 16-1. Stylized diagram of Class I and Class II major histocompatibility complex molecules showing α and β polypeptide chains, their structural domains, and attached carbohydrate units.

Class II antigens (HLA-DR, -DQ, and -DP) have a molecular weight of approximately 63,000 Daltons and consist of two structurally similar glycoprotein chains (α and β), both of which traverse the membrane. (See Fig 16-1.) The extramembranous portion of each chain has two amino acid domains, of which the outermost contains the variable regions of the Class II alleles. The expression of Class II antigens is more restricted than that of Class I antigens. Class II antigens are expressed constitutively on B lymphocytes, monocytes, macrophages, dendritic cells, intestinal epithelium, and early hematopoietic cells. There is also constitutive expression of Class II antigens on some endothelial cells, especially those lining the microvasculature. However, in general, endothelium, particularly that of larger blood vessels, is negative for Class II antigen expression, although Class II antigen expression can be readily induced (for instance, by interferon-gamma during immune activation). Resting T lymphocytes are normally negative for Class II antigen expression and become positive when activated.

Soluble HLA Class I and Class II antigens shed from cells are present in blood and body fluids and may play a role in modulating immune reactivity.[3] Levels of soluble HLA increase with infection [including with human immunodeficiency virus (HIV)], inflammatory disease, and transplant rejection, but HLA levels decline with progression of some malignancies. Levels of soluble HLA in blood components are proportional to the number of residual donor leukocytes and the duration of storage. Soluble HLA in blood components may be involved in the immunomodulatory effect of blood transfusion.

Configuration

A representative three-dimensional structure of Class I and Class II molecules can be obtained by x-ray crystallographic analysis of purified HLA antigens. (See Fig 16-2.) The outer domains, which contain the regions of greatest amino acid variability and the antigenic epitopes of the molecules, form a structure known as the "peptide-binding groove." Alleles that are defined by polymorphisms in the HLA gene sequences encode unique amino acid sequences and therefore form unique binding grooves, each of which is able to bind peptides of different sequences. The peptide-binding groove is critical for the functional aspects of HLA molecules. (See "Biologic Function" section below.)

Nomenclature for HLA Antigens

An international committee sponsored by the World Health Organization (WHO) establishes

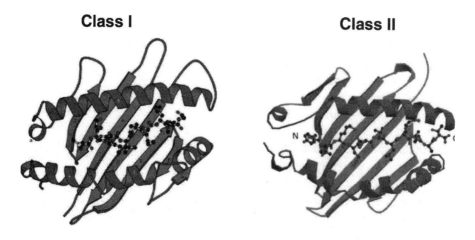

Class I   **Class II**

FIGURE 16-2. Ribbon diagram of HLA Class I and Class II molecules. Note the peptide in the groove of each molecule.

the nomenclature of the HLA system. This nomenclature is updated regularly to incorporate new HLA alleles.[2] HLA antigens are designated by a number following the letter that denotes the HLA series (eg, HLA-A1 or HLA-B8). Previously, antigenic specificities that were not fully confirmed carried the prefix "w" (eg, HLA-Aw33) for "workshop." When the antigen's identification became definitive, the WHO Nomenclature Committee dropped the "w" from the designation. (The committee meets regularly to update nomenclature by recognizing new specificities or genetic loci.) The "w" prefix is no longer applied in this manner and is now used only for the following: 1) Bw4 and Bw6, to distinguish such "public" antigens (see "Public" Antigens section below) from other B-locus alleles; 2) all serologically defined C-locus specificities, to avoid confusion with components of the complement system; and 3) Dw specificities that were defined by mixed leukocyte reactions but are now known to be caused by *HLA-DR, HLA-DQ,* and *HLA-DP* polymorphisms. The numeric designations for the HLA-A and HLA-B specificities were assigned according to the order of their discovery.

Splits and Cross-Reactive Groups

Refinement of serologic methods permitted antigens that were previously believed to represent a single specificity to be "split" into specificities that were recognized as serologically (and, later, genetically) distinct. The designation for an individual antigen that was split from an earlier recognized antigen often includes the number of the parent antigen in parentheses [eg, HLA-B44 (12)].

In addition to "splits," certain apparently distinct HLA antigens may have other epitopes in common. Antibodies that are reactive with these shared determinants often cause cross-reactions in serologic testing. The collective term for a group of HLA antigens that exhibit such cross-reactivity is "cross-reactive epitope group" (CREG).

"Public" Antigens

In addition to splits and CREGs, HLA proteins have reactivity that is common to many different HLA specificities. Called "public" antigens, these common amino acid sequences appear to represent the less variable portion of the HLA molecule. Two well-characterized public antigens, HLA-Bw4 and HLA-Bw6, are present in almost all HLA-B molecules.[4] The *HLA-A* locus molecules A23, A24, A25, and A32 also have a Bw4-like epitope.

Public antigens are clinically important because patients exposed to them through pregnancy, transfusion, or transplantation can make antibodies to these antigens if the patients do not express the epitopes themselves. A single antibody, when directed against a public antigen, can resemble multiple discrete alloantibodies, and this has significant consequences for identifying compatible donors for transplantation and platelet transfusion.

Nomenclature for HLA Alleles

Nucleotide sequencing has largely replaced serologic methods to investigate the HLA system, and increasing numbers of HLA alleles are being identified, many of which share common serologic phenotypes. The minimum requirement for designation of a new allele is the sequence of exons 2 and 3 for HLA Class I and exon 2 for HLA Class II. These exons encode the variable amino acids that confer HLA antigen specificity and much of the biologic function of the HLA molecule.

A uniform nomenclature has been adopted that takes into account the locus, major serologic specificity, and allele group determined by molecular typing techniques. For example, although many alleles have been sequenced only for exon 2, nucleotide sequencing has identified at least 300 unique amino acid sequence variants (alleles) of HLA-DR4 as of December 2016 (see http://hla.alleles.org/alleles/class2.html).[2] The first HLA-DR4 variant is designated *"DRB1*04:01,"* indicating the locus (DR), protein (β1 chain), major serologic specificity (04 for HLA-DR4), and sequence 2 variation allele number (variant 01). The asterisk indicates that an allele name follows (and that the typing was determined by molecular techniques).

A similar system is used for naming Class I alleles. The name of the locus—for example, "*HLA-B*"—is followed by an asterisk and then by several digits separated by colons. The first two digits correspond to the antigen's serologic specificity in most cases. The next group of digits makes up the code for a unique amino acid sequence in exons 2 and 3, with numbers being assigned in the order in which the DNA sequences were determined. Therefore, "*B*27:04*" represents the *HLA-B* locus, has a serologic specificity of B27, and was the fourth unique sequence 2 and 3 allele described in this family. (See Table 16-1.) A third "place" in the allele name is added for alleles that differ only by synonymous ("silent") nucleotide substitutions in exons 2 and 3 for Class I or in exon 2 for Class II. For example, *A*01:01:02* differs from *A*01:01:01* only in that the codon for isoleucine in position 142 is ATT instead of ATC. A fourth "place" in the allele name can be added for alleles that differ only in sequences within introns or in 3′ or 5′ untranslated regions. Finally, the nomenclature accommodates alleles with null or low expression or other characteristics by the addition of an "N" or "L," respectively, or another letter as appropriate to the end of the allele name. The other official expression modifiers are as follows: S (secreted, not on cell surface), Q (expression level questionable), A (unknown but aberrant expression, perhaps null), and C (cytoplasmic expression only). The last two have not been used to date.

Biologic Function

The essential function of the HLA system is self/nonself discrimination, which is accomplished by the interaction of T lymphocytes with peptide antigens presented by HLA proteins. T lymphocytes interact with peptide antigens only when the T-cell receptor (TCR) for antigen engages both an HLA molecule and the antigenic peptide contained within the TCR's peptide-binding groove. This limitation is referred to as "MHC restriction."[5]

In the thymus, T lymphocytes with TCRs that bind to a self HLA molecule are selected (positive selection), with the exception of those with TCRs that also bind to a peptide derived from a self-antigen, in which case the T lymphocytes are deleted (negative selection). Some self-reactive T cells escape negative selection, and if not functionally inactivated (for instance, by the mechanism of anergy), may become involved in an autoimmune process.

Role of Class I Molecules

Class I molecules are synthesized, and peptide antigens are inserted into the peptide-binding groove, in the endoplasmic reticulum. Peptide

TABLE 16-1.   Current HLA Nomenclature

Species	Locus		Antigen Equivalent		Allele		Silent Mutation		Outside Exon	Expression Modifier
HLA	DRB1	*	04	:	01	:	01	:	02	N,L,S,Q

Examples:
DR4   - Serology
DRB1*04:xx   - Serologic Equivalent
DRB1*04:02   - Allele
DRB1*04:01:01; DRB1*04:01:02 - Silent Mutations
A*02:15N;   DRB4*01:03:01:02N - Null Alleles (exon, intron)
A*24:02:01:02L
B*44:02:01:02   > - Expression Modifiers
B*32:11Q

antigens that fit into the Class I peptide-binding groove are typically eight or nine amino acids in length and are derived from proteins made by the cell (endogenous proteins). Such endogenous proteins—which may be normal self-proteins; altered self-proteins, such as those in cancer cells; or viral proteins, such as those in virus-infected cells—are degraded in the cytosol by a large multifunctional protease (LMP) and are transported to the endoplasmic reticulum by a transporter associated with antigen processing (TAP). The LMP and TAP genes are both localized to the MHC.

Class I molecules are transported to the cell surface, where the molecules are available to interact with CD8-positive T lymphocytes. If the TCR of a CD8 cell can bind the antigenic peptide in the context of the specific Class I molecule displaying it, then TCR binding activates the cytotoxic properties of the T cell, which attacks the cell, characteristically eliciting an inflammatory response. The presentation of antigen by Class I molecules is especially important in host defense against viral pathogens and malignant transformation. Tumor cells that do not express Class I antigens escape this form of immune surveillance.

Role of Class II Molecules

Like Class I molecules, Class II molecules are synthesized in the endoplasmic reticulum, but peptide antigens are not inserted into the peptide-binding groove there. Instead, an invariant chain (Ii) is inserted as a placeholder. The Class II-invariant chain complex is transported to an endosome, where the invariant chain is removed by a specialized Class II molecule called "DM." The DM locus is also localized to the MHC. A Class II antigenic peptide is then inserted into the peptide-binding groove.

Peptide antigens that fit into the Class II peptide-binding groove are typically 12 to 25 amino acids in length and are derived from proteins that are taken up by the cell through endocytosis (of exogenous proteins). Exogenous proteins, which may be normal self-proteins or proteins derived from pathogens, such as bacteria, are degraded to peptides by enzymes in the endosomal pathway. Class II molecules are then transported to the cell surface, where the molecules are available to interact with CD4-positive T lymphocytes, which secrete immunostimulatory cytokines in response. That mechanism is especially important for the production of antibodies.

GENETICS OF THE MHC

Class I and II HLA antigens are cell-surface glycoproteins that are products of closely linked genes mapped to the p21.3 band on the short arm of chromosome 6 (Fig 16-3). That genomic region, the MHC, is usually inherited en bloc as a haplotype. Each of the many loci has multiple alleles with codominant expression of the products from each chromosome. The HLA system is the most polymorphic genetic system described in humans.[6]

The genes HLA-A, HLA-B, and HLA-C encode the corresponding Class I A, B, and C antigens. The genes HLA-DRA1, -DRB1, -DRB3, -DRB4, -DRB5; HLA-DQA1, -DQB1; and HLA-DPA1, -DPB1 encode the corresponding Class II antigens. Located between the Class I and Class II genes is a group of non-HLA genes that code for molecules that include the complement proteins C2, Bf, C4A, and C4B; a steroid enzyme (21-hydroxylase); and a cytokine (tumor necrosis factor) and other genes involved in immune responses. This non-HLA region is referred to as "MHC Class III" even though it does not contain any HLA genes.

Organization of HLA Genetic Regions

The HLA Class I region contains (in addition to the "classical" genes HLA-A, HLA-B, and HLA-C) other gene loci designated HLA-E, HLA-F, HLA-G, HLA-H, HFE, HLA-J, HLA-K, HLA-L, MICA, and MICB. The latter genes encode nonclassical, or Class Ib, HLA proteins, which have limited polymorphism, low levels of expression, and limited distribution of tissue expression.[7] Some Class Ib genes express nonfunctional proteins or no proteins whatsoever. Genes that are unable to express a functional protein product are termed "pseudogenes" and presumably represent an evolutionary

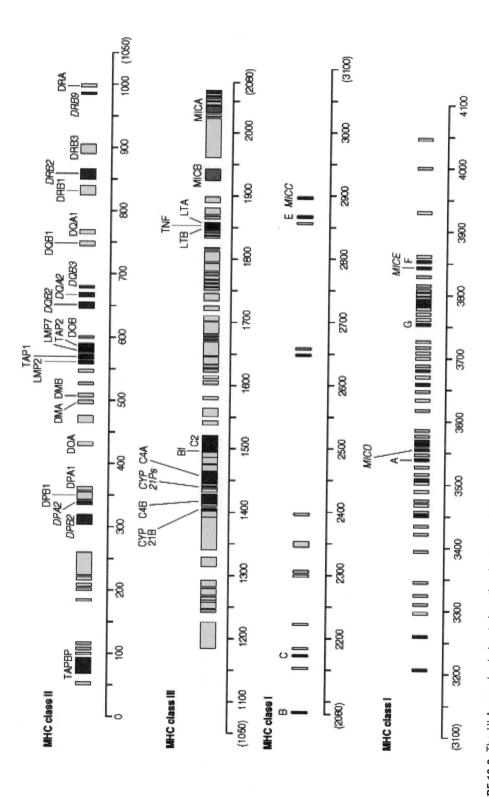

FIGURE 16-3. The HLA complex is located on the short arm of chromosome 6. The centromere is to the top left of the figure, the telomere to the bottom right. The organization of the Class I, II, and III regions is shown. (See also http://hla.alleles.org/alleles/index.html.) Used with permission from Janeway CA, Travers P, Walport M, et al. The immune system in health and disease. 5th ed. New York: Garland Science, 2001.

dead end. In contrast, other nonclassical HLA proteins that are expressed have been associated with a variety of functions. For example, HLA-E is associated with the surveillance system of one subset of natural killer cells. HLA-G is expressed by the trophoblast and may be involved in the development of maternal immune tolerance of the fetus. Hereditary hemochromatosis (HH), an iron overload disorder with a 10% carrier frequency in people of Northern European ancestry, is associated with two missense mutations in a Class I-like gene.[8] The gene that causes HH was initially named "*HLA-H*"; however, the *HLA-H* designation had already been assigned to an HLA Class I pseudogene by the WHO Nomenclature Committee.[9] The gene that is responsible for HH is now called "*HFE*." Additional Class I-like genes that code for molecules, such as CD1, are also located outside the MHC. These molecules present nonprotein antigens (such as lipids) to T cells.

The genomic organization of the MHC Class II (*HLA-D*) region is more complex. An MHC Class II molecule consists of a noncovalent complex of two structurally similar chains: the α-chain and the β-chain. Both of these chains are encoded within the MHC. The polymorphism of HLA Class II molecules results from differences in both the α-chain and the β-chain; this polymorphism depends on the Class II isoform. For example, with HLA-DR, the α-chain is essentially monomorphic, but the β-chain is very polymorphic. Multiple loci code for the α- and β-chains of the Class II MHC proteins.

Different haplotypes have different numbers of Class II genes and pseudogenes. The proteins coded by *DRA1* and *DRB1* result in HLA-DR1 through HLA-DR18 antigens. The products of *DRA1* and *DRB3* (if present) express HLA-DR52; those of *DRA1* and *DRB4* (if present) express HLA-DR53; and those of *DRA1* and *DRB5* (if present) express HLA-DR51. The HLA-DQ1 through DQ9 antigens are expressed on the glycoproteins coded by *DQA1* and *DQB1* in the DQ cluster. Many of the other genes of the DQ cluster are likely pseudogenes. A similar organization is found in the HLA-DP gene cluster.

Although not generally considered part of the HLA system, the MHC Class III region contains four complement genes with alleles that are typically inherited together as a unit, termed a "complotype." More than 10 different complotypes are inherited in humans. Two of the Class III genes, *C4A* and *C4B*, encode for variants of the C4 molecule and antigens of the Chido/Rodgers blood group system. These variants have distinct protein structures and functions; the C4A molecule (if present) carries the Rg antigen, and the C4B molecule (if present) carries the Ch antigen. Both of these antigens are adsorbed onto the red cells of individuals who possess the gene(s).

Patterns of Inheritance

Although MHC organization is complicated, its inheritance follows the established principles of Mendelian genetics. Every person has two different copies of chromosome 6 and possesses two HLA haplotypes, one from each parent. The expressed gene products constitute the phenotype, which can be determined by typing for HLA antigens or alleles. Because HLA genes are autosomal and codominant, the phenotype represents the combined expression of both haplotypes. However, to define haplotypes, parents (and possibly other family members) must also be typed to determine which alleles are inherited together. Figure 16-4 illustrates inheritance of haplotypes.

Finding HLA-Identical Siblings

A child inherits one copy of chromosome 6 from each parent; hence, one MHC haplotype is inherited from each parent. Because each parent has two different copies of chromosome 6, four different combinations of haplotypes are possible in the offspring (assuming that no recombination occurs). The inheritance pattern is important in predicting whether family members will be compatible donors for transplantation. The chance that two siblings will be genotypically HLA identical is 25%. The chance that any one patient with "n" siblings will have at least one HLA-identical sibling is $1 - (3/4)^n$. Having two siblings provides a 44% chance, and having three

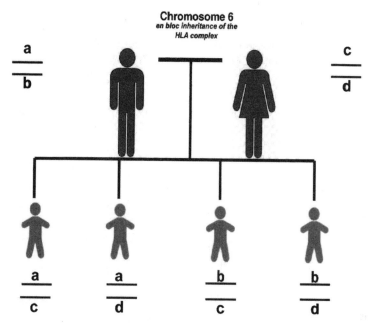

FIGURE 16-4. The designations a/b and c/d represent paternal and maternal HLA haplotypes, respectively. Except for crossovers, the HLA complex is transmitted en bloc from parent to offspring.

siblings provides a 58% chance that one sibling will be HLA identical. Moreover, each time a new sibling is tested, that new sibling has (only) a 25% chance of being a match, no matter how many siblings have previously been tested.

Absence of Antigens

Before the advent of molecular-based HLA typing, the absence of an antigen in serologic phenotyping results was attributed to homozygosity at a locus (eg, inheritance of A1 from both parents, which in reality represented only an apparent absence of the antigen as a result of limitations of phenotyping methods) or to a null (nonexpressed) allele. With DNA sequencing and other molecular HLA typing methods, homozygosity can now be presumed with a higher degree of confidence. However, homozygosity still can be proven only through family studies or methods permitting hemizygous typing (ie, typing of an individual haplotype). A null allele is characterized by one or more DNA sequence changes, within or outside the gene's coding region, that prevent expression

of a functional protein at the cell surface. Such inactivation of a gene may be caused by nucleotide substitutions, deletions, or insertions that lead to a premature cessation in the protein's synthesis. In the absence of a family study, a phenotyping study revealing a single allele at any locus offers only presumptive evidence for homozygosity. In this situation, the allele should be listed only once because it is unknown whether that allele is present twice (a true homozygote) or there is another allele not detected by the available method.

Crossovers

The genes of the HLA region occasionally demonstrate chromosome crossover, in which segments containing linked genetic material are exchanged between the two chromosomes during meiosis or gametogenesis. The recombinant chromosomes are then transmitted as new haplotypes to the offspring. Crossover frequency is related partly to the physical distance between the genes and partly to the resistance or susceptibility of specific A, B, and DR antigens to recombination. (See below.)

The *HLA-A*, *HLA-B*, and *HLA-DR* loci are close together, with 0.8% crossover between the *A* and *B* loci and 0.5% between the *B* and *DR* loci. Crossovers between the *HLA-B* and *HLA-C* loci or between the *HLA-DR* and *HLA-DQ* loci are extremely rare, whereas crossovers between the *DQ* and *DP* loci are relatively common.[10] In family studies and relationship evaluations, the possibility of recombination should always be considered.

Linkage Disequilibrium

The MHC system is so polymorphic that the number of possible unique HLA phenotypes is theoretically greater than that of the global human population. Moreover, new HLA alleles are constantly being discovered and characterized. As of January 2017, 3830 HLA-A alleles, 4647 HLA-B alleles, 2011 DRB1 alleles, and 1054 DQB1 alleles had been identified.[11] Usually, HLA genes are inherited as an entire chromosome. Many HLA haplotypes are overrepresented compared with what would be expected if the distribution of HLA genes were random. The phenomenon of linkage disequilibrium accounts for the discrepancy between expected and observed HLA haplotype frequencies.

Expected frequencies for HLA haplotypes are derived by multiplication of the frequencies of each allele. For example, in individuals of European ancestry, the overall frequency of HLA-A1 is 0.15 and that for HLA-B8 is 0.10; therefore, 3.0% (0.15 × 0.10 × 2) of all HLA haplotypes in people of European ethnicity would be expected to contain both HLA-A1 and HLA-B8 if the haplotypes were randomly distributed. The actual haplotype frequency of the A1 and B8 combination, however, is 7% to 8% in that population.

Certain allelic combinations occur with increased frequency in different racial groups and constitute common haplotypes in those populations. These common haplotypes are called "ancestral haplotypes" because they appear to be inherited from a single common ancestor or to be conserved within the population, because of either survival advantage of carriers or resistance to recombination. The most common ancestral haplotype in people of Northern European ancestry—*A1, B8, DR17 (DRB1*03:01), DQ2*—includes both Class I and Class II regions.

Some haplotypes in apparent linkage disequilibrium may represent relatively young haplotypes that have not had sufficient time to undergo recombination, whereas some old haplotypes are resistant to recombination because of selection or physical limitations. For example, the *A1, B8, DRB1*03:01* haplotype appears to be resistant to recombination because of deletion of the complement C4A gene, which results in decreased distance between HLA-B and HLA-DRB1 in those individuals. Linkage disequilibrium in the HLA system is important in relationship studies because haplotype frequencies in the relevant population make the transmission of certain gene combinations more likely than others. Linkage disequilibrium also affects the likelihood of finding suitable unrelated donors for HLA-matched platelet transfusions and HPC transplantation.

IDENTIFICATION OF HLA ANTIGENS AND ALLELES

Methods for the identification of HLA antigens and alleles fall into two categories: 1) molecular (DNA based) and 2) serologic (antibody based). Historically, cell-based assays were also used.

Detailed procedures for commonly used assays are available from reagent and kit manufacturers and have been summarized in reviews of available methodology.[12] Depending on the clinical situation, a particular HLA antigen/allele detection or typing method may be preferable. (See Table 16-2.)

DNA-Based Assays

DNA-based typing has several advantages over serologic assays: 1) high sensitivity and specificity, 2) use of small sample volumes, and 3) no need for cell-surface-antigen expression or cell viability. Although serologic methods can distinguish among a limited number of HLA specificities, high-resolution DNA-based

TABLE 16-2.   HLA Typing Methods and Appropriate Applications

Method	Clinical Application	Resolution
SSP (PCR)	Solid-organ and related and unrelated HPC transplantation	Serologic to allele level, higher resolution with large number of primers
Forward SSOP hybridization	Solid-organ and HPC transplantation (can accommodate high-volume testing)	Serologic to allele level
Reverse SSOP hybridization	Solid-organ and related and unrelated HPC transplantation	Serologic, higher resolution with larger number of probes
DNA sequencing	Unrelated HPC transplantation, resolution of typing problems with other methods, characterization of new alleles	Allele level
Lymphocytotoxicity	Supplemental testing for DNA-based HLA typings without defined HLA antigen assignments and research support for HLA allele and antigen designation	Serologic specificity

SSP = sequence-specific primer; PCR = polymerase chain reaction; HPC = hematopoietic progenitor cell; SSOP = sequence-specific oligonucleotide probe.

methods have the potential capability to identify all known alleles.

Polymerase Chain Reaction Testing

Polymerase chain reaction (PCR) technology allows amplification of large quantities of a particular target segment of genomic DNA. Low- to intermediate-resolution typing detects the HLA serologic equivalents with great accuracy (eg, it distinguishes DR15 from DR16), whereas high-resolution typing distinguishes individual alleles (eg, *DRB1*01:01:01* from *DRB1*01:02:01*). Several PCR-based methods have been developed; three general approaches are described below.

Oligonucleotide Probes. Sequence-specific oligonucleotide probes (SSO or SSOP) use arrays of labeled oligonucleotide probes to detect HLA nucleotide sequences present in immobilized DNA.[12] Reverse SSO (rSSO) has become more widely used and uses probes individually attached to a solid-phase matrix (for example, each probe may be attached to a dif-

ferent microbead). DNA from a target locus is then amplified by PCR, and the binding to the different probes is evaluated. Commercially available microbead array assays use rSSO methods for HLA Class I and Class II low-to-high-resolution tissue typing. This method has been widely adopted and allows rapid molecular typing using computer algorithms to match binding patterns to allele databases.[13]

Sequence-Specific Primers. A second major technique uses sequence-specific primer (SSP) pairs that target and amplify a particular DNA sequence.[12] This sequence-specific method requires the performance of multiple PCR assays in which each reaction is selected for a particular allele or group of alleles. The amplification products are directly visualized after agarose gel electrophoresis. Because SSPs have specific targets, the amplified material indicates the presence of the allele or alleles that have that sequence. The pattern of positive and negative PCR amplifications is examined to determine the HLA allele(s) present. Primer pair sets are commercially available that can determine HLA-A, -B, -C, -DR, -DQA1, -DQB1, and -DPB1 phenotypes and may be combined to determine common alleles.

Sequence-Based Typing ("Sequencing"). High-resolution typing is necessary for assignment of HLA alleles.[14] Sanger-chemistry sequence-based typing (SBT) can be used to identify known alleles and characterize new alleles.[12] Although SBT is considered the "gold standard" for HLA typing, ambiguities occur when two different base pairs are found at the same position and can result in two different possible combinations of alleles. These ambiguities occur because SBT evaluates both maternal and paternal HLA genes (haplotypes) simultaneously. Pairs of single nucleotide substitutions can be encountered in which *cis* (same parental haplotype) or *trans* (nucleotide assignment of the second polymorphic site is on the other haplotype) can give ambiguous results when those nucleotide combinations are assigned to different alleles. The haplotype to assign individual base pairs in polymorphic combinations may be determined with additional results from selected SSP or SSO reactions.

Next-Generation Sequencing. Massively parallel sequencing ("next-generation sequencing," or NGS) has allowed for sequencing of whole genes and improved resolution of the ambiguities that occur with Sanger-chemistry SBT because NGS is sequencing of single strands of DNA. The method has been applied to HLA typing,[15] and kits are commercially available for both clinical and research instruments. NGS methods obtain sequences from libraries formed from fractured pre- or post-PCR cellular DNA. The very large number of sequences obtained allow for identification of overlapping sequences and arrangement of the resulting sequences through computer analysis (requiring very powerful processors, large sequence databases, and complex programming).

Two families of NGS are sequencing by synthesis and sequencing by hybridization and ligation. Sequencing by synthesis has three methodologies: pyrosequencing; ion semiconductor sequencing; and fluorescently labeled, reversible nucleotide terminator chemistry. Nucleotide sequence detection is by photon release from dideoxynucleotide incorporation, detection of hydrogen ion release, or laser interrogation of dye terminator incorporation. A much less common method is matrix-assisted laser desorption/ionization time-of-flight mass spectrometry (MALDI-TOF MS). NGS is rapidly evolving, and selection of methods and instrumentation should be determined by individual laboratory needs.

Serologic (Lymphocytotoxicity) Assays

The microlymphocytotoxicity test[12] [now commonly referred to as "lymphocytotoxicity" or "complement-dependent cytotoxicity" (CDC), or incorrectly as "cell-dependent cytotoxicity"] has largely been replaced by molecular typing and solid-phase antibody detection for clinical laboratory testing. Molecular typing methods are required by accrediting organizations and regulatory agencies in the United States for solid-organ and hematopoietic stem cell transplantation. Solid-phase antibody detection and identification is required in the United States for solid-organ transplantion candidates. The reader is referred to previous editions of the AABB *Technical Manual* and Bontadini[12] for detailed descriptions of the use of the lymphocytotoxicity method.

Cellular Assays

Historically, the MLC and primed lymphocyte typing (PLT) assays were used to detect genetic differences in the Class II region. In MLC, the ability of one population of cells (the responder) to recognize the HLA-D (combined DR, DQ, and DP) antigens/alleles of the other (the target) as foreign can be detected by measuring the proliferation of the responding cells. In PLT, reagent cells previously stimulated by specific Class II mismatched types allow the identification of those types by their accelerated proliferative responses to stimulator cells sharing the original mismatches.

MLC and PLT have become obsolete as a result of the use of molecular HLA typing methods for clinical typing and better immunosuppression. These assays are still used in some clinical laboratories to monitor immune function or assess relative functional compatibility.

CROSSMATCHING AND DETECTION OF HLA ANTIBODIES

Cell-Based Assays

As noted above, lymphocytotoxicity testing has been used in the past for antibody detection. Compatibility testing similar to the red cell crossmatch has been performed by lymphocytotoxicity for almost 50 years[16] and is best referred to as "lymphocyte crossmatching." Crossmatching consists of incubating serum from a potential recipient with lymphocytes (unfractionated or separated into T and B lymphocytes) from prospective donors. Variations of the lymphocytotoxicity test include extended incubations, inclusion of wash steps, and use of an antiglobulin reagent. Flow cytometry has largely replaced the cytotoxicity crossmatch method with an even greater sensitivity than the antiglobulin-enhanced crossmatch.

Solid-Phase Assays

The current approach to identify HLA antibodies relies on the use of beads or microparticles (ie, solid-phase methodology) coated either with clusters of HLA Class I or Class II antigens from cultured lymphocytes (ie, an HLA phenotype) or with individually purified or recombinant HLA antigens (single-antigen beads).[16] Antibody binding is detected by staining with fluorescently labeled antihuman globulin (AHG). The presence of antibody is detected with flow cytometry, flow microarrays or enzyme-linked immunosorbent assay (ELISA). Flow cytometry and flow microarray methods are more sensitive than lymphocytotoxicity and focus on the detection of IgG antibodies. The use of single-antigen bead assays are of particular importance for highly sensitized patients where multiple HLA antibody specificities cannot be reliably distinguished and identified with either cell-based cytotoxic assays or solid-phase assays using clusters of HLA molecules.

Although HLA antibody has been demonstrated in transplant population studies to be detrimental to transplanted organ and patient survival, the clinical significance of low-level antibodies only detectable by solid-phase assays cannot be predicted for individual patients. Newer adaptations of the solid-phase technology can determine whether the antibodies do or do not fix complement and may improve the predictive value of testing for individual patients.

THE HLA SYSTEM AND TRANSFUSION

HLA system antigens and antibodies play important roles in a number of transfusion-related events, including platelet refractoriness, FNHTRs, TRALI, and TA-GVHD. HLA antigens are highly immunogenic. In response to pregnancy, transfusion, or transplantation, immunologically competent individuals are more likely to form antibodies to HLA antigens than to any other antigens.

Platelet Refractoriness

The incidence of HLA alloimmunization and platelet refractoriness has been substantially reduced by the implementation of nearly universal transfusion of leukocyte-reduced cellular blood components in Canada and the United States.[17] The refractory state exists when a transfusion of suitably preserved platelets fails to increase the recipient's platelet count. Platelet refractoriness may be caused by clinical factors, such as sepsis, high fever, disseminated intravascular coagulopathy, bleeding, medications, hypersplenism, complement-mediated destruction, or a combination of these factors; alternatively, it may have an immune basis.

Antibody Development

Antibodies against HLA Class I antigens are a common cause of immune-mediated platelet refractoriness, but antibodies to platelet-specific or ABH antigens may also be involved. Although platelets express HLA Class I antigens, the most likely cause of HLA sensitization from transfusion is the leukocytes in the blood component. This is demonstrated by the development of antibodies to HLA Class II antigens, which are not expressed on platelets. Leukocyte reduction to $<5 \times 10^6$ per component was shown to reduce alloimmunization from 19% to 7% and alloimmune platelet refractoriness from 14% to 4% in patients undergoing chemotherapy for acute leukemia or stem cell transplantation.[17]

Identifying Compatible Donors

The HLA antibodies present in transfused individuals may be directed against individual specificities or public alloantigens and are best characterized by solid-phase single-antigen assay, as described above. Platelet-refractory patients with broadly reactive antibodies may be difficult to support with platelet transfusions.

Selection of donors is based on avoiding donors with antigens to which the patient has antibody (selection of "antigen-negative" donors) and observing which donors provide acceptable corrected count increments (CCIs) after transfusion.

Alternatively, some HLA-alloimmunized patients respond to crossmatch-compatible platelets selected by using patient serum and samples of apheresis platelets in a platelet antibody assay. Commercially available crossmatching methods assess compatibility for both HLA and platelet-specific antibodies.[18] For additional information on platelet refractoriness, see Chapter 19.

Febrile Nonhemolytic Transfusion Reactions

HLA, granulocyte, and platelet-specific antibodies have been implicated in the pathogenesis of FNHTRs. The recipient's antibodies, reacting with transfused antigens, elicit the release of cytokines (eg, interleukin-1) that are capable of causing fever. Serologic investigation, if undertaken, may require multiple techniques and target cells from a number of different donors. (See Chapter 22.)

TRALI

In TRALI, a potentially fatal transfusion reaction that may occur with transfusion of plasma-containing blood components, acute noncardiogenic pulmonary edema develops in response to transfusion. (See Chapter 22.) The pathogenesis of TRALI appears to reflect the presence of HLA or neutrophil antibodies in donor blood that react with the target antigens in the recipient. Studies have shown that 2% (male donors) to 17% (female donors) of blood components can contain detectable amounts of HLA antibodies.[19] If present, such antibodies can be reactive with and fix complement to the recipient's granulocytes, leading to severe capillary leakage and pulmonary edema. Rarely, the recipient's HLA antibodies are reactive with transfused leukocytes from the donor.

Cases of TRALI have been reported that appear to be caused by donor antibodies against Class I or Class II antigens in recipients. HLA Class II antigens are not expressed on resting neutrophils but are expressed on alveolar macrophages and are inflammation-inducible in both neutrophils and alveolar endothelial cells. In the presence of preexisting inflammation, HLA Class II antibodies will bind directly to the target antigens on the recipient's neutrophils, macrophages, and endothelium. Without preexisting inflammation, the antibodies may bind to the alveolar macrophages and stimulate release of cytokines and chemokines, resulting in the recruitment and activation of neutrophils in the lungs.[20,21]

Chimerism and TA-GVHD

"Chimerism" refers to the presence of two cell populations, such as transfused or transplanted donor cells and recipient cells, in an individual. Persistent chimerism after blood transfusion may lead to the development of TA-GVHD in the recipient. The development of TA-GVHD depends on the following factors: 1) the degree to which the recipient is immunocompromised, 2) the number and viability of lymphocytes in the transfused component, and 3) the number of HLA alleles shared by the donor and recipient. The development of TA-GVHD with the use of fresh blood components from blood relatives has highlighted the pathogenic role of the HLA system.

Figure 16-5 illustrates the conditions for increased risk of TA-GVHD. The parents have one HLA haplotype in common. Each child, therefore, has one chance in four of inheriting the same haplotype from each parent, and child 1 is homozygous for the shared parental HLA haplotype. Transfusion of blood from child 1 to an unrelated recipient with different haplotypes would have no untoward consequences. If, however, child 1 were a directed donor for a relative who was heterozygous for that haplotype (eg, one of the parents or child 3), the recipient's body would fail to recognize the antigens on the transfused lymphocytes as

foreign and would not eliminate them. The donor cells would recognize the recipient's other haplotype as foreign and would become activated, proliferate, and attack the host.

To avoid this situation, it is recommended that all cellular components from blood relatives be irradiated before transfusion. Other specially chosen donor units, including HLA-matched platelets, may also present an increased risk of TA-GVHD and should be irradiated. Rarely, TA-GVHD has occurred after the transfusion of blood from an unrelated donor, usually within populations in which shared HLA haplotypes are common.

Chimerism is proposed to be responsible for the maintenance of tolerance in some organ transplant recipients as well as for the maintenance of HLA sensitization.[22] It has been postulated that scleroderma is a form of

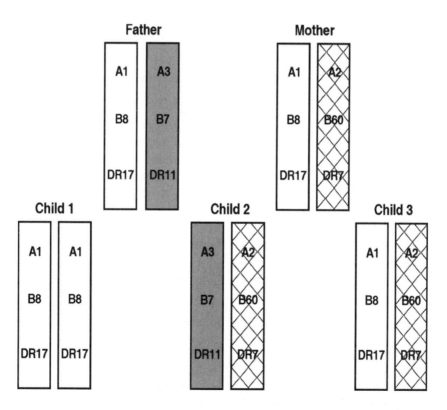

FIGURE 16-5. HLA haplotypes in a family at risk for transfusion-associated graft-vs-host disease (GVHD). In contrast to the family shown in Fig 16-4, each parent shares a common HLA haplotype, *HLA-A1,B8,DR17.* Child 1 is homozygous for the haplotype shared by the parents and by child 3. The lymphocytes of child 1 are capable of producing posttransfusion GVHD if they are transfused to either parent or to child 3.

GVHD resulting from chimeric cells derived from fetal cells transferred across the placenta during pregnancy.[23] Furthermore, the persistence of donor lymphocytes originally present in and transplanted with a solid-organ allograft has been documented to cause fatal GVHD in recipients of these organs.[24] Although donor lymphocytes are potentially detectable by molecular typing for HLA in all but HLA-identical transplants, current standards require chimerism testing for marrow engraftment monitoring using a different method. The test for chimerism after transplantation involves identifying the genetic profiles of the recipient and donor and then evaluating the extent of mixture in the recipient after transplantation. The technique commonly employed uses DNA analysis of short tandem repeat (STR) sequences that are amplified, separated by capillary electrophoresis, and evaluated by the DNA fragment sizes.[25]

HLA incompatibility has rarely been implicated in shortened red cell survival in patients with antibodies to HLA antigens, such as Bg^a (B7), Bg^b (B17-B57 or B58), and Bg^c (A28-A68 or A69). These antigens are expressed, although weakly, on red cells. Such incompatibility may not be detected by conventional pretransfusion testing.

HLA TESTING AND TRANSPLANTATION

HLA testing is an integral part of solid-organ and HPC transplantation. The extent of testing differs depending on the type of transplantation. (See Chapter 26.)

Hematopoietic Progenitor Cell Transplants

It has long been recognized that disparity within the HLA system is an important barrier to successful HPC transplantation.[26] HLA similarity and compatibility between the donor and the recipient are required for engraftment and to reduce the risk of GVHD. However, some degree of rejection or GVHD is a common problem for recipients of

allogeneic HPCs, despite immunosuppressive conditioning.

The goal of HLA typing is to match the alleles of the prospective donor and recipient at the HLA-A, -B, -C, -DRB1, and -DQB1 loci.[27] Some transplant programs also attempt to match donors and recipients for HLA-DP alleles. When matched stem cell donors are unavailable, haploidentical stem cell transplants are considered for patients with high-risk hematologic malignancies.[28]

Although HLA-identical sibling donors remain the best choice for HPC transplantation, there is increasing use of unrelated donors identified by searching the files of more than 20 million HPC donors listed in the National Marrow Donor Program's registry of volunteer donors, cord blood registries, and international registries.[27]

Kidney Transplants

ABO compatibility is the most important factor in determining the immediate outcomes of kidney transplants. Because ABH antigens are expressed in varying amounts on all of the body's cells, transplanted ABO-incompatible tissue comes into continuous contact with the recipient's ABO antibodies. Of particular importance is the expression of ABH antigens on vascular endothelial cells because the vascular supply in the transplant is the primary site of rejection. The use of non-A$_1$ blood group A organs for group B and group O recipients with low anti-A blood group titers has become acceptable for populations with prolonged wait times.[29,30] In addition, ABO-incompatible transplants may be facilitated using protocols that include various combinations of antibody suppression, splenectomy, plasmapheresis, infusion of intravenous immune globulin (IVIG), and other treatments to remove preexisting antibodies and promote accommodation of the transplanted organ.

Unlike HPC transplantation, renal transplants are not routinely HLA matched. Analogous to red cell transfusions, in renal transplantation the donor and recipient need to be compatible; meaning that the donor does not express preformed antibodies (ABH or HLA) directed against antigens on the donor kidney. Recipients and donors are routinely typed for ABO and HLA. Recipients are typed for HLA-A, -B, and -DR at a minimum. Donors are typed for HLA-A, -B, -C, -DRB, -DQA, -DQB, and -DPB antigens by molecular methods. Before transplantation, a crossmatch between recipient serum and donor lymphocytes is required. Clinical Laboratory Improvement Amendments (CLIA) regulations [*Code of Federal Regulations* (CFR) Title 42, Part 493.1448(e)] and US federal Organ Procurement and Transplant Network (OPTN) regulations require a sensitive crossmatch method.[31] Flow cytometry is the most sensitive method and has been credited with predicting early acute rejection and delayed graft function, both of which are strong predictors of chronic rejection (if results are positive) and long-term allograft survival (if results are negative).[32]

HLA antibody levels are dynamic and change with new immunologic challenges, including inflammatory conditions. Serum used for crossmatching is often obtained within 48 hours of surgery for sensitized potential recipients and may be retained in the frozen state for any subsequent testing. An incompatible crossmatch with unfractionated or T lymphocytes is typically a contraindication to kidney transplantation. A positive B-cell crossmatch is significant when caused by donor-specific HLA Class I or Class II antibodies.

Sera from patients awaiting deceased-donor kidney transplant surgery are tested at regular intervals to screen for HLA antibodies and to determine the specificities of the detected antibodies. A measure of sensitization is given by the proportion of HLA antigen phenotype beads (solid-phase array) to which a patient's serum reacts ["panel-reactive antibody" (PRA) level; historically performed with preselected panels of lymphocytes]. If an antibody with a defined HLA specificity is identified in a recipient, a common practice is to avoid donors who express the corresponding HLA antigen(s). Such antigens are deemed "unacceptable." Using a standardized algorithm involving the HLA frequencies from 12,000 HLA-typed donors, a calculated PRA (cPRA) is obtained and is a more specific measure of the sensitization of the patient and the percentage of probability of encountering incompatible or "unacceptable" random donors.[33] Frozen serum samples used for periodic antibody testing are often stored so that "historic" samples with the greatest reactivity can be used in addition to a preoperative sample for pretransplantation crossmatching.

Prospective crossmatching is often not performed for recipients who are conclusively devoid of HLA antibodies (ie, cPRA = 0%). Prompt transplantation with reduced cold-ischemia time for the renal allograft may provide greater benefit to the patient than prospective crossmatching, provided that 1) a very sensitive method for antibody detection, such as flow cytometry or microarrays, has been used, and 2) it is certain that the patient has had no additional sensitizing event (ie, immunizations or transfusions in the 2 weeks before or at any time after the serum was screened).[34] "Virtual crossmatching" for renal transplantation requires careful review of the patient history and HLA antibody test results and is similar to the concept of an "electronic crossmatch" for red cell transfusion. In other words, a virtual crossmatch is an inferred crossmatch that involves a determination of the presence or absence of donor HLA-specific antibodies in a patient by comparing the patient's HLA antibody specificity profile to the HLA type of the proposed donor without carrying out a physical crossmatch such as a CDC or flow-cytometric crossmatch.

Long-term allograft survival is longer with living donors than deceased organ donors. One-year graft survival rates from living and deceased renal donors were 97% and 91.3%, respectively, and the half-lives of living-donor and deceased-donor renal allograft recipients were 14.2 years and 9.9 years, respectively.[35]

The significantly better graft survival rate for recipients of living- vs deceased-donor renal allografts, even when donors and recipients are completely unrelated, coupled with inadequate numbers of deceased-organ donors has led to kidney paired donations (KPD), which permit patients with an ABO- or HLA-incompatible potential living donor to exchange their donor for the donor of other patients in the same situation.[36] KPDs have been facilitated through local and national registries. As a simple example, a blood group A transplant candidate with an incompatible blood group B potential living kidney donor could exchange that donor for the incompatible blood group A living kidney donor of a blood group B transplant candidate. Patients with HLA-incompatible potential donors have similar possibilities for donor exchange, and multiple "pairs" can be involved in one continuous exchange (chain) process.

The introduction of altruistic donors (ie, individuals who choose to donate a kidney without having a specific intended recipient) can significantly expand KPD options. Briefly, an altruistic donor donates a kidney to a patient with an incompatible potential living donor, who then donates to a different recipient with an incompatible donor, starting a chain with the possibility of a large number of living-donor transplants. A chain of 10 transplants has been reported.[37]

Other Solid-Organ Transplants

For liver, heart, lung, and heart/lung transplants, ABO compatibility remains the primary immunologic concern for donor selection, and pretransplant determination of ABO compatibility between the donor and recipient is required. Young pediatric heart or liver transplant recipients, who have low levels of ABO isoagglutinins, have had successful outcomes with ABO-incompatible hearts or livers.[38,39] HLA antibody screening and typing of potential recipients of nonrenal organs is recommended to improve deceased-donor organ transplantation outcomes. Likewise, a crossmatch should be available before transplantation when the recipient has demonstrated HLA antibody, except for emergency situations. Although the degree of HLA compatibility correlates with graft survival after heart, lung, small-intestine, and liver transplantations, prospective HLA matching is generally not performed for these procedures because of the relative scarcity of donors. Pancreas transplantation generally follows the same guidelines as kidney transplantation.

Relationship and Other Forensic Testing

HLA typing has been replaced by analysis of STR polymorphisms at numerous well-defined polymorphic loci for relationship and other forensic testing. STR analysis is sometimes used to confirm that an apparent twin who is HLA-identical to the recipient is a true monozygotic twin through an analysis of these loci on other chromosomes. These reliable methods and established population databases allow exclusion or identification of individuals using extremely small samples of DNA-containing biologic material such as body fluids and tissues. STR analysis may also be used to identify unlabeled or mislabeled surgical pathology samples.

OTHER CLINICALLY SIGNIFICANT ASPECTS OF HLA

For some conditions, especially those believed to have an autoimmune etiology, an association exists between HLA phenotype and the occurrence of, or resistance to, clinical disease.[40-43] (See Table 16-3.) HLA-associated disease susceptibilities are known or suspected to be inherited, display a clinical course with acute exacerbations and remissions, and

TABLE 16-3. HLA-Associated Diseases

Disease	HLA	RR[40-43]
Celiac disease	DQ2	>250
Ankylosing spondylitis	B27	>150
Narcolepsy	DQ6	>38
Subacute thyroiditis	B35	14
Type 1 diabetes	DQ8	14
Multiple sclerosis	DR15, DQ6	12
Rheumatoid arthritis	DR4	9
Juvenile rheumatoid arthritis	DR8	8
Grave disease	DR17	4

RR = relative risk.

usually have characteristics of autoimmune disorders.

Although linkage to disease-susceptibility genes was favored as an explanation for the HLA associations with individual diseases, evidence has been accumulating that implicates the HLA molecules themselves. The most frequently stated hypothesis is abnormal presentation of peptides by particular HLA molecules that result in autoreactivity from presentation of cross-reactive non-self peptides or improper presentation of self peptides. The ancestral haplotype *HLA-A1, B8, DR17 (DRB1*03:01), DQ2*, discussed in the "Linkage Disequilibrium" section above, is associated with susceptibility to type 1 diabetes, systemic lupus erythematosus, celiac disease, common variable immunodeficiency, IgA deficiency, and myasthenia gravis.[42] This haplotype is also associated with an accelerated course of HIV infection. A problem with the abnormal peptide presentation hypothesis is the lack of commonality in the associated disease processes.[43]

One of the first disease associations identified was between HLA-B27 and ankylosing spondylitis. Although >90% of patients of European ancestry with ankylosing spondylitis express HLA-B27 (most commonly *HLA-B*27:02* or *-B*27:05*), the test's specificity is low; only 20% of individuals with B27 develop ankylosing spondylitis. One of the strongest associations between an HLA allele and a medical condition is narcolepsy and the HLA allele *DQB1*06:02*.[44] As with HLA-B27 and ankylosing spondylitis, >90% of individuals with narcolepsy are positive for *HLA-DQB1*06:02*, but only a minority of the individuals with the allele develop the disease. For some autoimmune diseases, the specific peptide that might trigger the autoimmune response has been at least tentatively identified: a gluten peptide, gliadin, for celiac disease; cyclic citrullinated peptides for rheumatoid arthritis; and a peptide from glutamic acid decarboxylase for type 1 diabetes.[45-47] Resistance to cerebral malaria seems to result from a strong cytotoxic T-cell response to particular malarial peptides that are restricted by (ie, fit into the peptide-binding grooves of) two specific HLA molecules.[48]

Peptide-binding specificity is important to consider in the development of vaccines. For example, a vaccine to enhance immune responses to melanoma using a melanoma-specific peptide that binds only to the cells of individuals with the HLA type *HLA-A*02:01* was selected for development because *A*02:01* is the most common allele in virtually all populations.[49]

Some HLA alleles have been noted to be associated with increased risk for hypersensitivity reactions, such as toxic epidermal necrolysis (TEN), with certain drugs. Among the growing list of associations are *HLA-B*57:01* with abacavir, *HLA-B*15:02* with carbamazepine, and *HLA-B*58:01* with allopurinol.[50] The use of molecular genetics in pharmacology is called pharmacogenetics.

The degree of association between a given HLA type and a disease is often described in terms of relative risk (RR), which is a measure of how much more frequently a disease occurs in individuals with a specific HLA type than in individuals not having that HLA type. Calculation of RR is usually based on the cross-product ratio of a 2 × 2 contingency table. However, because the HLA system is so polymorphic, there is an increased possibility of finding an association between an HLA antigen and a disease by chance alone. Therefore, calculating RRs for HLA disease associations is more complex and is typically accomplished by use of Haldane's modification of Woolf's formula.[51,52] The RR values for some diseases associated with HLA types are shown in Table 16-3.

SUMMARY

In conclusion, the HLA system is a complex and highly polymorphic set of genes that are collectively involved in all aspects of the immune response. The recent development of molecular tools to explore this genetic oasis is providing additional information, such as the elucidation of unrecognized polymorphisms within the HLA complex (ie, single nucleotide polymorphisms, or SNPs). In the future, the translation of this basic information will undoubtedly lead to new clinical applications in transplantation, autoimmune diseases, vaccine development, pharmacogenetics, and infectious diseases.

ACKNOWLEDGMENT

The authors of the current version of the chapter gratefully acknowledge the previous au-thors of the chapter, Drs. Robert A. Bray, Marilyn S. Pollack, and Howard M. Gebel. Because of their definitive review of this topic, we have attempted only to revise and update where appropriate.

KEY POINTS

1. Genes encoded by the major histocompatibility complex (HLA complex in humans) are critical components of the immune system and play a major role in distinguishing self from nonself.
2. HLA genes are located within multiple highly polymorphic loci on the short arm of chromosome 6.
3. HLA genes encode multiple Class I (eg, HLA-A, -B, and -C) and Class II (eg, HLA-DR, -DQ, and -DP) cell-surface proteins.
4. Class I proteins are expressed ubiquitously; Class II proteins have restricted tissue distribution.
5. Everyone inherits a set of HLA genes from her or his mother and father, referred to as the "maternal haplotype" and "paternal haplotype," respectively.
6. Together, the maternal and paternal haplotypes are referred to as the genotype. The cell-surface expression of proteins encoded by the HLA genes is referred to as the phenotype.
7. Class I and Class II HLA proteins are strongly immunogenic and can induce an immune response—for example, formation of HLA antibodies and reactive T cells.
8. Donor-directed HLA antibodies are associated with graft dysfunction and/or loss.
9. Solid-phase assays (eg, flow cytometry and flow microarrays) have become the gold standard for detecting and identifying HLA antibodies.
10. Identification of donor-directed HLA antibodies can be used to perform a virtual (in-silico) crossmatch.

REFERENCES

1. Marsh SGE, Albert ED, Bodmer WF, et al. Nomenclature for factors of the HLA system, 2010. Tissue Antigens 2010;75:291-455.
2. Robinson J, Halliwell JA, Hayhurst JH, et al. The IPD and IMGT/HLA database: Allele variant databases. Nucleic Acids Res 2015; 43:D423-31. [See also http://hla.alleles.org/ (accessed February 21, 2017).]
3. Tabayoyong WB, Zavazava N. Soluble HLA revisited. Leuk Res 2007;31:121-5.
4. Voorter CE, van der Vlies S, Kik M, van den Berg-Loonen EM. Unexpected Bw4 and Bw6 reactivity patterns in new alleles. Tissue Antigens 2000;56:363-70.
5. Zinkernagel RM, Doherty PC. The discovery of MHC restriction. Immunol Today 1997;18:1417.
6. Mungall AJ, Palmer SA, Sims SK, et al. The DNA sequence and analysis of human chromosome 6. Nature 2003;425:805-11.
7. Horton R, Wilming L, Rand Vikki, et al. Gene map of the extended human MHC. Nat Rev Genet 2004;5:889-99.
8. Feder JN, Gnirke A, Thomas W, et al. A novel MHC class I-like gene is mutated in patients with hereditary haemochromatosis. Nat Genet 1996;13:399-408.
9. Bodmer JG, Parham P, Albert ED, Marsh SG. Putting a hold on "HLA-H." Nat Genet 1997;15: 234-5.
10. Buchler T, Gallardo D, Rodriguez-Luaces M, et al. Frequency of HLA-DPB1 disparities

detected by reference strand-mediated conformation analysis in HLA-A, -B, and -DRB1 matched siblings. Hum Immunol 2002;63: 13942.

11. IMGT/HLA Statistics. Hinxton, UK: European Molecular Biology Laboratory/European Bioinformatics Institute, 2017. [Available at http://www.ebi.ac.uk/ipd/imgt/hla/stats.html (accessed February 21, 2017).]

12. Bontadini A. HLA techniques: Typing and antibody detection in the laboratory of immunogenetics. Methods 2012;56:471-6.

13. Erlich H. HLA DNA typing: Past, present and future. Tissue Antigens 2012;80:1-11.

14. Nunes E, Heslop H, Fernandez-Vina M, et al. Definitions of histocompatibility typing terms. Blood 2011;118:e180-3.

15. De Santis D, Dinauer D, Duke J, et al. 16th IHIW: Review of HLA typing by NGS. Int J Immunogenet 2013;40:72-6.

16. Terasaki PI. A personal perspective: 100-Year history of the humoral theory of transplantation. Transplantation 2012;93:751-6.

17. Klein HG, Anstee DJ. Immunology of leukocytes, platelets and plasma components. In: Mollison's blood transfusion in clinical medicine. 11th ed. Malden, MA: Blackwell Publishing, 2005:546-610.

18. Kopko PM, Warner P, Kresie L, Pancoska C. Methods for the selection of platelet products for alloimmune-refractory patients. Transfusion 2015;55:235-44.

19. Triulzi DJ, Kleinman S, Kakaiya RM, et al. The effect of previous pregnancy and transfusion on HLA alloimmunization in blood donors: Implications for a transfusion-related acute lung injury risk reduction strategy. Transfusion 2009;49:1825-35.

20. Kopko PM, Popovsky MA, MacKenzie MR, et al. HLA class II antibodies in transfusion-related acute lung injury. Transfusion 2001; 41:1244-8.

21. Sachs UJH, Wasel W, Bayat B, et al. Mechanism of transfusion-related acute lung injury induced by HLA class II antibodies. Blood 2011;117:669-77.

22. Sivasai KSR, Jendrisak M, Duffy BF, et al. Chimerism in peripheral blood of sensitized patients waiting for renal transplantation. Transplantation 2000;69:538-44.

23. Artlett CM, Smith JB, Jimenez SA. Identification of fetal DNA and cells in skin lesions from women with system sclerosis. N Engl J Med 1998;338:1186-91.

24. Pollack MS, Speeg KV, Callander NS, et al. Severe, late-onset graft vs host disease in a liver transplant recipient documented by chimerism analysis. Hum Immunol 2005;66:28-31.

25. Clark JR, Scott SD, Jack AL, et al. Monitoring of chimerism following allogeneic haematopoietic stem cell transplantation (HSCT): Technical recommendations for the use of Short Tandem Repeat (STR) based techniques, on behalf of the United Kingdom National External Quality Assessment Service for Leucocyte Immunophenotyping Chimerism Working Group. Br J Haematol 2015;68:26-37.

26. Thomas ED. Bone marrow transplantation: A review. Semin Hematol 1999;36:95-103.

27. Petersdorf EW. Optimal HLA matching in hematopoietic cell transplantation. Curr Opin Immunol 2008;20:588-93.

28. Ricci MJ, Medin JA, Foley RS. Advances in haplo-identical stem cell transplantation in adults with high-risk hematological malignancies. World J Stem Cells 2014;6:380-90.

29. Bryan CF, Winklhofer FT, Murillo D, et al. Improving access to kidney transplantation without decreasing graft survival: Long-term outcomes of blood group A2/A2B deceased donor kidneys in B recipients. Transplantation 2005;80:75-80.

30. Tyden G, Donauer J, Wadstrom J, et al. Implementation of a protocol for ABO-incompatible kidney transplantation—a three-center experience with 60 consecutive transplantations. Transplantation 2007;83:1153-5.

31. Organ Procurement and Transplantation Network. Policy 4: Histocompatibility. Rockville, MD: Health Resources and Services Administration, 2017. [Available at https://optn.transplant.hrsa.gov/media/1200/optn_policies.pdf#nameddest=Policy_04 (accessed March 13, 2017).]

32. Bryan CF, Baier KA, Nelson PW, et al. Long-term graft survival is improved in cadaveric renal retransplantation by flow cytometric crossmatching. Transplantation 2000;66:1827-32.

33. Cecka JM. Calculated PRA (CPRA): The new measure of sensitization for transplant candidates. Am J Transplant 2010;10:26-9.

34. Gebel HM, Bray RA. Sensitization and sensitivity: Defining the unsensitized patient. Transplantation 2000;69:1370-4.

35. Scientific Registry of Transplant Recipients; Organ Procurement and Transplantation Network. SRTR/OPTN 2012 annual data report. [Available at http://srtr.transplant.hrsa.gov/ (accessed February 21, 2017).]

36. Terasaki PI, Cecka JM, Gjertson DW, Takemoto S. High survival rates of kidney transplants from spousal and living unrelated donors. N Engl J Med 1995;333:333-6.

37. Rees MA, Kopke JE, Pelletier RP, et al. A nonsimultaneous, extended, altruistic-donor chain. N Engl J Med 2009;360:1096-101.

38. Daebritz SH, Schmoeckel M, Mair H, et al. Blood type incompatible cardiac transplantation in young infants. Eur J Cardiothorac Surg 2007;31:339-43.

39. Heffron T, Welch D, Pillen T, et al. Successful ABO-incompatible pediatric liver transplantation utilizing standard immunosuppression with selective postoperative plasmapheresis. Liver Transpl 2006;12:972-8.

40. Thorsby E. Invited anniversary review: HLA associated diseases. Hum Immunol 1997;53:1-11.

41. Pile KS. HLA and disease associations. Pathology 1999;31:202-12.

42. Price P, Witt C, Allcock R, et al. The genetic basis for the association of the 8.1 ancestral haplotype (A1, B8, DR3) with multiple immunopathological diseases. Immunol Rev 1999; 167:257-74.

43. Holoshitz J. The quest for better understanding of HLA-disease association: Scenes from a road less traveled by. Discov Med 2013;16:93-101.

44. Pelin Z, Guilleminault C, Risch N, et al. HLAD-QB1*0602 homozygosity increases relative risk for narcolepsy but not for disease severity in two ethnic groups. US Modafinil in Narcolepsy Multicenter Study Group. Tissue Antigens 1998;51:96-100.

45. Cinova J, Palova-Jelinkova L, Smythies LE, et al. Gliadin peptides activate blood monocytes from patients with celiac disease. J Clin Immunol 2007;27:201-9.

46. Van Gaalen FA, van Aken J, Huizinga TW, et al. Association between HLA class II genes and autoantibodies to cyclic citrullinated peptides (CCPs) influences the severity of rheumatoid arthritis. Arthritis Rheum 2004;50:2113-21.

47. Mayr A, Schlosser M, Grober N, et al. GAD autoantibody affinity and epitope specificity identify distinct immunization profiles in children at risk for type 1 diabetes. Diabetes 2007; 56:1527-33.

48. Hill AV. The immunogenetics of resistance to malaria. Proc Assoc Am Physicians 1999;111: 272-7.

49. Slingluff CL Jr, Yamshchikov G, Neese P, et al. Phase I trial of a melanoma vaccine with gp100(280-288) peptide and tetanus helper peptide I adjuvant: Immunologic and clinical outcomes. Clin Cancer Res 2001;7:3012-24.

50. Pavlos R, Mallal S, Phillips E. HLA and pharmacogenetics of drug hypersensitivity. Pharmacogenomics 2012;13:1285-306.

51. Haldane JBS. The estimation and significance of the logarithm of a ratio of frequencies. Ann Hum Genet 1956;20:309-11.

52. Woolf B. On estimating the relation between blood groups and disease. Ann Hum Genet 1955;19:251-3.

Chapter 17

Transfusion-Service-Related Activities: Pretransfusion Testing and Storage, Monitoring, Processing, Distribution, and Inventory Management of Blood Components

• • •

Sarah K. Harm, MD, and Nancy M. Dunbar, MD

HOSPITAL-BASED TRANSFUSION service activities ensure transfusion of pure, potent, safe, and efficacious blood components to recipients needing this life-sustaining therapy. Safe transfusion practice begins at the bedside with proper recipient identification, sample collection, and labeling; continues with pretransfusion testing; and culminates in the selection and distribution of compatible blood and blood components that have been appropriately processed, tested, monitored, and stored.

SAMPLES AND REQUESTS

Transfusion Requests

All requests for blood and blood components must be complete, accurate, and legible and contain two independent identifiers for accurate recipient identification.[1(p34)] Requests should include the type and amount of component requested, any special needs (eg, irradiation) or special processing required (eg, volume reduction) and the name of the ordering physician or authorized health professional.

Sarah K. Harm, MD, Medical Director of Blood Bank, University of Vermont Medical Center, and Assistant Professor, Department of Pathology, Robert Larner, MD, College of Medicine, Burlington, Vermont; and Nancy M. Dunbar, MD, Medical Director of Blood Bank, Dartmouth-Hitchcock-Medical Center, Lebanon, New Hampshire, and Associate Professor, Department of Pathology and Laboratory Medicine, Geisel School of Medicine at Dartmouth, Hanover, New Hampshire
The authors have disclosed no conflicts of interest.

Additional useful information to guide testing and/or product/component selection may include the recipient's gender, age, weight, diagnosis, and transfusion and/or pregnancy history.

Recipient Identification and Sample Labeling

Collection of a properly labeled pretransfusion blood sample from the intended recipient is critical to safe blood transfusion. At the time of sample collection, the phlebotomist must accurately identify the potential transfusion recipient before collecting the pretransfusion sample and must ensure that the correct recipient information is placed on the sample label before the sample leaves the side of the recipient.[1(p35)] There must be a mechanism to identify the phlebotomist and the date of sample collection.[1(p35)] ABO-incompatible Red Blood Cell (RBC) transfusions should never occur, but when they do, they most commonly result from misidentification of recipients or pretransfusion sample labeling errors.[2] These errors may result in wrong blood in tube (WBIT), a situation where the blood in the tube is not that of the recipient identified on the sample label.[3] The risk of WBIT is about 1 in 2000 samples.[4]

Because of the risk for WBIT, when a computer system is used as the method to detect ABO incompatibility (ie, "electronic crossmatch"), two determinations of a transfusion recipient's ABO group are required. Compliance with this requirement may be accomplished by 1) testing a second current sample; 2) comparison with previous records; or 3) retesting the same sample if recipient identification was verified using an electronic identification system or process validated to reduce the risk of misidentification.[1(p38)] Electronic identification systems that use machine-readable information (eg, bar codes or embedded radio-frequency-emitting chips) are available to perform and integrate many functions, including recipient identification, sample labeling, blood unit identification, and linkage of blood components to their intended recipient(s).[5-7]

Confirming Sample Linkage

When a pretransfusion sample is received in the laboratory, laboratory personnel must confirm that the information on the sample label and the information on the pretransfusion testing request are in agreement. If there is any doubt about the identity of the recipient or the labeling of the sample, a new sample must be obtained.[1(p35)] One study found that samples that failed to meet acceptability criteria were 40 times more likely to have a blood grouping discrepancy.[8] Thus, a strict policy of canceling the testing of incorrectly labeled samples should help avoid blood grouping errors and decrease the risk for transfusion of ABO-incompatible blood components.

PRETRANSFUSION TESTING OF RECIPIENT BLOOD

Serologic Testing Overview

The recipient's ABO group and Rh type must be determined before transfusion. In addition, testing for unexpected antibodies to red cell antigens (eg, antibody screen) is required before transfusion of Whole Blood, RBCs, and granulocytes.[1(p36)] Results of testing on the current sample must be compared with previous transfusion service records to identify any discrepancy between previous and current ABO group and Rh type on file.[1(p37)] Current testing results must also be compared to previous records to identify any history of clinically significant antibodies, any previous adverse events to transfusion, or any special transfusion requirements.[1(p37)] Crossmatch is required on any blood component containing ≥2 mL of red cells. Unless the need for blood is urgent, a crossmatch must be performed before a Whole Blood or an RBC transfusion. Crossmatch is also required before granulocyte transfusion and platelet transfusions unless the component is prepared by a method known to result in a component containing <2 mL of red cells.[1(p37)] When clinically significant antibodies are not detected using current antibody detection tests and there is no record of previous detection of such antibodies, then a method must be used to detect ABO incompatibility.[1(p38)] The advantages and limitations of various pretransfusion testing schemes are shown in Table 17-1.

Serologic Testing Principles

The basis of pretransfusion testing is the detection of in-vitro red cell antigen-and-antibody reactions by observing either agglutination or hemolysis. Agglutination is a reversible chemical reaction that occurs in two stages: 1) sensitization when the antibody attaches to the red cell antigen, and 2) agglutination when the sensitized red cells are bridged to form a macroscopically detectable lattice. The antiglobulin phase, or Coombs test, detects bound red cell antibodies that do not produce direct agglutination.[9] This test uses antihuman globulin (AHG) sera produced by injecting animals with human globulins to stimulate antibody production against the foreign human protein. This antisera attaches to and causes agglutination of red cells sensitized with human globulins, as illustrated in Fig 17-1. Causes of false-positive and false-negative results

in antiglobulin tests are found in Appendices 17-1 and 17-2.

Various factors may enhance or decrease sensitization and agglutination, including temperature, immunoglobulin (Ig) class, and interactions between antigen configuration and the antigen-binding fragment site of the antibody. These factors affect the incubation time necessary to achieve the detectable end point. The strength of agglutination or degree of hemolysis, or both, observed during serologic testing should be recorded immediately after reading. Refer to Method 1-9 for details on the grading and scoring of serologic test reactions.

Sample Requirements

Pretransfusion testing uses recipient red cells and either serum or plasma. Because the end point of pretransfusion testing is the visualization of agglutination, the use of hemolyzed or lipemic samples may create difficulties in evaluating test results. Plasma is often the preferred sample, as incompletely clotted serum samples may contain small fibrin clots that

TABLE 17-1.   Pretransfusion Testing Schemes

Test Scheme	Tests Performed	Advantages	Limitations
Hold	None	A sample has been collected.	ABO, Rh, and antibody detection testing are *not* performed.
Type and hold	ABO and Rh	A sample has been collected; the recipient's ABO group and Rh type are known.	Antibody detection testing is *not* performed.
Type and screen	ABO, Rh, and antibody detection test/identification	Most of the pretransfusion testing has been performed; compatible blood can be provided in most situations.	Does not include crossmatch.
Type and screen with crossmatch*	ABO, Rh, antibody detection test/identification, Red Blood Cell unit selection or phenotyping, and crossmatch	Routine pretransfusion testing has been performed; compatible blood can be provided in most situations.	Units are removed from general inventory and may not be available for timely use by other recipients.

*"Prepare" (or other term) may be used instead of the word "crossmatch" by some hospital electronic ordering systems.

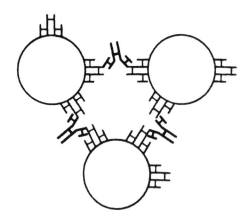

FIGURE 17-1. The antiglobulin reaction. Antihuman immunoglobulin G (IgG) molecules are shown reacting with the Fc portion of human IgG coating adjacent red cells (eg, D-positive red cells coated with anti-D).

trap red cells into aggregates, which may cause false-positive results. In addition, clotting may be incomplete in anticoagulated serum samples, such as those from recipients who have been treated with heparin. Adding thrombin or protamine sulfate to the sample may correct the problem. (See Method 1-3.) At times, it may be necessary to obtain a pretransfusion blood sample from the same extremity in which there is an intravenous infusion. If this is the case, steps should be taken to avoid dilution of the sample, which might result in a failure to detect unexpected red cell antibodies.

Sample Age

When pretransfusion testing is performed for a recipient who has been pregnant or transfused within the previous 3 months, or when pregnancy and/or transfusion history are uncertain, the pretransfusion sample used for testing must be no more than 3 days old at the time of the intended transfusion because a recent transfusion or pregnancy may stimulate production of unexpected antibodies. The day of collection is counted as day 0; therefore, a sample collected on a Monday can be used for a transfusion until 11:59 pm on Thursday of the same week.[1(p36)] Although the specification

of 3 days is arbitrary, the 3-day requirement was created as a practical approach to ensure that the sample used for testing reflects the recipient's current immunologic status.[10] If the histories of transfusion and pregnancy are known with certainty and if no transfusion or pregnancy has occurred in the previous 3 months, pretransfusion testing may be completed in advance of a scheduled surgical procedure. Pretransfusion testing is performed at some centers up to 45 days before a scheduled surgical procedure to reduce delays and cancellations associated with unexpected antibodies identified when samples are drawn on the day of surgery.[11]

Testing Methodologies

Pretransfusion testing may be performed using the traditional tube method or using automated and semi-automated testing platforms that use column-agglutination, microplate solid-phase, or hemagglutination-microplate technologies. Fluid-phase and solid-phase assays are discussed in greater detail in Chapter 8. Automated testing systems require validation before implementation and after any alteration in software functionality. Molecular testing is not routinely performed for pretransfusion testing but may be employed to resolve ABO group and/or Rh typing discrepancies and determine red cell antigen genotyping when serologic typing cannot be performed. Molecular testing is also discussed in greater detail in Chapter 8.

ABO Group and Rh Typing

To determine the recipient's ABO group, red cells must be tested with anti-A and anti-B reagent (forward or front typing). In addition, the recipient's serum or plasma must be tested against A_1 and B red cells (reverse or back typing). (See Method 2-2.) Donor red cells must be ABO compatible with the recipient's plasma. Any discrepant ABO typing results must be resolved before type-specific blood can be given (Method 2-4). If urgent transfusion is necessary, the recipient should receive group O red cells.[1(p36)] Routine testing for ABO and resolution of ABO discrepancies are described in greater detail in Chapter 10. Table 17-2 lists selection criteria for ABO groups of blood components when ABO-identical components are not available.

To determine the recipient's Rh type, the recipient's red cells must be tested for the D antigen using anti-D reagent (Method 2-13).[1(p36)] Weak D testing is not required for recipient samples except when assessing the red cells of an infant born to an Rh-negative mother (Method 2-15).[1(p46)] If problems in D typing arise, especially if the recipient is a female of childbearing potential, it is prudent to limit transfusion of blood components containing red cells to those that are D negative, at least until the problem is resolved. Testing for the D antigen is described in greater detail in Chapter 11.

Detection of Unexpected Antibodies

Antibody screening is designed to detect clinically significant antibodies, including those associated with hemolytic disease of the fetus and newborn (HDFN), hemolytic transfusion reactions, or notably decreased survival of transfused red cells.[1(p36)] The procedure uses the indirect antiglobulin test (IAT) method to demonstrate in-vitro reactions between red cells and antibodies. The recipient serum or plasma is incubated with unpooled reagent antibody screening cells. Panels of two, three, or four screening cells may be used. Following incubation at 37 C, the cells are then washed to remove unbound globulins. The presence of agglutination with the addition of AHG reagent indicates antibody binding to a specific red cell antigen.

When reactivity is identified in the antibody screen, additional testing is performed to identify the target red cell antigen(s). Additional testing strategies used for antibody identification may include use of enhancement media [albumin additive, low-ionic-strength saline (LISS), polyethylene glycol (PEG)] and/or enzyme or chemical treatment of the panel screening cells. Antibody identification is discussed in greater detail in Chapter 13.

Recipients with clinically significant red cell antibodies or a history of such antibodies must receive crossmatch-compatible Whole Blood and/or RBCs that lack the corresponding antigen. Clinically significant red cell alloantibodies may become undetectable in a recipient's plasma over time. Between 30% and 35% of antibodies are undetectable within 1 year, and nearly 50% are undetectable after 10 or more years.[12] The failure to detect a weakly reactive red cell alloantibody can be followed by a rapid anamnestic production of antibody and then by a delayed hemolytic transfusion reaction.[13]

Immediate-Spin Crossmatch

The immediate-spin (IS) crossmatch method is the serologic method used to detect ABO

TABLE 17-2. Blood Component ABO Requirements

Whole Blood	Must be identical to that of the recipient.
Red Blood Cells	Must be compatible with the recipient's plasma.
Granulocytes	Must be compatible with the recipient's plasma.
Plasma	Selected to be compatible with the recipient's red cells. Some centers are using thawed group A plasma for emergent transfusions.
Platelets	All ABO groups are acceptable. Although ABO-identical platelets are preferred, components that are compatible with the recipient's red cells are recommended.
Cryoprecipitated antihemophilic factor	All ABO groups are acceptable.

incompatibility between donor red cells and recipient serum. This method can be used as the sole crossmatch method *only* if the recipient has no present or previously detected, clinically significant antibodies.[1(p38)] When the IS crossmatch result is used for recipients with a negative antibody detection test result, the risk of an overt hemolytic reaction from an undetected alloantibody is low.[14] The potential benefits in using an IS crossmatch instead of a full AHG crossmatch in recipients with a negative antibody screen include reductions in turnaround time, workload, and reagent costs.

In the IS saline technique, recipient serum or plasma is mixed with saline-suspended donor red cells at room temperature. The tube is centrifuged immediately and observed for the presence of agglutination. Failure to properly perform the IS crossmatch test can lead to false-negative results and the failure to detect ABO-incompatible RBC units.[15] This technique is described in greater detail in Method 3-1.

Computer/Electronic Crossmatch

ABO compatibility may alternatively be verified by using computerized/electronic crossmatch, provided that the following conditions have been met[1(pp38-39)]:

- The computer system has been validated on site to ensure that only ABO-compatible Whole Blood or RBCs are selected for transfusion.
- Two determinations of the recipient's ABO group are made—one on a current sample and a second by one of the following methods:
  – Testing a second current sample.
  – Comparison with previous records.
  – Retesting the same sample if recipient identification was verified using an electronic identification system or another process validated to reduce the risk of misidentification.
- The computer system contains the donation identification number (DIN), compo-

nent name, ABO group, and Rh type of the component; the confirmed donor unit's ABO group; the two unique recipient identifiers; the recipient ABO group, Rh type, and antibody screen results; and interpretation of compatibility.

- A method exists to verify correct entry of data before the release of blood components.
- The system contains logic to alert the user 1) to discrepancies between the donor ABO group/Rh type on the unit label and ABO group/Rh type determined by blood group confirmatory tests and 2) to ABO incompatibility between the recipient and donor unit.

This method can be used as the sole crossmatch method *only* if the recipient has no present or previously detected, clinically significant antibodies.[1(p38)] Potential advantages of a computer crossmatch include decreased workload, reduced sample volume required for testing, reduced exposure of personnel to blood samples, and better use of blood inventory.[16]

Antiglobulin Crossmatch

Blood lacking relevant antigens should be selected for transfusion in a recipient with a clinically significant antibody identified currently or historically, even if the antibody is presently nonreactive.[1(p37)] This crossmatch includes incubation at 37 C and the AHG test. The AHG crossmatch may be performed using tube, column-agglutination, or solid-phase systems. For a routine tube AHG crossmatch, the donor red cells obtained from a segment of tubing that was originally attached to the unit to be transfused are washed and resuspended to between 2% and 5% in saline. Recipient serum or plasma is then mixed with the washed donor red cells. Following incubation at 37 C, the cells are again washed to remove unbound immunoglobulins. The presence of agglutination with the addition of AHG reagent indicates incompatibility (Method 3-2).

Interpretation of Antibody Screening and Crossmatch Results

Most samples tested have a negative antibody screening result and are crossmatch compatible with the donor RBC units selected. A negative antibody screening result, however, does not guarantee that the serum or plasma does not have clinically significant red cell antibodies. Such a result shows only that the sample contains no detectable antibodies that are reactive with the screening cells or techniques used. Furthermore, a compatible crossmatch does not guarantee normal red cell survival. See Appendix 3 for a summary of positive pretransfusion test results and their possible causes. Requirements for compatibility testing for neonates/infants <4 months of age are discussed in Chapter 24.

BLOOD AND BLOOD COMPONENT STORAGE AND MONITORING

General Considerations

Transport and storage requirements must be followed when blood components are transferred from the collection site to the processing facility, from the supplier to the blood bank, or from the blood bank to the recipient. Storage requirements and expiration dates vary by component type and are based on factors such as in-vitro red cell metabolism for RBC components in various storage solutions or coagulation protein stabilization for plasma products (Table 17-3). Failure to adhere to these storage and expiration requirements can result in decreased component potency and/or safety.

Temperature requirements during transport of blood components differ from those during storage.[17] (See Table 17-3.) Shipping from the supplier to the hospital blood bank is considered transport, and applicable temperature requirements must be met. When blood components are issued from the blood bank to the recipient-care area, maintenance of appropriate temperature requirements allows for the possibility of returning the components to inventory if they are not transfused.

Refrigerators, freezers, and platelet incubators for blood and blood component storage can be equipped with continuous-temperature-monitoring devices to allow detection of temperature deviations before components are affected. Automated electronic monitoring devices that are available include: 1) weekly pen-and-chart recorders, 2) sets of hard-wired or radio-frequency temperature-recording devices, and 3) centralized temperature-monitoring systems.

Thermometers or thermocouples should be strategically placed in the equipment for optimal temperature monitoring. If an automated temperature-recording device is not used, temperatures of the blood storage environment must be recorded manually every 4 hours.[1(p14)] This requirement includes ambient room temperature monitoring of platelets that are not stored in a platelet chamber or incubator.

The recorded temperatures should be checked daily to ensure proper operation of the equipment and recorder. Deviations from acceptable temperature ranges should be documented and explained (including any actions taken), dated, and initialed by the person noting the deviation.

Most component-storage devices are equipped with audible alarms to alert personnel that temperature ranges are approaching unacceptable levels. Central alarm monitoring allows facilities that do not have personnel in the vicinity of the equipment to alert designated staff at another location when an alarm is activated. Because platelets must be gently agitated during storage, typically using horizontal flatbed or elliptical rotators, alarm systems should also emit alerts when the platelet agitator has malfunctioned.

Transfusion services may locate blood storage refrigerators in other areas of the hospital to allow immediate access to blood in emergency situations. Such a practice requires that the same blood component storage monitoring standards be met in these other areas.

If an equipment failure occurs and prevents acceptable temperature ranges from being maintained, the facility should have

TABLE 17-3. Reference Standard 5.1.8A—Requirements for Storage, Transportation, and Expiration[*][1]

Item No.	Component	Storage	Transport	Expiration[†]	Additional Criteria
Whole Blood Components					
1	Whole Blood	1-6 C. If intended for room temperature components, then store at 1-6 C within 8 hours after collection	Cooling toward 1-10 C. If intended for room temperature components, cooling toward 20-24 C	ACD/CPD/CP2D: 21 days CPDA-1: 35 days	
2	Whole Blood Irradiated	1-6 C	1-10 C	Original expiration or 28 days from date of irradiation, whichever is sooner	
Red Blood Cell Components					
3	Red Blood Cells (RBCs)	1-6 C	1-10 C	ACD/CPD/CP2D: 21 days CPDA-1: 35 days Additive solution: 42 days Open system: 24 hours	
4	Deglycerolized RBCs	1-6 C	1-10 C	Open system: 24 hours Closed system: 14 days or as FDA approved	
5	Frozen RBCs 40% Glycerol	≤−65 C if 40% glycerol or as FDA approved	Maintain frozen state	10 years (A policy shall be developed if rare frozen units are to be retained beyond this time)	Frozen within 6 days of collection unless rejuvenated Frozen before Red Blood Cell expiration if rare unit
6	RBCs Irradiated	1-6 C	1-10 C	Original expiration or 28 days from date of irradiation, whichever is sooner	

#	Component	Storage	Transport	Expiration	Notes
7	RBCs Leukocytes Reduced	1-6 C	1-10 C	ACD/CPD/CP2D: 21 days CPDA-1: 35 days Additive solution: 42 days Open system: 24 hours	
8	Rejuvenated RBCs	1-6 C	1-10 C	CPD, CPDA-1: 24 hours	AS-1: freeze after rejuvenation
9	Deglycerolized Rejuvenated RBCs	1-6 C	1-10 C	24 hours or as approved by FDA	
10	Frozen Rejuvenated RBCs	≤-65 C	Maintain frozen state	CPD, CPDA-1: 10 years AS-1: 3 years (A policy shall be developed if rare frozen units are to be retained beyond this time)	
11	Washed RBCs	1-6 C	1-10 C	24 hours	
12	Apheresis RBCs	1-6 C	1-10 C	Additive solution: 42 days Open system: 24 hours	
13	Apheresis RBCs Leukocytes Reduced	1-6 C	1-10 C	Additive solution: 42 days Open system: 24 hours	
Platelet Components					
14	Platelets	20-24 C with continuous gentle agitation	As close as possible to 20-24 C‡	24 hours to 5 days, depending on collection system	Maximum time without agitation: 24 hours
15	Platelets—Irradiated	20-24 C with continuous gentle agitation	As close as possible to 20-24 C‡	No change from original expiration date	Maximum time without agitation: 24 hours
16	Platelets—Leukocytes Reduced	20-24 C with continuous gentle agitation	As close as possible to 20-24 C‡	Open system: 4 hours Closed system: No change in expiration	Maximum time without agitation: 24 hours

(Continued)

TABLE 17-3. Requirements for Storage, Transportation, and Expiration*[1] (Continued)

Item No.	Component	Storage	Transport	Expiration†	Additional Criteria
17	Pooled Platelets Leukocytes Reduced	20-24 C with continuous gentle agitation	As close as possible to 20-24 C‡	4 hours after pooling or 5 days following collection of the oldest unit in the pool‡	Maximum time without agitation: 24 hours
18	Pooled Platelets (in open system)	20-24 C with continuous gentle agitation	As close as possible to 20-24 C‡	Open system: 4 hours	
19	Apheresis Platelets	20-24 C with continuous gentle agitation	As close as possible to 20-24 C‡	24 hours or 5 days, depending on collection system	Maximum time without agitation: 24 hours
20	Apheresis Platelets Irradiated	20-24 C with continuous gentle agitation	As close as possible to 20-24 C‡	No change from original expiration date	Maximum time without agitation: 24 hours
21	Apheresis Platelets Leukocytes Reduced	20-24 C with continuous gentle agitation	As close as possible to 20-24 C‡	Open system: within 4 hours of opening the system Closed system: 5 days	Maximum time without agitation: 24 hours
22	Apheresis Platelets Platelet Additive Solution Added Leukocytes Reduced	20-24 C with continuous gentle agitation	As close as possible to 20-24 C‡	5 days	Maximum time without agitation: 24 hours
Granulocyte Components					
23	Apheresis Granulocytes	20-24 C	As close as possible to 20-24 C	24 hours	Transfuse as soon as possible; Standard 5.28.10 applies
24	Apheresis Granulocytes Irradiated	20-24 C	As close as possible to 20-24 C	No change from original expiration date	Transfuse as soon as possible; Standard 5.28.10 applies
Plasma Components					
25	Cryoprecipitated AHF	≤−18 C	Maintain frozen state	12 months from original collection	Thaw the FFP at 1-6 C Place cryoprecipitate in the freezer within 1 hour after removal from refrigerated centrifuge

26	Cryoprecipitated AHF (after thawing)	20-24 C	As close as possible to 20-24 C	Single unit: 6 hours	Thaw at 30-37 C
27	Pooled Cryoprecipitated AHF (pooled before freezing)	≤-18 C	Maintain frozen state	12 months from earliest date of collection of product in pool	Thaw the FFP at 1-6 C. Place cryoprecipitate in the freezer within 1 hour after removal from refrigerated centrifuge
28	Pooled Cryoprecipitated AHF (after thawing)	20-24 C	As close as possible to 20-24 C	Pooled in an open system: 4 hours. If pooled using a sterile connection device: 6 hours	Thaw at 30-37 C
29	Fresh Frozen Plasma (FFP)◊,¶	≤-18 C or ≤-65 C	Maintain frozen state	≤-18 C: 12 months from collection. ≤-65 C: 7 years from collection	Place in freezer within 8 hours of collection or as stated in FDA-cleared operator's manuals/package inserts. Storage at ≤-65 C requires FDA approval if product is stored >12 months
30	FFP (after thawing)¶	1-6 C	1-10 C	If issued as FFP: 24 hours	Thaw at 30-37 C or using an FDA-cleared device
31	Plasma Frozen Within 24 Hours After Phlebotomy (PF24)◊,¶	≤-18 C	Maintain frozen state	12 months from collection	
32	Plasma Frozen Within 24 Hours After Phlebotomy (after thawing)◊,¶	1-6 C	1-10 C	If issued as PF24: 24 hours	Thaw at 30-37 C or using an FDA-cleared device

(Continued)

TABLE 17-3. Reference Standard 5.1.8A—Requirements for Storage, Transportation, and Expiration*[1] (Continued)

Item No.	Component	Storage	Transport	Expiration[2]	Additional Criteria
33	Plasma Frozen Within 24 Hours After Phlebotomy Held At Room Temperature Up To 24 Hours After Phlebotomy (PF24RT24)◊	≤−18 C	Maintain frozen state	12 months from collection	
34	Plasma Frozen Within 24 Hours After Phlebotomy Held At Room Temperature Up To 24 Hours After Phlebotomy (after thawing)◊	1-6 C	1-10 C	If issued as PF24RT24: 24 hours	Thaw at 30-37 C or using an FDA-cleared device
35	Thawed Plasma¶	1-6 C	1-10 C	5 days from date product was thawed or original expiration, whichever is sooner	Shall have been collected and processed in a closed system
36	Plasma Cryoprecipitate Reduced	≤−18 C	Maintain frozen state	12 months from collection	
37	Plasma Cryoprecipitate Reduced (after thawing)	1-6 C	1-10 C	If issued as Plasma Cryoprecipitate Reduced: 24 hours	Thaw at 30-37 C
38	Thawed Plasma Cryoprecipitate Reduced	1-6 C	1-10 C	If issued as Thawed Plasma Cryoprecipitate Reduced: 5 days from date product was thawed or original expiration, whichever is sooner	Shall have been collected and processed in a closed system
39	Liquid Plasma	1-6 C	1-10 C	5 days after expiration of Whole Blood	21 CFR 610.53(c) applies

40	Recovered Plasma, liquid or frozen	Refer to short supply agreement	Refer to short supply agreement	Refer to short supply agreement	Requires a short supply agreement§

Tissue and Derivatives

41	Tissue	Conform to source manufacturer's written instructions	Conform to manufacturer's written instructions	Conform to manufacturer's written instructions	21 CFR 1271.3(b), 1271.3(bb), and 21 CFR 1271.15(d) apply
42	Derivatives	Conform to manufacturer's written instructions	Conform to manufacturer's written instructions	Conform to manufacturer's written instructions	

*Products may be pathogen reduced if approved by the FDA.

†If the seal is broken during processing, components stored at 1 to 6 C shall have an expiration time of 24 hours, and components stored at 20 to 24 C shall have an expiration time of 4 hours, unless otherwise indicated. This expiration shall not exceed the original expiration date or time.

‡21 CFR 600.15(a).

§21 CFR 601.22.

◊If a liquid freezing bath is used, the container shall be protected from chemical alteration.

¶These lines could apply to apheresis plasma or whole-blood-derived plasma.

policies, processes, and procedures in place to relocate blood and blood components. The secondary storage location may be another on- or off-site refrigerator or freezer, qualified storage boxes, or coolers used with a validated process that has been shown to maintain required storage temperatures during storage. Because the safety, purity, potency, and quality of the blood components could be affected by delays in relocation to a secondary storage location, it is recommended that the relocation occur *before* upper or lower acceptable storage temperatures are exceeded. This can be accomplished by setting the alarm points of the storage devices so that an alarm sounds before the unacceptable temperature limit is reached.

Some facilities may use temperature-monitoring indicators for each blood component container. Such indicators monitor the liquid temperature of the immediate inner bag, not the liquid core temperature in the unit, which may be cooler. Policies, processes, and procedures should specify how the facility will determine the disposition of blood components when using temperature-monitoring indicators.

Specific Considerations

Holding blood components that have been dispensed from the blood bank in other hospital areas before transfusion is considered to be "storage." If the blood components are not kept in a monitored device, they must be stored in containers (eg, boxes or coolers) validated to maintain the correct temperature during storage.

Red Blood Cells

RBC components are stored in plastic bags of different types with a variety of added anticoagulants and additive solutions that modify the cellular and protein environment. The storage temperature must be maintained at 1 to 6 C throughout the duration of storage (Table 17-3).

During storage of RBC units, biochemical and morphologic changes to the red cells occur that have been termed the "storage lesion." These changes include cell membrane shape change and microvesiculation; decreased pH, adenosine triphosphate, and 2,3-diphosphoglycerate; and increased lysophospholipids, potassium, and free hemoglobin.[18] In addition to posttransfusion in-vivo red cell recovery, the red cell storage lesion directly affects how long RBC units may be stored. Product approval by the Food and Drug Administration (FDA) requires in-vivo labeling studies demonstrating that at least 75% of the transfused red cells are present in circulation 24 hours after transfusion with less than 1% hemolysis. Although the in-vitro observations of the storage lesion are well described, there is emerging evidence that red cell storage duration does not correlate with worse clinical outcomes.[19-21] One situation where evidence supports the use of fresher RBC units is large-volume transfusions (>25 mL/kg) in neonates.[22]

Platelets

Platelet metabolic, morphologic, and functional changes associated with storage define the shelf life and storage conditions of platelet components. Metabolic changes include the glycolytic production of lactic acid and the oxidative metabolism of free fatty acids, which results in the production of carbon dioxide. Platelet pH is maintained above 6.2 via buffering of lactic acid by bicarbonate and promotion of oxidative metabolism facilitated by the diffusion of oxygen and carbon dioxide across a gas-permeable storage bag during gentle agitation.[23] The maximum time for platelets to be without agitation is 24 hours (Table 17-3). Platelets are stored at 20 to 24 C. Investigation of cold-stored and cryopreserved platelets is ongoing.

Platelet shelf life is limited also because of an increased risk of bacterial growth due to room-temperature storage. Blood banks and transfusion services are required to have methods to detect or inactivate bacteria in all platelet components.[1(p11)] Recent changes have allowed platelet shelf life to be extended from 5 days to 7 days if the platelets are stored in bags approved for 7-day storage, are stored in 100% plasma, and have screened negative for bacterial contamination with an FDA-approved "safety measure" test. At the time of writing, the shelf life of platelets stored in platelet additive solution or pathogen inactivation systems in the United States cannot exceed 5 days.

Plasma and Cryoprecipitate

Plasma and cryoprecipitate storage conditions and shelf life affect coagulation factor activity.[24,25] Fresh Frozen Plasma (FFP), Plasma Frozen Within 24 Hours After Phlebotomy (PF24), Plasma Frozen Within 24 Hours After Phlebotomy Held At Room Temperature Up To 24 Hours After Phlebotomy (PF24RT24), and Plasma Cryoprecipitate Reduced must be stored at –18 C or colder (Table 17-3). Frozen plasma and cryoprecipitate must be thawed before transfusion as described in the "Pretransfusion Processing" section below.

Granulocytes

Granulocytes are fragile, deteriorate rapidly in vitro, and should be transfused as soon as possible after receipt from the supplier. Granulocytes are stored at 20 to 24 C (Table 17-3), should not be agitated, and must never be leukocyte reduced. In addition, granulocyte components should be irradiated because recipients who require granulocytes are severely immunocompromised.

PRETRANSFUSION PROCESSING

Thawing Plasma and Cryoprecipitate

Frozen plasma (FFP, PF24, PF24RT24, Plasma Cryoprecipitate Reduced) must be thawed at 30 to 37 C using a waterbath or other FDA-approved device. Thawing in a waterbath requires the frozen component to be in a plastic overwrap before insertion into the water to prevent contamination of the container entry ports. Once thawed, plasma is stored at 1 to 6 C and expires 24 hours after thawing (Table 17-3).

Thawed FFP, PF24, and PF24RT24 must be relabeled as "Thawed Plasma" if stored for longer than 24 hours. Although not licensed by the FDA, Thawed Plasma is included in the AABB *Standards for Blood Banks and Transfusion Services*[1(p28)] and the *Circular of Information for the Use of Human Blood and Blood Components.*[25] Thawed Plasma is stored at 1 to 6 C and expires 5 days after it was originally thawed. Facilities may label such components as "Thawed Plasma" at the initial time of thawing. By maintaining a Thawed Plasma inventory, transfusion services may decrease wastage of thawed plasma components and have plasma immediately available for emergent need such as for trauma recipients.[26]

Levels of labile coagulation factors (Factor V and Factor VIII) and stable factors are well above 50% of immediate postthaw levels in Thawed Plasma that has been stored for up to 5 days.[27] Thawed Plasma does, however, contain reduced concentrations of Factor V, Factor VII, and Factor VIII. For this reason, Thawed Plasma is not suitable for single-factor replacement when antihemophilic factor derivatives are unavailable.

Cryoprecipitate is thawed at 30 to 37 C and gently resuspended; it can be pooled for ease of transfusion using small quantities of 0.9% sodium chloride injection (USP) to rinse the contents of the bag into the final container (Method 6-11). Thawed cryoprecipitate is stored at 20 to 24 C and expires within 4 hours of pooling if it is pooled in an open system or within 6 hours for single units or units pooled using an FDA-cleared sterile connecting device.[25]

Thawing and Deglycerolizing RBCs

RBC units may be frozen and stored for up to 10 years following the addition of glycerol as a cryopreservation agent (Methods 6-6 and 6-7).[28,29] Frozen units can be thawed using a 37 C dry heater or 37 C waterbath. After units are thawed, the glycerol must be removed before the component is transfused. Commercial instruments for batch or continuous-flow washing are available for deglycerolization. The manufacturer's instructions should be followed to ensure maximal red cell recovery and minimal hemolysis. Measurement of free hemoglobin in the final wash can be used to confirm adequate free hemoglobin removal and as a surrogate marker for adequate deglycerolization (Method 6-8).

Integrally attached tubing must be filled with the deglycerolized red cells and sealed appropriately so that a segment may be detached and available for crossmatch testing.

The shelf life of Deglycerolized RBCs depends on the type of system used. Closed-system devices allow storage for up to 14 days, while components prepared using open systems expire within 24 hours of the start of the deglycerolization process.

Platelet Gel Production

Platelet gel is produced when thrombin and calcium are added to platelet-rich plasma to produce a glue-like substance for surgical application.[30] This product is typically prepared at the bedside immediately before use. Facilities involved in the production of this component should refer to the current edition of the AABB *Standards for Perioperative Autologous Blood Collection and Administration* for guidance and quality oversight of this manufacturing process.

Irradiation

Irradiation of cellular components is intended to prevent transfusion-associated graft-vs-host disease (TA-GVHD), which is caused by proliferation of donor T lymphocytes. People at increased risk of TA-GVHD include profoundly immunocompromised recipients; recipients of intrauterine transfusion; recipients undergoing marrow, umbilical cord blood, or peripheral blood stem cell transplantation; and recipients of cellular components from blood relatives or donors selected for HLA compatibility or platelet crossmatch compatibility.

Sources of radiation include gamma rays (cesium-137 or cobalt-60 radioisotopes) and x-rays. The required gamma-radiation dose needed to prevent proliferation of donor T lymphocytes in the recipient is a minimum of 25 Gy (2500 cGy/rad) to the central point of the blood container and 15 Gy (1500 cGy/rad) to

any other part of the container. Confirmation that the blood container has received an adequate radiation dose can be achieved with the use of commercially available radiographic film labels.

Irradiation is associated with damage to the red cell membrane, which may result in increases in extracellular free hemoglobin and potassium during component storage. For this reason, the expiration date of irradiated RBCs is 28 days after irradiation or the original expiration date, whichever is earlier.

Hospital transfusion services may purchase irradiated blood components from their supplier or perform irradiation within the blood bank using approved and monitored radiation devices. Hospitals that perform their own irradiation may irradiate their inventory on demand or in batches. Maintenance of a dual inventory (irradiated and nonirradiated) requires policies and procedures to ensure that transfusion recipients receive the appropriate component for their clinical situation.

Poststorage Leukocyte Reduction

Poststorage leukocyte reduction can be performed by the blood bank before issuing a component using a leukocyte reduction filter attached by a sterile connection. It can also be performed at the bedside during transfusion using a blood-administration filter designed for this purpose. Leukocyte reduction filters are designed to remove >99.9% of white cells (3-log reduction) and meet the AABB standard of $<5 \times 10^6$ leukocytes in 95% of sampled units for RBCs and Apheresis Platelets, and $<8.3 \times 10^5$ leukocytes in 95% of sampled units for whole-blood-derived platelets.[1(p24)] The manufacturer's instructions must be followed for the filtration device used to achieve acceptable leukocyte reduction.

Prestorage leukocyte reduction is the preferred method for leukocyte reduction because it prevents accumulation of cytokines during component storage. Quality control of bedside filtration is challenging, and the process has been associated with hypotensive transfusion reactions.[31]

Volume Reduction

Volume reduction results when plasma and additive solutions are partially removed from RBC or platelet components typically following centrifugation. This process may be used to aggressively manage volume in recipients at risk of transfusion-associated circulatory overload, reduce exposure to plasma proteins or additives, or achieve a target hematocrit level.

Volume reduction of platelets is described in Method 6-13. The speed of centrifugation may affect the degree of platelet loss. Higher *g* forces are associated with better platelet retention but raise the theoretical concern of platelet damage and activation as platelets are forced against the container wall. When platelet volumes are reduced, platelets should rest at room temperature for 20 to 60 minutes following centrifugation and before resuspension in remaining plasma or added saline. The manufacturer's instructions must be followed regarding the minimum volume necessary to maintain proper air exchange across the gas-permeable platelet-storage bag. The shelf life of volume-reduced platelets is 4 hours. In addition to centrifugation, RBC components can be volume reduced through settling by gravity overnight with the ports of the unit facing upward and simple removal of the overlying plasma and preservative solution. The shelf life of volume-reduced RBC components is 24 hours.

Washing

Cellular components are typically washed to remove plasma proteins. Washing can also be performed to remove glycerol from frozen RBC units after thawing. Indications for washing RBC or platelet components include a recipient history of severe allergic reactions to components containing plasma, the presence of antibodies against immunoglobulin A (IgA) in an IgA-deficient recipient when IgA-deficient cellular components are not available, the presence of maternal antibodies to human platelet antigen (HPA)-1a (eg, when using maternal blood for a neonatal transfusion), and the need for complement removal for recipients experiencing posttransfusion purpura. RBC units for intrauterine transfusions are typically washed to remove some of the preservative solutions and excess potassium that accumulates during storage.

Washing is accomplished with the use of 1 to 2 L of sterile normal saline (preferably using automated equipment). As with volume reduction, washed platelets should rest at room temperature without agitation between centrifugation and resuspension with normal saline. Up to 20% of the red cell yield or 33% of the platelet yield may be lost during washing. Because washing creates an "open system" and removes anticoagulant-preservative solutions, washed RBC units expire 24 hours after the start of washing, and washed platelet units expire 4 hours after the start of washing. It is recommended that hospitals performing washing comply with the manufacturer's recommendations regarding minimum volumes needed for component storage bags to maintain optimal storage conditions unless the component is used shortly thereafter.

Pooling

Certain blood components (whole-blood-derived platelets, cryoprecipitate, or RBCs and plasma to produce reconstituted Whole Blood) may need to be pooled to provide clinically effective transfusion therapy without the need to transfuse multiple single components.

Pooled whole-blood-derived platelets may contain a significant number of red cells, and therefore ABO compatibility and risk for RhD alloimmunization are recipient factors that must be considered. If whole-blood-derived platelets are pooled using an open system, the expiration time is 4 hours from the start of pooling. A commercially available, FDA-cleared, prestorage, whole-blood-derived platelet pooling system allows storage for up to 5 days and the ability to perform culture-based bacteria testing.[32] When this system is used, the pool maintains the expiration date of the earliest collected component in the pool.

Single cryoprecipitate units are pooled after thawing in a manner similar to that used for platelets (Method 6-11). The expiration time of cryoprecipitate pools depends on the method used for pooling. Cryoprecipitate pooled in an open system expires within 4 hours of the start of pooling. Thawed single concentrates and pooled concentrates using sterile connecting devices expire 6 hours after thawing. Thawed cryoprecipitate is stored at 20 to 24 C. As an alternative, the blood center may pool single concentrates before freezing.

Reconstituted Whole Blood consists of RBCs combined with ABO-compatible plasma. This product can be used for neonatal exchange transfusion. The conventional approach is to combine group O RBCs (Rh compatible with the neonate) and group AB plasma to achieve a 50% ± 5% hematocrit of the final product. The volumes of the two components before pooling can be adjusted to achieve a desired hematocrit level. Following recombination, the product can be stored at 1 to 6 C for up to 24 hours.

Current FDA uniform guidelines should be followed when pooled components are labeled.[33] A unique pool number should be affixed to the final container, and all units in the pool must be documented in electronic or manual records.

Aliquoting

Recipients requiring low-volume transfusions may receive aliquots of smaller volumes derived from the original unit via an FDA-cleared sterile connecting device or integrated transfer bags. Available products designed for use with sterile connecting devices include transfer packs, smaller-volume bags, and tubing with integrally attached syringes.

The expiration date of the aliquot and minimum residual volumes that must be maintained depend on the storage container used. Hospital transfusion services must develop policies and procedures for aliquot preparation and storage that comply with manufacturer specifications. The use of aliquots for neonatal transfusion has been shown to result in a decreased number of donor exposures.[34] The process of preparing aliquots for small-volume transfusion in neonates and children is discussed in greater detail in Chapter 24. Lower-volume components (split units) may also be prepared for adult recipients who require slow rates of transfusion because of concerns about fluid overload. Split units are recommended when the component volume cannot be transfused at a rate that ensures completion of the transfusion within 4 hours.

DISTRIBUTION

Inspection

Inspection is a critical control point in blood component manufacturing and must occur before shipping, upon receipt, and before issue for transfusion. Proper documentation of this process includes 1) date of inspection, 2) DIN, 3) description of any visual abnormalities, 4) action(s) taken, and 5) identity of the staff member performing the inspection. Visible abnormalities may include discoloration of the segments, component, or supernatant fluid or the presence of visible clots, particulate matter, or other foreign bodies. Detection of any such abnormalities should result in component quarantine for further investigation that may include returning the component to the supplier.

If a component is determined to be bacterially contaminated, the component manufacturer must be notified so that an immediate investigation can take place. Other components prepared from that collection should be quarantined until the investigation is complete. If the component (or co-component) has been transfused, the recipient's attending physician should be notified, and consultation with the medical director is recommended.

Shipping

Blood components may be transported between blood centers, between hospitals, and between blood centers and hospitals. All containers used to transport blood components must be qualified before use to ensure that the proper component transport temperature is maintained. The shipping transit time, mode of transport, and climate conditions must also be validated. All components should be inspected upon receipt to confirm appropriate transport conditions, component appearance, and expiration date. Any deviation from routine shipping or component conditions should be reported to the shipping facility and documented according to each location's policies, processes, and procedures.

Whole Blood, RBCs, and Thawed Plasma Components

Whole Blood, RBCs, and thawed plasma components must be transported at a temperature of 1 to 10 C. A variety of options exist for maintaining transport temperature, including bagged wet ice, commercial cooling packs, and specially designed containers. All transport coolers must be qualified to maintain the transport temperature when packed using a validated process.

Blood components transported at 1 to 10 C and stored at 1 to 6 C may need to be temporarily removed from those temperatures for entry into inventory, irradiation, or other processing. The maximum number of units that can be manipulated before the component reaches an unacceptable temperature should be determined and not exceeded. Validation of this process may be accomplished using manual temperature monitoring indicators affixed to the blood components or electronic devices that can measure the temperature of the blood components.

Platelets, Thawed Cryoprecipitate, and Granulocytes

Platelets, thawed cryoprecipitate, and granulocytes must be transported at a temperature as close to 20 to 24 C as possible (Table 17-3). All transport coolers must be qualified to maintain this transport temperature when packed using a validated process. For platelets, the maximum time without agitation is 24 hours.

Frozen Components

Frozen components should be packaged to minimize breakage and maintain a frozen state. Dry ice in a suitable container has historically been used for shipping these components. Recent concerns about shipping with dry ice and CO_2 release in enclosed vehicles has led to the use of dry ice alternatives that can maintain frozen components. Any dry ice alternative should be qualified in the properly packed shipping container. All transport coolers must be qualified to maintain the transport temperature when packed using a validated process.

Receiving

The receiving facility should notify the shipping facility and document any deviation from usual shipping container packing or appearance of the shipped blood components. Any blood component not in compliance with the facility's policies, processes, and procedures should be quarantined. Only after investigation of the deviation and determination that the component meets acceptance criteria may the component be removed from quarantine and released into the general inventory.

Blood components should be fully traceable from collection to final disposition. Electronic or manual records indicating compliance with policies, processes, and procedures should be generated and maintained for the applicable record-retention time. Any deviation must be recorded, and blood components not meeting requirements should be quarantined. Deviations must be investigated to determine appropriate component disposition and possible corrective action. The results of any corrective action should be reported to the blood supplier as needed. Inventory management should consist of routine determination that all blood components are accounted for and transfused or appropriately discarded.

Component Testing

Before transfusion, the ABO group of all units and Rh type of any units labeled "Rh negative" must be confirmed by serologic testing for all red-cell-containing components (RBCs, Whole Blood, and granulocytes). Any typing discrepancies identified must be reported immediately to the supplier and resolved before the component is issued for transfusion.[1(p35)]

Retention and Storage of Donor Samples

IS crossmatch and AHG-phase crossmatch are both performed using the recipient's serum or plasma and donor red cells, which must be obtained from a segment of tubing that was integrally attached to the unit to be transfused.

The recipient's sample and a segment from any red-cell-containing component must be stored at refrigerated temperatures for at least 7 days after each transfusion.[1(p35)] Retaining both the recipient's sample and donor's red cells allows for repeat or additional testing if the recipient has a transfusion reaction. Testing of stored samples should be based on the sample storage limitations in the reagent manufacturer's package insert.

Lack of appropriate storage space may limit the length of time that samples are stored. Institutions that limit the use of pretransfusion recipient samples to those that have been stored for no more than 3 days frequently store these samples for 10 days (ie, 3 days + 7 days). Institutions that permit the testing of pretransfusion samples that have been stored for >3 days need to ensure that each pretransfusion sample is retained for at least 7 additional days after the transfusion for which the sample was used for donor selection.

Donor red cells may be obtained from the remainder of the segment used in the crossmatching or from a segment removed before the blood was issued. If the opened crossmatching segment is saved, it should be placed in a tube labeled with the unit number and then sealed or stoppered.

ISSUING OF COMPONENTS

Donor RBC Unit Selection

The results of compatibility testing, as well as a visual inspection, should guide donor unit selection (see "Transfusion Documentation and Recipient Identification" section below). Compatibility considerations vary according to ABO, Rh, and other blood group status.

ABO Group Compatibility

Whenever possible, recipients should receive ABO-identical blood components; however, it may occasionally be necessary to select alternative components. If the component to be transfused contains ≥2 mL of red cells, the donor's red cells must be ABO compatible with the recipient's plasma.[1(pp37-38)] Because plasma-containing components can also affect the recipient's red cells, anti-A and/or anti-B antibodies in plasma for routine transfusions should be compatible with the recipient's red cells when feasible.[35] Some centers use thawed group A plasma for emergent transfusions because of the relative scarcity of group AB plasma.[36] As a result of frequent platelet shortages, ABO-incompatible platelet components are often transfused. Requirements for components and acceptable alternative choices are summarized in Table 17-2.

Rh Type

D-positive blood components should be routinely selected for D-positive recipients. D-negative units are compatible with D-positive recipients but should be reserved for D-negative recipients. D-negative recipients (especially females of childbearing potential) should receive red-cell-containing components that are D negative to avoid alloimmunization to the D antigen and prevent possible HDFN. When ABO-compatible, D-negative components are not available for a D-negative recipient, the blood bank physician and the recipient's physician should weigh alternative courses of action. The risk of alloimmunization to the D antigen in hospitalized D-negative recipients of D-positive RBC units is approximately 22%, while the incidence of alloimmunization after apheresis platelet transfusion is <2% in the hematology-oncology recipient population.[37,38] Depending on the clinical situation (especially childbearing potential) of the recipient and the volume of red cells transfused, it may be desirable to administer Rh Immune Globulin to a D-negative recipient who is given D-positive blood.[39]

Other Blood Groups

Antigens other than ABO and D are not routinely considered in the selection of units of blood for transfusion to nonalloimmunized recipients. However, for recipients with certain medical conditions, such as sickle cell disease, some institutions may elect to transfuse phenotypically matched RBC units to prevent alloimmunization in a frequently transfused population.[40] One study showed that North American hospital transfusion service laboratories most commonly match for the C, E, and K antigens when phenotype-matched RBCs are transfused to nonalloimmunized recipients with sickle cell disease.[41] Matching for more than three antigens may be of incremental benefit, although sustaining an inventory of such components may be extremely challenging.

If the recipient has clinically significant and unexpected antibody(ies), blood lacking the corresponding antigen(s) should be selected for crossmatching. If there is an adequate quantity of the recipient's serum or if another recipient's serum with the same antibody specificity is available, and if that antibody reacts well with antigen-positive red cells, that serum may be used to screen for antigen-negative donor RBC units. When red cells are found to be antigen negative, this result must be confirmed with an FDA-licensed reagent when such a reagent is available. When licensed reagents are not available (eg, anti-Lan or anti-Yt^a), expired reagents or stored serum samples from recipients or donors may be used, provided that the results of controls tested on the day of use are acceptable.[42] When crossmatch-compatible units cannot be found, the transfusion service's attending physician should be involved in the decision about how to manage the recipient. Antigen-negative donor RBC units are not usually provided for recipients whose antibodies are not clinically significant.

Transfusion Documentation and Recipient Identification

The recipient's medical record must include proper documentation of all transfusions. For each transfusion, this documentation must contain the transfusion order, consent for transfusion, component name, DIN, date and time of transfusion, pre- and posttransfusion vital signs, volume transfused, identification of the transfusionist, and, if applicable, any transfusion-related adverse events.

Ensuring that the correct blood component is transfused to the correct recipient is paramount for transfusion safety. All requests for blood components must contain at least two independent identifiers so that the intended recipient can be uniquely identified. Recipient compatibility-testing records must also be reviewed. Current testing results must be compared with historical records, if available, and any discrepancies must be resolved before component selection.

Personnel must visually inspect and document that the selected component is acceptable for use. This inspection must include confirmation that the component does not have an abnormal color or appearance and that the container is intact. Once selected for transfusion, the blood component must have an attached label or tie tag that contains the intended recipient's two independent identifiers, DIN, and compatibility test result interpretation, if performed. At the time of issue, there must be a final check of each unit that includes the following[1(p42)]:

- The intended recipient's two independent identifiers, ABO group, and Rh type.
- The DIN, donor ABO group, and, if required, Rh type.
- The interpretation of the crossmatch test results, if performed.
- Special transfusion requirements [eg, cytomegalovirus (CMV)-reduced-risk, irradiated, or antigen-negative components], if applicable.
- The expiration date and, if applicable, time.
- The date and time of issue.

The transfusion service must confirm that the recipient identifying information, transfusion request, testing records, and blood component labeling and compatibility are accurate and in agreement. Any discrepancies identified must be resolved before issue. Additional records that may be useful include those that identify the person issuing the blood, the person to whom the blood was issued, and the unit's destination. After the transfusion, a record of the transfusion becomes part of the recipient's permanent electronic or paper medical record. Records must contain the identity of the person(s) performing the crossmatch and, if blood is issued before the resolution of compatibility problems, the final serologic findings.

Final identification of the transfusion recipient and blood component rests with the transfusionist(s). The Joint Commission requires hospitals to use a two-person verification process before initiating a blood or blood component transfusion. If two individuals are not available, an automated ID technology (eg, bar coding) may be used in place of one of the individuals.[43] The individual(s) must identify the recipient and donor unit and certify that the identifying information on forms, tags, and labels are in agreement.

Special Clinical Situations

Emergent Transfusion

When blood is urgently needed, the recipient's physician must weigh the risk of transfusing uncrossmatched or partially compatible blood against the risk of delaying transfusion until compatibility testing is complete or fully compatible blood components are identified. A transfusion service physician should be available for consultation as needed.

If transfusion is deemed medically necessary and blood is released before pretransfusion testing is complete, the records must contain a signed statement from the requesting physician indicating that the clinical situation was sufficiently urgent to require release of blood components before completion of compatibility testing.[1(p43)] Such a statement does not need to be obtained before a lifesaving

transfusion takes place, and it does not absolve blood bank personnel from their responsibility to issue properly labeled donor blood that is ABO compatible with the recipient.

When emergency release is requested, blood bank personnel should take the following actions:

- Issue uncrossmatched group O RBCs if the recipient's ABO group is unknown. It is preferable to give D-negative RBCs if the recipient is a female of childbearing potential, while other recipients may receive group O, D-positive RBCs.
- Issue blood that is ABO and Rh compatible if there has been time to test a current sample.
- Indicate in a conspicuous fashion on the tag or label attached to the unit that compatibility testing was *not* completed at the time the unit was issued.
- Begin compatibility tests and complete them promptly (for massive transfusion, see below). If incompatibility is detected, the recipient's physician and the transfusion service physician should be notified as soon as possible.

Massive Transfusion

There are several different definitions of massive transfusion. In this chapter, "massive transfusion" is defined as the administration of 8 to 10 RBC units in an adult recipient in <24 hours or acute administration of 4 to 5 RBC units within 1 hour. Exchange transfusion of a neonate/infant is also considered a massive transfusion.

Many hospitals have developed massive transfusion protocols to standardize the response to hemorrhage.[44,45] Massive transfusion protocols are designed to rapidly provide blood components in a balanced ratio of plasma and platelets to RBCs, particularly when laboratory testing is not rapid enough to guide transfusion support. Typical ratios of plasma and platelets to RBCs range from 1:2 to 1:1, with evidence that there is no statistically significant difference in recipient survival in the trauma setting if a 1:2 or a 1:1 ratio is used.[46]

Additional studies are needed to clarify whether the use of these protocols is associated with improved recipient outcomes.

To ensure the ability to accurately interpret ABO group testing results, the recipient sample should be obtained for testing as early as possible during massive transfusion. If the recipient ABO group cannot be determined, continued support with group O RBCs is required, and consideration can be given to using A plasma rather than AB plasma. Unexpected and significant usage of group O RBCs in the setting of massive transfusion should be considered when determining component inventory levels. In massive transfusion situations where large amounts of blood may be required, policies may be developed to provide D-positive RBCs to select D-negative recipients, such as all adult males and postmenopausal females.

If possible, in the massive transfusion setting, an abbreviated crossmatch, such as IS crossmatch, should be performed to confirm the ABO compatibility of the units administered. If the recipient has no transfusion testing history, collection of a second sample is recommended to verify the ABO group and Rh type, which may allow for the use of electronic/computer crossmatching. If the recipient qualifies for electronic/computer crossmatching (two separate ABO group and Rh typings, current negative antibody screen, no history of clinically significant antibodies), electronic crossmatching can save significant amounts of time when issuing blood components in an emergency. If a more limited pretransfusion testing protocol is used, the protocol should be described in a written standard operating procedure. The transfusion service should have a policy that addresses compatibility testing in massively transfused recipients, such as abbreviation or omission of crossmatching.[1(p41)]

Blood Administration after Non-Group-Specific Transfusion

Once a sample is received and the recipient's ABO group and Rh type are determined, the recipient can begin receiving transfusions of group-specific components. Group O RBC units stored in additive solution contain minimal residual plasma, which minimizes concerns regarding passive transfusion of anti-A and anti-B. Therefore, switching to ABO-identical RBC components can be done safely, although an occasional recipient may exhibit a transient positive direct antiglobulin test (DAT) result. In some cases, such as when large volumes of RBCs are transfused or small children or infants receive transfusions, passively acquired anti-A and/or anti-B may be detected in the recipient's serum or plasma.[47] If so, transfusion with RBCs that lack the corresponding A and/or B antigen(s) should be continued.

D-negative RBC units should be selected if the recipient is a female of childbearing potential and Rh type is unknown, or if the recipient, regardless of gender, has anti-D or a history of anti-D. In massive transfusion situations where large amounts of blood may be required, policies may be developed to provide D-positive RBCs to select recipients. If a recipient receives blood of an Rh type that is different from that of his or her own blood, it may become difficult to determine the recipient's true Rh type. If there is any question about the recipient's true Rh type, it may be prudent to administer D-negative blood, especially if the recipient is a female of childbearing potential.

INVENTORY MANAGEMENT

General Considerations

A sufficient number of units of varying ABO and Rh specificities should be available to meet routine hospital needs, allow for unanticipated increases in utilization from emergency situations, and minimize component outdating. Factors that influence determination of blood bank component inventory levels include historic usage patterns, outdate rates, and distance from suppliers. Inventory levels should be periodically evaluated in response to institutional changes that may affect component usage, including expansion of inpatient beds or operating rooms; implementation of new surgical procedures; or changes in hospital guidelines or medical practice that may influence transfusion behavior.

The blood bank should also maintain a reserve of universally compatible RBCs for emergency use and have a reliable emergency delivery system to ensure adequate availability of blood components in unexpected situations when demand exceeds supply. A disaster plan should be developed and tested periodically.

Inventory levels should be monitored daily to facilitate timely ordering from blood suppliers and maintain adequate inventory levels. This can be particularly challenging for platelets because of their limited shelf life. Inventory-management plans should also take into consideration desirable inventory levels of special products, such as leukocyte-reduced (ie, CMV-reduced-risk) and irradiated components. Antigen-negative RBC units and HLA-matched/HLA-selected platelets/crossmatched platelets are typically ordered on an as-needed basis from suppliers.

Surgical Blood Ordering Practices

Component outdate rates are influenced by surgical ordering practices. For example, when RBC units are crossmatched for surgical recipients, they are unavailable to other recipients and have a greater likelihood of outdating if the component is not promptly returned to the uncrossmatched inventory. The crossmatch-to-transfusion (C:T) ratio is the number of RBC units crossmatched divided by the number of RBC units actually transfused and is most useful in determining individual physician or specialty-specific ordering practices. When C:T ratios are monitored, a C:T ratio of >2.0 may indicate excessive ordering of crossmatched blood and may identify instances when a preoperative type and screen order is more appropriate.

One approach to reducing excessive C:T ratios is to identify procedures that do not typically require blood, and use this information to develop guidelines for the use of type and screen orders or hold-sample orders (samples that are received in the transfusion service but do not have any testing orders) instead of crossmatch orders. Maximum surgical blood

order schedules (MSBOSs) for common elective procedures can also be developed based on local transfusion utilization patterns.[48] The MSBOS serves as a guideline not only for how many units should be available, but also for which surgical procedures require a type and screen or not. The advent of IS and electronic crossmatching have decreased the utility of MSBOS, and this practice is primarily useful now in hospital transfusion services that lack the ability to perform electronic crossmatching. A discussion with the clinician and the blood bank staff should occur to determine how many units to crossmatch for recipients undergoing elective surgery who are known to have clinically significant alloantibodies and require crossmatch-compatible, antigen-negative blood. If an MSBOS has been established, the transfusion service routinely crossmatches the predicted number of units for each recipient undergoing the designated procedures. Routine orders may need to be modified for recipients with anemia, bleeding disorders, or other conditions in which increased blood use is anticipated. As with other circumstances that require rapid availability of blood components, the transfusion service staff should be prepared to provide additional blood components if the need arises.

Unfortunately, it is not uncommon for an initial pretransfusion sample to be received by the transfusion service laboratory on the morning of a same-day-admission surgical procedure, which gives the laboratory limited time to complete pretransfusion red cell compatibility testing.[49] Up to 9% of type and screen samples may not be tested completely until *after* the recipient's surgery has begun. Such testing may offer the first and only opportunity for a laboratory to determine a recipient's ABO group and Rh type. In addition, approximately 3% of samples received have a serologic finding that requires further investigation.[50] The discovery of a serologic finding requiring further investigation at the last minute may cause dangerous delays in blood availability for a recipient. Thus, each recipient's blood sample should be received in the laboratory in advance of the scheduled procedure, and sufficient time must be available to complete all preoperative pretransfusion testing before surgery begins. Collection of a type-and-screen sample days or even weeks in advance of surgery, with collection of a second sample on the morning of a scheduled surgery, is one approach to mitigate the problem.

Return of Blood Components and Reissue

The transfusion service may receive back into inventory units that meet acceptance specifications. These conditions include the following[1(p43)]:

- The container closure has not been disturbed.
- The component has been maintained at the appropriate temperature.
- At least one sealed segment remains integrally attached to the container, if RBCs.
- Documentation indicates that the component has been inspected and is acceptable for reissue.

Individual-unit temperature indicators or temperature-reading devices can be used to determine the acceptability of components for return to inventory. Blood and blood components may also be transported or stored in qualified containers using a validated process that has been shown to maintain acceptable temperatures for a defined interval. If time frames are used to determine the acceptability of a component's return to inventory, the time frame must be validated by the individual facility. The validation should demonstrate that for the defined period, the appropriate temperature of the component has been maintained.

Components meeting the acceptance criteria may be returned to the general blood inventory and reissued. Components not meeting the acceptance criteria must be quarantined for further investigation or discarded in a biohazard container to prevent inadvertent return to inventory.

KEY POINTS

1. Two independent recipient identifiers are required for pretransfusion samples. The phlebotomist must label each blood sample tube, in the recipient's presence, with the two independent recipient identifiers and the date of collection.
2. Laboratory personnel must confirm that the information on the pretransfusion testing sample label and the information on the pretransfusion testing request are in agreement. If there is any doubt about the identity of the recipient or about the labeling of the sample, a new sample must be obtained.
3. Pretransfusion testing, including ABO group, Rh type, antibody detection, and crossmatching, is performed in order to prevent transfusion of incompatible RBCs. ABO and Rh test results on a current sample must be compared with previous transfusion service records if available. Discrepant ABO group results should be resolved before blood is given. If transfusion is necessary before resolution, the recipient should receive group O RBCs.
4. If a recipient has been pregnant or transfused within the previous 3 months, or if the pregnancy history and transfusion history are uncertain, the pretransfusion sample used for testing must be no more than 3 days old at the time of intended transfusion, because recent transfusion or pregnancy may stimulate production of unexpected antibodies.
5. At the time of blood component issue, labeling information must be complete and be checked against blood bank records. Any discrepancies identified must be resolved before components are issued or transfused.
6. Visual inspection of the blood component is a critical control point in the manufacturing process and must occur before labeling, before shipping, upon receipt, and before issue for transfusion.

7. Refrigerators, freezers, and platelet incubators for blood component storage must be monitored to ensure that proper storage conditions are maintained. Because the safety, purity, potency, and quality of the blood components may be affected by improper storage, alarm settings should be configured to notify necessary personnel *before* the upper or lower acceptable storage temperatures are exceeded.

8. Temperature requirements during transport of blood components differ from those during storage. Blood components held outside the blood bank before transfusion are considered to be in storage. Validated processes must ensure that acceptable storage temperatures are maintained.

9. Acceptable time frames for returning blood components to inventory after issue should be validated by individual facilities. Individual-unit temperature indicators or temperature-reading devices may be used to determine component acceptability for return to inventory.

10. Thawed FFP, PF24, and PF24RT24 expire within 24 hours of thawing. These components may be labeled as "Thawed Plasma" to allow for a 5-day shelf life (from the date the component was thawed) if they were originally collected in a closed system.

REFERENCES

1. Ooley PW, ed. Standards for blood banks and transfusion services. 30th ed. Bethesda, MD: AABB, 2016.
2. Linden JV, Wagner K, Voytovich AE, Sheehan J. Transfusion errors in New York state: An analysis of 10 years' experience. Transfusion 2000; 40:1207-13.
3. Bolton-Maggs PH, Wood EM, Wiersum-Osselton JC. Wrong blood in tube—potential for serious outcomes: Can it be prevented? Br J Haematol 2015;168:3-13.
4. Figueroa PI, Ziman A, Wheeler C, et al. Nearly two decades using the check-type to prevent ABO incompatible transfusions: One institution's experience. Am J Clin Pathol 2006;126: 422-6.
5. Knels R, Ashford P, Bidet F, et al for the Task Force on RFID of the Working Party on Information Technology; International Society of Blood Transfusion. Guidelines for the use of RFID technology in transfusion medicine. Vox Sang 2010;98(Suppl 2):1-24.
6. Askeland RW, McGrane S, Levitt JS, et al. Improving transfusion safety: Implementation of a comprehensive computerized bar code-based tracking system for detecting and preventing errors. Transfusion 2008;48:1308-17.
7. Murphy MF, Fraser E, Miles D, et al. How do we monitor hospital transfusion practice using an end-to-end electronic transfusion management system? Transfusion 2012;52:2502-12.
8. Lumadue JA, Boyd JS, Ness PM. Adherence to a strict specimen-labeling policy decreases the incidence of erroneous blood grouping of blood bank specimens. Transfusion 1997; 37:1169-72.
9. Coombs RRA, Mourant AE, Race RR. A new test for the detection of weak and "incomplete" Rh agglutinins. Br J Exp Pathol 1945;26:255-66.
10. Shulman IA. When should antibody screening tests be done for recently transfused recipients? Transfusion 1990;30:39-41.
11. Boisen ML, Collins RA, Yazer MH, Waters JH. Pretransfusion testing and transfusion of uncrossmatched erythrocytes. Anesthesiology 2015;122:191-5.
12. Ramsey G, Smietana SJ. Long-term follow-up testing of red cell alloantibodies. Transfusion 1994;34:122-4.
13. Hendrickson JE, Hillyer CD. Noninfectious serious hazards of transfusion. Anesth Analg 2009;108:759-69.
14. Shulman IA, Odono V. The risk of overt acute hemolytic transfusion reaction following the use of an immediate-spin crossmatch. Transfusion 1994;34:87-8.
15. Shulman IA, Calderon C. Effect of delayed centrifugation or reading on the detection of ABO incompatibility by the immediate-spin crossmatch. Transfusion 1991;31:197-200.
16. Mazepa MA, Raval JS, Park YA; Education Committee of the Academy of Clinical Laboratory Physicians and Scientists. Pathology consultation on electronic crossmatch. Am J Clin Pathol 2014;141:618-24.
17. Nunes E. Transport versus storage: What is the difference? AABB News 2013;15(2):4-5.

18. Klein HG, Spahn DR, Carson JL. Red blood cell transfusion in clinical practice. Lancet 2007; 370:415-26.

19. Fergusson DA, Hebert P, Hogan DL, et al. Effect of fresh red blood cell transfusions on clinical outcomes in premature, very-low-birth-weight infants: The ARIPI randomized trial. JAMA 2012;308:1443-51.

20. Lacroix J, Hebert P, Fergusson DA, et al. Age of transfused blood in critically ill adults. N Engl J Med 2015;372:1410-18.

21. Steiner ME, Ness PM, Assmann SF, et al. Effects of red-cell storage duration on recipients undergoing cardiac surgery. N Engl J Med 2015; 372:1419-29.

22. Strauss RG. Data-driven blood banking practices for neonatal RBC transfusions. Transfusion 2000;40:1528-40.

23. Shrivastava M. The platelet storage lesion. Transfus Apher Sci 2009;41:105-13.

24. Scott E, Puca K, Heraly JC, et al. Evaluation and comparison of coagulation factor activity in fresh-frozen plasma and 24-hour plasma at thaw and after 120 hours of 1 to 6 C storage. Transfusion 2009;49:1584-91.

25. AABB, American Red Cross, America's Blood Centers, Armed Services Blood Program. Circular of information for the use of human blood and blood components. Bethesda, MD: AABB, 2017.

26. Werhli G, Taylor NE, Haines, AL, et al. Instituting a thawed plasma procedure: It just makes sense and saves cents. Transfusion 2009;49: 2625-30.

27. Tholpady A, Monson J, Radovancevic R, et al. Analysis of prolonged storage on coagulation Factor (F)V, FVII, and FVIII in thawed plasma: Is it time to extend the expiration date beyond 5 days? Transfusion 2013;53:645-50.

28. Meryman HT, Hornblower M. A method for freezing and washing RBCs using a high glycerol concentration. Transfusion 1972;12:145-56.

29. Valeri CR, Ragno G, Pivacek LE, et al. A multicenter study of in vitro and in vivo values in human RBCs frozen with 40-percent (wt/vol) glycerol and stored after deglycerolization for 15 days at 4 degrees C in AS-3: Assessment of RBC processing in the ACP 215. Transfusion 2001;41:933-9.

30. Borzini P, Mazzucco L. Platelet gels and releasates. Curr Opin Hematol 2005;12:473-9.

31. Cyr M, Hume H, Sweeney JD, et al. Anomaly of the des-Arg9-bradykinin metabolism associat-ed with severe hypotensive reactions during blood transfusions: A preliminary report. Transfusion 1999;39:1084-8.

32. Benjamin RJ, Kline L, Dy BA, et al. Bacterial contamination of whole-blood-derived platelets: The introduction of sample diversion and prestorage pooling with culture testing in the American Red Cross. Transfusion 2008;48: 2348-55.

33. Food and Drug Administration. Guidance: Industry consensus standard for the uniform labeling of blood and blood components using ISBT 128 version 2.0.0, November 2005. (September 22, 2006) Silver Spring, MD: CBER Office of Communication, Outreach, and Development, 2006.

34. Liu EA, Mannino FL, Lane TA. Prospective, randomized trial of the safety and efficacy of a limited donor exposure transfusion program for premature neonates. J Pediatr 1994;125:92-6.

35. Fung M, Downes KA, Shulman IA. Transfusion of platelets containing ABO-incompatible plasma: A survey of 3,156 North American laboratories. Arch Pathol Lab Med 2007;131:909-16.

36. Dunbar NM, Yazer MH; Biomedical Excellence for Safer Transfusion Collaborative. A possible new paradigm? A survey-based assessment of the use of thawed group A plasma for trauma resuscitation in the United States. Transfusion 2016;56:125-9.

37. Yazer MH, Triulzi DJ. Detection of anti-D in D-recipients transfused with D+ red blood cells. Transfusion 2007;47:2197-201.

38. Cid J, Lozano M, Ziman A, et al. Low frequency of anti-D alloimmunization following D+ platelet transfusion: The Anti-D Alloimmunization after D-incompatible Platelet Transfusions (ADAPT) study. Br J Haematol 2015;168: 598-603.

39. Pollack W, Ascari WQ, Crispen JF, et al. Studies on Rh prophylaxis II: Rh immune prophylaxis after transfusion with Rh-positive blood. Transfusion 1971;11:340-4.

40. Afenyi-Annan A, Brecher ME. Pre-transfusion phenotype matching for sickle cell disease recipients. Transfusion 2004;44:619-20.

41. Osby M, Shulman IA. Phenotype matching of donor red blood cell units for nonalloimmunized sickle cell disease recipients: A survey of 1182 North American laboratories. Arch Pathol Lab Med 2005;129:190-3.

42. Food and Drug Administration. Compliance Program guidance manual. Chapter 42 - Blood and Blood Products. Silver Spring, MD: FDA, 2013. [Available at http://www.fda.gov/downloads/BiologicsBloodVaccines/Guidance ComplianceRegulatoryInformation/Compli anceActivities/Enforcement/CompliancePro grams/UCM239615.pdf (accessed February 9, 2017).]

43. 2017 National patient safety goals. Oakbrook Terrace, IL: The Joint Commission, 2017. [Available at http://www.jointcommission. org/standards_information/npsgs.aspx (accessed February 9, 2017).]

44. Young PP, Cotton BA, Goodnough LT. Massive transfusion protocols for recipients with substantial hemorrhage. Transfus Med Rev 2011; 25:293-303.

45. Hendrickson JE, Shaz BH, Pereira G, et al. Implementation of a pediatric trauma massive transfusion protocol: One institution's experience. Transfusion 2012;52:1228-36.

46. Holcomb JB, Tilley BC, Baraniuk S, et al. Transfusion of plasma, platelets, and red blood cells in a 1:1:1 vs a 1:1:2 ratio and mortality in recipients with severe trauma: The PROPPR randomized clinical trial. JAMA 2015;313:471-82.

47. Garratty G. Problems associated with passively transfused blood group alloantibodies. Am J Clin Pathol 1998;109:169-77.

48. Boral LI, Dannemiller FJ, Standard W, et al. A guideline for anticipated blood usage during elective surgical procedures. Am J Clin Pathol 1979;71:680-4.

49. Friedberg RC, Jones BA, Walsh MK. Type and screen completion for scheduled surgical procedures: A College of American Pathologists Q-Probes study of 8941 type and screen tests in 108 institutions. Arch Pathol Lab Med 2003; 127:533-40.

50. Saxena S, Nelson JM, Osby M, et al. Ensuring timely completion of type and screen testing and the verification of ABO/Rh status for elective surgical recipients. Arch Pathol Lab Med 2007;131:576-81.

● **APPENDIX 17-1**
Sources of False-Positive Results in Antiglobulin Testing

Cells Agglutinated Before Washing

If potent agglutinins are present, agglutinates may not disperse during washing. Observe red cells before the addition of antihuman globulin (AHG) or use a control tube and substitute saline for AHG. Reactivity before the addition of AHG or in the saline control invalidates AHG results.

Particles of Contaminants

Dust or dirt in glassware may cause clumping (not agglutination) of red cells. Fibrin or precipitates in test serum may produce red cell clumps that mimic agglutination.

Improper Procedures

Overcentrifugation may pack cells so tightly that they do not easily disperse and they appear to be positive.

Centrifugation of the sample with polyethylene glycol or positively charged polymers before washing may create clumps that do not disperse.

Cells That Have a Positive Direct Antiglobulin Test (DAT) Result

Cells that are positive by DAT will be positive in any indirect antiglobulin test. Procedures for removing IgG from DAT-positive cells are given in Methods 2-20 and 2-21.

Complement

Complement components, primarily C4, may bind to cells from clots or from citrate-phosphate-dextrose-adenine-1 donor segments during storage at 4 C and occasionally at higher temperatures. For DAT, use red cells anticoagulated with EDTA, acid-citrate-dextrose, or citrate-phosphate-dextrose.

Samples collected in tubes containing silicone gel may have spurious complement attachment.[1]

Complement may attach to red cells in samples collected from infusion lines used to administer dextrose-containing solutions. Reactions are strongest when large-bore needles are used or sample volume is <0.5 mL.[2]

1. Geisland JR, Milam JD. Spuriously positive direct antiglobulin tests caused by silicone gel. Transfusion 1980;20:711-13.
2. Grindon AJ, Wilson MJ. False-positive DAT caused by variables in sample procurement. Transfusion 1981;21:313-14.

● **APPENDIX 17-2**
Sources of False-Negative Results in Antiglobulin Testing

Neutralization of Antihuman Globulin (AHG) Reagent
Neutralization of AHG reagent may result from failure to wash cells adequately to remove all serum or plasma. Fill tube at least three-quarters full of saline for each wash. Check volume dispensed by automated washers.
If increased serum volumes are used, routine washing may be inadequate. Wash additional times or remove serum before washing.
The AHG might be contaminated by extraneous protein. Using contaminated droppers or the wrong reagent dropper can neutralize an entire bottle of AHG. Do not use a finger or hand to cover the tube.
If the concentration of IgG paraproteins in test serum is high, protein may remain even after multiple washes.[1]

Interruption in Testing
Bound IgG may dissociate from red cells and leave too little IgG to detect or neutralize AHG reagent.
Agglutination of IgG-coated red cells will weaken. Centrifuge and read results immediately.

Improper Reagent Storage
AHG reagent may lose reactivity if it is frozen.
Excessive heat or repeated freezing or thawing may cause loss of reactivity of test serum.
Reagent red cells may lose antigen strength during storage. Other subtle cell changes may cause loss of reactivity.

Improper Procedures
Overcentrifugation may pack red cells so tightly that the agitation required to resuspend red cells breaks up agglutinates. Undercentrifugation may not be optimal for agglutination.
Failure to add test serum, enhancement medium, or AHG may cause a negative test result.
Red cell suspensions that are too heavy may mask weak agglutination. Suspensions that are too light may be difficult to read.
Improper or insufficient serum:cell ratios can adversely affect results.

Complement
Rare antibodies, notably some anti-Jk^a or anti-Jk^b, may be detected only when polyspecific AHG is used and active complement is present.

Saline
The low pH of saline solution can decrease the sensitivity of the test.[2] The optimal pH of saline wash solution for most antibodies is 7.0 to 7.2.
Some antibodies may require saline to be at a specific temperature to retain antibody on the cell. Use 37 C or 4 C saline.

1. Ylagen ES, Curtis BR, Wildgen ME, et al. Invalidation of antiglobulin tests by a high thermal amplitude cryoglobulin. Transfusion 1990;30:154-7.
2. Rolih S, Thomas R, Fisher E, Talbot J. Antibody detection errors due to acidic or unbuffered saline. Immunohematology 1993;9:15-18.

● **APPENDIX 17-3**
Causes of Positive Pretransfusion Test Results*

Negative Antibody Screening Result and Incompatible Immediate-Spin Crossmatch
Donor red cells are ABO incompatible.
Donor red cells are polyagglutinable.
Anti-A_1 is in the serum of an individual with A_2 or A_2B.
Other alloantibodies (eg, anti-M) are reactive at room temperature.
Rouleaux have formed.
Autoantibodies (eg, anti-I) are cold.
Anti-A or anti-B has been passively acquired.
Negative Antibody Screen Result and Incompatible Antiglobulin Crossmatch
Donor red cells have a positive direct antiglobulin test result.
Antibody is reactive only with red cells having strong expression of a particular antigen (eg, dosage) or variation in antigen strength (eg, P1).
An antibody to a low-incidence antigen is present on the donor red cells.
Anti-A or anti-B has been passively acquired.
Positive Antibody Screen Result and Compatible Crossmatches
Autoanti-IH (-H) or anti-Le^{bH} and non-group-O units are selected.
Antibodies are dependent on the reagent red cell diluent used.
Antibodies demonstrating dosage and donor red cells are from heterozygotes (ie, expressing a single dose of antigen).
Donor unit lacks corresponding antigen.
Positive Antibody Screen Result, Incompatible Crossmatches, and Negative Autocontrol
Alloantibody(ies) are present.
Positive Antibody Screen Result, Incompatible Crossmatches, Positive Autocontrol, and Negative Direct Antiglobulin Test Result
An antibody is present to an ingredient in the enhancement media or enhancement-dependent autoantibody.
Rouleaux have formed.
Positive Antibody Screen Result, Incompatible Crossmatches, Positive Autocontrol, and Positive Direct Antiglobulin Test Result
Alloantibody causes a delayed serologic or hemolytic transfusion reaction.
Passively acquired autoantibody (eg, intravenous immune globulin) is present.
Cold- or warm-reactive autoantibody is present.

*Causes depend on serologic methods used.

Chapter 18

Administration of Blood Components

• ● •

Melanie Jorgenson, RN, BSN, LSSGB

T HE SAFE ADMINISTRATION of blood and its components requires a multidisciplinary collaboration among clinical and ancillary services and clinicians. Policies and procedures should be developed with input from transfusionists, the transfusion service, surgeons, anesthesiology care providers, primary-care physicians, and transport personnel. The transfusionist typically provides the last line of defense in the detection of errors before the transfusion commences. All personnel involved in preparing, delivering, and administering a transfusion should be given appropriate training to ensure the provision of the safest transfusion possible.

EVENTS AND CONSIDERATIONS BEFORE DISPENSING COMPONENTS

Before a transfusion begins, thoughtful consideration, planning, and preparation are required. The following areas will be discussed in detail throughout this chapter.

1. Recipient consent.
2. Recipient education and history.
3. Baseline assessment of recipient.
4. Order for blood component and administration.
5. Pretransfusion sample.
6. Preparation of ordered units for transfusion.
7. Prophylactic medications.
8. Equipment.
9. Intravenous (IV) access.
10. Readiness to transfuse.
11. Delivery of blood components.
12. Infusion sets and compatible IV solutions.
13. Recipient and other verifications at the time of administration.
14. Rates of transfusion.
15. Monitoring during the transfusion.
16. Suspected transfusion reactions.
17. Documentation of the transfusion.
18. Unique transfusion settings.

Recipient Consent

The AABB *Standards for Blood Banks and Transfusion Services (Standards)* states, "The blood bank or transfusion service medical di-

Melanie Jorgenson, RN, BSN, LSSGB, Client Delivery Lead, Accumen, San Diego, California
The author has disclosed no conflicts of interest.

rector shall participate in the development of policies, processes, and procedures regarding recipient consent for transfusion."[1(p44)] Recipient informed consent should address indications for; risks, benefits, and possible side effects of; and alternatives to transfusions of allogeneic blood components. Some state laws require certain additional elements in the recipient consent.

The recipient has the right to choose or refuse a transfusion and must have an opportunity to ask questions of a learned professional before providing consent. Documentation of the consent process must be entered into the recipient's medical record. Some facilities require an institution-approved signed consent form to document that the consent process has occurred and that the risks, benefits, and alternatives of transfusion were discussed with the recipient or legal representative. Each institution should have a process for recording a patient's refusal to receive blood or blood components in the patient's medical record. Institutional policies should identify healthcare providers who are allowed to obtain consent and the length of time and range of patient care (eg, in- and outpatient) for which a consent remains valid.

Consent for transfusion must be obtained from patients who have the requisite capacity to make such decisions. If a patient is unable to give consent, a legally authorized representative or surrogate may do so (depending on local and state laws). If no one is available to provide consent and the need for transfusion is considered a medical emergency, the blood component may be administered based on the doctrine of implied consent. Individual state and local laws governing requirements for implied consent may vary, but the emergent need for transfusion should be carefully documented in the medical record.[2] Informed consent for transfusion may or may not include the name of the health-care provider who obtained consent, but the hospital policy may require that the consenter include an entry into the medical record that documents the conversation.

Recipient Education and History

The transfusionist should educate the recipient about reporting any symptoms that may be indicative of a reaction and how long the transfusion will take. The recipient's questions should be answered before the transfusion is started. It is important to collect a history from the recipient before the component is ordered to assess whether the recipient is at increased risk of a transfusion reaction. This history includes previous transfusions and any adverse reactions. If the recipient has had previous reactions to transfusion, the medical team should determine whether the recipient needs to receive prophylactic medications before the transfusion or whether special processing of the component is indicated to mitigate the risk of an adverse reaction.

Baseline Assessment of Recipient

A baseline physical assessment should include measurement of vital signs that include blood pressure, heart rate, temperature, and respirations. Many institutions also routinely measure oxygen saturation using oximetry. The pretransfusion assessment should include symptoms, such as shortness of breath, rash, pruritus, wheezing, and chills, as a basis for comparison after the transfusion is initiated.

A recipient with renal or cardiopulmonary disease may require a slower infusion rate to prevent fluid overload. A patient with an elevated temperature may destroy cellular components at an increased rate.[3] Moreover, if the patient presents with an elevated temperature before the transfusion, it may be difficult to determine later whether an additional increase in temperature was caused by a transfusion reaction. Administration of an antipyretic should be considered in such cases.

Order for Blood Component and Administration

A licensed provider often writes two orders for the components to be administered. The first order requests appropriate laboratory testing and preparation of the ordered blood component and notes special processing requirements. The second order explains to the transfusionist how to administer the components, including the transfusion rate. Both of these orders should specify:

- Recipient name and other independent identifier (eg, date of birth or medical record number).
- Component [eg, Red Blood Cells (RBCs) or Apheresis Platelets] to prepare or to administer.
- Special processing required (eg, leukocyte reduction, irradiation, or washing).
- Number of units or volume to administer.
- Date and time for the infusion.
- Flow rate or period for administering the component.
- Indication for transfusion.

Note: It is appropriate for the rate and duration of the transfusion (eg, not to exceed 4 hours from the time that the container is entered until completion)[4] to be described in a policy approved by the hospital's medical staff.

When the health-care team is considering transfusion, several orders may be written by the health-care provider. To prepare for a possible transfusion, there may be laboratory testing, including ABO/Rh testing, type and screen, or type and crossmatch. To administer the intended blood components, administration orders are written. The transfusionist has the responsibility, as with any other order, to critically think through the order. As with medication orders, the transfusionist must determine that the orders are for the right recipient, for the right product, for the right reasons, in the right amount, at the appropriate rate. The ordering provider and the transfusionist should also ensure that the order does not conflict with any facility-specific transfusion guidelines. If the transfusionist has concern about any of these areas, a conversation with the ordering provider is essential before carrying out the order.

Pretransfusion Sample

In nonemergent situations, a pretransfusion blood sample is required before all RBC trans-

fusions. In some hospitals where a historical ABO type is known, a pretransfusion sample might not be required for plasma and platelet transfusions, which do not require a crossmatch except in rare cases (excessively bloody unit of platelets). In emergent cases, blood components may be dispensed, and retrospective testing may be performed once sample collection can be achieved. Typically, the sample is obtained within 3 days of transfusion, with the draw date considered to be day 0.[1(p36)] Institutional policies may vary regarding the sample outdate. If the recipient has not had a transfusion or been pregnant in the preceeding 90 days, the sample may be acceptable for longer than 3 days for testing purposes.

According to The Joint Commission, containers used for blood specimens must be labeled in the presence of the recipient.[5] The sample must be labeled at the recipient's side with at least two unique identifiers (eg, the recipient's name, date of birth, or identification number). The identification of the person collecting the sample and the date on which the sample was collected must be traceable.[1(p35)]

All those involved in the pretransfusion sample collection and recipient verification must be taught that their utmost attention is absolutely necessary to avoid mislabeling of samples that may lead to ABO mismatches with potentially fatal outcomes. In some institutions, computer-assisted positive patient identification and collection of confirmatory ABO samples are additional methods used to further mitigate patient identification errors.

Preparation of Ordered Units for Transfusion

Pretransfusion testing of the recipient's blood sample, including evaluation for unexpected antibodies to red cell antigens, is described in detail in Chapters 13 and 17. The time interval from sample receipt to availability of the requested component can vary greatly. A positive antibody screen requires further investigation, and the time to definitive identification of clinically significant red cell antibodies extends the time it takes to complete the testing. If clinically significant red cell antibodies are present, identification of corresponding antigen-negative or crossmatch-compatible units may require additional time, especially when external suppliers must be consulted to locate an appropriate unit. For recipients with multiple or rare antibodies, additional hours and sometimes days may be required to find a crossmatch-compatible unit. If the need for transfusion is urgent, the ordering licensed provider must weigh the risks and benefits of administering least-incompatible or uncrossmatched units, ideally in consultation with the transfusion service's medical staff.

Some components require thawing, pooling, relabeling, or other preparation before release. All of these factors necessitate timely communication between transfusion service staff and transfusionists. Components that are pooled or require thawing may also have a shortened shelf life after being prepared (4-24 hours); transfusionists should be made aware when the time available to complete a transfusion of such components is decreased.[1(pp51-59)]

Prophylactic Medications Given Before Transfusion

Although antipyretics (eg, acetaminophen) are commonly ordered to reduce the risk of febrile nonhemolytic transfusion reactions (FNHTRs), indications for their use are controversial.[6] Some providers use antipyretics routinely in a prophylactic manner, some order them prophylactically only after the recipient has experienced at least one febrile transfusion reaction, and others believe that prophylactic use of antipyretics may mask the elevated temperature that results from a transfusion reaction.

Recent evidence indicates that use of premedication does not minimize transfusion-related reactions. Leukocyte reduction was found to reduce the incidence of febrile reactions but not allergic reactions.[7] Some experts recommend that "in the absence of definitive evidence-based studies, pretransfusion medication to prevent transfusion reactions should not be encouraged."[6]

In a Cochrane review[7] of studies on premedication to prevent allergic reactions and FNHTRs, the authors stated that current evidence from three randomized controlled trials (RCTs) involving 462 recipients indicated that no pretransfusion medication regimen reduces the risk of allergic reaction or FNHTR. However, the conclusion is based on the evidence from a review of three trials of low to moderate quality. A better-powered RCT is necessary to evaluate the role of pretransfusion medication in the prevention of allergic reactions and FNHTR.

Antihistamines (diphenhydramine and/or H2 blockers) may be ordered as premedication for individuals who have had allergic reactions to transfusions in the past. Meperidine or corticosteroids are occasionally ordered for recipients who have experienced severe rigors during transfusion.[8] Corticosteroids have also been used to premedicate recipients who have had prior anaphylactoid reactions or recurrent FNHTRs. Significant time is required for the onset of corticosteroid immunosuppression. The efficacy of premedication with corticosteroids has not been adequately assessed, and the optimal timing and efficacy of corticosteroids have not been established in the transfusion setting.[9,10]

If premedication is required, it should be administered before obtaining the component from the transfusion service. Oral premedications should be administered 30 minutes before the start of the transfusion. Intravenous medications should be given 10 minutes before the transfusion is initiated.

Equipment

Blood Warmers

Infusions of cold components can cause hypothermia and cardiac complications, increasing morbidity and mortality.[11] The likelihood of clinically important hypothermia is increased when blood is transfused through a central venous device directly into the right atrium.

Blood warmers are rarely needed during routine transfusions. However, they are used when rapid transfusion of components is required, especially in trauma or surgery settings. Blood warmers are also advantageous during transfusions to neonates, where hypothermia can cause serious adverse effects. Opinions vary on the utility of blood warmers in recipients with cold agglutinins.[12,13]

AABB *Standards*[1(p6)] states that "warming devices shall be equipped with a temperature-sensing device and a warning system to detect malfunctions and prevent hemolysis or other damage to blood or blood components." Warming blood to temperatures >42 C may cause hemolysis.[14] The transfusion service should collaborate with departments that use blood warmers to ensure that the devices are approved by the Food and Drug Administration (FDA) for infusion of components. Warming devices should be validated; maintenance and testing of alarms should be performed according to the manufacturer's suggestions. Blood components should not be warmed by placing them in a microwave, on a heat source, or in hot water, or by using devices that are not approved by the FDA specifically for blood warming.

Infusion Systems

Infusion pumps or systems are used to administer fluids, medications, blood, and blood components through clinically accepted routes of administration. These devices allow for a controlled infusion rate over a desired period; they also provide an alarm system to notify clinicians of problems with the infusion. Consequently, the use of infusion pumps or systems may be preferred over simple gravity-based administration. However, there is a potential for hemolysis of the cellular components infused through these pumps. The manufacturer of the pump should be consulted to determine whether the pump is approved for the infusion of blood components. If it is not approved, the institution should establish a validation plan to confirm that the pump will not damage cellular components before their use. The majority of infusion devices require the use of a compatible blood administration set with an in-line filter.

Syringe Infusion Pumps

A syringe infusion pump may be used for small-volume transfusions to neonatal or pediatric recipients. The transfusion service should have established policies for preparing blood in syringes for administration. For more details, see Chapter 24.

Pressure Devices

The use of an externally applied pneumatic pressure device may achieve flow rates of 70 to 300 mL per minute, depending on the pressure applied. The device should have a gauge to monitor the pressure, which should be applied evenly over the entire bag. Any pressure >300 mm Hg may cause the seams of the blood component bag to leak or rupture. When a pressure device is used, a large-gauge cannula should be employed to prevent hemolysis.

The application of an external pressure device to the blood bag to expedite the transfusion of RBC units causes minimal damage to the red cells and is a safe practice in the majority of recipients.[15] However, the use of pressure devices has been reported to provide only a small increase in component flow rates. When rapid infusion is desired, an increase in IV catheter cannula size typically provides better results.

Availability of Emergency Equipment

The transfusionist should be prepared to obtain and initiate emergency interventions when needed. Items used to respond to a transfusion reaction include the following:

- A 0.9% sodium chloride IV solution and administration set to keep an IV line open.
- Medications to treat a reaction, along with a mechanism to obtain emergency medications prescribed to treat the sequelae of transfusion reactions.
- A mechanism to activate emergency resuscitation measures in the event of a severe reaction.
- Ventilatory assistance and an oxygen source.

Intravenous Access

Acceptable IV catheter sizes for use in transfusing cellular blood components range from 22 to 14 gauge.[16,17] A 20- to 18-gauge IV catheter is suitable for the general adult population and provides adequate flow rates without excessive discomfort to the recipient. When an infant or a toddler is transfused, a 25- to 24-gauge IV catheter may be suitable, but a constant flow rate using an infusion device should be applied.[18] (See Chapter 24.)

When using smaller-gauge catheters, it is recommended that the rate be slowed. The pressure or force used during the transfusion is more likely than the needle gauge to cause hemolysis of red cells.[19]

In some circumstances when IV access cannot be achieved, intraosseous infusions may be warranted.

Readiness to Transfuse

After notification that the ordered units are available, in order to reduce the time the blood component is outside of the controlled laboratory environment, the transfusionist should request components for delivery to the patient location only after the following items have been addressed:

1. The ordered component is available.
2. Informed consent for transfusion has been completed and documented.
3. IV access is available, patent, and appropriate for transfusion.
4. The ordering provider's order is appropriate for the clinical situation of the recipient.
5. A transfusionist or an appropriate designee is available to properly monitor the recipient throughout the transfusion in accordance with the institutional policy.
6. The recipient has received any ordered prophylactic medications.
7. The necessary equipment is available and functioning.

Occasionally, despite the best attempts at planning, the blood component arrives at the patient's bedside but there is a significant delay in the start of transfusion due to unanticipated circumstances. There should be a process for prompt return of the blood component. Transfusion services should ensure that other departments of the hospital are aware of the requirement for returning components if a transfusion is delayed.

BLOOD COMPONENT TRANSPORTATION AND DISPENSING

There must be a process to correctly identify the intended recipient and component at the time of the request to issue the component. To verify that the correct unit is being issued to the correct recipient, transfusion services should allow the issue of only 1 unit at a time unless it is an emergent or large-volume transfusion. Upon dispensation, a final clerical check of transfusion service records with each unit or component must be performed. Verification must include[1(p42)]:

1. The type of component (red cells, plasma, platelets, cryoprecipitate, granulocytes).
2. The intended recipient's two independent identifiers (name, date of birth, or recipient identification number and/or unique identifier given at the time the crossmatch sample is drawn), ABO group, and Rh type.
3. The donation identification number (DIN), donor ABO group, and if required, donor Rh type.
4. The interpretation of results of crossmatch tests, if performed.
5. Special transfusion or blood component processing requirements.
6. The component's expiration date and, if applicable, time.
7. The date and time of issue.

Before issuing the unit, transfusion service personnel should inspect it for abnormal appearance (significant color change, cloudiness, clots, clumps, or loss of bag integrity).

The component must not be used if any of these are noted.[4]

Institutions may use dedicated personnel or automated delivery systems (eg, pneumatic tube systems, validated transport coolers, automated blood delivery robots, or blood dispensing kiosks in remote sites) to facilitate the delivery of components to their final destination. Provision of RBCs via automated blood vending machines (remote, automated, computer-controlled blood storage and dispensing refrigerators) at the point of care may help prevent delays in transportation. The use of a remote dispensing solution employs an electronic issuance process and requires confirmation of the absence of clots, clumps, or loss of bag integrity before stocking the dispensing refrigerator.

ADMINISTRATION

Infusion Sets

Components must be administered through special IV tubing with a filter designed to remove blood clots and particles that are potentially harmful to the recipient.[1(p45)] Standard blood administration tubing typically has a 170- to 260-micron (macroaggregate) filter, but this micron size is not mandated or required. The tubing can be primed with either 0.9% sodium chloride or the component itself. The manufacturer's instructions should be reviewed for proper use.

Microaggregate Filters

Microaggregate filters are not used for routine blood administration. These second-generation filters were originally developed to remove leukocytes and to complement or replace the clot screen in the 1970s.[20] They have since been replaced by more efficient leukocyte reduction filters.[21] Microaggregate filters have a screen filter depth of 20 to 40 microns and retain fibrin strands and clumps of dead cells. Red cells, which are 8 microns in diameter, can flow through the filters. Microaggregate filters are typically used for the reinfusion of shed autologous blood collected during or after surgery.

Leukocyte Reduction Filters

Leukocyte reduction filters are designed to reduce the number of leukocytes to <5×10^6 per RBC unit, resulting in the removal of >99.9% of the leukocytes. Leukocyte reduction decreases the incidence of febrile transfusion reactions, risk of HLA alloimmunization, and transmission of cytomegalovirus (CMV) by cellular blood components.[20,21] (See Chapter 7.) These filters are provided by various manufacturers for prestorage use shortly after collection of the units or for poststorage use at the recipient's bedside.

Prestorage leukocyte reduction is more effective than bedside leukocyte reduction, results in lower levels of cytokines in storage, and can promote ready access to an adequate inventory of leukocyte-reduced components.[22] Use of bedside leukocyte reduction filters has been associated with dramatic hypotension in some individuals, often in the absence of other symptoms. This happens more frequently with recipients taking angiotensin-converting enzyme inhibitors. The use of components that were filtered in the blood center or transfusion service before storage decreases the incidence of such reactions.[23] Incorporating prestorage leukocyte reduction into the blood component manufacturing process has greatly reduced the need for bedside leukocyte reduction. Some institutions have noted a decrease in the rate of FNHTRs when leukocyte-reduced components are used.

It is important to verify that the leukocyte reduction filter used is compatible with the component transfused (RBCs or platelets) and to note the maximum number of units that can be administered through one filter. Filters designed for RBCs or platelets may not be used interchangeably. The manufacturer's instructions should be followed for priming and administering blood components through the filter. Otherwise, leukocyte removal may be ineffective or an air lock may develop, preventing passage of the component through the filter. Leukocyte filters should never be used to administer granulocytes or hematopoietic progenitor cells.

Compatible IV Solutions

No medications or solutions other than 0.9% sodium chloride injection, USP, should be administered with blood components through the same tubing at the same time. Solutions containing dextrose alone may cause red cells to swell and lyse. Lactated Ringer solution or other solutions containing high levels of calcium may overcome the buffering capacity of the citrate anticoagulant in the blood preservative solution and cause clotting of the component.[24] The tubing should be flushed with 0.9% sodium chloride solution before or after transfusion if it is used for other medications or solutions.

AABB *Standards* allows exceptions to the above restrictions when 1) the drug or solution has been approved by the FDA for use with blood administration, or 2) there is documentation available to show that the addition is safe and does not adversely affect the blood or component.[1(p45)]

Acceptable solutions according to these criteria include ABO-compatible plasma, 5% albumin, or plasma protein fraction. Certain solutions are compatible with blood or blood components as noted in the package inserts reviewed by the FDA, including Normosol-R pH 7.4 (Hospira, Lake Forest, IL), Plasma-Lyte-A injection pH 7.4 (Baxter Healthcare, Deerfield, IL), and Plasma-Lyte 148 injection (Multiple Electrolytes Injection, Type 1, USP, Baxter Healthcare). There are several formulations of Plasma-Lyte that are not isotonic or that contain calcium; package inserts must be checked to confirm their compatibility with blood components.

Recipient Verification at the Time of Administration

Proper bedside identification of the recipient is the final step to prevent the administration of an incorrect blood component to a recipient. Although individuals are often concerned about the possibility of exposure to infectious agents from transfusion, equal concern should focus on the inadvertent transfusion of incompatible blood. Approximately 1 in every 19,000 units of RBCs is transfused to the wrong recipient each year; 1 in 76,000 transfusions results in an acute hemolytic transfusion reaction, and 1 in 1.8 million units of transfused RBCs results in death from an acute hemolytic transfusion reaction.[25]

To prevent the potentially fatal consequences of misidentification, specific systems have been developed and marketed, including identification bracelets with bar codes and/or radio frequency identification devices, biometric scanning, mechanical or electronic locks that prevent access to bags assigned to unintended recipients, and handheld computers suitable for transferring blood request and administration data from the recipient's bedside to the transfusion service information system in real time. Each system provides a method to bring staff toward self-correction during the procedure.[26,27] Studies show that rates of positive recipient identification can be increased by such systems. However, none of these systems negates the need for good quality management, such as standard operating procedures, regular training, periodic competency assessment, and system monitoring.

Verifications before the Start of Transfusion

- **Identification of recipient and unit.** The recipient's two independent identifiers (eg, name and identification number) must match the information on the unit label or attached tag. The requirements of the institution for recipient identification must be satisfied.
- **Donation identification number.** The DIN and donor ABO/Rh type on the blood component label must match the attached tag.
- **Blood type.** The recipient's ABO group (and Rh type if required) should be compatible with that of the unit. Interpretation of any crossmatch tests (if performed) is also verified.
- **Medical order.** The transfusionist should verify that the component matches the

product ordered and that any special processing in the order was performed.

- **Expiration date (and time, if applicable).** Transfusion of the unit need only start before the expiration date or time has passed.

The transfusion should not be initiated if any discrepancy or abnormality is found.

Starting the Transfusion

The unit identifiers should never be removed during the transfusion. Once the identification of the unit and the recipient is verified, the unit is spiked using an aseptic technique. At institutions that use Joint Commission hospital accreditation, Joint Commission requirements for the transfusionist (HR.01.02.01) apply: "If blood transfusions and intravenous medications are administered by staff other than doctors of medicine or osteopathy, the staff members must have special training for this duty."[28]

The blood administration tubing should be primed with either 0.9% sodium chloride or the blood component itself. If any solution or medication other than 0.9% sodium chloride is infused before component administration, the tubing should be flushed with 0.9% sodium chloride immediately before the blood infusion.

The infusion should start slowly, at approximately 2 mL per minute, for the first 15 minutes while the transfusionist remains near the recipient. Some policies may require "direct observation of the recipient" during this time. Severe reactions may occur after as little as 10 mL has been transfused. Potentially life-threatening reactions most commonly occur within 10 to 15 minutes of the start of a transfusion. The recipient should be reassessed, and vital signs should be obtained to assess the recipient's tolerance of the transfusion.[29]

Rates of Transfusion

The rate of transfusion should be increased after 15 minutes to ensure the unit is administered within the 4-hour window. The advantages of using relatively rapid transfusion rates (eg, 240 mL/hour) include correction of defi-

ciency as rapidly as possible as well as reduced recipient and nursing time dedicated to transfusion. Disadvantages include the potential to cause reactions (eg, volume overload) or increase the severity of a reaction (eg, FNHTRs, septic reactions, or allergic reactions). Many FNHTRs as well as septic, allergic, and even some hemolytic reactions may not be evident within the first 15 minutes.

If there is no sign of a reaction after the first 15 minutes, the flow rate can be increased to the designated infusion rate, taking into consideration the recipient's size, blood volume, and hemodynamic condition in determining the flow rate. (See Table 18-1.) Careful attention should be paid to avoid transfusing the unit too rapidly in relation to the recipient's cardiac and/or respiratory status. Transfusions of a blood component must be completed within 4 hours of the start of transfusion.[4] If the patient is unable to tolerate completion of the entire transfusion dose in the 4-hour timeframe, a request to the blood bank can be made to issue an aliquot or a split product of a smaller volume, allowing for the entire transfusion dose to be transfused over two separate transfusions.

Monitoring during the Transfusion

The transfusionist should continue to periodically monitor the recipient throughout the infusion, including the IV site and flow rate. If the IV rate has slowed down, the transfusionist should take one or more of the following actions: 1) verify that the IV is patent and there are no signs of infiltration; 2) raise or elevate the unit; 3) examine the filter for air, excessive debris, or clots; 4) attempt to administer the component through an infusion pump; or 5) consider the addition of 0.9% sodium chloride as a diluent if the unit is too viscous.

Frequent recipient monitoring during the infusion helps alert the transfusionist to a possible transfusion reaction and allows for early intervention.

Vital signs should be taken within 15 minutes of beginning the transfusion and then according to institutional policy. There is little evidence to support a best practice related to

TABLE 18-1. Blood Component Transfusions in Nonemergent Settings

Component	Suggested Adult Flow Rates		Special Considerations	ABO Compatibility	Filter
	First 15 Minutes	After 15 Minutes			
Red Blood Cells (RBCs)	1-2 mL/min (60-120 mL/hour)	As rapidly as tolerated; approximately 4 mL/minute or 240 mL/hour	Infusion duration should not exceed 4 hours. Generally administered over 1-2 hours for hemodynamically stable recipients. For recipients at risk of fluid overload, may adjust flow rate to as low as 1 mL/kg/hour.	Whole blood: ABO identical RBCs: ABO compatible with recipient's plasma Crossmatch required	In-line (170-260 micron) Leukocyte reduction if indicated
Platelets	2-5 mL/min (120-300 mL/hour)	300 mL/hour or as tolerated	Usually given over 1-2 hours. For recipients at risk of fluid overload, use slower flow rate (see RBCs).	Crossmatch not required ABO/Rh compatibility preferable but not required May be HLA matched	In-line (170-260 micron) Leukocyte reduction if indicated
Plasma	2-5 mL/min (120-300 mL/hour)	As rapidly as tolerated; approximately 300 mL/hour	Time for thawing may be needed before issue. For recipients at risk of fluid overload, use slower flow rate (see RBCs).	Crossmatch not required ABO compatibility with recipient red cells	In-line (170-260 micron)
Granulocytes	1-2 mL/min (60-120 mL/hour)	120-150 mL/hour or as tolerated	Over approximately 2 hours. Infuse as soon as possible after collection/release of component; irradiate.	Crossmatch required ABO/Rh compatibility required May be HLA matched	In-line (170-260 micron) Do not use leukocyte reduction or microaggregate filters
Cryoprecipitated AHF	As rapidly as tolerated		Infuse as soon as possible after thawing; pooling is preferred.	Crossmatch and ABO compatibility not required	In-line (170-260 micron)

the frequency of vital-sign monitoring other than at baseline, soon after the start of the transfusion, and after transfusion.[30] AABB *Standards* requires that the medical record include pre- and posttransfusion vital signs.[1(p45)] Vital signs should be taken at once if there is a suspected transfusion reaction or a change in the clinical condition of the recipient.

Suspected Transfusion Reactions

The transfusionist should be knowledgeable about signs and symptoms indicative of an adverse reaction and be able to act quickly. (See Chapter 22.) Visual observation and recipient reporting of any changes should be used to determine if a reaction has occurred because the recipient may experience symptoms before changes occur in vital signs. If a transfusion reaction is suspected, the transfusion should be stopped. The patency of the IV should be maintained with new IV tubing and 0.9% saline attached near the IV insertion site to prevent infusion of any residual blood component to the recipient.

The component unit identification information should be rechecked. Prompt notification of the licensed provider for treatment of suspected transfusion reactions is needed. For serious adverse events, notification of the hospital rapid response team should be considered. Institutions should provide ready access to descriptions of common transfusion reactions, including signs and symptoms as well as immediate steps to be taken or interventions to anticipate.

As soon as possible, the transfusion service should be notified of a suspected transfusion reaction, and institutional policy should be followed for returning the component bag and/or to order the laboratory studies needed to evaluate the reaction. Documentation of the suspected transfusion reaction should be completed per institution policy.

Completing the Transfusion

The recipient is assessed at the completion of the transfusion, and his or her vital signs are obtained. The blood unit bag and tubing are discarded in a biohazard container if the trans-

fusion was uneventful. The 0.9% saline bag should be discarded per institution policy.

Because recipients can experience transfusion reactions several hours to days after the transfusion is complete, clinical staff should continue to monitor the recipient periodically for 4 to 6 hours after the end of the transfusion to detect febrile or pulmonary reactions that may be associated with blood administration. If the recipient is not under direct clinical supervision after a transfusion, clinical staff should provide written instructions to the recipient and caregiver regarding signs and symptoms to report and a phone number to call or a person to contact should a reaction occur later.

DOCUMENTATION OF THE TRANSFUSION

The transfusion should be documented in the recipient's medical record. At a minimum, AABB *Standards* requires documentation of the following[1(p45)]:

1. Transfusion order.
2. Recipient consent.
3. Component name.
4. Donation identification number.
5. Date and time of transfusion.
6. Pre- and posttransfusion vital signs.
7. Volume transfused.
8. Identification of the transfusionist.
9. Transfusion-related adverse events, if applicable.

Please note that although the AABB *Standards* does not specify documentation of start and end times for transfusions, the *Circular of Information for the Use of Human Blood and Blood Components* requires that transfusions be completed within 4 hours.[4] Documentation would be necessary to demonstrate compliance with this requirement. If additional units are to be transfused, the institution's policy and/or manufacturer's recommendations should be followed to determine whether the same blood administration tubing may be used. If there are no contraindications from the manufacturer, institutions frequently allow additional units to be transfused with the same blood administration set within 4 hours of the start of the initial transfusion.

UNIQUE TRANSFUSION SETTINGS

See Chapter 24 for information about transfusion in pediatric and neonatal recipients.

Operating Room and Trauma: Rapid Infusions

If components need to be administered rapidly, the use of rapid infusion/warming devices, large-bore administration tubing, and large-bore IV catheters, including central venous or intraosseous access, can decrease the infusion time without inducing hemolysis.[31-33] Some tubing sets with appropriate filters are specifically designed for rapid blood administration and may be used alone or with specific devices. Flow rates as fast as 10 to 25 mL/second (600-1500 mL/minute) have been reported with such tubing. Rapid infusion of multiple blood components can lead to hypothermia, coagulopathy, and electrolyte imbalances. Use of a blood/fluid warming device can lessen the incidence of hypothermia.[34]

Hypocalcemia has been noted with rapid transfusions. This is usually transient and dependent on the amount and rate of citrate infused. Calcium replacement may be administered based on the recipient's ionized serum calcium level and the rate of citrate administration.[35] Transfusion-associated hyperkalemic cardiac arrest has been reported with rapid administration of RBCs. It may develop with rapid RBC administration even with a modest transfusion volume such as 1 unit (in a neonate). Contributing factors are acidosis, hypoglycemia, hypocalcemia, and hypothermia at the time of cardiac arrest.[35]

If components are urgently needed and a delay in transfusion could be detrimental to the recipient, the transfusion service should have a process to provide components before all pretransfusion compatibility testing is completed. In such cases, uncrossmatched units are released with a signed statement from the requesting physician indicating that the clinical situation requires urgent release before the completion of testing.[1(p43)]

If components in the transfusion service inventory are not immediately accessible to a trauma unit or operating room, a supply of group O red cells may be maintained in an appropriate remote storage device in these areas. The transfusion service must ensure proper storage of components at these satellite storage sites.

Out-of-Hospital Transfusion

Transfusion of blood in a non-hospital setting requires a well-planned program that incorporates all the relevant aspects of the hospital setting and emphasizes safety considerations.[36]

Out-of-hospital settings for blood transfusion can include dialysis centers, medical transport vehicles, skilled nursing facilities, outpatient surgery centers, and even recipients' homes. The proper documentation and maintenance of records is part of a well-designed program. Transfusionists should be competent in performing blood administration procedures, recipient monitoring, and recognition and reporting of suspected transfusion reactions. To optimize the care of these recipients, proper arrangements for treatment of suspected transfusion reactions must be made. Blood administration outside the hospital should be performed by personnel with substantial experience in blood administration in this setting.

Transfusion in the home generally allows close monitoring of the transfusion event because the personnel-to-recipient ratio is 1:1. The disadvantage is that there is no trained assistant available in the event of a severe adverse reaction. Issues to consider when preparing for a transfusion in the home include availability of the following[36]:

- A competent adult in the home to assist in recipient identification and to summon medical assistance if needed.

- A mechanism to obtain immediate physician consultation.
- A telephone to contact emergency personnel, and easy access for emergency vehicles.
- Documentation of prior transfusions with no history of severe reactions.
- A way to properly dispose of medical waste.

CONCLUSIONS

Transfusion of blood components and the creation of blood administration procedures and policies should be recipient centric. Policies and procedures should follow evidence-based best practice and provide the transfusionist with information to competently perform transfusions and recognize and report suspected transfusion reactions. Close monitoring and early intervention when transfusion reactions occur can make a critical difference in recipient outcomes. Audits of the blood administration process to identify areas for improvement, instances of nonconformance, and analysis of their causes are needed for optimal transfusion safety.

KEY POINTS

1. Blood administration involves the process of informed consent, preparation of the recipient, administration of the appropriate component to the correct recipient, and careful observation of the recipient during and after the transfusion for any adverse reaction. All steps must be appropriately documented in the recipient's medical record.
2. The recipient should be informed of the need for a transfusion and educated about the transfusion of the blood component. Informed consent for the transfusion must be obtained from the recipient.
3. A licensed care provider should initiate requests for blood administration with an order for the appropriate blood component testing and preparation and an order for the administration of the component(s).
4. Transfusionists should be educated on appropriate clinical indications for transfusion and proper safety steps involved in a successful transfusion process.
5. Before planned transfusion, the transfusionist should verify available, appropriate, and patent venous access; administer any ordered prophylactic medications; and gather required equipment (eg, blood warmer, infusion pump, pressure devices, and emergency equipment).
6. Vital signs and a baseline assessment of the recipient should be performed for subsequent comparison.
7. Institutions should identify appropriate blood and blood component issue and delivery mechanisms to ensure that the transfusionist receives the components in a timely manner.
8. Transfusion services should ensure that other departments are aware of the requirement for returning components if a transfusion is delayed.
9. At the recipient's bedside, verification of recipient and component identification should be performed. The following items should be verified: 1) identity of the recipient and unit, 2) DIN and donor ABO/Rh type, 3) recipient blood type, 4) medical order, and 5) expiration date/time of the component.
10. Components must be administered through the appropriate infusion sets and filters. Only compatible IV solutions (usually 0.9% sodium chloride injection, USP) should be administered through the same tubing unless the tubing has been flushed with 0.9% sodium chloride, USP, immediately before and after the transfusion.
11. The infusion should start slowly at approximately 2 mL per minute for the first 15 minutes.

12. During this time, the transfusionist should remain near the recipient. If no sign of reaction appears, the infusion rate can be increased. The transfusionist monitors the recipient throughout the infusion and stops the infusion in the event of an adverse reaction.

13. Infusions must be completed within 4 hours of start of transfusion. After completion, the transfusionist takes the recipient's vital signs. If the recipient will not be under direct clinical supervision after the transfusion, the recipient and caregiver should receive instructions regarding signs and symptoms to report and to whom to report these reactions.

14. The following information, at a minimum, regarding the transfusion must be documented in the recipient's medical record: 1) the transfusion order, 2) recipient consent for transfusion, 3) name of component, 4) DIN, 5) date and time of infusion, 6) pre- and posttransfusion vital signs, 7) volume transfused, 8) identity of the transfusionist, and 9) any adverse reaction.

REFERENCES

1. Ooley PW, ed. Standards for blood banks and transfusion services. 30th ed. Bethesda, MD: AABB, 2016.

2. Stowell CP, Sazama, K, eds. Informed consent in blood transfusion and cellular therapies: Patients, donors, and research subjects. Bethesda, MD: AABB Press, 2007.

3. Klein H, Anstee D. Mollison's blood transfusion in clinical medicine. 12th ed. Oxford: Wiley-Blackwell, 2014.

4. AABB, American Red Cross, America's Blood Centers, Armed Services Blood Program. Circular of information for the use of human blood and blood components. Bethesda, MD: AABB, 2017.

5. 2017 National patient safety goals. Oakbrook Terrace, IL: The Joint Commission, 2017. [Available at http://www.jointcommission.org/standards_information/npsgs.aspx (accessed February 9, 2017).]

6. Duran J. Effects of leukoreduction and premedication with acetaminophen. J Pediatr Oncol Nurs 2014;31:223-9.

7. Marti-Carvajal AJ, Sola I, Gonzalez LE, et al. Pharmacological interventions for the prevention of allergic and febrile non-haemolytic transfusion reactions. Cochrane Database Syst Rev 2010;(6):CD007539.

8. Patterson BJ, Freedman J, Blanchette V, et al. Effect of premedication guidelines and leukoreduction on the rate of febrile nonhaemolytic platelet transfusion reactions. Transfus Med 2000;10:199-206.

9. Goss JE, Chambers CE, Heupler FA, et al. Systemic anaphylactoid reactions to iodinated contrast media during cardiac catheterization procedures: Guidelines for prevention, diagnosis, and treatment. Cath Cardiovasc Diagn 1995;34:99-104.

10. Tramer MR, von Elm E, Loubeyre P, Hauser C. Pharmacological prevention of serious anaphylactic reactions due to iodinated contrast media: Systematic review. Br Med J 2006;333:675-81.

11. Boyan CP, Howland WS. Cardiac arrest and temperature of bank blood. JAMA 1963;183:58-60.

12. Donham JA, Denning V. Cold agglutinin syndrome: Nursing management. Heart Lung 1985;14:59-67.

13. Iserson KV, Huestis DW. Blood warming: Current applications and techniques. Transfusion 1991;31:558-71.

14. Hirsch J, Menzebach A, Welters ID, et al. Indicators of erythrocyte damage after microwave warming of packed red blood cells. Clin Chem 2003;49:792-9.

15. Frelich R, Ellis MH. The effect of external pressure, catheter gauge, and storage time on hemolysis in RBC transfusion. Transfusion 2001;41:799-802.

16. Acquillo G. Blood transfusion flow rate. J Assoc Vasc Access 2007;124:225-6.

17. Makic MB, Martin SA, Burns S, et al. Putting evidence into nursing practice: Four traditional practices not supported by evidence. Crit Care Nurse 2013;33:28-42.

18. Barcelona SL, Vilich F, Coté CJ. A comparison of flow rates and warming capabilities of the Level 1 and Rapid Infusion System with various-size intravenous catheters. Anesth Analg 2003;97:358-63.

19. Miller MA, Schlueter AJ. Transfusions via hand-held syringes and small-gauge needles

as risk factors for hyperkalemia. Transfusion 2004;44:373-81.

20. Wortham ST, Ortolano GA, Wenz B. A brief history of blood filtration: Clot screens, microaggregate removal, and leukocyte reduction. Transfus Med Rev 2003;17:216-22.

21. Lane TA. Leukocyte reduction of cellular blood components: Effectiveness, benefits, quality control, and costs. Arch Pathol Lab Med 1994; 118:392-404.

22. Bandarenko N, King K, eds. Blood transfusion therapy: A physician's handbook. 12th ed. Bethesda, MD: AABB, 2017.

23. Zoon KC, Jacobson ED, Woodcock J. Hypotension and bedside leukocyte reduction filters. Int J Trauma Nurs 1999;5:121-2.

24. Dickson DN, Gregory MA. Compatibility of blood with solutions containing calcium. S Afr Med J 1980;57:785-7.

25. Vamvakas EC, Blajchman MA. Transfusion related mortality: The ongoing risks of allogeneic blood transfusion and the available strategies for their prevention. Blood 2009;113: 3406-17.

26. Pagliaro P, Rebulla P. Transfusion recipient identification. Vox Sang 2006;91:97-101.

27. Koshy R. Navigating the information technology highway: Computer solutions to reduce errors and enhance patient safety. Transfusion 2005;45(Suppl 4):189S-205S.

28. Comprehensive accreditation manual for hospitals. Oakbrook Terrace, IL: The Joint Commission, 2017.

29. Bradbury M, Cruickshank JP. Blood transfusion: Crucial steps in maintaining safe practice. Br J Nurs 2000;9:134-8.

30. Oldham J, Sinclair L, Hendry C. Right patient, right blood, right care: Safe transfusion practice. Br J Nurs 2009;18:312, 314, 316-20.

31. Davis DT, Johannigman JA, Pritts TA. New strategies for massive transfusion in the bleeding trauma patient. J Trauma Nurs 2012;19:69-75.

32. ASC TQIP massive transfusion in trauma guidelines. Chicago, IL: American College of Surgeons, 2014.

33. Shaz B, Hillyer C. Massive transfusion. In: Shaz B, Hillyer C, Roshal M, Abrams C, eds. Transfusion medicine and hemostasis. 2nd ed. London: Elsevier Science, 2013.

34. Hrovat TM, Passwater M, Palmer RN, for the Scientific Section Coordinating Committee. Guidelines for the use of blood warming devices. Bethesda, MD: AABB, 2002.

35. Hayter MA, Pavenski K, Baker J. Massive transfusion in the trauma patient: Continuing professional development. Can J Anaesth 2012: 59:1130-45.

36. Benson K. Home is where the heart is: Do blood transfusions belong there too? Transfus Med Rev 2006;20:218-29.

Hemotherapy Decisions and Their Outcomes

• ● •

Richard M. Kaufman, MD, and Nadine Shehata, MD, FRCP

AS WITH ALL medical interventions, the risks and benefits of blood transfusion must be weighed carefully. This chapter provides an overview of the scientific literature supporting the use of transfusion therapy in adult patients.

RED BLOOD CELL TRANSFUSION

Red Blood Cells (RBCs) are transfused to increase oxygen-carrying capacity in patients with anemia in whom physiologic compensatory mechanisms are inadequate to maintain normal tissue oxygenation. There are myriad causes of anemia; one classification scheme is shown in Table 19-1. In patients with chronic, stable anemia, RBC transfusion is often unnecessary. In a patient with well-compensated anemia from iron deficiency, for example, simply replacing iron may be the appropriate maneuver to correct the anemia. Conversely, RBC transfusion may be lifesaving in cases of anemia where, as mentioned, physiologic compensatory mechanisms are inadequate to maintain tissue oxygenation. Signs and symptoms of anemia that should prompt consideration of RBC transfusion include hemodynamic instability, chest pain of cardiac origin, shortness of breath, and tachycardia at rest. In nonbleeding patients, the hemoglobin concentration (Hb) is used to help guide RBC transfusion decisions. Because 98% of blood oxygen is hemoglobin bound, the Hb is easy to measure, and no better physiologic measurements to support RBC transfusion are currently available. As discussed below, current RBC transfusion thresholds are based on lower Hb levels than those used previously.

Liberal vs Restrictive Transfusion Strategies

The first high-quality study investigating the clinical use of RBC transfusions was the Canadian Transfusion Requirements in Critical Care (TRICC) trial.[1] In the TRICC trial, 838 hemodynamically stable, critically ill patients

Richard M. Kaufman, MD, Medical Director, Adult Transfusion Service, Brigham and Women's Hospital, Boston, Massachusetts; and Nadine Shehata, MD, FRCP, Division of Hematology and Oncology, Mount Sinai Hospital, Toronto, Ontario, Canada
R. Kaufman has disclosed a financial relationship with Janssen, Inc. N. Shehata has disclosed no conflicts of interest.

19

TABLE 19-1. Classification of Anemia

Blood Loss	
Increased Red Cell Destruction (hemolysis)	**Decreased Red Cell Production**
Extrinsic to Red Cells	**Microcytic**
Immune	Iron deficiency
Alloantibody-mediated hemolytic anemia	Thalassemia
Warm autoimmune hemolytic anemia	Lead poisoning
Cold agglutinin disease	Anemia of chronic disease
Paroxysmal cold hemoglobinuria	Sideroblastic anemia
Drug-related hemolytic anemia	
Nonimmune	**Normocytic**
Mechanical cause	Myelophthisic anemia
Microangiopathic anemia	Renal/low erythropoietin
	Anemia of chronic disease
Intrinsic to Red Cells	Marrow hypo/aplasia
Hemoglobinopathies	
Membrane defects	**Macrocytic**
Enzyme defects	*Megaloblastic*
	B12
	Folate
	Medication
	Nonmegaloblastic
	Marrow hypo/aplasia

with a Hb <9 g/dL were randomly assigned to receive RBC transfusion for a Hb <10 g/dL (liberal group) or a Hb <7 g/dL (restrictive group). The primary endpoint, 30-day all-cause mortality, did not significantly differ between the study groups. Significantly better survival was observed in the restrictive group in younger patients (<55 years old) and in less acutely ill patients [Acute Physiology and Chronic Health Evaluation (APACHE) II score <20]. The 2011 trial known as "FOCUS"[2] was the second large randomized controlled trial (RCT) to examine the clinical consequences of adhering to a liberal vs restrictive RBC transfusion strategy in adult patients. In this study, 2016 patients at age 50 or older having hip-fracture surgery with a history of (or risk factors for) cardiovascular disease were randomly assigned to receive postoperative RBC transfusion for a Hb <10 g/dL (liberal group) vs 8 g/dL (restrictive group). FOCUS was designed as a superiority trial; the aim was to determine whether transfusing RBCs more liberally was associated with better functional outcomes following hip-fracture repair. There was no difference in the primary endpoint of death or the inability to walk across a room unassisted at 60 days after randomization. Smaller trials of liberal vs restrictive postoperative RBC transfusion in orthopedic surgical patients similarly failed to show a benefit of liberal transfusion.[3,4]

RCTs of various sizes comparing liberal vs restrictive RBC transfusion strategies have now been performed in several populations of hospitalized adult patients,[5,6] including cardiac surgery,[7-10] septic shock,[11] acute upper gastrointestinal bleeding,[12,13] surgical oncology,[14] postpartum hemorrhage,[15] and traumatic brain injury.[16] More RCTs are in various stages of development. With a few exceptions,[14] these studies overwhelmingly failed to demonstrate any clinical benefits of a liberal transfusion strategy. A 2016 meta-analysis[17] evaluated 31 trials comparing liberal vs restrictive transfusion strategies. A total of 12,587 patients in various clinical settings (eg, surgery, critical care) were included. Overall, using a restrictive RBC transfusion threshold (typically a Hb of 7.0-8.0 g/dL) reduced the proportion of exposed patients by 43%, without causing either harm or benefit as compared with a liberal transfusion strategy. On this basis, clinical practice guidelines, including a 2016 AABB guideline,[18] recommended that a restrictive RBC strategy should be used for hospitalized inpatients. A few points merit emphasis. First, clinical practice guidelines are not standards, nor can they substitute for clinical judgment. The RCTs in this area have tended to simplify the decision to transfuse RBCs by basing it on a single parameter, the patient's Hb level. For individual patients, clinical signs and symptoms, comorbidities, and other factors should be integrated into the transfusion decision. That said, if an individual patient is clinically stable, and the *only* factor driving the decision to transfuse RBCs is the patient's Hb, then a restrictive approach should be followed. Second, the RCTs conducted to date have almost exclusively included hemodynamically stable, hospitalized, adult patients. Hb levels may be of limited utility in patients who are actively bleeding inside or outside the operating room. Also, it is often appropriate for providers to transfuse ambulatory outpatients more liberally, for logistical reasons (eg, fewer clinic visits). Subjective quality-of-life (QOL) measures may vary based on a patient's Hb, although a consistent relationship between Hb and functional activity/QOL has been difficult to demonstrate.[19]

Acute coronary syndromes represent an indication distinct from those mentioned. Currently, the best approach to transfuse patients having acute myocardial infarction (MI) or unstable angina remains unclear. In the TRICC study, patients with acute coronary syndromes were the only subgroup in which survival was poorer among patients assigned to the restrictive transfusion strategy. However, the survival advantage seen in the liberal transfusion group was not statistically significant.[1,20] In the 2015 Transfusion Indication Threshold Reduction (TITRe2) trial,[9] 2007 adult patients having elective cardiac surgery were randomly assigned to a liberal (Hb <9 g/dL) vs restrictive (Hb <7.5 g/dL) RBC transfusion strategy. There was no significant difference in the primary outcome of serious infection or ischemic events (eg, stroke or MI). A secondary analysis, however, revealed higher 90-day all-cause mortality among subjects in the restrictive group [4.2% vs 2.6%; hazard ratio, 1.64 (1.00-2.67)]. Thus, the existing data may suggest that a more liberal transfusion approach may be appropriate in patients with acute coronary syndromes or having cardiac surgery. This area will surely be the subject of further studies. The AABB guideline noted that there was insufficient evidence to recommend a restrictive RBC transfusion strategy for patients with acute coronary syndrome, severe thrombocytopenia, or chronic transfusion-dependent anemia.[18]

Thalassemia and Sickle Cell Syndromes

The hemoglobinopathies thalassemia and sickle cell disease are among the most commonly inherited syndromes. The thalassemia syndromes refer to the reduced production of α or β globin as a result of gene mutations. β-thalassemia major is characterized by severe anemia, ineffective erythropoiesis, and extramedullary hematopoiesis. The sickle cell syndromes include hemoglobin SS, hemoglobin SC, and hemoglobin Sβ^0. Hemoglobin S results from a single amino acid substitution (valine for glutamic acid) in position 6 of the β globin protein. Hemoglobin S polymerizes in relatively deoxygenated regions of the circulation, causing abnormal red cell morphology, subsequent occlusion of the microvasculature, and acute and chronic organ dysfunction.

Individuals with thalassemia major often begin a regular RBC transfusion program in childhood if there is poor growth or evidence of extramedullary hematopoiesis resulting in bony abnormalities, and/or if the hemoglobin level is <7 to 9 g/dL.[21,22] RBC transfusion is used to treat anemia and reduce the risk of morbidity from extramedullary hematopoiesis. RBCs are provided every 2 to 4 weeks to maintain a pretransfusion Hb of 9 to 10 g/dL.[21]

Sickle red cells cause microvasculature occlusion not only because of their rigidity but also because sickle cells tend to adhere to other blood cells and the endothelium.[23,24] RBC transfusions in patients with sickle cell disease decrease the incidence of acute and chronic complications by reducing the proportion of circulating sickle cells. However, allogeneic RBCs are also associated with risk, and RBC transfusion requires balancing risks and benefits. In patients with sickle cell disease, the overall risk of alloimmunization remains ~20%.[25,26] Alloimmunization rates are high in sickle cell disease partially because of antigen disparity between donors and sickle cell disease patients and because of variant Rh alleles.[27] Additionally, the inflammatory response that occurs with vaso-occlusive crises may predispose to alloimmunization.[28] In addition to alloimmunization, the risks of hemolytic transfusion reactions secondary to hyperhemolysis and iron overload also need to be balanced against the benefits of transfusion. Hyperhemolysis refers to the development of severe anemia where the Hb following transfusion is lower than that before transfusion. Hyperhemolysis is often, although not always, associated with a delayed hemolytic reaction to a clinically significant red cell alloantibody. It is accompanied by fever, pain, laboratory evidence of hemolysis (eg, elevated lactate dehydrogenase and indirect bilirubin and reduced haptoglobin levels), and a reduction in reticulocyte counts. RBC transfusion often exacerbates the anemia, and hyperhemolysis may

also occur with future RBC transfusions.[29] Transfusion avoidance and potentially the use of intravenous immune globulin (IVIG) and corticosteroids can be used to treat hyperhemolysis.[30]

To reduce the alloimmunization risk, patients with sickle cell disease often receive RBCs selected through an extended match (ie, units matched for C, E, K, and other antigens) in addition to the usual matching for ABO and RhD.[31,32] Nonetheless, phenotyping may not match the Rh haplotypes that often occur in these patients.[27,33] Genotyping for red cell antigens is costly; however, the cost of genotyping needs to be balanced against the need to avoid alloimmunization in those at high risk who require frequent transfusions.

RBCs can be administered as a simple transfusion, by manual exchange, or by automated exchange. Automated exchange transfusion can readily deliver more volume, thereby significantly reducing hemoglobin S levels and reducing the risk of iron overload. RBCs are administered acutely or chronically as prophylaxis or for various indications, such as pulmonary hypertension.[24] Clear indications for the use of RBCs are provided by RCT evidence and, in the absence of RCTs, as evidence-based clinical guidelines. Table 19-2 summarizes RBC transfusion recommendations in sickle cell disease from a recent National Heart, Lung, and Blood Institute (NHLBI) guideline.[24] The 1998 Stroke Prevention Trial in Sickle Cell Anemia (STOP trial) showed that chronic RBC transfusions significantly reduce the incidence of stroke in sickle cell patients determined to be at high risk based on transcranial Doppler (TCD) ultrasonography (middle cerebral artery flow velocity >200 cm/sec).[34] The subsequent STOP2 trial showed that discontinuing chronic transfusion in this patient population results in a reversion to baseline risk of abnormal flow velocities and stroke.[35] In the recent TCD With Transfusions Changing to Hydroxyurea (TWITCH) trial, children with sickle cell disease and abnormal TCD velocities were randomly assigned to monthly transfusion or hydroxycarbamide (hydroxyurea) for 1 year. Hydroxycarbamide was found to be noninferi-

TABLE 19-2. The Use of RBC Transfusion for Sickle Cell Disease Complications*

Complication	Transfusion Method (strength of recommendation)
Symptomatic severe acute chest syndrome (defined by an oxygen saturation <90% despite supplemental oxygen)	Exchange (strong)
Acute splenic sequestration and severe anemia	Simple (strong)
Acute stroke in children and adults: Initiate a program of monthly transfusions	Simple or exchange (strong)
Hepatic sequestration	Simple or exchange (moderate)
Intrahepatic cholestasis	Exchange or simple (consensus)
Multisystem organ failure	Exchange or simple (consensus)
Aplastic crisis	Simple (consensus)
Symptomatic anemia	Simple (consensus)
Child with transcranial Doppler reading >200 cm/s	Exchange or simple (strong)
Adults or children with previous clinically overt stroke	Exchange or simple (moderate)

*Adapted from Yawn et al.[24]

or to chronic transfusion, thereby providing a potential alternative to chronic transfusion.[36] RBCs are not generally indicated in an uncomplicated painful vaso-occlusive crisis, priapism, asymptomatic anemia, or acute kidney injury. Guidance from sickle cell experts is recommended for patients with sickle cell disease requiring surgery with general anesthesia, as these individuals may require simple or exchange transfusion.[24]

RBC Storage Duration

As described above, clinical trials have typically failed to demonstrate a benefit of RBC transfusion for most patients with moderate anemia. Likely, this reflects the ability of physiologic compensatory mechanisms to ensure adequate tissue oxygenation at Hb levels in the range where transfusion is often considered. An alternate hypothesis potentially explaining the apparent lack of benefit of RBC transfusion relates to the RBC "storage lesion." In the United States, RBCs may be refrigerator stored for up to 42 days, and various biochemical and morphologic changes are known to

occur. As examples, extracellular potassium increases; 2,3-diphosphoglycerate (DPG), a key regulator of oxygen offloading, declines; and free hemoglobin and free iron increase. Observational studies suggested that RBCs stored for longer durations might be associated with adverse clinical outcomes.[37] The impact of RBC storage duration on clinical outcomes in various patient populations has been examined in several RCTs, including ARIPI[38] (neonates), ABLE[39] (patients in intensive care), RECESS[40] (cardiac surgical patients), TOTAL[41] (children with severe anemia, mainly from malaria), and INFORM[42] (hospitalized adult patients). No differences in clinical outcomes were seen in any of these trials. At this time, no clinical practice changes based on RBC storage duration are indicated.

Emergency Transfusion of RBCs

RBC transfusions are typically matched for ABO (Table 19-3) as well as RhD blood group antigens. In bleeding emergencies, there may be insufficient time to complete standard

TABLE 19-3. ABO Matching

Recipient ABO Type	ABO-Compatible RBC Units	ABO-Compatible Plasma or Platelet Units
O	O	A, B, O, AB
A	A, O	A, AB
B	B, O	B, AB
AB	A, B, O, AB	AB

RBC = Red Blood Cell.

pretransfusion testing. Uncrossmatched type O RBC units are used in situations where RBCs must be transfused immediately, before any patient testing is completed. Group O, RhD-negative units are the component of choice for females of childbearing potential, often defined as <50 years old. Group O, RhD-positive units are used for men and for postmenopausal women. Approximately 3% of recipients are expected to have one or more non-ABO red cell alloantibodies; nonetheless, in practice, clinically significant hemolytic reactions to uncrossmatched type O units are rare. Occasionally, for bleeding emergencies, patients with known red cell alloantibodies may need RBC transfusion before antigen-negative units can be identified and crossmatched. Close communication between the primary service (eg, the operating room staff) and a transfusion medicine physician is important in such cases. Clinicians may have concerns about transfusing units that are not proven to be "fully compatible." However, most non-ABO antibodies will not cause immediate, intravascular hemolysis, as can occur with a major-ABO-mismatched transfusion. Rather, most non-ABO red cell alloantibodies will cause delayed, extravascular hemolysis. Thus, transfusing units known to be incompatible is still preferable to exsanguination or life-threatening severe anemia. Finally, a brief summary of approaches to massive transfusion is provided below in the section on plasma transfusion.

RBC Transfusion in Autoimmune Hemolytic Anemia

The mainstay of therapy for warm autoimmune hemolytic anemia (WAIHA) is immunosuppression, but RBC transfusions play a key supportive role. Red cell autoantibodies are broadly reactive; thus, finding compatible RBCs for patients with WAIHA is problematic.[43] Characteristically panreactive in vitro, autoantibodies may also mask the presence of one or more clinically significant alloantibodies. Alloantibodies have been reported to occur in 20% to 40% of patients with warm autoantibodies.[44,45] For patients who have not been recently transfused, autologous adsorption is the preferred method of removing the autoantibody to permit alloantibody identification so that antigen-negative RBC units may be provided. For recently transfused patients, allogeneic (heterologous) adsorptions may be performed to identify underlying alloantibodies. Providing either phenotypically or genotypically matched RBCs is another option to reduce the risks of both alloimmunization and hemolytic transfusion reactions in these patients.[46,47] In some WAIHA cases, the autoantibody will demonstrate a relative antigenic specificity. For example, the autoantibody may appear to react more strongly in vitro with RhD-positive units as compared with RhD-negative units. In such cases, there may be some benefit, in terms of survival of transfused red cells, in providing units that are negative for the "mimicking" autoantibody specificity.[48] However, it is more important to avoid preformed underlying alloantibodies than to provide units matched for the relative specificity of the autoantibody.

In many WAIHA cases, fully crossmatch-compatible RBC units will never be available; that is, the patient's autoantibody will react in vitro with all tested red cells. However, hemolysis in some cases of WAIHA progresses extremely rapidly, and RBC transfusions should not be withheld from patients with potentially life-threatening anemia. Clinicians should be reassured that even if RBCs are incompatible in vitro, the transfused units will be no more "incompatible" than the patient's own red cells. Sufficient RBCs should be transfused to relieve signs and symptoms of anemia (eg, air hunger, tachycardia at rest, chest pain). These transfusions, which are considered lifesaving, should not be avoided, particularly for patients who have not been transfused or pregnant and thus are highly unlikely to have alloantibodies. Frequent monitoring of the transfused patient is warranted, and close communication between the transfusion service and primary clinical service is critical.[43]

PLATELET TRANSFUSION

Prophylactic Platelet Transfusions for Therapy-Induced Hypoproliferative Thrombocytopenia

Most platelet transfusions are administered to nonbleeding patients with hypoproliferative thrombocytopenia resulting from chemotherapy or stem cell transplantation. This practice began in the 1960s, at a time when fatal intracerebral hemorrhage was a frequent cause of death among severely thrombocytopenic patients receiving chemotherapy. A seminal study[49] demonstrated that days of gross hemorrhage increased at lower platelet counts, although a clear threshold for increased bleeding risk was not identified. Nevertheless, it became standard practice to transfuse platelets prophylactically for a platelet count <20,000/μL. The threshold for platelet prophylaxis was subsequently lowered to 10,000/μL on the basis of both observational studies[50,51] and randomized trials.[52-54] An observational study suggested that an even lower platelet count threshold, 5000/μL, would be safe,[55] but the threshold of 10,000/μL has been used most commonly and is currently recommended by several clinical practice guidelines.[56,57] Several RCTs have been performed in this area, as described below. In many cases, the primary endpoint used has been bleeding at World Health Organization (WHO) Grade 2 or higher. A summary of the WHO scale is provided in Table 19-4.

There have been tremendous advances in the care of patients with cancer since the 1960s, and severe bleeding is now extremely rare. Consequently, two recent RCTs challenged the necessity of providing prophylactic platelet transfusions at all.[58-60] In a study by Wandt and colleagues,[60] 391 patients receiving chemotherapy for acute myelogenous leukemia (AML) or undergoing autologous hematopoietic progenitor cell transplantation (HPCT) were randomly assigned to receive or not receive prophylactic platelet transfusions for a morning platelet count at or below 10,000/μL. Subjects in the no-prophylaxis arm were transfused with platelets only if bleeding occurred. WHO Grade 2 or higher bleeding was observed among 42% of subjects in the no-prophylaxis arm vs 19% of subjects receiving prophylactic platelet transfusions (p <0.0001). The risk of bleeding was much higher among patients receiving chemotherapy for AML compared with the autologous HPCT patients: 27 out of 28 (96%) Grade 3 or Grade 4 bleeds occurred among patients receiving chemotherapy for AML. In the Trial of Prophylactic Platelets (TOPPS) study,[58,59] 600 patients receiving chemotherapy or autologous HPCT were randomized to platelet prophylaxis or no-prophylaxis for a morning platelet count <10,000/μL. Grade 2 or higher bleeding occurred in 50% of the no-prophylaxis subjects vs 43% of those receiving prophylaxis. As in the study of Wandt et al, the benefits of platelet prophylaxis were much stronger among patients receiving chemotherapy compared with autologous HPCT recipients. These two RCTs were included in a recent meta-analysis that concluded that providing platelet prophylaxis in the setting of hypoproliferative thrombocytopenia is associated with a significant reduction in Grade 2 or higher bleeding [odds ratio, 0.53; 95% confidence interval (CI), 0.32-0.87)].[61] Thus, prophylactic platelet transfusions continue to be standard, although some individual facilities are contemplating a therapeutic-platelet-transfusion-only strategy for autologous HPCT recipients. It needs to be emphasized that the usual platelet transfusion threshold used, 10,000/μL, is intended for hospitalized patients only. Outpatients are typically transfused with platelets more liberally, for practical reasons (ie, to permit fewer clinic visits).

TABLE 19-4. Summary of WHO Bleeding Scale*

WHO Bleeding Grade	Examples
1	Oropharyngeal bleeding ≤30 minutes in 24 hours
	Epistaxis ≤30 minutes in previous 24 hours
	Petechiae of oral mucosa or skin
	Purpura ≤1 inch in diameter
	Positive stool occult blood test
2	Epistaxis >30 minutes in 24 hours
	Purpura >1 inch in diameter
	Hemoptysis
	Melanotic stool
	Gross/visible hematuria
	Visible blood in body cavity fluid
	Bleeding at invasive sites
3	Bleeding requiring RBC transfusion over routine needs
	Bleeding associated with moderate hemodynamic instability
4	Bleeding associated with severe hemodynamic instability
	CNS bleeding on imaging study
	Fatal bleeding

*Modified from Kaufman et al.[56]
WHO = World Health Organization; RBC = Red Blood Cell; CNS = central nervous system.

Nonetheless, the optimal approach to prophylaxis in outpatients has not yet been formally studied.

A provocative 1985 study[62] suggested that while most platelets will circulate for their normal life span (approximately 8-10 days), a relatively small, fixed number of platelets, estimated to be approximately 7100 per μL per day, are used to promote vascular integrity. This population of platelets is thought to be cleared in an age-independent fashion. With this hypothesis in mind, Hersh et al[63] proposed that perhaps only a low dose of platelets is all that is needed for prophylaxis and published a mathematical model suggesting that providing low-dose platelets (3 units of platelet concentrates vs 6) would, over time, result in an overall 22% savings in the number of platelets

transfused. Subsequently, a small number of RCTs examined the question of the optimal dose of platelets to transfuse for prophylaxis in the setting of therapy-related hypoproliferative thrombocytopenia.[61] The largest of these was the Platelet Dosing (PLADO) study,[64] in which 1272 hospitalized hematology-oncology patients with hypoproliferative thrombocytopenia were randomly assigned to receive low-dose (1.1×10^{11} platelets/m^2), medium-dose (2.2×10^{11} platelets/m^2), or high-dose platelets (4.4×10^{11} platelets/m^2) for a morning platelet count of 10,000/μL. The medium-dose arm was meant to approximate one apheresis platelet unit, the current standard at the time. The primary endpoint, the proportion of patients in each arm with Grade 2 or higher bleeding, was not significantly different (71%,

69%, 70%, respectively), demonstrating that low-dose platelets are a safe alternative to the standard dose. Consistent with the prediction from the Hersh model, fewer overall platelets were transfused in the low-dose arm. However, because patients receiving low-dose platelets had a lower increment, it was necessary for them to be transfused more often (average of five transfusions per patient vs three for patients in the medium- or high-dose arms.) To date, low-dose platelets have not been widely adopted, although low-dose platelets are sometimes used to stretch inventories during shortages. When low-dose platelets are used, it is necessary to consider not only the number of platelets being transfused but also the recipient's body surface area.[64]

Platelet Transfusions as Prophylaxis for Invasive Procedures

Platelet transfusions are often administered before minor (ie, bedside) and major invasive (ie, surgical) procedures to try to reduce the bleeding risk in patients with quantitative or qualitative platelet deficiencies. The published evidence supporting the use of platelet transfusions in these settings is limited. In 2015, AABB published a clinical practice guideline on platelet transfusion; these recommendations are summarized in Table 19-5.[56] This guideline was based on a systematic review of the literature.[61] Except for its Recommendation 1 (platelet prophylaxis for therapy-related hypoproliferative thrombocytopenia), all other recommendations are weak and based on low- or very-low-quality evidence. For central venous catheter placement, AABB suggests that prophylactic platelet transfusion may be considered for a platelet count <20,000 cells/μL. A prophylactic platelet count threshold of 50,000/μL is suggested for lumbar puncture and for major elective nonneuraxial surgery. Although the platelet count is important to consider, it is also relevant to note that this does not provide information on platelet function. Clinical judgment, rather than a specific platelet count threshold, is of primary importance when deciding whether to transfuse platelets in these settings.

TABLE 19-5. Summary of AABB Recommendations for Prophylactic Platelet Transfusion in Adults[56]

Clinical Setting	PLT Transfusion May Be Indicated for:	Strength of Recommendation	Quality of Evidence
Therapy-related hypoproliferative thrombocytopenia	PLT count ≤10,000/μL	Strong	Moderate
Central venous catheter placement	PLT count <20,000/μL	Weak	Low
Diagnostic lumbar puncture	PLT count <50,000/μL*	Weak	Very low
Major elective nonneuraxial surgery	PLT count <50,000/μL	Weak	Very low
Cardiac surgery with bypass	Perioperative bleeding with thrombocytopenia and/or evidence of PLT dysfunction. Routine PLT prophylaxis not recommended.	Weak	Very low
Intracranial hemorrhage on anti-PLT therapy	Insufficient evidence for recommendation	Uncertain	Very low

*Clinical judgment should be used for patients with PLT counts between 20,000 and 50,000/μL.
PLT = platelet.

Platelet Transfusions to Treat Active Bleeding

In thrombocytopenic patients who are bleeding, it is often recommended that platelets should be transfused to maintain a platelet count above >50,000/μL. In bleeding patients with qualitative platelet dysfunction (eg, patients on antiplatelet medications or after cardiopulmonary bypass), platelet transfusions may be appropriate even at a normal platelet count. Currently, no high-quality evidence is available to help guide platelet transfusion in the setting of active bleeding.

ABO and Rh Matching for Platelets

ABO matching is not an absolute requirement for platelets (or plasma) as it is for RBCs. But platelets do express ABH antigens, often at high levels.[65,66] Preformed anti-A or anti-B in the recipient may destroy transfused major-mismatched platelets (eg, A donor, O recipient).[65,67,68] Transfusion of major-mismatched platelets usually results in lower platelet increments.[69] Conversely, transfusing ABO minor-mismatched platelets (eg, O donor, B recipient) can cause hemolytic transfusion reactions, albeit rarely, resulting from passive administration of anti-A or anti-B in the plasma.[70] Providing ABO-identical platelet transfusions to all patients is often not feasible because of inventory limitations. Several studies have investigated the impact of ABO matching on various outcomes,[67,70-72] including mortality, bleeding, transfusion reactions, platelet count increment, and refractoriness. Mortality, bleeding, and transfusion reaction rates were not definitively shown to be improved by ABO matching, whereas the platelet count increment does increase with ABO matching. Two controlled trials[73,74] demonstrated a 40% to 60% reduction in refractoriness with ABO matching, but because definitions of refractoriness differed, the absolute benefit could not be determined. Overall, when available, ABO-identical platelets should be transfused.

Platelets do not express Rh antigens,[75] but platelet units do contain some "contaminating" red cells. Small volumes of RhD-positive red cells can cause alloimmunization resulting in anti-D. Apheresis platelet units now typically contain only microliter quantities of red cells,[76-78] and platelets are often administered to immunocompromised patients who may be less capable of becoming alloimmunized. Thus, the overall frequency of alloimmunization from RhD-positive platelet units is very low.[79] This low risk can essentially be eliminated by administering Rh Immune Globulin (RhIG) within 72 hours of transfusion of RhD-positive platelets to an RhD-negative recipient. Nonetheless, the decision to administer RhIG to prevent RhD alloimmunization in this setting should include consideration of risks and benefits and the potential clinical impact of alloimmunization (ie, in females of childbearing potential).

Platelet Refractoriness

Platelet refractoriness represents a consistent failure to achieve an appropriate platelet count increment following platelet transfusion. In most cases, platelet refractoriness is thought to have a nonimmune cause such as sepsis, disseminated intravascular coagulation (DIC), bleeding, hypersplenism, drug effects, or other platelet-consumptive states. Approximately 20% of cases of platelet refractoriness are thought to have an immune etiology.[80] Some possible causes of platelet refractoriness are listed in Table 19-6.

If a typical apheresis platelet unit (~4×10^{11} platelets) is transfused to an average-sized, relatively healthy recipient, the expected 1-hour posttransfusion increment is ~30,000 to 60,000/μL. In severely thrombocytopenic patients receiving platelet prophylaxis, it is common for the observed platelet increment to be smaller and for the transfused platelets to have a shorter survival. The prevailing hypothesis explaining this observation is that the lower the pretransfusion platelet count, the higher the proportion of platelets needed to maintain vascular integrity.[62]

There has not been agreement on a precise definition of platelet refractoriness. Published studies of platelet transfusion have often used a platelet refractoriness definition of

TABLE 19-6. Causes of Platelet Refractoriness[81]

Nonimmune	Immune
Fever	HLA antibodies
Medications (eg, amphotericin, vancomycin)	ABO incompatibility
Splenomegaly	Human platelet antigen (HPA) antibodies
Sepsis	Drug-dependent autoantibodies
Disseminated intravascular coagulation	
Hemorrhage	
Veno-occlusive disease	
Graft-vs-host disease	
Prolonged platelet storage	

repeated 1-hour corrected count increments (CCIs) <7.5. The CCI attempts to adjust the absolute platelet increment observed for the number of platelets transfused ($\times 10^{11}$) and the size of the recipient as reflected by body surface area [BSA (m^2)]:

$$CCI = \frac{\text{Platelet increment} \times BSA \text{ (m}^2)}{\text{Platelets transfused } (\times 10^{11})}$$

Example: A patient with a BSA of 2.0 m^2 and a platelet count of 5000/μL receives a unit of apheresis platelets containing 4×10^{11} platelets, and the posttransfusion platelet count is 25,000/μL. The CCI may be calculated as follows:

$$CCI = \frac{20 \times 2.0}{4.0} = 10$$

CCIs are not used in routine clinical practice, because the number of platelets transfused is usually unavailable. Rather, the unadjusted platelet count increment is used to judge whether the patient's platelet count increased appropriately. To evaluate a patient for immune refractoriness, platelet counts should be obtained between 10 and 60 minutes after transfusion. Poor increments (eg, <10,000/μL) on at least two early posttransfusion counts may be attributable to immune refractori-

ness.[81] Alternatively, if the platelet count increases appropriately 1 hour after transfusion but then declines to baseline at 24 hours, a nonimmune cause of platelet refractoriness is likely (eg, consumption).

Immune refractoriness is usually caused by antibodies that target HLA[82,83] and cause rapid clearance of transfused platelets. Less commonly, immune refractoriness is attributable to antibodies directed against human platelet antigens (HPAs). Transfusion recipients may become alloimmunized to platelet HLA antigens either by prior pregnancy, organ transplantation, or transfusion. Platelets express HLA Class I antigens, but they are relatively poor immunogens. When immune refractoriness occurs in platelet transfusion recipients, the HLA antibody response is mainly provoked by contaminating white blood cells in the unit rather than the platelets themselves.[84] The Trial to Reduce Alloimmunization to Platelets (TRAP) confirmed that leukocyte reduction significantly reduces the risk of HLA alloimmunization. Pregnancy is by far the most important risk factor for primary HLA sensitization.[85] In the era of leukocyte-reduced blood components, immune refractoriness, often reflecting a secondary immune response to HLA antigens, is a particular problem in multiparous women.[86]

Identifying HLA antibodies is a second important step in approaching immune refractoriness. HLA antibody detection is most commonly performed using flow cytometry of multiantigen-coated beads, although other methods (eg, lymphocytotoxicity assays, enzyme-linked immunosorbent assays) are also used. Laboratories report a panel-reactive antibody (PRA) score reflecting the degree of HLA allo-immunization; for example, a PRA of 20% has been used as a threshold consistent with immune refractoriness.[64] However, anti-HLA assays vary considerably across laboratories, and there is no standard definition of a meaningful PRA score.

Maneuvers to mitigate platelet immune refractoriness were recently reviewed.[87,88] Options to manage immune refractoriness include providing HLA-matched platelets, HLA-antibody avoidance (ie, identifying HLA-antibody specificity and providing antigen-negative platelet units, analogous to similar strategies with RBC units), and platelet cross-matching.[89] When providing HLA-matched platelet units, grade A or BU matches provide the best chance for success, although a failure to achieve a good increment is still seen in 20% of cases.[89] A recent systematic review[87] examined the efficacy of providing HLA-matched platelet units for refractory patients receiving prophylaxis. Most of the existing data come from observational studies performed before 2000, prior to the routine use of current HLA antibody testing methods. Most of these studies report posttransfusion increments among immune-refractory patients receiving HLA-matched platelets, with varying degrees of success. A 2014 single-center observational study[90] found that providing HLA-matched units (grade A, B1U, or B1X) was associated with a successful increment in only 29% of transfusions to refractory patients. Although better than providing random units, transfusing HLA-matched platelets was of only limited utility. Studies powered to examine the effect of HLA-selected platelets on bleeding outcomes have not yet been performed.

PLASMA TRANSFUSION

Plasma Prophylaxis for Invasive Procedures

Before performing invasive procedures, physicians often transfuse plasma to patients with modest abnormalities in coagulation tests [eg, the prothrombin time/international normalized ratio (PT/INR) or activated partial thromboplastin time (aPTT)], with the goal of reducing the bleeding risk. In most cases, this practice exposes patients to all the risks of plasma transfusion without providing a real benefit. This is because 1) mild-to-moderate abnormalities in test results like the INR fail to predict bleeding in nonbleeding individuals[91]; 2) modest elevations in the INR are usually not corrected to normal by plasma transfusion[92]; and 3) prior RCTs and observational studies failed to show that prophylactic plasma transfusions affect bleeding outcomes.[93-97]

Plasma Transfusions to Treat Bleeding

Plasma transfusion is indicated for bleeding patients with multiple coagulation deficiencies (eg, liver disease, DIC). It is also indicated to manage patients with specific plasma-protein deficiencies (eg, Factor XI deficiency) for which a licensed coagulation factor concentrate is not available.

Massive Transfusion Protocols

"Massive transfusion" is most often defined as transfusion of adults with 10 or more RBC units in a 24-hour period, although other definitions (eg, 4 RBC units in 1 hour) are also used.[98] In the past, trauma patients with substantial blood loss were typically treated with RBC transfusions plus crystalloid, with hemostatic products such as platelets, plasma, and cryoprecipitate administered based on laboratory test results. In recent years, this approach was largely superseded by a more aggressive and empiric approach, whereby the initial resuscitation of trauma patients is focused on early transfusion with plasma, platelets, and RBCs in a fixed ratio (eg, 1:1:1; note: for platelets, the "1" refers to a single whole-blood-derived platelet concentrate and not 1 apheresis platelet unit). These fixed ratios are intended to approximate the transfusion of whole blood through a combination of components in order to prevent dilutional coagulopathy. The fixed ratio or "formula-based" approach was devised by military physicians during the Iraq and Afghanistan wars of the 2000s. The publication credited with sparking interest in this approach[99] described 246 injured soldiers in Iraq who were retrospectively grouped by the ratio of plasma to RBCs received. Patients in the low plasma-to-RBC group (median of 1 unit of plasma for every 8 RBC units) had a 65% mortality rate, as compared with a 19% mortality rate among patients in the high plasma-to-RBC group (median of 1 unit of plasma for every 1.4 RBC units). Although striking, this study and multiple other subsequent retrospective studies were highly confounded. Trauma patients who die from their injuries due to blood loss tend to do so very early (ie, often in less than an hour after hospital arrival).[100] It was unclear whether early and aggressive plasma transfusion led to better survival, or whether plasma transfusion was available for the less-severely injured patients who survived (ie, there was time to thaw and transfuse frozen plasma in cases where patients did not die rapidly on arrival).[101,102]

Two recent multicenter studies examined transfusion management of massively bleeding trauma patients. The Prospective, Observational, Multicenter, Major Trauma Transfusion (PROMMTT) study[103] was a prospective observational study of adult trauma patients treated at 1 of 10 civilian trauma centers in the United States. Study staff performed direct bedside observation as patients were resuscitated. To reduce potential survivor bias, patients dying within the first 30 minutes of arrival were excluded. Patients who received plasma to RBCs in a 1:1 ratio had significantly better 6-hour survival than patients receiving a lower ratio of plasma to RBCs. However, survival at later time points did not differ significantly. A subsequent RCT, called the Pragmatic Randomized Optimal Platelet and Plasma Ratios (PROPPR) trial,[104] compared outcomes among 680 adult civilian trauma patients who were randomly assigned to be resuscitated using a 1:1:1 vs 1:1:2 ratio of plasma to platelets to RBCs. The primary outcomes, 24-hour and 30-day survival, did not significantly differ between the study groups. Currently, it is common for blood banks to incorporate fixed ratios of blood components (ie, 1:1:1 or 1:1:2) into their local massive transfusion protocols (MTPs). Although it is difficult to judge the effectiveness of this approach from the published data, it does improve the speed and simplicity of the initial response. Laboratory-based, targeted transfusion of specific components is often used after the patient has stabilized. It is important to note that although much of the data on MTPs relates to trauma, in civilian hospitals, massive transfusions are actually more likely to occur among other patient populations (eg, solid-organ transplant patients and cardiac surgical patients).[105,106]

Group AB plasma is a preferred blood component in trauma MTPs before blood group determination because it lacks anti-A and anti-B. However, because AB plasma is in short supply due to the low frequency of type AB donors (~4%), group A plasma has been used in several centers as an alternate to AB plasma. Studies of group B and AB trauma patients who have received group A plasma support the safety of this practice, although the data are limited.[107]

Warfarin Reversal

During clot formation, several coagulation factors such as Factors II, VII, IX, and X associate with the surface of activated platelets via hydrophobic protein domains called gamma-carboxyglutamic acid (Gla) domains. Gla domains help ensure that when activated, coagulation factors localize where they are needed to provide full hemostatic function. To form Gla domains, specific glutamic acid (Glu) residues must undergo posttranslational gamma-carboxylation. The reduced form of vitamin K is required to contribute electrons to these carboxylation reactions. In the process, vitamin K becomes oxidized. Enzymes called vitamin K epoxide reductases serve to recycle vitamin K back to its "useful" reduced form so that it can participate in subsequent gamma-carboxylation reactions. Warfarin, which is structurally similar to vitamin K, competitively inhibits the epoxide reductases. Thus, warfarin intake causes a deficiency of reduced vitamin K, which in turn causes decreases in the functional activity of Factors II (thrombin), VII, IX, and X, as well as antithrombotic factors: proteins C and S.[108]

There are several methods available to reverse the effect of warfarin. For warfarinized patients in whom urgent reversal is needed (eg, bleeding or requiring emergency surgery), the treatment of choice is a four-factor prothrombin complex concentrate (PCC). PCCs contain high levels of Factors II, VII, IX, and X in the nonactivated state, as well as proteins C and S. A recent RCT demonstrated that warfarin reversal was more rapid and reliable in bleeding patients taking warfarin who received a PCC as compared with patients receiving plasma.[109,110] Vitamin K administration is also recommended when reversing warfarin, to ensure a sustained effect. Plasma can also be used if PCCs are contraindicated, such as in patients who have had heparin-induced thrombocytopenia, because some PCCs contain heparin.

Types of Plasma

Several varieties of plasma are available for transfusion, including Fresh Frozen Plasma (FFP), Plasma Frozen Within 24 Hours After Phlebotomy (FP24), and solvent/detergent-treated plasma (SD plasma). By definition, FFP is frozen within 8 hours of collection and transfused within 24 hours of thawing, to preserve levels of the most heat-labile coagulation factors, Factors VIII and V. Many transfusion services provide Thawed Plasma, which is plasma that has been thawed and maintained in a closed system at 1 to 6 C for up to 5 days. (Thawed Plasma is not currently regulated by the US Food and Drug Administration but is recognized in both the *Circular of Information for the Use of Blood and Blood Components* and AABB *Standards for Blood Banks and Transfusion Services.*) Advantages of Thawed Plasma are that it is available to be issued im-

mediately in bleeding emergencies and, because of its longer shelf life, it reduces wastage. The activity of individual coagulation factors, such as Factor VIII, can variably decline over time, but overall factor activities have been shown to remain within the normal range during 5-day refrigerated storage.[111-113] Differences in clinical outcome among recipients of various types of plasma have not been demonstrated, and many transfusion services currently use Thawed Plasma from any original source (FFP, PF24, SD plasma, etc) interchangeably with freshly thawed FFP. SD plasma provides an extra measure of safety with respect to transmission of enveloped viruses and other pathogens[114]; the main disadvantage is cost.

CRYOPRECIPITATE TRANSFUSION

Cryoprecipitate is a plasma derivative that is relatively enriched for fibrinogen, Factor VIII, von Willebrand Factor (vWF), fibronectin, and Factor XIII. There are limited indications for cryoprecipitate, as there are pathogen-reduced products and recombinant products available for several of the indications where cryoprecipitate was used previously. Cryoprecipitate is suggested for fibrinogen replacement for acquired hypofibrinogenemic conditions such as liver transplantation and postpartum hemorrhage.[115-117] Pathogen-reduced concentrates are standard-of-care to treat Factor VIII deficiency, congenital hypofibrinogenemia, dysfibrinogenemia, and von Willebrand disease. Congenital Factor XIII deficiency, associated with a delayed bleeding phenotype, is extremely rare, and there is now a recombinant Factor XIII concentrate available. Fibronectin is not currently used as a therapeutic agent. Thus, cryoprecipitate is primarily used to replace fibrinogen in patients who are bleeding or having invasive procedures.

Pregnancy is associated with an increase in fibrinogen concentration above the laboratory levels of normal (approximately 6 g/L in the third trimester compared to 2-4 g/L in the nonpregnant state).[118] A low fibrinogen concentration among women with postpartum hemorrhage has been reported to be independently associated with severe bleeding.[119,120] To restore hemostasis, fibrinogen replacement has been advocated.[121] Plasma, cryoprecipitate, and fibrinogen concentrate are all sources of fibrinogen. However, the volume of plasma needed is considerably larger than that of cryoprecipitate to achieve the same replacement dose of fibrinogen (eg, 300-400 mg of fibrinogen can be replaced with 250 mL of plasma or with only 10-15 mL of cryoprecipitate). Fibrinogen concentrate is also a low-volume option, and it has the additional advantages of being pathogen reduced and requiring no thawing time. To date, cryoprecipitate and fibrinogen concentrate have not been directly compared in clinical studies. In a small retrospective study of women with postpartum hemorrhage, similar outcomes were achieved among patients receiving either cryoprecipitate or fibrinogen concentrate.[116] In the 2015 Fibrinogen Concentrate as Initial Treatment for Postpartum Haemorrhage (FIB-PPH) trial,[122] women with postpartum hemorrhage were randomly assigned to receive 2 g of fibrinogen concentrate or placebo. No difference in clinical outcomes was observed (20% of patients in the fibrinogen concentrate group received RBCs vs 22% of controls). However, only a small proportion of patients had severe postpartum hemorrhage in this trial.

Cardiac surgery is associated with acquired hemostatic defects secondary to cardiopulmonary bypass that lead to excess bleeding.[123-125] Individuals having cardiac surgery are at high risk of receiving blood transfusion.[126] The use of prophylactic fibrinogen is intended to reduce the risk of bleeding and consequently the exposure to blood components, because a lower fibrinogen concentration following cardiac surgery was associated with a higher bleeding risk.[127] In a small, single-center, placebo-controlled, double-blinded RCT, prophylactic fibrinogen concentrate administered after protamine administration reduced blood component usage among nonanemic cardiac surgery patients. Patients randomly assigned to fibrinogen

concentrate, as compared with placebo, were significantly less likely to be transfused with any allogeneic blood component (67% vs 45%; p = 0.015). Postoperative bleeding was significantly (although modestly) lower in the fibrinogen concentrate group (median blood loss of 300 mL vs 355 mL; p = 0.042).[128] Nonetheless, further studies are needed to define the role of fibrinogen replacement and the effects on bleeding, mortality, blood component utilization, and adverse events.[129] A more recent placebo-controlled multicenter RCT of fibrinogen concentrate in postoperative cardiac surgery patients showed no benefit; patients receiving fibrinogen concentrate actually received significantly more allogeneic blood components.[130]

GRANULOCYTE TRANSFUSION

Prolonged severe neutropenia (defined as an absolute neutrophil count of <500/μL) predisposes patients to life-threatening bacterial and fungal infections despite aggressive antimicrobial therapy.[131] Prolonged severe neutropenia usually occurs with intensive chemotherapy for hematologic malignancies or in the setting of hematopoietic stem cell transplantation. Providing granulocytes is thought to reduce the risk of morbidity and mortality associated with the related infections. Donors are stimulated with corticosteroids and/or granulocyte colony-stimulating factor (G-CSF), allowing high numbers of granulocytes to be collected by apheresis. Granulocyte components are stored at room temperature and must be transfused as soon as possible and within 24 hours of collection. Granulocyte components contain several milliliters of red cells. To prevent acute hemolytic reactions, granulocyte components are matched to the recipient according to RBC ABO-matching rules (Table 19-3). Also, it is necessary to irradiate all granulocyte components to prevent transfusion-associated graft-vs-host disease.

However, a survival benefit of transfusing septic, neutropenic patients with granulocytes has not been definitively demonstrated.[132] This lack of benefit may be due to the inability to provide an adequate number of granulocytes for transfusion.[131,133] In a systematic review of 10 RCTs, prophylactic granulocyte transfusion was not associated with a difference in morbidity or mortality secondary to infections; however, intermediate-dose granulocyte transfusions ($1\text{-}4 \times 10^{10}$ granulocytes per day) were associated with a reduction in the number of patients with infections after 30 days [relative risk (RR), 0.4; 95% CI, 0.26 to 0.63] and the number of patients with bacteremia and fungemia (RR, 0.45; 95% CI, 0.30 to 0.65).[133] Trials of therapeutic granulocyte transfusion in septic immunocompromised patients have also shown inconsistent results.[131] For example, in the multicenter Resolving Infection in Neutropenia with Granulocytes (RING) trial,[132] neutropenic patients with proven or likely infection were randomly assigned to receive standard antimicrobial therapy or standard antimicrobial therapy plus granulocytes collected from donors stimulated with G-CSF and dexamethasone. Overall, no benefit was observed from transfusing granulocytes. Nonetheless, the RING study was underpowered, having enrolled only 50% of the predefined sample size required to detect a difference in the primary composite outcome of survival and microbial clearance after 42 days. Also, the target dose of $>4 \times 10^{10}$ granulocytes per transfusion (0.6×10^9 cells/kg) was achieved in only 70% of transfusions.[134] A secondary analysis suggested that patients who received higher doses of granulocytes tended to have better outcomes than patients who received lower doses.[132] Currently, the role of granulocyte transfusion remains undefined, and clinical judgment is required. If granulocyte transfusions are used, a high dose of granulocytes should be provided whenever possible.

KEY POINTS

1. In deciding to transfuse RBCs, it is important to consider the patient's clinical status, comorbidities, etiology and time course of anemia, and Hb level. In hemodynamically stable inpatients, when Hb level is the sole consideration, then a restrictive transfusion approach (Hb threshold of 7-8 g/dL) should be used.

2. Currently, insufficient evidence is available to recommend a restrictive RBC transfusion approach for patients with acute coronary syndrome, severe thrombocytopenia, or chronic transfusion-dependent anemia.

3. In patients with sickle cell disease at high risk for stroke based on transcranial Doppler ultrasonography, chronic RBC transfusion (or hydroxyurea) reduces stroke risk. RBC transfusion is not recommended to treat patients with sickle cell disease with uncomplicated painful vaso-occlusive crises, priapism, asymptomatic anemia, or acute kidney injury.

4. Neonatal, pediatric, and adult patients may receive RBC units of any storage age within the licensed storage period.

5. When clinically indicated, RBC transfusion should not be withheld in cases of WAIHA, even though units are incompatible because of the autoantibody. Efforts should be made to detect and avoid underlying clinically significant alloantibodies, and sufficient RBCs should be transfused to relieve signs and symptoms of anemia.

6. In hospitalized patients with therapy-related hypoproliferative thrombocytopenia, prophylactic platelet transfusions reduce the risk of spontaneous bleeding. For this patient group, a prophylactic platelet transfusion threshold of 10,000/μL is appropriate.

7. Most cases of platelet refractoriness are nonimmune in origin. Patients with immune refractoriness may benefit from a trial of HLA-matched, antigen-negative, or crossmatched platelet units.

8. Plasma transfusion is indicated for bleeding patients with multiple coagulation factor deficiencies and in massive transfusion protocols. Urgent warfarin reversal is best achieved using a four-factor prothrombin complex concentrate (PCC).

9. Cryoprecipitate is used for fibrinogen replacement. Fibrinogen concentrate may be used as an alternative.

10. Granulocytes are sometimes transfused to treat severe refractory bacterial or fungal infections in neutropenic patients. The utility of granulocyte transfusions remains unclear. If granulocytes are used, high doses should be administered.

REFERENCES

1. Hébert PC, Wells G, Blajchman MA, et al. A multicenter, randomized, controlled clinical trial of transfusion requirements in critical care. Transfusion Requirements in Critical Care Investigators, Canadian Critical Care Trials Group. N Engl J Med 1999;340:409-17.

2. Carson JL, Terrin ML, Noveck H, et al. Liberal or restrictive transfusion in high-risk patients after hip surgery. N Engl J Med 2011;365:2453-62.

3. Grover M, Talwalkar S, Casbard A, et al. Silent myocardial ischaemia and haemoglobin concentration: A randomized controlled trial of transfusion strategy in lower limb arthroplasty. Vox Sang 2006;90:105-12.

4. So-Osman C, Nelissen R, Te Slaa R, et al. A randomized comparison of transfusion triggers in elective orthopaedic surgery using leucocyte-depleted red blood cells. Vox Sang 2010;98:56-64.

5. Carson JL, Carless PA, Hébert PC. Transfusion thresholds and other strategies for guiding allogeneic red blood cell transfusion. Cochrane Database Syst Rev 2012;(4):CD002042.

6. Holst LB, Petersen MW, Haase N, et al. Restrictive versus liberal transfusion strategy for red blood cell transfusion: Systematic review of randomised trials with meta-analysis and trial sequential analysis. BMJ 2015;350:h1354. doi: 10.1136/bmj.h1354.

7. Bracey AW, Radovancevic R, Riggs SA, et al. Lowering the hemoglobin threshold for transfusion in coronary artery bypass procedures: Effect on patient outcome. Transfusion 1999;39:1070-7.

8. Hajjar LA, Vincent JL, Galas FR, et al. Transfusion requirements after cardiac surgery: The TRACS randomized controlled trial. JAMA 2010;304:1559-67.

9. Murphy GJ, Pike K, Rogers CA, et al. Liberal or restrictive transfusion after cardiac surgery. N Engl J Med 2015;372:997-1008.

10. Shehata N, Burns LA, Nathan H, et al. A randomized controlled pilot study of adherence to transfusion strategies in cardiac surgery. Transfusion 2012;52:91-9.

11. Holst LB, Haase N, Wetterslev J, et al. Lower versus higher hemoglobin threshold for transfusion in septic shock. N Engl J Med 2014;371:1381-91.

12. Villanueva C, Colomo A, Bosch A, et al. Transfusion strategies for acute upper gastrointestinal bleeding. N Engl J Med 2013;368:11-21.

13. Jairath V, Kahan BC, Gray A, et al. Restrictive versus liberal blood transfusion for acute upper gastrointestinal bleeding (TRIGGER): A pragmatic, open-label, cluster randomised feasibility trial. Lancet 2015;386:137-44.

14. de Almeida JP, Vincent J-L, Galas FRBG, et al. Transfusion requirements in surgical oncology patients: A prospective, randomized controlled trial. Anesthesiology 2015;122:29-38.

15. Prick BW, Jansen A, Steegers E, et al. Transfusion policy after severe postpartum haemorrhage: A randomised non-inferiority trial. BJOG 2014;121:1005-14.

16. Robertson CS, Hannay HJ, Yamal J-M, et al. Effect of erythropoietin and transfusion threshold on neurological recovery after traumatic brain injury. JAMA 2014;312:36-47.

17. Carson JL, Stanworth SJ, Roubinian N, et al. Transfusion thresholds and other strategies for guiding allogeneic red blood cell transfusion. Cochrane Database Syst Rev 2016;10: CD002042.

18. Carson JL, Guyatt G, Heddle NM, et al. Clinical practice guidelines from the AABB: Red Blood Cell transfusion thresholds and storage. JAMA 2016;316:2025-35.

19. So-Osman C, Nelissen R, Brand R, et al. Postoperative anemia after joint replacement surgery is not related to quality of life during the first two weeks postoperatively. Transfusion 2011;51:71-81.

20. Hébert PC, Yetisir E, Martin C, et al. Is a low transfusion threshold safe in critically ill patients with cardiovascular diseases? Crit Care Med 2001;29:227-34.

21. Rachmilewitz EA, Giardina PJ. How I treat thalassemia. Blood 2011;118:3479-88.

22. Goss C, Giardina P, Degtyaryova D, et al. Red blood cell transfusions for thalassemia: Results of a survey assessing current practice and proposal of evidence-based guidelines. Transfusion 2014;54:1773-81.

23. Bunn HF. Pathogenesis and treatment of sickle cell disease. N Engl J Med 1997;337:762-9.

24. Yawn BP, Buchanan GR, Afenyi-Annan AN, et al. Management of sickle cell disease: Summary of the 2014 evidence-based report by expert panel members. JAMA 2014;312:1033-48.

25. Rosse WF, Gallagher D, Kinney TR, et al. Transfusion and alloimmunization in sickle cell disease. The Cooperative Study of Sickle Cell Disease. Blood 1990;76:1431-7.

26. Yazdanbakhsh K, Ware RE, Noizat-Pirenne F. Red blood cell alloimmunization in sickle cell disease: Pathophysiology, risk factors, and transfusion management. Blood 2012;120:528-37.

27. Chou ST, Jackson T, Vege S, et al. High prevalence of red blood cell alloimmunization in sickle cell disease despite transfusion from Rh-matched minority donors. Blood 2013;122:1062-71.

28. Fasano RM, Booth GS, Miles M, et al. Red blood cell alloimmunization is influenced by recipient inflammatory state at time of transfusion in patients with sickle cell disease. Br J Haematol 2015;168:291-300.

29. Win N. Hyperhemolysis syndrome in sickle cell disease. Expert Rev Hematol 2009;2:111-15.

30. Win N, Sinha S, Lee E, Mills W. Treatment with intravenous immunoglobulin and steroids may correct severe anemia in hyperhemolytic transfusion reactions: Case report and literature review. Transfus Med Rev 2010;24:64-7.

31. Kacker S, Ness PM, Savage WJ, et al. Cost-effectiveness of prospective red blood cell antigen matching to prevent alloimmunization among sickle cell patients. Transfusion 2014;54:86-97.

32. Vichinsky EP, Luban NL, Wright E, et al. Prospective RBC phenotype matching in a stroke-prevention trial in sickle cell anemia: A multi-center transfusion trial. Transfusion 2001;41:1086-92.

33. Tournamille C, Meunier-Costes N, Costes B, et al. Partial C antigen in sickle cell disease patients: Clinical relevance and prevention of alloimmunization. Transfusion 2010;50:13-19.

34. Adams RJ, McKie VC, Hsu L, et al. Prevention of a first stroke by transfusions in children with sickle cell anemia and abnormal results on transcranial Doppler ultrasonography. N Engl J Med 1998;339:5-11.

35. Adams RJ, Brambilla D, STOP2 Trial investigators. Discontinuing prophylactic transfusions used to prevent stroke in sickle cell disease. N Engl J Med 2005;353:2769-78.

36. Ware RE, Davis BR, Schultz WH, et al. Hydroxycarbamide versus chronic transfusion for maintenance of transcranial doppler flow velocities in children with sickle cell anaemia—TCD With Transfusions Changing to Hydroxyurea (TWiTCH): A multicentre, open-label, phase 3, non-inferiority trial. Lancet 2016;387:661-70.

37. Koch CG, Li L, Sessler DI, et al. Duration of red-cell storage and complications after cardiac surgery. N Engl J Med 2008;358:1229-39.

38. Fergusson DA, Hébert P, Hogan DL, et al. Effect of fresh red blood cell transfusions on clinical outcomes in premature, very low-birth-weight infants: The ARIPI randomized trial. JAMA 2012;308:1443-51.

39. Lacroix J, Hébert PC, Fergusson DA, et al. Age of transfused blood in critically ill adults. N Engl J Med 2015;372:1410-18.

40. Steiner ME, Ness PM, Assmann SF, et al. Effects of red-cell storage duration on patients undergoing cardiac surgery. N Engl J Med 2015;372:1419-29.

41. Dhabangi A, Ainomugisha B, Cserti-Gazdewich C, et al. Effect of transfusion of Red Blood Cells with longer vs shorter storage duration on elevated blood lactate levels in children with severe anemia. JAMA 2015;314:2514-23.

42. Heddle NM, Cook RJ, Arnold DM, et al. Effect of short-term vs. long-term blood storage on mortality after transfusion. N Engl J Med 2016;375:1937-45.

43. Petz LD. A physician's guide to transfusion in autoimmune haemolytic anaemia. Br J Haematol 2004;124:712-16.

44. Issitt PD, Combs MR, Bumgarner DJ, et al. Studies of antibodies in the sera of patients who have made red cell autoantibodies. Transfusion 1996;36:481-6.

45. Laine ML, Beattie KM. Frequency of alloantibodies accompanying autoantibodies. Transfusion 1985;25:545-6.

46. Shirey RS, Boyd JS, Parwani AV, et al. Prophylactic antigen-matched donor blood for

patients with warm autoantibodies: An algorithm for transfusion management. Transfusion 2002;42:1435-41.

47. El Kenz H, Efira A, Le PQ, et al. Transfusion support of autoimmune hemolytic anemia: How could the blood group genotyping help? Transl Res 2014;163:36-42.

48. Petz LD, Garratty G. Immune hemolytic anemias. Philadelphia: Churchill Livingstone, 2004.

49. Gaydos LA, Freireich EJ, Mantel N. The quantitative relation between platelet count and hemorrhage in patients with acute leukemia. N Engl J Med 1962;266:905-9.

50. Wandt H, Frank M, Ehninger G, et al. Safety and cost effectiveness of a 10 x 10(9)/L trigger for prophylactic platelet transfusions compared with the traditional 20 x 10(9)/L trigger: A prospective comparative trial in 105 patients with acute myeloid leukemia. Blood 1998; 91:3601-6.

51. Slichter SJ, Harker LA. Thrombocytopenia: Mechanisms and management of defects in platelet production. Clin Haematol 1978; 7:523-39.

52. Heckman KD, Weiner GJ, Davis CS, et al. Randomized study of prophylactic platelet transfusion threshold during induction therapy for adult acute leukemia: 10,000/microL versus 20,000/microL. J Clin Oncol 1997;15:1143-9.

53. Rebulla P, Finazzi G, Marangoni F, et al. The threshold for prophylactic platelet transfusions in adults with acute myeloid leukemia. Gruppo Italiano Malattie Ematologiche Maligne dell'Adulto. N Engl J Med 1997;337:1870-5.

54. Zumberg MS, del Rosario MLU, Nejame CF, et al. A prospective randomized trial of prophylactic platelet transfusion and bleeding incidence in hematopoietic stem cell transplant recipients: 10,000/L versus 20,000/microL trigger. Biol Blood Marrow Transplant 2002;8:569-76.

55. Gmür J, Burger J, Schanz U, et al. Safety of stringent prophylactic platelet transfusion policy for patients with acute leukaemia. The Lancet 1991;338:1223-6.

56. Kaufman RM, Djulbegovic B, Gernsheimer T, et al. Platelet transfusion: A clinical practice guideline from the AABB. Ann Intern Med 2015;162:205-13.

57. Nahirniak S, Slichter SJ, Tanael S, et al. Guidance on platelet transfusion for patients with hypoproliferative thrombocytopenia. Transfus Med Rev 2015;29:3-13.

58. Stanworth SJ, Estcourt LJ, Llewelyn CA, et al. Impact of prophylactic platelet transfusions on bleeding events in patients with hematologic malignancies: A subgroup analysis of a randomized trial. Transfusion 2014;54:2385-93.

59. Stanworth SJ, Estcourt LJ, Powter G, et al. A no-prophylaxis platelet-transfusion strategy for hematologic cancers. N Engl J Med 2013;368: 1771-80.

60. Wandt H, Schaefer-Eckart K, Wendelin K, et al. Therapeutic platelet transfusion versus routine prophylactic transfusion in patients with haematological malignancies: An open-label, multicentre, randomised study. The Lancet 2012;380:1309-16.

61. Kumar A, Mhaskar R, Grossman BJ, et al. Platelet transfusion: A systematic review of the clinical evidence. Transfusion 2014;55:1116-27.

62. Hanson SR, Slichter SJ. Platelet kinetics in patients with bone marrow hypoplasia: Evidence for a fixed platelet requirement. Blood 1985; 66:1105-9.

63. Hersh JK, Hom EG, Brecher ME. Mathematical modeling of platelet survival with implications for optimal transfusion practice in the chronically platelet transfusion-dependent patient. Transfusion 1998;38:637-44.

64. Slichter SJ, Kaufman RM, Assmann SF, et al. Dose of prophylactic platelet transfusions and prevention of hemorrhage. N Engl J Med 2010; 362:600-13.

65. Cooling L. ABO and platelet transfusion therapy. Immunohematology 2007;23:20-33.

66. Kelton JG, Hamid C, Aker S, Blajchman MA. The amount of blood group A substance on platelets is proportional to the amount in the plasma. Blood 1982;59:980-5.

67. Julmy F, Ammann RA, Taleghani BM, et al. Transfusion efficacy of ABO major-mismatched platelets (PLTs) in children is inferior to that of ABO-identical PLTs. Transfusion 2009;49:21-33.

68. Aster RH. Effect of anticoagulant and ABO incompatibility on recovery of transfused human platelets. Blood 1965;26:732-43.

69. Lee EJ, Schiffer CA. ABO compatibility can influence the results of platelet transfusion. Results of a randomized trial. Transfusion 1989; 29:384-9.

70. Kaufman RM. Platelet ABO matters. Transfusion 2009;49:5-7.

71. Triulzi DJ, Assmann SF, Strauss RG, et al. The impact of platelet transfusion characteristics on posttransfusion platelet increments and clinical bleeding in patients with hypoproliferative thrombocytopenia. Blood 2012;119: 5553-62.

72. Kaufman RM, Assmann SF, Triulzi DJ, et al. Transfusion-related adverse events in the Platelet Dose study. Transfusion 2015;55:144-53.

73. Heal J, Rowe J, McMican A, et al. The role of ABO matching in platelet transfusion. Eur J Haematol 1993;50:110-17.

74. Carr R, Hutton J, Jenkins J, et al. Transfusion of ABO-mismatched platelets leads to early platelet refractoriness. Br J Haematol 1990;75: 408-13.

75. Dunstan RA, Simpson MB, Rosse WF. Erythrocyte antigens on human platelets: Absence of Rh, Duffy, Kell, Kidd, and Lutheran antigens. Transfusion 1984;24:243-6.

76. Molnar R, Johnson R, Geiger TL. Absence of D alloimmunization in D- pediatric oncology patients receiving D-incompatible single-donor platelets. Transfusion 2002;42:177-82.

77. Culibrk B, Stone E, Levin E, et al. Application of the ADVIA cerebrospinal fluid assay to count residual red blood cells in blood components. Vox Sang 2012;103:186-93.

78. Santana JM, Dumont LJ. A flow cytometric method for detection and enumeration of low-level, residual red blood cells in platelets and mononuclear cell products. Transfusion 2006;46:966-72.

79. Cid J, Lozano M, Ziman A, et al. Low frequency of anti-D alloimmunization following D+ platelet transfusion: The Anti-D Alloimmunization after D-incompatible Platelet Transfusions (ADAPT) study. Br J Haematol 2015;168: 598-603.

80. Doughty HA, Murphy MF, Metcalfe P, et al. Relative importance of immune and non-immune causes of platelet refractoriness. Vox Sang 1994;66:200-5.

81. Hod E, Schwartz J. Platelet transfusion refractoriness. Br J Haematol 2008;142:348-60.

82. Yankee RA, Grumet FC, Rogentine GN. Platelet transfusion: The selection of compatible platelet donors for refractory patients by lymphocyte HL-A typing. N Engl J Med 1969;281: 1208-12.

83. Slichter SJ. Factors affecting posttransfusion platelet increments, platelet refractoriness, and platelet transfusion intervals in thrombocytopenic patients. Blood 2005;105:4106-14.

84. Claas FH, Smeenk RJ, Schmidt R, et al. Alloimmunization against the MHC antigens after platelet transfusions is due to contaminating leukocytes in the platelet suspension. Exp Hematol 1981;9:84-9.

85. Triulzi DJ, Kleinman S, Kakaiya RM, et al. The effect of previous pregnancy and transfusion on HLA alloimmunization in blood donors: Implications for a transfusion-related acute lung injury risk reduction strategy. Transfusion 2009;49:1825-35.

86. Slichter SJ. Leukocyte reduction and ultraviolet B irradiation of platelets to prevent alloimmunization and refractoriness to platelet transfusions. The Trial to Reduce Alloimmunization to Platelets Study Group. N Engl J Med 1997;337:1861-9.

87. Pavenski K, Rebulla P, Duquesnoy R, et al. Efficacy of HLA-matched platelet transfusions for patients with hypoproliferative thrombocytopenia: A systematic review. Transfusion 2013;53:2230-42.

88. Stanworth SJ, Navarrete C, Estcourt L, Marsh J. Platelet refractoriness - practical approaches and ongoing dilemmas in patient management. Br J Haematol 2015;171:297-305.

89. Moroff G, Garratty G, Heal JM, et al. Selection of platelets for refractory patients by HLA matching and prospective crossmatching. Transfusion 1992;32:633-40.

90. Rioux-Massé B, Cohn C, Lindgren B, et al. Utilization of cross-matched or HLA-matched platelets for patients refractory to platelet transfusion. Transfusion 2014;54:3080-7.

91. Holland L, Sarode R. Should plasma be transfused prophylactically before invasive procedures? Curr Opin Hematol 2006;13:447-51.

92. Abdel-Wahab O, Healy B, Dzik W. Effect of fresh-frozen plasma transfusion on prothrombin time and bleeding in patients with mild coagulation abnormalities. Transfusion 2006; 46:1279-85.

93. Karam O, Tucci M, Combescure C, et al. Plasma transfusion strategies for critically ill patients. Cochrane Database Syst Rev 2013;12: CD010654.

94. Murad MH, Stubbs JR, Gandhi MJ, et al. The effect of plasma transfusion on morbidity and mortality: A systematic review and meta-analysis. Transfusion 2010;50:1370-83.

95. Segal JB, Dzik WH. Paucity of studies to support that abnormal coagulation test results

predict bleeding in the setting of invasive procedures: An evidence-based review. Transfusion 2005;45:1413-25.

96. Yang L, Stanworth S, Hopewell S, et al. Is fresh-frozen plasma clinically effective? An update of a systematic review of randomized controlled trials. Transfusion 2012;52:1673-86.

97. Jia Q, Brown MJ, Clifford L, et al. Prophylactic plasma transfusion for surgical patients with abnormal preoperative coagulation tests: A single-institution propensity-adjusted cohort study. Lancet Haematol 2016;3:e139-48.

98. Moren AM, Hamptom D, Diggs B, et al. Recursive partitioning identifies greater than 4 U of packed red blood cells per hour as an improved massive transfusion definition. J Trauma Acute Care Surg 2015;79:920-4.

99. Borgman M, Spinella P, Perkins J, et al. The ratio of blood products transfused affects mortality in patients receiving massive transfusions at a combat support hospital. J Trauma 2007;63:805-13.

100. Acosta JA, Yang JC, Winchell RJ, et al. Lethal injuries and time to death in a level I trauma center. J Am Coll Surg 1998;186:528-33.

101. Stansbury LG, Dutton RP, Stein DM, et al. Controversy in trauma resuscitation: Do ratios of plasma to red blood cells matter? Transfus Med Rev 2009;23:255-65.

102. Callum JL, Nascimento B, Tien H, Rizoli S. "Formula-driven" versus "lab-driven" massive transfusion protocols: At a state of clinical equipoise (editorial). Transfus Med Rev 2009;23:247-54.

103. Holcomb JB, del Junco DJ, Fox EE, et al. The Prospective, Observational, Multicenter, Major Trauma Transfusion (PROMMTT) study. JAMA Surgery 2013;148:127-36.

104. Holcomb JB, Tilley BC, Baraniuk S, et al. Transfusion of plasma, platelets, and red blood cells in a 1:1:1 vs a 1:1:2 ratio and mortality in patients with severe trauma: the PROPPR randomized clinical trial. JAMA 2015;313:471-82.

105. Dzik WS, Ziman A, Cohen C, et al. Survival after ultramassive transfusion: A review of 1360 cases. Transfusion 2016;56:558-63.

106. Johnson DJ, Scott AV, Barodka VM, et al. Morbidity and mortality after high-dose transfusion. Anesthesiology 2016;124:387-95.

107. Chhibber V, Greene M, Vauthrin M, et al. Is group A thawed plasma suitable as the first option for emergency release transfusion? Transfusion 2014;54:1751-5.

108. Presnell SR, Stafford DW. The vitamin K-dependent carboxylase. Thromb Haemost 2002;87:937-46.

109. Sarode R, Milling TJ, Refaai MA, et al. Efficacy and safety of a four-factor prothrombin complex concentrate (4F-PCC) in patients on vitamin K antagonists presenting with major bleeding: A randomized, plasma-controlled, Phase IIIb study. Circulation 2013;128:1234-43.

110. Goldstein JN, Refaai MA, Milling TJ Jr, et al. Four-factor prothrombin complex concentrate versus plasma for rapid vitamin K antagonist reversal in patients needing urgent surgical or invasive interventions: A phase 3b, open-label, non-inferiority, randomised trial. Lancet 2015;385:2077-87.

111. Yazer MH, Cortese-Hassett A, Triulzi DJ. Coagulation factor levels in plasma frozen within 24 hours of phlebotomy over 5 days of storage at 1 to 6°C. Transfusion 2008;48:2525-30.

112. Neisser-Svae A, Trawnicek L, Heger A, et al. Five-day stability of thawed plasma: Solvent/detergent-treated plasma comparable with fresh-frozen plasma and plasma frozen within 24 hours. Transfusion 2016;56:404-9.

113. Downes KA, Wilson E, Yomtovian R, Sarode R. Serial measurement of clotting factors in thawed plasma stored for 5 days. Transfusion 2001;41:570.

114. Benjamin RJ, McLaughlin LS. Plasma components: Properties, differences, and uses. Transfusion 2012;52(Suppl 1):9S-19S.

115. Levy JH, Goodnough LT. How I use fibrinogen replacement therapy in acquired bleeding. Blood 2015;125:1387-93.

116. Ahmed S, Harrity C, Johnson S, et al. The efficacy of fibrinogen concentrate compared with cryoprecipitate in major obstetric haemorrhage—an observational study. Transfus Med 2012;22:344-9.

117. Pavord S, Maybury H. How I treat postpartum hemorrhage. Blood 2015;125:2759-70.

118. Reger B, Peterfalvi A, Litter I, et al. Challenges in the evaluation of D-dimer and fibrinogen levels in pregnant women. Thromb Res 2013;131:e183-7.

119. Charbit B, Mandelbrot L, Samain E, et al. The decrease of fibrinogen is an early predictor of the severity of postpartum hemorrhage. J Thromb Haemost 2007;5:266-73.

120. Cortet M, Deneux-Tharaux C, Dupont C, et al. Association between fibrinogen level and severity of postpartum haemorrhage: Secondary

analysis of a prospective trial. Br J Anaesth 2012;108:984-9.

121. Abdul-Kadir R, McLintock C, Ducloy A-S, et al. Evaluation and management of postpartum hemorrhage: Consensus from an international expert panel. Transfusion 2014;54:1756-68.

122. Wikkelso AJ, Edwards HM, Afshari A, et al. Preemptive treatment with fibrinogen concentrate for postpartum haemorrhage: Randomized controlled trial. Br J Anaesth 2015;114:623-33.

123. Besser MW, Klein AA. The coagulopathy of cardiopulmonary bypass. Crit Rev Clin Lab Sci 2010;47:197-212.

124. Besser MW, Ortmann E, Klein AA. Haemostatic management of cardiac surgical haemorrhage. Anaesthesia 2014;70:87-e31.

125. Woodman R, Harker LA. Bleeding complications associated with cardiopulmonary bypass. Blood 2003;76:1680-97.

126. Bennett-Guerrero E, Zhao Y, O'Brien SM, et al. Variation in use of blood transfusion in coronary artery bypass graft surgery. JAMA 2010; 304:1568-75.

127. Kindo M, Hoang Minh T, Gerelli S, et al. Plasma fibrinogen level on admission to the intensive care unit is a powerful predictor of postoperative bleeding after cardiac surgery with cardiopulmonary bypass. Thromb Res 2014; 134:360-8.

128. Ranucci M, Baryshnikova E, Crapelli GB, et al. Randomized, double-blinded, placebo-controlled trial of fibrinogen concentrate supplementation after complex cardiac surgery. J Am Heart Assoc 2015;4:e002066.

129. Wikkelso A, Lunde J, Johansen M, et al. Fibrinogen concentrate in bleeding patients. Cochrane Database Syst Rev 2013;8:CD008864.

130. Rahe-Meyer N, Levy JH, Mazer CD, et al. Randomized evaluation of fibrinogen vs placebo in complex cardiovascular surgery (REPLACE): A double-blind Phase III study of haemostatic therapy. Br J Anaesth 2016;117:41-51.

131. Strauss RG. Role of granulocyte/neutrophil transfusions for haematology/oncology patients in the modern era. Br J Haematol 2012; 158:299-306.

132. Price TH, Boeckh M, Harrison RW, et al. Efficacy of transfusion with granulocytes from G-CSF/dexamethasone-treated donors in neutropenic patients with infection. Blood 2015; 126:2153-61.

133. Estcourt LJ, Stanworth S, Doree C, et al. Granulocyte transfusions for preventing infections in people with neutropenia or neutrophil dysfunction. Cochrane Database Syst Rev 2015; 6:CD005341.

134. Cancelas JA. Granulocyte transfusion: Questions remain. Blood 2015;126:2082-3.

Chapter 20

Patient Blood Management

• • •

Kathleen E. Puca, MD, MT(ASCP)SBB

BLOOD TRANSFUSIONS CAN be lifesaving, but they can also be associated with complications. A seemingly endless number of observational studies published over the last several years has linked unnecessary blood transfusion with worse patient outcomes. In addition, growing attention by professional associations and healthcare organizations on the wide variation in transfusion practice and overuse of blood has intensified the need for more appropriate utilization.[1-3] Furthermore, efforts to lower health-care costs and improve quality of care and patient safety have led to increased focus on the part of care providers and hospital administrators on the stewardship and utilization of blood components within their organizations.

Accordingly, many institutions have implemented patient blood management (PBM) strategies and related activities. In reports from both the 2013 and 2015 National Blood Collection and Utilization Surveys and the 2013 AABB Blood Collection, Utilization, and Patient Blood Management Survey, more than one-third of hospitals had a PBM program, and even more facilities had implemented one or more interventions to improve care and reduce transfusions. These initiatives have resulted in a steady decline in Red Blood Cell (RBC) transfusions in the United States of approximately 16% annually since 2008.[4,5]

DEFINITION AND SCOPE OF PATIENT BLOOD MANAGEMENT

PBM is an evidence-based, multidisciplinary approach to optimize the care of patients who might need a transfusion. Although evidence-based transfusion guidelines are fundamental, PBM goes beyond appropriate blood component utilization. It encompasses the entire course of care, from before the patient enters the hospital to after treatment is completed. The primary aim of PBM is to improve patient safety and clinical outcomes by appropriately managing the patient's "own blood." PBM entails a proactive approach, employing evidence-based pharmacological, medical, and surgical modalities to manage anemia, optimize hemostasis, and minimize blood loss in a patient-specific manner to reduce or avoid unnecessary transfusions. In addition, when a transfusion is the only appropriate intervention, PBM requires that transfusion decisions be based on best practices and the amount given is the minimum to improve care.

Although the term "patient blood management" may be fairly new, the concepts have developed over time in parallel with medical

---

Kathleen E. Puca, MD, MT(ASCP)SBB, Medical Director, BloodCenter of Wisconsin, Milwaukee, Wisconsin
The author has disclosed no conflicts of interest.

20

advances. A full discussion of this history is beyond the scope of this chapter. However, two examples illustrate the shared "drivers" of blood transfusion and PBM. One example is the influence of wartime injuries. The discoveries of blood groups, crossmatching, and blood preservation in the early years of the 20th century enabled the use of banked blood in the treatment of exsanguinating wounds suffered in armed conflicts of the same period. Yet transporting blood was difficult, and battlefield surgeons developed techniques to treat casualties when no transfusion was possible. A second example is the influence of Jehovah's Witnesses, who cite biblical passages as the foundation for their refusal of blood transfusion. By the middle of the 20th century, blood transfusion had become universally accepted as a medical treatment for a wide range of indications. Jehovah's Witness patients had to seek out those few physicians and hospitals that would provide medical and surgical care without blood transfusion. These surgeons and hospitals became increasingly used by Jehovah's Witnesses and other patients who refuse blood, and blood conservation programs began to flourish. With an emphasis on an individualized, patient-centric approach, these programs led the way toward the PBM movement seen today.

Although the focus is frequently on surgical patients, PBM encompasses the entire scope of any patient's hospital experience. It includes:

1. Efforts to identify and manage anemia and bleeding risks before any treatment begins.
2. Use of blood-sparing surgical techniques and intraoperative blood recovery methods.
3. Adjunctive strategies during intensive care unit (ICU) and postoperative care that decrease the need for transfusion.
4. Blood utilization review and feedback to ordering physicians.
5. PBM education of all health-care providers involved in patient care.

The scope of PBM activities is discussed in detail in the section "Basic Elements of a PBM Program."

THE RATIONALE FOR PBM

Although the reasons for PBM are many, the most compelling are those that align with the Institute for Healthcare Improvement's "Triple Aim" initiative[6]—safe and quality care, improved patient experience and outcomes, and reduced health-care costs.

1. **Safety.** Although viral infections transmitted by blood transfusion are rare today, allogeneic transfusions are not without risk. For example, emerging pathogens remain a concern. In addition, noninfectious adverse events, such as transfusion-related acute lung injury, transfusion-associated circulatory overload, wrong blood component transfused, and hemolytic transfusion reactions, are the leading causes of transfusion-related death and serious morbidity.[7] Transfusing blood only when appropriate and at the minimum amount necessary can reduce these risks.
2. **Quality of Care.** The wide variation in transfusion practice suggests that a significant number of transfusions may be inappropriate and avoidable. In the last 15 years, several randomized controlled trials on restrictive vs liberal RBC transfusion thresholds have been published. These showed no harm with a restrictive strategy, which results in a reduced number of units transfused and patients transfused.[8] Applying evidence-based transfusion practices promotes appropriate use of blood components and enhances patient safety. A PBM program can provide protocols and education to avoid unnecessary transfusions and the associated risks.
3. **Better Outcomes.** Patients who get less blood often do better. The use of restrictive transfusion strategies results in fewer transfusions, with patient outcomes that

are similar to, and sometimes better than, those associated with more liberal transfusion strategies. Lower risks of mortality, cardiac and respiratory complications, and serious infections in surgical and critically ill patients are clear benefits of PBM.[9,10]

4. **Patient Need.** The increasing age of the population and the diminishing donor pool may have significant impacts on future blood availability. Today, 40% of the US population aged 16 to 64 is eligible to donate, but only about 4% does so. Moreover, current estimates indicate that patients who are 65 or older receive 55% to 60% of all blood donated.[11] In the next 10 to 20 years, the number of individuals in the United States who are older than 65 will increase at a faster rate than those aged 16 to 64. By 2030, older adults will comprise roughly 20% of the US population, and by 2060 the number will be more than double that in 2014.[12] Undoubtedly, this shift in the population dynamics will increase the number of older individuals undergoing complex surgical procedures for which transfusions will still be necessary. Conservation of already constrained resources allows blood to be available for those patients who are truly in need.

5. **Patient Autonomy and Satisfaction.** Religious beliefs, individual concerns, and cultural differences may influence a patient's decision for or against blood transfusion. PBM presents a patient-centered decision-making approach where the risks and benefits of not only the transfusion option but also alternatives to transfusion and avoidance of treatment are presented for the patient to make a more informed choice. By respecting patient wishes and needs related to the treatment options, PBM strategies not only provide a "right fit" but also improve patient outcomes and satisfaction.

6. **Reduced Health-Care Costs.** Blood transfusion was identified as one of the top five overused procedures in hospitalized patients.[2,3] This overuse undoubtedly leads to increased costs. In addition, the total cost of an RBC transfusion is three to four times higher than that of the blood component alone.[13] PBM programs, where evidence-based practices reduce or even avoid the need for transfusion, have the potential for substantial cost savings while improving patient outcomes.[14,15]

BASIC ELEMENTS OF A PBM PROGRAM

As noted above, several PBM strategies can be implemented to decrease allogeneic blood transfusions and improve patient outcomes. They encompass all aspects of the patient's evaluation and clinical management. A PBM approach is typically implemented in elective surgical patients in the preoperative, intraoperative, and postoperative phases of care as outlined in Table 20-1[16] and in the following sections. PBM strategies are also relevant for medical patients. Although any one of the strategies used individually can successfully decrease the use of allogeneic blood transfusion, they are most effective, and have the greatest potential for improved outcomes, when combined and individualized for a specific patient.

Preoperative Strategies

Patient evaluation and planning is the cornerstone of a PBM program. A detailed medical history and physical examination, with special attention to family and personal history of spontaneous or postoperative bleeding and anemia, are vital for assessing patients at risk and identifying correctable factors. Structured questions can help with the evaluation, which should be performed sufficiently ahead of the planned surgery (eg, 30 days) to allow for diagnostic testing and therapeutic interventions, as needed.[17]

TABLE 20-1. Scope of PBM*

Nonsurgical or Preoperative	Intraoperative	ICU and Postoperative	Blood Utilization Review	Medical Education
● Anemia screening and management – iron therapy – cautious use of EPO ● Screen for bleeding risks and optimize coagulation – discontinue anticoagulants and antiplatelet drugs – discontinue herbal supplements, some vitamins – address genetic coagulation abnormalities ● Minimize crystalloids in acute bleeding ● Limit phlebotomy ● Preoperative autologous donation	● Replacement fluids – crystalloid – colloid ● Surgical techniques – meticulous suturing – harmonic scalpel – suction control – rinsing swabs ● Acute normovolemic hemodilution ● Intraoperative blood recovery ● Hemostatics – topical thrombin – fibrin sealant – platelet gel ● Point-of-care testing ● Monitor acute bleeding and manage coagulation ● Tolerate low hemoglobin ● Avoid hypothermia ● Tolerate low blood pressure ● Positioning	● Replacement fluids – crystalloid – colloid ● Limit phlebotomy ● Tolerate low hemoglobin ● Monitor bleeding ● Wound drainage ● Iron therapy ● Hyperbaric oxygen ● Point-of-care testing	● Clinical practice guidelines – indications – thresholds – restrictive strategies ● Blood utilization or transfusion committee ● Audits – prospective – concurrent – retrospective ● Patient blood management coordinator or transfusion safety officer	● In-service – grand rounds – conferences – reminders (posters, data cards, etc) – journal club ● Continuing education – certification – CME/CE credit – online tools (webinars, interactive modules) ● Medical and nursing school curricula

*Modified with permission from Becker and Shaz.[16]

ICU = intensive care unit; EPO = erythropoietin; CME = continuing medical education; CE = continuing education.

Anemia Assessment and Management

Recognition and management of anemia in medical and surgical patients is a core principle of PBM. Anemia, defined by the World Health Organization (WHO) as a hemoglobin level <13 g/dL in men and <12 g/dL in premenopausal, nonpregnant women,[18] is common and often underdiagnosed and undertreated. The prevalence of preoperative anemia is generally estimated at 20% to 40% but depends on patient age, coexisting conditions, the reason for surgery, and the definition of anemia used. In colorectal surgery, preoperative anemia can be as high as 75%.[19,20]

Preoperative anemia is an important modifiable risk factor for postoperative complications. In patients undergoing cardiac and noncardiac surgeries, preexisting anemia has been associated with increased risk of infection, cardiac events, renal failure, higher transfusion rates, longer hospital stays, and decreased survival.[20-23] In a study of 227,425 patients undergoing various general and vascular surgical procedures reported in the American College of Surgeons' National Surgical Quality Improvement Program database, 69,229 (30.4%) had preoperative anemia. After adjusting for confounders, anemic patients had a 35% higher risk of one or more postoperative complications and 42% higher risk of death at 30 days.[23] Similarly, in a retrospective study of more than 300,000 elderly veterans undergoing major noncardiac surgery, the more severe the anemia, the higher the risk of 30-day mortality and cardiac events.[24] Even mild anemia is an independent risk factor for adverse outcomes in patients undergoing surgery.[22,23] Moreover, anemia is one of the strongest predictors of the need for perioperative blood transfusion. Both anemia and exposure to transfusion can have an additive effect for worse outcomes.

Screening for anemia should be performed as early as 30 days before a scheduled surgery to allow time for investigation and appropriate therapy. If anemia is detected, additional laboratory testing, such as creatinine, reticulocyte count, iron and iron-binding capacity, ferritin, vitamin B12, and folate, should be considered to aid in diagnosis. Several published guidelines can assist the PBM program in developing algorithms for identifying and treating anemia in medical and preoperative patients.[25,26] Whenever possible, an elective, high-blood-loss surgery should be delayed until the anemia is explained and appropriately treated.

Pharmacologic agents for anemia may include iron (both oral and intravenous preparations), folic acid, vitamin B12, or erythropoiesis-stimulating agents [(ESAs), see Appendix 20-1.] The choice of therapeutic agent should be guided by the underlying etiology of the anemia, the patient's other medical conditions, and available time to treat before any surgery.

Intravenous (IV) iron is safe and can quickly correct iron-deficiency anemia. It may be the preferred route over oral preparations when there is intolerance of oral iron, short time to surgery, or use of ESAs, or in the postoperative period.[27] The efficacy of IV iron therapy in treating anemia has been consistently proven. A recent systematic review showed IV iron reduced the need for allogeneic RBC transfusions in many clinical settings.[28] ESAs also effectively increase hemoglobin levels if sufficient iron stores are present. A short preoperative regimen of ESA or a single dose of ESA plus IV iron in the preoperative or intraoperative period may significantly reduce transfusion rates.[27] However, because of the risk of thromboembolic events, tumor growth, and death associated with ESAs, further safety and efficacy trials in high-blood-loss surgeries that routinely require transfusion are required to make evidence-based conclusions. Conservative dosing and strict monitoring of ESAs is recommended.[29]

Preoperative "anemia clinics" are therapeutically effective and cost-effective in improving patient hemoglobin levels before surgery and decreasing overall transfusion rates.[14,30,31] Developing the delivery model and putting it into operation to serve and manage preoperative patients requires in-depth planning, which is described in detail elsewhere.[32,33]

Addressing Bleeding Risk

A second important aspect of preoperative optimization is assessing a patient's risk for bleeding in relation to the type and complexity of surgery and anticipated blood loss. Addressing current medications and the presence of any preexisting anemia and/or coagulopathy can help formulate an individualized plan. Screening questionnaires and protocols for discontinuation or dose adjustment of antiplatelet, anticoagulant, and herbal medicines are essential preoperative planning tools. Published guidelines, such as those developed by the American Society for Anesthesiologists, the Society for Thoracic Surgery, and the American College of Chest Physicians can provide a basis for developing such protocols to guide best practices.[34-37]

Preoperative evaluation is paramount for improving postoperative outcomes. Appropriate patient preparation for surgery decreases surgical delays and cancellations and enables a dialogue between patients, family, and health-care providers, so that patients can make informed decisions and the health-care team understands their preferences. Such engagement truly exemplifies the patient-centered PBM approach.

Preoperative Autologous Blood Donation

Historically, preoperative autologous blood donation (PAD) was the primary means to reduce the use of allogeneic blood. However, over the last several years, there has been a significant downward trend in the number of autologous units collected in the United States. In 2015, only 25,000 units were collected, representing approximately 0.2% of the total allogeneic RBC/whole blood collection and 60% fewer units than were collected in 2013.[4,38] Major factors contributing to this decline include the increased safety of and public confidence in the blood supply, adoption of intraoperative blood-conserving techniques, high wastage of PAD blood ($\geq$45% discarded), and a higher risk for preoperative anemia after donation.[38,39] Studies showed that although patients partici-pating in a PAD program had lower exposure to allogeneic transfusions as compared to patients who did not participate, they had a higher likelihood of receiving any transfusions (allogeneic and/or autologous) as a result of donation-induced anemia.[38,40] Errors related to production and handling, delays in receipt of the units at the designated hospital, and increasing acquisition costs also added to the decrease in PAD.[41]

Despite these concerns, PAD can be a reasonable option for patients with rare blood types or multiple red cell alloantibodies, or for patients who refuse allogeneic blood. In these situations, advanced planning and patient evaluation are crucial before PAD is attempted. To mitigate the anemia induced by PAD and avoid allogeneic transfusions, efforts should focus on 1) timing of collections to allow 3 to 4 weeks between the last donation and planned surgery, 2) collecting the minimal amount, and 3) prescribing iron-replacement therapy with or without an ESA before donation.

Intraoperative Strategies

Acute Normovolemic Hemodilution

Acute normovolemic hemodilution (ANH) is the removal of whole blood from the patient into a standard blood bag containing anticoagulant immediately before or shortly after the beginning of the surgical procedure. Crystalloid or colloid solutions, or both, are reinfused to maintain adequate circulatory volume. Any blood lost from the patient during surgery is thereby diluted and has a reduced red cell content.

The patient's fresh whole blood is typically stored at room temperature (for up to 8 hours) and is often reinfused near the end of the procedure, or whenever transfusion is needed.[42] An added value of ANH is that platelets and coagulation factors remain viable when the product is stored at room temperature. Although ANH is relatively safe and can lower the likelihood of allogeneic transfusion, reports on its clinical efficacy and benefits are mixed.[43,44]

ANH is more likely to be beneficial in patients who undergo high-blood-loss procedures (≥1500 mL), have a relatively high preoperative hematocrit, and can have the maximum-allowable units removed.[45] Planning and coordination by the surgical team are critical for a successful outcome.

Intraoperative Blood Recovery

Intraoperative blood recovery can also reduce the use of allogeneic transfusions. Use of recovered shed blood is most efficacious in high-blood-loss procedures, such as cardiothoracic, vascular, orthopedic, and trauma surgery. The shed blood is collected from the surgical site, centrifuged, and washed with normal saline. During centrifugation and washing, plasma, platelets, red cell stroma, contaminants, and anticoagulant are removed. The washed red cells are transferred to a separate bag and then reinfused to the same patient. Ideally, washed recovered blood should have a hematocrit of at least 45% to 60%.

In a systematic review of the use of intraoperative blood recovery in cardiac and orthopedic surgery, allogeneic RBC transfusions were reduced by 38% with an average savings of 0.68 unit of allogeneic RBCs per patient.[46] However, recent advances in other intraoperative strategies to decrease blood loss, such as use of antifibrinolytic agents, may diminish the effectiveness of autologous blood recovery in certain surgical procedures. Nonetheless, the use of intraoperative blood recovery should be individualized and considered when the anticipated surgical blood loss is ≥20% of the patient's estimated blood volume (typically approximately 1000 mL in adults).

Concerns about the safety of blood recovery arise regarding cancer and obstetric surgery and when there is bacterial contamination of the surgical field. In these settings, unwanted material and cells (eg, tumor cells, bacteria, amniotic fluid) may be reinfused into the patient. However, a double-suction setup and leukocyte reduction filters reduce these risks.[47] In addition, recent reviews do not support the theoretical concern for increased risks of amniotic fluid embolism or cancer recurrence.[48,49] To date, intraoperative blood recovery in obstetrics has not led to poor maternal outcomes, and the American College of Obstetricians and Gynecologists and the American Society of Anesthesiology endorse its use in postpartum hemorrhage.[49,50]

For many hospitals, limited experience, constrained resources, and other challenges may hinder development of a fully comprehensive quality system approach for collecting, preparing, and administering these intraoperative blood components. Formalized PBM programs provide an opportunity for collaboration between the transfusion service and surgery, perfusion, anesthesia, and nursing departments to improve and advance the hospital blood recovery program. Guidelines and regulatory requirements for establishing, enhancing, and maintaining quality and safety for these particular transfusion practices are well described in various AABB publications.[42,51,52]

Anesthesia and Surgical Techniques

Minimizing intraoperative bleeding is critical for reducing the need for allogeneic transfusion. Measures include meticulous surgical technique and rapid and rigorous control of bleeding. Minimally invasive approaches, such as laparoscopy and robotic-assisted surgery, are also associated with reduced bleeding. Proper positioning of the patient can reduce blood loss and is guided by two basic principles: elevating the surgical site above the level of the heart and avoiding obstruction of venous drainage at the surgical site. The deliberate reduction of mean arterial pressure, known as "controlled or deliberate hypotension," in selected patients can reduce blood flow to the surgical site, thereby decreasing blood loss; however, the benefits must be balanced against potential risk for organ ischemia.[53,54]

Maintaining normothermia is important for optimal coagulation and hemostasis. Keeping the patient warm by using warm IV fluids and air-warming blankets, and keeping the surgical suite warm, can help avoid hypothermia, thereby decreasing surgical blood loss.

Optimal fluid management, including the choice of infusion fluids, volume, and timing of administration, also affects surgical blood loss and transfusion requirements. Modern tissue dissection devices minimize tissue damage and provide better hemostasis at the incision site. Other measures influencing surgical blood loss include tourniquets, direct control of bleeding, infiltration of vasoconstrictors into the surgical wound, choice of ventilation patterns, and choice of anesthesia.[55,56]

Point-of-Care Testing and Transfusion Algorithms

Point-of-care testing (POCT) has several advantages over conventional laboratory testing, including availability for use whenever necessary, more rapid turnaround time, and minimal sample volumes required for testing. POCT can help avoid iatrogenic anemia and provide timely information for transfusion decisions. Various POCT devices provide information on coagulation, platelet function, and clot stability; these are most often used in surgical and critical care settings.[57,58]

Transfusions based on clinical observation of bleeding and blood loss are highly variable. POCT systems linked to transfusion algorithms can affect blood component use by providing timely results to inform and guide clinical transfusion decisions. In particular, whole blood global viscoelastic tests [eg, thromboelastography (TEG) or rotational thromboelastometry (ROTEM)] are gaining in popularity for monitoring the complex coagulopathies that can occur in cardiac surgery, trauma, and liver disease. These assays measure clot formation dynamics, from initiation to fibrinolysis, and provide real-time information to guide transfusion therapy.

In cardiac surgery, TEG- or ROTEM-based transfusion algorithms significantly reduce the proportion of patients transfused with not only plasma and platelets but also RBCs, when compared to clinician-directed and/or standard laboratory-based transfusion algorithms. The incidence of surgical reexploration also decreased in cohorts managed with TEG- or ROTEM-based algorithms.[59,60]

TEG and ROTEM are routinely used in liver transplant surgery, and these assays are increasingly viewed as an appropriate tool to assess the unique coagulation alterations occurring in liver disease patients.[61] Control of bleeding is central in any surgery, but managing hemostasis in liver transplantation can be exceptionally challenging. Although current evidence is limited, TEG/ROTEM-based algorithms during liver transplantation lower blood loss and transfusion requirements, particularly plasma.[62] Likewise, fewer plasma and platelet transfusions were given when using a TEG-guided algorithm in cirrhotic patients with severe coagulopathy before invasive procedures, without increasing the risk for periprocedural bleeding.[63]

Massive transfusion protocols (MTPs) are associated with increased survival of trauma patients as a result of rapid and early delivery of plasma and platelets. TEG/ROTEM-based algorithms can detect trauma-induced coagulopathy and fibrinolysis during MTPs and facilitate goal-directed therapy; in addition, they may provide an advantage over conventional laboratory tests.[64,65] In a systematic review of 55 observational studies, the evidence supporting TEG/ROTEM for reducing transfusion needs and mortality in trauma was uncertain.[66] However, in a recent randomized controlled trial,[65] fewer plasma and platelet transfusions were required in the early phase of resuscitation, and improved survival was seen when an MTP directed by TEG was used, as compared to conventional coagulation tests. Although the total amount of blood components transfused at 24 hours did not differ between the two groups, the authors claim that incorporating a TEG-based algorithm in the MTP promoted delivery of the most appropriate component at the optimal time. Although further research is needed to assess the clinical effectiveness of TEG/ROTEM-based algorithms in trauma, recent guidelines recommend that, when available, viscoelastic methods be performed along with standard laboratory testing to help characterize the coagulopathy and guide transfusion therapy.[67,68]

Goal-directed TEG/ROTEM-based transfusion algorithms may reduce transfusion requirements and lower costs by optimizing bleeding management.[60] Because these viscoelastic assays are not available everywhere, it is important for institutions to establish their own algorithms based on available coagulation assays and therapeutic options.

Pharmacologic Agents

Antifibrinolytics are increasingly used in various surgical settings to reduce blood loss and the need for transfusion. Aminocaproic acid and tranexamic acid (TXA) both inhibit fibrinolytic activity, preventing premature breakdown of blood clots, although TXA is more commonly used. In a systematic review involving 7838 patients undergoing cardiac, orthopedic, and other surgical procedures, TXA reduced the risk for blood transfusion by 38%.[69] During cardiopulmonary bypass, there is increased potential for activation of the fibrinolytic system, and both agents effectively reduce surgical blood loss and allogeneic transfusions.[70] In this surgical setting with the potential for high doses, TXA has been associated with seizures.[71] Adopting TXA as a blood conservation strategy in joint replacement surgery is becoming common and cost-effective.[72,73] In trauma patients with significant bleeding, TXA also improved survival when given within 3 hours of injury.[74] Similarly, TXA may reduce the risk of death from bleeding if administered within 3 hours of postpartum hemorrhage.[75] In addition, the safety of these drugs in patients at risk for vaso-occlusive events remains unclear.[74]

Desmopressin (DDAVP) stimulates release of stored von Willebrand factor (vWF) and Factor VIII from endothelium, which increases the circulating levels of these factors and platelet adhesion to endothelial cells. DDAVP is commonly used to control bleeding associated with minor surgical procedures in patients with mild hemophilia A and Type I von Willebrand disease. Although routine prophylaxis with DDAVP is not recommended for surgical patients without congenital bleeding disorders, patients with uremia, liver cirrhosis, or drug-induced platelet dysfunction may benefit.[76] In cardiac surgery, only patients who ingested aspirin or experienced prolonged extracorporeal cardiopulmonary bypass have benefited from perioperative use of DDAVP with regard to reduced postoperative blood loss and transfusion.[77]

Topical agents, such as hemostatics, sealants, and adhesives, are gaining importance as useful tools that can reduce surgical bleeding by enhancing clotting, sealing vessels, or gluing tissues. Focused reviews on these topical agents and other pharmacologic agents are available.[78,79]

Postoperative Strategies

Postoperative Blood Recovery

Postoperative blood recovery involves collecting and reinfusing blood from surgical drains and/or wounds. Adequate amounts of blood need to be collected and processed for this to be effective. Thus, it is used mainly in trauma, vascular, cardiac, and complex orthopedic surgical cases where the shed blood volume can be significant (≥ 500 mL). Postoperative recovered blood can be unwashed or washed. When unwashed, shed blood is collected and filtered in a device until sufficient volume is reached; then it is transferred to an infusion bag for reinfusion. For the washed product, once sufficient shed blood is collected, it is processed by washing and then transferred to a bag for reinfusion.

In the past, reinfusion of unwashed shed blood was popular as a blood conservation technique in joint replacement surgery. However, the growing use of antifibrinolytics has led to a decline in surgical bleeding, making postoperative blood recovery unnecessary.[80,81] In addition, unwashed shed blood is less desirable because it has a hematocrit of 20% to 30% and contains activated clotting and complement factors, inflammatory mediators, cytokines, and fat particles that can increase the risk for febrile reactions.[82,83]

For patients with substantial postoperative blood loss, improved product quality and safety (eg, hematocrit of 60% to 80% with removal of contaminants) can be achieved with devices that wash and concentrate the postoperative wound-drainage blood. Maintaining competency of nursing staff and the higher cost for these devices may be disadvantageous for some hospitals. However, for those centers engaged in complex, high-risk surgical cases, using postoperative autologous washed blood can reduce the need for allogeneic blood.

Limiting Phlebotomy-Related Blood Loss

Minimizing the impact of phlebotomy on the development of iatrogenic anemia is important for reducing transfusion requirements. Blood loss from routine laboratory testing contributes significantly to anemia in critically ill patients. In a study of 145 Western European ICUs, the mean number of blood draws per patient was 4.6, and blood loss from phlebotomy averaged 41.1 mL per day per patient.[84] For an ICU stay of ≥7 days this can equate to the loss of a unit of blood or more. In a US retrospective database study of more than 17,000 patients with acute myocardial infarction, every 50 mL of blood drawn increased the risk of moderate to severe anemia by 18%.[85] Not unexpectedly, total phlebotomy volume is an independent predictor of subsequent transfusions.[86,87] Moreover, there appears to be a positive correlation between the severity of illness and both the number of blood draws and the total volume of blood taken for diagnostic testing, placing the sickest patients at the highest risk for anemia and subsequent blood transfusion.[84,87]

Reducing the quantity and frequency of laboratory testing should logically reduce the amount of blood loss related to phlebotomy. Although routine standing orders are common, laboratory testing should be ordered only when clinically justified and when the results are likely to change clinical management. Laboratory test requests should also be consolidated to minimize the number of tubes collected. Pediatric or small-volume tubes could also be used for sample collection; this can reduce blood loss from laboratory testing by up to 70%.[88] Smaller sample volumes, often <0.5 mL, can also be used with POCT devices.

Even the phlebotomy process can be a significant cause of blood loss. Patients with invasive lines (eg, central venous or arterial catheters) provide a threefold increase in phlebotomy volume as compared to patients without them.[86] The ease with which samples can be obtained, and the added requirement to discard the first few milliliters (up to 10 mL) each time the line is accessed, can contribute to greater blood loss. Such catheters should be discontinued as soon as they are no longer required. Orders for specimens drawn from these catheters should be consolidated to minimize the amount of "discard" blood. Use of a closed blood sampling device may even have a larger impact on reducing blood "lost" to phlebotomy. These devices, whereby the initial volume of blood is reinfused back to the patient instead of discarded, can reduce mean phlebotomy volume by 50%, lower the decline in hemoglobin between ICU admission and discharge, and result in fewer RBC transfusions, even when a restrictive transfusion practice is followed.[86,89]

Increasing Tolerance of Anemia and Transfusion Thresholds

A patient's response to anemia is highly individualized and depends on ability to maintain adequate oxygen delivery to tissues. Tolerance depends on the patient's volume status, physiologic reserve (including cardiac, pulmonary, and renal function), and the dynamics of the anemia. The response becomes one of the most important factors in determining the need for transfusion.[90]

Patients with chronic anemia due to chronic renal failure or slow gastrointestinal bleeding often physiologically adapt to a lower hemoglobin level by increasing cardiac output, heart rate, or stroke volume. However, rapid blood loss from surgical bleeding or trauma often results in hemodynamic instability, shock, and other symptoms that require more rapid volume replacement.

Increasing a patient's tolerance for lower hemoglobin includes increasing oxygen delivery or decreasing oxygen consumption, thereby limiting the need for RBC transfusion. Strategies to optimize hemodynamic status and oxygenation include maintaining normovolemia with intravenous fluids, using appropriate vasopressor agents, using supplemental oxygen or mechanical ventilation, providing adequate pain control and/or sedation, maintaining normothermia, and promptly treating infections.[91]

Incorporating evidence-based transfusion protocols is the foundation for reducing unnecessary transfusions. Historically, hemoglobin levels of ≤10 g/dL were used as the transfusion threshold. Several recent randomized controlled trials and consensus guidelines provide RBC transfusion thresholds that are more evidence-based.[34,36,92-96] In most patient populations, a more restrictive transfusion threshold (eg, hemoglobin of 7-8 g/dL) is safe and reduces the number of patients transfused and the total amount of RBC transfusions without increasing morbidity or mortality.[8] However, evidence is lacking for applying a restrictive threshold in patients with active bleeding, ongoing cardiac ischemia, or traumatic brain injury. More importantly, an arbitrary hemoglobin level or "trigger" should not be the sole driver for transfusion. Transfusion decisions should be individualized and based not only on the hemoglobin level but also on the patient's clinical signs and symptoms of anemia and ability to tolerate and compensate for the anemia.[93]

Traditionally, physicians ordered 2 units for RBC transfusion, a practice that evolved several decades ago when single-unit transfusions were extensively criticized.[97,98] A unit of blood can have varying effects on hemoglobin and hematocrit, depending on patient total blood volume and fluid shifts. Often a single RBC unit provides an adequate response and relieves symptoms. In the nonbleeding patient, single-unit RBC transfusion followed with clinical reassessment is advocated.[95] The impact of implementing a single-unit transfusion policy can be significant. Based on a transfusion hemoglobin threshold of 8 g/dL and adoption of a single-unit strategy, one center predicted a 60% reduction in RBC usage.[99] More recently, a single-unit transfusion

policy in hospitalized chemotherapy and stem cell transplant patients led to a 25% reduction in RBC usage with no associated increase in outpatient transfusion frequency.[100] Depending on the institution's baseline practices, implementing a single-unit transfusion policy can substantially decrease RBC transfusions.

Blood Utilization Review and Changing Physician Behavior

Changing the behavior of physicians whose transfusion practices are embedded in tradition and habit is challenging. The elements required to create a cultural change in the physician's practice include: 1) a desire for change, 2) providing a new behavior practice, 3) a perception that the new practice is safe and straightforward, and 4) a presentation of change that is nonthreatening to autonomy.[101]

Hospital administrators increasingly recognize that the unnecessary use of blood components can affect patient safety and outcomes, and increase cost. Thus, a desire for change is already under way. Strategies focused on education regarding appropriate transfusion practices, providing sound alternatives to transfusion, and communication and feedback by respected colleagues or "champions" are fundamental elements in changing transfusion practices. Building a team of dedicated stakeholders and champions as the network for change management is crucial for the success of any change and a key element for a successful PBM program.

Studies show several interventions can change transfusion practice, although no one intervention appears superior. Even simple interventions can be effective.[102] These can be broadly grouped into 1) education, 2) adoption of guidelines, 3) reminders, and 4) audits with feedback.

Education is integral to any PBM initiative. Because behavioral change is sometimes difficult to achieve, repetition and reinforcement over time are typically required for success. Because PBM is multidisciplinary, different audiences may respond to different approaches and more favorably to their peers.

One-on-one education with physicians, although more time consuming, is likely to have a more sustained effect. The educational content needs to be evidence-based, provided by respected colleagues or opinion leaders, and be ongoing. Providing repeated sessions and easy access to educational information, such as on the hospital website, can help support physicians as they consider changing their practices.

Evidence-based transfusion guidelines are the basis for improving transfusion practice. Key physicians from various specialties should be involved in formulating these guidelines. For successful implementation, the guidelines must be combined with committed educational efforts. Issuing a memo of the transfusion guidelines to physicians without follow-up typically fails to reduce blood usage.

Concurrent reminders at the point of transfusion decision, such as pretransfusion checklists or order sets with the institution's transfusion indications, can improve practice. Using computerized provider order entry (CPOE) systems with the capability of clinical decision support (CDS), and requiring physicians to document the indication when outside of guidelines, facilitates adoption and improves transfusion practice.[103]

Auditing or monitoring physician practice is another intervention that is useful and reinforces evidence-based transfusion guidelines. Audits occurring at the time of the transfusion order, or during the 12 to 24 hours after transfusion, and accompanied with education provide clear opportunities for changing behavior.[104] Prospective or "real-time" audits (approval before issuing the component), where the review is performed manually by laboratory staff, may be the most effective; but such reviews can be labor intensive and time consuming, and can create animosity. The use of CPOE transfusion order sets with CDS, where "hard stops" or "alerts" and patient-specific information (eg, hemoglobin level, vital signs) can support the clinical decision process, is more practical and provides an interactive means to increase physician awareness of best practices. These CPOE/CDS systems vary in their effectiveness in reducing

TABLE 20-2. General Strategy for Implementing a PBM Program

1.	Education
	a. A knowledgeable advocate
	b. Executives
	c. Core group (pharmacy, nursing, blood bank)
	d. Any department involved in PBM activities (ordering clinicians, finance, information technology)
2.	Buy-in from executives
	a. "C" suite (CEO, COO, CFO, CMO)
	b. Medical executive committee
	c. Blood utilization/transfusion committee
	d. Surgical services committee
3.	Business proposal
	a. Background/current environment
	b. Program description
	c. Financial aspects
	d. Risk/benefit analysis
	e. Summary/conclusion
4.	Teamwork
	a. Broad-based stakeholder group of those affected by PBM program (multidisciplinary emphasis, identification of concerns, details to be addressed, enhanced buy-in)
	b. Smaller, more focused steering committee (baseline usage data, relationship to strategic plan, implementation steps, timeline, policy review, monitor progress checks)
	c. Effective meetings
	d. Milestone celebrations
5.	Evaluation
	a. Possible improvements/lessons learned
	b. Study of metrics/outcome data
	c. Analysis/report of program success
	d. Possible program expansion

blood utilization and are likely influenced by configuration, existing practice at baseline, concurrent education, and feedback.[103,105,106] Employing CPOE with CDS standardizes practice and helps sustain compliance. (See Chapter 21 for more on auditing.)

Blood utilization reports that incorporate benchmarking with the goal of continuous quality improvement are powerful tools for changing physician practice. Providing physicians with outcome data regarding their transfusion rates for a surgical procedure or specific treatment, as well as comparisons to their peers, is more likely to motivate change. Providing physicians with timely regular reports helps maintain awareness and interest in identifying additional strategies for reducing avoidable transfusions.[107,108]

A recent initiative to improve transfusion practice involves employing transfusion safety officers or patient blood management coordinators. As change agents, they can provide regular education to all staff involved in transfusion practice, increase awareness of and access to transfusion alternatives, develop a network of caregivers and "champions" for the promotion of optimal transfusions, and provide utilization reports for continuous improvement. Partnering with local physician "champions," these coordinators can be instrumental in changing the culture and reducing allogeneic transfusions.[109,110]

Program Development

Successfully implementing a PBM program requires planning, education, and teamwork. It is important to first analyze current transfusion practices within the hospital. A needs assessment can help evaluate current behaviors and understand the hospital culture and readiness for change.

Demonstrating the clinical benefits and potential cost savings with a PBM program is key to ensuring support and buy-in at all levels. Care must be taken to ensure that clinical staff understand that the primary objective of a PBM program is to improve patient outcomes, even though hospital administrators may focus on cost savings.

The specific activities performed by a PBM program can vary by institution and are defined by the executive management team of the facility. Guidance is available from various professional organizations. The Society for the Advancement of Blood Management offers *Administrative and Clinical Standards for Patient Blood Management Programs,* which outlines 12 standards related to the activities of a formal, comprehensive, organizational-wide PBM program.[111] A PBM program can be designated as an activity level 1, 2, or 3 program, as outlined in AABB's *Standards for a Patient Blood Management Program.*[112] The responsibilities for oversight and monitoring at each activity level are described in Appendix 20-2. In addition, a hospital certification program for PBM based on the AABB *Standards* has been developed jointly by AABB and The Joint Commission. Information on this program and many other PBM resources may be found on the AABB website (aabb.org/pbm).

An effective hospitalwide PBM program involves a multidisciplinary effort with acceptance and input from nursing and physician leadership, along with collaboration and participation from multiple departments, including pharmacy, laboratory, transfusion medicine, nursing, ethics, surgery, and information technology departments. Identifying champions who understand PBM principles and are willing to take "ownership" and drive the program is essential for starting and maintaining the program. Once established, PBM programs often gain momentum from the improved outcomes attained. A general strategy for implementing a PBM program is summarized in Table 20-2, and more detailed descriptions are available.[113,114]

KEY POINTS

1. PBM is an evidence-based, multidisciplinary approach to optimizing the care of patients who might need transfusion.
2. Several factors have been drivers of PBM, including transfusion-associated risks, demand for improved quality of care, promotion of evidence-based practice, economic pressures, overutilization of blood components, patient autonomy and satisfaction, and a projected shrinking of the blood supply.
3. Elements of a PBM program may include: a) management of anemia and bleeding risks before treatment begins; b) intraoperative blood recovery, hemostatic pharmacologic agents, blood-sparing surgical techniques, and POCT-based transfusion algorithms; c) ICU and postoperative strategies to reduce the need for transfusion; d) blood utilization review; and e) education of health-care providers.
4. PBM can provide benefit to medical as well as surgical patients.
5. Preoperative anemia is common. Identifying and treating preoperative anemia is one of the fundamentals of PBM.
6. PBM is more than just transfusion avoidance. It involves the use of pharmaceutical agents, blood recovery techniques, surgical tools to limit blood loss, limiting phlebotomy for laboratory testing, adherence to transfusion guidelines, and medical education.
7. A multidisciplinary team with "champions" is critical for the success, growth, and sustainability of the PBM program.
8. Ongoing blood utilization reviews with benchmarking and emphasis on patient outcomes are powerful tools for a successful program.

REFERENCES

1. Best practices in blood utilization (white paper). Charlotte, NC: Premier Healthcare Alliance, 2012. [Available at https://www.premier inc.com/transforming-healthcare/healthcare-performance-improvement/healthcare-consulting/resource-utilization/ (accessed March 1, 2017).]
2. Proceedings from the National Summit on Overuse, September 24, 2012: Organized by The Joint Commission and the American Medical Association-Convened Physician Consortium for Performance Improvement (PCPI). Oakbrook Terrace, IL: The Joint Commission, 2012. [Available at http://www.jointcommis sion.org/assets/1/6/national_summit_over use.pdf (accessed March 1, 2017).]
3. Combes JR, Arespacochaga E. Appropriate use of medical resources. American Hospital Association's Physician Leadership Forum, Chicago, IL, November 2013. Chicago, IL: AHA, 2013. [Available at http://www.aha.org/content/13/ appropusewhiteppr.pdf (accessed March 1, 2017).]

4. US Department of Health and Human Services. Supplemental findings from the national blood collection and utilization surveys, 2013 and 2015. Transfusion 2017;57(Suppl): 1599-624.
5. Whitaker BI, Rajbhandary S, Harris A. The 2013 AABB blood collection, utilization, and patient blood management survey report. Bethesda, MD: AABB, 2015. [Available at http:// www.aabb.org/research/hemovigilance/ bloodsurvey/Docs/2013-AABB-Blood-Survey-Report.pdf (accessed March 1, 2017).]
6. Berwick DM, Nolan TW, Whittington J. The Triple Aim: Care, health, and cost. Health Affairs 2008;27:759-69. [Available at: http:// www.ihi.org/resources/Pages/Publications/ TripleAimCareHealthandCost.aspx (accessed March 1, 2017).]
7. Food and Drug Administration. Fatalities reported to FDA following blood collection and transfusion: Annual summary for fiscal year 2015. Silver Spring, MD: CBER Office of Communication, Outreach, and Development, 2016. [Available at https://www.fda.gov/

downloads/BiologicsBloodVaccines/Safety Availability/ReportaProblem/TransfusionDonationFatalities/UCM518148.pdf (accessed March 1, 2017).]

8. Holst LB, Petersen MW, Haase N, et al. Restrictive versus liberal transfusion strategy for red blood cell transfusion: Systematic review of randomised trials with meta-analysis and trial sequential analysis. BMJ 2015;350:h1354. doi: 10.1136/bmj.h1354.

9. Rohde JM, Dimcheff DE, Blumberg N, et al. Health care-associated infection after red cell transfusion: A systematic review and meta-analysis. JAMA 2014;311:1317-26.

10. Salpeter SR, Buckley JS, Chatterjee S. Impact of more restrictive blood transfusion strategies on clinical outcomes: A meta-analysis and systematic review. Am J Med 2014;127;124-31.

11. Benjamin RJ, Whitaker BJ. Boom or bust? Estimating blood demand and supply as the baby boomers age (editorial). Transfusion 2011;51: 670-3.

12. Colby SL, Ortman JM. Projections of the size and composition of the US population: 2014 to 2060. Population estimates and projections. Current population reports. (March 2015) Washington, DC: US Census Bureau, 2015. [Available at https://www.census.gov/content/dam/Census/library/publications/2015/demo/p25-1143.pdf (accessed March 1, 2017).]

13. Shander A, Hofmann A, Ozawa S, et al. Activity-based costs of blood transfusions in surgical patients at four hospitals. Transfusion 2010;50:753-65.

14. Freedman J. The ONTraC Ontario program in blood conservation. Transfus Apher Sci 2014; 50:32-6.

15. Gross I, Seifert B, Hofmann A, Spahn DR. Patient blood management in cardiac surgery results in fewer transfusions and better outcomes. Transfusion 2015;55:1075-81.

16. Becker J, Shaz B, for the Clinical Transfusion Medicine Committee and the Transfusion Section Coordinating Committee. Guidelines for patient blood management and blood utilization. Bethesda, MD: AABB, 2011.

17. Liumbruno GM, Bennardello F, Lattanzio A, et al for the Italian Society of Transfusion Medicine and Immunohaematology (SIMTI) Working Party. Recommendations for the transfusion management of patients in the perioperative period. I. The pre-operative period. Blood Transfus 2011;9:19-40.

18. World Health Organization. Haemoglobin concentrations for the diagnosis of anaemia and assessment of severity. WHO/NMH/NHD/MNM/11.1. Geneva, Switzerland: WHO, 2011. [Available at http://www.who.int/vmnis/indicators/haemoglobin.pdf (accessed March 1, 2017).]

19. Spahn DR. Anemia and patient blood management in hip and knee surgery: A systematic review of the literature. Anesthesiology 2010; 113:482-95.

20. Shander A, Knight K, Thurer R, et al. Prevalence and outcomes of anemia in surgery: A systematic review of the literature. Am J Med 2004;116(Suppl 7A):58S-69S.

21. Hogan M, Klein AA, Richards T. The impact of anaemia and intravenous iron replacement therapy on outcomes in cardiac surgery. Eur J Cardiothorac Surg 2015;47:218-26.

22. Leichtle SW, Mouawad NJ, Lampman R, et al. Does preoperative anemia adversely affect colon and rectal surgery outcomes? J Am Coll Surg 2011;212:187-94.

23. Musallam KM, Tamim HM, Richards T, et al. Preoperative anaemia and postoperative outcomes in non-cardiac surgery: A retrospective cohort study. Lancet 2011;378:1396-407.

24. Wu WC, Schifftner TL, Henderson WG, et al. Preoperative hematocrit levels and postoperative outcomes in older patients undergoing noncardiac sugery. JAMA 2007;297:2481-8.

25. Goodnough LT, Shander A, Spivak JL, et al. Detection, evaluation, and management of anemia in the elective surgical patient. Anesth Analg 2005;101:1858-61.

26. Goodnough LT, Maniatis A, Earnshaw P, et al. Detection, evaluation, and management of preoperative anemia in the elective orthopaedic surgical patient: NATA guidelines. Br J Anaesthesia 2011;106:13-22.

27. Lin DM, Lin ES, Tran MH. Efficacy and safety of erythropoietin and intravenous iron in perioperative blood management: A systematic review. Transfus Med Rev 2013;27:221-34.

28. Litton E, Xiao J, Ho KM. Safety and efficacy of intravenous iron therapy in reducing requirement for allogeneic blood transfusion: Systematic review and meta-analysis of randomized clinical trials. BMJ 2013;347:f4822.

29. Food and Drug Administration. FDA drug safety communication: Erythropoiesis-stimulating agents (ESAs): Procrit, Epogen, and Aranesp. Silver Spring, MD: CDER Office of Communications, 2010. [Available at http://

www.fda.gov/Drugs/DrugSafety/Postmarket DrugSafetyInformationforPatientsandProviders/ucm200297.htm (accessed March 1, 2017).]

30. Shuvy M, Mewa J, Wolff R, et al. Preprocedure anemia management decreases transfusion rates in patients undergoing transcatheter aortic valve implantation. Can J Cardiol 2016; 32:732-8.

31. Kotze A, Carter LA, Scally AJ. Effect of a patient blood management programme on preoperative anaemia, transfusion rate, and outcome after primary hip and knee arthroplasty: A quality improvement cycle. Br J Anaesth 2012; 108:943-52.

32. Bader AM, Sweitzer B, Kumar A. Nuts and bolts of preoperative anemia clinics: The view from three institutions. Cleve Clin J Med 2009;76: S104-11.

33. Guinn NR, Guercio JR, Hopkins TJ, et al. How do we develop and implement a preoperative anemia clinic designed to improve perioperative outcomes and reduce cost? Transfusion 2016;56:297-303.

34. Apfelbaum JL, Nuttall GA, Connis RT, et al. American Society of Anesthesiologists Task Force on Perioperative Blood Management. Practice guidelines for perioperative blood management: An updated report by the American Society of Anesthesiologists Task Force on Perioperative Blood Management. Anesthesiology 2015;122:241-75.

35. Douketis JD, Spyropoulos AC, Spencer FA, et al. Perioperative management of antithrombotic therapy: Antithrombotic therapy and prevention of thrombosis. 9th ed. American College of Chest Physicians evidence-based clinical practice guidelines. Chest 2012;141(2 Suppl):e326S-50S.

36. Ferraris VA, Brown JR, Despotis GJ, et al. Society of Thoracic Surgeons Blood Conservation Guideline Task Force; Society of Cardiovascular Anesthesiologists Special Task Force on Blood Transfusion; International Consortium for Evidence Based Perfusion. 2011 update to the Society of Thoracic Surgeons and the Society of Cardiovascular Anesthesiologists blood conservation clinical practice guidelines. Ann Thorac Surg 2011;91:944-82.

37. Ferraris VA, Saha SF, Oesterich JH. 2012 update to the Society of Thoracic Surgeons guidelines on use of antiplatelet drugs in patients having cardiac and noncardiac operations. Ann Thorac Surg 2012;94:1761-81.

38. Vassallo R, Goldman M, Germain M, Lozano M, for the BEST Collaborative. Preoperative autologous blood donation: Waning indications in an era of improved blood safety. Transfus Med Rev 2015;29:268-75.

39. Lee GC, Cushner FD. The effects of preoperative autologous donations on perioperative blood levels. J Knee Surg 2007;20:205-9.

40. Kennedy C, Leonard M, Devitt A, et al. Efficacy of preoperative autologous blood donation for elective posterior lumbar spinal surgery. Spine (Phila Pa 1976) 2011;36:E1736-43.

41. Goldman M, Remy-Prince S, Trepanier A, Decary F. Autologous donation error rate in Canada. Transfusion 1997;37:523-7.

42. Berg MP, ed. Standards for perioperative autologous blood collection and administration. 7th ed. Bethesda, MD: AABB, 2016.

43. Zhou X, Zhang C, Wang Y, et al. Preoperative acute normovolemic hemodilution for minimizing allogeneic blood transfusion: A meta-analysis. Anesth Analg 2015;121:1443-55.

44. Grant MC, Resar LMS, Frank SM. The efficacy and utility of acute normovolemic hemodilution (editorial). Anesth Analg 2015;121:1412-14.

45. Shander A, Rijhwani TS. Acute normovolemic hemodilution. Transfusion 2004;44:26S-34S.

46. Carless PA, Henry DA, Moxey AJ, et al. Cell salvage for minimising perioperative allogeneic blood transfusion. Cochrane Database Syst Rev 2010;(4):CD001888.

47. Esper SA, Waters JH. Intra-operative cell salvage: A fresh look at the indications and contraindications. Blood Transfus 2011;9:139-47.

48. Waters JH, Yazer M, Chen YF, Kloke J. Blood salvage and cancer surgery: A meta analysis of available studies. Transfusion 2012;52:2167-73.

49. Liumbruno GM, Meschini A, Liumbruno C, Rafanelli D. The introduction of intra-operative cell salvage in obstetric clinical practice: A review of the available evidence. Eur J Obstet Gynecol Reprod Biol 2011;159:19-25.

50. Goucher H, Wong CA, Patel SK, Toledo P. Cell salvage in obstetrics. Anesth Analg 2015;121: 465-8.

51. Waters JH, Shander A, eds. Perioperative blood management: A physician's handbook. 3rd ed. Bethesda, MD: AABB, 2014.

52. Berte L. Quality manual preparation workbook for perioperative autologous collection and administration. Bethesda, MD: AABB Press, 2007.

53. Anesthesia – more than sleeping. In: Seeber P, Shander A. Basics of blood management. 2nd ed. Chichester, West Sussex, UK: Wiley-Blackwell, 2013:191-200.

54. Nuttall GA, Oliver WC. Ancillary techniques. In: Waters JH, ed. Blood management: Options for better patient care. Bethesda, MD: AABB Press, 2008:281-99.

55. Physical methods of hemostasis. In: Seeber P, Shander A. Basics of blood management. 2nd ed. Chichester, West Sussex, UK: Wiley-Blackwell, 2013:173-190.

56. Gombotz H. Patient blood management: A patient-orientated approach to blood replacement with the goal of reducing anemia, blood loss and the need for blood transfusion in elective surgery. Transfus Med Hemother 2012; 39:67-72.

57. Enriquez LJ, Shore-Lesserson L. Point-of-care coagulation testing and transfusion algorithms. Br J Anaesth 2009;103(Suppl 1):i14-22.

58. Perry DJ, Fitzmaurice DA, Kitchen S, et al. Point-of-care testing in haemostasis. Br J Haematol 2010;150:501-14.

59. Bollinger D, Tanaka KA. Roles of thrombelastography and thromboelastometry for patient blood management in cardiac surgery. Transfus Med Rev 2013;27:213-20.

60. Whiting P, Al M, Westwood M, et al. Viscoelastic point-of-care testing to assist with the diagnosis, management and monitoring of haemostasis: A systematic review and cost-effectiveness analysis. Health Technol Assess 2015;19:1-228.

61. Mallett SV. Clinical utility of viscoelastic tests of coagulation (TEG/ROTEM) in patients with liver disease and during liver transplantation. Semin Thromb Hemost 2015;41:527-37.

62. Gurusamy KS, Pissanou T, Pikhart H, et al. Methods to decrease blood loss and transfusion requirements for liver transplantation. Cochrane Database Syst Rev 2011;12: CD009052.

63. Pietri LD, Bianchini M, Montalti R, et al. Thrombelastography-guided blood product use before invasive procedures in cirrhosis with severe coagulopathy: A randomized, controlled trial. Hepatology 2016;63:566-73.

64. Holcomb JB, Minei KM, Scerbo ML, et al. Admission rapid thrombelastography can replace conventional coagulation tests in the emergency department: Experience with 1974 consecutive trauma patients. Ann Surg 2012; 256:476-86.

65. Gonzalez E, Moore EE, Moore HB, et al. Goal-directed hemostatic resuscitation of trauma-induced coagulopathy: A pragmatic randomized clinical trial comparing a viscoelastic assay to conventional coagulation assays. Ann Surg 2016;263:1051-9.

66. Da Luz LT, Nascimento B, Shankarakutty AK, et al. Effect of thromboelastography (TEG) and rotational thromboelastometry (ROTEM) on diagnosis of coagulopathy, transfusion guidance and mortality in trauma: Descriptive systematic review. Crit Care 2014;18:518.

67. American College of Surgeons Trauma Quality Improvement Program. ACS TQIP massive transfusion in trauma guidelines. [Available at https://www.facs.org/~/media/files/quality%20programs/trauma/tqip/massive%20transfusion%20in%20trauma%20guilde lines.ashx (accessed March 2, 2017).]

68. Spahn DR, Bouillon B, Cerny V, et al. Management of bleeding and coagulopathy following major trauma: An updated European guideline. Crit Care 2013;17:R76. [Available at http://ccforum.com/content/17/2/R76 (accessed March 2, 2017).]

69. Ker K, Edwards P, Perel P, et al. Effect of tranexamic acid on surgical bleeding: Systematic review and cumulative meta-analysis. BMJ 2012;344:e3054.

70. Henry DA, Carless PA, Moxey AJ, et al. Antifibrinolytic use for minimising perioperative allogeneic blood transfusion. Cochrane Database Syst Rev 2011;(3):CD001886.

71. Manji RA, Grocott HP, Leake J, et al. Seizures following cardiac surgery: The impact of tranexamic acid and other risk factors. Can J Anaesth 2012;59:6-13.

72. Harris RN, Moskal JT, Capps SG. Does tranexamic acid reduce blood transfusion cost for primary total hip arthroplasty? A case-control study. J Arthroplasty 2015;30:192-5.

73. Moskal JT, Harris RN, Capps SG. Transfusion cost savings with tranexamic acid in primary total knee arthroplasty from 2009 to 2012. J Arthroplasty 2015;30:365-8.

74. Ker K, Roberts I, Shakur H, Coats TJ. Antifibrinolytic drugs for acute traumatic injury. Cochrane Database Syst Rev 2015;5: CD004896.

75. Shakur H, Roberts I, Fawole B, et al for the WOMAN Trial Collaborators. Effect of early tranexamic acid administration on mortality, hysterectomy, and other morbidities in women with post-partum haemorrhage (WOMAN):

An international, randomised, double-blind, placebo-controlled trial. Lancet 2017;389: 2105-16.

76. Svensson PJ, Bergqvist PB, Juul KV, Berntorp E. Desmopressin in treatment of haematological disorders and in prevention of surgical bleeding. Blood Rev 2014;28:95-102.

77. Wademan BH, Galvin SD. Desmopressin for reducing postoperative blood loss and transfusion requirements following cardiac surgery in adults. Interact Cardiovasc Thorac Surg 2014;18:360-70.

78. Shander A, Kaplan LJ, Harris MT, et al. Topical hemostatic therapy in surgery: Bridging the knowledge and practice gap. J Am Coll Surg 2014;219:570-9.e4.

79. Goodnough LT, Shander A. Current status of pharmacologic therapies in patient blood management. Anesth Analg 2013;116:15-34.

80. Oremus K, Sostaric S, Trkulja V, Haspl M. Influence of tranexamic acid on postoperative autologous blood retransfusion in primary total hip and knee arthroplasty: A randomized controlled trial. Transfusion 2014;54:31-41.

81. Springer BD, Odum SM, Fehring TK. What is the benefit of tranexamic acid vs. reinfusion drains in total joint arthroplasty? J Arthroplasty 2016;31:76-80.

82. Munoz M, Garcia-Vallejo JJ, Ruiz MD, et al. Transfusion of postoperative shed blood: Laboratory characteristics and clinical utility. Eur Spine J 2004;13(Suppl 1):S107-13.

83. Sinardi D, Marino A, Chillemi S, et al. Composition of the blood sampled from surgical drainage after joint arthroplasty: Quality of return. Transfusion 2005;45:202-7.

84. Vincent JL, Baron JF, Reinhart K, et al. Anemia and blood transfusion in critically ill patients. JAMA 2002;288:1499-507.

85. Salisbury AC, Reid KJ, Alexander KP, et al. Diagnostic blood loss from phlebotomy and hospital-acquired anemia during acute myocardial infarction. Arch Intern Med 2011;171: 1646-53.

86. Fowler RA, Berenson M. Blood conservation in the intensive care unit. Crit Care Med 2003; 31(Suppl):S715-20.

87. Chant C, Wilson G, Friedrich JO. Anemia, transfusion, and phlebotomy practices in critically ill patients with prolonged ICU length of stay: A cohort study. Crit Care 2006;10:R140.

88. Sanchez-Giron F, Alvarez-Mora F. Reduction of blood loss from laboratory testing in hospitalized adult patients using small-volume (pediatric) tubes. Arch Pathol Lab Med 2008;132: 1916-19.

89. Mukhopadhyay A, Yip HS, Prabhuswamy D, et al. The use of a blood conservation device to reduce red blood cell transfusion requirements: A before and after study. Crit Care 2010; 14:R7.

90. Lelubre C, Vincet JL. Red blood cell transfusion in the critically ill patient. Ann Intensive Care 2011;1:43.

91. Physiology of anemia and oxygen transport. In: Seeber P, Shander A. Basics of blood management. 2nd ed. Chichester, West Sussex, UK: Wiley-Blackwell, 2013:9-20.

92. Carson JL, Carless PA, Hébert PC. Transfusion thresholds and other strategies for guiding allogeneic red blood cell transfusion. Cochrane Database Syst Rev 2012;(4):CD002042.

93. Carson JL, Guyatt G, Heddle NM, et al. Clinical practice guidelines from the AABB: Red blood cell transfusion thresholds and storage. JAMA 2016:2025-35.

94. National Clinical Guideline Centre. Blood transfusion. NICE guideline no. 24 (November 18, 2015). London: National Institute for Health and Care Excellence (NICE), 2015. [Available at http://www.guideline.gov/content.aspx?id=49905&search=red+cell+transfusion+thresholds (accessed March 1, 2017).]

95. Retter A, Wyncoll D, Pearse R, et al. British Committee for Standards in Haematology. Guidelines on the management of anaemia and red cell transfusion in adult critically ill patients. Br J Haematol 2013;160:445-64.

96. American Academy of Orthopaedic Surgeons clinical practice guideline on management of hip fractures in the elderly. Rosemont, IL: American Academy of Orthopaedic Surgeons (AAOS), 2014. [Available at http://www.guideline.gov/content.aspx?id=48518&search=red+cell+transfusion+thresholds (accessed March 1, 2017).]

97. Crispen JF. The single-unit transfusion: A continuing problem. Pa Med 1966;69:44-8.

98. Domen RE. The single-unit transfusion. J Fla Med Assoc 1986;73:855-7.

99. Ma M, Eckert K, Ralley F, Chin-Yee I. A retrospective study evaluating single-unit red blood cell transfusions in reducing allogeneic blood exposure. Transfus Med 2005;15:307-12.

100. Berger MD, Gerber B, Arn K, et al. Significant reduction of red blood cell transfusion requirements by changing from a double-unit to a single-unit transfusion policy in patients re-

ceiving intensive chemotherapy or stem cell transplantation. Haematologica 2012;97:116-22.

101. Tinmouth A. Reducing the amount of blood transfused by changing clinicians' transfusion practices. Transfusion 2007;47:132S-6S.

102. Tinmouth A, MacDougall L, Fergusson D, et al. Reducing the amount of blood transfused: A systematic review of behavioral interventions to change physicians' transfusion practices. Arch Intern Med 2005;165:845-52.

103. Hibbs SP, Nielsen ND, Brunskill S, et al. The impact of electronic decision support on transfusion practice: A systematic review. Transfus Med Rev 2015;29:14-23.

104. Toy P. Effectiveness of transfusion audits and practice guidelines. Arch Pathol Lab Med 1994; 118:435-7.

105. Dunbar NM, Szczepiorkowski ZM. Hardwiring patient blood management: Harnessing information technology to optimize transfusion practice. Curr Opin Hematol 2014;21:515-20.

106. Butler CE, Noel S, Hibbs SP, et al. Implementation of a clinical decision support system improves compliance with restrictive transfusion policies in hematology patients. Transfusion 2015;55:1964-71.

107. Bradley EH, Holmboe ES, Mattera JA, et al. Data feedback efforts in quality improvement: Lessons learned from US hospitals. Qual Saf Health Care 2004;13:26-31.

108. Beaty CA, Haggerty KA, Moser MG, et al. Disclosure of physician specific behavior improves blood utilization protocol adherence in cardiac surgery. Ann Thorac Surg 2013;96: 2168-74.

109. Freedman J, Luke K, Escobar M, et al. Experience of a network of transfusion coordinators for blood conservation (Ontario Transfusion Coordinators [OnTraC]). Transfusion 2008; 48:237-50.

110. Maynard KJ. Review of roles: Transfusion safety officer and patient blood management coordinator. In: Johnson ST, Puca K eds. Transfusion medicine's emerging positions: Transfusion safety officers and patient blood management coordinators. Bethesda, MD: AABB Press, 2013:37-46.

111. SABM administrative and clinical standards for patient blood management programs. 3rd ed. Richmond, VA: Society for the Advancement of Blood Management, 2014. [Available at http://www.sabm.org/sites/default/files/ SABM_Admin-Standards3rdEdition.pdf (accessed March 2, 2017).]

112. Frey K, ed. Standards for a patient blood management program. 2nd ed. Bethesda, MD: AABB, 2017.

113. Building a better patient blood management program: Identifying tools, solving problems and promoting patient safety (white paper). Bethesda, MD: AABB, 2015.

114. Frank SM, Johnson DJ, Resar LMS. Development of a patient blood management program. In: Waters JH, Frank SM, eds. Patient blood management: Multidisciplinary approaches to optimizing care. Bethesda, MD: AABB Press/SABM, 2016:13-38.

● **APPENDIX 20-1**

Pharmacologic Therapies for Supporting Patient Blood Management*

Pharmacologic Agent	Specific Drug	Primary Use	Mechanism of Action	Considerations
Intravenous (IV) iron therapy	Iron high-molecular-weight dextran; iron low-molecular-weight dextran; ferric gluconate; iron sucrose; ferumoxytol; ferric carboxymaltose	Treating iron deficiency and iron-deficiency anemia.	• Iron is an essential element of hemoglobin and the site of oxygen binding. It helps transport oxygen to tissues. • There is substantial evidence that IV iron effectively treats iron-deficiency anemia in many chronic conditions.	• Blood loss is a major cause of iron deficiency. • Even under the best circumstances, oral iron is not well tolerated, and patients are often noncompliant due to gastrointestinal (GI) symptoms.[1] • IV iron given concurrently with ESAs provides better responses than oral iron and allows lowering of ESA dose in certain patient populations.[1] • High-molecular-weight dextran is associated with serious side effects.[1]
Erythropoiesis-stimulating agents (ESAs)	Epoetin alfa; darbepoetin alfa	• Approved for treating anemia resulting from chronic kidney failure, chemotherapy, certain treatments for human immunodeficiency virus, and also to reduce the number of blood transfusions during and after certain elective noncardiac, nonvascular surgeries (hemoglobin >10 g/dL but <13 g/dL).	• ESAs stimulate differentiation of stem cells into immature red cells; increase rate of mitosis and release of reticulocytes into the circulation; and induce hemoglobin formation. • A glycoprotein hormone produced in the kidney, a growth factor for red cell precursors in marrow.	• Response seen by day 5-7 in iron-replete patients. • One unit equivalent hematocrit increase by day 7; 3-5 units by day 28. • Darbepoetin is an alternative used in renal and oncology settings.[2,3]

Category	Agent	Description	Clinical Notes
		Synthetic erythropoietin produced by recombinant DNA technology.	• Society for Thoracic Surgery 2011 guidelines report: "It is reasonable to use preoperative erythropoietin plus iron, given several days before cardiac surgery, for preoperative anemia, in candidates who refuse transfusion (eg, Jehovah's Witnesses), or in patients who are at high risk for postoperative anemia."[4] • Black box warning due to increased risk for death, myocardial infarction, stroke, venous thromboembolism, thrombosis of vascular access, and tumor progression or recurrence.[5]
Antifibrinolytics	Epsilon-aminocaproic acid (EACA)	Enhances hemostasis associated with surgical complications following heart surgery; orthopedic surgery; some hematologic disorders associated with thrombocytopenia; and massive traumatic bleeding in the presence of fibrinolysis.	
	Tranexamic acid (TXA)[6]	• Blocks fibrinolysis by inhibiting activation of plasminogen to plasmin, which is responsible for limiting and dissolving clots. • TXA provides equivalent antifibrinolytic effect as EACA but at only 1/10 the concentration and has a slower renal clearance (6-8 hours vs <3 hours with EACA).[7] • Dysfunctional uterine bleeding, menorrhagia associated with intrauterine device, conization of cervix, post-/antepartum hemorrhage, uterine/vaginal surgery.	• Reduces blood loss and transfusion requirements in cardiac and orthopedic surgeries.[8] • Early administration of TXA to trauma patients with significant bleeding (within 3 hrs from onset of injury) has been shown to reduce mortality.[9] • Rapid intravenous administration should be avoided; may induce hypotension, bradycardia, and/or arrhythmia. • Use with caution in hematuria of upper urinary tract origin, unless the possible benefits outweigh risk. • Contraindicated in patients with disseminated intravascular coagulation. • Must use renal dosing guidelines for patients with impaired renal function. • Adverse effects: nausea, vomiting, diarrhea, dizziness, headache, stuffy nose, skin rash, theoretic risk of thrombosis.[6,7]

(Continued)

● **APPENDIX 20-1**
Pharmacologic Therapies for Supporting Patient Blood Management* (Continued)

Pharmacologic Agent	Specific Drug	Primary Use	Mechanism of Action	Considerations
Antifibrinolytics (Continued)		• Oral bleeding, post-dental-extraction bleeding in patients with hemophilia, von Willebrand disease (vWD), or thrombocytopenia.		
Reversal agents	Vitamin K	Reverses the anticoagulant effect of warfarin.	Vitamin K is necessary for hepatic synthesis of coagulation factors (Factors II, VII, IX, and X) and anticoagulant proteins (protein C and S).	See clinical practice guidelines outlining the evidence-based management of vitamin K antagonist initiation, monitoring, and treatment of complications.[10,11]
	Protamine	• Neutralizes unfractionated heparin (UFH) after cardiac surgery. • Antidote when bleeding complications are associated with excessive heparin anticoagulation.	Binds to heparin and displaces antithrombin from heparin-antithrombin complex.[12]	• Adverse events may include hypotension, pulmonary edema, and anaphylaxis. • Excess protamine can lead to an anticoagulation effect. • In cardiac surgery, dosing based on point-of-care testing allows more appropriate dose and reduces postoperative bleeding.[12] • May be used for reversal of low-molecular-weight heparin, but less effective.[13]

Coagulation factor concentrates	Prothrombin complex concentrate (PCC)	• 3-factor PCCs have only one approved indication: preventing and controlling bleeding related to hemophilia B.[1] • 4-factor PCCs are approved for urgent reversal of vitamin K antagonist (warfarin) in acute major bleeding or when needed for urgent surgery or invasive procedures.[1,14]	• PCCs are derived from pooled human plasma. • 3-factor PCCs contain three vitamin-K-dependent coagulation factors (Factors II, IX, and X) and a small amount of Factor VII. • 4-factor PCCs contain therapeutic levels of Factor VII, in addition to Factors II, IX, and X.	• 3-factor PCCs do not effectively lower the international normalized ratio (INR); addition of a small amount of Fresh Frozen Plasma (mean 2 units) increases the likelihood of satisfactory INR lowering.[15] • 4-factor PCCs contain heparin and should not be used in patients with heparin allergies or heparin-induced thrombocytopenia.[14] • Efficacy and safety of 3-factor PCCs or 4-factor PCCs in the setting of patients with severe or life-threatening bleeding associated with target-specific oral anticoagulants (eg, dabigatran, rivaroxaban, apixaban, edoxaban) is unclear.[16]
	Recombinant Factor VIIa (rFVIIa)	• Approved by the Food and Drug Administration (FDA) for treating hemophilia A and B with inhibitors.[1] • Acceptable in patients with congenital Factor VII deficiency or patients with Glanzmann thrombasthenia with antibodies to glycoprotein IIb/IIIa.[1]	Enhances thrombin generation at the site of vascular injury.	• Black box warning issued in 2005 regarding the risk of arterial thromboembolic complications.[1] • Efficacy of rFVIIa as a general hemostatic drug remains unproven.[17] • Although there are anecdotal cases of resolution of bleeding with rFVIIa administration in certain conditions, such as blunt trauma and after complex cardiac surgery, clinical trial data has generally not shown efficacy, and there are data suggesting increased thrombotic risk. Therefore, off-label use of rFVIIa should be restricted to settings of ongoing refractory bleeding despite administration of all available therapies, when the benefit clearly outweighs the risk, and at the lowest dose.

(Continued)

● **APPENDIX 20-1**
Pharmacologic Therapies for Supporting Patient Blood Management* (Continued)

Pharmacologic Agent	Specific Drug	Primary Use	Mechanism of Action	Considerations
Coagulation factor concentrates (Continued)	Fibrinogen concentrate	Approved by FDA for treating bleeding only in patients with congenital fibrinogen deficiency.[18]	• Derived from pooled human plasma. • Precursor to fibrin; thrombin converts fibrinogen to fibrin to form soluble fibrin clot, which is then stabilized by activated Factor XIII.	• Adverse reactions include allergic and hypersensitivity reactions.[18] • Thromboembolic events were reported.[18] • Use in obstetric hemorrhage, trauma, and cardiac surgery was reported but is considered off-label, and future studies are needed to prove efficacy.[1]
Topical hemostatic agents	Mechanical hemostatics (porcine gelatin, bovine collagen, oxidized regenerated cellulose); biologically active hemostatics (bovine thrombin, human thrombin, recombinant human thrombin); fibrin sealants; polyethylene glycol polymer sealants; synthetic adhesives	Hemostatics, sealants, and adhesives are primarily used during surgery for various applications to aid hemostasis when ligation, sutures, compression, or cautery are not effective. The types of bleeding where topical agents may be used include: diffuse raw surface bleeding, oozing venous-type bleeding, bone bleeding, and needle-hole bleeding.	Agents generally act by compressing the bleeding vessel, activating/ aggregating platelets, and/or providing a scaffold for clot formation. Some applications include thrombin, which speeds clot formation.	• Topical hemostatic agents can be highly effective, but must be used carefully to avoid systemic reactions.[1] • Full descriptions of these agents, including uses, are available.[19]

Category	Drug	Mechanism	Uses	Notes
Pharmaceuticals used primarily in obstetrics to control bleeding	Oxytocin	Stimulates uterine contractions.	• Obstetric hemorrhage. • Used to treat uterine atony.	Oxytocin is the treatment of choice for preventing and treating postpartum hemorrhage.[20,21]
	Methergine	Increases the strength, duration, and frequency of uterine contractions.	• Obstetric hemorrhage. • Used to treat uterine atony.	• Second-line therapy for treating uterine atony and postpartum hemorrhage.[21] • Hypertension and toxemia are contraindications.
	Carboprost	Stimulates uterine contractions.	• Obstetric hemorrhage. • FDA-approved to treat uterine atony that does not respond to conventional treatment.	• Second-line therapy for treating postpartum hemorrhage.[21] • Contraindicated in patients with pulmonary, cardiac, renal, and hepatic disease. • Asthma is a relative contraindication.[20,21]
	Misoprostol	Synthetic prostaglandin.	• Obstetric hemorrhage. • Used to treat uterine atony.	• Studies of the efficacy of misoprostol for preventing and treating obstetric hemorrhage show mixed results.[21] • Works most effectively when used with other medications listed in this table (synergistic action).[20]
Other pharmaceuticals that can help with hemostasis	Desmopressin (DDAVP; synthetic analog of vasopressin)[22]	• Raises circulating Factor VIII and vWF; unidentified effect on platelets and endothelium.[12,22] • Synthetic analog of the natural pituitary hormone 8-arginine vasopressin, an antidiuretic hormone affecting renal water conservation.[22]	• Useful in patients with mild hemophilia A or Type I vWD (DDAVP is contraindicated in Type 2B and platelet-type vWD).[22] • May be useful in patients with uremia or cirrhosis; these patients have prolonged bleeding times due to complex disorders of hemostasis.[22]	• Responsiveness to DDAVP in mild hemophilia A and Type I vWD is usually confirmed by elective challenge (trial). • Should be used with caution in patients with fluid or electrolyte imbalance, as with cystic fibrosis; patients may develop hyponatremia. • Patients who may benefit from DDAVP include[12,22,23]: – Patients undergoing prolonged surgery with cardiopulmonary bypass. – Patients experiencing excessive postoperative bleeding or those who are at high risk for bleeding. – Patients taking platelet-inhibiting drugs. – Patients with chronic renal failure or liver dysfunction.

(Continued)

APPENDIX 20-1
Pharmacologic Therapies for Supporting Patient Blood Management* (Continued)

Pharmacologic Agent	Specific Drug	Primary Use	Mechanism of Action	Considerations
Other pharmaceuticals that can help with hemostasis (Continued)	Conjugated estrogen	• Dysfunctional uterine bleeding. • Uremia.	• Precise mechanism of action not known. • May involve effect on mucopolysaccharide content of vessel wall; increased synthesis of vWF by endothelial cells.[12]	• Possible alternative or adjunct for cryoprecipitate or desmopressin for the treatment of bleeding associated with renal failure. • Effectiveness of use in uremia patients is mixed.
	Proton pump inhibitors	• Peptic ulcer. • Upper GI hemorrhage.	Reduces incidence of upper GI rebleeding after sclerotherapy by increasing pH to >4, which is necessary for clot formation and stabilization.	Proton pump inhibitors are more effective than H2-antagonists in preventing persistent or recurrent bleeding from peptic ulcer, although this seems to be more evident in patients not having adjunct sclerotherapy.[24]
	Octreotide	• Variceal hemorrhage. • Acute nonvariceal upper GI bleeding.	• An octapeptide that mimics natural somatostatin pharmacologically. • Long-acting analog of somatostatin (half-life of ~90 minutes, as compared to 2-3 minutes for somatostatin).	Octreotide and somatostatin are at least as effective as conventional vasoactive drugs and balloon tamponade in treating variceal hemorrhage, with the advantage of fewer side effects.[25]

- Reduces splanchnic blood flow via a multifactorial mechanism.
- Most effective when combined with sclerotherapy.
- Eliminates vasospasm complications seen with vasopressin.

*Drugs approved for use in the United States as of April 2016. The table is intended to provide general information. Professionals seeking additional information and individuals seeking personal medical advice should consult a qualified physician.

1. Goodnough LT, Shander A. Current status of pharmacologic therapies in patient blood management. Anesth Analg 2013;116:15-34.
2. Goodnough LT, Monk TG, Andriole GL. Erythropoietin therapy. N Engl J Med 1997;336:933-8.
3. Ross SD, Allen IE, Henry DH, et al. Clinical benefits and risk associated with epoetin and darbepoetin in patient with chemotherapy-induced anemia: A systematic review of the literature. Clin Ther 2006;28:801-31.
4. Ferraris VA, Brown JR, Despotis GJ, et al. Society of Cardiovascular Anesthesiologists Special Task Force on Blood Transfusion; International Consortium for Evidence Based Perfusion. 2011 update to the Society of Thoracic Surgeons and the Society of Cardiovascular Anesthesiologists blood conservation clinical practice guidelines. Ann Thorac Surg 2011;91:944-82.
5. Epogen (epoetin alfa) injection for intravenous or subcutaneous use package insert. Thousand Oaks, CA: Amgen, 2016. [Available at http://pi.amgen.com/united_states/epogen/epogen_pi_hcp_english.pdf (accessed March 2, 2017).]
6. Cyklokapron tranexamic acid injection package insert. New York, NY: Pfizer, 2014. [Available at http://labeling.pfizer.com/ShowLabeling.aspx?id=556 (accessed March 2, 2017).]
7. Use of desmopressin, antifibrinolytics, and conjugated estrogens in hemostasis. In: Goodnight SH, Hathaway WE. Disorders of hemostasis and thrombosis: A clinical guide. 2nd ed. New York: McGraw-Hill, 2001:528-42.
8. Henry DA, Carless PA, Moxey AJ, et al. Anti-fibrinolytic use for minimising perioperative allogeneic blood transfusion. Cochrane Database Syst Rev 2011;(3):CD001886.
9. CRASH-2 trial collaborators. Effect of tranexamic acid on death, vascular occlusive events, and blood transfusion in trauma patients with significant hemorrhage (CRASH-2): A randomized, placebo-controlled trial. Lancet 2010;376:23-32.
10. Holbrook A, Schulman S, Witt DM, et al. Evidence-based management of anticoagulant therapy. Antithrombotic therapy and prevention of thrombosis. 9th ed. American College of Chest Physicians evidence-based clinical practice guidelines. Chest 2012;141(Suppl):e152S-e184S.
11. Patriquin C, Crowther M. Treatment of warfarin-associated coagulopathy with vitamin K. Expert Rev Hematol 2011;4:657-67.
12. Bolan CD, Klein HG. Blood component and pharmacologic therapy for hemostatic disorders. In: Kitchens CS, Kessler CM, Konkle BA, eds. Consultative hemostasis and thrombosis. 3rd ed. Philadelphia: Elsevier Saunders, 2013:496-525.
13. Garcia DA, Baglin TP, Weitz JI, et al. Parenteral anticoagulants. Antithrombotic therapy and prevention of thrombosis. 9th ed. American College of Chest Physicians evidence-based clinical practice guidelines. Chest 2012;141(Suppl):e24S-e43S.
14. Kcentra (prothrombin complex concentrate, human) for intravenous use, lyophilized powder for reconstitution. Package insert. (Revised September 2014) Kankakee, IL: CSL Behring, 2014. [Available at http://labeling.cslbehring.com/PI/US/Kcentra/EN/Kcentra-Prescribing-Information.pdf (accessed March 2, 2017).]

APPENDIX 20-1
Pharmacologic Therapies for Supporting Patient Blood Management* (Continued)

15. Holland L, Warkentin TE, Refaai M, et al. Suboptimal effect of a three-factor prothrombin complex concentrate (Profilnine-SD) in correcting supratherapeutic international normalized ratio due to warfarin overdose. Transfusion 2009;49:1171-7.

16. Siegal DM, Garcia DA, Crowther MA. How I treat target-specific oral anticoagulant-associated bleeding. Blood 2014;123:1153-8.

17. Simpson E, Lin Y, Stanworth S, et al. Recombinant factor VIIa for the prevention and treatment of bleeding in patients without haemophilia. Cochrane Database Syst Rev 2012;(3):CD005011.

18. RiaSTAP, fibrinogen concentrate (human) for intravenous use, lyophilized powder for reconstitution. Package insert. Kankakee, IL: CSL Behring, 2011. [Available at http://labeling.cslbehring.com/PI/US/Ria STAP/EN/RiaSTAP-Prescribing-Information.pdf (accessed March 2, 2017).]

19. Spotnitz WD. Hemostats, sealant, and adhesives: A practical guide for the surgeon. Am Surg 2012;78:1305-21.

20. Esler MD, Douglas JM. Planning for hemorrhage: Steps an anesthesiologist can take to limit and treat hemorrhage in the obstetric patient. Anesthesiol Clin North Am 2003;21:127-44.

21. Shields L, Lagrew D, Lyndon A. Uterotonic medications for prevention and treatment of postpartum hemorrhage. CMQCC obstetric hemorrhage toolkit version 2.0. (March 24, 2015) Stanford, CA: California Maternal Quality Care Collaborative, 2015. [Available at: http://www.cmqcc.org/resources-tool-kits/toolkits/ob-hemorrhage-toolkit (accessed March 2, 2017).]

22. Svensson PJ, Bergqvist PBF, Juul KV, Berntorp E. Desmopressin in treatment of haematological disorders and in prevention of surgical bleeding. Blood Rev 2014;28:95-102.

23. Wademan BH, Galvin SD. Desmopressin for reducing postoperative blood loss and transfusion requirements following cardiac surgery in adults. Interact Cardiovasc Thorac Surg 2014;18:360-70.

24. Gisbert JP, González L, Calvert X, et al. Proton pump inhibitors versus H2-antagonists: A meta-analysis of their efficacy in treating bleeding peptic ulcers. Aliment Pharmacol Ther 2001;15:917-26.

25. Abid S, Jafri W, Hamid S, et al. Terlipressin vs. octreotide in bleeding oesophageal varices as an adjuvant therapy with endoscopic band ligation: A randomized double-blind placebo-controlled trial. Am J Gastroenterol 2009;104:617-23.

● **APPENDIX 20-2**
Responsibilities for Activity Levels 1, 2, and 3 PBM Programs*

Item	Responsibility	Activity Level 1	Activity Level 2	Activity Level 3
1	Evidence of institutional support for the patient blood management program at the hospital administration level.	X	X	X
2	Patient outcomes related to transfusion.	X	X	X
3	Budgeting to the level of care required by the implementation of these *Standards*.	X	X	X
4	Pretransfusion patient testing and evaluation.	X	X	X
5	Patient or case specific assessment of potential blood usage.	X	X	X
6	Ordering of blood, including completion of type and antibody testing before procedure start time with a plan for antibody positive patients.	X	X	X
7	Preprocedure optimization of patient coagulation function including discontinuation of medications and herbal supplements that impair hemostasis.	X	X	X
8	Percentage of blood components wasted by component type (such as RBC, rare unit RBCs, platelets, matched platelets, plasma, AB plasma, cryoprecipitate, and granulocytes) and cause for wastage (misordering, mishandling, not released in a timely manner, outdating in stock, etc).	X	X	X
9	Minimize blood loss due to laboratory testing.	X	X	X
10	Process for managing the blood needs of unidentified patients and resolving their identification.	X	X	X
11	Processes to identify, prior to or upon admission, patients who may refuse transfusion under any circumstances	X	X	X
12	Adverse events and incidents related to transfusion.	X	X	X
13	Evidenced based massive transfusion protocol.	X	X	X
14	Treatment of massive blood loss (massive transfusion).	X	X	X
15	Processes and/or equipment to facilitate rapid decision making with regard to anemia and coagulation management.	X	X	N/A
16	Plan by each service line to reduce perioperative blood loss.	X	X	N/A
17	Strategies to reduce blood loss and manage anemia and coagulopathy in nonoperative patients.	X	X	N/A

(Continued)

● **APPENDIX 20-2**

Responsibilities for Activity Levels 1, 2, and 3 PBM Programs* (Continued)

Item	Responsibility	Activity Level 1	Activity Level 2	Activity Level 3
18	Formal program to care for patients who decline use of blood or blood-derived products.	X	N/A	N/A
19	Identification and management of presurgical anemia before elective procedures for which type and screen or type and crossmatch is recommended.	X	N/A	N/A
20	Use of perioperative techniques consistent with current AABB *Standards for Perioperative Autologous Blood Collection and Administration.*	X	N/A	N/A
21	Active program with evidence-based metrics and clinician feedback to ensure compliance with transfusion guidelines.	X	N/A	N/A

Frey K, ed. Standards for a patient blood management program. 2nd ed. Bethesda, MD: AABB, 2017:2-4.

Approaches to Blood Utilization Auditing

● ● ●

Irina Maramica, MD, PhD, MBA, and Ira A. Shulman, MD

BLOOD TRANSFUSIONS ARE among the most common procedures performed in hospitals in the United States, but are also associated with significant risk for the patients. With millions of units of blood components transfused annually, quality organizations have focused on appropriate blood management as an area of opportunity to improve clinical outcomes through evidence-based standardization. Transfusion of blood components is also identified as one of the most overused therapeutic interventions performed during patient hospitalizations.[1-4] Several clinical trials provide evidence that patient outcomes associated with a restrictive transfusion strategy are similar, if not better, than patient outcomes associated with more liberal transfusion strategies.[5-7] Specifically, patients receiving fewer transfusions have a shorter length of stay, a lower incidence of infection, and lower readmission rates for postoperative complications.[8-10] With a growing evidence base linking transfusions with adverse clinical outcomes, a significant proportion of transfusions may be unwarranted.[11-13] In addi-

tion, the optimal use of blood components means not only avoiding overtransfusion or inappropriate transfusions but also making better transfusion decisions that would avoid undertransfusion.

To curtail inappropriate transfusions, several accreditation agencies have endorsed patient blood management (PBM) programs, which are based on multidisciplinary approaches to optimize safety and outcomes in patients who are candidates for transfusion. By integrating evidence-based steps to reduce the probability of transfusions, PBM programs can reduce health-care costs while ensuring that blood components are available for patients who need them.[14] However, successful implementation of a comprehensive PBM program requires the support of administrative and clinical leadership, who can remove obstacles to achieving interdepartmental consensus regarding existing gaps and goals of the program. This support is best achieved by developing a clear business case and enlisting clinical champions to highlight patient care benefits of the program. Central to this effort is

Ira A. Shulman, MD, Director, USC Transfusion Medicine Services Group, Department of Pathology, University of Southern California, Los Angeles, California; and Irina Maramica, MD, PhD, MBA, Medical Director, Transfusion Medicine, Department of Pathology and Laboratory Medicine, University of California Irvine Health, Orange, California

The authors have disclosed no conflicts of interest.

the ability to audit transfusion practices and demonstrate measurable improvements in blood component utilization.[15] Furthermore, hospitals are required by accrediting agencies, such as The Joint Commission and AABB, to have blood utilization audit programs that monitor transfusions of all types of blood components.

THE AUDITING PROCESS

Hospitals are allowed flexibility in designing the scope of the audit process; however, to satisfy this requirement, the review must be based on objective guidelines for assessing blood utilization and transfusion effectiveness. Institutional transfusion committees can provide oversight of PBM programs and take the first step in the development of the blood utilization review process by developing or adopting evidence-based guidelines for blood component use. This committee can also create auditing criteria for detecting outliers and targeting those practices requiring further evaluation. Audit criteria are designed to flag potentially inappropriate or questionable transfusion decisions. Such criteria are often institution-specific and commonly differ from clinical transfusion guidelines. The 2013 AABB Blood Collection, Utilization, and Patient Blood Management Survey reports that transfusion guidelines were used by 78.2% of reporting hospitals.[16] Of the hospitals using transfusion guidelines, 89.5% used one or more national guidelines, with most hospitals using guidelines from AABB (76.4%) and the College of American Pathologists (29.2%). Other sources included the American Society of Anesthesiologists, American Red Cross, Food and Drug Administration, National Institutes of Health, The Joint Commission, New York State Department of Health, internal transfusion committees, and/or multiple sources of evidence-based practice literature.[16]

Monitoring of blood component ordering, transfusion, return, and wastage provides data for assessing an institution's transfusion efficiency.[17,18] Data must be collected, tabulated, and analyzed at regular, specified times. Blood utilization review ideally should be per-

formed for all services that use blood, but the greatest impact of such a review is likely to be seen when auditing clinical services with high transfusion volumes (eg, surgery) and/or providing transfusion support to high-risk patients (eg, trauma victims, liver transplant recipients). Metrics reflecting the ordering and transfusion of all types of blood components used within the institution should form the basis for review of blood utilization. Data analysis should include trends in blood use throughout the institution, by department, by patient population, by protocol (eg, massive transfusion protocol), and by physician.

Data sources include electronic patient records, transfusion service records, and reports from the blood supplier(s). Clerical staff from the hospital's quality assurance department can be trained to process transfusion data and generate reports. Alternatively, with the help of the information systems department, hospitals can develop a blood transfusion dashboard to capture specific trends in transfusion practices and allow benchmarking with less effort and cost. These data should be further analyzed by members of the transfusion committee for inappropriate trends, with the goal of identifying areas for improvement. Processes that may benefit from monitoring by the transfusion committee include the appropriateness of blood component ordering, specific quality indicators related to handling and dispensing blood components in both blood banks and satellite blood storage areas (including storage in or near the operating rooms), steps in blood component administration, and adverse events related to transfusions.[18,19] Metrics should also monitor undertransfusion of patients.[20] Hospital-based transfusion safety officers (TSOs) are utilized by some institutions. The TSO is a key person who supports the PBM program outside the laboratory through education, active surveillance of transfusion practices, and blood utilization review.[21]

In 2011, The Joint Commission published a performance measure set for PBM that focuses on transfusion appropriateness and clinical decision-making regarding blood component transfusion, as well as optimization of patient clinical status to reduce blood transfusion requirements.[22] Hospitals are encouraged to perform objective gap-analysis of The Joint Commission PBM measures and identify areas for improvements.[23] More recently, AABB and The Joint Commission started offering a joint PBM certification program that is based on the AABB *Standards for a Patient Blood Management Program*.[24,25] Certified programs are required to obtain and review at least quarterly (unless noted) the data summarized in Table 21-1.

In addition to any combined programs between AABB and The Joint Commission, institutions may adopt one or more of the following specific quality improvement objectives under the rubric of blood component stewardship:

- Promote reduced wastage of blood components that have been dispensed to the patient care area.

TABLE 21-1. Review Items Required by AABB and The Joint Commission for the PBM Certification Program

Data Review*
• Blood component use
• Blood component wastage and outdate
• Crossmatch/transfusion (C/T) ratio
• Deviation from transfusion practices and protocols
• Transfusion reactions
• Intraoperative blood recovery use and quality control
• Informed consent for blood transfusion documentation
• Massive transfusion protocol effectiveness
• Blood infusion equipment and warmers maintenance program (annually)
• External assessment results (biannually)

*Quarterly except as noted.

- Promote reduced wastage of blood components that are in the hospital inventory but never dispensed.
- Identify, develop, and promote implementation of PBM to improve appropriate use of blood and blood components by health providers.
- Improve clinical outcomes and reduce adverse events from transfusion.

TYPES OF BLOOD UTILIZATION REVIEW

AABB guidelines describe three methods of blood utilization review, which can be used individually or in combination depending on the institution's needs: prospective, concurrent, and retrospective.[18] Each method has advantages and shortcomings, which are summarized in Table 21-2.[26]

Prospective Review

Prospective review of individual blood component orders occurs in real time, before the component is distributed from the blood bank and immediately before transfusion. This proactive approach to blood utilization review provides an opportunity to intercept unnecessary transfusion and modify both component selection, as appropriate, and timing of administration. In academic institutions, prospective review is often performed by clinical pathology residents under the supervision of a transfusion medicine physician. It requires vigilance by the blood bank staff to bring to the attention of residents all orders for blood components that fall outside established transfusion guidelines. Ideally, this review incorporates both laboratory values and clinical data obtained from patient records and/or direct communication with the clinical team. Prospective review improves patient care and saves blood components but is labor-intensive and can cause delays in situations requiring urgent transfusion support. Furthermore, increasing use of point-of-care testing in operating rooms allows clinicians to make real-time transfusion decisions based on results that are usually not available to transfusion services at

TABLE 21-2. Types of Blood Utilization Review

Type of Review	Temporal Relation to Transfusion Event	Reviewer	Advantage	Disadvantage
Prospective	Real-time	● Residents ● Medical director ● Blood bank staff ● CPOE	● Proactive ● Improves patient care and saves blood in real time	● Labor-intensive ● Potential to cause delays in issuing blood
Concurrent	Within 12-24 hours	● Residents ● TSO	● Consultative opportunity ● Training tool for residents	● Labor-intensive ● Ineffective if no MD involvement
Retrospective internal	Days to weeks	● Quality assurance personnel ● Medical director ● Clinical peers	● Easiest approach ● Provides data for trending and benchmarking	● Nonstandardized review ● Difficult to use data for direct physician comparison
Retrospective external	Days to weeks	Network of trained peer reviewers	● Objective, thorough, and standard-ized review ● Produces directly comparable data	● Up-front expense that can be offset by savings in reduced blood usage

CPOE = computerized provider (physician) order entry; TSO = transfusion safety officer; MD = physician.

the time of request for blood components. Because of these considerations, most hospitals exempt the emergency department, labor and delivery departments, and operating rooms from prospective review.

Examples of orders subject to prospective reviews include the following: requests for multiple doses of platelets without checking posttransfusion platelet counts in patients without acute hemorrhage, orders of inadequate doses of plasma components or cryoprecipitate, and orders for cytomegalovirus (CMV)-negative or irradiated components. In case of a disagreement between the ordering and reviewing physicians about the appropriateness of a blood order, the usual practice is to defer to the ordering physician, as they are more familiar with the patient's clinical condition, as long as transfusion of the requested component does not have the potential for an immediate adverse effect on the patient. However, questionable blood component requests such as these may be subsequently referred to the transfusion committee for further review. Sometimes, the transfusion service physician may request additional testing to be performed before subsequent transfusions (eg, CMV testing for requests for CMV-negative blood).

Concurrent Review

The concurrent review process involves review of transfusions administered within the previous 12 to 24 hours, thus avoiding the risk of delaying patient care. This allows the reviewer to judge the appropriateness of blood component use based on all pertinent laboratory and clinical data. If the transfusion episode appears to be out of line with good clinical practice, the review leads to an interaction with the transfusing clinician, who is still likely to remember events surrounding the transfusion. Concurrent review is a consultative opportunity, and the consultant should not be perceived as a gatekeeper. Rather, if properly conducted, this interaction can promote cooperative relationships between the transfusion service and medical staff, and influence transfusion practices.[27] Furthermore, performing these audits

in academic institutions represents an excellent training tool for clinical pathology residents. Residents should be encouraged to document these reviews, evaluate them for efficacy, and present them in an educational format to other residents.

An example of concurrent review that can result in consultative opportunity is daily review of platelet transfusions along with pre- and posttransfusion platelet counts. In their audits of transfusion events that fall outside audit criteria, residents should evaluate patient records for the presence of bleeding, deficiencies in platelet function, and the presence of medications known to affect platelet number or function. This review allows the identification of not only patients who may be receiving platelets outside of transfusion guidelines but also those who might be refractory.[28] Similarly, residents can perform plasma audits from daily reports that include pre- and posttransfusion prothrombin time/international normalized ratio (PT/INR) and activated partial thromboplastin time (aPTT) levels, using evidence-based guidelines for plasma transfusion and evaluating additional information, such as the degree of abnormal result correction by plasma transfusion and the presence of drugs that may interfere with the coagulation system.[18,29,30] For example, cryoprecipitate audits can be based on fibrinogen levels, presence of bleeding, or Factor XIII deficiency.[26] In the aforementioned 2013 AABB survey, questions were added to evaluate policies for using hemoglobin, platelet, PT/INR, aPTT, and fibrinogen thresholds for determining when to transfuse components.[16]

However, in nonacademic institutions, if there is no TSO, concurrent review might be too labor-intensive for the blood bank staff and allow only for review based on laboratory transfusion thresholds without the ability to evaluate the patient's clinical condition. Moreover, concurrent review is effective only when the transfusion service physician or TSO is directly involved, resulting in a significant reduction in transfusions.[27,31-33] In contrast, concurrent review without physician involvement has failed to reduce blood usage.[34]

Retrospective Review

Retrospective review can be performed by those internal to, or external to, the organization. Such reviews are performed days to weeks following the transfusion event, usually at specified time intervals, using preset audit criteria that might differ from transfusion guidelines.

Internal Retrospective Review

Quality assurance personnel can perform the initial review. Cases that fall outside audit criteria can be referred to a transfusion medicine physician or a clinical peer of the physician whose transfusion decision is under review; this allows closer evaluation to determine whether the patient's clinical condition justified the component request. This is the easiest approach to utilization review, providing valuable information about overall institutional transfusion practices and data for trending and benchmarking. However, one limitation of internal retrospective review is that patient data are often generated in a nonstandardized and inconsistent manner; thus, direct comparison of care provided by any two physicians can be difficult.

External Retrospective Review

This process uses an external third party that provides a network of trained physicians to serve as peer reviewers. Patient charts and transfusion decisions are evaluated using objective criteria in a thorough, critical, and standardized way, to produce directly comparable data. To be successful, it must allow review of all medical records, including all forms of paper and electronic data, and not require additional work on the part of the hospitals. Because a network of trained physicians provides anonymous review of colleagues whose identity is blinded to the reviewers, the reviews are less likely to be biased; physicians often find it challenging to perform unbiased critical reviews of colleagues with whom they have social, economic, and political relationships.

Although retrospective reviews cannot change blood component usage in real time,

or effectively involve transfusing clinicians in the review process, they are excellent models of peer review.[26,27] They provide opportunities to mentor physicians on proper transfusion practices, such as correction of anemia, blood loss control, iron supplementation, evaluation of vital sign monitoring, and avoiding 2-unit transfusions without checking the response.[35] One effective indicator for retrospective monitoring of transfusion appropriateness is the transfused patient's discharge hemoglobin value.[36] Furthermore, if trends are identified in certain departments indicating frequent transfusion outside of transfusion guidelines, letters can be sent to clinicians and department heads, and representatives can be invited to transfusion committee meetings.

BLOOD UTILIZATION REVIEW OF TRANSFUSIONS TO HIGH-RISK PATIENTS

Uncontrolled hemorrhage requiring massive transfusion in patients with trauma or postpartum hemorrhage remains one of the leading causes of preventable death. It is now recognized that severe trauma-induced coagulopathy increases morbidity and mortality in these patients and that early, aggressive, and ratio-based blood component resuscitation provides improved outcomes.[30] This is best achieved by protocol-driven care, now recommended by the National Partnership for Maternal Safety, National Institute for Health and Care Excellence policy, and Trauma Quality Improvement Program guidelines.[37,38] Development of massive transfusion protocols that include point-of-care testing and hemostatic resuscitation require careful planning and cooperation between various clinical teams, including surgery, anesthesia, and transfusion medicine. Review of transfusions is especially important in this high-risk patient population, as it offers an opportunity for continuous improvement of both the protocol and the delivery of care by the multidisciplinary team. Such reviews can yield important results as measured by improved patient outcomes and improved blood utilization. Because of the acuity of transfusion requirements, performing prospective review of massive transfusions in real time can lead to delays in patient care and is often not feasible. This review is best achieved by concurrent or retrospective review of data on massive transfusion protocol availability, criteria for activation, timeliness of provision of components, and protocol effectiveness.[25,37,38]

THE ROLE OF A COMPUTERIZED PROVIDER ORDER ENTRY SYSTEM IN BLOOD UTILIZATION REVIEW

Application of health-care information technology (IT) to transfusion medicine provides PBM programs with new tools for blood utilization review and for influencing physician ordering practices. Blood component order entry screens incorporate clinical guidelines designed to guide physicians regarding the appropriateness of component ordering.[39] Implementation of computerized provider order entry (CPOE) allows creation of electronic reports that can be used for order auditing, assessment of blood utilization, and compliance monitoring.[5] In the 2013 AABB survey, 77.5% of institutions with transfusion guidelines incorporated them into paper or electronic order sets. Sixty-five percent reported that their CPOE system included transfusion guidelines. Of these, approximately half had guidelines with "hard stops," where the physician/provider must select a transfusion rationale before the order is accepted. Only 45.9% of these CPOE systems included an algorithm or clinical decision support to warn or alert the physician/provider if they are ordering a blood component outside of guidelines. Most reporting hospitals (71.9%) required that a physician document the reason or clinical justification for transfusion in the medical record based on guidelines developed by the hospital transfusion or quality committee.[16]

In some hospitals, guidelines incorporated into the CPOE system do not result in hard stops, but rather, the indication for a blood component order is captured electronically and stored for later review. If the most recent laboratory value does not match the indication, an automatic message is provided to the clinician, requesting an indication for the "override." Component orders with overrides are collated electronically with other relevant information and are reviewed by transfusion committee members.[26]

CPOE alone does not always improve blood use if only laboratory parameters are used for determining transfusion appropriateness, or if clinical users record inaccurate reasons for transfusion. Therefore, retrospective review remains important, even with CPOE, to evaluate transfusion appropriateness by reviewing clinical information. Additional functionality is achieved by incorporating a clinical decision support system (CDSS) into CPOE to guide transfusion ordering by providing clinicians with tailored treatment recommendations based on individual laboratory and clinical information, along with local transfusion guidelines.[1,40,41] For example, based on the clinical reason for transfusion selected by the clinician from a menu of choices, and the most recent laboratory values, the system could provide adaptive alerts, allowing the clinician to modify orders that do not fall within guidelines. This system is particularly useful if it requires physicians to enter the reason for overriding the system's recommendation. Subsequent analysis of reports, with reasons for override, can be used to audit individual physician ordering practices. Systematic reviews of the impact of an electronic CDSS found that it is a useful educational tool, and its implementation improves RBC usage, increases provider compliance with guidelines, and results in cost savings.[41-43] Additional studies are needed to assess the effectiveness of the CDSS on ordering practices for other components and patient outcomes.[42,44]

USE OF "BIG DATA" TO ASSESS PERFORMANCE AND PROGRESS MEASURES IN TRANSFUSION MEDICINE

The advent of electronic health records (EHR) is opening up the field of "big data" in health care. Data collection and data mining through linkage of different data sets within the EHR can provide a plethora of information, which can drive improvements in patient outcomes.[44,45] Examples of using big data in transfusion medicine are described below.

Benchmarking

Comparisons of blood usage between institutions and/or countries, performed with the aim of identifying best practices in transfusion medicine, were recently introduced.[46] Major challenges in developing meaningful benchmarking processes include defining best practices and developing cost-effective data collection methods. Often, hospitals do not have adequate IT support to develop data mining tools that enable transfusion services to collect uniform data across different hospitals. In the 2013 AABB survey, 41.9% of responding hospitals participated in performance benchmarking programs relating to transfusion medicine.[16]

Implementing benchmarking principles in transfusion medicine has improved practices on individual and organizational levels. Benchmarking can identify existing gaps that can become PBM program improvement targets and represents an instrument of learning, as it relies on communication, collaboration, and sharing of experiences. Benchmarking can identify opportunities for savings in presentations to hospital leadership. Furthermore, after implementation of new practices, performance should be reevaluated, preferably by continuous data collection.

Benchmarking data can come from various sources, including medical record reviews, third-party gap assessments, blood bank inventory management, financial systems (eg, patient billing and budget), patient morbidity and mortality data, and observa-

tions or supportive statements from key stakeholders.[14] Several benchmarking databases exist that allow comparisons of PBM metrics with member hospitals nationwide or with other similarly sized hospitals.[47] Commonly used metrics are summarized in Table 21-3.

In the AABB survey, the two most common metrics used by institutions to measure transfusion rate were the total number of RBCs, platelets, and plasma units transfused (71.5%), and the total number of components transfused (57.3%).[16] Other measures included the percentage of patients transfused per hospital admission; the number of RBC units per patient transfused; transfused RBC units per 100 hospital admissions or discharges, per 1000 patient days, per adjusted patient-days, or per adjusted or case mix index (CMI)-adjusted discharges; transfusions per surgical case; and transfusions per medical/surgical admission. For meaningful comparison of transfusion rates between different institutions, it is important to use metrics that capture transfusions in both inpatient and outpatient settings and account for the institution's CMI (eg, CMI-adjusted discharges).

Three possible models of benchmarking in transfusion medicine have been described by Apelseth et al.[46] The ideal model according to these authors would be a regional benchmarking model, which requires a central coordinator who facilitates communication between institutions and manages the information flow to participants. In a sentinel model, data from a limited number of sites are

TABLE 21-3. PBM Metrics Used for Benchmarking

Metrics
● Overall transfusion rate compared with that of comparably sized hospitals
● Percentage of transfusions that fall outside of hospital or professional transfusion guidelines
● Transfusion administration compliance
● Reviews of wasted blood components
● Budget for transfusion services

collected into a central database, preferably by web-based reporting. This model is less costly and easier to implement and can be applied nationally and internationally. These two models gather information into a centralized database, whereas in a third, institutional model, all data are collected for the institution initiating the benchmarking process. The latter is least likely to succeed, because it requires individual initiative, volunteer collaboration, and resources to be successful. Benchmarking can contribute to evidence-based guidelines, especially when randomized controlled trials may be difficult or costly to perform. Examples of countries that reduced blood utilization using national PBM and benchmarking programs include Finland, Scotland, Spain, the Netherlands, Germany, the United Kingdom, Canada, and Australia.

Active Surveillance of Transfusion-Related Complications

Examples of this type of surveillance include searching large Medicare databases by linking the procedure code for transfusion with diagnostic codes to determine the rate of a recognized complication such as posttransfusion purpura, or using an automated electronic algorithm to detect transfusion-associated circulatory overload or transfusion-related acute lung injury, and linking this to the transfusion episode.[45,48] Transfusion reaction tracking can help identify underrecognition or underreporting of transfusion-related adverse events. Once a problem is identified, education can be developed and implemented to improve staff knowledge and compliance with reporting of adverse events.[14]

Monitoring Patterns of Blood Use by Procedure over Time

Linking transfusion episode data with diagnostic and procedure codes allows monitoring of transfusion rates for specific types of cases (eg, hip replacement, cardiac surgery). These rates can be compared to national data or data in the literature. In the AABB survey, some hospitals reported using the percentage of patients transfused per selected ICD-9 code, or average blood component use per surgical case category (eg, coronary artery bypass graft only or knee/hip replacement).[16]

Definition of Blood Order Schedules

A maximum surgical blood ordering schedule (MSBOS) for surgery can be developed by using data held within the anesthetic electronic management system.[49] Creating a data-driven MSBOS is useful in optimizing transfusion-ordering practices.[50] One metric used for assessing and benchmarking transfusion ordering practices is the crossmatch/transfusion (C/T) ratio, which reflects overordering of blood as compared with actual transfusion.[51] This overordering of high-volume activities, such as unnecessary crossmatches, represents a waste of transfusion service resources. However, it is important to emphasize that the incidence of patients undergoing elective surgery without available crossmatched blood represents one of the main indicators of quality and safety in transfusion medicine.[52]

KEY POINTS

1. Data-driven and multidisciplinary blood utilization auditing is central to establishing successful institutional and national evidence-based PBM programs.
2. Optimizing blood transfusions requires comprehensive review not only of transfusion appropriateness but also of processes for ensuring patient safety, best patient outcomes, and blood component stewardship.
3. Transfusion auditing can be performed as a prospective, concurrent, or retrospective review. Retrospective reviews may use either internal or external resources.
4. Different metrics have evolved over time to assess various aspects of transfusions and allow benchmarking of transfusion practices at different levels.

5. Various national organizations have developed educational resources and campaigns to promote wise use of blood components. AABB and The Joint Commission, for example, have joined forces to produce a PBM certification program. These tools enable physicians to eliminate unnecessary blood transfusions and optimize transfusions in high-risk patients while reducing health-care costs and improving patient outcomes.

REFERENCES

1. Goodnough LT, Shah N. The next chapter in patient blood management: Real-time clinical decision support. Am J Clin Pathol 2014;142: 741-7.

2. Morton J, Anastassopoulos KP, Patel ST, et al. Frequency and outcomes of blood products transfusion across procedures and clinical conditions warranting inpatient care: An analysis of the 2004 healthcare cost and utilization project nationwide inpatient sample database. Am J Med Qual 2010;25:289-96.

3. Ferraris VA, Davenport DL, Saha SP, et al. Surgical outcomes and transfusion of minimal amounts of blood in the operating room. Arch Surg 2012;147:49-55.

4. Carson JL, Carless PA, Hébert PC. Outcomes using lower vs higher hemoglobin thresholds for red blood cell transfusion. JAMA 2013;309: 83-4.

5. Goodnough LT, Shah N. Is there a "magic" hemoglobin number? Clinical decision support promoting restrictive blood transfusion practices. Am J Hematol 2015;90:927-33.

6. Hébert PC, Wells G, Blajchman MA, et al. A multicenter, randomized, controlled clinical trial of transfusion requirements in critical care. Transfusion requirements in critical care investigators, Canadian Critical Care Trials Group. N Engl J Med 1999;340:409-17.

7. Carson JL, Brooks MM, Abbott JD, et al. Liberal or restrictive transfusion in high-risk patients after hip surgery. N Engl J Med 2011;365:2453-62.

8. Salpeter SR, Buckley JS, Chatterjee S. Impact of more restrictive blood transfusion strategies on clinical outcomes: A meta-analysis and systematic review. Am J Med 2014;127:124-31.

9. Goodnough LT, Maggio P, Hadhazy E, et al. Restrictive blood transfusion practices are associated with improved patient outcomes. Transfusion 2014;54(Pt 2):2753-9.

10. Rohde JM, Dimcheff DE, Blumberg N, et al. Health care-associated infection after red blood cell transfusion: A systematic review and meta-analysis. JAMA 2014;311:1317-26.

11. Goodnough LT, Verbrugge D, Vizmeg K, Riddell J. Identifying elective orthopedic surgical patients transfused with amounts of blood in excess of need: The transfusion trigger revisited. Transfusion 1992;32:648-53.

12. Shander A, Fink A, Javidroozi M, et al. Appropriateness of allogeneic red blood cell transfusion: The international consensus conference on transfusion outcomes. Transfus Med Rev 2011;25:232-46.

13. Spahn DR, Shander A, Hofmann A. The chiasm: Transfusion practice versus patient blood management. Best Pract Res Clin Anaesthesiol 2013;27:37-42.

14. Building a better patient blood management program: Identifying tools, solving problems and promoting patient safety (white paper). Bethesda, MD: AABB, 2015. [Available at http://www.aabb.org/pbm/Documents/AABB-PBM-Whitepaper.pdf (accessed February 7, 2017).]

15. Murphy MF, Yazer MH. Measuring and monitoring blood utilization. Transfusion 2013;53: 3025-8.

16. Whitaker BI, Rajbhandary S, Harris A. The 2013 AABB blood collection, utilization, and patient blood management survey report. Bethesda, MD: AABB, 2015. [Available at http://www.aabb.org/research/hemovigilance/bloodsurvey/Pages/default.aspx (accessed February 7, 2017).]

17. Wagner J, AuBuchon JP, Saxena S, Shulman IA, for the Clinical Transfusion Medicine Committee. Guidelines for the quality assessment of transfusion. Bethesda, MD: AABB, 2006.

18. Becker J, Shaz B, for the Clinical Transfusion Medicine Committee and the Transfusion Medicine Section Coordinating Committee. Guidelines for patient blood management and blood utilization. Bethesda, MD: AABB, 2011.

19. Saxena S, ed. The transfusion committee: Putting patient safety first. 2nd ed. Bethesda, MD: AABB Press, 2013.

20. Mair B, Agosti SJ, Foulis PR, et al. Monitoring for undertransfusion. Transfusion 1996;36: 533-35.

21. Dunbar NM, Szczepiorkowski ZM. How do we utilize a transfusion safety officer? Transfusion 2015;55:2064-8.

22. Patient blood management performance measures project - 2011. Oakbrook Terrace, IL: The Joint Commission, 2016. [Available at http://www.jointcommission.org/patient_blood_management_performance_measures_project/ (accessed February 7, 2017).]

23. De Leon EM, Szallasi A. "Transfusion indication RBC (PBM-02)": Gap analysis of a Joint Commission Patient Blood Management Performance Measure at a community hospital. Blood Transfus 2014;12(Suppl 1):187-90.

24. Holcomb J, ed. Standards for a patient blood management program. Bethesda, MD: AABB, 2014.

25. AABB, The Joint Commission. Patient blood management certification review process guide for health care organizations 2017. Oakbrook Terrace, IL: The Joint Commission, 2017. [Available at https://www.jointcommission.org/assets/1/18/2017_PBM_Org_ RPG.pdf (accessed April 4, 2017).]

26. Haspel RL, Uhl L. How do I audit hospital blood product utilization? Transfusion 2012; 52:227-30.

27. Toy P, Eberhard F. Blood utilization review. In: Saxena S, Shulman IA, eds. The transfusion committee: Putting patient safety first. 1st ed. Bethesda, MD: AABB, 2006.

28. Kaufman RM, Djulbegovic B, Gernsheimer T, et al. Platelet transfusion: A clinical practice guideline from the AABB. Ann Intern Med 2015;162:205-13.

29. Roback JD, Caldwell S, Carson J, et al. Evidence-based practice guidelines for plasma transfusion. Transfusion 2010;50:1227-39.

30. Murad MH, Slubbs JR, Gandhi MJ, et al. The effect of plasma transfusion on morbidity and mortality: A systematic review and meta-analysis. Transfusion 2010;50:1370-83.

31. Silver H, Tahha HR, Anderson J, et al. A non-computer-dependent prospective review of blood and blood component utilization. Transfusion 1992;32:260-5.

32. Simpson MB. Prospective-concurrent audits and medical consultation for platelet transfusions. Transfusion 1987;27:192-5.

33. Hawkins TE, Carter JM, Hunter PM. Can mandatory pretransfusion approval programmes be improved? Transfus Med 1994;4:45-50.

34. Lam HT, Schweitzer SO, Petz L, et al. Effectiveness of a prospective physician self-audit transfusion-monitoring system. Transfusion 1997;37:577-84.

35. Paone G, Brewer R, Likosky DS, et al. Transfusion rate as a quality metric: Is blood conservation a learnable skill? Ann Thorac Surg 2013;96:1279-86.

36. Edwards J, Morrison C, Mohluddin M, et al. Patient blood transfusion management: Discharge hemoglobin level as a surrogate marker for red blood cell utilization appropriateness. Transfusion 2012;52:2445-51.

37. Stephens CT, Gumbert S, Holcomb JB. Trauma-associated bleeding: Management of massive transfusion. Curr Opin Anaesthesiol 2016;29:250-5.

38. Kacmar RM, Mhyre JM, Scavone BM, et al. The use of postpartum hemorrhage protocols in United States academic obstetric anesthesia units. Anesth Analg 2014;119:906-10.

39. Dzik S. Use of a computer-assisted system for blood utilization review. Transfusion 2007;47(2 Suppl):142S-4S.

40. Goodnough LT, Shieh L, Hadhazy E, et al. Improved blood utilization using real-time clinical decision support. Transfusion 2014;54:1358-65.

41. Rothschild JM, McGurk S, Honour M, et al. Assessment of education and computerized decision support interventions for improving transfusion practice. Transfusion 2007;47:228-39.

42. Hibbs SP, Nielsen ND, Brunskill S, et al. The impact of electronic decision support on transfusion practice: A systematic review. Transfus Med Rev 2015;29:14-23.

43. Cohn CS, Welbig J, Bowman R, et al. A data-driven approach to patient blood management. Transfusion 2014;54:316-22.

44. Dunbar NM, Szczepiorkowski ZM. Hardwiring patient blood management: Harnessing information technology to optimize transfusion practice. Curr Opin Hematol 2014;21:515-20.

45. Pendry K. The use of big data in transfusion medicine. Transfus Med 2015;25:129-37.

46. Apelseth TO, Molnar L, Arnold E, Heddle NM. Benchmarking: Applications to transfusion medicine. Transfus Med Rev 2012;26:321-32.

47. Carson JL, Guyatt G, Heddle NM, et al. Clinical practice guidelines from the AABB: Red blood cell transfusion thresholds and storage. JAMA 2016;316:2025-35.

48. Clifford L, Singh A, Wilson GA, Toy P. Electronic health record surveillance algorithms facilitate the detection of transfusion-related

pulmonary complications. Transfusion 2013;53: 1205-16.

49. Frank SM, Rothschild JA, Masear CG, Rivers RJ. Optimizing preoperative blood ordering with data acquired from an anesthesia information management system. Anesthesiology 2013; 118:1286-97.

50. Cheng CK, Trethewey D, Brousseau P, Sadek I. Creation of a maximum surgical blood order-ing schedule via novel low-overhead database method. Transfusion 2008;48:2268-9.

51. Dexter F, Ledolter J, Davis E, Witkowski TA. Systematic criteria for type and screen based on procedure's probability of erythrocyte transfusion. Anesthesiology 2012;116:768-78.

52. Goodnough LT. Operational, quality, and risk management in the transfusion service: Lessons learned. Transfus Med Rev 2012;26:252-61.

Chapter 22

Noninfectious Complications of Blood Transfusion

• ● •

William J. Savage, MD, PhD, and Eldad A. Hod, MD

STATISTICALLY, THE GREATEST risk of morbidity and mortality from transfusion is from the noninfectious complications of blood transfusion. In fact, transfusion-related acute lung injury (TRALI), hemolytic transfusion reactions (HTRs), and transfusion-associated circulatory overload (TACO) are the three most commonly reported causes of transfusion-related mortality.[1]

HEMOVIGILANCE

Hemovigilance involves the collection of information on the complications of transfusion, analysis of these data, and subsequent data-driven improvements in transfusion practices. One of the main purposes of developing a hemovigilance program is to improve reporting of transfusion-related adverse events. It is widely believed that the major noninfectious complications of transfusion are both under-recognized and underreported.

The National Healthcare Safety Network Hemovigilance Module was created through a collaboration between government and non-

government organizations to implement a national surveillance of transfusion-associated adverse events aimed at improving patient safety. Definitions and classification schemes are detailed in the appendices of the Hemovigilance Module Surveillance Protocol.[2] (See Chapter 4.)

RECOGNITION AND EVALUATION OF A SUSPECTED TRANSFUSION REACTION

Identification of a Transfusion Reaction

As with many medical therapies, adverse effects of transfusion usually cannot be accurately predicted or the risks completely avoided. Transfusing clinicians should be aware of such risks when discussing the need for transfusion with a patient. Informed consent for transfusion may include a discussion of the risks of infectious disease and serious noninfectious complications, such as TRALI and

William J. Savage, MD, PhD, Associate Medical Director, Department of Pathology, Brigham and Women's Hospital, Boston, Massachusetts; and Eldad A. Hod, MD, Associate Professor, Department of Pathology and Cell Biology, Columbia University Medical Center, New York, New York
W. Savage has disclosed a financial relationship with Fresenius Kabi and Momenta Pharmaceuticals. E. Hod has disclosed no conflicts of interest.

HTRs. Furthermore, medical staff administering blood components should be well aware of the signs and symptoms of possible reactions. Staff should be prepared to mitigate any immediate episodes and prevent future similar reactions when possible.

Many common clinical signs and symptoms are associated with more than one type of adverse reaction. (See Table 22-1.) Early recognition, prompt cessation of the transfusion, and further evaluation are key to a successful outcome. The signs and symptoms that may be indicators of a transfusion reaction include the following:

- Fever, generally defined as a ≥1 C rise in temperature to ≥38 C (the most common sign of an acute HTR).
- Chills with or without rigors.
- Respiratory distress, including wheezing, coughing, hypoxia, and dyspnea.
- Hyper- or hypotension.
- Abdominal, chest, flank, or back pain.
- Pain at the infusion site.
- Skin manifestations, including rash, flushing, urticaria, pruritus, and localized edema.
- Jaundice or hemoglobinuria.
- Nausea/vomiting.
- Abnormal bleeding.
- Oliguria/anuria.

Clinical Evaluation and Management of a Transfusion Reaction

The evaluation of a suspected transfusion reaction involves a two-pronged investigation combining clinical evaluation of the patient with laboratory verification and testing. The clinical team should discontinue the transfusion of the implicated component, and contact the blood bank for directions on the investigation. When an acute transfusion reaction is suspected, several steps must be taken immediately (below).

Patient-Focused Steps

1. Stop the transfusion immediately but keep the line open with normal saline.

2. Document the clerical recheck between the patient and the component. The labels on the component, on patient records, and on patient identification should be examined for identification errors. Transfusing facilities may require repeat ABO and Rh typing of the patient using a new sample. (See "Standard Laboratory Investigation of a Transfusion Reaction" section below.)

3. Identify the appropriate diagnostic tests to work up the case.

4. Consult the clinical team for a plan of care.

Component-Focused Steps

1. Contact the transfusion service for directions on investigating and documenting the potential causes of the reaction.

2. Obtain instructions concerning the return of any remaining component, associated intravenous fluid bags, and tubing.

3. The transfusion service determines whether the blood donor center should be notified of the acute transfusion reaction. The Food and Drug Administration (FDA) requires reporting to the blood center when the component is at fault for causing the reaction (eg, suspected problem with labeling or manufacturing or suspected bacterial contamination of the component). The FDA must be notified when a complication of transfusion is confirmed to be fatal [Code of Federal Regulations (CFR) Title 21, Part 606.170].

Standard Laboratory Investigation of a Transfusion Reaction

When the laboratory receives notice of a possible transfusion reaction, the technologist should perform several steps:

1. Clerical check of the component bag, label, paperwork, and patient sample.

2. Request for return of any remaining component, associated intravenous fluid bags,

TABLE 22-1. Categories of Adverse Transfusion Reactions and Their Management*

Type	Incidence	Etiology	Presentation	Diagnostic Testing	Therapeutic/Prophylactic Approaches[†]
Acute (<24 hours) Transfusion Reactions—Immunologic					
Hemolytic	ABO/Rh mismatch: 1 in 40,000 AHTR: 1 in 76,000 Fatal HTR: 1 in 1.8 million	Red cell incompatibility	Chills, fever, hemoglobinuria, hypotension, renal failure with oliguria, hemorrhage (DIC), back pain, pain along infusion vein, anxiety	Clerical check DAT Visual inspection (free Hb) Repeat patient ABO, pre- and posttransfusion sample Further tests as indicated to define possible incompatibility Further tests as indicated to detect hemolysis (LDH, bilirubin, etc)	Stop transfusion Keep urine output >1 mL/kg/hr with fluids and IV diuretic Analgesics Pressors for hypotension Hemostatic components (platelets, cryoprecipitate, or plasma) for bleeding
Febrile, nonhemolytic	0.1% to 1% with universal leukocyte reduction	Accumulated cytokines in platelet unit Antibody to donor WBCs	Fever, chills/rigors, headache, vomiting	Rule out hemolysis (DAT, inspect for hemoglobinemia, repeat patient ABO) Rule out bacterial contamination HLA antibody screen	Leukocyte-reduced blood Antipyretic premedication (acetaminophen, no aspirin) Washed cellular components if severe
Urticarial	1:100-1:33 (1%-3%)	Antibody to donor plasma proteins	Urticaria, pruritis, flushing, angioedema	None	Antihistamine In some cases after stopping transfusion, unit may be restarted slowly after antihistamine if symptoms resolve

(Continued)

TABLE 22-1. Categories of Adverse Transfusion Reactions and Their Management* (Continued)

Type	Incidence	Etiology	Presentation	Diagnostic Testing	Therapeutic/Prophylactic Approaches
Anaphylactic	1:20,000-1:50,000	Usually idiopathic and idiosyncratic Rarely, antibody to donor plasma proteins (includes IgA, haptoglobin, C4)	Hypotension, urticaria, angioedema, bronchospasm, stridor, abdominal pain	In appropriate setting, IgA and haptoglobin concentrations, anti-IgA, serum IgE concentrations if passively transfused	Stop transfusion IV fluids Epinephrine (0.5 mg or 0.01 mg/kg) Antihistamines, corticosteroids, beta-2 agonists Modified components (eg, washed RBCs and platelets, SD plasma, IgA-deficient blood components if indicated)
TRALI	1:1200-1:190,000	WBC antibodies in donor (occasionally in recipient), other WBC-activating agents in components	Hypoxemia, respiratory failure, hypotension, fever, bilateral pulmonary edema	Rule out hemolysis (DAT, inspect for hemoglobinemia, repeat patient ABO) Rule out cardiogenic pulmonary edema HLA, HNA typing Anti-HLA, anti-HNA antibody screening Chest x-ray	Supportive care until recovery Deferral of implicated donors

Acute (<24 hours) Transfusion Reactions—Nonimmunologic

Transfusion-associated sepsis	Varies by component (see "Infectious Disease Screening, Chapter 7," for discussion of platelets)	Bacterial contamination	Fever, chills, hypotension	Gram stain Culture of component Patient culture Rule out hemolysis (DAT, inspect for hemoglobinemia, repeat patient ABO)	Broad-spectrum antibiotics
Hypotension associated with ACE inhibition	Dependent on clinical setting	Inhibited metabolism of bradykinin with infusion of bradykinin (negatively charged filters) or activators of prekallikrein	Flushing, hypotension	Rule out hemolysis (DAT, inspect for hemoglobinemia, repeat patient ABO)	Withdraw ACE inhibition Avoid albumin volume replacement for plasmapheresis Avoid bedside leukocyte filtration
Circulatory overload	1%	Volume overload	Dyspnea, orthopnea, cough, tachycardia, hypertension, headache	Chest x-ray Rule out TRALI	Upright posture Oxygen IV diuretic Phlebotomy (250-mL increments)
Nonimmune hemolysis	Rare	Physical or chemical destruction of blood (heating, freezing, hemolytic drug or solution added to blood)	Hemoglobinuria, hemoglobinemia	Rule out patient hemolysis (DAT, inspect for hemoglobinemia, repeat patient ABO) Test unit for hemolysis	Identify and eliminate cause if related to blood administration
Air embolus	Rare	Air infusion via line	Sudden shortness of breath, acute cyanosis, pain, cough, hypotension, cardiac arrhythmia	X-ray for intravascular air	Place patient on left side with legs elevated above chest and head

(Continued)

TABLE 22-1. Categories of Adverse Transfusion Reactions and Their Management* (Continued)

Type	Incidence	Etiology	Presentation	Diagnostic Testing	Therapeutic/Prophylactic Approach
Hypocalcemia (ionized calcium; citrate toxicity)	Dependent on clinical setting	Rapid citrate infusion (massive transfusion of citrated blood, delayed metabolism of citrate, apheresis procedures)	Paresthesia, tetany, arrhythmia	Ionized calcium Prolonged Q-T interval on electrocardiogram	Pause/reduce transfusion rate Calcium supplementation
Hypothermia	Dependent on clinical setting	Rapid infusion of cold blood	Cardiac arrhythmia	Central body temperature	Employ blood warmer
Delayed (>24 hours) Transfusion Reactions—Immunologic					
Alloimmunization, red cell antigens	1:100 (1%)	Immune response to foreign antigens on red cells	Positive blood group antibody screening test, delayed serologic or hemolytic transfusion reaction, hemolytic disease of the newborn (maternal alloimmunization)	Antibody screen DAT	Avoid unnecessary transfusions
Alloimmunization, HLA antigens	1:10 (10%)	WBCs and platelets (HLA)	Platelet refractoriness	Platelet antibody screen HLA antibody screen	Avoid unnecessary transfusions Leukocyte-reduced blood
Hemolytic	1:2500-11,000	Anamnestic immune response to red cell antigens	Fever, decreasing hemoglobin, new positive antibody screening test, mild jaundice	Antibody screen DAT Tests for hemolysis (visual inspection for hemoglobinemia, LDH, bilirubin, urinary hemosiderin as clinically indicated)	Identify antibody Transfuse compatible RBCs as needed

Graft-vs-host disease	Rare	Donor lymphocytes engraft in recipient and mount attack on host tissues	Erythroderma, vomiting, diarrhea, hepatitis, pancytopenia, fever	Skin biopsy, HLA typing, Molecular analysis for chimerism	Immunosuppression, Irradiation of blood components for patients at risk (including components from related donors and HLA-selected components)
Posttransfusion purpura	Rare	Recipient platelet antibodies (apparent alloantibody, usually anti-HPA-1a) destroy autologous platelets	Thrombocytopenic purpura, bleeding 8-10 days after transfusion	Platelet antibody screen and identification	IVIG, HPA-1a-negative platelets, Plasmapheresis
Delayed (>24 hours) Transfusion Reactions—Nonimmunologic					
Iron overload	After >20 RBC units	Multiple transfusions with obligate iron load in transfusion-dependent patient	Diabetes, cirrhosis, cardiomyopathy	Liver and cardiac iron concentration (MRI), Serum ferritin, Liver enzymes, Endocrine function tests	Iron chelators

*For platelet refractoriness, see chapter on platelet and granulocyte antigens and antibodies; for septic transfusion reactions, see chapter on transfusion-transmitted diseases.

†For all acute reactions, the transfusion should be stopped to allow investigation, as explained in the text. The approaches listed do not represemt comprehensive treatment recommendations.

AHTR = acute hemolytic transfusion reaction; HTR = hemolytic transfusion reaction; DIC = disseminated intravascular coagulation; DAT = direct antiglobulin test; Hb = hemoglobin; LDH = lactate dehydrogenase; IV = intravenous; WBCs = white blood cells; IgA = immunoglobulin A; RBCs = Red Blood Cells; SD plasma = solvent/detergent-treated plasma; TRALI = transfusion-related acute lung injury; HNA = human neutrophil antigen; ACE = angiotensin-converting enzyme; HPA = human platelet antigen; IVIG = intravenous immune globulin; MRI = magnetic resonance imaging.

and tubing for possible bacteria culture or Gram staining.

3. Request for a posttransfusion blood sample to be collected.

4. Repeat ABO testing on the posttransfusion sample.

5. Visual check of pre- and posttransfusion samples for evidence of hemolysis (which may not be visible if <50 mg/dL of hemoglobin is present).

6. Direct antiglobulin test (DAT) on a posttransfusion sample.

7. Report of findings to the blood bank supervisor or medical director, who may request additional studies or tests, request quarantine of co-components generated from the same donor collection, or impose transfusion restrictions/instructions.

The transfusion service must retain any patient records that are related to transfusion reactions, clinically significant antibodies, or special transfusion requirements. Transfusion services are able to share medical information on patient transfusion history. When a patient is cared for by different transfusion services, medical warning bracelets or wallet identification cards may benefit patients with red cell alloantibodies.

Specialized Laboratory Investigations for Selected Reactions

Additional laboratory evaluation may be required for investigations of some nonhemolytic transfusion reactions, such as anaphylaxis, sepsis, or TRALI, as described in their respective sections below.

ACUTE OR IMMEDIATE TRANSFUSION REACTIONS

Acute or immediate transfusion reactions occur within 24 hours of the administration of a component and often during the transfusion. Acute transfusion reactions include immune and nonimmune-mediated hemolysis, transfusion-related sepsis, TRALI, allergic reactions, TACO, sequelae of massive transfusion, air embolism, hypotensive reactions, and febrile nonhemolytic transfusion reactions (FNHTRs). The clinical significance of an acute transfusion reaction often cannot be determined by the patient's clinical history or signs and symptoms alone but requires laboratory evaluation.

Acute Hemolytic Transfusion Reactions

Presentation

Rapid hemolysis of as little as 10 mL of incompatible blood can produce symptoms of acute HTR (AHTR). The most common presenting symptom is fever with or without accompanying chills or rigors. A patient with a mild reaction may have abdominal, chest, flank, or back pain. If a patient has a severe AHTR, hypotension, dyspnea, and flank pain may be present and, in some cases, progress to shock with or without accompanying disseminated intravascular coagulation (DIC). Red or dark urine may be the first sign of intravascular hemolysis, particularly in an anesthetized or unconscious patient, who may also present with oliguria or, in rare cases, DIC. The severity of the symptoms of this reaction is related to the amount of incompatible blood transfused. Prompt recognition of the reaction and immediate cessation of the transfusion can prevent grave consequences.

Differential Diagnosis

Many of the signs and symptoms of an immune-mediated AHTR also occur in other acute transfusion reactions. Fever with or without chills and accompanied by hypotension may also develop in transfusion-related sepsis and TRALI. However, hemolysis is not associated with TRALI, and respiratory difficulty is not typically a symptom of an AHTR. Fever or chills are more commonly caused by a febrile nonhemolytic reaction but cannot be distinguished symptomatically from the more serious AHTR without an assessment of hemolysis. The patient's underlying disease process can also make the diagnosis of an AHTR difficult. Alternatively, acute hemolysis may result from nonimmune mechanisms, as described in the "Nonimmune-Mediated Hemolysis" section below.

Pathophysiology

The interaction of preformed antibodies with red cell antigens is the immunologic basis for AHTRs. The most severe reactions are associated with transfusions of red cells that are ABO incompatible with the recipient, resulting in acute intravascular destruction of the transfused cells. Transfusion of ABO-incompatible antibodies, as can happen with minor-incompatible apheresis platelets or intravenous immune globulin (IVIG) infusion, may also cause hemolysis. The most common circumstance for platelet transfusion is when group O platelets from donors with high titers of anti-A are transfused to group A recipients.[3] Although these forms of acute hemolysis are not usually clinically significant or characterized by typical hemolytic symptoms, they can be severe if the transfused components have high titers of ABO antibodies.

When preformed immunoglobulin M (IgM) or IgG antibodies recognize corresponding red cell antigens, complement activation may occur, resulting in intravascular hemolysis, hemoglobinemia, and hemoglobinuria. IgM antibodies are strong activators of complement, and IgG antibodies, when present at sufficient concentrations and of the relevant subclass, may activate complement as well.

Complement activation involves C3 cleavage with the ensuing production of C3a, an anaphylatoxin, which is released into the plasma, and C3b, which coats the red cells. If complement activation proceeds to completion, membrane attack complexes are assembled on the red cell surface, and intravascular lysis occurs. C5a, an anaphylatoxin that is 100 times more potent than C3a, is produced as part of this hemolysis. C3a and C5a promote the release of histamine and serotonin from mast cells, leading to vasodilation and smooth-muscle contraction, particularly of bronchial and intestinal muscles. C3a and C5a

are recognized by many other cell types and are involved in the production and release of cytokines, leukotrienes, free radicals, and nitric oxide.[4] The end result may include wheezing, flushing, chest pain or tightness, and gastrointestinal symptoms. These symptoms may also be caused by release of bradykinin and norepinephrine resulting from antigen-antibody complex stimulation.

If complement activation does not proceed to completion, which is usually the case with non-ABO antibodies, the red cells can undergo extravascular hemolysis where cells coated with C3b and/or IgG are rapidly removed from the circulation by phagocytes.[5] In extravascular hemolysis, the consequences of complement activation, including release of anaphylatoxins and opsonization of red cells, may still have adverse effects. Furthermore, extravascular hemolysis can lead to cytokine release, which may play a role in producing the effects of acute hemolysis.[6]

Coagulation abnormalities that are associated with AHTRs may be caused by various mechanisms. The intrinsic pathway of the clotting cascade may be activated by antigen-antibody interaction, resulting in activation of Factor XII, also known as Hageman factor. Activation of the Hageman factor can result in hypotension through its effect on the kinin system. The kinin system produces bradykinin, which in turn increases vascular permeability and causes vasodilation.[7] Activated complement, tumor necrosis factor alpha (TNFα), and interleukin 1 (IL-1) may increase the expression of tissue factor. Tissue factor can activate the extrinsic pathway and is associated with the development of DIC. DIC is an often life-threatening consumptive coagulopathy. Its characteristics include microvascular thrombi formation with ischemic organ and tissue damage; consumption of platelets, fibrinogen, and coagulation factors; and activation of fibrinolysis with production of fibrin-degradation products. The end result of these activations can vary from generalized oozing to uncontrolled bleeding.

Shock may also accompany AHTRs. Hypotension, caused by the release of vasoactive amines, kinins, and other mediators, produces a compensatory vasoconstrictive response that further aggravates organ and tissue damage. Renal failure may occur as well. Free hemoglobin impairs renal function, but compromised renal cortical supply is thought to be the major contributing factor in renal failure. In addition, antigen-antibody complex deposition, vasoconstriction, and thrombi formation contribute to the development of renal vascular compromise.

Frequency

The frequency of AHTRs is not easy to determine. The authors of a review article based on data from several surveillance systems estimated the risk of clinical or laboratory evidence of ABO HTR to be 1 in 80,000 and the risk of a fatal ABO HTR to be 1 in 1.8 million.[8] Of the transfusion-related fatalities reported to the FDA from 2010 to 2014, 21% (38 patients) were caused by HTRs.[1]

Treatment

Prompt recognition of an AHTR and immediate cessation of the transfusion are crucial. The unit of blood should be returned to the blood bank for investigation. Saline should be infused to maintain venous access, treat hypotension, and maintain renal blood flow, with a goal of a urine flow rate at >1 mL/kg/hour. Consultation with critical care, renal, and hematology experts should be considered.

The addition of the diuretic furosemide promotes increased urine output and further enhances renal cortical blood flow. If urine output remains diminished after a liter of saline has been infused, acute tubular necrosis may have occurred, and the patient may be at risk of developing pulmonary edema. Oliguric renal failure may be complicated by hyperkalemia and subsequent cardiac arrest. Metabolic acidosis and uremia often necessitate the institution of dialysis.

DIC is an equally serious component of an AHTR. DIC is difficult to treat and may be the first indication that hemolysis has occurred in an anuric or anesthetized patient. Traditional therapy for DIC includes treating or removing the underlying cause and providing supportive care via the administration of platelets, plasma, and cryoprecipitate.

Unconscious or anesthetized patients may receive multiple units of incompatible blood before acute hemolysis is recognized. Because the severity of an AHTR is related to the amount of incompatible red cells transfused, red cell exchange transfusion may be considered. Some severe reactions to a single unit of strongly incompatible blood may require exchange transfusion as well. Antigen-negative blood must be used for the red cell exchange. Likewise, plasma and platelets that will not contribute to hemolysis should be chosen.

Finally, inhibiting the complement cascade may be beneficial, especially early in the hemolytic transfusion reaction. A single case report on the use of eculizumab, a monoclonal antibody that blocks the cleavage of complement component C5, suggests that this may be a useful strategy for preventing hemolysis of incompatible red cells.[9]

Prompt initiation of therapy to aggressively manage hypotension, renal blood flow, and DIC provides the greatest chance of a successful outcome. Furthermore, consultation with appropriate medical specialists early in the course of treatment will ensure that the patient receives hemodialysis, cardiac monitoring, and mechanical ventilation when needed.

Prevention

Clerical and human errors involving patient, sample, and blood unit identification are the most common causes of mistransfusion and, therefore, AHTRs. Reported estimates place the risk of a near miss at 1:1000, wrong blood given at 1:15,000, ABO-incompatible transfusion at 1:40,000, and error that results in harm at 1:4500.[8,10] Institutional policies and procedures must be in place to minimize the likelihood of such errors, and corrective and preventive action programs should target continual reduction of such errors. However, no one method for reducing the number of errors is foolproof.[11] Products available to increase patient safety include technology-based solutions, such as radiofrequency identification chips, handheld bar-code scanners, and "smart" refrigerators similar to systems used for pharmacologic agents.

The prevention of potential hemolysis from the administration of minor-ABO-incompatible platelets remains a challenge with constrained platelet inventories. A number of options, including anti-A or anti-B titration of the component, limiting the total amount of incompatible plasma transfused from platelets, and volume reduction may offer some benefit.[12] The use of platelet additive solutions for reducing minor-incompatible hemolysis risk has not been clinically studied.

Nonimmune-Mediated Hemolysis

Transfusion-associated hemolysis can also result from several nonimmune-mediated causes. Longer duration of storage before issue is associated with increased hemolysis of storage-damaged red cells.[13] Furthermore, improper shipping or storage temperatures, as well as incomplete deglycerolization of frozen red cells, can lead to hemolysis. At the time of transfusion, using a needle with an inappropriately small bore size or employing a rapid pressure infuser can cause mechanical hemolysis, which may be related to the use of roller pumps. Improper use of blood warmers or the use of microwave ovens or hot water-baths can cause temperature-related hemolysis. AABB *Standards* allow for 0.9% sodium chloride to be added to blood during infusion.[14(p45)] Other fluids need FDA approval for transfusion with red cells. Infusion of red cells simultaneously through the same tubing with hypotonic solutions or with certain pharmacologic agents may cause osmotic hemolysis. For safe administration, red cells and these solutions or agents should be given via alternate venous access locations. In rare cases, hemolysis may be caused by bacterial contamination of the Red Blood Cell (RBC) unit. Patients may also experience hemolysis as part of their underlying disease process. Although a negative DAT result usually indicates no evidence of an immune-mediated cause of hemolysis, complete destruction of incompatible transfused red cells may be associated with a negative DAT result.

When both immune and nonimmune causes of hemolysis have been excluded, the possibility of an intrinsic red cell membrane defect in the recipient or even in the transfused cells should be considered. Cells with these defects, such as G6PD deficiency, have increased fragility when challenged with particular stressors and may undergo coincidental hemolysis.

Treatment

Hemolysis of nonimmune etiology may cause symptoms whose severity depends on the degree of hemolysis and amount of component transfused. In all cases, the transfusion should be discontinued and appropriate care should be administered. (See the earlier section on the treatment of AHTRs for details on managing hypotension and declining renal function.)

Prevention

Written procedures for all aspects of the manufacture and transfusion of blood and components should always be followed. Prompt recognition of nonimmune hemolysis and robust root cause analysis may prevent additional occurrences.

Transfusion-Related Sepsis

Presentation

Fever (particularly a temperature of $\geq$38.5 C or 101 F), chills, rigors, and hypotension during or shortly after transfusion are the most frequent presenting symptoms of transfusion-related sepsis. Gram-negative bacteria typically cause more severe symptoms, including shock, renal failure, and DIC. Gram-positive organisms may present with isolated fever in the patient and may present hours after the completion of transfusion.

Differential Diagnosis

The abruptness of onset and severity of the signs and symptoms associated with transfusion-related sepsis may be very similar to those of AHTRs. Mild cases may be confused with FNHTRs. Fever or bacteremia unrelated to transfusion may confound the diagnosis. The key to diagnosing transfusion-related sepsis is culturing the same organism from both the patient and the remainder of the component. The returned component should be visually examined in suspected cases of posttransfusion sepsis. Attention should be paid to any color changes, especially brown or purple discoloration in an RBC component and bubbles/frothiness in a platelet component. A Gram stain should be performed on the returned component.

Treatment

If transfusion-related sepsis is suspected, the transfusion should be stopped immediately, and supportive care and antibiotics should be initiated.

Prevention

Suspected septic transfusion reactions should be immediately reported to the blood collector so that co-componenents from the same donation can be intercepted to avoid exposing other patients to contaminated blood components.[15] Any co-components or aliquots from the same donation that are in the hospital's inventory should be immediately quarantined, pending investigation results. Bacteria detection tests and pathogen inactivation technologies are discussed in Chapter 7.

Febrile Nonhemolytic Transfusion Reactions

Presentation

An FNHTR is usually defined as the occurrence of a ≥1 C rise in temperature ≥38 C that is associated with transfusion and for which no other cause is identifiable. Accompanying symptoms may include rigors, chills, and respiratory changes. In some instances, the patient may be afebrile but have the remaining constellation of symptoms. Symptoms usually occur during transfusion but may occur up to 4 hours after. Although FNHTRs are self-limited, they may cause significant discomfort.

Differential Diagnosis

Recognition of an FNHTR requires diagnosis by exclusion. The symptoms associated with an FNHTR may be present in several other types of transfusion reactions, the most serious of which are HTRs, sepsis, and TRALI. Each of these other reactions has signs, symptoms, and associated laboratory results that help distinguish them from an FNHTR once an investigation is begun. Hemolysis must be ruled out in a patient who experiences fever associated with transfusion. Fever may commonly occur as a manifestation of a patient's underlying illness. In a patient who has been experiencing spiking fevers during the course of admission, it may be difficult to rule out an FNHTR. Bacterial contamination of the component must always be considered to be a potential cause of a febrile reaction.

Pathophysiology

Recipient leukocyte antibodies may cause febrile transfusion reactions.[16] HLA antibodies in particular can react with cognate antigens on transfused lymphocytes, granulocytes, or platelets. FNHTRs may also be the result of accumulated cytokines in a cellular blood component. This mechanism may be particularly relevant in reactions that occur after the transfusion of platelets.[17] Whether passively transfused or generated by leukocytes in the recipient, pyrogenic cytokine release is the common event leading to symptoms of FNHTR.

Treatment

When an FNHTR is suspected, the transfusion should be discontinued and a transfusion reaction workup initiated. Antipyretics (eg, acetaminophen) may be administered. For more severe reactions that include rigors, meperidine may be administered, although its efficacy has not been rigorously studied.

When fever develops during transfusion, the remainder of the implicated component should not be transfused. Among the few situations in which transfusion of the remainder of the component should be considered is when the component is a medically indicated rare unit. If a portion of the component remains, the laboratory workup to exclude hemolysis must be completed and a discussion with the patient's clinical care team regarding the likelihood of transfusion-transmitted sepsis must be held before the transfusion is resumed.

Prevention

Prestorage leukocyte reduction decreases the frequency of FNHTRs.[18,19] Premedication with acetaminophen has limited benefit in preventing febrile reactions, without impairing the ability to detect serious complications of transfusion.[20] Plasma reduction reduces the rate of FNHTRs to platelets.[21]

Allergic Reactions

Presentation

Most allergic transfusion reactions (ATRs) are mild, but their spectrum can range from a simple allergic reaction (urticaria) to life-threatening anaphylaxis. Symptoms generally occur within minutes after the start of the transfusion. If symptoms do not appear until >4 hours later, they may represent an allergic reaction that is unrelated to the blood transfusion.

Hives usually cause itching (pruritus) but may also burn or sting. Hives can appear anywhere on the body and can coalesce over large areas. They can last from hours to several days before fading, but most respond quickly to treatment with antihistamines. More extensive cases may be accompanied by angioedema, which is a deep tissue swelling, often around the eyes and lips. Angioedema can involve the throat, tongue, or lungs, causing respiratory distress, although feeling throat fullness or dyspnea without respiratory insufficiency is more common.

Anaphylactic transfusion reactions can be generally defined as the presentation of mucocutaneous signs of urticaria and angioedema in combination with other organ system involvement (cardiovascular, respiratory, gastrointestinal).[22] Manifestations of anaphylaxis are hypotension, loss of consciousness, dyspnea, wheezing, stridor, abdominal pain, and vomiting.

Differential Diagnosis

It can be difficult to distinguish anaphylaxis from other reactions characterized by hypotension, dyspnea, and/or loss of consciousness. Reactions that may be mistaken for anaphylactic shock are vasovagal and hypotensive reactions. Urticaria, angioedema, pruritus, and respiratory symptoms, such as wheezing or stridor, are symptoms of anaphylaxis but do not occur in vasovagal or hypotensive reactions. The respiratory symptoms of anaphylaxis may be suggestive of asthma exacerbations or TRALI. However, the classic symptoms of allergy, including urticaria, angioedema, and pruritus, do not occur in asthma or TRALI. Fever, a prominent symptom of HTR and bacterial contamination, is not a feature of anaphylaxis. Patients who take angiotensin-converting enzyme (ACE) inhibitors and undergo plasma exchange sometimes develop hypotensive reactions that mimic anaphylaxis.

Pathophysiology

The pathophysiology of nearly all ATRs is not understood. Extrapolating from a small number of case reports, ATRs are attributed to hypersensitivity reactions to allergens in the component caused by preformed IgE antibody in the recipient. A combination of recipient and donor factors is likely involved, as recipients with an atopic predisposition appear to have a higher rate of ATRs, and certain donors' platelets are associated with an increased risk.[22,23] Clinical transfusion parameters have not been associated with ATRs.[24]

Selective protein deficiency, classically IgA deficiency, is a rare cause of ATRs. These reactions are caused by anti-IgA in the recipient.[25] Although IgA deficiency is present in approximately 1:700 people of European ancestry, only a small percentage of these people ever make antibodies against IgA. People with absolute IgA deficiency (<0.05 mg/dL) may form class-specific antibodies that are associated with anaphylactic reactions. Those with decreased but detectable amounts of IgA, or relative IgA deficiency, can form subclass-specific antibodies (eg, anti-IgA1 or anti-IgA2) that typically result in less severe reactions.[26]

Although precautions should be taken when transfusing an IgA-deficient patient, it must be kept in mind that the majority of ATRs are caused by substances other than IgA.[27] Most of these allergens are not identified but rarely may include haptoglobin[28] or the complement protein C4.[29] Transfusion can passively sensitize patients to donor antibodies, resulting in transient allergy (eg, to peanuts).[30]

Frequency

ATRs are common, with an overall frequency of approximately 2% with traditional platelet and plasma components.[31] The incidence is about 10-fold lower with RBCs.[32] Platelet additive solution platelets and pooled plasma components have lower rates of ATRs. Life-threatening anaphylactic reactions account for <1% of all ATRs. Of the transfusion-associated fatalities reported to the FDA from 2010 to 2014, 6% (10 of 176) were caused by anaphylaxis, and most are not caused by IgA deficiency.[1,27]

Treatment

Urticaria is the only transfusion reaction in which the administration of the component may be routinely resumed after prompt treatment. When a patient develops symptoms, the transfusion should be paused so that an antihistamine may be administered. Once the symptoms have dissipated, the transfusion may be resumed, and a laboratory workup need not be initiated.

Severe urticarial reactions may be treated with H1 and H2 receptor antagonists and corticosteroids. Epinephrine 0.5 mg intramuscularly (pediatric dose of 0.01 mg/kg) is the consensus first-line treatment for anaphylaxis; the dose may be repeated up to every 5 minutes.[33]

Prevention

Evidence does not support routine premedication to prevent ATRs.[34] Antihistamines (diphenhydramine or a nonsedating antihistamine, eg, cetirizine) are useful to treat allergic symptoms once they arise. If H1 receptor antihistamines are not sufficient, an H2 receptor antagonist (eg, ranitidine) or corticosteroids may be beneficial. For patients whose reactions are severe or recurrent, washed RBCs or platelets, platelet additive solution platelets, or pooled solvent/detergent-treated plasma may be considered.

Recipient IgA or haptoglobin concentrations are often not available by the time a subsequent transfusion is needed; however, most cases of anaphylaxis are idiosyncratic to a specific unit and not the result of selective protein deficiency. Tolerance of prior plasma and platelet transfusions is a reasonable indicator that subsequent plasma transfusions may be acceptable from unselected donors. Pooled solvent/detergent-treated plasma has a lower risk of allergic reactions, but its use in prevention of recurrent anaphylactic reactions has not been established. At some institutions, the plasma used for transfusions for patients with a history of severe ATRs and diagnosed IgA deficiency with anti-IgA is requested to come from IgA-deficient donors (<0.05 mg/dL). If IgA-deficient plasma is not available, desensitization with IgA-containing plasma may be possible.[35] Cellular components (RBCs and platelets) can be depleted of plasma proteins through washing. IgA deficiency without the presence of anti-IgA or without a history of an ATR does not clearly warrant the use of IgA-deficient or plasma-depleted components.

Transfusion-Related Acute Lung Injury

Presentation

TRALI is a syndrome that is clinically similar to adult respiratory distress syndrome (ARDS), but it usually resolves within 96 hours. Clinical signs and symptoms of TRALI include fever, chills, dyspnea, cyanosis, hypotension, and new-onset bilateral pulmonary edema.[36] A dramatic transient neutropenia or leukopenia may also be observed.[37] Symptoms arise within 6 hours of transfusion, with most cases becoming evident within 1 to 2 hours.

All plasma-containing components, including whole blood, RBCs, platelets, cryoprecipitate, and Fresh Frozen Plasma (FFP), have been implicated in TRALI. Transfusion volumes as small as 15 mL have led to TRALI.

TRALI is a form of acute lung injury (ALI). The American-European Consensus Conference[38] defined ALI as acute hypoxemia with a PaO_2/FiO_2 (partial pressure of oxygen in arterial blood/inspired oxygen concentration) ratio of ≤300 mm Hg and bilateral pulmonary edema on frontal chest radiograph. The Canadian Consensus Conference[39] relied on this definition of ALI when creating its diagnostic criteria for TRALI: 1) ALI with hypoxemia and PaO_2/FiO_2 ≤300 or SpO_2 (blood oxygen saturation) <90% on room air, 2) no preexisting ALI before transfusion, 3) onset of symptoms within 6 hours of transfusion, and 4) no temporal relationship with an alternative risk factor for ALI. The panel also defined "possible TRALI" using the same criteria as for TRALI, except allowing for the presence of an alternative risk factor for ALI.

Although the lung injury in ALI is usually irreversible, the lung injury in TRALI is most often transient. Approximately 80% of patients with TRALI improve within 48 to 96 hours. The remaining 20% of patients who do not improve rapidly have either a protracted clinical course or a fatal outcome. In one TRALI study, 100% of the patients required oxygen support and 72% required mechanical ventilation.[40]

Differential Diagnosis

The three main conditions that need to be distinguished from TRALI are 1) anaphylactic transfusion reactions, 2) TACO, and 3) transfusion-related sepsis. In anaphylactic transfusion reactions, bronchospasm, laryngeal edema, severe hypotension, erythema (often confluent), and urticaria are prominent symptoms. Fever and pulmonary edema are not associated with anaphylactic reactions. The clinical presentation of TACO is very similar to that of TRALI, with respiratory distress, tachypnea, and cyanosis as the most prominent features. Key distinctions between TACO and TRALI are that the pulmonary edema in TACO is cardiogenic and responsive to diuretics, whereas it is noncardiogenic and not responsive to diuretics in TRALI. High fever with hypotension and vascular collapse are prominent features of transfusion-related sepsis. Respiratory distress is infrequently associated with septic reactions. Finally, other possible causes of ALI should be considered, such as coincident myocardial infarction and pulmonary embolus.

Pathophysiology

Several mechanisms for the pulmonary manifestations of TRALI have been proposed. The primary effector cell is the neutrophil, with lung histology from fatal cases showing predominantly neutrophilic infiltrates and alveolar edema.[41] TRALI has been associated with the infusion of antibodies to leukocyte antigens and of biologic response modifiers (BRMs).[42] Infusions of these antibodies or BRMs are thought to initiate cellular activation and damage of the basement membrane in the lungs, leading to leakage of protein-rich fluid into the alveolar space.

A two-event model of the mechanism of TRALI has been hypothesized.[43] In the first event, generation of biologically active compounds activates pulmonary vascular endothelial cells and primes neutrophils, resulting in sequestration of neutrophils in the pulmonary microvasculature. This first event predisposes the recipient to develop TRALI and can result from a variety of physiologic stressors, including sepsis, surgery, and massive transfusion. The infusion of BRMs or antibodies is the second event. BRMs consist of a mixture of lysophosphatidylcholines that accumulate in some cellular components during storage. The transfused antibodies may be to HLA Class I, HLA Class II, or human neutrophil antigens (HNAs). These stimuli activate the primed neutrophils in the pulmonary microvasculature, resulting in pulmonary endothelial damage, capillary leakage, and pulmonary edema.

Frequency

TRALI occurs in about 1 in 10,000 units transfused.[42] TRALI is the leading cause of transfusion-related mortality reported to the FDA. Because HLA or HNA antibodies are more common in multiparous women, efforts to decrease the amount of transfusable plasma collected from female donors has decreased the number of TRALI fatalities.[44] In 2006, the year before many blood centers implemented measures to reduce the risk of TRALI from plasma transfusions, 35 fatal cases of TRALI, 22 of which were associated with transfusion of FFP, were reported to the FDA. Since 2008, the year after many blood centers implemented such measures, the numbers of TRALI fatalities have decreased by over half.

Treatment

Treatment of TRALI consists of respiratory and circulatory support. Oxygen supplementation with or without mechanical ventilation is required in almost all cases. Pressor agents may be needed to support blood pressure. Because TRALI is not associated with volume overload, diuretics are typically not indicated. Administration of corticosteroids has not been shown to improve clinical outcome in TRALI or ARDS.[45]

Prevention

There is no method to predict which patients will develop TRALI. Donors whose collections are linked to cases of TRALI are permanently deferred. Although approximately 10% of blood donations contain HLA and/or HNA antibodies, TRALI is much rarer. Nevertheless, an important mitigation strategy is to collect plasma components, whole blood, and platelets from male donors, never-pregnant female donors, or females who have been tested since their last pregnancy and found to be negative for HLA antibodies. Although these measures reduce the risk of TRALI, it is important to recognize that they do not eliminate TRALI completely because they do not address the risk of TRALI from RBC or cryoprecipitate components, and required donor testing in previously pregnant females does not screen for HNA antibodies and BRMs.

Transfusion-Associated Circulatory Overload

Presentation

It is well known that transfusion can precipitate acute pulmonary edema caused by volume overload. Patients >70 years and infants are at greatest risk, as well as patients with compromised ability to regulate fluid balance (eg, those with congestive heart failure and end-stage renal disease), although all transfusion recipients are susceptible to some degree. Whereas large volumes of components and nonblood fluids are most frequently implicated, modest volumes can also precipitate TACO in susceptible patients. A high flow rate is frequently a cofactor.

TACO has no pathognomonic signs or symptoms. Within 1 to 2 hours of transfusion, patients may develop any or all of the following: gallop, jugular venous distension, elevated central venous pressure, dyspnea, orthopnea, new ST-segment and T-wave changes on electrocardiogram, elevated serum troponin, and elevated brain natriuretic peptide (BNP).[46] Increased blood pressure characterized by a widening of the pulse pressure is characteristic of TACO. Radiographs show a widened cardiothoracic ratio.

Differential Diagnosis

TACO is frequently confused with TRALI because both types of reactions produce pulmonary edema. It is also possible for TACO and TRALI to occur concurrently in the same patient. The timelines and the clinical presentation are similar, but hypertension is a typical feature of TACO, whereas it is only an infrequent and transient manifestation of TRALI. Furthermore, rapid improvement with diuresis is consistent with TACO.

In congestive heart failure, BNP levels are elevated. A posttransfusion-to-pretransfusion

BNP ratio of 1.5 with a posttransfusion level of at least 100 pg/mL as a cutoff yields a sensitivity and specificity >80% in TACO.[46] However, in the intensive care setting, BNP is only of moderate value for distinguishing TACO from TRALI.[47] Some clinical laboratories measure the N-terminal propeptide BNP (NT-proBNP), which has a longer half-life than BNP. NT-proBNP is also predictive of TACO.[48] With rapid onset of respiratory distress, possible causes of ALI, such as coincident myocardial infarction, pulmonary embolus, and others, should be considered in addition to TACO and TRALI.

Frequency

TACO is an underreported adverse reaction to transfusion, and hemovigilance and retrospective studies underestimate the incidence. Furthermore, the incidence differs across patient populations with different comorbidities.[49] From 2010 to 2014, 22% of the transfusion-associated fatalities reported to the FDA (38 patients) were a consequence of TACO.[1] Platelet and plasma components are associated with a TACO incidence of approximately 1%,[50,51] and RBCs, with an incidence of up to 2.7%.[49]

Treatment

As soon as symptoms suggest TACO, the transfusion should be stopped. The symptoms should be treated by placing the patient in a seated position (if possible), providing supplementary oxygen, and reducing the intravascular volume with diuretics. If symptoms persist in confirmed TACO, administration of additional diuretics or therapeutic phlebotomy is appropriate.

Prevention

In the absence of ongoing and rapid blood loss, components should be administered slowly, particularly in patients at risk of TACO (ie, pediatric patients, patients with severe anemia, and patients with congestive heart failure). Rates of 2 to 4 mL/minute and 1 mL/kg of body weight per hour are the most frequently cited, despite a paucity of data on appropriate infusion rates. Total fluid input and output must be monitored.

Hypotensive Reactions

Presentation

Hypotensive transfusion reactions (HyTRs) are defined as the sudden and unexpected onset of clinically significant hypotension associated with the transfusion of blood or blood components that resolves shortly after the transfusion is stopped. Systolic blood pressure (SBP) drops by >30 mm Hg or to <80 mm Hg in adults. In children, an SBP drop of >25% is consistent with a HyTR. Another characteristic is that HyTRs usually start within the first 15 minutes of transfusion. All types of patients can be affected with any blood component.[52] One study found 1% of platelet transfusions can be complicated by HyTRs.[53]

Differential Diagnosis

Hypotension can be a primary manifestation of HyTR, anaphylaxis, septic transfusion, AHTR, TRALI, or underlying disease/medication. All may present within the first 15 minutes of transfusion, but the absence of concomitant signs and symptoms and the prompt resolution of hypotension upon discontinuation of transfusion distinguish HyTRs from other reactions. Anaphylactic shock usually is accompanied by mucocutaneous allergic manifestations (eg, flushing, angioedema, urticaria). Septic shock from transfusion is often accompanied by fever. AHTRs are associated with hemoglobinuria, pain, and fever. A minority of TRALI cases involve clinically significant hypotension, but TRALI cases have acute pulmonary insufficiency, a finding that is atypical for HyTRs.

Pathophysiology

Bradykinin is thought to have a causal role in HyTRs.[54] Bradykinin is a vasoactive peptide generated via activation of the kinin-kallikrein system from its precursor, high-molecular-weight kininogen. Factors that increase concentrations of bradykinin in blood components include storage, filtration, and ACE activity in donors and recipients. ACE activity can be affected by ACE-inhibitor medication and cardiopulmonary bypass circuits, because the lungs are a primary site of ACE activity.[55] Recent prostatectomy may increase bradykinin concentrations in patients as a result of kallikreins released from the prostate.

Treatment

The primary treatment intervention is to stop the transfusion. Blood pressure usually increases within minutes after cessation of transfusion, but circulatory support with intravenous fluids and vasopressors may be needed. With acute onset of hypotension, the etiology is often not immediately clear. Treatments for anaphylaxis and sepsis may be initiated as the clinical presentation unfolds.

Prevention

If a patient who experienced a HyTR is taking ACE-inhibitor medication that is not discontinued, subsequent transfusions should be given as slowly as is feasible to prevent a recurrence. Because HyTRs are typically idiosyncratic to a specific unit, patients without risk factors for a HyTR typically tolerate subsequent transfusions well. Washing cellular blood components will reduce accumulated bradykinin, but washed component protocols are seldom needed, as most cases are not recurrent.

Complications of Massive Transfusion

The potential complications of massive transfusion, usually defined as the receipt of >10 RBC units within 24 hours, include metabolic and hemostatic abnormalities, immune hemolysis, and air embolism. Metabolic abnormalities can depress cardiac function. Hypothermia from refrigerated blood, citrate toxicity, and lactic acidosis from underperfusion and tissue ischemia, which are often complicated by hyperkalemia, can contribute to this effect. Although metabolic alkalosis caused by citrate metabolism may occur, it is not likely to be clinically significant. Patients who lose blood rapidly may have preexisting or coexisting hemostatic abnormalities or develop them during resuscitation. Hemostatic abnormalities may include dilutional coagulopathy, DIC, and liver and platelet dysfunction.[56]

Citrate Toxicity

Pathophysiology and Manifestations. When large volumes of citrated blood components are transfused rapidly, particularly in the presence of liver disease, plasma citrate levels may rise, binding calcium, resulting in hypocalcemia. In patients with a normally functioning liver, citrate is rapidly metabolized; thus, these symptoms are transient.[57] Hypocalcemia is more likely to cause manifestations in patients who are hypothermic or in shock.

A decrease in ionized calcium levels increases neuronal excitability, which in the conscious patient leads to symptoms of perioral and peripheral tingling, shivering, and lightheadedness, followed by a diffuse sense of vibration, muscle cramps, fasciculations, spasm, and nausea. In the central nervous system, hypocalcemia is thought to increase the respiratory center sensitivity to carbon dioxide, causing hyperventilation. Because myocardial contraction is dependent on the intracellular movement of ionized calcium, hypocalcemia depresses cardiac function.

Treatment and Prevention. Unless the patient has a predisposing condition that hinders citrate metabolism, hypocalcemia caused by citrate overload during massive transfusion can usually be treated by slowing the infusion. Intravenous calcium replacement with calcium gluconate or calcium chloride should be considered early, as hypocalcemia contributes to a hypocoagulable state in massive transfusion.[58]

Hyperkalemia and Hypokalemia

Pathophysiology. When red cells are stored at 1 to 6 C, the intracellular potassium gradually leaks into the supernatant plasma or additive solution. Although the concentration in the supernatant may be high, because of the small volume, the total extracellular potassium load is <0.5 mEq for fresh RBC units and only 5 to 7 mEq for units at expiration. These potassium concentrations rarely cause problems in the recipient because rapid dilution, redistribution into cells, and excretion blunt the effect.[59] However, hyperkalemia can be a problem in patients with renal failure, in premature infants, and in newborns receiving large transfusions, such as in cardiac surgery or exchange transfusion; otherwise, hyperkalemia is typically a transient effect during very rapid transfusions.[60]

Hypokalemia occurs more frequently than hyperkalemia after transfusion because potassium-depleted donor red cells reaccumulate this ion intracellularly, and citrate metabolism causes further movement of potassium into the cells in response to the consumption of protons. Catecholamine release and aldosterone-induced urinary loss can also trigger hypokalemia in the setting of massive transfusion.[59]

Treatment and Prevention. No treatment or preventive strategy for hypokalemia and hyperkalemia is usually necessary, provided that the patient is adequately resuscitated from the underlying condition that required massive transfusion. For infants receiving routine transfusions, units infused up to 0.5 cc/kg/min may be used safely until the expiration date.[61] Although washing of RBC units results in very low levels of potassium, there is no evidence that this is indicated for routine RBC transfusions, even in patients with impaired renal function.[62]

Hemostatic Abnormalities in Massive Transfusion

Pathophysiology. Coagulopathy can occur in massive transfusion, particularly when the lost blood is initially replaced with RBCs and crystalloids. Coagulopathy in massive transfusion is frequently ascribed to the dilution of platelets and clotting factors as patients lose hemostatically active blood, and enzymatic activity is reduced as the core body temperature lowers if a blood warmer is not used. Mortality rates associated with hemostatic abnormalities range from 20% to 50%.[63] The high rate of

mortality results from hypothermia, metabolic acidosis, and coagulopathy.[64]

Studies of military and civilian trauma patients demonstrated a progressive increase in the incidence of microvascular bleeding (MVB) characteristic of a coagulopathy with increasing transfusion volumes that typically occurs after replacement of 2 to 3 blood volumes (20 to 30 units).[65] Although platelet counts, coagulation parameters, and levels of selected clotting parameters correlate with the volume transfused, contrary to expectations from a simple dilutional model, the relationship is marked by tremendous variability. Moreover, there is frequently discordance between the laboratory assessment and the clinical evidence of bleeding.

MVB increases with platelet counts below ~50,000/μL; however, no simple relationship can be determined between a patient's coagulation test results and the onset of bleeding. The etiology of bleeding (elective surgery vs massive trauma) may play a role as well.[66]

Subsequent studies have refined these observations. Significant platelet dysfunction has been demonstrated in massively transfused patients.[67] Low fibrinogen and platelet counts are better predictors of hemostatic failure than elevations of prothrombin time (PT) and partial thromboplastin time (PTT), suggesting that consumptive coagulopathy is an important factor in MVB in addition to dilution.[68] The degree of platelet and clotting abnormalities correlates with the length of time that the patient is hypotensive, suggesting that shock is the most important cause of DIC. In aggregate, hypoperfusion is a major risk factor for coagulopathy in heavily transfused patients.[69]

These data may not be generalizable to patients undergoing massive transfusion in the controlled setting of the operating room, where hypotension caused by volume loss is prevented. In this context, coagulation factor levels may be more significant than platelet problems. Murray and colleagues documented that excessive bleeding in elective surgery patients transfused with >1 blood volume (RBCs and crystalloid) corresponded to a prolongation in PT and PPT compared to patients with normal hemostasis.[66]

Treatment and Prevention. The dilutional model of coagulopathy in massive transfusion suggests that prophylactic replacement of hemostatic components based on the volume of RBCs or whole blood transfused prevents the development of a bleeding diathesis. No specific regimen has yet been shown to be superior to any other in prospective studies. Although there was no statistically significant difference in mortality, the Pragmatic Randomized Optimal Platelet and Plasma Ratios (PROPPR) trial indicated improvement in hemorrhage control using a 1:1:1 plasma/platelet/RBC unit ratio vs a 1:1:2 ratio.[70]

Although the optimal transfusion ratio in trauma resuscitation is still debated, institutions should develop a massive transfusion protocol. Replacement of platelets and coagulation factors in the massively transfused surgical and trauma patient should be based on the identification of a specific abnormality using platelet counts, international normalized ratio, activated PTT, and fibrinogen levels, as clinically indicated. Frequent monitoring of these laboratory values serves to avoid overuse of platelets and plasma components by anticipating the specific components needed while avoiding dilutional coagulopathy. It is imperative that the laboratory provide results of these tests rapidly. Intraoperative and postoperative laboratory testing, such as thromboelastography, may be useful.

Antifibrinolytics have a role in controlling massive bleeding from trauma. The Clinical Randomization of an Antifibrinolytic in Significant Hemorrhage 2 (CRASH-2) and other studies conclude that tranexamic acid should be given as early as possible in the trauma patient.[71] Activated clotting factors do not have a defined role in massive transfusion.

Air Embolism

Air embolism can occur if blood in an open system is infused under pressure or if air enters a central catheter while containers or blood administration sets are being changed. Air embolism has been reported in association with intraoperative and perioperative blood recovery systems that allow air into the blood infusion bag. The minimum volume of air embolism that is potentially fatal for an adult is approximately 100 mL.[72] Symptoms include cough, dyspnea, chest pain, and shock. If air embolism is suspected, the patient should be placed on the left side with the head down to displace the air bubble from the pulmonic valve. Aspiration of the air is sometimes attempted.[73]

Hypothermia

Blood warmers may be used to prevent hypothermia. Proper procedures for the use of blood warmers should be followed because overheating may induce hemolysis and serious transfusion reactions, including fatalities.

DELAYED TRANSFUSION REACTIONS

Delayed Hemolytic Transfusion Reactions

Presentation

Development of an alloantibody following transfusion can result in an asymptomatic delayed serologic transfusion reaction (DSTR) or in a delayed HTR (DHTR). Fever and anemia occurring days to weeks after transfusion of an RBC component are characteristic of a DHTR. The hemolysis associated with a DHTR is more protracted than an AHTR and typically does not precipitate the acute signs and symptoms of an AHTR, although some patients may develop jaundice and leukocytosis. In a DHTR, the hemolysis is primarily extravascular, so although hemoglobinuria may occur in rare cases, acute renal failure and DIC are not generally present. In some cases, the hemolysis occurs without causing clinical symptoms. These patients present with unexplained anemia or do not experience the expected increase in hemoglobin concentrations following transfusion.

Differential Diagnosis

Fever with hemolysis may also occur well after transfusion when the component has been contaminated with an intracellular red cell parasite, such as malaria or babesia. Fever without hemolysis may be an indication of graft-vs-host disease (GVHD) [described in the transfusion-associated (TA)-GVHD section below] or transfusion-transmitted viral disease (eg, cytomegalovirus). Hemolysis resulting from antibody production by donor passenger lymphocytes may occur after transplantation of a minor-ABO-incompatible organ (eg, transplantation of a group O liver in a group A patient).

In a DHTR/DSTR, antibodies may be found in the serum, on transfused red cells, or both. Diagnosis by routine antibody screening and antibody identification should be possible. If transfused red cells are still present in the patient's circulation, the DAT result may be positive. When the DAT result is positive, an eluate should be performed and the antibody identified. If a segment from the unit is available, antigen typing may confirm the diagnosis.

Pathophysiology

After transfusion, transplantation, or pregnancy, a patient may make an antibody to a red cell antigen that he or she lacks. Red cell antibodies may cause a delayed transfusion reaction if the patient subsequently receives a unit of blood expressing the corresponding red cell antigen. Primary alloimmunization occurs anywhere from days to months after a transfusion of antigen-positive red cells, depending on the immunogenicity and dose of the antigen.

Approximately 1% to 1.6% of RBC transfusions are associated with antibody formation, excluding antibodies to antigens in the Rh system. D-negative blood is usually transfused to D-negative patients, so the frequency attributable to anti-D is relatively low. Newly formed alloantibodies are routinely detected during pretransfusion screening. (See Chapters 13 and 17.) Recently transfused or pregnant patients must have samples drawn for compatibility testing within 3 days of the scheduled transfusion to ensure identification of any potential new alloantibodies. A 5-year retrospective study of alloimmunization showed that 11 of 2932 patients (0.4%) had developed new antibodies, including anti-E, anti-K, and anti-Jkª, within 3 days after their transfusion.[74]

DHTRs and DSTRs rarely, if ever, occur as a result of primary immunization and are generally associated with subsequent transfusions. Antibody titers may slowly decrease after the initial immune response, a phenomenon termed evanescence,[75] with as many as 30% to 60% of alloantibodies becoming undetectable over months to years. Antibodies against antigens of some blood group systems, such as the Kidd system, frequently exhibit this behavior. Subsequent transfusion of an antigen-positive unit triggers an anamnestic response, with production of antibody occurring over the next several days to weeks after the transfusion. The rapidity of antibody production and hemolytic potential of the antibody combine to influence the clinical presentation. Blood group antibodies associated with DHTRs/DSTRs include those of the Kidd, Duffy, Kell, and MNS systems.

Frequency

As with AHTRs, the estimated rate of DHTRs varies widely from study to study. Some of this variation is the result of the practice of considering DSTRs and DHTRs as one category. Also, improvements in laboratory techniques have contributed to an increased number of DSTRs detected. Nonetheless, delayed reactions occur much more frequently than AHTRs, with estimates of approximately 1:2500 for either type of delayed reaction, and DSTRs twice as common as DHTRs.[76] These reactions are likely to be greatly underrecognized because most patients do not undergo red cell antibody screening following transfusion.[77]

Treatment

The treatment of DHTRs consists of monitoring the patient and providing supportive care. Correction of the anemia by transfusing antigen-negative RBCs may be needed.

Prevention

DHTRs/DSTRs caused by known antibody specificities can be prevented by the transfusion of antigen-negative RBCs. It is essential to obtain prior transfusion records for the recipient because of antibody evanescence. Many institutions have programs to provide prophylactic, partial phenotype-matching of blood for patients with sickle cell disease or other chronic anemias. Patients with sickle cell disease may develop a life-threatening complication known as hyperhemolysis, even after crossmatch-compatible RBC transfusion, in which autologous and allogeneic cells are destroyed. (See Chapter 24.)

Transfusion-Associated Graft-vs-Host Disease

Presentation

TA-GVHD occurs in <1 per million transfusions. The clinical manifestations of TA-GVHD typically begin 8 to 10 days after transfusion, although symptoms can occur as early as 3 days and as late as 30 days. Signs and symptoms include rash, fever, enterocolitis with watery diarrhea, elevated liver function test results, and pancytopenia. The rash begins on the trunk and progresses to the extremities. In severe cases, bullae may develop.[78] Unlike GVHD after allogeneic hematopoietic stem cell transplantation, TA-GVHD leads to profound marrow aplasia, with a mortality rate higher than 90%. The time course of the reaction is very rapid; death typically occurs within 1 to 3 weeks of the first symptoms.

Differential Diagnosis

Because the clinical manifestations of TA-GVHD appear several days after a transfusion, it may be difficult to associate the patient's symptoms with the transfusion. The symptoms can easily be attributed to other conditions, including drug reactions and viral illness. In cases of TA-GVHD, a skin biopsy reveals a superficial perivascular lymphocytic infiltrate, necrotic keratinocytes, compact orthokeratosis, and bullae formation. Molecular techniques, including HLA typing, cytogenetics, and chimerism assessment, can be used to make the diagnosis.

Pathophysiology

There are three requirements for GVHD to develop in a patient. First, there must be differences in the HLA antigens expressed between the donor and the recipient. Second, immunocompetent cells must be present in the component. Finally, the host must be incapable of rejecting the immunocompetent cells. The three primary factors that determine the risk of developing TA-GVHD are the degree of recipient immunodeficiency, number of viable T lymphocytes in the transfusion, and degree of a population's genetic diversity. The number of viable lymphocytes in a transfusion can be affected by the age, leukocyte reduction status, and irradiation status of the component.[79] Although current leukocyte-reduction technologies significantly reduce the number of lymphocytes in a component, leukocyte reduction does not eliminate the risk of TA-GVHD.

Clinical risk factors for developing TA-GVHD include leukemia, lymphoma, use of immunosuppressive drugs administered for transplant or myeloablative chemotherapy, congenital immunodeficiency disorders, and neonatal age, although immunodeficiency is not required for TA-GVHD.[80] TA-GVHD can occur after a transfusion from a donor who is homozygous for an HLA haplotype to a heterozygous recipient (one-way haplotype match). In this circumstance, the recipient's immune system does not reject the HLA-homozygous transfused lymphocytes as foreign. The transfused lymphocytes are able to recognize the host cells as foreign and are able to mount an immunologic attack on the host. As mentioned, the degree of genetic diversity in a population affects the risk of developing TA-GVHD.

Treatment

Treatment of TA-GVHD has been attempted with a variety of immunosuppressive agents. Unfortunately, the disorder is almost uniformly fatal; only rare cases of successful treatment, many involving stem cell transplant, have been reported. Therefore, emphasis is placed on prevention of the disorder.

Prevention

The only reliable way to prevent TA-GVHD is by irradiation of cellular blood components. AABB *Standards* requires a minimum dose of 25 Gy (2500 cGy) delivered to the central portion of the container and a minimum of 15 Gy (1500 cGy) elsewhere.[14(pp24-25)] AABB *Standards* requires irradiation of cellular blood components when 1) the patient is identified as being at risk of TA-GVHD, 2) the donor is a blood relative of the recipient, and 3) the donor is selected for HLA compatibility by typing or crossmatching.[14(pp40-41)] These standards are minimum requirements for irradiation of cellular blood components, and institutions may choose to administer irradiated components to other categories of patients. (See Table 22-2.)

Posttransfusion Purpura

Presentation

Posttransfusion purpura (PTP) is a relatively uncommon complication of transfusion, and its true incidence is therefore difficult to estimate. Nonetheless, >200 cases have been reported in the literature, and data from the Serious Hazards of Transfusion (SHOT) program in the United Kingdom suggest that the disorder may be more common than previously believed.[81]

Patients typically present with wet purpura and thrombocytopenia within 2 weeks after a transfusion. The thrombocytopenia is often profound, with platelet counts of <10,000/μL.[82] Bleeding from mucous membranes and the gastrointestinal and urinary tract is common. Mortality rates in large case series range up to 16%, primarily due to intracranial hemorrhage.[83]

PTP has most commonly been associated with transfusions of RBCs or whole blood; however, the disorder has also been associated with transfusions of platelets or plasma.

Differential Diagnosis

The differential diagnosis of PTP includes alternative causes of thrombocytopenia, such as autoimmune thrombocytopenic purpura, thrombotic thrombocytopenic purpura, heparin-induced thrombocytopenia, DIC, and drug-induced thrombocytopenia. Although the diagnosis of PTP can be obvious in patients with previously normal platelet counts and no other significant medical abnormalities, it can be a challenge in patients with multiple medical problems. Platelet serology studies may aid in the diagnosis.

Pathophysiology

The pathogenesis of PTP is related to the presence of platelet-specific alloantibodies in a patient who has previously been exposed to platelet antigens via pregnancy or transfusion. The female-to-male ratio of affected patients

TABLE 22-2. Well-Documented Indications for Irradiated Components

Intrauterine transfusions
Prematurity, low birthweight, or erythroblastosis fetalis in newborns
Congenital immunodeficiencies
Hematologic malignancies or solid tumors (neuroblastoma, sarcoma, Hodgkin disease)
Peripheral blood stem cell/marrow transplantation
Components that are crossmatched or HLA matched, or from directed donations (from family members or other related donors)
Fludarabine therapy
Granulocyte components

is 5 to 1. Antibodies against human platelet antigen 1a (HPA-1a), located on glycoprotein II-Ia, are identified in about 70% of PTP cases. Antibodies to HPA-1b, other platelet antigens, and HLA antigens have also been implicated in PTP.[84]

The reason for the concomitant destruction of autologous platelets in this disorder is unknown. The theory that the platelet alloantibody has autoreactivity that develops when a patient is reexposed to a foreign platelet-specific antigen currently has the most support.

Treatment

Because the duration of thrombocytopenia in untreated patients is about 2 weeks, it can be difficult to assess the effectiveness of therapies for PTP. Steroids, whole-blood exchange, and plasma exchange have all been used to treat PTP. The current treatment of choice for PTP is IVIG.[85] Patients respond within 4 days, on average, and some respond within hours.

Prevention

The use of prestorage leukocyte-reduction filters may decrease the incidence of PTP. In the 3 years before the implementation of universal leukocyte reduction in the United Kingdom, there were 10.3 cases of PTP per year, compared to 2.3 cases per year after universal leukocyte reduction (p <0.001).[81]

PTP typically does not recur with subsequent transfusions. However, there are case reports of PTP recurrence. Therefore, for patients with previously documented PTP, efforts should be made to obtain components from antigen-matched donors. Autologous donations and directed donations from antigen-matched donors and family members may also be appropriate. Because PTP has also occurred after transfusions of deglycerolized rejuvenated or washed RBCs, such manipulations are not indicated to prevent recurrence.

Iron Overload

A unit of RBCs contains approximately 200 to 250 mg of iron. Because humans lack a physiologic means to excrete excess iron, persistent increase in iron influx from transfusions can result in iron overload. When the accumulation of iron overwhelms the capacity for safe storage, tissue damage can ensue. As iron accumulates in the reticuloendothelial system, liver, heart, spleen, and endocrine organs, tissue damage leading to heart failure, liver failure, diabetes, and hypothyroidism may occur. Patients who are chronically transfused for diseases such as thalassemia, sickle cell disease, and other chronic anemias are at greatest risk for iron overload. Cumulative doses of as few as 20 or more RBC units are associated with increased morbidity and mortality.[86,87] Preventing the accumulation of toxic iron levels by reducing iron stores through the use of iron chelators or therapeutic phlebotomy can reduce these complications.

FATALITY REPORTING REQUIREMENTS

When the death of a patient results from a reaction to or complication of a transfusion, current regulations require that the fatality be reported to the FDA by the facility that performed the compatibility testing. The director of the Office of Compliance and Biologics Quality at the FDA Center for Biologics Evaluation and Research must be notified as soon as possible, followed by the submission of a written report within 7 days. Table 22-3 lists the contact information for the FDA. The report should contain the pertinent medical record, including laboratory reports, and the autopsy results when available. The patient's underlying illness may make determination of the cause of death difficult. If there is any clinical suspicion that the transfusion may have contributed to the patient's death, that possibility should be investigated. Most transfusion-associated fatalities are caused by acute hemolysis, TRALI, or TACO. Investigations of these cases must attempt to rule out laboratory, transfusion service, or blood administration errors.

TABLE 22-3. How to Contact the FDA[88]

Method	Contact Details
E-mail	fatalities2@fda.hhs.gov
Telephone/voicemail	240-402-9160
Fax	301-595-1304, Attn: CBER Fatality Program Manager
Express mail	US Food and Drug Administration CBER Office of Compliance and Biologics Quality Document Control Center 10903 New Hampshire Avenue WO71, G112 Silver Spring, MD 20993-0002

FDA = Food and Drug Administration; CBER = Center for Biologics Evaluation and Research.

KEY POINTS

1. The blood supply is safer today than at any time in history, but adverse sequelae to transfusion still occur.
2. Many transfusion reactions have signs or symptoms that may be present in more than one type of reaction. Early recognition of the reaction, prompt cessation of the transfusion, and further evaluation are key to the successful resolution of a reaction.
3. Acute intravascular hemolytic reactions are often caused by sample or patient misidentification and are therefore usually preventable.
4. Allergic reactions range from urticaria (hives) to anaphylaxis. Most severe reactions are idiosyncratic and not due to selective protein deficiencies (eg, IgA and haptoglobin).
5. TRALI is often caused by HLA and HNA antibodies in donor components. TRALI is the leading cause of transfusion-related mortality reported to the FDA.
6. Recognition of TRALI requires diagnosis by exclusion. Most patients recover from TRALI with supportive care.
7. TACO can be confused with TRALI because both feature pulmonary edema. TACO should be suspected in patients with positive fluid balance and patients who have difficulty regulating fluid balance; for example, those with congestive heart failure and end-stage renal disease.
8. The most common complications of massive transfusion are hemostatic abnormalities. Each institution should develop its own massive transfusion protocol that takes into account the availability of appropriate laboratory testing.
9. TA-GVHD has a much more acute and severe course than GVHD after marrow or stem cell transplantation. TA-GVHD is fatal in >90% of cases and can be prevented by irradiation of blood components.
10. PTP is a serious but rare complication in which antibodies to human platelet antigens result in destruction of autologous and allogeneic platelets.
11. Iron overload is perhaps the longest-lasting long-term noninfectious complication of transfusion. Chelation and therapeutic phlebotomy are the primary treatments.
12. Recipient fatalities must be reported to the FDA by the compatibility testing facility as soon as possible after a fatal complication of transfusion has been confirmed.

REFERENCES

1. Food and Drug Administration. Fatalities reported to FDA following blood collection and transfusion: Annual summary for fiscal year 2015. Silver Spring, MD: CBER Office of Communication, Outreach, and Development, 2016. [Available at https://www.fda.gov/downloads/BiologicsBloodVaccines/Safety Availability/ReportaProblem/TransfusionDo nationFatalities/UCM518148.pdf (accessed February 7, 2017).]

2. Centers for Disease Control and Prevention. National Healthcare Safety Network manual: Biovigilance Component v2.4 Hemovigilance Module surveillance protocol. Atlanta, GA: Division of Healthcare Quality Promotion, National Center for Emerging and Zoonotic Infectious Diseases, 2017. [Available at https://www.cdc.gov/nhsn/pdfs/biovigilance/bv-hv-protocol-current.pdf (accessed February 28, 2017).]

3. Berseus O, Boman K, Nessen SC, Westerberg LA. Risks of hemolysis due to anti-A and anti-B caused by the transfusion of blood or blood components containing ABO-incompatible plasma. Transfusion 2013;53(Suppl 1):114S-23S.

4. Stowell SR, Winkler AM, Maier CL, et al. Initiation and regulation of complement during hemolytic transfusion reactions. Clin Dev Immunol 2012;2012:307093.

5. Brodsky RA. Complement in hemolytic anemia. Blood 2015;126:2459-65.

6. Hod EA, Cadwell CM, Liepkalns JS, et al. Cytokine storm in a mouse model of IgG-mediated hemolytic transfusion reactions. Blood 2008; 112:891-4.

7. Long AT, Kenne E, Jung R, et al. Contact system revisited: An interface between inflammation, coagulation, and innate immunity. J Thromb Haemost 2016;14:427-37.

8. Vamvakas EC, Blajchman MA. Transfusion-related mortality: The ongoing risks of allogeneic blood transfusion and the available strategies for their prevention. Blood 2009;113: 3406-17.

9. Weinstock C, Mohle R, Dorn C, et al. Successful use of eculizumab for treatment of an acute hemolytic reaction after ABO-incompatible red blood cell transfusion. Transfusion 2015; 55:605-10.

10. Maskens C, Downie H, Wendt A, et al. Hospital-based transfusion error tracking from 2005 to 2010: Identifying the key errors threatening patient transfusion safety. Transfusion 2014;54:66-73; quiz 65.

11. Heddle NM, Fung M, Hervig T, et al. Challenges and opportunities to prevent transfusion errors: A Qualitative Evaluation for Safer Transfusion (QUEST). Transfusion 2012;52: 1687-95.

12. Dunbar NM, Ornstein DL, Dumont LJ. ABO incompatible platelets: Risks versus benefit. Curr Opin Hematol 2012;19:475-9.

13. Hod EA, Brittenham GM, Billote GB, et al. Transfusion of human volunteers with older, stored red blood cells produces extravascular hemolysis and circulating non-transferrin-bound iron. Blood 2011;118:6675-82.

14. Ooley PW, ed. Standards for blood banks and transfusion services. 30th ed. Bethesda, MD: AABB, 2016.

15. Eder AF, Meena-Leist CE, Hapip CA, et al. Clostridium perfringens in apheresis platelets: An unusual contaminant underscores the importance of clinical vigilance for septic transfusion reactions (CME). Transfusion 2014;54:857-62; quiz 6.

16. Brubaker DB. Clinical significance of white cell antibodies in febrile nonhemolytic transfusion reactions. Transfusion 1990;30:733-7.

17. Heddle NM, Klama L, Singer J, et al. The role of the plasma from platelet concentrates in transfusion reactions. N Eng J Med 1994;331: 625-8.

18. King KE, Shirey RS, Thoman SK, et al. Universal leukoreduction decreases the incidence of febrile nonhemolytic transfusion reactions to RBCs. Transfusion 2004;44:25-9.

19. Paglino JC, Pomper GJ, Fisch GS, et al. Reduction of febrile but not allergic reactions to RBCs and platelets after conversion to universal prestorage leukoreduction. Transfusion 2004;44:16-24.

20. Ezidiegwu CN, Lauenstein KJ, Rosales LG, et al. Febrile nonhemolytic transfusion reactions. Management by premedication and cost implications in adult patients. Arch Pathol Lab Med 2004;128:991-5.

21. Heddle NM, Blajchman MA, Meyer RM, et al. A randomized controlled trial comparing the frequency of acute reactions to plasma-removed platelets and prestorage WBC-reduced platelets. Transfusion 2002;42:556-66.

22. Savage WJ, Tobian AA, Fuller AK, et al. Allergic transfusion reactions to platelets are associated more with recipient and donor factors than with product attributes. Transfusion 2011;51:1716-22.

23. Savage WJ, Hamilton RG, Tobian AA, et al. Defining risk factors and presentations of allergic reactions to platelet transfusion. J Allergy Clin Immunol 2014;133:1772-5.e9.

24. Savage WJ, Tobian AA, Savage JH, et al. Transfusion and component characteristics are not associated with allergic transfusion reactions to apheresis platelets. Transfusion 2015;55:296-300.

25. Vyas GN, Fudenberg HH. Isoimmune anti-IgA causing anaphylactoid transfusion reactions. N Engl J Med 1969;280:1073-4.

26. Vyas GN, Holmdahl L, Perkins HA, Fudenberg HH. Serologic specificity of human anti-IgA and its significance in transfusion. Blood 1969; 34:573-81.

27. Sandler SG, Eder AF, Goldman M, Winters JL. The entity of immunoglobulin A-related anaphylactic transfusion reactions is not evidence based. Transfusion 2015;55:199-204.

28. Shimada E, Tadokoro K, Watanabe Y, et al. Anaphylactic transfusion reactions in haptoglobin-deficient patients with IgE and IgG haptoglobin antibodies. Transfusion 2002; 42:766-73.

29. Westhoff CM, Sipherd BD, Wylie DE, Toalson LD. Severe anaphylactic reactions following transfusions of platelets to a patient with anti-Ch. Transfusion 1992;32:576-9.

30. Poisson JL, Riedo FX, AuBuchon JP. Acquired peanut hypersensitivity after transfusion. Transfusion 2014;54:256-7.

31. Kaufman RM, Assmann SF, Triulzi DJ, et al. Transfusion-related adverse events in the Platelet Dose study. Transfusion 2015;55:144-53.

32. Kleinman S, Chan P, Robillard P. Risks associated with transfusion of cellular blood components in Canada. Transfus Med Rev 2003;17:120-62.

33. Kemp SF, Lockey RF, Simons FE. Epinephrine: The drug of choice for anaphylaxis. A statement of the World Allergy Organization. Allergy 2008;63:1061-70.

34. Tobian AA, King KE, Ness PM. Transfusion premedications: A growing practice not based on evidence. Transfusion 2007;47:1089-96.

35. Kiani-Alikhan S, Yong PF, Grosse-Kreul D, et al. Successful desensitization to immunoglob-

ulin A in a case of transfusion-related anaphylaxis. Transfusion 2010;50:1897-901.

36. Popovsky MA, Haley NR. Further characterization of transfusion-related acute lung injury: Demographics, clinical and laboratory features, and morbidity. Immunohematology 2000;16:157-9.

37. Nakagawa M, Toy P. Acute and transient decrease in neutrophil count in transfusion-related acute lung injury: Cases at one hospital. Transfusion 2004;44:1689-94.

38. Bernard GR, Artigas A, Brigham KL, et al. Report of the American-European Consensus conference on acute respiratory distress syndrome: Definitions, mechanisms, relevant outcomes, and clinical trial coordination. Consensus Committee. J Crit Care 1994;9:72-81.

39. Kleinman S, Caulfield T, Chan P, et al. Toward an understanding of transfusion-related acute lung injury: Statement of a consensus panel. Transfusion 2004;44:1774-89.

40. Popovsky MA, Moore SB. Diagnostic and pathogenetic considerations in transfusion-related acute lung injury. Transfusion 1985;25:573-7.

41. Cherry T, Steciuk M, Reddy VV, Marques MB. Transfusion-related acute lung injury: Past, present, and future. Am J Clin Pathol 2008;129:287-97.

42. Toy P, Gajic O, Bacchetti P, et al. Transfusion-related acute lung injury: Incidence and risk factors. Blood 2012;119:1757-67.

43. Silliman CC, Boshkov LK, Mehdizadehkashi Z, et al. Transfusion-related acute lung injury: Epidemiology and a prospective analysis of etiologic factors. Blood 2003;101:454-62.

44. Eder AF, Dy BA, Perez JM, et al. The residual risk of transfusion-related acute lung injury at the American Red Cross (2008-2011): Limitations of a predominantly male-donor plasma mitigation strategy. Transfusion 2013;53:1442-9.

45. Steinberg KP, Hudson LD, Goodman RB, et al. Efficacy and safety of corticosteroids for persistent acute respiratory distress syndrome. N Engl J Med 2006;354:1671-84.

46. Zhou L, Giacherio D, Cooling L, Davenport RD. Use of B-natriuretic peptide as a diagnostic marker in the differential diagnosis of transfusion-associated circulatory overload. Transfusion 2005;45:1056-63.

47. Li G, Daniels CE, Kojicic M, et al. The accuracy of natriuretic peptides (brain natriuretic pep-

tide and N-terminal pro-brain natriuretic) in the differentiation between transfusion-related acute lung injury and transfusion-related circulatory overload in the critically ill. Transfusion 2009;49:13-20.

48. Tobian A, Sokoll L, Tisch D, et al. N-terminal pro-brain natriuretic peptide is a useful diagnostic marker for transfusion-associated circulatory overload. Transfusion 2008;48:1143-50.

49. Clifford L, Jia Q, Yadav H, et al. Characterizing the epidemiology of perioperative transfusion-associated circulatory overload. Anesthesiology 2015;122:21-8.

50. Narick C, Triulzi DJ, Yazer MH. Transfusion-associated circulatory overload after plasma transfusion. Transfusion 2012;52:160-5.

51. Raval JS, Mazepa MA, Russell SL, et al. Passive reporting greatly underestimates the rate of transfusion-associated circulatory overload after platelet transfusion. Vox Sang 2015;108:387-92.

52. Pagano M, Ness P, Chajewski O, et al. Hypotensive transfusion reactions in the era of prestorage leukoreduction. Transfusion 2015;55:1668-74.

53. Li N, Williams L, Zhou Z, Wu Y. Incidence of acute transfusion reactions to platelets in hospitalized pediatric patients based on the US hemovigilance reporting system. Transfusion 2014;54:1666-72.

54. Cyr M, Hume H, Champagne M, et al. Anomaly of the des-Arg9-bradykinin metabolism associated with severe hypotensive reactions during blood transfusions: A preliminary study. Transfusion 1999;39:1084-8.

55. Cugno M, Nussberger J, Biglioli P, et al. Increase of bradykinin in plasma of patients undergoing cardiopulmonary bypass: The importance of lung exclusion. Chest 2001;120:1776-82.

56. Sihler KC, Napolitano LM. Complications of massive transfusion. Chest 2010;137:209-20.

57. Dzik WH, Kirkley SA. Citrate toxicity during massive blood transfusion. Transfus Med Rev 1988;2:76-94.

58. Spinella PC, Holcomb JB. Resuscitation and transfusion principles for traumatic hemorrhagic shock. Blood Rev 2009;23:231-40.

59. Wilson RF, Binkley LE, Sabo FM Jr, et al. Electrolyte and acid-base changes with massive blood transfusions. Am Surg 1992;58:535-44; discussion, 44-5.

60. Strauss RG. RBC storage and avoiding hyperkalemia from transfusions to neonates and infants. Transfusion 2010;50:1862-5.

61. Liu EA, Mannino FL, Lane TA. Prospective, randomized trial of the safety and efficacy of a limited donor exposure transfusion program for premature neonates. J Pediatr 1994;125:92-6.

62. Bansal I, Calhoun BW, Joseph C, et al. A comparative study of reducing the extracellular potassium concentration in red blood cells by washing and by reduction of additive solution. Transfusion 2007;47:248-50.

63. Malone DL, Hess JR, Fingerhut A. Massive transfusion practices around the globe and a suggestion for a common massive transfusion protocol. J Trauma 2006;60:S91-6.

64. Engstrom M, Schott U, Romner B, Reinstrup P. Acidosis impairs the coagulation: A thromboelastographic study. J Trauma 2006;61:624-8.

65. Counts RB, Haisch C, Simon TL, et al. Hemostasis in massively transfused trauma patients. Ann Surg 1979;190:91-9.

66. Murray DJ, Pennell BJ, Weinstein SL, Olson JD. Packed red cells in acute blood loss: Dilutional coagulopathy as a cause of surgical bleeding. Anesth Analg 1995;80:336-42.

67. Harrigan C, Lucas CE, Ledgerwood AM, et al. Serial changes in primary hemostasis after massive transfusion. Surgery 1985;98:836-44.

68. Martini WZ. Coagulopathy by hypothermia and acidosis: Mechanisms of thrombin generation and fibrinogen availability. J Trauma 2009;67:202-8; discussion, 8-9.

69. Collins JA. Recent developments in the area of massive transfusion. World J Surg 1987;11:75-81.

70. Holcomb JB, Tilley BC, Baraniuk S, et al. Transfusion of plasma, platelets, and red blood cells in a 1:1:1 vs a 1:1:2 ratio and mortality in patients with severe trauma: The PROPPR randomized clinical trial. JAMA 2015;313:471-82.

71. Roberts I, Shakur H, Ker K, et al. Antifibrinolytic drugs for acute traumatic injury. Cochrane Database Syst Rev 2012;12:CD004896.

72. O'Quin RJ, Lakshminarayan S. Venous air embolism. Arch Intern Med 1982;142:2173-6.

73. Mirski MA, Lele AV, Fitzsimmons L, Toung TJ. Diagnosis and treatment of vascular air embolism. Anesthesiology 2007;106:164-77.

74. Schonewille H, van de Watering LM, Loomans DS, Brand A. Red blood cell alloantibodies after transfusion: Factors influencing incidence and specificity. Transfusion 2006;46: 250-6.

75. Tormey CA, Stack G. The persistence and evanescence of blood group alloantibodies in men. Transfusion 2009;49:505-12.

76. Vamvakas EC, Pineda AA, Reisner R, et al. The differentiation of delayed hemolytic and delayed serologic transfusion reactions: Incidence and predictors of hemolysis. Transfusion 1995;35:26-32.

77. Schonewille H, van de Watering LM, Brand A. Additional red blood cell alloantibodies after blood transfusions in a nonhematologic alloimmunized patient cohort: Is it time to take precautionary measures? Transfusion 2006;46: 630-5.

78. Ruhl H, Bein G, Sachs UJ. Transfusion-associated graft-versus-host disease. Transfus Med Rev 2009;23:62-71.

79. Klein HG. Transfusion-associated graft-versus-host disease: Less fresh blood and more gray (Gy) for an aging population. Transfusion 2006;46:878-80.

80. Kopolovic I, Ostro J, Tsubota H, et al. A systematic review of transfusion-associated graft-versus-host disease. Blood 2015;126:406-14.

81. Williamson LM, Stainsby D, Jones H, et al. The impact of universal leukodepletion of the blood supply on hemovigilance reports of posttransfusion purpura and transfusion-associated graft-versus-host disease. Transfusion 2007;47:1455-67.

82. Taaning E, Svejgaard A. Post-transfusion purpura: A survey of 12 Danish cases with special reference to immunoglobulin G subclasses of the platelet antibodies. Transfus Med 1994; 4:1-8.

83. Shtalrid M, Shvidel L, Vorst E, et al. Post-transfusion purpura: A challenging diagnosis. Isr Med Assoc J 2006;8:672-4.

84. Hayashi T, Hirayama F. Advances in alloimmune thrombocytopenia: Perspectives on current concepts of human platelet antigens, antibody detection strategies, and genotyping. Blood Transfus 2015;13:380-90.

85. Ziman A, Klapper E, Pepkowitz S, et al. A second case of post-transfusion purpura caused by HPA-5a antibodies: Successful treatment with intravenous immunoglobulin. Vox Sang 2002;83:165-6.

86. Alessandrino EP, Della Porta MG, Bacigalupo A, et al. Prognostic impact of pre-transplantation transfusion history and secondary iron overload in patients with myelodysplastic syndrome undergoing allogeneic stem cell transplantation: A GITMO study. Haematologica 2010;95:476-84.

87. Fung EB, Harmatz P, Milet M, et al. Morbidity and mortality in chronically transfused subjects with thalassemia and sickle cell disease: A report from the multi-center study of iron overload. Am J Hematol 2007;82:255-65.

88. Food and Drug Administration. Guidance for industry: Notifying FDA of fatalities related to blood collection or transfusion. (September 2003) Silver Spring, MD: CBER Office of Communication, Outreach, and Development, 2003. [Available at http://www.fda.gov/BiologicsBloodVaccines/GuidanceCompliance RegulatoryInformation/Guidances/Blood/ucm074947.htm (accessed February 7, 2017).]

Chapter 23

Perinatal Issues in Transfusion Practice

• • •

Meghan Delaney, DO, MPH; Annika M. Svensson, MD, PhD;
Lani Lieberman, MD, MSc

HEMOLYTIC DISEASE OF the fetus and newborn (HDFN), fetal/neonatal alloimmune thrombocytopenia (FNAIT), and immune thrombocytopenia (ITP) affect pregnant women, their fetuses, and newborns. The blood bank and transfusion service play critical roles in supporting the diagnosis and treatment of these conditions, including the appropriate provision of Rh Immune Globulin (RhIG).

HEMOLYTIC DISEASE OF THE FETUS AND NEWBORN

HDFN is the destruction of fetal and newborn red cells by maternal red cell antibodies specific for red cell antigens that are paternally inherited. HDFN can range from a clinically unaffected newborn with a positive direct antiglobulin test (DAT) result to severe anemia and occasionally fetal demise.

Pathophysiology

Maternal immunoglobulin G (IgG) antibody is transported across the placenta into the fetal circulation, where it binds to fetal red cells. The subclasses IgG1 and IgG3 are more efficient in causing hemolysis than IgG2 or IgG4.[1,2] The hemolysis increases hematopoietic drive in a condition known as erythroblastosis fetalis, which can cause liver and spleen enlargement secondary to extramedullary hematopoiesis, and portal hypertension. Liver enlargement can lead to decreased production of albumin, which leads to decreased plasma oncotic pressure, generalized edema, ascites, and effusions known as hydrops fetalis. Severe HDFN can occur as early as 18 to 20 weeks' gestation; severity usually increases in subsequent pregnancies. Untreated, hydrops fetalis, with its associated high-output cardiovascular failure secondary to anemia, can lead to fetal

Meghan Delaney, DO, MPH, Associate Professor, Departments of Laboratory Medicine and Pediatrics (adjunct), University of Washington, and Medical Director, Immunohematology Reference Laboratory, Bloodworks NW, and Medical Director, Transfusion Services, Seattle Children's Hospital, Seattle, Washington; Annika M. Svensson, MD, PhD, Transfusion Medicine Consultant, Denver, Colorado; and Lani Lieberman, MD, MSc, Assistant Professor, Department of Laboratory Medicine and Pathobiology, University of Toronto, and Department of Clinical Pathology, University Health Network, Toronto, Ontario, Canada

L. Lieberman has disclosed financial relationships with Octapharma and Grifols. M. Delaney and A. Svensson have disclosed no conflicts of interest.

death. The destruction of red cells also leads to elevated bilirubin levels. While in utero, the maternal liver clears the bilirubin, preventing the accumulation of bilirubin in the fetus. After birth, the infant's immature liver enzymatic pathways cannot metabolize the unconjugated bilirubin, which can increase to dangerous levels and cause permanent damage to the newborn's brain, known as kernicterus.[3] The maternal antibody decreases in the neonate over 12 weeks, with a half-life of about 25 days. Al-Alaiyan et al found that prolonged (mean postnatal age of 43.3 ± 15.7 days) hyporegenerative anemia (hemoglobin <8 g/dL) is common among Rh-isoimmunized infants, regardless of the use of intravascular intrauterine transfusion (IUT), in term and late-preterm infants.[4]

Because of the widespread prophylactic use of RhIG in industrialized nations, ABO incompatibility is currently the most common cause of HDFN. When present, ABO HDFN is typically clinically mild.[5] If treatment is needed, phototherapy is usually sufficient; neonatal exchange transfusion is uncommonly required. The incidence of ABO HDFN ranges from 1% to 4% depending on the ethnicity of the population. It develops when naturally occurring IgG anti-A and/or -B are transported across the placenta and bind to fetal A and/or B antigens on red cells. A meta-analysis found that maternal IgG anti-A and/or -B titers are significantly associated with the risk of ABO HDFN. Compared with maternal titers of <64, the pooled odds ratio for the risk of ABO HDFN is 2.86 for titers between 128 and 256, and 4.67 for titers of >512. Group O mothers of European or Asian ancestry with group A infants are most commonly affected; in populations of African ancestry, group B infants with group O mothers are most likely to be affected. ABO HDFN rarely leads to severe anemia, because fetal ABO antigens are poorly developed and isohemaglutinins are neutralized by tissue and soluble antigens. If a cord blood DAT result is negative, clinically significant ABO HDFN is unlikely.[5]

Maternal Alloimmunization

The biological characteristics that make certain individuals responsive to immunogenic stimuli have not been clearly elucidated. Females can be alloimmunized to red cell antigens by blood component transfusion, transplantation, or pregnancy. Minor fetomaternal hemorrhage (FMH) occurs spontaneously in a high proportion of women during gestation. The likelihood of FMH increases with gestational age (from 3% in trimester I to 12% and 45% in trimesters II and III, respectively) and is at the highest risk at delivery. After exposure, the maternal immune system must form the red cell antibody and switch its class from IgM to IgG before FMH becomes possibly clinically significant. For all of these reasons, the first pregnancy is rarely affected by HDFN.[6,7] FMH risk factors include abdominal trauma, placenta previa, abruptio placentae, ectopic pregnancy, threatened termination, or fetal death, and procedures such as amniocentesis, fetal blood sampling, intrauterine manipulation, or abortion.

Rh(D) is the most potent immunogenic red cell antigen. It remains the most important cause of HDFN in nations without robust access to prenatal care.[8] As little as 0.1 to 1 mL of D-positive red cells can stimulate alloantibody production.[9] Before RhD immunoprophylaxis, 16% of ABO-compatible, D-negative mothers with D-positive infants became immunized; in contrast, the rate was ≤2% in ABO-incompatible, D-negative mothers, thus demonstrating a partially protective effect of ABO incompatibility.[10,11] The level of hemolysis caused by the presence of anti-K is less than that caused by anti-D, because the K antigen is expressed on the early red cell precursors leading to decreased reticulocytosis and significant anemia.[12] Other antibodies that have been less commonly reported to cause moderate or severe disease include antibodies against E, c, C, k, Kp[a], Kp[b], Ku, Js[a], Js[b], Jk[a], Fy[a], Fy[b], S, s, and U.[13,14] The presence of multiple antibodies may lead to more severe HDFN.[15]

Diagnosis and Monitoring

The diagnosis of HDFN and ongoing laboratory assessments involve the cooperation of the patient, provider, and blood bank/laboratory personnel. The patient's obstetric and transfusion history should be obtained; a previously affected pregnancy alerts the provider of the potential for future problems.[16] During the first prenatal visit, the maternal ABO and Rh type and an antibody detection test to detect IgG-phase antibodies [37 C with antihuman globulin (AHG)] should be performed. If a D-negative woman is negative for anti-D, she is a candidate for RhIG administration to prevent RhD alloimmunization. (See below.) A positive antibody detection test requires antibody identification and titration. Antibodies against the carbohydrate blood groups such as anti-I, -P1, -Le^a, and -Le^b, whether IgM or IgG, may be ignored because these antigens are poorly developed at birth. Treatment of the mother's plasma with dithiothreitol (DTT) preferentially destroys IgM antibodies and can help distinguish IgG from IgM antibodies for cases of anti-M with increasing titer.[17] After identifying a clinically significant red cell antibody, the father should be tested for the corresponding red cell antigen, if possible, to stratify risk of fetal inheritance. Homozygous fathers have a 100% chance of offspring expressing the red cell antigen; heterozygous fathers portend a 50% chance. For women sensitized to RhD, serologic methods cannot readily determine paternal zygosity; when possible, a predicted genotype using paternal DNA testing is indicated.[18] Alternatively, fetal risk stratification can also be accomplished by directly genotyping fetal DNA, either using amniocytes or noninvasively with cell-free fetal DNA (cffDNA) present in a maternal peripheral blood specimen.[19]

During a sensitized pregnancy, monthly maternal antibody titers can be used to deduce if the fetus is the source of ongoing maternal immune stimulation and at risk for clinically significant HDFN. The AABB-recommended method is the use of saline AHG incubated for 60 minutes at 37 C (Method 5-3). Other methods, such as using albumin AHG or gel, may result in higher titers than the recommended method and should be validated with clinical findings and laboratory data to ensure appropriate interpretation. Because of the poor reproducibility of red cell antibody titers, individual blood banks should validate their testing internally and keep previous specimens for subsequent comparison.[20] The critical titer for anti-D (the level below which HDFN and hydrops fetalis are unlikely and no invasive procedures are needed) is 16 in the AHG phase. Because Kell sensitization may lead to hypoproliferative anemia, a titer of 8 is generally accepted as the critical level, although some centers regard any K sensitization as critical. Once a critical titer is reached, Doppler fetal ultrasound of the middle cerebral artery (MCA) is a noninvasive way to assess fetal anemia.[16] Decisions about when to intervene are based on the degree of fetal anemia and gestational age; an increase in the velocity of the end systolic MCA blood flow to >1.5 multiples of the mean (MoM) on the ultrasound denotes moderate to severe anemia. The provider may perform IUT or delivery, depending on the gestational age.[16]

Treatment

In cases of severe anemia, fetal transfusion is indicated to treat the anemia, which will suppress the fetal erythropoiesis and thus the production of red cells with the corresponding antigen for the maternal alloantibody. After birth, neonatal therapies such as phototherapy, simple transfusion, and exchange transfusion may be indicated.

Fetal Transfusion

Red Blood Cell (RBC) units for IUT should be 1) crossmatch compatible with the mother's plasma and lack the implicated antigen(s), 2) irradiated to prevent transfusion-associated graft-vs-host disease (TA-GVHD), 3) cytomegalovirus (CMV) reduced-risk (leukocyte reduced or from a CMV-seronegative donor), and 4) known to lack hemoglobin S to prevent sickling under low oxygen tension. RBC units collected within 5-7 days are preferred, if available, because of the large transfusion volume.

RBC units may be washed or concentrated to a hematocrit of 70%-85%. Most institutions will routinely use group O, D-negative units for IUT, but type-specific (D positive) units may be used if anti-D is not causative and/or if the fetus is known to be D positive. If the maternal antibody is directed at a high-prevalence antigen and no compatible blood is available, the mother's washed or frozen and deglycerolized irradiated red cells can be used.[21] Testing the mother's siblings or searching rare donor registries may provide additional sources of compatible RBC units in these situations.

The volume of blood to be transfused can be calculated by 1) multiplying the ultrasound-estimated fetal weight in grams by the factor 0.14 mL/g to determine the fetal and placental total blood volume, 2) multiplying this amount by the difference in posttransfusion (desired) and pretransfusion hematocrit, and 3) dividing the resulting amount by the hematocrit of the RBC unit to be transfused. For example: with an estimated fetal weight of 1000 g, a desired posttransfusion hematocrit of 40% (0.4), a pretransfusion hematocrit of 15% (0.15), and a measured hematocrit of the RBC unit of 85% (0.85), the volume to transfuse is 41.2 mL, as shown below.

$$[1000 \text{ g} \times 0.14 \text{ mL/g} \times (0.40 - 0.15)]/0.85 = 41.2 \text{ mL}$$

The volume and rate of the transfusion should be adjusted to accommodate the clinical status of the fetus.[22] When delivery is not imminent, IUT is repeated according to the severity of the disease or based on an estimated decline in hematocrit of 1% per day to maintain the fetal hematocrit at about 30%. Transfusion into the peritoneal cavity can be used in cases where the umbilical cord artery cannot be accessed, particularly when IUT is required in early pregnancy. In the absence of severe hydrops fetalis, the outcome of a successful IUT treatment is generally excellent, with a low incidence of neurodevelopmental impairment.[23]

Maternal Treatment

During pregnancy, alternative or adjunctive therapies to IUT include maternal plasma exchange and the administration of intravenous immune globulin (IVIG). Both have been used early in gestation before IUT can be accomplished, or as alternatives to IUT, with the goal of blunting the effect of the maternal antibody.[4] IVIG infusion has been shown to stabilize anti-D titers, and results were best when the procedure was started before 28 weeks' gestation.[24] Plasma exchange can temporarily reduce antibody levels by as much as 75% and has been shown to reduce the risk of fetal death and/or morbidity in a mother with a previous severe course of HDFN.[25] The American Society for Apheresis classifies plasma exchange as a Category III treatment (Chapter 25) based on weak (grade 2C) evidence for this indication.[26]

Neonatal Treatment

After delivery, hemoglobin and bilirubin must be closely monitored. The threat of kernicterus can be high in HDFN, especially in premature neonates.[27] Phototherapy oxidizes elevated unconjugated bilirubin, allowing the oxidation products to be excreted in the urine. For severe jaundice unresponsive to phototherapy, some recommend IVIG with the goal to avoid an exchange transfusion (American Academy of Pediatrics), while other studies question its efficacy, particularly given side effects such as hemolysis and necrotizing enterocolitis.[28-30] In neonates who are unresponsive to phototherapy and IVIG, a double-volume exchange transfusion replaces approximately 85%-90% of the blood volume and removes 50% of the bilirubin. Exchange transfusion (Chapter 24) is generally unnecessary if the infant received IUTs; however, small-volume "top-up" transfusions are generally required until the neonate's erythropoiesis is able to support the hemoglobin requirement and residual maternal antibodies have disappeared.

Prevention

Rh Immune Globulin

D-negative and some variant D-positive females are candidates for RhIG prophylaxis during pregnancy to prevent RhD alloimmunization. RhIG is made from pooled human plasma from individuals either naturally or intentionally immunized to the D antigen; recombinant products are in development. The product contains IgG subtype anti-D. It is available in 300-, 120-, and 50-µg doses. Appropriate ante- and postpartum administration of RhIG reduces the risk of a D-negative mother becoming immunized by a D-positive fetus from about 16% to <0.1%. The American College of Obstetricians and Gynecologists recommends the first dose of RhIG be given at 28 weeks' gestation because 92% of women who develop anti-D during pregnancy do so at or after 28 weeks.[31] Outside of the United States, RhIG prophylactic protocols may differ. RhIG is indicated after any event that increases the risk for FMH. cffDNA obtained from maternal blood samples can identify pregnancies with D-negative fetuses, for which RhIG is not indicated.[32,33] D-negative females who have been previously immunized to the D antigen, D-positive females, and D-negative females whose infants are known to be D negative are not candidates for RhIG. Women with apparent antibodies to both D and C should be investigated to determine the presence of anti-G before determining their candidacy for RhIG. Unless specific reactivity to D is demonstrated, a pregnant D-negative female with anti-G should receive RhIG. Administration of RhIG during pregnancy may produce a positive antibody screening result in the mother, but the anti-D titer is low and thus poses no risk to the fetus. Occasionally, it will cause a positive DAT result in the newborn. The mechanism of action of RhIG has not been completely elucidated. D-positive red cells are opsonized by RhIG and cleared by macrophages in the spleen, which results in cytokine secretion and immunomodulation.[34,35] Similar antigen-specific suppression of the immune response has been observed in a murine system where anti-K prevented immunization against transfused K-positive cells but not against other antigens.[36]

Historically, when serologic weak D testing (Chapter 11) was performed in pregnant women, those found to be positive were classified as D negative and given RhIG.[37] However, in populations of European ancestry, a majority of individuals with the serologic weak D phenotype may not benefit from the administration of RhIG, because they have underlying *RHD* genotypes of weak D types 1, 2, or 3, which have not been reported to form D alloantibody after exposure to conventional D epitopes.[38,39] Genotyping pregnant women with serologic weak D phenotype early in their pregnancy to identify weak D genotypes 1, 2, and 3 allows for more precise administration of RhIG to those who will benefit and avoids unnecessary treatment of women who will not. The practice of weak D genotyping in this population is becoming more standard. If a woman is found to have serologic weak D phenotype for the first time at the time of delivery, *RHD* genotyping often cannot practically be completed before the close of the 72-hour window for RhIG administration. Thus, in such cases, administration of RhIG is the prudent choice, with subsequent *RHD* genotyping for weak D types to guide care for future pregnancies. For women proven to have weak D types 1, 2, or 3, it is also possible to manage them as D-positive for the purpose of transfusion.[38,40,41] Counseling female patients found to have weak D genotypes 1, 2, or 3 about their *RHD* status is important for their peace of mind and to minimize confusion about the need for RhIG in the future. At this time, there is not enough experience to determine if other variant *RHD* genotypes can form anti-D; thus, women with other *RHD* genotypes (not found to have weak D types 1, 2, or 3) should be considered D negative for the purposes of transfusion and RhIG administration.

After delivery of a D-positive infant, D-negative mothers without alloanti-D should receive RhIG. About 10% of the RhIG dose at 28-weeks' gestation will be present in the mother when the infant is delivered at term. (The half-life of IgG is about 25 days.) To determine the correct RhIG dose for postpartum administration, a maternal blood sample is screened for FMH. The rosette screening test is used to detect ≥10 mL fetal red cells (99.5% sensitive test). It is performed by incubating the D-negative maternal blood sample with D antisera and subsequently adding D-positive indicator red cells, which form agglutinates (rosettes) with any fetal D-positive red cells in the maternal sample. The sample is read microscopically and rosettes (agglutinates) are counted. If the screening test result is negative, a standard dose of 300-µg RhIG is given, which is sufficient to prevent immunization by 15 mL of fetal red cells or 30 mL of whole blood. A positive screening test result indicates that the FMH may be ≥30 mL, which requires further quantification. (See below.) Mothers with variant RHD genes can cause false-positive rosette screening results. To quantify the larger FMH volumes, a quantitative assay, such as the Kleihauer-Betke (KB) test or flow-cytometric assessment, is used. Flow cytometry measures fetal hemoglobin and/or D-positive red cells with higher precision than the KB test, although the requirement for rapid turnaround time leads many laboratories to continue using the KB method.[42]

The KB test is an acid elution test that capitalizes on the resistance of fetal hemoglobin to acid treatment (Method 5-2). A thin smear of maternal blood is placed on a slide, treated with acid, rinsed, counterstained, and read microscopically by counting 1000 to 2000 cells to estimate the ratio of fetal to maternal red cells. The maternal red cells appear as pale "ghost" cells, and the fetal red cells are pink. The presence of fetal hemoglobin in the maternal cells, such as in hereditary persistence of fetal hemoglobin or sickle cell disease, can confound the results. The volume of fetal red cells is estimated as follows:

(Fetal cells/total cell counted) × maternal blood volume (mL) = FMH, whole blood (mL)

For example: For 6 fetal cells counted out of 2000 cells, and an estimated maternal blood volume of 5000 mL, the FMH is calculated to be 15 mL. Maternal obesity should be taken

into account when calculating the maternal blood volume and for the route of administration.[43,44]

The estimated FMH volume is used to calculate the dose of RhIG. A 300-µg dose of RhIG will suppress alloimmunization by 30 mL of fetal whole blood. The risk of excessive FMH >30 mL at the time of delivery is approximately 1 in 1250.[7] In the above example, the FMH is 15 mL, so the number of RhIG vials to administer can be calculated as 15 mL/30 mL RhIG/vial = 0.5 vial. Because of the subjective nature of the KB test performance and interpretation, the RhIG dose is rounded up to the next whole number if the number to the right of the decimal point is ≥5 (if <5, it should be rounded down). An additional vial should be added to all calculations. (See Table 23-1.) For example, the dose is calculated as follows: 0.5 vial is rounded up to 1 vial, then 1 extra vial is added, resulting in a total of 2 vials to be administered.

1.6 vials calculated from formula =
  2 (rounded up) + 1 (one vial added) =
  3 vials

1.4 vials calculated from formula =
  1 (rounded down) + 1 (one vial added) =
  2 vials

Postpartum RhIG should be given to the mother within 72 hours of delivery. If prophylaxis is delayed, the American College of Obstetricians and Gynecologists recommends that treatment should still be administered. If the RhD type of the newborn is unknown or undetermined (eg, for a stillborn infant), RhIG should be administered. RhIG can be given by the intramuscular (IM) or intravenous (IV) route. RhIG consists almost entirely of IgG, with only small amounts of other immunoglobulins. Active D immunization has a significant IgM component; thus, new anti-D produced by the mother is often detected in the saline phase and can be completely or partially inactivated by 2-mercaptoethanol or DTT treatment, whereas reactivity derived from RhIG IgG remains. Passively acquired anti-D rarely achieves a titer >4. Risk for anti-D im-

TABLE 23-1. Examples of RhIG Dose Selection Based on Differing Volumes of Fetomaternal Hemorrhage in a 70-kg Female Using Vial Size of 300 μg

% Fetal Cells	Vials to Inject	Dose	
		μg (mcg)	IU
0.3-0.8	2	600	3000
0.9-1.4	3	900	4500
1.5-2.0	4	1200	6000
2.1-2.6	5	1500	7500

Notes:
1. Table reflects calculations based on an example maternal blood volume of 5000 mL.
2. In the United States, 1 vial of 300 μg (1500 IU) is needed for each 15 mL of fetal red cells or 30 mL of fetal whole blood. Other vial sizes are available.

munization despite RhIG administration appears to be affected by increased FMH volumes, although in many cases, a cause cannot be determined.[45]

Red Cell Selection

Primary prevention of HDFN aims to reduce exposure of females of childbearing potential to red cell alloantigens. In life-threatening hemorrhage when uncrossmatched RBCs are needed, it is standard to use D-negative RBCs for such females.[46] In some countries, more extensive matching (K, C, c, E, or e) is undertaken for transfusion to these females.[47] Secondary prevention of HDFN involves administration of RhIG as described above.

Selection of RBC units for IUT constitutes tertiary prevention for HDFN because the mother has already demonstrated immune responsiveness to red cells. Studies have shown that IUT can pose an immunization risk that may affect future pregnancies.[48] Providing RBCs matched for the K, Rh (C, c, E, e), as well as Duffy, Kidd, and S antigens decreased immunization to Duffy, Kidd, and S antigens by 60% when matching between mother and donor was accomplished; however, as the level of match increases, locating appropriate RBC units becomes more difficult.[49]

THROMBOCYTOPENIA

Maternal IgG antibodies to platelets can cross the placenta and cause fetal thrombocytopenia. Two categories of immune thrombocytopenia are recognized, FNAIT and ITP, caused by alloantibodies and autoantibodies, respectively. The diagnostic distinction between them is important for therapy selection.

Fetal and Neonatal Alloimmune Thrombocytopenia

Pathophysiology

FNAIT occurs when the maternal immune system forms platelet-specific antibodies that cross the placenta and destroy fetal platelets. Platelet antigens represent specific polymorphisms in platelet membrane glycoproteins. In people of European ancestry, approximately 80% of FNAIT cases are caused by human platelet antigen HPA-1a, which is present in about 98% of the US population.[50,51] About 10% of cases are caused by anti-HPA-5b, 4% by anti-HPA-1b, 2% by anti-HPA-3a, and 6% by other antibodies (including multiple antibodies).[50] In people of Asian ancestry, HPA-4b is more often implicated than HPA-1a.[52]

The reported incidence of affected pregnancies ranges from 1:350 to 1:1000.[53-55] In 25%

of FNAIT cases, the platelet antibody develops during the first pregnancy and affects the first pregnancy. In fact, the maternal antibody has been detected as early as 17 weeks' gestation, and the fetus may develop thrombocytopenia as early as 20 weeks' gestation. However, FNAIT is often not discovered until birth, when the newborn presents with petechiae, ecchymoses, gastrointestinal bleeding, and/or intracranial hemorrhage (ICH). Clinically significant ICH due to FNAIT occurs in 3 and 10 per 100,000 pregnancies. Eighty percent of the ICHs occur in utero and approximately 50% before 30 weeks gestation.[56] One-third of ICH events are fatal; nonfatal events can be associated with significant neurologic consequences.[57]

Diagnosis

A history of antenatal ICH or FNAIT in a sibling is one of the most important predictors of thrombocytopenia in a subsequent fetus.[58] The mother and father should be typed for platelet antigens, and the mother should be screened for alloantibodies. DNA testing of the father can determine the zygosity of the antigen involved.[31] Direct fetal platelet genotyping can be determined via amniotic fluid (18-20 weeks), chorionic villus material (8-10 weeks), or fetal DNA present in a maternal blood sample.[59,60] Genetic counseling of maternal siblings should be considered.

Treatment

Antenatal intervention should be offered to all mothers of affected fetuses who have had a previous pregnancy with FNAIT. Assessment of the fetus should begin at or before 20 weeks' gestation. Mainstay antenatal treatment includes close monitoring at a high-risk obstetrical center, with or without IVIG, and with or without corticosteroids.[61] The optimal dose, schedule, and gestational age to initiate IVIG is not known; treatment options include weekly doses of 1 or 2 g/kg starting as early as 12 weeks' gestation. The estimated rate of IVIG

effectiveness is nearly 100%, with success defined as absence of ICH.[62]

When a fetus is at risk for FNAIT, an estimate of the likely severity should be made. The most direct method is to assess a platelet count on a fetal blood sample. However, invasive strategies of fetal blood sampling and intrauterine platelet transfusions are associated with a high risk of adverse events, including exsanguination. Some experts recommend that these procedures be abandoned and suggest using noninvasive clues (previous fetus with early in-utero ICH) to assess whether and when to give IVIG earlier instead.[63] If fetal blood sampling and intrauterine platelet transfusions are performed, irradiated, CMV-reduced-risk (safe), antigen-negative platelets should be available at the time of the procedure. Many blood suppliers have identified donors who are negative for HPA-1a. The goal of treatment is to avoid a fetal or neonatal ICH. There is currently no consensus regarding the optimal mode of delivery. Although cesarean section is routinely used to deliver neonates at risk of FNAIT, evidence to support a protective effect is lacking. There is a theoretical risk of increased bleeding with a vaginal delivery. If a neonate will be delivered vaginally, the fetal platelet count should be >50,000/µL, although this information is not always available. Regardless of the route of delivery, irradiated, CMV-reduced-risk, antigen-negative platelets should be available.

After delivery, the greatest risk of infant bleeding is present during the first 96 hours of life.[64,65] The primary goal of management is to prevent or stop bleeding. A platelet count of 50,000 to 100,000/µL is suggested as a transfusion threshold for newborns with bleeding symptoms, and 30,000/µL is suggested as an appropriate threshold in the nonbleeding, asymptomatic newborn.[66,67] For bleeding or thrombocytopenic infants, platelets should be ordered urgently.[68,69] One retrospective study reported that in 89% of cases, platelet counts increased to >40,000/µL; in 59% of cases, a count of >80,000/µL was achieved with random whole-blood-derived platelets.[68] Transfusion of HPA antigen matched or antigen negative platelets, if available, will be effective in

>95% of cases seen in populations of European ancestry.[70] Irradiated maternal platelets are another option, although logistically these can be challenging in terms of collection and component manipulation. The typical platelet nadir occurs within 48 hours of delivery and majority of infants respond within 1 week of life when the maternal antibody has been cleared by the newborn. In rare cases, thrombocytopenia may persist for up to 8-12 weeks.

Immune Thrombocytopenia

Maternal thrombocytopenia of pregnancy is common; 75% of cases are typically secondary to gestational thrombocytopenia; only 4% of cases have an immunologic cause.[71] Infants of mothers with thrombocytopenia from ITP, systemic lupus erythematosus (SLE), or other autoimmune disorders may be thrombocytopenic because of placental transfer of maternal autoantibodies. In general, thrombocytopenia and sequelae in neonates born to mothers with ITP is less severe than in FNAIT: 10% of neonates have platelet counts <50,000/μL, and 5% <20,000/μL; ICH has been found in 0 to 1.5%.[72,73] Although clinically significant bleeding episodes are rare, newborns should be followed closely, as platelet counts often decrease after birth.

There are no high-quality prospective studies to guide management of mother or delivery of the infant; recommendations are based on expert opinion. Older guidelines suggest 1) asymptomatic women do not require treatment until platelet count is <10,000 to 30,000/μL; 2) a platelet count of >50,000/μL is recommended for vaginal delivery; and 3) platelet counts of >80,000/μL are safe for epidural, cesarean section, or spinal procedures.[74,75] More recent American Society of Hematology (ASH) guidelines state that there is no evidence to support the routine use of intrapartum fetal platelet counts and that data are limited to support specific platelet count thresholds that are "safe" in the ante- or peripartum period.[74] For women who require treatment, both IVIG and oral corticosteroids provide a good response. The mode of delivery should be based on obstetrician and patient preference; there is no strong evidence to suggest cesarean section over a vaginal delivery.[76,77] Procedures during labor associated with increased hemorrhagic risk should be avoided.[78]

Although the maternal platelet count is often monitored in ITP, it does not correlate with the newborn's platelet count.[73] The best predictor of severe thrombocytopenia at birth is a previously affected sibling with thrombocytopenia.[79] Fetal blood sampling to determine platelet count is not recommended, because the risk of morbidity and mortality from the procedure is greater than or equal to the risk of severe bleeding in utero or at delivery. However, if fetal sampling is performed, a platelet transfusion should be administered at the same time.[76]

All infants from mothers with a history of an autoimmune disease should have an early postnatal platelet count taken. Intramuscular injections such as vitamin K should be avoided until the platelet count is known to be low. If the platelet count is below the normal range, it should be followed, because the platelet count may fall during the first 3 to 5 days before recovering spontaneously. A head ultrasound is needed to rule out ICH in thrombocytopenic infants. If the platelet count remains <30,000/μL, IVIG (1 g/kg for 2 days, or 0.5 g/kg for 4 days) may be ordered. Neonates with life-threatening hemorrhage should be treated with immediate platelet transfusion and IVIG or IVIG and steroids.[76,77]

Maternal thrombocytopenia secondary to SLE is usually less severe than thrombocytopenia of ITP. If the newborn's platelet count drops to <30,000/μL and/or symptomatic bleeding is noted, the approach to treatment with use of IVIG with or without corticosteroids is similar to the approach for an ITP patient.

KEY POINTS

1. HDFN is caused by maternal red cell antibodies that are specific to a paternal red cell antigen. The maternal IgG antibody is transported across the placenta, where it destroys fetal red cells, causing fetal anemia and hyperbilirubinemia.
2. Some antibodies, such as anti-I, -P1, -Le^a, and -Le^b, can be ignored in pregnancy. The most common clinically significant antibodies that cause HDFN are anti-D, -C, -K, -E, and -c. ABO HDFN is common but usually only causes mild to moderate anemia.
3. Molecular typing of cffDNA can be performed on maternal plasma as early as 12 weeks to determine the fetal red cell antigens. Paternal testing can also predict fetal inheritance. Molecular methods are required to determine paternal *RHD* zygosity.
4. The recommended titer method is saline AHG with 60-minute incubation at 37 C. Other methods, such as those using albumin AHG or gel, may result in higher titers that may lead to misinterpretation by the obstetrician.
5. For IUT, the RBCs should be irradiated, CMV reduced-risk, hemoglobin S negative, group O (in most cases), and <7 days old.
6. The rosette test is a sensitive method for detecting FMH of approximately 10 mL or more. The KB test is used to quantify FMH levels that are >10 mL. Flow cytometry can more precisely measure hemoglobin F and/or D-positive red cells compared to KB testing.
7. The calculated RhIG dose should be rounded up if the number to the right of the decimal point is ≥0.5, or rounded down if the number is <0.5. In either case, an additional vial should be added to the result.
8. In FNAIT, the maternal platelet antibody may develop at around 17 weeks of gestation in the first pregnancy, and fetal thrombocytopenia may develop as early as 20 weeks. Previous pregnancy outcomes predict future outcomes.
9. Irradiated, CMV-reduced-risk, antigen-negative platelets should be given to treat neonatal thrombocytopenia and avoid hemorrhage. Platelets are efficacious.

REFERENCES

1. Firan M, Bawdon R, Radu C, et al. The MHC class I-related receptor, FcRn, plays an essential role in the maternofetal transfer of gamma-globulin in humans. Int Immunol 2001;13:993-1002.
2. Pollock JM, Bowman JM. Anti-Rh(D) IgG subclasses and severity of Rh hemolytic disease of the newborn. Vox Sang 1990;59:176-9.
3. Dennery PA, Seidman DS, Stevenson DK. Neonatal hyperbilirubinemia. N Eng J Med 2001; 344:581-90.
4. al-Alaiyan S, al Omran A. Late hyporegenerative anemia in neonates with rhesus hemolytic disease. J Perinat Med 1999;27:112-15.
5. Herschel M, Karrison T, Wen M, et al. Isoimmunization is unlikely to be the cause of hemolysis in ABO-incompatible but direct antiglobulin test-negative neonates. Pediatrics 2002;110:127-30.
6. Bowman JM, Pollock JM, Penston LE. Fetomaternal transplacental hemorrhage during pregnancy and after delivery. Vox Sang 1986; 51:117-21.
7. Sebring ES, Polesky HF. Fetomaternal hemorrhage: Incidence, risk factors, time of occurrence, and clinical effects. Transfusion 1990; 30:344-57.
8. Bhutani VK, Zipursky A, Blencowe H, et al. Neonatal hyperbilirubinemia and Rhesus disease of the newborn: Incidence and impairment estimates for 2010 at regional and global levels. Pediatr Res 2013;74(Suppl 1):86-100.
9. Bowman JM. The prevention of Rh immunization. Transfus Med Rev 1988;2:129-50.
10. Bowman JM. Controversies in Rh prophylaxis. Who needs Rh immune globulin and when should it be given? Am J Obstet Gynecol 1985; 151:289-94.

11. Ayache S, Herman JH. Prevention of D sensitization after mismatched transfusion of blood components: Toward optimal use of RhIG. Transfusion 2008;48:1990-9.

12. Vaughan JI, Manning M, Warwick RM, et al. Inhibition of erythroid progenitor cells by anti-Kell antibodies in fetal alloimmune anemia. N Eng J Med 1998;338:798-803.

13. Reid ME, Lomas-Francis C, Olsson ML. The blood group antigen factsbook. 3rd ed. San Diego, CA: Academic Press, 2012.

14. Koelewijn JM, Vrijkotte TG, van der Schoot CE, et al. Effect of screening for red cell antibodies, other than anti-D, to detect hemolytic disease of the fetus and newborn: A population study in the Netherlands. Transfusion 2008;48:941.

15. Markham KB, Rossi KQ, Nagaraja HN, O'Shaughnessy RW. Hemolytic disease of the fetus and newborn due to multiple maternal antibodies. Am J Obstet Gynecol 2015;213: 68.e61-5.

16. Moise KJ Jr, Argoti PS. Management and prevention of red cell alloimmunization in pregnancy: A systematic review. Obstet Gynecol 2012;120:1132-9.

17. De Young-Owens A, Kennedy M, Rose RL, et al. Anti-M isoimmunization: Management and outcome at the Ohio State University from 1969 to 1995. Obstet Gynecol 1997;90:962-6.

18. Wagner FF, Flegel WA. RHD gene deletion occurred in the Rhesus box. Blood 2000;95:3662.

19. Finning KM, Martin PG, Soothill PW, Avent ND. Prediction of fetal D status from maternal plasma: Introduction of a new noninvasive fetal RHD genotyping service. Transfusion 2002; 42:1079.

20. Bachegowda LS, Cheng YH, Long T, Shaz BH. Impact of uniform methods on interlaboratory antibody titration variability: Antibody titration and uniform methods. Arch Pathol Lab Med 2017;141:131-8.

21. Biale Y, Dvilansky A. Management of pregnancies with rare blood types. Acta Obstet Gynecol Scand 1982;61:219.

22. Radunovic N, Lockwood CJ, Alvarez M, et al. The severely anemic and hydropic isoimmune fetus: Changes in fetal hematocrit associated with intrauterine death. Obstet Gynecol 1992; 79:390-3.

23. Lindenburg IT, Smits-Wintjens VE, van Klink JM, et al. Long-term neurodevelopmental outcome after intrauterine transfusion for hemolytic disease of the fetus/newborn: The LOTUS

study. Am J Obstet Gynecol 2012;206:141.e141-8.

24. Margulies M, Voto LS, Mathet E, Margulies M. High-dose intravenous IgG for the treatment of severe rhesus alloimmunization. Vox Sang 1991;61:181-9.

25. Ruma MS, Moise KJ Jr, Kim E, et al. Combined plasmapheresis and intravenous immune globulin for the treatment of severe maternal red cell alloimmunization. Am J Obstet Gynecol 2007;196:138.e131-6.

26. Schwartz J, Padmanabhan A, Aqui N, et al. Guidelines on the use of therapeutic apheresis in clinical practice—evidence-based approach from the Writing Committee of the American Society for Apheresis: The seventh special issue. J Clin Apher 2016;31:149-338.

27. Management of hyperbilirubinemia in the newborn infant 35 or more weeks of gestation. Pediatrics 2004;114:297-316.

28. Smits-Wintjens VE, Walther FJ, Rath ME, et al. Intravenous immunoglobulin in neonates with rhesus hemolytic disease: A randomized controlled trial. Pediatrics 2011;127:680-6.

29. Figueras-Aloy J, Rodriguez-Miguelez JM, Iriondo-Sanz M, et al. Intravenous immunoglobulin and necrotizing enterocolitis in newborns with hemolytic disease. Pediatrics 2010;125:139-44.

30. Christensen RD, Ilstrup SJ, Baer VL, Lambert DK. Increased hemolysis after administering intravenous immunoglobulin to a neonate with erythroblastosis fetalis due to Rh hemolytic disease. Transfusion 2015;55:1365-6.

31. ACOG practice bulletin. Prevention of Rh D alloimmunization. Number 4, May 1999 (replaces educational bulletin Number 147, October 1990). Clinical management guidelines for obstetrician-gynecologists. American College of Obstetrics and Gynecology. Int J Gynaecol Obstet 1999;66:63-70.

32. Daniels G, Finning K, Martin P, Massey E. Noninvasive prenatal diagnosis of fetal blood group phenotypes: Current practice and future prospects. Prenat Diagn 2009;29:101-7.

33. Clausen FB. Integration of noninvasive prenatal prediction of fetal blood group into clinical prenatal care. Prenat Diagn 2014;34:409-15.

34. Kumpel BM. On the immunologic basis of Rh immune globulin (anti-D) prophylaxis. Transfusion 2006;46:1652-6.

35. Brinc D, Lazarus AH. Mechanisms of anti-D action in the prevention of hemolytic disease

of the fetus and newborn. Hematology Am Soc Hematol Educ Program 2009:185-91.

36. Stowell SR, Arthur CM, Girard-Pierce KR, et al. Anti-KEL sera prevents alloimmunization to transfused KEL RBCs in a murine model. Haematologica 2015;100:e394-7.

37. Sandler SG, Roseff SD, Domen RE, et al. Policies and procedures related to testing for weak D phenotypes and administration of Rh immune globulin: Results and recommendations related to supplemental questions in the Comprehensive Transfusion Medicine survey of the College of American Pathologists. Arch Pathol Lab Med 2014;138:620-5.

38. Sandler SG, Flegel WA, Westhoff CM, et al. It's time to phase in RHD genotyping for patients with a serologic weak D phenotype. Transfusion 2015;55:680-9.

39. Pham BN, Roussel M, Peyrard T, et al. Anti-D investigations in individuals expressing weak D Type 1 or weak D Type 2: Allo- or autoantibodies? Transfusion 2011;51:2679-85.

40. Kacker S, Vassallo R, Keller MA, et al. Financial implications of RHD genotyping of pregnant women with a serologic weak D phenotype. Transfusion 2015;55:2095-103.

41. Haspel RL, Westhoff CM. How do I manage Rh typing in obstetric patients? Transfusion 2015; 55:470-4.

42. Sandler SG, Delaney M, Gottschall JL. Proficiency tests reveal the need to improve laboratory assays for fetomaternal hemorrhage for Rh immunoprophylaxis. Transfusion 2013; 53:2098-102.

43. Pham HP, Marques MB, Williams LA 3rd. Rhesus Immune Globulin dosing in the obesity epidemic era (letter). Arch Pathol Lab Med 2015;139:1084.

44. Woo EJ, Kaushal M. Rhesus Immunoglobulin dosage and administration in obese individuals (comment). Arch Pathol Lab Med 2017; 141:17.

45. Koelewijn JM, de Haas M, Vrijkotte TG, et al. Risk factors for RhD immunisation despite antenatal and postnatal anti-D prophylaxis. BJOG 2009;116:1307-14.

46. Callum JL, Waters JH, Shaz BH, et al. The AABB recommendations for the Choosing Wisely campaign of the American Board of Internal Medicine. Transfusion 2014;54:2344.

47. Delaney MWA, Wikman A, van de Watering L, et al for the BEST Collaborative. Blood Group Antigen Matching Influence on Gestational Outcomes (AMIGO) study. Transfusion 2017; 57:525-32.

48. Schonewille H, Klumper FJ, van de Watering LM, et al. High additional maternal red cell alloimmunization after Rhesus- and K-matched intrauterine intravascular transfusions for hemolytic disease of the fetus. Am J Obstet Gynecol 2007;196:143.e141.

49. Schonewille H, Prinsen-Zander KJ, Reijnart M, et al. Extended matched intrauterine transfusions reduce maternal Duffy, Kidd, and S antibody formation. Transfusion 2015;55:2912-19.

50. Davoren A, Curtis BR, Aster RH, McFarland JG. Human platelet antigen-specific alloantibodies implicated in 1162 cases of neonatal alloimmune thrombocytopenia. Transfusion 2004;44:1220-5.

51. Blanchette VS, Chen L, de Friedberg ZS, et al. Alloimmunization to the PlA1 platelet antigen: Results of a prospective study. Br J Haematol 1990;74:209-15.

52. Feng ML, Liu DZ, Shen W, et al. Establishment of an HPA-1- to -16-typed platelet donor registry in China. Transfus Med 2006;16:369-74.

53. Turner ML, Bessos H, Fagge T, et al. Prospective epidemiologic study of the outcome and cost-effectiveness of antenatal screening to detect neonatal alloimmune thrombocytopenia due to anti-HPA-1a. Transfusion 2005;45: 1945-56.

54. Bussel JB, Zacharoulis S, Kramer K, et al. Clinical and diagnostic comparison of neonatal alloimmune thrombocytopenia to non-immune cases of thrombocytopenia. Pediatr Blood Cancer 2005;45:176-83.

55. Williamson LM, Hackett G, Rennie J, et al. The natural history of fetomaternal alloimmunization to the platelet-specific antigen HPA-1a (PlA1, Zwa) as determined by antenatal screening. Blood 1998;92:2280-7.

56. Tiller H, Kamphuis MM, Flodmark O, et al. Fetal intracranial haemorrhages caused by fetal and neonatal alloimmune thrombocytopenia: An observational cohort study of 43 cases from an international multicentre registry. BMJ Open 2013;3; pii: e002490; doi: 10.1136/bmj open-2012-002490.

57. Spencer JA, Burrows RF. Feto-maternal alloimmune thrombocytopenia: A literature review and statistical analysis. Aust N Z J Obstet Gynaecol 2001;41:45-55.

58. Bussel JB, Zabusky MR, Berkowitz RL, McFarland JG. Fetal alloimmune thrombocytopenia. N Engl J Med 1997;337:22-6.

59. Le Toriellec E, Chenet C, Kaplan C. Safe fetal platelet genotyping: New developments. Transfusion. 2013;53:1755-62.

60. Scheffer PG, Ait Soussan A, Verhagen OJ, et al. Noninvasive fetal genotyping of human platelet antigen-1a. BJOG 2011;118:1392-5.

61. Arnold DM, Smith JW, Kelton JG. Diagnosis and management of neonatal alloimmune thrombocytopenia. Transfus Med Rev 2008;22:255-67.

62. Kamphuis MM, Oepkes D. Fetal and neonatal alloimmune thrombocytopenia: Prenatal interventions. Prenat Diagn 2011;31:712-19.

63. Winkelhorst D, Murphy MF, Greinacher A, et al. Antenatal management in fetal and neonatal alloimmune thrombocytopenia: A systematic review. Blood 2017;129:1538-47.

64. Peterson JA, McFarland JG, Curtis BR, Aster RH. Neonatal alloimmune thrombocytopenia: Pathogenesis, diagnosis and management. Br J Haematol 2013;161:3-14.

65. Delbos F, Bertrand G, Croisille L, et al. Fetal and neonatal alloimmune thrombocytopenia: Predictive factors of intracranial hemorrhage. Transfusion 2016;56:59-66.

66. Chakravorty S, Roberts I. How I manage neonatal thrombocytopenia. Br J Haematol 2012;156:155-62.

67. Josephson CD, Su LL, Christensen RD, et al. Platelet transfusion practices among neonatologists in the United States and Canada: Results of a survey. Pediatrics 2009;123:278-85.

68. Kiefel V, Bassler D, Kroll H, et al. Antigen-positive platelet transfusion in neonatal alloimmune thrombocytopenia (NAIT). Blood 2006;107:3761-63.

69. Bakchoul T, Bassler D, Heckmann M, et al. Management of infants born with severe neonatal alloimmune thrombocytopenia: The role of platelet transfusions and intravenous immunoglobulin. Transfusion 2014;54:640-5.

70. Blanchette VS, Johnson J, Rand M. The management of alloimmune neonatal thrombocytopenia. Baillieres Best Pract Res Clin Haematol 2000;13:365-90.

71. Kelton JG. Idiopathic thrombocytopenic purpura complicating pregnancy. Blood Rev 2002;16:43-6.

72. Gill KK, Kelton JG. Management of idiopathic thrombocytopenic purpura in pregnancy. Semin Hematol 2000;37:275-89.

73. Webert KE, Mittal R, Sigouin C, et al. A retrospective 11-year analysis of obstetric patients with idiopathic thrombocytopenic purpura. Blood 2003;102:4306-11.

74. Neunert C, Lim W, Crowther M, et al. The American Society of Hematology 2011 evidence-based practice guideline for immune thrombocytopenia. Blood 2011;117:4190-207.

75. Guidelines for the investigation and management of idiopathic thrombocytopenic purpura in adults, children and in pregnancy. Br J Haematol 2003;120:574-96.

76. Birchall JE, Murphy MF, Kaplan C, Kroll H. European collaborative study of the antenatal management of feto-maternal alloimmune thrombocytopenia. Br J Haematol 2003;122:275-88.

77. George JN, Woolf SH, Raskob GE, et al. Idiopathic thrombocytopenic purpura: A practice guideline developed by explicit methods for the American Society of Hematology. Blood 1996;88:3-40.

78. Provan D, Stasi R, Newland AC, et al. International consensus report on the investigation and management of primary immune thrombocytopenia. Blood 2010;115:168.

79. Samuels P, Bussel JB, Braitman LE, et al. Estimation of the risk of thrombocytopenia in the offspring of pregnant women with presumed immune thrombocytopenic purpura. N Engl J Med 1990;323:229-35.

Chapter 24

Neonatal and Pediatric Transfusion Practice

• ● •

Edward C.C. Wong, MD, and Rowena C. Punzalan, MD

TRANSFUSION PRACTICE IN pediatric patients, particularly in neonates, differs from that in adults.[1] The differences are related to physiologic changes occurring during the transition from fetus to adolescent, blood volume, hematologic norms, immune system maturity, and physiologic response to hypovolemia and hypoxia that are variable in this heterogeneous population, contributing to the complexity and intricacies of pediatric transfusion practice. Advances in neonatology now permit the survival of extremely premature infants, and most neonatal transfusions are now given to very low birthweight (VLBW) infants.[2] This chapter discusses neonatal and pediatric transfusion practice during two distinct periods: the newborn period (birth to 4 months), and infancy (after 4 months) through childhood. Transfusion practices relevant to special pediatric populations are also described.

TRANSFUSION IN INFANTS YOUNGER THAN 4 MONTHS

Patients younger than 4 months have small blood/plasma volumes and immature organ system function, which necessitate special approaches to component therapy. This is especially important for VLBW infants (<1500 g) and extremely low-birthweight infants (<1000 g). The mean cord blood hemoglobin level of healthy neonates is 16.9 ± 1.6 g/dL, whereas that of preterm neonates is 15.9 ± 2.4 g/dL. The hemoglobin concentration normally declines during the first few weeks of life, resulting in physiologic anemia of infancy, a condition that is self-limited and usually tolerated without harmful effects in term infants but potentially more worrisome in preterm infants.[3]

The rate of decline in hemoglobin levels is a function of gestational age at birth. At 4 to 8 weeks after birth, hemoglobin decreases to as low as 8.0 g/dL in preterm infants weighing

Edward C.C. Wong, MD, Former Associate Director of Transfusion Medicine, Children's National Health System, and Adjunct Associate Professor, Pediatrics and Pathology, George Washington School of Medicine and Health Sciences, Washington, District of Columbia; and Rowena C. Punzalan, MD, Medical Director, Transfusion Service, BloodCenter of Wisconsin and Children's Hospital of Wisconsin, and Associate Professor, Pediatrics (Hematology), Medical College of Wisconsin, Milwaukee, Wisconsin

E. Wong has disclosed a financial relationship with Comprehensive Care Services and is an employee of Quest Diagnostics Nichols Institute. R. Punzalan has disclosed no conflicts of interest.

1000 to 1500 g, and 7.0 g/dL in neonates weighing <1000 g at birth.[4] The physiologic decrease in hemoglobin concentration is caused by several factors: 1) a decrease in erythropoietin (EPO) that is more prolonged in preterm infants, resulting in diminished red cell production; 2) decreased survival of fetal red cells; and 3) increasing blood volume due to rapid growth. Reduced EPO production results from increased oxygen delivery to tissues because of increased pulmonary blood flow, elevated arterial pO_2 levels, increased red cell 2,3-diphosphoglycerate (2,3-DPG), and increased hemoglobin A levels. The reduction in EPO production is greatest in preterm infants because of persistent liver-based EPO production, which is normally regulated in the more hypoxic in-utero state. Kidney-based EPO production, which is regulated at higher pO_2 levels, does not normally occur until after a term delivery.[5]

Considerations for Transfusion

Body Size and Blood Volume

Full-term newborns have a blood volume of approximately 85 mL/kg; preterm newborns, about 100 mL/kg. Because of the small total blood volumes of preterm infants (≤250 mL),[6] to avoid waste, blood banks must be capable of providing appropriately sized blood components.[7] The vast majority of preterm infants needing transfusions weigh <1.0 kg (28 weeks' gestational age).

Many factors, including iatrogenic blood loss from repeated phlebotomy, can lead to frequent transfusions in sick newborns. Hypovolemia (>10% blood volume) is not tolerated well in newborns because of their limited ability to compensate with increased heart rate. In such situations, the decreased cardiac output (along with increased peripheral vascular resistance to maintain blood pressure) ultimately results in poor tissue perfusion and oxygenation, and metabolic acidosis.[8] As described later in more detail, red cell transfusions are often administered to maintain a target hemoglobin level in certain clinical situations and for symptomatic anemia.[2,9,10]

Erythropoietic Response and Therapy

In contrast to older children and adults, newborns have decreased EPO production in response to hypoxia, likely to prevent polycythemia in the hypoxic intrauterine environment. Most premature infants produce the smallest amount of EPO expected for any degree of anemia.[11,12] As an alternative to transfusion, the use of recombinant human EPO and the longer half-life form darbepoetin has been studied and shown to reduce donor exposures in premature infants and minimize the severity of anemia.[13] However, the reductions in donor exposure and transfusions are small relative to the costs and potential adverse effects of EPO therapy,[14,15] including possible increased severity of retinopathy of prematurity[16] and increased incidence of infantile hemangiomas.[17] As compliance with strict transfusion threshold criteria has increased, clinicians have decreased their phlebotomy rates and draw volumes as well as utilized point-of-care testing in VLBW infants, reducing the rates of iatrogenically induced anemia and the number of transfusions.[18,19] Thus, in most cases, this approach combined with the use of aliquots from a single-donor blood component unit for multiple transfusions achieves the same goal (ie, decreases the use of transfusions and the number of donor exposures) without the need for EPO therapy.

Cold Stress

Hypothermia in the neonate can trigger or exaggerate several responses, including 1) an increase in metabolic rate, 2) hypoglycemia, 3) metabolic acidosis, and 4) potential apneic events that may lead to hypoxia, hypotension, and cardiac arrest.[20] In-line blood warmers are required for all red cell exchange transfusions to combat the effects of hypothermia. A radiant heater should never be used to warm the blood being transfused because of the risk of hemolysis. Furthermore, to prevent hemolysis in neonates undergoing phototherapy, the blood-administration tubing should be positioned to minimize exposure to phototherapy light.[21]

Immunologic Status

Much of the special processing of components for preterm infants and neonates is directly related to their underdeveloped immune function. Unexpected red cell alloantibodies of either IgM or IgG class are rarely produced by the infant during the neonatal period. This lack of red cell alloantibody production is not well understood but has been postulated to be caused by deficient T-helper-cell function, enhanced T-suppressor-cell activity, and poor antigen-presenting-cell function.[22] Because of this poor humoral immunity and the desire to reduce the number of blood draws from a neonate, AABB *Standards for Blood Banks and Transfusion Services (Standards)* allows waiving of repeat ABO group and Rh type testing and repeat antibody screening for the remainder of the neonate's hospitalization or until the neonate reaches 4 months of age, whichever is sooner.[23(p39)] (See "Compatibility Testing" under "RBC Transfusion" below.)

Cellular immune responses are also incompletely developed during this early period and may make infants susceptible to transfusion-associated graft-vs-host disease (TA-GVHD). TA-GVHD has been reported most frequently in newborns with confirmed or suspected congenital immunodeficiency. The majority of TA-GVHD cases reported in nonimmunocompromised infants have occurred after intrauterine transfusion and subsequent postnatal exchange transfusion.[24,25] There have also been rare cases of TA-GVHD associated with extreme prematurity, neonatal alloimmune thrombocytopenia, or extracorporeal membrane oxygenation (ECMO).[24,26] Once an infant develops TA-GVHD, the chance of associated mortality is >90%. TA-GVHD can be prevented by pretransfusion irradiation of cellular blood components[26,27] or possibly by the use of pathogen-reduced components.[28]

Immature Metabolic Pathways

In infants younger than 4 months, large-volume transfusions of reconstituted whole blood or plasma may result in acidosis and/or hypocalcemia because of the immature liver's inability to effectively metabolize citrate. The immature kidneys also contribute to these complications because of lower glomerular filtration rates and concentrating ability than in older infants and children, leading to difficulties in excreting excess potassium, acid, and/or calcium. In addition, in infants <3 days old, parathyroid hormone secretion in response to decreased ionized calcium resulting from citrate exposure during whole blood exchange is blunted in comparison to infants >3 days old.[29]

Potassium. Small-volume, simple transfusions administered slowly have been shown to have little effect on serum potassium concentrations in infants younger than 4 months despite the high potassium levels in the plasma of stored Red Blood Cells (RBCs). In calculating levels of infused potassium, Strauss mathematically determined that transfusion of an aliquot from an RBC unit that is sedimented by gravity (80% hematocrit) and stored in an extended storage medium for 42 days would deliver 2 mL of plasma containing only 0.1 mmol/L of potassium when transfused at 10 mL/kg.[27,30] This amount of potassium is much less than the daily requirement of 2 to 3 mmol/L for a patient weighing 1 kg. It must be stressed that this calculation does not apply to the transfusion of large volumes of RBCs (>20 mL/kg). Serum potassium can rise rapidly in these small patients—particularly during surgery, exchange transfusion, or ECMO—and is dependent on the plasma potassium levels in the blood and manipulation of the blood components.[31,32]

The type of anticoagulant-preservative solution used to store RBCs at collection determines the amount of potassium delivered. For instance, a unit of RBCs preserved in an additive solution (AS)—which involves removal of plasma and addition of additives such as AS-1, AS-3, AS-5, AS-7, or saline-adenine-glucose-mannitol (SAGM)—delivers less extracellular potassium than RBCs stored in citrate-phosphate-dextrose-adenine (CPDA)-1.[27,33] In addition, special component processing, such as irradiation, can potentiate potassium leakage from the red cell membrane. If irradiated components are stored for more than 24 hours, washing may be required to remove the excess potassium before transfusion.[26] There are reports of severe adverse effects, including cardiac arrest and death, in infants who received via central line or intracardiac line either older RBC units or units that had been irradiated (>1 day before transfusion).[34,35] Alternatively, and more practically, several institutions accept AS units for low-volume neonatal transfusions without washing as long as these units do not exceed a certain storage age or time after irradiation.[36]

2,3-DPG. Levels of 2,3-DPG in red cells are known to decline rapidly after 1 to 2 weeks of storage. This deficit does not affect older children and adult recipients negatively because of their ability to replenish the missing 2,3-DPG in vivo and to compensate for hypoxia by increasing their heart rate. Infants younger than 4 months are not able to do this as effectively as a result of their low levels of intracellular 2,3-DPG that reach even lower levels with respiratory distress syndrome or septic shock. Thus, if a large proportion of the neonate's blood volume is composed of transfused 2,3-DPG-depleted blood, the resulting shift in the hemoglobin oxygen dissociation curve further increases oxygen affinity for hemoglobin and reduces oxygen availability to the tissues.[37] However, this shift in the hemoglobin dissociation curve might be minimized by opposing shifts to the curve from decreased pH and increased pCO_2 that is associated with hypoxia.

Therefore, the recommended therapy for newborns requiring red cell exchange is that usually the RBC units selected should be <14 days old, although this practice is variable and dependent on institutional standard operating procedures (SOPs). The medical need for fresh RBC units for small-volume transfusions has not been established, and these transfusions have even been characterized as unnecessary.[2,27,32] Prospective randomized controlled trials to assess the outcomes of longer vs shorter storage times of RBCs have been performed in this population and found that small-volume transfusion comparing older AS-1 or AS-3 units to fresher CPDA units were equivalent in terms of safety and efficacy.[38,39] (See "RBC Age" section below.)

RBC Transfusion

Ill neonates are more likely to receive RBC transfusions than any other patient age group, and RBCs are the component most often transfused during the neonatal period.[2] RBC replacement is considered for sick neonates when approximately 10% of blood volume has been lost or they have symptomatic anemia.

Indications

Several guidelines have been published over the past 15 years regarding the indications for RBC transfusions in neonates.[9,10,40-42] Most of the recommendations are based on experience acquired in clinical practice rather than published evidence. To this end, a critical need exists for clinical studies in this area. Table 24-1 lists the indications from one of these guidelines.[9]

Compatibility Testing

AABB *Standards* allows limited pretransfusion serologic testing for infants younger than 4 months.[23(p39)] Initial patient testing must include ABO and D typing of the patient's red cells and screening for unexpected red cell antibodies using either plasma or serum from the infant or mother. During any hospitalization, crossmatch-compatibility testing and repeat ABO and D typing need not be conducted as long as all of the following criteria are met: 1) the antibody screening result is negative; 2) transfused RBCs are group O, ABO identical, or ABO compatible; and 3) transfused cells are either D negative or the same D type as the patient. Testing the infant's reverse type for anti-A and/or anti-B is not necessary. However, before non-group-O RBCs can be issued, testing of the infant's plasma or serum is required to detect passively acquired maternal anti-A or anti-B and should include antiglobulin phase. If antibody is present, ABO-compatible RBCs must be transfused until the acquired antibody is no longer detected.

If an unexpected non-ABO alloantibody is detected in the infant's or mother's specimen, the infant must be transfused with RBC units

TABLE 24-1. Transfusion Guidelines for RBCs in Infants Younger than 4 Months[9]

1.	Hematocrit <20% with low reticulocyte count and symptomatic anemia (tachycardia, tachypnea, poor feeding).
2.	Hematocrit <30% and any of the following:
a.	On <35% oxygen hood.
b.	On oxygen by nasal cannula.
c.	On continuous positive airway pressure and/or intermittent mandatory ventilation or mechanical ventilation with mean airway pressure <6 cm of water.
d.	With significant tachycardia or tachypnea (heart rate >180 beats/minute for 24 hours, respiratory rate >80 beats/minute for 24 hours).
e.	With significant apnea or bradycardia (>6 episodes in 12 hours or 2 episodes in 24 hours requiring bag and mask ventilation while receiving therapeutic doses of methylxanthines).
f.	With low weight gain (<10 g/day observed over 4 days while receiving ≥100 kcal/kg/day).
3.	Hematocrit <35% and either of the following:
a.	On >35% oxygen hood.
b.	On continuous positive airway pressure/intermittent mandatory ventilation with mean airway pressure ≥6-8 cm of water.
4.	Hematocrit <45% and either of the following:
a.	On extracorporeal membrane oxygenation.
b.	With congenital cyanotic heart disease.

lacking the corresponding antigen(s) or units that are compatible by antiglobulin crossmatch. This regimen should continue until the maternal antibody is no longer detected in the infant's plasma or serum. The policy of the hospital transfusion service determines the frequency for reevaluating the patient's antibodies. Once a negative antibody screening result is obtained, crossmatches and use of antigen-negative blood are no longer required in infants younger than 4 months because of their immature immunologic status.

Multiple observational studies have shown that alloimmunization to red cell antigens is rare during the neonatal period.[22,43,44] For this reason, repeated typing and screening, which are required for adults and children older than 4 months, is unnecessary in younger infants and also contributes to significant iatrogenic blood loss. Also, the transfusion service should avoid transfusing any components that may passively transfer unexpected alloantibodies or ABO-incompatible antibodies to recipients.[45]

Aliquoting for Small-Volume Transfusion

The purpose of creating small-volume aliquots is to limit donor exposures, prevent circulatory overload, and potentially decrease donor-related risks.[38,46-49] Several technical approaches can be used to accomplish these goals and minimize blood wastage.[42]

Small-volume RBC transfusion aliquots are commonly made with a multiple-pack system.[42,50] Quad packs, employed mostly by blood centers, are produced from a single unit of whole blood that is diverted into a primary bag with three integrally attached smaller bags. The plasma is then separated and diverted into one bag during component preparation. The remaining red cells are drawn into the smaller bags as needed for transfusion. Each of the smaller units has the same expiration date as the original unit because the system's original seal has remained intact and a "closed system" is maintained. A hospital transfusion service can then remove (either by heat sealer or metal clips) each aliquot as needed. For hospital transfusion services that do not have a sterile connecting device (Fig 24-1), this method provides three aliquots from a single unit.[42]

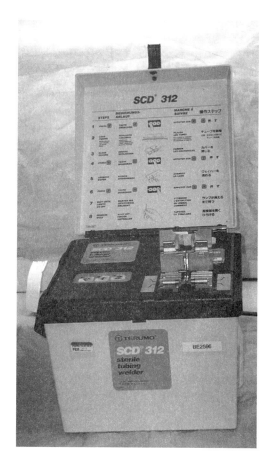

FIGURE 24-1. A sterile tubing welder. (Reproduced with permission from Terumo Medical Corp., Somerset, NJ.)

However, blood components may still be wasted when used in aliquots that are larger than the dose selected for each patient based on body weight.

Hospital transfusion services that have a sterile connecting device have multiple options to produce aliquots, such as transfer packs [eg, PEDI-PAK system (Charter Medical, Ltd, Winston-Salem, NC), Fig 24-2], small-volume bags, or tubing that has integrally attached syringes. Syringe sets (Fig 24-3) offer the greatest accuracy for obtaining the desired volume to be transfused based on volume-per-weight calculations. Some syringe sets have an attached 150-micron in-line filter for use during the aliquoting process so that, when issued by the blood bank, the cells are ready to be placed on a syringe pump without further manipulation of the component at the bedside. This process eliminates the need for the nurse to transfer blood from the pack to a syringe at the bedside for delivery by a syringe pump. Removing this additional step reduces the risk of contamination, mislabeling, or damage to the unit that results in blood loss or spillage.[42]

Reducing donor exposures is readily accomplished by aliquoting, which enables a recipient to receive multiple small-volume transfusions from a single unit until it reaches its expiration date.[39,51] Some hospital transfusion services assign a single unit of RBCs to one or more infants based on their weight.[48-50]

Once an aliquot is produced at either the blood center or hospital blood bank, it must be labeled with the expiration date, and the origin and disposition of each smaller unit must be recorded. Aliquot expiration dates vary from institution to institution, and local SOPs should always be followed.

RBC Additive Solutions

Historically, transfused RBCs for children contained CPDA-1 anticoagulant-preservative solution.[38,39] However, as the use of additive solutions containing adenine and mannitol (Chapter 6) evolved to extend the shelf life of RBCs, many experts began to question their

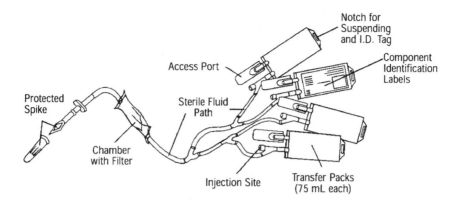

FIGURE 24-2. Diagram of PEDI-PAK. (Reproduced with permission from Charter Medical, Ltd, Winston-Salem, NC.)

safety in neonates. One concern is the dose of adenine in AS and its relation to renal toxicity. Mannitol is a potent diuretic with effects on fluid dynamics that can result in fluctuations in the cerebral blood flow of preterm infants.

Most evidence suggests that small-volume transfusions (up to 15 mL/kg) containing AS are safe for this patient population. Specifically, when AS-1 and AS-3 were compared, no harmful effects were observed in neonates receiving small-volume, simple transfusions.[38,39,51,52] These transfusions were as effective as CPDA-1 RBCs in increasing hemoglobin levels in recipients. Luban and colleagues used theoretical calculations in a variety of clinical settings to demonstrate that red cells preserved in extended storage media present no major risk when used for small-volume transfusions.[53] Because the use of AS extends shelf life, the number of aliquots that can be used from a single RBC unit is increased, which may reduce the overall donor exposure to a patient further.

Because it is unknown whether these theoretical concerns for AS are significant for patients with renal or hepatic insufficiency, some facilities may remove the AS from RBC units, particularly if multiple transfusions from the same unit are expected; however, this is technically challenging and not possible in

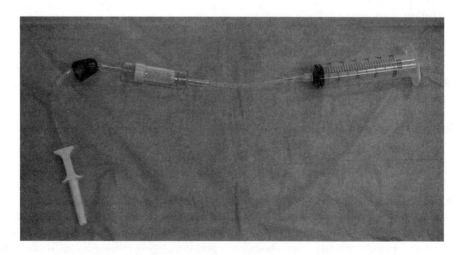

FIGURE 24-3. Syringe with filter. (Reproduced with permission from Charter Medical, Ltd, Winston-Salem, NC.)

many facilities. The safety of AS-preserved RBCs in trauma-related massive transfusions, in extracorporeal membrane oxygenation, cardiac surgery, or exchange transfusions is unknown. Therefore, AS-preserved RBC units should be used with caution in settings where large volumes are being transfused.[52-54]

RBC Age

The age of RBC units and its impact on patient outcomes has become a concern, although clinical confirmation of the basis for this concern is controversial. A randomized controlled trial conducted in Canada, Age of Red Blood Cells in Premature Infants (ARIPI), randomly assigned low-birthweight infants to receive RBCs that were ≤7 days old (mean = 5.1 days; n = 188) or standard-issue RBCs divided into aliquots and stored for 2 to 42 days (mean = 14.6 days; n = 189).[55] The primary composite endpoints included necrotizing enterocolitis (NEC), intraventricular hemorrhage (IVH), and bronchopulmonary dysplasia. The ARIPI trial found no differences in the primary endpoints between infants in the two arms, suggesting that in the study population, the age of RBCs does not affect these common morbidities of prematurity.

ARIPI's external validity has been questioned because of the study's liberal transfusion strategy, use of SAGM units, and average duration of blood storage. These practices do not reflect the transfusion practices, storage solution, and ages of RBCs used in many centers in the United States.[56] Thus, it has not been firmly established if there is a causal relationship between morbidities and transfusion of older RBC units in premature infants.

Transfusion Thresholds for RBCs

In neonates, symptomatic anemia is the major indication for simple transfusion. Specifically, a venous hemoglobin of <13 g/dL in the first 24 hours of life necessitates consideration of RBC transfusion.[9,10,40] RBC transfusions are also considered when approximately 10% of a sick neonate's blood volume has been removed or lost. When 10 mL/kg of RBCs with a hematocrit of >80% (achieved by allowing an RBC unit to sediment by gravity undisturbed with aliquot ports on the bottom) is transfused, the expected increase in hemoglobin concentration in a neonate is approximately 3 g/dL. A similar volume of RBCs with AS usually has a hematocrit of 65%, and its transfusion results in a projected posttransfusion hemoglobin increase of 2 g/dL. (See Table 24-2 for blood component dosing recommendations and the expected results.[57])

Two randomized controlled trials have compared the outcomes of restrictive (hemoglobin = 7 g/dL) vs liberal (hemoglobin = 10 g/dL) RBC transfusion thresholds in VLBW infants. The Iowa trial revealed a lower rate of transfusion events (3.3 vs 5.2; p = 0.025) with the restrictive compared to the liberal strategy.[58] However, rates of periventricular leukomalacia and death were higher in the restrictive arm. The Premature Infants in Need of Transfusion (PINT) study from Canada found no significant difference between the two arms, which had similar thresholds as the Iowa study, in the composite endpoint of death or bronchopulmonary dysplasia, retinopathy of prematurity (stage >3), or brain injury (periventricular leukomalacia, intracranial hemorrhage Grade 4, or ventriculomegaly).[59] The follow-up of the PINT study revealed that at 18 to 24 months after birth, infants in the restrictive arm had more cognitive delay than those in the liberal arm.[60] On the other hand, follow-up studies on the patients in the Iowa trial showed decreased brain structure and function at ages 7 to 10 years in the liberal arm, suggesting an opposite effect in long-term neurocognitive outcomes.[61,62]

The contradictory findings of these studies make it unclear whether a restrictive or liberal RBC transfusion strategy should be adopted in this population. The Transfusion of Premature Infants Study (TOPS), currently being conducted in the United States, looks at whether death and neurodevelopmental outcome at 22-26 months corrected age is less common among premature infants transfused with high hemoglobin thresholds.[63]

TABLE 24-2.   Blood Components and Dosing of Small Volumes in Neonatal and Pediatric Patients[57]

Component	Dose	Expected Increment
Red Blood Cells	10-15 mL/kg	Hemoglobin increase: 2-3 g/dL*
Fresh Frozen Plasma	10-15 mL/kg	15%-20% rise in factor levels (assuming 100% recovery)
Platelets [whole-blood-derived (WBD) or apheresis]	5-10 mL/kg or 1 WBD unit/10 kg (patients ≥10 kg)	50,000/μL rise in platelet count (assuming 100% recovery)[†]
Cryoprecipitated AHF	1-2 units/10 kg	60-100 mg/dL rise in fibrinogen (assuming 100% recovery)

*Dependent on anticoagulant-preservative solution, with 3 g/dL increment for CPD and CPDA-1, and 2 g/dL for AS-1, AS-3, AS-5, AS-7, and SAGM.
[†]Assumes ≥5.5 × 10¹⁰ platelets in 50 mL of plasma (WBD) and ≥3.0 × 10¹¹ platelets in 250 to 300 mL plasma (apheresis).
CPD = citrate-phosphate-dextrose; CPDA-1 = citrate-phosphate-dextrose-adenine-1; AS = additive solution; SAGM = saline-adenine-glucose-mannitol; AHF = antihemophilic factor.

Exchange Transfusion

The most common indication for exchange transfusion in neonates is hyperbilirubinemia. Occasionally, it is used to eliminate toxins, drugs, or chemicals administered to the mother near the time of delivery. Exchange transfusion is also used when toxic doses have been administered to the infant or accumulate at high levels in the infant as a result of prematurity and/or an inborn error of metabolism.[64,65]

Physiology

In neonates, excessively high levels of unconjugated bilirubin may cross the blood-brain barrier, concentrate in the basal ganglia and cerebellum and cause irreversible damage, known as kernicterus. Infants are susceptible to hyperbilirubinemia because their immature liver conjugates bilirubin poorly and because their incompletely developed blood-brain barrier allows bilirubin transit. Phototherapy (blue/green light in the range of 460-490 nm, which converts unconjugated bilirubin into a water-soluble isomer, aiding excretion) is the current treatment of choice for hyperbilirubinemia; exchange transfusion is reserved for patients who fail phototherapy.[66]

Two critical objectives of exchange transfusion are the removal of unconjugated bilirubin and maximization of albumin binding of residual bilirubin. In addition, in antibody-mediated hemolytic processes, exchange transfusion removes both free antibody and antibody-coated red cells, replacing these with antigen-negative red cells.

Exchange transfusion needs to be performed before the development of kernicterus. In full-term infants, kernicterus rarely develops at bilirubin levels <25 mg/dL. However, in sick VLBW infants, kernicterus can occur at bilirubin levels as low as 8 to 12 mg/dL.[67]

A double-volume exchange transfusion (two 85-mL/kg transfusions for full-term infants and two 100-mL/kg transfusions for VLBW infants) removes approximately 70% to 90% of circulating red cells and approximately 50% of total bilirubin.[68] After the first exchange transfusion, bilirubin may reequilibrate between extravascular tissue and plasma, which may necessitate another exchange transfusion.

Component Choice

Typically, RBCs are resuspended in ABO-compatible thawed Fresh Frozen Plasma (FFP) for an exchange transfusion. No single method of combining components has been shown to be superior to another. Most often, RBCs <5 to 7 days old and stored in CPDA-1 are used to avoid high levels of potassium and to maximize red cell survival.[69] When using AS-RBC units, some blood banks elect to remove the additive-containing plasma to reduce the volume transfused.

Most transfusion services provide RBC units that are hemoglobin S negative, cytomegalovirus (CMV) reduced-risk (leukocyte reduced and/or CMV seronegative), and irradiated. Irradiation should be performed just before the exchange to prevent potentiation of the potassium storage lesion. If units are not irradiated immediately before use, some experts recommend washing or removing the supernatant of red cells that have been irradiated to avoid the complications of hyperkalemic cardiac arrhythmias.[70]

The glucose load administered during exchange transfusion can be high in some cases, which stimulates the infant's pancreas to release insulin and results in rebound hypoglycemia.[71] Therefore, infant plasma glucose levels should be monitored during the first few hours following exchange transfusion. Because resuspended RBCs do not include platelets, the platelet count should be assessed after completion of the exchange transfusion.

A double-volume exchange transfusion in neonates rarely necessitates the infusion of >1 RBC unit. The unit's hematocrit should be approximately 45% to 60%, and the unit should have sufficient plasma (based on estimated blood volume) to provide clotting factors.[70] If the neonate's condition requires a higher postexchange transfusion hematocrit, a small-volume RBC transfusion may be given or a unit with a higher hematocrit can be used for the initial exchange transfusion. The reconstituted blood should be well mixed to sustain the intended hematocrit throughout the exchange. The infant's hematocrit and bilirubin can be measured by removing the last aliquot of the exchange unit.

Vascular Access

Umbilical venous catheters are used for exchange transfusions in preterm and full-term infants just after birth. If umbilical venous catheters are not available, small saphenous catheters may be used. Two exchange-transfusion techniques are commonly employed: isovolumetric and manual push-pull. In isovolumetric exchange transfusion, two catheters of identical size provide vascular access. The catheters allow simultaneous withdrawal and infusion of blood and are regulated by a single peristaltic pump. The umbilical vein is typically used for infusion, and the umbilical artery is used for withdrawal. The manual push-pull technique uses a single vascular access portal with a three-way stopcock attached to the unit of blood, the patient, and a graduated discard container. A standard filter and in-line blood warmer are recommended.

With both techniques, the absolute maximum volume of each withdrawal and infusion depend on the infant's body weight and hemodynamic status. Usually, no more than 5 mL/kg body weight or 5% of the infant's blood volume is removed and replaced during a 3- to 5-minute cycle.[69] The exchange transfusion should not be performed rapidly because sudden hemodynamic changes may affect cerebral blood flow and shift intracranial pressure, contributing to IVH.[72] A total double-volume exchange transfusion typically takes 90 to 120 minutes.[69]

Platelet Transfusion

Mild-to-moderate thrombocytopenia (platelet count <150,000/μL) is the most common hemostatic abnormality in ill preterm and full-term infants, affecting approximately 20% of infants in neonatal intensive care units (ICUs).[73] The most common cause is increased destruction of platelets that is generally associated with a variety of self-limited conditions.[74] Other causes of thrombocytopenia include impaired platelet production, abnormal platelet distribution, and/or platelet dilution secondary to massive transfusion. In rare instances, thrombocytopenia may be the result of in-utero destruction associated with maternal alloimmunization to paternally inherited platelet antigens. (See Chapter 23.)

Indications

Most platelet transfusions in preterm and full-term infants are performed for platelet counts <50,000/μL to treat active bleeding or prevent occurrence or extension of IVH.[75,76]

Prophylactic platelet transfusions in this population are controversial.[77,78] (See Table 24-3 for transfusion indications and thresholds.) Unlike adult patients who rarely have severe bleeding complications until platelet counts decline to <10,000/μL, preterm infants with other complicating illnesses may bleed at higher platelet counts.[75] This increased risk may be attributable to 1) lower concentrations of plasma coagulation factors, 2) circulation of an anticoagulant that potentiates thrombin inhibition, 3) intrinsic or extrinsic platelet dysfunction/hyperreactivity, or 4) increased vascular fragility.

A severe complication of prematurity is IVH, which occurs in approximately 40% of preterm neonates in the first 72 hours after birth. Although prophylactic platelet transfusions may increase platelet counts and shorten bleeding times, this approach has not been shown to reduce the incidence of IVH, and the severity of thrombocytopenia appears to be independent of the risk of IVH Grade >2.[79] Hence, the use of platelets in this situation and the appropriate platelet dose remain controversial.[80] Thus, although posttransfusion platelet counts at 15 to 60 minutes after transfusion can help evaluate platelet survival, these counts are not necessarily a good predictor of hemostatic efficacy.

The current Platelets for Neonatal Transfusion study (Study 2) aims to compare mortality and major bleeding in premature neonates who are randomly assigned to receive platelet transfusion at thresholds of

TABLE 24-3. Transfusion Guidelines for Platelets in Neonates and Older Children[9,10]

With Thrombocytopenia
1. Platelet count <10,000/μL with failure of platelet production.
2. Platelet count <30,000/μL in neonate with failure of platelet production.
3. Platelet count <50,000/μL in stable premature infant:
a. With active bleeding, or
b. Before an invasive procedure, with failure of platelet production.
4. Platelet count <100,000/μL in sick premature infant:
a. With active bleeding, or
b. Before an invasive procedure in patient with DIC.
Without Thrombocytopenia
1. Active bleeding in association with qualitative platelet defect.
2. Unexplained excessive bleeding in a patient undergoing cardiopulmonary bypass.
3. Patient undergoing ECMO with:
a. A platelet count of <100,000/μL, or
b. Higher platelet counts and bleeding.

DIC = disseminated intravascular coagulation; ECMO = extracorporeal membrane oxygenation.

25,000/μL vs 50,000/μL and may provide evidence for use of a lower platelet threshold in these patients.[81]

Components and Dose

The use of whole-blood-derived platelets at doses of 5 to 10 mL/kg body weight have been demonstrated to raise the platelet count of an average full-term newborn by 50,000 to 100,000/μL, depending on the concentration of the platelet component used.[30,73] A similar dosing regimen is typically used with apheresis platelets.

When possible, the platelet component should be ABO group-specific/compatible and should not contain clinically significant red cell antibodies. Transfusion of ABO-incompatible plasma should be avoided in children, and especially in infants, because of their small blood and plasma volumes.[45] If it becomes necessary to administer ABO-incompatible platelets in an infant, plasma may be removed either by volume reduction or washing with saline resuspension. (Please refer to local protocols.) However, routine centrifugation to remove plasma from the platelets should be avoided because it has been shown to decrease the posttransfuion platelet count increment.[82]

In addition, when platelets are stored in a syringe, the pH has been shown to decrease rapidly, a potential problem for an already ill and acidotic recipient.[83,84] Therefore, when volume reduction in an open system is used and the component is placed in a syringe, the processing should be performed as close to the time of issuance as possible, and the component should be infused within 4 hours of processing.

Plasma Transfusion

In neonates, low levels of vitamin K-dependent factors (Factors II, VII, IX, and X) and contact factors (Factor XI, Factor XII, prekallikrein, and high-molecular-weight kininogen) contribute to altered coagulation test results.[85,86] (See Table 24-4.) The naturally occurring anticoagulants (proteins C and S

TABLE 24-4. Screening Laboratory Tests for Hemostasis: Neonates vs Adults*

	Preterm Neonates vs Full-Term Neonates	Neonates vs Older Children/Adults	Approximate Age Adult Values Are Reached[†]
aPTT	Longer	Longer	16 years
Prothrombin time	Longer	Same or longer	16 years
Thrombin time	Longer	Same or longer	5 years
Bleeding time	Longer[‡]	Shorter	1 month
PFA-100	Longer[‡]	Shorter	1 month
ROTEM/TEG			
Clotting time	Same	Shorter	3 months
Clot formation time	Same	Shorter	3 months
Maximal clot firmness	Stronger	Stronger	3 months

*Modified with permission from Revel-Vilk.[87]

[†]Maximum age reported.

[‡]In samples drawn in the first 7 to 10 days of life.

aPTT = activated partial thromboplastin time; PFA = platelet function analyzer; ROTEM = rotating thromboelastometry; TEG = thromboelastography.

and antithrombin) are also decreased.[86] In spite of these issues, the procoagulant and anticoagulant systems are usually in balance in healthy newborns, so spontaneous bleeding and thrombosis are rare.[87] (See Table 24-4.) However, the reserve capacity for both systems is limited. Therefore, serious bleeding, and less commonly, thrombosis, may occur in sick premature infants during the first week of life. Cryoprecipitate and FFP are transfused to treat bleeding or clotting complications, such as disseminated intravascular coagulation (DIC).[78,88]

Plasma

FFP is frequently used to replace coagulation factors in preterm and full-term infants with hemorrhage or before surgery, particularly if multiple factor deficiencies are present, such as in hemorrhagic disease of the newborn due to vitamin K deficiency. (See Table 24-5.) It is occasionally used to replace anticoagulant factors when anticoagulation is contraindicated in infants with life-threatening thrombosis. The usual dose of FFP is 10 to 15 mL/kg, which is expected to increase all factor activity levels by 15%-20% unless there is a marked consumptive coagulopathy.[73,78] The evidence for use of plasma to correct the coagulopathy without bleeding is weak.[78,88]

To limit donor exposure for each recipient while minimizing plasma wastage, blood can be collected into a system with multiple,

TABLE 24-5. Transfusion Guidelines for Plasma Products in Neonates and Older Children[9,10]

Fresh Frozen Plasma (FFP)
1   Support during treatment of disseminated intravascular dissemination.
2.   Replacement therapy:
a.   When specific factor concentrates are not available, including, but not limited to, antithrombin; protein C or S; and Factor II, Factor V, Factor X, and Factor XI.
b.   During therapeutic plasma exchange when FFP is indicated (cryopoor plasma, plasma from which the cryoprecipitate has been removed).
3.   Reversal of warfarin in an emergency situation may also be an alternative, such as before an invasive procedure with active bleeding.
Note: FFP is not indicated for volume expansion or enhancement of wound healing.
Cryoprecipitated AHF
1.   Hypofibrinogenemia or dysfibrinogenemia with active bleeding.
2.   Hypofibrinogenemia or dysfibrinogenemia while undergoing an invasive procedure.
3.   Factor XIII deficiency with active bleeding or while undergoing an invasive procedure in the absence of Factor XIII concentrate.
4.   Limited directed-donor cryoprecipitate for bleeding episodes in small children with hemophilia A (when recombinant and plasma-derived Factor VIII products are not available).
5.   In the preparation of fibrin sealant.
6.   Von Willebrand disease with active bleeding, but only when both of the following are true:
a.   Deamino-D-arginine vasopressin (DDAVP) is contraindicated, not available, or does not elicit response.
b.   Virus-inactivated plasma-derived Factor VIII concentrate (which contains von Willebrand factor) or von Willebrand recombinant concentrate is not available.

integrally attached bags that create ready-to-freeze aliquots.[69] Once thawed, the aliquots can be subdivided further for several patients if they can be used within a 24-hour period. In some institutions, after the initial 24-hour period, the plasma is relabeled as Thawed Plasma and is considered an acceptable substitute that can be used over the next 4 days. (See Chapter 6.)

FFP for infants must be ABO compatible and free of clinically significant antibodies. Transfused antibodies can reach high concentrations in infants and children with very small plasma volumes. A common practice at some institutions is to use group AB FFP because a single unit can provide multiple small-volume doses for several neonates.

Cryoprecipitated Antihemophilic Factor

Cryoprecipitate transfusions are primarily used to treat conditions resulting from decreased or dysfunctional fibrinogen (congenital or acquired), or Factor XIII deficiency if Factor XIII concentrate (eg, Corifact) is not available. Cryoprecipitate is usually given in conjunction with platelets and FFP to treat DIC in newborns. Typically, 1 unit is sufficient to achieve hemostatic levels in an infant.

ABO-compatible cryoprecipitate is preferred because transfusion of a large volume of ABO-incompatible cryoprecipitate may result in a positive direct antiglobulin test result and, in very rare cases, mild hemolysis.[89,90]

Cryoprecipitate transfusion is not recommended for patients with Factor VIII deficiency because the standard therapy is to treat this condition with recombinant or virus-inactivated, monoclonal-antibody-purified, plasma-derived Factor VIII products.[91,92] Furthermore, cryoprecipitate should be used only to treat von Willebrand disease if plasma-derived, virus-inactivated concentrates or recombinant products containing von Willebrand factor are not available.[92] Recombinant von Willebrand factor recently became available but has not been studied in neonates. See Table 24-5 for other guidelines regarding cryoprecipitate use.[73]

Granulocyte Transfusion

Indications

The role of granulocyte transfusion for sepsis in neonates is unclear, and this treatment is rarely used, although dose appears to correlate with efficacy. It is important to establish the following factors before the transfusion of granulocytes: 1) evidence of bacterial or fungal septicemia; 2) absolute neutrophil count $<500/\mu L$, chronic granulomatous disease, or leuko-cyte adhesion deficiency; and 3) diminishing storage pool (such that 7% of nucleated cells in the marrow are granulocytes that are metamyelocytes or more mature).[93,94]

Components and Dose

Granulocyte concentrates are produced by standard apheresis techniques or by pooling buffy coats from whole blood. A typical dose for infants is 10 to 15 mL/kg body weight, which is approximately 1×10^9 to 2×10^9 polymorphonuclear cells/kg.[9,93] Treatment is usually administered daily until an adequate neutrophil count is maintained and/or the patient shows clinical improvement.

Granulocytes must be irradiated, given that recipients are neonates with immature T-cell function and they are at increased risk for TA-GVHD, and obtained from CMV-seronegative donors to prevent virus transmission if the recipient is CMV seronegative.[23(p40)] Granulocytes must also be ABO compatible with the red cells of the recipient infant because of the significant red cell content in these components.[23(p37)] Many institutions also provide D-compatible components to decrease Rh alloimmunization.

Transfusion Administration

Vascular Access

Vascular access is the most difficult aspect of transfusion administration in patients younger than 4 months, particularly in preterm infants who require long-term or continuous intravenous infusions. The umbilical vein is most frequently cannulated after birth to facilitate administration of fluids and transfusions and to monitor central venous pressure. Vascular catheters (24-gauge) and small needles (25-gauge) generally can be safely used for RBC transfusions without causing hemolysis if constant flow rates are applied. The outcomes of transfusions using smaller-gauge needles and catheters or intra-osseous catheters in neonates have not been evaluated.

Filters and Transfusion Sets

For standard filter requirements, see Chapter 18.

The plastic tubing in the administration sets can add a significant amount of dead-space volume to the transfusion and may need to be accounted for when preparing a transfusion dose. Pediatric infusion sets created for platelets and other small-volume components have less dead space than standard sets. When using normal saline (NS) to flush blood components into the patient, ceasing the flush before the NS reaches the patient may decrease the risk of dilution.

Administration Rates

The rate of blood component administration is dictated by the clinical needs of the pediatric patient. Despite concerns from neonatologists that rapid blood infusion rates may adversely affect intravascular volume and electrolyte levels, an increased risk of IVH in these small and fragile patients has not been clearly demonstrated. Therefore, administering a simple transfusion over 2 to 4 hours is adequate in nonemergent situations. However, in states of shock or severe bleeding, a rapid infusion is often required.

Unique Therapies and Situations in Neonates

Polycythemia

Neonatal polycythemia is defined as venous hematocrit >65% or hemoglobin >22 g/dL at any time during the first week after birth. Approximately 5% of all newborns develop polycythemia, and this risk may be higher in neonates who are small for their gestational age and infants of diabetic mothers. Once the hematocrit rises above 65%, viscosity increases and oxygen transport decreases. However, in neonates, the exponential rise in viscosity can occur at a hematocrit as low as 40%.[95] Congestive heart failure can result because infants have limited capability to increase their cardiac output to compensate for hyperviscosity. Central nervous system abnormalities, pulmonary and renal failure, and NEC can occur from the resultant decreased blood flow.

A partial exchange is used to normalize the hematocrit to between 55% and 60% and improve tissue perfusion while maintaining blood volume. This exchange is accomplished by removing whole blood and replacing it with normal saline or other crystalloid solutions. Plasma is not used to replace whole blood because NEC has been reported as a complication of plasma transfusion.[92]

The formula below can be used to approximate the volume of replacement fluid required and the volume of whole blood that must be withdrawn for the partial exchange:

$$\text{Volume of replacement fluid} = \frac{(\text{Blood volume}) \times (\text{Observed Hct} - \text{Desired Hct})}{\text{Observed Hct}}$$

Extracorporeal Membrane Oxygenation

ECMO is a prolonged treatment whereby blood is removed from the patient's venous circulation, circulated through a machine to remove CO_2 and replenish O_2, and then returned to the patient. In neonates and children, ECMO has become a lifesaving treatment for meconium aspiration syndrome, persistent pulmonary hypertension of the newborn, congenital diaphragmatic hernia, and respiratory failure due to sepsis. It is also used for postoperative support following cardiac surgery. Because the standardized guidelines for transfusion practice in ECMO have not been established, centers typically establish their own criteria. Table 24-6 provides some guidelines for ECMO.[96]

Bleeding complications are frequent during ECMO treatment and are usually multifactorial. Causes include 1) systemic heparinization, 2) platelet dysfunction, 3) thrombocytopenia, 4) other coagulation defects, and/or 5) the nonendothelial ECMO circuit. Hospital blood banks and transfusion services must be in close communication with the ECMO staff and observe local protocols to ensure safe, efficient, and consistent care. Thrombotic complications are also common.

ECMO initiation typically requires 1 to 2 units of ABO and Rh group-compatible and crossmatch-compatible RBCs for blood priming. In addition, a single unit of group-compatible FFP should be allocated to the ECMO patient. RBC units are usually negative for hemoglobin S, relatively fresh (<5 to 7 days old), irradiated (many patients requiring ECMO are neonates and/or potential transplant recipients), and CMV seronegative and/or leukocyte reduced.[70] Because the ECMO circuit consumes platelets, higher platelet counts are often maintained. However, there are no evidence-based guidelines for transfusion to patients on ECMO.

Necrotizing Enterocolitis

NEC, a serious condition in neonates, is characterized by ischemic necrosis of the intestinal mucosa, associated with inflammation, invasion of enteric-gas-forming organisms, and dissection of gas into the abdominal cavity. Small studies have suggested the possibility of RBC transfusion as an independent risk factor for development of NEC in neonates, and a meta-analysis showed an increased risk of NEC (odds ratio = 2) in transfused neonates.[97] However, more recent and prospective studies have indicated otherwise, including a prospective, multicenter observational cohort study of VLBW infants that found that severe anemia (rather than transfusion) was independently associated with NEC.[98]

TRANSFUSION IN INFANTS OLDER THAN 4 MONTHS AND CHILDREN

RBC Transfusion

The most significant differences between RBC transfusions in infants older than 4 months and adults are 1) blood volume, 2) the ability

TABLE 24-6. Blood Component Preparation Protocols for ECMO[96]

Clinical Scenario	Urgency	Components	Blood Groups	Storage
Cardiac arrest	5-10 min	2 units RBCs	O-neg RBCs	<14 days, AS
ECMO circuit disruption	5-10 min	2 units RBCs	O-neg RBCs	<14 days, AS
Progressive septic shock (nonneonate)	30 min	2 units RBCs	O-neg RBCs or type specific	<10 days, any preservative
Neonate transferred for ECMO	1-2 hours	2 units RBCs 1 unit FFP 1 unit platelets	O-neg RBCs AB plasma	<10 days, CPD or CPDA
Cardiac ICU	30-60 min	2 units RBCs	Type specific	<7 days, AS
Gradual respiratory or cardiac failure on conventional support	Hours to days	2 units RBCs	Type specific	<10 days, CPD

ECMO = extracorporeal membrane oxygenation; RBCs = Red Blood Cells; AS = additive solution; FFP = Fresh Frozen Plasma; CPD = citrate-phosphate-dextrose; CPDA = citrate-phosphate-dextrose-adenine; ICU = intensive care unit.

to tolerate blood loss, and 3) age-appropriate hemoglobin and hematocrit levels. In this age group, the most common indication for RBC transfusion is to treat or prevent tissue hypoxia caused by decreased red cell mass, typically because of surgery, anemia of chronic disease, or hematologic malignancies. Chronic RBC transfusions are administered to combat tissue hypoxia and suppress endogenous hemoglobin production in children with hemoglobinopathies. Table 24-7 can help guide transfusion decisions in patients older than 4 months.

Before receiving any RBC transfusion, all pediatric patients older than 4 months require ABO and Rh testing and screening for the presence of clinically significant antibodies. Compatibility testing should be performed according to AABB *Standards*.[23]

Sickle Cell Disease

Chronic transfusion in patients with sickle cell disease (SCD) decreases the proportion of red cells containing hemoglobin S, reduces sickling, and prevents blood viscosity increase. It has been shown that the risk of recurrent stroke is reduced to <10% if hemoglobin levels are maintained between 8 and 9 g/dL and the percentage of hemoglobin S stays <30%.[99,100] In children with SCD and silent cerebral infarcts (SCIs), transfusion therapy is more effective at preventing stroke and SCI recurrence than hydroxyurea and phlebotomy[101] or observation.[102,103]

Simple or partial manual exchange transfusions can be administered every 3 to 4 weeks. Automated red cell exchange has also been used to prevent iron overload in patients

TABLE 24-7. Transfusion Guidelines for RBCs in Patients Older than 4 Months[9,10]

1.	Emergency surgical procedure in patient with significant postoperative anemia.
2.	Preoperative anemia when other corrective therapy is not available.
3.	Intraoperative blood loss >15% total blood volume.
4.	Hematocrit <24% and:
	a. In perioperative period, with signs and symptoms of anemia.
	b. While on chemotherapy/radiotherapy.
	c. Chronic congenital or acquired symptomatic anemia.
5.	Acute blood loss with hypovolemia not responsive to other therapy.
6.	Hematocrit <40% and:
	a. With severe pulmonary disease.
	b. On extracorporeal membrane oxygenation.
7.	Sickle cell disease and:
	a. Cerebrovascular accident.
	b. Acute chest syndrome.
	c. Splenic sequestration.
	d. Aplastic crisis.
	e. Recurrent priapism.
	f. Preoperatively when general anesthesia is planned (target hemoglobin = 10 mg/dL).
8.	Chronic transfusion programs for disorders of red cell production (eg, β-thalassemia major and Diamond-Blackfan syndrome unresponsive to therapy).

with SCD.[104] See Table 24-7 for a list of other indications for simple or chronic RBC transfusion in SCD. Of note, RBCs for patients with SCD should be screened for hemoglobin S and, ideally, leukocyte reduced to prevent HLA alloimmunization and decrease platelet refractoriness in preparation for possible stem cell transplantation.

RBC Alloimmunization in SCD. Patients with SCD have the highest rates of alloimmunization of any patient group.[105,106] These antibodies are produced against common Rh, Kell, Duffy, and Kidd system antigens. Many SCD treatment centers perform an extended phenotype or genotype analysis of a patient's red cells before beginning transfusion therapy and preferentially transfuse red cell antigen-matched (Rh and Kell) units to reduce the rate of red cell alloimmunization.[107,108] Red cell genotyping can identify extended phenotype, provide information about variant Rh alleles that may appear phenotypically negative but form antibodies against Rh antigens, and provide results about common silencing mutations.[109] However, particularly for patients who are not yet alloimmunized, this process of matching for red cell antigens remains controversial because phenotypically compatible units are considerably more costly[110] and may be difficult to obtain.[111]

In academic institutions in the United States and Canada, the most common protocol for prevention of red cell alloimmunization in nonalloimmunized patients with SCD is transfusion of ABO/Rh-compatible units that are additionally matched for C, E, and K antigens.[112] Once patients have developed a red cell antibody, extension of matching to additional red cell antigens (Fy, Jk, S) is often used to prevent further alloimmunization.[113]

Other Complications of RBC Transfusions in SCD. Although the benefits of chronic transfusion therapy in patients with SCD have been demonstrated, it is not without risks, such as iron overload (that can cause organ dysfunction)[114] and minor red cell antigen alloimmunization, as well as the risks of increased donor exposure during erythrocytapheresis. Patients with SCD may also be at risk of life-threatening, delayed hemolytic transfu-

sion reactions. Early hydroxyurea therapy has been shown to decrease transfusions, hospitalizations, vaso-occlusive pain crises, and acute chest syndrome, and is now standard of care in children with hemoglobin SS or Sβ+-thalassemia.[112,115] The optimal clinical circumstances for hematopoietic progenitor cell transplantation in SCD have not been determined.[116] If a patient's hemoglobin level decreases after transfusion, the patient might have developed "hyperhemolytic" syndrome. This poorly understood phenomenon is characterized by destruction of the patient's own red cells along with transfused cells. If hyperhemolytic syndrome is suspected, case reports suggest that stopping transfusion and administering corticosteroids in combination with intravenous immune globulin may be beneficial.[117,118] These patients should also be monitored closely for the formation of autoantibodies.[108,119]

Thalassemia

Thalassemia with severe anemia is treated with transfusion to improve tissue oxygenation and suppress extramedullary erythropoiesis in the liver, spleen, and marrow, decreasing long-term associated complications. Most protocols aim for target hemoglobin between 8 to 10 g/dL to allow normal growth and development. Iron overload can occur even without transfusion and is treated with chelation therapy beginning early in childhood.[120]

Platelet and Plasma Transfusion

In older infants and children, platelets are most often prophylactically administered for chemotherapy-induced thrombocytopenia. The transfusion threshold for these patients is usually a platelet count between 10,000 and 20,000/μL, although the platelet count should not be the sole determinant for transfusion. The Prophylactic Platelet Dose (PLADO) study showed that in patients with hypoproliferative thrombocytopenia, the dose of prophylactic platelets administered had no effect on the incidence of moderate to severe bleeding.[121] A subgroup analysis of the 198 children in this study showed that children were at a higher risk of bleeding over a wider range of platelet counts than adults.[122] Therefore, prophylactic platelet transfusions at a platelet count of 10,000/µL in concert with different doses of platelets do not seem to affect the bleeding rates of children or adults. See Table 24-1 for platelet dosing for desired increment.

The indications for platelet and plasma transfusion support are similar for older infants, children, and adults. Tables 24-3 and 24-5 provide the indications for the transfusion of platelets, FFP, and cryoprecipitate. A recent prospective observational study showed that plasma transfusions were independently associated with an increased risk of new or progressive multiple organ dysfunction, nosocomial infections, and prolonged length of stay in 831 children admitted to one institution's pediatric critical care unit.[123] Plasma transfusions should be considered with caution in this population. Indications for transfusion of cryoprecipitate are the same as those in neonates. (See "Cryoprecipitated Antihemophilic Factor," above.)

Granulocyte Transfusion

For children older than 4 months, the indications for granulocyte transfusions—persistent neutropenia or granulocyte dysfunction in conjunction with bacterial and/or fungal infections—are similar to those previously mentioned for younger (<4 months) infants. (See "Granulocyte Transfusion," above.) For larger children and adults a minimum dose of 1 × 10E+10 is suggested, with a dose of 4-8 × 10E+10 granulocytes collected by using donors stimulated with G-CSF and steroids, is preferred.[9,91,93] If a patient weighs over 20 kg, either one-half unit or the whole unit can be transfused, depending on its volume and the volume status of the patient.

To obtain higher doses of granulocytes for larger patients, donors can be mobilized with steroids, growth factors [eg, granulocyte colony-stimulating factor (G-CSF)], or a combination. A multicenter study that randomly assigned neutropenic adults and children with systemic bacterial or fungal infection to receive standard antimicrobials with or without granulocytes (from donors stimulated with G-CSF and steroid) showed no benefit in mortality or microbial response in the granulocyte group. However the study closed early because of poor accrual and it was insufficiently powered to adequately address the efficacy of granulocyte transfusions.[93] Therefore, there remains no definitive evidence for benefit of granulocyte transfusions obtained from donors stimulated with steroids and G-CSF.

Whole Blood Transfusion

There are limited indications for transfusion of whole blood in children. Since the early 1990s, after Manno et al[124] studied the hemostatic effects of fresh whole blood vs stored whole blood following open-heart surgery in children, RBCs in the form of fresh whole blood have been advocated in order to improve hemostasis and decrease systemic inflammation. In that study, children <2 years undergoing cardiopulmonary bypass (CPB) surgery who received whole blood <48 hours old had significantly decreased mean 24-hour postoperative blood loss compared to children who received reconstituted whole blood. Of note, children >2 years of age undergoing simpler defect repairs did not have a greater benefit from fresh whole blood <48 hours old over reconstituted whole blood. Improved hemostasis was attributed to better platelet function in fresh whole blood. In 2004, another study examined fresh whole blood (<48 hours old) vs reconstituted blood (RBCs and FFP) for priming of the CPB circuit in children <1 year old. Neither postoperative bleeding nor inflammatory markers were significantly different between groups. Interestingly, circuit priming with whole blood was associated with a longer ICU stay and greater fluid balance (overload).[125] Thus, the use of fresh whole blood after CPB may be warranted if it can be obtained from the local blood center or hospital blood center to use in the postoperative setting, but it may not be as useful for the CPB prime.

PREVENTION OF ADVERSE EFFECTS OF TRANSFUSION IN THE PEDIATRIC POPULATION

CMV Prevention

The manifestation of CMV infection in susceptible individuals (eg, neonates, immuno-compromised patients) is variable, ranging from asymptomatic seroconversion to multi-organ involvement, viremia, and death. CMV may be transmitted transplacentally, during the birth process, during breastfeeding, as a result of personal contact with infected persons, or from transfusion. With current technologies, the risk of acquiring CMV from transfusion is likely lower than the historically reported 1% to 3%.[126] The risk of transfusion-transmitted CMV infection may be higher in multitransfused low-birthweight infants (<1200 g) born to seronegative mothers.[27,127]

Reduction of CMV transmission from transfusion is achieved by leukocyte reduction or provision of blood from CMV-seronegative donors, with evidence in adults of similar efficacy.[126] Using both approaches has been shown in a nonrandomized study to completely prevent CMV transmission by transfusion in VLBW neonates.[128] However, in the absence of superior benefit of using both approaches, providing leukocyte-reduced components is generally felt to be adequate to prevent transfusion-transmitted CMV.[129]

Leukocyte Reduction

The benefits of transfusing leukocyte-reduced components include reducing the risk of transfusion-transmitted CMV, prevention of febrile nonhemolytic transfusion reactions, and decreasing the risk of HLA allo-immunization.[130]

Irradiation

Cellular blood components are irradiated to prevent TA-GVHD in immunocompromised recipients. (See Table 24-8.) Expert opinions and practices differ on this topic. Therefore, protocols should be based on the patient populations served, equipment available, and best practices. The processes of irradiation, irradiator quality control, and quality assurance are addressed in Chapters 1 and 17.[131]

Volume Reduction and Washing

The plasma volume of the component (usually platelets, because RBCs have little plasma) is usually reduced in transfusions to patients who cannot tolerate increased intravascular volume (eg, patient with renal ischemia or compromised cardiac function). In 1993, the AABB Committee on Pediatric Hemotherapy stated that volume reduction of platelet concentrates should be reserved for infants who have total body fluid restrictions.[75] Methods for platelet volume reduction have been published.[132] (See Method 6-13). However,

TABLE 24-8. Irradiation Guidelines for Children Who Require Cellular Blood Components[9,10]

1.	Premature neonates weighing <1200 g at birth.
2.	Any patient with:
	a. Known or suspected cellular immune deficiency.
	b. Significant immunosuppression related to chemotherapy or radiation treatment.
3.	Any patient receiving:
	a. Components from blood relatives.
	b. HLA-matched or crossmatched platelet components.
	c. Granulocyte transfusion.

there is not an optimal centrifugation rate and preparation method. As with any platelet modification, the total number of platelets typically decreases, and platelet activation may occur with these procedures.[133]

Saline-washed RBCs and platelets are administered in an effort to reduce the risk of severe allergic reactions from plasma. Other uses may include removal of anticoagulant-preservative solutions and removal of high levels of potassium in RBCs, although centrifugation alone may be adequate. Maternal cells should be washed to remove maternal antibodies and irradiated if they are being used for fetal or neonatal transfusion.

Pathogen Inactivation

Pathogen inactivation techniques have been approved by the US Food and Drug Administration for several blood components and have been used in several European countries for many years, including in children.[134,135] Nonetheless, studies describing the potential of the technology to improve safety for pediatric patients, especially with regard to infectious disease transmission and to prevent TA-GVHD, have yet to be published. (See Chapter 7.)

Age of RBCs

To avoid hyperkalemia in patients with renal failure or anuria or who receive RBCs rapidly (ie, for ECMO), RBCs <7 days old may be provided. The practice of providing fresh RBCs for all pediatric patients is based on less evidence than for adults in whom the evidence from randomized control trials is weak.

In the TOTAL randomized noninferiority trial of 290 children (aged 6-60 months), most with malaria or SCD, with a hemoglobin level of ≤5 g/dL and a lactate level of ≥5 mmol/L, older RBCs (25 to 35 days) did not result in statistically different reductions in lactate levels 24 hours after transfusion compared to fresher RBCs (1 to 10 days). There were also no differences in clinical assessment, cerebral

oxygen saturation, electrolyte abnormalities, adverse events, survival, and 30-day recovery between the groups.[136]

While there is an ongoing multicenter trial (ABC PICU study) comparing clinical outcomes in children in the ICU who receive RBCs stored <7 days or those of standard age,[137] there is currently no evidence to support the transfusion of fresh RBCs in the pediatric population.

Massive Transfusion in the Pediatric Setting

Trauma is the leading cause of death in infants, children, and young adults aged 1 to 21 years. Although trauma rarely leads to hemorrhagic shock and massive transfusion, resuscitation after trauma can be challenging.

The evidence to support a pediatric massive transfusion protocol (MTP) is limited, but several pediatric institutions use MTPs to improve the outcomes of patients who have massive bleeding with trauma.[138] The appropriate ratios of RBCs to plasma and platelets have not been well-defined in pediatric patients because a large trial has not been undertaken and, given the rarity of patients, would be difficult to accomplish.[139-143] In a recently published multicenter trial, adults with severe trauma and major bleeding who received early administration of plasma, platelets, and RBCs in a 1:1:1 ratio compared with a 1:1:2 ratio did not have significant difference in mortality at 24 hours or at 30 days. However, there was less death from bleeding at 24 hours in the 1:1:1 group, so this ratio has been adapted in many trauma centers, including for older children.[144]

Although studies indicate that an MTP in the pediatric setting is feasible not only for providing rapid and balanced blood component support but also for decreasing the risk of thromboembolic events, the role of the MTP and the optimal ratio of components is not specifically defined in the pediatric setting.[140,142,143]

KEY POINTS

1. RBCs are the most frequently transfused blood component in neonates.
2. Frequent blood loss, including iatrogenic losses from repeated phlebotomy, contribute to the need for RBC transfusions in neonates.
3. A full-term newborn has a blood volume of approximately 85 mL/kg; a preterm infant has a total approximate blood volume of 100 mL/kg.
4. In infants <4 months of age, initial patient testing must include ABO and D typing of the infant's red cells and a screen for unexpected red cell antibodies, using either plasma or serum from the infant or mother. During any one hospitalization, crossmatch-compatibility testing and repeat ABO and D typing may be omitted as long as all of the following criteria are met: The antibody screen is negative; transfused red cells are group O, ABO identical, or ABO compatible; and transfused cells are either D negative or the same D type as the patient. Testing the infant's reverse type for anti-A and/or anti-B is not necessary.
5. Small-volume (10-15 mL/kg) simple transfusions of RBCs (regardless of storage solution), when administered slowly, have been shown to have little effect on serum potassium concentrations in infants <4 months of age despite elevated potassium levels in the plasma of stored RBCs.
6. During component preparation, if aliquots are made with a sterile connecting device, they are considered to have been prepared within a "closed system," and the original unit's expiration date can be used for the new aliquot.
7. Transfusion of ABO-incompatible plasma should be avoided in infants and children because of their small blood and plasma volumes. If ABO out-of-group platelet transfusion becomes necessary, plasma may be removed by volume reduction.
8. Chronic RBC transfusion therapy of indefinite duration to maintain hemoglobin S levels below 30% is the therapy of choice to reduce the risk of stroke recurrence in patients with SCD. SCD patients have the highest rates of alloimmunization to red cell minor antigens of any patient group. The most commonly formed antibodies are to Rh, Kell, Duffy, and Kidd system antigens. Many SCD treatment centers try to prevent red cell alloimmunization by matching for phenotypically similar antigen profiles on recipients. This strategy is not the same at all centers and is controversial because obtaining enough phenotypically similar units may be difficult and costly.
9. To decrease the risk of transfusion-transmitted CMV infection in susceptible populations such as low-birthweight neonates and immunocompromised children, these patients should receive blood components that either have been leukocyte reduced or are from CMV-seronegative donors.

REFERENCES

1. Hillyer CD, Mondoro TH, Josephson CD, et al. Pediatric transfusion medicine: Development of a critical mass. Transfusion 2009;49:596-601.
2. Hume H, Bard H. Small volume red blood cell transfusions for neonatal patients. Transfus Med Rev 1995;9:187-99.
3. Blanchette V, Doyle J, Schmidt B, et al. Hematology. In: Avery G, Fletcher M, MacDonald M, eds. Neonatology: Pathophysiology and management of the newborn. 4th ed. Philadelphia: JB Lippincott, 1994:952-99.
4. Brugnara C, Platt OS. The neonatal erythrocyte and its disorders. In: Nathan DG, Orkin SH, eds. Nathan and Oski's hematology of infancy and childhood. 7th ed. Philadelphia: WB Saunders, 2009:21-66.
5. Dame C, Fahnenstich H, Freitag P, et al. Erythropoietin mRNA expression in human fetal and neonatal tissue. Blood 1998;92:3218-25.

6. Sisson TR, Whalen LE, Telek A. The blood volume of infants. II. The premature infant during the first year of life. J Pediatr 1959; 55:430-46.

7. Fabres J, Wehrli G, Marques MB, et al. Estimating blood needs for very-low-birth-weight infants. Transfusion 2006;46:1915-20.

8. Wallgren G, Hanson JS, Lind J. Quantitative studies of the human neonatal circulation. 3. Observations on the newborn infants central circulatory responses to moderate hypovolemia. Acta Paediatr Scand 1967;(Suppl 179):45.

9. Roseff SD, Luban NL, Manno CS. Guidelines for assessing appropriateness of pediatric transfusion. Transfusion 2002;42:1398-413.

10. Wong EC, Paul W. Intrauterine, neonatal, and pediatric transfusion. In: Mintz PD, ed. Transfusion therapy: Clinical principles and practice. 3rd ed. Bethesda, MD: AABB Press, 2010: 209-51.

11. Ohls RK. Evaluation and treatment of anemia in the neonate. In: Christensen RD, ed. Hematologic problems of the neonate. Philadelphia: WB Saunders, 2000:137-69.

12. Halvorsen S, Bechensteen AG. Physiology of erythropoietin during mammalian development. Acta Paediatr Suppl 2002;91:17-26.

13. Ohls RK, Christensen RD, Kamath-Rayne BD, et al. A randomized, masked, placebo-controlled study of darbepoetin alfa in preterm infants. Pediatrics 2013;132:e119-27.

14. Ohlsson A, Aher SM. Early erythropoietin for preventing red blood cell transfusion in preterm and/or low birth weight infants. Cochrane Database Syst Rev 2014;(4): CD004863.

15. Aher SM, Ohlsson A. Late erythropoietin for preventing red blood cell transfusion in preterm and/or low birth weight infants. Cochrane Database Syst Rev 2014;(4): CD004868.

16. Kandasamy Y, Kumar P, Hartley L. The effect of erythropoietin on the severity of retinopathy of prematurity. Eye 2014;28:814-18.

17. Doege C, Pritsch M, Fruhwald MC, et al. An association between infantile haemangiomas and erythropoietin treatment in preterm infants. Arch Dis Child Fetal Neonatal Ed 2012; 97:F45-9.

18. Henry E, Christensen RD, Sheffield MJ, et al. Why do four NICUs using identical RBC transfusion guidelines have different gestational age-adjusted RBC transfusion rates? J Perinatol 2015;35:132-6.

19. Carroll PD, Widness JA. Nonpharmacological, blood conservation techniques for preventing neonatal anemia—effective and promising strategies for reducing transfusion. Semin Perinatol 2012;36:232-43.

20. Barcelona SL, Cote CJ. Pediatric resuscitation in the operating room. Anesthesiol Clin North Am 2001;19:339-65.

21. Luban NL, Mikesell G, Sacher RA. Techniques for warming red blood cells packaged in different containers for neonatal use. Clin Pediatr 1985;24:642-4.

22. DePalma L. Review: Red cell alloantibody formation in the neonate and infant: Considerations for current immunohematologic practice. Immunohematology 1992;8:33-7.

23. Ooley PW, ed. Standards for blood banks and transfusion services. 30th ed. Bethesda, MD: AABB, 2016.

24. Sanders MR, Graeber JE. Posttransfusion graft-versus-host disease in infancy. J Pediatr 1990; 117:159-63.

25. Ruhl H, Bein G, Sachs UJH. Transfusion-associated graft-versus-host disease. Transfus Med Rev 2009;23:62-71.

26. Ohto H, Anderson KC. Posttransfusion graft-versus-host disease in Japanese newborns. Transfusion 1996;36:117-23.

27. Strauss RG. Data-driven blood banking practices for neonatal RBC transfusions. Transfusion 2000;40:1528-40.

28. Devine DV, Schubert P. Pathogen inactivation technologies: The advent of pathogen-reduced blood components to reduce blood safety risk. Hematol Oncol Clin North Am 2016;30:609-17.

29. Dincsoy MY, Tsang RC, Laskarzewski P, et al. The role of postnatal age and magnesium on parathyroid hormone responses during "exchange" blood transfusion in the newborn period. J Pediatr 1982;100:277-83.

30. Strauss RG. Transfusion therapy in neonates. Am J Dis Child 1991;145:904-11.

31. Strauss RG. Neonatal transfusion. In: Anderson KC, Ness PN, eds. Scientific basis of transfusion medicine: Implications for clinical practice. 2nd ed. Philadelphia: WB Saunders, 2000:321-6.

32. Strauss RG. Routinely washing irradiated red cells before transfusion seems unwarranted. Transfusion 1990;30:675-7.

33. McDonald TB, Berkowitz RA. Massive transfusion in children. In: Jefferies LC, Brecher ME,

eds. Massive transfusion. Bethesda, MD: AABB, 1994:97-119.

34. Lee AC, Reduque LL, Luban NLC, et al. Transfusion-associated hyperkalemic cardiac arrest in pediatric patients receiving massive transfusion. Transfusion 2014;54:244-54.

35. Hall TL, Barnes A, Miller JR, et al. Neonatal mortality following transfusion of red cells with high plasma potassium levels. Transfusion 1993;33:606-9.

36. Fung MK, Roseff SD, Vermoch KL. Blood component preferences of transfusion services supporting infant transfusions: A University HealthSystem Consortium benchmarking study. Transfusion 2010;50:1921-5.

37. Wong EC, Luban NL. Hematology and oncology. In: Slonim AD, Pollack MM, eds. Pediatric critical care medicine. Philadelphia: Lippincott, Williams and Wilkins, 2006:157-95.

38. Strauss RG, Burmeister LF, Johnson K, et al. AS-1 red cells for neonatal transfusions: A randomized trial assessing donor exposure and safety. Transfusion 1996;36:873-8.

39. Strauss RG, Burmeister LF, Johnson K, et al. Feasibility and safety of AS-3 red blood cells for neonatal transfusions. J Pediatr 2000;136:215-19.

40. New HV, Berryman J, Bolton-Maggs PHB, et al. Guidelines on transfusion for fetuses, neonates and older children. Br J Haematol 2016;175:784-828.

41. Girelli G, Antoncecchi S, Casadei AM, et al. Recommendations for transfusion therapy in neonatology. Blood Transfus 2015;13:484-97.

42. Roseff SD. Pediatric blood collection and transfusion technology. In: Herman JK, Manno CS, eds. Pediatric transfusion therapy. Bethesda, MD: AABB Press, 2002:217-47.

43. Strauss RG. Selection of white cell-reduced blood components for transfusions during early infancy. Transfusion 1993;33:352-7.

44. Ludvigsen CWJ, Swanson JL, Thompson TR, et al. The failure of neonates to form red blood cell alloantibodies in response to multiple transfusions. Am J Clin Pathol 1987;87:250-1.

45. Josephson CD, Castillejo M, Grima K, et al. ABO-mismatched platelet transfusions: Strategies to mitigate patient exposure to naturally occurring hemolytic antibodies. Transfus Apher Sci 2010;42:83-8.

46. Wang-Rodriguez J, Mannino FL, Liu E, et al. A novel strategy to limit blood donor exposure and blood waste in multiply transfused premature infants. Transfusion 1996;36:64-70.

47. Liu EA, Mannino FL, Lane TA. Prospective, randomized trial of the safety and efficacy of a limited donor exposure transfusion program for premature neonates. J Pediatr 1994;125:92-6.

48. Bednarek FJ, Weisberger S, Richardson DK, et al. Variations in blood transfusions among newborn intensive care units. SNAP II study group. J Pediatr 1998;133:601-7.

49. Maier RF, Sonntag J, Walka MM, et al. Changing practices of red blood cell transfusions in infants with birth weights less than 1000 g. J Pediatr 2000;136:220-4.

50. Levy GJ, Strauss RG, Hume H, et al. National survey of neonatal transfusion practices: I. Red blood cell therapy. Pediatrics 1993;91:523-9.

51. Goodstein MH, Herman JH, Smith JF, et al. Metabolic consequences in very low birth weight infants transfused with older AS-1 preserved erythrocytes. Pediatr Pathol Lab Med 1999;18:173-85.

52. Rock G, Poon A, Haddad S, et al. Nutricel as an additive solution for neonatal transfusion. Transfus Sci 1999;20:29-36.

53. Luban NL, Strauss RG, Hume HA. Commentary on the safety of red cells preserved in extended-storage media for neonatal transfusions. Transfusion 1991;31:229-35.

54. Tuchschmid P, Mieth D, Burger R, et al. Potential hazard of hypoalbuminemia in newborn babies after exchange transfusions with ADSOL red blood cell concentrates. Pediatrics 1990;85:234-5.

55. Fergusson DA, Hébert P, Hogan DL, et al. Effect of fresh red blood cell transfusions on clinical outcomes in premature, very low-birth-weight infants: The ARIPI randomized trial. JAMA 2012;308:1443-51.

56. Patel RM, Josephson CD. Storage age of red blood cells for transfusion of premature infants. JAMA 2013;309:544-5.

57. Wong E, Roseff SD, eds. Pediatric hemotherapy data card. Bethesda, MD: AABB, 2015.

58. Bell EF, Strauss RG, Widness JA, et al. Randomized trial of liberal versus restrictive guidelines for red blood cell transfusion in preterm infants. Pediatrics 2005;115:1685-91.

59. Kirpalani H, Whyte RK, Andersen C, et al. The premature infants in need of transfusion (PINT) study: A randomized, controlled trial of a restrictive (low) versus liberal (high) transfusion threshold for extremely low birth weight infants. J Pediatr 2006;149:301-7.

60. Whyte RK, Kirpalani H, Asztalos EV, et al. Neurodevelopmental outcome of extremely low birth weight infants randomly assigned to restrictive or liberal hemoglobin thresholds for blood transfusion. Pediatrics 2009;123:207-13.

61. McCoy TE, Conrad AL, Richman LC, et al. Neurocognitive profiles of preterm infants randomly assigned to lower or higher hematocrit thresholds for transfusion. Child Neuropsychol 2011;17:347-67.

62. Nopoulos PC, Conrad AL, Bell EF, et al. Long-term outcome of brain structure in premature infants: Effects of liberal vs restricted red blood cell transfusions. Arch Pediatr Adolesc Med 2011;165:443-50.

63. Kirpalani H, Bell E, D'Angio C, et al. Transfusion of prematures (TOP) trial: Does a liberal red blood cell transfusion strategy improve neurologically-intact survival of extremely-low-birth-weight infants as compared to a restrictive strategy? Version 1.0 (October 8, 2012). Bethesda, MD: National Institutes of Health, 2012. [Available at https://www.nichd.nih.gov/about/Documents/TOP_protocal.pdf (accessed April 6, 2017).]

64. Ballard RA, Vinocur B, Reynolds JW, et al. Transient hyperammonemia of the preterm infant. N Engl J Med 1978;299:920-5.

65. Leonard JV. The early detection and management of inborn errors presenting acutely in the neonatal period. Eur J Pediatr 1985;143:253-7.

66. American Academy of Pediatrics Subcommittee on Hyperbilirubinemia. Management of hyperbilirubinemia in the newborn infant 35 or more weeks of gestation. Pediatrics 2004;114:297-316.

67. Kliegman RM, Stanton BMD, St. Geme J, Schor NF, eds. Nelson's textbook of pediatrics. 20th ed. Philadelphia: WB Saunders, 2016.

68. Valaes T. Bilirubin distribution and dynamics of bilirubin removal by exchange transfusion. Acta Paediatr Scand 1963;52:604.

69. Wong EC, Pisciotto PT. Technical considerations/mechanical devices. In: Hillyer CD, Strauss RG, Luban NLC, eds. Handbook of pediatric transfusion medicine. London: Elsevier Academic Press, 2004:121-8.

70. Luban NL. Massive transfusion in the neonate. Transfus Med Rev 1995;9:200-14.

71. Weisz B, Belson A, Milbauer B, et al. [Complications of exchange transfusion in term and preterm newborns]. Harefuah 1996;130:170-3.

72. Bada HS, Chua C, Salmon JH, et al. Changes in intracranial pressure during exchange transfusion. J Pediatr 1979;94:129-32.

73. Blanchette VS, Kuhne T, Hume H, et al. Platelet transfusion therapy in newborn infants. Transfus Med Rev 1995;9:215-30.

74. Castle V, Andrew M, Kelton J, et al. Frequency and mechanism of neonatal thrombocytopenia. J Pediatr 1986;108:749-55.

75. Andrew M, Vegh P, Caco C, et al. A randomized, controlled trial of platelet transfusions in thrombocytopenic premature infants. J Pediatr 1993;123:285-91.

76. Honohan A, van't Ende E, Hulzebos C, et al. Posttransfusion platelet increments after different platelet products in neonates: A retrospective cohort study. Transfusion 2013;53:3100-9.

77. New HV, Stanworth SJ, Engelfriet CP, et al. Neonatal transfusions. Vox Sang 2009;96:62-85.

78. Poterjoy BS, Josephson CD. Platelets, frozen plasma, and cryoprecipitate: What is the clinical evidence for their use in the neonatal intensive care unit? Semin Perinatol 2009;33:66-74.

79. von Lindern JS, van den Bruele T, Lopriore E, et al. Thrombocytopenia in neonates and the risk of intraventricular hemorrhage: A retrospective cohort study. BMC Pediatrics 2011;11:16.

80. Josephson CD, Su LL, Christensen RD, et al. Platelet transfusion practices among neonatologists in the United States and Canada: Results of a survey. Pediatrics 2009;123:278-85.

81. Curley A, Venkatesh V, Stanworth S, et al. Platelets for neonatal transfusion - study 2: A randomised controlled trial to compare two different platelet count thresholds for prophylactic platelet transfusion to preterm neonates. Neonatology 2014;106:102-6.

82. Honohan A, Tomson B, van der Bom J, et al. A comparison of volume-reduced versus standard HLA/HPA-matched apheresis platelets in alloimmunized adult patients. Transfusion 2012;52:742-51.

83. Pisciotto PT, Snyder EL, Snyder JA, et al. In vitro characteristics of white cell-reduced single-unit platelet concentrates stored in syringes. Transfusion 1994;34:407-11.

84. Diab Y, Wong E, Criss VR, et al. Storage of aliquots of apheresis platelets for neonatal use in syringes with and without agitation. Transfusion 2011;51:2642-6.

85. Andrew M, Paes B, Johnston M. Development of the hemostatic system in the neonate and young infant. Am J Pediatr Hematol 1990;12: 95-104.

86. Monagle P, Barnes C, Ignjatovic V, et al. Developmental haemostasis: Impact for clinical haemostasis laboratories. Thromb Haemost 2006;95:362-72.

87. Revel-Vilk S. The conundrum of neonatal coagulopathy. Hematology Am Soc Hematol Educ Program 2012;2012:450-4.

88. Motta M, Del Vecchio A, Radicioni M. Clinical use of fresh-frozen plasma and cryoprecipitate in neonatal intensive care unit. J Matern Fetal Neonatal Med 2011;24:129-31.

89. AABB, America's Blood Centers, American Red Cross, Armed Services Blood Program. Circular of information for the use of human blood and blood components. Bethesda, MD: AABB, 2017.

90. Bandarenko N, King K, eds. Blood transfusion therapy: A physician's handbook. 12th ed. Bethesda, MD: AABB, 2017.

91. Wong ECC, Roseff SD, King KE, eds. Pediatric transfusion: A physician's handbook. 4th ed. Bethesda, MD: AABB, 2015.

92. Di Paola J, Montgomery RR, Gill JC, Flood V. Hemophilia and von Willebrand disease. In: Orkin SH, Fisher DE, Ginsburg D, et al, eds. Nathan and Oski's hematology and oncology of infancy and childhood. 8th ed. Philadelphia: Elsevier Saunders, 2015:1028-54.

93. Price TH, Boeckh M, Harrison RW, et al. Efficacy of transfusion with granulocytes from G-CSF/dexamethasone-treated donors in neutropenic patients with infection. Blood 2015; 126:2153-61.

94. Marfin AA, Price TH. Granulocyte transfusion therapy. J Intensive Care Med 2015;30:79-88.

95. Maheshwari A, Carlo WA. Plethora in the newborn infant (polycythemia). In: Kliegman RM, Stanton BF, Schor NF, et al, eds. Nelson textbook of pediatrics. 20th ed. Philadelphia: Elsevier, 2015:887-8.

96. Friedman DF, Montenegro LM. Extracorporeal membrane oxygenation and cardiopulmonary bypass. In: Hillyer CD, Strauss RG, Luban NLC, eds. Handbook of pediatric transfusion medicine. London: Elsevier Academic Press, 2004: 181-9.

97. Mohamed A, Shah PS. Transfusion associated necrotizing enterocolitis: A meta-analysis of observational data. Pediatrics 2012;129:529-40.

98. Patel RM, Knezevic A, Shenvi N, et al. Association of red blood cell transfusion, anemia, and necrotizing enterocolitis in very low-birth-weight infants. JAMA 2016;315:889-97.

99. Ware RE, Helms RW, SWiTCH Investigators. Stroke with transfusions changing to hydroxyurea (SWiTCH). Blood 2012;119:3925-32.

100. Estcourt LJ, Fortin PM, Hopewell S, et al. Blood transfusion for preventing primary and secondary stroke in people with sickle cell disease. Cochrane Database Syst Rev 2017;1: 003146.

101. Ware RE, Davis BR, Schultz WH, et al. Hydroxycarbamide versus chronic transfusion for maintenance of transcranial doppler flow velocities in children with sickle cell anaemia—TCD with transfusions changing to hydroxyurea (TWiTCH): A multicentre, open-label, phase 3, non-inferiority trial. Lancet 2016;387:661-70.

102. DeBaun MR, Gordon M, McKinstry RC, et al. Controlled trial of transfusions for silent cerebral infarcts in sickle cell anemia. N Engl J Med 2014;371:699-710.

103. Adams RJ, McKie VC, Hsu L, et al. Prevention of a first stroke by transfusions in children with sickle cell anemia and abnormal results on transcranial doppler ultrasonography. N Engl J Med 1998;339:5-11.

104. Kelly S, Quirolo K, Marsh A, et al. Erythrocytapheresis for chronic transfusion therapy in sickle cell disease: Survey of current practices and review of the literature. Transfusion 2016;56:2877-88.

105. Rosse WF, Gallagher D, Kinney TR, et al. Transfusion and alloimmunization in sickle cell disease: The cooperative study of sickle cell disease. Blood 1990;76:1431-7.

106. Rosse WF, Telen M, Ware RE. Transfusion support for patients with sickle cell disease. Bethesda, MD: AABB Press, 1998.

107. Vichinsky EP, Luban NL, Wright E, et al. Prospective RBC phenotype matching in a stroke-prevention trial in sickle cell anemia: A multicenter transfusion trial. Transfusion 2001;41: 1086-92.

108. Yazdanbakhsh K, Ware RE, Noizat-Pirenne F. Red blood cell alloimmunization in sickle cell disease: Pathophysiology, risk factors, and transfusion management. Blood 2012;120: 528-37.

109. Chou ST, Jackson T, Vege S, et al. High prevalence of red blood cell alloimmunization in

sickle cell disease despite transfusion from Rh-matched minority donors. Blood 2013;122: 1062-71.

110. Kacker S, Ness PM, Savage WJ, et al. Cost-effectiveness of prospective red blood cell antigen matching to prevent alloimmunization among sickle cell patients. Transfusion 2014;54:86-97.

111. Hillyer KL, Hare VW, Josephson CD, et al. Partners for life: The transfusion program for patients with sickle cell disease offered at the American Red Cross Blood Services, Southern Region, Atlanta, Georgia. Immunohematology 2006;22:108-11.

112. Yawn BP, Buchanan GR, Afenyi-Annan AN, et al. Management of sickle cell disease: Summary of the 2014 evidence-based report by expert panel members. JAMA 2014;312:1033-48.

113. Tahhan HR, Holbrook CT, Braddy LR, et al. Antigen-matched donor blood in the transfusion management of patients with sickle cell disease. Transfusion 1994;34:562-9.

114. Wood JC, Cohen AR, Pressel SL, et al. Organ iron accumulation in chronically transfused children with sickle cell anaemia: Baseline results from the TWiTCH trial. Br J Haematol 2016;172:122-30.

115. Wong TE, Brandow AM, Lim W, et al. Update on the use of hydroxyurea therapy in sickle cell disease. Blood 2014;124:3850-7.

116. Arnold SD, Bhatia M, Horan J, et al. Haematopoietic stem cell transplantation for sickle cell disease—current practice and new approaches. Br J Haematol 2016;174:515-25.

117. Petz LD, Calhoun L, Shulman IA, et al. The sickle cell hemolytic transfusion reaction syndrome. Transfusion 1997;37:382-92.

118. Win N, Doughty H, Telfer P, et al. Hyperhemolytic transfusion reaction in sickle cell disease. Transfusion 2001;41:323-8.

119. Garratty G. Autoantibodies induced by blood transfusion. Transfusion 2004;44:5-9.

120. Olivieri NF, Brittenham GM. Iron-chelating therapy and the treatment of thalassemia. Blood 1997;89:739-61.

121. Slichter SJ, Kaufman RM, Assmann SF, et al. Dose of prophylactic platelet transfusions and prevention of hemorrhage. N Engl J Med 2010; 362:600-13.

122. Josephson CD, Granger S, Assmann SF, et al. Bleeding risks are higher in children versus adults given prophylactic platelet transfusions for treatment-induced hypoproliferative thrombocytopenia. Blood 2012;120:748-60.

123. Karam O, Lacroix J, Robitaille N, et al. Association between plasma transfusions and clinical outcome in critically ill children: A prospective observational study. Vox Sang 2013;104:342-9.

124. Manno CS, Hedberg KW, Kim HC, et al. Comparison of the hemostatic effects of fresh whole blood, stored whole blood, and components after open heart surgery in children. Blood 1991;77:930-6.

125. Mou SS, Giroir BP, Molitor-Kirsch EA, et al. Fresh whole blood versus reconstituted blood for pump priming in heart surgery in infants. N Engl J Med 2004;351:1635-44.

126. Bowden RA, Slichter SJ, Sayers M, et al. A comparison of filtered leukocyte-reduced and cytomegalovirus (CMV) seronegative blood products for the prevention of transfusion-associated CMV infection after marrow transplant. Blood 1995;86:3598-603.

127. Brady MT, Milam JD, Anderson DC, et al. Use of deglycerolized red blood cells to prevent posttransfusion infection with cytomegalovirus in neonates. J Infect Dis 1984;150:334-9.

128. Josephson CD, Caliendo AM, Easley KA, et al. Blood transfusion and breast milk transmission of cytomegalovirus in very low-birth-weight infants: A prospective cohort study. JAMA Pediatr 2014;168:1054-62.

129. AABB, Clinical Transfusion Medicine Committee, Heddle NM, et al. AABB committee report: Reducing transfusion-transmitted cytomegalovirus infections. Transfusion 2016;56:1581-7.

130. Trial to reduce alloimmunization to platelets study group. Leukocyte reduction and ultraviolet B irradiation of platelets to prevent alloimmunization and refractoriness to platelet transfusions. N Engl J Med 1997;337:1861-9.

131. Delaney M, Wendel S, Bercovitz RS, et al. Transfusion reactions: Prevention, diagnosis, and treatment. Lancet 2016;388:2825-36.

132. Moroff G, Friedman A, Robkin-Kline L, et al. Reduction of the volume of stored platelet concentrates for use in neonatal patients. Transfusion 1984;24:144-6.

133. Schoenfeld H, Muhm M, Doepfmer UR, et al. The functional integrity of platelets in volume-reduced platelet concentrates. Anesth Analg 2005;100:78-81.

134. Knutson F, Osselaer J, Pierelli L, et al. A prospective, active haemovigilance study with combined cohort analysis of 19,175 transfusions of platelet components prepared with amotosalen-UVA photochemical treatment. Vox Sang 2015;109:343-52.

135. McCullough J, Vesole DH, Benjamin RJ, et al. Therapeutic efficacy and safety of platelets treated with a photochemical process for pathogen inactivation: The SPRINT trial. Blood 2004;104:1534-41.

136. Dhabangi A, Ainomugisha B, Cserti-Gazdewich C, et al. Effect of transfusion of red blood cells with longer vs shorter storage duration on elevated blood lactate levels in children with severe anemia: The TOTAL randomized clinical trial. JAMA 2015;314:2514-23.

137. Age of blood in children in pediatric intensive care units (ABC PICU). St. Louis, MO: Washington University School of Medicine, 2015. [Available at https://clinicaltrials.gov/ct2/show/NCT01977547 (accessed April 7, 2017).]

138. Horst J, Leonard JC, Vogel A, et al. A survey of US and Canadian hospitals' paediatric massive transfusion protocol policies. Transfus Med 2016;26:49-56.

139. Dehmer JJ, Adamson WT. Massive transfusion and blood product use in the pediatric trauma patient. Semin Pediatr Surg 2010;19:286-91.

140. Hendrickson JE, Shaz BH, Pereira G, et al. Implementation of a pediatric trauma massive transfusion protocol: One institution's experience. Transfusion 2012;52:1228-36.

141. Chidester SJ, Williams N, Wang W, et al. A pediatric massive transfusion protocol. J Trauma Acute Care Surg 2012;73:1273-7.

142. Nosanov L, Inaba K, Okoye O, et al. The impact of blood product ratios in massively transfused pediatric trauma patients. Am J Surg 2013;206:655-60.

143. Hwu RS, Spinella PC, Keller MS, et al. The effect of massive transfusion protocol implementation on pediatric trauma care. Transfusion 2016;56:2712-19.

144. Holcomb JB, Tilley BC, Baraniuk S, et al. Transfusion of plasma, platelets, and red blood cells in a 1:1:1 vs a 1:1:2 ratio and mortality in patients with severe trauma: The PROPPR randomized clinical trial. JAMA 2015; 313:471-82.

Chapter 25

Therapeutic Apheresis

• ● •

Chester Andrzejewski Jr, PhD, MD, and
Robertson D. Davenport, MD

THERAPEUTIC APHERESIS (TA) is an extracorporeal therapy used in the treatment and management of various diseases and is accomplished either through the removal and discarding of selected blood constituents or via the collection of selected blood elements with their subsequent ex-vivo manipulation and return to the patient. It is related to but distinct from "preparative apheresis," in which blood components are collected from blood donors for therapeutic uses (covered in Chapter 6). Standards and guidelines for TA performance, health-care provider education, qualifications and clinical privileging, and procedural documentation have been promulgated by AABB, the American Society for Apheresis (ASFA), and the College of American Pathologists (CAP).[1-7] In 2012, the National Heart, Lung, and Blood Institute (NHLBI) sponsored a National Institutes of Health (NIH) State of the Science Symposium in Therapeutic Apheresis exploring various aspects related to TA, including scientific opportunities in TA, what challenges/barriers exist to increasing TA research, and prioritization of TA research activities.[8]

GENERAL PRINCIPLES

The major goals of TA are: 1) to remove a pathologic cellular and/or humoral element(s) from a patient's blood; 2) to replace a deficient substance(s), typically in the context of the removal of a pathologic constituent; 3) to modulate cellular functionality (eg, via further extracorporeal manipulations and the return of those cellular elements, such as encountered through ultraviolet light exposure in photopheresis); and/or 4) to collect various autologous nonpathologic cellular populations for further manipulation and therapeutic uses (eg, cellular therapies involving stem cells, dendritic cells, and chimeric antigen receptor T-cell production).

The various types of apheresis procedures are listed in Table 25-1. In the most commonly performed clinical apheresis procedure, therapeutic plasma exchange (TPE), 1.0 or 1.5

Chester Andrzejewski Jr, PhD, MD, Medical Director, System Blood Banking/Transfusion and Apheresis Medicine Services, Baystate Health, Assistant Professor, Department of Pathology, University of Massachusetts Medical School-Baystate, Springfield, Massachusetts, Adjunct Assistant Professor, Department of Pathology, Tufts University School of Medicine, Boston, Massachusetts; and Robertson D. Davenport, MD, Medical Director, Blood Bank and Transfusion Service, and Associate Professor, University of Michigan Health System, Ann Arbor, Michigan

C. Andrzejewski has disclosed financial relationships with Amgen and Haemonetics. R. Davenport has disclosed no conflicts of interest.

TABLE 25-1. Therapeutic Apheresis Modalities

Procedure	Blood Component Removed	Typical Indication	Replacement Fluid*
Therapeutic plasma exchange	Plasma	Reduction of an abnormal plasma protein (eg, autoantibody)	Albumin or plasma
Red cell exchange	Red cells	Sickle cell disease-related complications	Red cells
Leukocytapheresis	Buffy coat	Leukemia with leukostasis	As needed
Thrombocytapheresis	Platelet-rich plasma	Thrombocytosis	As needed
Erythrocytapheresis	Red cells	Erythrocytosis	None
Extracorporeal photopheresis	Buffy coat (reinfused)	Chronic graft-vs-host disease	None
Selective adsorption	Specific plasma protein	Hypercholesterolemia	None
Rheopheresis	High-molecular-weight plasma proteins	Age-related macular degeneration	None

*Additional information appears in Table 25-3.

plasma volumes are typically removed in a single session. In the related but distinct procedure of plasmapheresis, used generally in the donor setting with its terminology often used interchangeably with TPE, lesser volumes of plasma (≤1 L) are removed, resulting in little to no need for fluid replacement. Targeting of larger volumes for removal increases the risk of coagulopathy, citrate toxicity, or electrolyte imbalances, depending on the replacement fluids used.

The effectiveness of apheresis in removing pathologic substances depends on the concentration of the substance in the blood, its volume of distribution into the extravascular space, the degree of protein binding of the targeted substance, the volume of blood processed and plasma removed, and the equilibrium between the substance's blood and extravascular concentrations. Most efficient at the procedure's beginning stages, component removal decreases exponentially and asymptotically with time because of the required addition of replacement fluids needed to maintain physiologic stability in the patient. Continued production or mobilization from the extravascular space will result in a less-

than-predicted decrease. In a 1.0 plasma volume exchange, approximately two-thirds of a targeted "idealized substance,"[9] such as IgM or fibrinogen, is typically removed, provided that the constituent does not diffuse significantly from the extravascular to the intravascular compartments.

DEVICE MODALITIES

Several technological platforms for performing apheresis exist. The most commonly available ones are described below.

Continuous-flow centrifugation apheresis devices have a rotating channel designed to introduce whole blood at one site, and the blood elements subsequently separate by density as blood flows through the channel. The resulting layers of plasma, platelets, leukocytes, and red cells can be selectively removed. The targeted constituent is diverted into a collection bag, while the remaining blood components are returned to the patient with appropriate replacement fluids. To achieve optimal separation and treatment blood volume, modern apheresis devices calculate and control blood withdrawal flow rates, amounts of anticoagulant solution and replacement fluids needed, and centrifuge speed.

Intermittent-flow centrifugation devices draw a specified volume of whole blood into a centrifugation bowl. Inlet flow is then stopped, and the extracorporeal blood product is processed. The rest of the procedure is similar to the continuous-flow process in that the blood is centrifuged, the selected component is diverted into a waste bag, and the remaining blood is returned to the patient with appropriate replacement fluid. The process can be repeated for several cycles.

Filtration devices also operate by continuous flow. Anticoagulated whole blood is passed through a microporous filter that allows plasma to pass through but retains the blood cells. The separated plasma can then be diverted into a waste bag, or as with selective adsorption, further processed and returned to the patient. This type of device is not suitable for the removal of select cellular components in circulation (cytapheresis). A variant of this technique is rheopheresis, or double-filtration TPE, in which high-molecular-weight molecules are removed, thereby reducing plasma viscosity.

In selective adsorption, blood or plasma is passed over a column that has a high affinity for a specific component, such as immune globulin G (IgG) or low-density lipoprotein (LDL), and the effluent is returned to the patient. This approach has the advantage of highly specific removal of the target of interest. However, it is restricted to the few conditions for which affinity adsorbents are available.

PATIENT EVALUATION AND MANAGEMENT

All patients should be evaluated by a physician familiar with apheresis before beginning any course of TA. General considerations in formulating an overall therapy plan are identified in Table 25-2. A more comprehensive evaluation of the patient is typically performed in this setting, with the clinical evaluation focusing on select elements at subsequent TPE encounters in stable patients receiving an extended series

of treatments, unless changes in the patient's clinical status dictate otherwise.

The indication, type of procedure, choice of replacement fluid (Table 25-3), vascular access, frequency and number of treatments, and the treatment goal or endpoint should be documented in the patient's record. During the initial evaluation, the nature of the procedure and its expected benefits, possible risks, and available alternatives must be explained to the patient, and informed consent must be documented. Depending on institutionally specific policies, these informed consent discussions should be repeated periodically (eg, annually) and documented in the medical record. Procedures should be performed only in settings where there is ready access to care for untoward reactions, including equipment, medications, and personnel trained in managing serious adverse events, such as anaphylaxis. Comorbidities that may affect the patient's ability to tolerate apheresis and concurrent medication reconciliation should be noted. Other specific points to consider when evaluating a patient include the following:

- **Transfusion/apheresis history:** Notation of prior transfusion/apheresis interventions and reactions, outcomes from such therapies, and special blood component requirements.
- **Neurologic status:** Mental status and the ability to consent and cooperate.
- **Cardiorespiratory status:** Adequate ventilation and oxygenation capabilities, presence of hyper- or hypovolemia, and any cardiac arrhythmias.
- **Renal and metabolic status:** Fluid balance, alkalosis, and electrolyte abnormalities, including hypocalcemia, hypokalemia, and hypomagnesemia.
- **Hematologic status:** Presence of clinically significant anemia, thrombocytopenia, coagulopathy, bleeding, or thrombosis.
- **Medications:** Recently administered intravenous immunoglobulin (IVIG) and antibody biologics, angiotensin-converting enzyme (ACE) inhibitors, drugs with high albumin-binding properties, and anticoagulants.

TABLE 25-2. Elements* in a Comprehensive Evaluation and Treatment Plan for Patients Being Considered for TA Interventions

Clinical diagnosis / chief complaint / clinical objective / reason for referral
History of the pertinent present illness
Patient's past / family medical histories, including prior TA and hemotherapies (eg, blood transfusions and IVIG infusions)
Pertinent review of systems and medication reconciliation
Pertinent physical examination, including vascular access assessment
TA indication / rationale / outcome objectives
Selection of apheresis equipment
Volume / duration / frequency targets
● Per procedure
● For entire series
Vascular access device considerations as needed
Choice of replacement fluids
Physiologic / adverse reaction / clinical outcomes monitoring
Coordination of pre- / intra- / post- and interprocedural laboratory testing and drug / blood administration
Use of ancillary equipment prn
● Blood warmers
● Fetal monitors
● Ventilatory support devices
● Separate IV access for calcium infusion
Patient educational materials and discharge instructions
Need for initial series extension / concurrent immunosuppressive therapies
Coagulopathies / anticoagulation medication when relevant

*Identified elements are typically considered in the clinical evaluation at the time of the initial consultation of all patients being assessed for TA. In stable individuals undergoing an extended series of TA, apheresis medicine specialists may elect to exclude select aspects (eg, patient's past/family medical histories, if obtained at time of initial consultation) from the patient's evaluation at each subsequent apheresis session unless changes in the clinical status of the patient warrant otherwise. Table adapted and modified from Andrzejewski.[10]

TA = therapeutic apheresis; IVIG = intravenous immune globulin; prn = as needed.

Appropriate laboratory monitoring is guided by the TA indication, the type and frequency of procedures, and concomitant medical conditions. In general, it is wise to obtain test results for a complete blood cell count, type and screen, coagulation profile, and electrolytes before starting treatment. Other diagnostic study results, such as tests for infectious diseases and pertinent specific disease markers, should be collected before the first treatment. Coagulation monitoring may be appropriate when albumin is used as the primary replacement fluid during frequently repeated procedures. The collection of an

TABLE 25-3. Comparison of Replacement Fluids

Replacement Solution	Advantages	Disadvantages
Crystalloids	Low cost Nonallergenic No viral risk	Two- to threefold more volume required Hypo-oncotic Lacking coagulation factors and immunoglobulins
Albumin	Iso-oncotic Low risk of reactions	Higher cost Lacking coagulation factors and immunoglobulins
Plasma	Iso-oncotic Normal levels of coagulation factors, immunoglobulins, and other plasma proteins	Viral transmission risk Increased citrate load ABO compatibility required Higher risk of allergic reactions
Cryoprecipitate-reduced plasma	Iso-oncotic Reduced high-molecular-weight von Willebrand factor and fibrinogen Normal levels of most other plasma proteins	Same as plasma

"archive specimen" before the initial apheresis session should also be considered, because concentrations of plasma constituents are altered by TA. Similarly, apheresis medicine practitioners should make colleagues and patients aware that diagnostic testing after apheresis can be differentially affected depending on the analyte of interest, the replacement fluids used, and the frequency of TPE sessions.

VASCULAR ACCESS

TA requires excellent vascular access to achieve adequate flow rates. Peripheral access is preferred and generally requires at least a 17-gauge needle for blood withdrawal and at least an 18-gauge catheter for return. Patients without adequate peripheral veins, those who require multiple frequent procedures, and those unable to provide hand compressions to maintain vascular flow may require placement of central venous catheters (CVCs). CVCs for apheresis must have rigid walls to accommodate the negative pressure generated in the withdrawal line. Peripherally inserted central

catheters (ie, PICC lines) typically do not support the high flow rates used in apheresis and should not be used. Dual-lumen catheters similar to the types used in hemodialysis are preferred, although single-lumen catheters can be used for intermittent-flow procedures. An implanted subcutaneous port may provide an option for some patients requiring long-term treatment, such as chronic red cell exchange.

The choice of placement site for a CVC is influenced by the anticipated duration of treatment. Subclavian or internal jugular access is generally preferable for TPE courses lasting up to several weeks. Femoral vein access should be used only temporarily because of the higher risk of infection. Patients requiring extended treatment courses usually have tunneled CVC placement. With proper care, tunneled catheters can be used for prolonged periods. Radiographic confirmation of non-femoral-vein CVC placement should be obtained before initiation of the first apheresis session and whenever a CVC replacement occurs.

Good catheter care is very important for patient safety and to maintain CVC patency. Responsibility for CVC maintenance needs to be clearly defined, and apheresis medicine services need to be actively involved in either directly providing this care or in its coordination with other parties involved in treating the patient. Catheters need to be flushed regularly. Heparin or 4% trisodium citrate is usually placed in each lumen after each use to prevent occlusion by clots. If a port becomes clotted, instillation of a fibrinolytic agent, such as urokinase or recombinant tissue plasminogen activator, may restore patency. Routine dressing care is essential to prevent insertion-site infections. An arteriovenous (AV) fistula may also be used for apheresis, but personnel should be suitably trained before attempting to access an AV fistula.

Venous access devices may cause thrombosis. Infrequently, their placement may result in severe complications, such as pneumothorax or perforation of the heart or great vessels. Other complications include arterial puncture, deep hematomas, and AV formation. Bacterial colonization may lead to catheter-associated bloodstream infection, especially in immunosuppressed patients. Inadvertent disconnection of catheters may produce hemorrhage or air embolism.

ANTICOAGULATION

Acid-citrate-dextrose solution A (ACD-A) is the most commonly used anticoagulant, although heparin combined with ACD-A is also used, particularly in the setting of large-volume leukapheresis for hematopoietic progenitor cell collection. Heparin anticoagulation is necessary for lipid apheresis and may be desirable for selected patients undergoing TPE who are particularly susceptible to hypocalcemia, such as small children, or in the setting of severe metabolic alkalosis or renal failure. With citrate anticoagulation, coagulation monitoring is generally not necessary, although knowledge and monitoring of ionized calcium levels may be helpful for selected patients. In patients with normal hepatic function, the infused citrate is rapidly metabolized and rarely causes systemic anticoagulation.

ADVERSE EFFECTS

Although TA is very safe, complications do occur; adverse events, mostly mild, occur in ~4% of procedures (Table 25-4).[11-14] Symptomatic hypocalcemia due to citrate anticoagulation is the most common adverse effect, typically characterized by perioral and digital paresthesiae. Nausea or other gastrointestinal symptoms may also occur, although tetany is rare. Cardiac arrhythmia is very rare, but patients with preexisting hypocalcemia or significant prolongation of the QT interval should be monitored carefully. Calcium supplementation may alleviate symptoms of citrate toxicity; a typical dose is 10 mL of 10% calcium gluconate per liter of albumin infused. Citrate also chelates ionized magnesium, so it is possible that hypomagnesemia contributes to the symptoms of citrate toxicity. However, one randomized clinical trial showed no benefit of adding magnesium during leukapheresis with

TABLE 25-4. Reported Frequency of Adverse Reactions to Apheresis*

Reaction	Frequency (%)
Paresthesia	1.30
Hypotension	0.91
Urticaria	0.63
Nausea	0.39
Shivering	0.29
Flushing	0.16
Dyspnea	0.15
Vertigo	0.17
Arrhythmia	0.11
Abdominal pain	0.12
Anaphylaxis	0.02
Total	4.25

*Adapted from Matsuzaki.[11]

continuous intravenous (IV) calcium supplementation.[15] Metabolism of citrate leads to a mild metabolic alkalosis, which can exacerbate hypocalcemia and may cause hypokalemia.[16]

Allergic reactions are most common with plasma replacement, although they may also occur with albumin. Most reactions are mild, characterized by urticaria or cutaneous flushing. More severe reactions can involve the respiratory tract with dyspnea, wheezing, and (rarely) stridor. Most allergic reactions respond quickly to IV diphenhydramine. Anaphylaxis is very rare but can occur. Patients receiving large volumes of plasma, such as those with thrombotic thrombocytopenic purpura (TTP), are most at risk for allergic reactions. Premedication with an antihistamine, or possibly steroids, is not necessary for routine apheresis but may be indicated for patients with repeated or previous severe reactions.

Respiratory difficulty during or immediately following apheresis can have many causes, such as pulmonary edema, pulmonary embolism, air embolism, leukostasis, anaphylactic reactions, and transfusion-related acute lung injury (TRALI).[17] Hemothorax or hemopericardium resulting from vascular erosion from a CVC is rare but may be fatal.[18] Pulmonary edema due to volume overload or cardiac failure is usually associated with dyspnea, an increase in diastolic blood pressure, and characteristic chest radiograph findings. Predominantly ocular reactions (periorbital edema, conjunctival swelling, and tearing) have occurred in individuals sensitized to the ethylene oxide gas used to sterilize disposable plastic apheresis kits.[19,20]

Hypotension during apheresis can be a sign of citrate toxicity, hypovolemia, or a vasovagal, allergic, drug, or transfusion reaction. Hypovolemia can occur early in treatments of small patients when the return fluid consists of the saline used to prime the apheresis circuit. Vasovagal reactions are characterized by bradycardia and hypotension. Such reactions usually respond well to a fluid bolus and placing the patient in the Trendelenburg position.

When hypotension occurs during plasma or red cell exchanges, potential transfusion reactions such as TRALI, acute hemolysis, bacterial contamination, or anti-IgA-related anaphylaxis should be considered. Hypotension is more frequent in children, the elderly, neurology patients, anemic patients, and those treated with intermittent-flow devices that have large extracorporeal volumes. Continuous-flow devices typically do not have large extracorporeal volumes but can produce hypovolemia if return flow is inadvertently diverted to a waste collection bag, either through operator oversight or device malfunction. Hypovolemia may also be secondary to inadequate volume or protein replacement. During all procedures, it is essential to carefully document and maintain records of the volumes processed, removed, and returned. (See Fig 25-1.)

When plasma is exposed to foreign surfaces such as plastic tubing or filtration devices, the kinin system can be activated, resulting in production of bradykinin. Infusion of plasma containing bradykinin can cause abrupt hypotension. Patients taking ACE inhibitors are more susceptible to these hypotensive reactions because these drugs block the enzymatic degradation of bradykinin.[21] Hypotensive reactions are more likely during selective adsorption procedures because these devices expose plasma to a very large surface area. Because some ACE inhibitors have a long duration of action, stopping the drug on the day before the procedure may not be sufficient to prevent a reaction.

Intensive TPE without plasma replacement depletes coagulation factors. A 1.0 plasma volume exchange typically reduces coagulation factor levels by 25% to 50%, although Factor VIII levels are less affected.[22] Levels of fibrinogen, a large intravascular molecule, are reduced by ~66%. If the patient has normal hepatic synthetic function, coagulation factor levels typically return to near normal within 2 days. Thus, many patients can tolerate TPE every other day for 1 to 2 weeks without developing significant coagulopathies requiring plasma replacement.

Bleeding due to coagulation factor depletion is rare. For patients at risk, plasma may be used for replacement at the end of the procedure. Apheresis can also cause

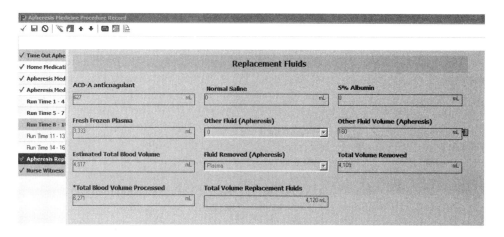

FIGURE 25-1. Computer-screen display of a select section of an apheresis procedural note detailing volumes and identities of fluids processed, removed, and replaced during a therapeutic plasma exchange for a patient with thrombotic thrombocytopenic purpura; these details are documented in the patient's electronic medical record used at Baystate Medical Center, Springfield, MA. See also Fig 25-2 (B).

thrombocytopenia. Intensive TPE can cause hypogammaglobulinemia. Serum levels of IgG and IgM recover to 40% to 50% of the pre-apheresis level by 48 hours.[22] The absolute immunoglobulin level at which a patient becomes at risk for infection has not been established.

Albumin-bound drugs are removed by TPE. This can produce subtherapeutic levels of medications unless dosages are adjusted. Biological therapeutics, such as IVIG, antithymocyte globulin, and monoclonal antibodies, have a long intravascular half-life and are readily removed by apheresis. TPE shortly after the administration of such drugs should be avoided because it may significantly impair their effectiveness.

Collapsed or kinked tubing, malfunctioning pinch valves, or improper threading of tubing may damage red cells in the extracorporeal circuit. Instrument-related hemolysis occurs in 0.06% of TA procedures.[12] Hemolysis can also occur with the use of hypotonic replacement fluids or ABO-incompatible plasma. The operator should carefully observe plasma collection lines for pink discoloration suggestive of hemolysis. Other types of equipment failure, such as problems with the rotating seal, leaks in plasticware, and roller pump failure, are rare.

Fatalities during apheresis are rare and are reportable to the Food and Drug Administration (FDA).[23] Death has been reported in 0.006% to 0.09% of therapeutic procedures, with most fatalities attributable to underlying medical conditions.[12,24]

THERAPEUTIC APHERESIS INDICATIONS

Although there are many case reports of successful treatment of various diseases and conditions by apheresis, there are few high-quality prospective case-control clinical trials. ASFA has published evidence-based clinical guidelines categorizing treatment indications.[2]

- **Category I:** Disorders for which apheresis is accepted as first-line therapy, either as a primary standalone treatment or in conjunction with other modes of treatment.
- **Category II:** Disorders for which apheresis is accepted as second-line therapy, either as a standalone treatment or in conjunction with other modes of treatment.

- **Category III:** Disorders in which the optimal role of apheresis therapy is not established. Decision-making for patients should be individualized.
- **Category IV:** Disorders in which published evidence demonstrates or suggests that apheresis is ineffective or harmful. Institutional review board approval is desirable if apheresis treatment is undertaken in these circumstances.

Fuller discussions of the conditions treated with TA may be found by consulting more comprehensive medical texts on the respective disorders. An overview of some of the more commonly encountered diseases treated by TA is provided below.

Therapeutic Plasma Exchange

In both alloimmune and autoimmune disorders, pathogenic factors that are circulating in the blood are targets for removal by TPE. Autoantibody-mediated diseases include acute and chronic inflammatory demyelinating polyneuropathies (AIDP and CIDP), antiglomerular basement membrane disease, and myasthenia gravis. Examples of conditions where the goal is to remove problematic alloantibodies include renal transplantation with presensitization and antibody-mediated organ transplant rejection. Diseases in which immune complexes may be pathogenic and can be removed by apheresis include rapidly progressive glomerulonephritis, cryoglobulinemia, and vasculitis. Other indications include conditions treated by removing protein-bound drugs, toxins, or high concentrations of lipoproteins. Indications for TPE are listed in Table 25-5.

In TTP, an absolute or functional deficiency of the von Willebrand factor (vWF)-cleaving metalloprotease ADAMTS13 results in the accumulation of high-molecular-weight vWF multimers, with subsequent intravascular platelet activation and platelet-rich thrombi in the microvasculature.[25] In many cases, an inhibitor of ADAMTS13 can be demonstrated. TPE is first-line treatment for TTP, with the goal of removing both the inhibitor and large vWF multimers while simultaneously replacing the deficient enzyme. TPE is typically performed daily until the platelet count and lactate dehydrogenase level normalize, typically with the former being >150,000/µL for 48 hours, but treatment duration should be guided by the individual patient's course. After response has been achieved, intermittent apheresis or plasma infusion tapers may be instituted, but the efficacy of these approaches in preventing relapse has not been established.[26] TPE results in greatly improved survival in TTP patients; however, treatment failures do occur.[27]

Hemolytic uremic syndrome (HUS) is a similar condition that occurs more commonly in children than in adults. HUS may follow diarrheal infections with verotoxin-secreting strains of *Escherichia coli* (strain 0157:H7) or *Shigella*. Compared to patients with classic TTP, those with HUS have more renal dysfunction and less prominent neurologic and hematologic findings. Most patients with HUS do not have antibodies to ADAMTS13 and have normal protease activity. Although diarrhea-associated HUS rarely responds to TPE, atypical HUS (aHUS) caused by complement factor deficiencies or autoantibodies to Factor H may respond; however, patients with aHUS caused by membrane cofactor protein mutations may not respond to TPE. Eculizumab, a monoclonal antibody directed against C5a, thereby inhibiting terminal complement activation, may be effective in treating individuals with aHUS.[28]

Secondary forms of microangiopathic hemolytic anemia (MAHA), associated with systemic lupus erythematosus, cancer, hematopoietic progenitor cell transplantation, chemotherapy, or immunosuppressive medications, may be clinically indistinguishable from classical TTP. In many of these cases, however, ADAMTS13 activity is normal or only moderately reduced, and the response to TPE is typically poor. Transplant-associated microangiopathic hemolysis rarely responds to apheresis and probably represents a different disease process.[29]

In multiple myeloma, where patients may exhibit hyperviscosity-related adverse

TABLE 25-5. Indications for Therapeutic Plasma Exchange[2]

Indication	Modifying Conditions	Category	Typical Course (number of treatments)
Acute disseminated encephalomyelitis	Steroid refractory	II	QOD (3-6)
Acute inflammatory demyelinating polyradiculoneuropathy/Guillain-Barré syndrome	Primary treatment	I	QOD (5-6)
	After IVIG	III	
Acute liver failure	Routine TPE	III	QD (variable)
	High-volume TPE	I	QD (3)
Amyloidosis, systemic		IV	
ANCA-associated rapidly progressive glomerulonephritis (granulomatosis with polyangiitis; and microscopic poly-angiitis)	Dialysis dependence	I	QD or QOD (6-9)
	DAH	I	
	Dialysis independence	III	
Antiglomerular basement membrane dis-ease (Goodpasture syndrome)	Dialysis dependence, no DAH	III	QD or QOD (variable)
	DAH	I	
	Dialysis independence	I	
Aplastic anemia, pure red cell aplasia	Aplastic anemia	III	QD or QOD (variable)
	Pure red cell aplasia	III	
Atopic (neuro-) dermatitis (atopic eczema), recalcitrant		III	Weekly (variable)
Autoimmune hemolytic anemia; WAIHA; cold agglutinin disease	Severe WAIHA	III	QD or QOD (variable)
	Severe cold agglutinin disease	II	
Burn shock resuscitation		III	1-3 within 24-36 hours
Cardiac neonatal lupus		III	Weekly to monthly
Cardiac transplantation	Desensitization	II	QD or QOD (variable)
	Antibody-mediated rejection	III	
Catastrophic antiphospholipid syndrome		II	QD or QOD (variable)
Chronic focal encephalitis (Rasmussen encephalitis)		III	QOD (3-6)
Chronic inflammatory demyelinating polyradiculoneuropathy		I	2-3/week
Coagulation factor inhibitors	Alloantibody	IV	QD (variable)
	Autoantibody	III	
Complex regional pain syndrome	Chronic	III	QOD (5-7)

TABLE 25-5.   Indications for Therapeutic Plasma Exchange[2] (Continued)

Indication	Modifying Conditions	Category	Typical Course (number of treatments)
Cryoglobulinemia	Symptomatic/severe	II	QOD (3-8)
Dermatomyositis/polymyositis		IV	
Dilated cardiomyopathy, idiopathic	NYHA II-IV	III	QOD (5)
Erythropoietic porphyria, liver disease		III	QOD (variable)
Familial hypercholesterolemia	Homozygotes with small blood volume	II	Once in 1-2 weeks (indefinite)
Focal segmental glomerulosclerosis	Recurrent in transplanted kidney	I	1-3/week (variable)
Hashimoto encephalopathy: Steroid-responsive encephalopathy associated with autoimmune thyroiditis		II	QD or QOD (3-9)
HELLP syndrome	Postpartum	III	QD (variable)
	Antepartum	IV	
Hematopoietic stem cell transplantation, ABO incompatible	Major—HPC, Marrow	II	QD (variable)
	Major—HPC, Apheresis	II	
Hematopoietic stem cell transplantation, HLA desensitization		III	QOD (variable)
Hemophagocytic lymphohistiocytosis; hemophagocytic syndrome; macrophage-activating syndrome		III	QD (variable)
Henoch-Schönlein purpura	Crescentic	III	QOD (4-11)
	Severe extrarenal disease	III	
Heparin-induced thrombocytopenia and thrombosis	Precardiopulmonary bypass	III	QD or QOD (variable)
	Thrombosis	III	
Hypertriglyceridemic pancreatitis		III	QD (1-3)
Hyperviscosity in monoclonal gammopathies	Symptomatic	I	QD (1-3)
	Prophylaxis for rituximab	I	QD (1-2)
Immune thrombocytopenia	Refractory	III	QOD (6)
Immunoglobulin A nephropathy	Crescentic	III	QOD (6-9)
	Chronic progressive	III	

(Continued)

TABLE 25-5. Indications for Therapeutic Plasma Exchange[2] (Continued)

Indication	Modifying Conditions	Category	Typical Course (number of treatments)
Lambert-Eaton myasthenic syndrome		II	QD or QOD (variable)
Liver transplantation	Desensitization, ABOi LD	I	QD or QOD (variable)
	Desensitization, ABOi DD	III	
	Antibody-mediated rejection (ABOi and HLA)	III	
Lung transplantation	Antibody-mediated rejection	III	QOD (variable)
	Desensitization	III	
Multiple sclerosis	Acute CNS inflammatory demyelinating	II	QOD (5-7)
	Chronic progressive	III	Weekly (variable)
Myasthenia gravis	Moderate/severe	I	QD or QOD (variable)
	Prethymectomy	I	
Myeloma cast nephropathy		II	QOD (10-12)
Nephrogenic systemic fibrosis		III	QD or QOD (5-14)
Neuromyelitis optica spectrum disorders	Acute	II	QOD (5-10)
	Maintenance	III	
N-methyl D-aspartate receptor antibody encephalitis		I	QOD (5-6)
Overdose, envenomation, and poisoning	Mushroom poisoning	II	QD (variable)
	Envenomation	III	
	Drug overdose/poisoning	III	
Paraneoplastic neurologic syndromes		III	QD or QOD (5-6)
Paraproteinemic demyelinating neuropathies/chronic acquired demyelinating polyneuropathies	Anti-MAG neuropathy	III	QOD (5-6)
	Multifocal motor neuropathy	IV	
	IgG/IgA	I	
	IgM	I	
	Multiple myeloma	III	
Pediatric autoimmune neuropsychiatric disorders associated with streptococcal infections (PANDAS); Sydenham chorea	PANDAS exacerbation	II	QD or QOD (3-6)
	Sydenham chorea, severe	III	

(Continued)

TABLE 25-5. Indications for Therapeutic Plasma Exchange[2] (Continued)

Indication	Modifying Conditions	Category	Typical Course (number of treatments)
Pemphigus vulgaris	Severe	III	QD or QOD (variable)
Phytanic acid storage disease (Refsum disease)		II	QD (variable)
Posttransfusion purpura		III	QD (variable)
Progressive multifocal leukoencephalopathy associated with natalizumab		I	QOD (variable)
Pruritus due to hepatobiliary diseases	Treatment resistant	III	1-2/week (variable)
Psoriasis		IV	
Red cell alloimmunization in pregnancy	Prior to IUT availability	III	1-3/week
Renal transplantation, ABO compatible	Antibody-mediated rejection	I	QD or QOD (variable)
	Desensitization, LD	I	
	Desensitization, DD	III	
Renal transplantation, ABO incompatible	Desensitization, LD	I	QD or QOD (variable)
	Antibody-mediated rejection	II	
	A_2/A_2B into B, DD	IV	
Scleroderma (systemic sclerosis)		III	2-3/week (6)
Sepsis with multiorgan failure		III	QD (variable)
Stiff-person syndrome		III	QOD (3-5)
Sudden sensorineural hearing loss		III	QOD (3)
Systemic lupus erythematosus	Severe	II	QD or QOD (3-6)
	Nephritis	IV	
Thrombotic microangiopathy, coagulation mediated	THBD mutation	III	QD or QOD (variable)
Thrombotic microangiopathy, complement mediated	Complement factor gene mutations	III	QD (variable)
	Factor H autoantibodies	I	
	MCP mutations	III	

(Continued)

TABLE 24-5. Indications for Therapeutic Plasma Exchange[2] (Continued)

Indication	Modifying Conditions	Category	Typical Course (number of treatments)
Thrombotic microangiopathy, drug associated	Ticlopidine	I	QD or QOD (variable)
	Clopidogrel	III	
	Calcineurin inhibitors	III	
	Gemcitabine	IV	
	Quinine	IV	
Thrombotic microangiopathy, hematopoietic stem cell transplantation associated		III	QD (variable)
Thrombotic microangiopathy, Shiga-toxin mediated	Severe neurologic symptoms	III	QD (variable)
	Streptococcus pneumoniae	III	
	Absence of severe neurologic symptoms	IV	
Thrombotic thrombocytopenic purpura		I	QD (variable)
Thyroid storm		III	QD or QOD (variable)
Toxic epidermal necrolysis	Refractory	III	QD or QOD (variable)
Vasculitis	HBV-PAN	II	QOD (9-12)
	Idiopathic PAN	IV	
	EGPA	III	
	Behçet disease	III	
Voltage-gated potassium channel antibodies		II	QOD (5-7)
Wilson disease	Fulminant	I	QD or QOD (variable)

QOD = every other day; IVIG = intravenous immunoglobulin; TPE = therapeutic plasma exchange; QD = daily; ANCA = antineutrophil cytoplasmic antibodies; DAH = diffuse alveolar hemorrhage; WAIHA = warm autoimmune hemolytic anemia; NYHA = New York Heart Association (class); HELLP = hemolysis, elevated liver enzymes, low platelet count (syndrome); HPC, Marrow = hematopoietic progenitor cells collected from marrow; HPC, Apheresis = HPCs from apheresis; ABOi = ABO incompatible; LD = living donor; DD = deceased donor; CNS = central nervous system; MAG = myelin-associated glycoprotein; IUT = intrauterine transfusion; THBD = thrombomodulin; MCP = membrane cofactor protein; HBV = hepatitis B virus; PAN = polyarteritis nodosa; EGPA = eosinophilic granulomatosis with polyangiitis.

sequelae, the goal is to remove excessive amounts of the tumor-associated paraprotein (M protein). Plasma viscosity measurements may not be useful in guiding therapy in some patients because they may not correlate with symptoms. Normal plasma viscosity is 1.4 to 1.8 centipoise (cP). Because most patients are asymptomatic until plasma viscosity is >4.0 to

5.0 cP, those with mild elevations may not require treatment. In general, hyperviscosity becomes a concern when M protein concentrations reach 3 g/dL for IgM, 4 g/dL for IgG, and 6 g/dL for IgA.[30] Nonetheless, symptomatic patients, regardless of plasma viscosity levels, especially those with visual and neurologic symptoms, are candidates for urgent apheresis treatments.

Conflicting data exist regarding the efficacy of TPE for treating acute renal failure in myeloma. A randomized controlled trial of TPE vs conventional care showed no difference in mortality or renal function at 6 months[31]; however, among dialysis-dependent patients, 43% in the TPE group and none in the control group recovered renal function. Another randomized clinical trial showed no benefit of TPE in a composite outcome measure of death, dialysis dependence, and glomerular filtration rate[32]; however, biopsy confirmation of the renal diagnosis was not required in this trial. Similarly, a retrospective cohort study showed no benefit of TPE in either reducing mortality or preserving renal function.[33] If TPE is to be undertaken, biopsy confirmation of cast nephropathy may be advisable. With the advent of new drugs to treat multiple myeloma patients, including proteosome inhibitors and monoclonal antibodies, and the determination to begin their use as soon as possible, the role for TPE in this setting continues to evolve.

Patients receiving rituximab (anti-CD20) for IgM Waldenström macroglobulinemia may experience a transient increase in M protein levels after drug initiation, and a short TPE series before starting this medication may be indicated in select patients. Patients with pretreatment IgM levels >5 g/dL are at particular risk of developing symptomatic hyperviscosity.[34]

TPE may be used to treat central nervous system (CNS) acute disseminated encephalomyelitis. Experience in treating chronic progressive multiple sclerosis with TPE has been discouraging. However, a randomized clinical trial in acute CNS inflammatory demyelinating diseases unresponsive to steroids showed that TPE was beneficial.[35] Early initiation of TPE may facilitate response, and some clinical responses may not manifest until later in follow-up.[36] TPE may also be effective in neuromyelitis optica (NMO), even in the absence of NMO antibodies.[37]

TPE to treat select peripheral nervous system diseases [eg, acute inflammatory demyelinating polyneuropathies like Guillain-Barré syndrome (GBS)] is well established, with randomized controlled clinical trials substantiating its efficacy in GBS patients not exhibiting spontaneous recovery.[2] IVIG infusions alone or following a course of TPE appear equally effective.[38] No biomarkers are currently known to distinguish between these different therapeutic strategies regarding which should be used initially. As a result of concomitant autonomic nervous system involvement, patients often exhibit blood pressure and pulse variability that can complicate initial sessions of TPE but typically becomes less pronounced during later TPE sessions. Given equivalent efficacy and similar severity and frequencies of adverse events with either TPE or IVIG, TPE appears to be a less expensive first-line therapy option for treating patients with GBS.[39]

In focal segmental glomerulosclerosis (FSGS), a circulating factor that increases glomerular permeability with resultant proteinuria was identified.[40,41] FSGS frequently recurs after renal transplantation and can produce allograft failure. TPE may effectively remove the permeability factor and induce remission in recurrent FSGS following renal transplantation. However, response to TPE in primary FSGS has not been well studied.

TPE may provide adjunctive immunosuppression in treating or preventing antibody-mediated rejection (AMR) of solid-organ transplants. AMR presenting in the early posttransplantation period may respond better to TPE than later AMR.[42] TPE before transplantation of an ABO-incompatible kidney may prevent hyperacute rejection, and posttransplantation TPE is often used to treat AMR in this setting.[43,44] TPE in conjunction with immunomodulatory therapies, such as IVIG, before transplantation can reduce the risk of rejection in HLA-alloimmunized patients.[45]

Cytapheresis

The goal of cytapheresis is to remove excessive or pathogenic leukocytes, platelets, or red cells. In addition, in red cell exchange, donor red cells are used to restore oxygen-carrying capacity. Indications for cytapheresis are listed in Table 25-6.

In leukemia, high cell counts (typically >100,000/μL) can produce microvascular stasis with headache, mental status changes, visual disturbances, or dyspnea. The leukocyte count at which a patient becomes symptomatic is variable. Typically, patients with acute or chronic lymphocytic leukemia tolerate higher cell counts than patients with myelogenous leukemia, and cytapheresis may not be required. Cytapheresis commonly results in a less-than-predicted reduction in leukocyte count, despite excellent collection, because of mobilization and reequilibration of marginated intravascular cells and cells from extravascular sites. Myelogenous leukemia cells commonly have a higher density than lymphocytic cells and can be difficult to separate from red cells by centrifugation. Use of hydroxyethyl starch enhances red cell sedimentation by rouleaux formation and can improve cytapheresis efficiency in acute myelogenous leukemia. Massive thrombocytosis, typically >1,000,000/μL, can occur in essential thrombocythemia, in polycythemia vera, or as a reactive phenomenon. Such patients may be at risk of thrombosis or hemorrhage. Reduction in platelet count is commonly less than predicted because of mobilization of platelets to the peripheral blood, primarily from the spleen.

Red cell exchange is most commonly performed in sickle cell disease (SCD). The goal is to reduce the burden of hemoglobin S and to provide donor red cells containing hemoglobin A. Acute chest syndrome, a serious complication of SCD, presents as dyspnea, chest pain, and cough, often accompanied by fever, leukocytosis, decreasing hematocrit, hypoxia, and pulmonary infiltrates. Respiratory failure can develop, and death occurs in ~3% of cases.[46] Red cell exchange is indicated for progressive infiltrates and hypoxemia refractory to conventional therapy and simple transfusion.[47,48] A common goal is to reduce hemoglobin S to <30%, with a final hematocrit not to exceed ~30%. Red cell exchange may also be indicated for preventing stroke in SCD. For patients with elevated cerebral blood flow velocity determined by transcranial Doppler imaging, transfusion reduces the risk of stroke.[49,50] Chronic red cell exchange, typically every 4-6 weeks, can normalize cerebral blood flow while minimizing iron overload. Red cell exchange may have a role in other sickle cell syndromes, including multiorgan failure, hepatic/splenic sequestration, priapism, and intrahepatic cholestasis. In addition, it may be used for preventing iron overload and for preventing or managing vaso-occlusive pain crises.

Red cells for replacement must be ABO compatible and negative for known, clinically significant, recipient alloantibodies. For SCD patients, red cells should be matched for C, E, and K, if possible.[51] It is desirable to use relatively fresh units to maximize posttransfusion red cell survival. Units containing either citrate-phosphate-dextrose-adenine (CPDA)-1 or additive solutions (AS) may be used. It is desirable that all units used in a given procedure contain the same anticoagulant solution so that they have similar hematocrits. Chronic red cell exchange may carry a lower risk of alloimmunization than simple transfusion in SCD patients.[52]

Extracorporeal Photopheresis

In extracorporeal photopheresis (ECP), the buffy-coat layer is collected from peripheral blood, treated with 8-methoxypsoralen and ultraviolet A light, and reinfused into the patient. The treatment causes crosslinking of leukocyte DNA, which prevents replication and induces apoptosis. ECP was developed to treat cutaneous T-cell lymphoma, although it is increasingly used for other indications (Table 25-7). ECP has complex immunomodulatory effects, including induction of monocyte differentiation into dendritic cells, alteration of T-cell subsets, and changes in cytokine profiles.[53] ECP may be effective in acute and chronic skin graft-vs-host disease (GVHD),

TABLE 25-6. Indications for Therapeutic Cytapheresis[2]

Indication	Modifying Conditions	Procedure	Category	Typical Course (number of treatments)
Babesiosis	Severe	Red cell exchange	II	Once
Erythropoietic porphyria, liver disease		Red cell exchange	III	QOD (variable)
Hematopoietic stem cell transplantation, ABO incompatible	Minor—HPC, Apheresis	Red cell exchange	III	Once
Hereditary hemachromatosis		Erythrocytapheresis	I	Every 2-4 weeks (variable)
Hyperleukocytosis	Symptomatic	Leukocytapheresis	II	QD (variable)
	Prophylactic or secondary		III	
Inflammatory bowel disease	Ulcerative colitis	Adsorptive cytapheresis	III/II	Weekly (5-10)
	Crohn disease		III	
Malaria	Severe	Red cell exchange	III	1-2 procedures
Polycythemia vera; erythrocytosis	Polycythemia vera	Erythrocytapheresis	I	Variable
	Secondary erythrocytosis		III	
Prevention of RhD alloimmunization after red cell exposure	Exposure to RhD(1) red cells	Red cell exchange	III	Once
Psoriasis	Disseminated pustular	Adsorptive cytapheresis	III	Weekly (5)
		Lymphocytapheresis	III	
Sickle cell disease, acute	Acute stroke	Red cell exchange	I	Once
	Acute chest syndrome, severe		II	
	Priapism		III	
	Multiorgan failure		III	
	Splenic/hepatic sequestration; intrahepatic cholestasis		III	
Sickle cell disease, nonacute	Stroke prophylaxis/iron overload prevention	Red cell exchange	I	Every 4-6 weeks (indefinite)
	Recurrent vaso-occlusive pain crisis		III	
	Preoperative management		III	Once
	Pregnancy		III	Every 4 weeks (until delivery)

(Continued)

TABLE 25-6. Indications for Therapeutic Cytapheresis[2] (Continued)

Indication	Modifying Conditions	Procedure	Category	Typical Course (number of treatments)
Thrombocytosis	Symptomatic	Thrombocytapheresis	II	QD (variable)
	Prophylactic or secondary		III	
Vasculitis	Behçet disease	Adsorption granulocytapheresis	II	Weekly (5)

QOD = every other day; QD = daily; HPC, Apheresis = hematopoietic progenitor cells collected from apheresis.

TABLE 25-7. Indications for Photopheresis[2]

Indication	Modifying Conditions	Category	Typical Course* (duration)
Atopic (neuro-) dermatitis (atopic eczema), recalcitrant		III	Every 2 weeks (12 weeks)
Cardiac transplantation	Cellular/recurrent rejection	II	Weekly or every 2-8 weeks (several months)
	Rejection prophylaxis	II	
Cutaneous T-cell lymphoma; mycosis fungoides; Sézary syndrome	Erythrodermic	I	Every 2-4 weeks (5-6 months)
	Nonerythrodermic	III	
Dermatomyositis/polymyositis		IV	
Graft-vs-host disease	Skin (chronic)	II	Every 1-2 weeks (8-12 weeks)
	Nonskin (chronic)	II	
	Skin (acute)	II	2-3 weekly, 2 weekly, then every 2 weeks
	Nonskin(acute)	II	
Inflammatory bowel disease	Crohn disease	III	Weekly (4), every 2 weeks (8)
Lung transplantation	Bronchiolitis obliterans syndrome	II	Weekly (5), every 2 weeks (4), every month (3)
Nephrogenic systemic fibrosis		III	Every 2-4 weeks (5)
Pemphigus vulgaris	Severe	III	Every 2-4 weeks (variable)
Psoriasis		III	Weekly (4 months)
Scleroderma (systemic sclerosis)		III	Every 4-6 weeks (6-12 months)

*One cycle typically consists of extracorporeal photopheresis on 2 consecutive days.

although its role in nonskin GVHD is less well defined.[54]

ECP for solid-organ transplant rejection was best studied in cardiac and lung transplantation. In a randomized clinical trial, prophylactic ECP, in conjunction with previous-generation immunosuppression (ie, not including calcineurin inhibitors or mycophenolate), resulted in fewer rejection episodes, decreased HLA antibodies, and reduced coronary artery intimal thickness; but no difference was found in time to first episode, incidence of hemodynamic compromise, or survival at 6 or 12 months.[55,56] In cardiac rejection, ECP may decrease rejection severity and allow for reduced immunosuppressive dosages.[57] ECP may have a role in cardiac rejection with hemodynamic compromise and in bronchiolitis obliterans syndrome after lung transplantation.[58,59]

Selective Adsorption

The currently established indications for selective adsorption of plasma proteins are listed in Table 25-8, although, in general, these are not widely used.

Selective removal of LDL can be accomplished by passing heparinized plasma over a dextran sulfate column or beads coated with anionic polyacrylate ligands, or by precipitation of heparin-LDL complexes in acidified plasma. Lipid apheresis treatments must be repeated indefinitely, typically at 2-week intervals. There is evidence that lipid apheresis reduces the incidence of major coronary events and stroke.[60] In addition, atherosclerotic plaque regression may occur in some patients.[11] Secondary, potentially beneficial, effects of lipid apheresis include reduction in levels of C-reactive protein, fibrinogen, tissue factor, and soluble adhesion molecules.[61,62] Lipid apheresis also may be used to treat primary or recurrent FSGS, although the mechanism of action is not well defined.[63]

IgG can be selectively removed by passing plasma over a column of staphylococcal protein A bound to silica. The putative mechanism of action is the removal of pathogenic autoantibodies or immune complexes, although an alternative mechanism has been proposed in immune thrombocytopenia (ITP).[64] Staphylococcal protein A adsorption treatment can

TABLE 25-8. Indications for Selective Adsorption[2]

Indication	Modifying Conditions	Treatment Modality	Category	Typical Course (number of treatments)
Age-related macular degeneration, dry		Rheopheresis	I	8-10 over 8-21 weeks
Amyloidosis, dialysis-related		β_2-microglobulin column	II	Each dialysis
Atopic (neuro-) dermatitis (atopic eczema), recalcitrant		IA	III	QD × 5 every 4 weeks
Coagulation factor inhibitors	Alloantibody Autoantibody	IA	III III	QD
Cryoglobulinemia	Symptomatic/severe	IA	II	QD or QOD (3-12)
Dilated cardiomyopathy, idiopathic	NYHA II-IV	IA	II	QD or QOD (5)

(Continued)

TABLE 25-8. Indications for Selective Adsorption[2] (Continued)

Indication	Modifying Conditions	Treatment Modality	Category	Typical Course (number of treatments)
Familial hypercholesterolemia	Homozygotes	Lipid apheresis	I	Once every 1-2 weeks (indefinite)
	Heterozygotes		II	
Focal segmental glomerulosclerosis	Steriod-resistant in native kidney	Lipid apheresis	III	Twice a week (12)
Immune thrombocytopenia	Refractory	IA	III	1-3/week (variable)
Lipoprotein (a) hyperlipoproteinemia		Lipid apheresis	II	Once every 1-2 weeks (indefinite)
Multiple sclerosis	Acute CNS inflammatory demyelinating	IA	III	QOD (5-7)
Paraneoplastic neurologic syndromes		IA	III	2/week (6)
Paraproteinemic demyelinating neuropathies/chronic acquired demyelinating polyneuropathies	IgG/IgA/IgM	IA	III	QOD (5-6)
Pemphigus vulgaris	Severe	IA	III	QD (3), then variable
Peripheral vascular disease		Lipid apheresis	II	1-2/week (variable)
Phytanic acid storage disease (Refsum disease)		Lipid apheresis	II	QD (variable)
Renal transplantation, ABO compatible	Antibody-mediated rejection	IA	I	QD or QOD (5-6)
	Desensitization, LD		I	
	Desensitization, DD		III	
Renal transplantation, ABO incompatible	Desensitization, LD	IA	I	QD or QOD (variable)
	Antibody-mediated rejection		II	
	A_2/A_2B into B, DD		IV	
Sudden sensorineural hearing loss		Rheopheresis	III	QD (1-2)
		Lipid apheresis	III	

IA = immunoadsorption; QD = daily; QOD = every other day; NYHA = New York Heart Association (class); CNS = central nervous system; IgG = immunoglobulin G; DD = deceased donor; LD = living donor.

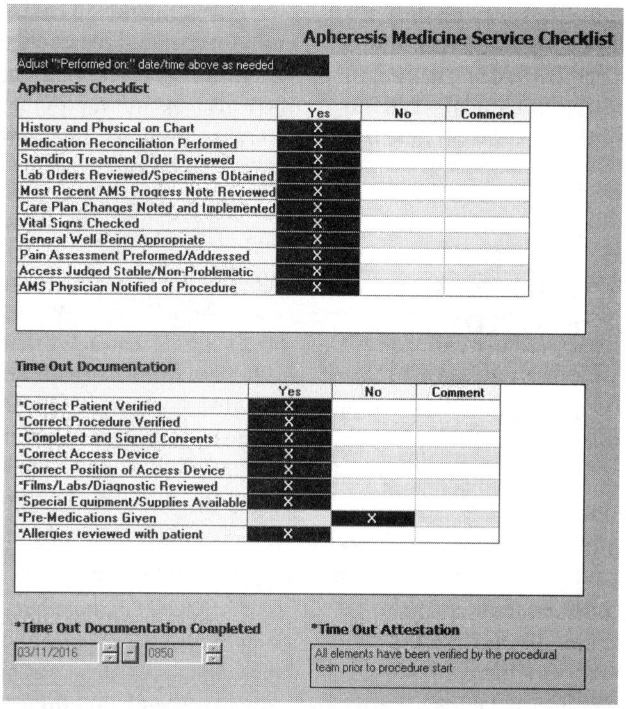

Apheresis Medicine Service Checklist

Adjust "*Performed on:" date/time above as needed

Apheresis Checklist

	Yes	No	Comment
History and Physical on Chart	X		
Medication Reconciliation Performed	X		
Standing Treatment Order Reviewed	X		
Lab Orders Reviewed/Specimens Obtained	X		
Most Recent AMS Progress Note Reviewed	X		
Care Plan Changes Noted and Implemented	X		
Vital Signs Checked	X		
General Well Being Appropriate	X		
Pain Assessment Preformed/Addressed	X		
Access Judged Stable/Non-Problematic	X		
AMS Physician Notified of Procedure	X		

Time Out Documentation

	Yes	No	Comment
*Correct Patient Verified	X		
*Correct Procedure Verified	X		
*Completed and Signed Consents	X		
*Correct Access Device	X		
*Correct Position of Access Device	X		
*Films/Labs/Diagnostic Reviewed	X		
*Special Equipment/Supplies Available	X		
*Pre-Medications Given		X	
*Allergies reviewed with patient	X		

***Time Out Documentation Completed**

03/11/2016 0850

***Time Out Attestation**

All elements have been verified by the procedural team prior to procedure start

(A)

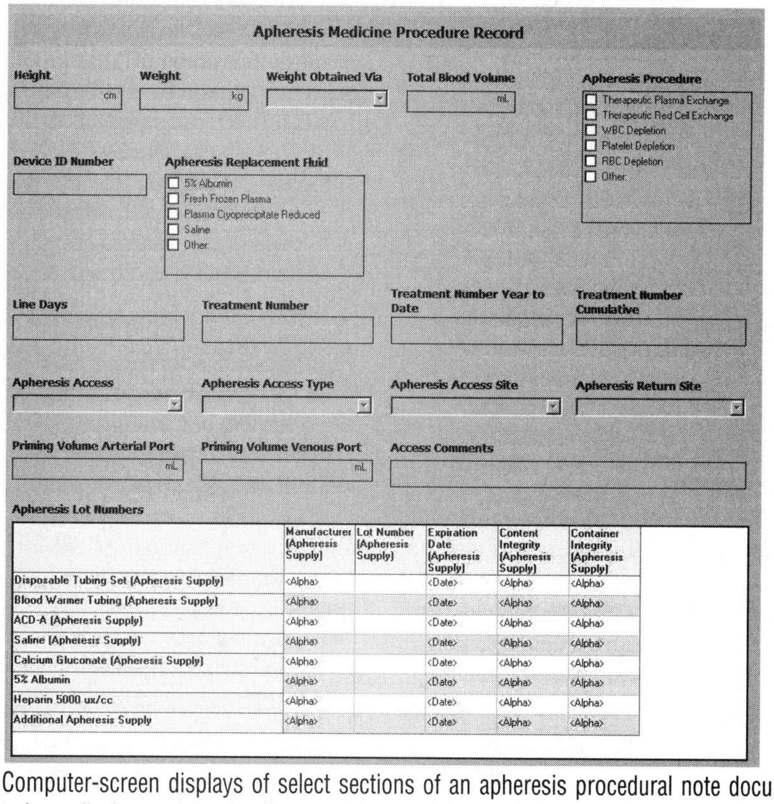

Apheresis Medicine Procedure Record

Height cm

Weight kg

Weight Obtained Via

Total Blood Volume mL

Apheresis Procedure

- Therapeutic Plasma Exchange
- Therapeutic Red Cell Exchange
- WBC Depletion
- Platelet Depletion
- RBC Depletion
- Other:

Device ID Number

Apheresis Replacement Fluid

- 5% Albumin
- Fresh Frozen Plasma
- Plasma Cryoprecipitate Reduced
- Saline
- Other:

Line Days

Treatment Number

Treatment Number Year to Date

Treatment Number Cumulative

Apheresis Access

Apheresis Access Type

Apheresis Access Site

Apheresis Return Site

Priming Volume Arterial Port mL

Priming Volume Venous Port mL

Access Comments

Apheresis Lot Numbers

	Manufacturer (Apheresis Supply)	Lot Number (Apheresis Supply)	Expiration Date (Apheresis Supply)	Content Integrity (Apheresis Supply)	Container Integrity (Apheresis Supply)
Disposable Tubing Set (Apheresis Supply)	<Alpha>		<Date>	<Alpha>	<Alpha>
Blood Warmer Tubing (Apheresis Supply)	<Alpha>		<Date>	<Alpha>	<Alpha>
ACD-A (Apheresis Supply)	<Alpha>		<Date>	<Alpha>	<Alpha>
Saline (Apheresis Supply)	<Alpha>		<Date>	<Alpha>	<Alpha>
Calcium Gluconate (Apheresis Supply)	<Alpha>		<Date>	<Alpha>	<Alpha>
5% Albumin	<Alpha>		<Date>	<Alpha>	<Alpha>
Heparin 5000 ux/cc	<Alpha>		<Date>	<Alpha>	<Alpha>
Additional Apheresis Supply	<Alpha>		<Date>	<Alpha>	<Alpha>

(B)

FIGURE 25-2. Computer-screen displays of select sections of an apheresis procedural note documented in a patient's electronic medical record used at Baystate Medical Center, Springfield, MA. Note checklist format and time-out review features incorporating various patient safety and regulatory/accreditation agencies' required documentation items (A) and information regarding disposables used in the procedure (B).

be performed manually or in conjunction with automated TPE. Affinity columns containing anti-IgG antibodies or ABO blood group substances have been tested in clinical trials, but are not currently approved for use in the United States.

THERAPEUTIC APHERESIS PROCEDURE DOCUMENTATION, PAYMENT, AND PROVIDER CREDENTIALING

Pertinent clinical documentation is essential for ensuring patient safety, health-care team communications, adherence to regulatory and accreditation agency requirements, monetary reimbursement of hospitals and providers, and medicolegal protections. Although no specific formats are mandated, inclusion of certain items in practitioners' written/electronic communications should occur. Some of these items related to the direct clinical care of the patient have been highlighted in earlier sections of this chapter. (See "Patient Evaluation and Management.") Other information regarding specific aspects of the apheresis in-tervention itself should be documented in nursing procedure records. Lot numbers of disposables, identification numbers of apheresis devices and related equipment (eg, blood warmers, medications, and blood components given during the procedure), and patient educational materials are some items that should be noted. Checklist approaches to such documentation are useful[65] (Fig 25-2, A and B).

Navigating payment systems for apheresis services in today's diverse health-care insurer environment can be challenging. Readers are referred to an ASFA annually updated guide for detailed information in this area.[66]

Apheresis medicine is a professionally diverse discipline involving specialists across a broad clinical spectrum. Hospital clinical privileging of both physicians and nurses involved in the delivery of apheresis medicine services is a topic of interest and discussion within professional societies and health-care institutions. Although no uniform approach has been mandated regarding practitioners' professional requirements, institutions interested in more formally addressing this subject may wish to review an ASFA commentary on the topic.[7]

KEY POINTS

1. Therapeutic apheresis treats diseases by removal of extracorporeal manipulation of pathologic plasma constituents, white cells, platelets, or red cells and may be accomplished by centrifugation, filtration, selective adsorption, or photopheresis.
2. Medical evaluation of the apheresis patient should focus on the disease indication; type of procedure; frequency, number, and duration of treatments; therapeutic goal; tolerance of the patient for apheresis; vascular access; replacement fluids; and medications. Appropriate laboratory monitoring is guided by the disease indication, type and frequency of procedures, duration of therapy, and concomitant medical conditions.
3. A solution of 5% albumin is the most commonly used replacement fluid for therapeutic plasma exchange, but plasma may be indicated for patients with TTP or coagulopathy.
4. Vascular access for apheresis may be accomplished through peripheral veins, but large-bore double-lumen central venous catheters or AV fistulas may be required for some patients.
5. Anticoagulation is usually accomplished with citrate, although heparin may be used, particularly for selective adsorption, hematopoietic progenitor cell collection, and photopheresis.
6. Adverse effects of apheresis are usually mild but may include symptomatic hypocalcemia, hypotension, urticaria, and nausea. Consequences of apheresis can include coagulopathy, hypogammaglobulinemia, and removal of certain drugs and biologics.
7. The American Society for Apheresis (ASFA) periodically publishes guidelines and recommendations for the use of therapeutic apheresis in clinical practice.

REFERENCES

1. Ooley PW, ed. Standards for blood banks and transfusion services. 30th ed. Bethesda, MD: AABB, 2016.

2. Schwartz J, Padmanabhan A, Aqui N, et al. Guidelines on the use of therapeutic apheresis in clinical practice—evidence-based approach from the Writing Committee of the American Society for Apheresis: The seventh special issue. J Clin Apher 2016;31:149-338.

3. American Society for Apheresis. Guidelines for therapeutic apheresis clinical privileges. J Clin Apher 2007;22:181-2.

4. American Society for Apheresis. Guidelines for documentation of therapeutic apheresis procedures in the medical record by apheresis physicians. J Clin Apher 2007;22:183.

5. College of American Pathologists, Commission on Laboratory Accreditation. Transfusion medicine checklist. July 28, 2015, ed. Northfield, IL: CAP, 2015.

6. Marshall C, Andrzejewski C, Carey P, et al. Milestones for apheresis education. J Clin Apher 2012;27:242-6.

7. Andrzejewski C Jr, Linz W, Hofman J, et al. American Society for Apheresis white paper: Considerations for medical staff apheresis medicine physician credentialing and privileging. J Clin Apher 2012;27:330-5.

8. National Institutes of Health. Therapeutic apheresis: Executive summary from an NHLBI working group, November 28 - 29, 2012. Bethesda, MD: National Heart, Lung, and Blood Institute, 2013. [Available at https://www.nhlbi.nih.gov/research/reports/therapeutic_apheresis (accessed February 3, 2017).]

9. Chopek M, McCullough J. Protein and biochemical changes during plasma exchange. In: Ulmas J, Berkman E, eds. Therapeutic hemapheresis: A technical workshop. Washington, DC: AABB, 1980:13-24.

10. Andrzejewski C Jr. Therapeutic plasma exchange: Rationales and indications. In: Hillyer CD, Hillyer KL, Strobl FJ, et al, eds. Handbook of transfusion medicine. San Diego, CA: Academic Press, 2001: 323-31.

11. Matsuzaki M, Hiramori K, Imaizumi T, et al. Intravascular ultrasound evaluation of coronary plaque regression by low density lipoprotein-apheresis in familial hypercholesterolemia: The Low Density Lipoprotein-Apheresis Coronary Morphology and Reserve Trial (LACMART). J Am Coll Cardiol 2002;40: 220-7.

12. McLeod BC, Sniecinski I, Ciavarella D, et al. Frequency of immediate adverse effects associated with therapeutic apheresis. Transfusion 1999;39:282-8.

13. Norda R, Berseus O, Stegmayr B. Adverse events and problems in therapeutic hemapheresis. A report from the Swedish registry. Transfus Apher Sci 2001;25:33-41.

14. Strauss RG, Crookston KP. Complications of therapeutic apheresis. In: Popovsky MA, ed. Transfusion reactions. 4th ed. Bethesda, MD: AABB Press, 2012:407-37.

15. Haddad S, Leitman SF, Wesley RA, et al. Placebo-controlled study of intravenous magnesium supplementation during large-volume leukapheresis in healthy allogeneic donors. Transfusion 2005;45:934-44.

16. Marques MB, Huang ST. Patients with thrombotic thrombocytopenic purpura commonly develop metabolic alkalosis during therapeutic plasma exchange. J Clin Apher 2001;16:120-4.

17. Askari S, Nollet K, Debol SM, et al. Transfusion-related acute lung injury during plasma exchange: Suspecting the unsuspected. J Clin Apher 2002;17:93-6.

18. Duntley P, Siever J, Korwes ML, et al. Vascular erosion by central venous catheters. Clinical features and outcome. Chest 1992;101:1633-8.

19. Leitman SF, Boltansky H, Alter HJ, et al. Allergic reactions in healthy plateletpheresis donors caused by sensitization to ethylene oxide gas. N Engl J Med 1986;315:1192-6.

20. Purello D'Ambrosio F, Savica V, Gangemi S, et al. Ethylene oxide allergy in dialysis patients. Nephrol Dial Transplant 1997;12:1461-3.

21. Owen HG, Brecher ME. Atypical reactions associated with use of angiotensin-converting enzyme inhibitors and apheresis. Transfusion 1994;34:891-4.

22. Orlin JB, Berkman EM. Partial plasma exchange using albumin replacement: Removal and recovery of normal plasma constituents. Blood 1980;56:1055-9.

23. Food and Drug Administration. Guidance for industry: Notifying FDA of fatalities related to blood collection or transfusion. (September 2003) Silver Spring, MD: CBER Office of Communication, Outreach, and Development, 2003. [Available at http://www.fda.gov/Biolog

icsBloodVaccines/GuidanceComplianceRegu latoryInformation/Guidances/Blood/ ucm074947.htm (accessed February 3, 2017).]

24. Kiprov DD, Golden P, Rohe R, et al. Adverse reactions associated with mobile therapeutic apheresis: Analysis of 17,940 procedures. J Clin Apher 2001;16:130-3.

25. Terrell DR, Williams LA, Vesely SK, et al. The incidence of thrombotic thrombocytopenic purpura-hemolytic uremic syndrome: All patients, idiopathic patients, and patients with severe ADAMTS-13 deficiency. J Thromb Haemost 2005;3:1432-6.

26. Bandarenko N, Brecher ME. United States thrombotic thrombocytopenic purpura apheresis study group (US TTP ASG): Multicenter survey and retrospective analysis of current efficacy of therapeutic plasma exchange. J Clin Apher 1998;13:133-41.

27. Howard MA, Williams LA, Terrell DR, et al. Complications of plasma exchange in patients treated for clinically suspected thrombotic thrombocytopenic purpura-hemolytic uremic syndrome. Transfusion 2006;46:154-6.

28. Legendre CM, Licht C, Muus P, et al. Terminal complement inhibitor eculizumab in atypical hemolytic-uremic syndrome. N Engl J Med 2013;368:2169-81.

29. George JN, Li X, McMinn JR, et al. Thrombotic thrombocytopenic purpura-hemolytic uremic syndrome following allogeneic HPC transplantation: A diagnostic dilemma. Transfusion 2004;44:294-304.

30. Somer T. Rheology of paraproteinaemias and the plasma hyperviscosity syndrome. Baillieres Clin Haematol 1987;1:695-723.

31. Johnson WJ, Kyle RA, Pineda AA, et al. Treatment of renal failure associated with multiple myeloma: Plasmapheresis, hemodialysis, and chemotherapy. Arch Intern Med 1990;150:863-9.

32. Clark WF, Stewart AK, Rock GA, et al. Plasma exchange when myeloma presents as acute renal failure: A randomized, controlled trial. Ann Intern Med 2005;143:777-84.

33. Movilli E, Guido J, Silvia T, et al. Plasma exchange in the treatment of acute renal failure of myeloma. Nephrol Dial Transplant 2007; 22:1270-1.

34. Treon SP, Branagan AR, Hunter Z, et al. Paradoxical increases in serum IgM and viscosity levels following rituximab in Waldenström's macroglobulinemia. Ann Oncol 2004;15:1481-3.

35. Weinshenker BG, O'Brien PC, Petterson TM, et al. A randomized trial of plasma exchange in acute central nervous system inflammatory demyelinating disease. Ann Neurol 1999;46: 878-86.

36. Llufriu S, Castillo J, Blanco Y, et al. Plasma exchange for acute attacks of CNS demyelination: Predictors of improvement. Neurology 2009;73:949-53.

37. Bonnan M, Valentino R, Olindo S, et al. Plasma exchange in severe spinal attacks associated with neuromyelitis optica spectrum disorder. Mult Scler 2009;15:487-92

38. Randomized trial of plasma exchange, intravenous immunoglobulin, and combined treatments in Guillain-Barré syndrome. Plasma Exchange/Sandoglobulin Guillain-Barré Syndrome Trial Group. Lancet 1997;349:225-30.

39. Winters JL, Brown D, Hazard E, et al. Cost-minimization analysis of the direct costs of TPE and IVIG in the treatment of Guillain-Barré syndrome. BMC Health Serv Res 2011; 11;101.

40. Savin VJ, Sharma R, Sharma M, et al. Circulating factor associated with increased glomerular permeability to albumin in recurrent focal segmental glomerulosclerosis. N Engl J Med 1996;334:878-83.

41. Wei C, El Hindi S, Li J, et al. Circulating urokinase receptor as a cause of focal segmental glomerulosclerosis. Nat Med 2011;17:952-60.

42. Al-Badr W, Kallogjeri D, Madaraty K, et al. A retrospective review of the outcome of plasma exchange and aggressive medical therapy in antibody mediated rejection of renal allografts: A single center experience. J Clin Apher 2008;23:178-82.

43. Sivakumaran P, Vo AA, Villicana R, et al. Therapeutic plasma exchange for desensitization before transplantation in ABO-incompatible renal allografts. J Clin Apher 2009;24:155-60.

44. Tobian AAR, Shirey RS, Montgomery RA, et al. Therapeutic plasma exchange reduces ABO titers to permit ABO incompatible renal transplantation. Transfusion 2009;49:1248-54.

45. Padmanabhan A, Ratner LE, Jhang JS, et al. Comparative outcome analysis of ABO-incompatible and positive crossmatch renal transplantation: A single-center experience. Transplantation 2009;87:1889-96.

46. Vichinsky EP, Neumayr LD, Earles AN, et al. Causes and outcomes of the acute chest syndrome in sickle cell disease. National Acute

Chest Syndrome Study Group. N Engl J Med 2000;342:1855-65.

47. Lawson SE, Oakley S, Smith NA, Bareford D. Red cell exchange in sickle cell disease. Clin Lab Haematol 1999;21:99-102.

48. Stuart MJ, Setty BN. Sickle cell acute chest syndrome: Pathogenesis and rationale for treatment. Blood 1999;94:1555-60.

49. Adams RJ, McKie VC, Hsu L, et al. Prevention of a first stroke by transfusions in children with sickle cell anemia and abnormal results on transcranial Doppler ultrasonography. N Engl J Med 1998;339:5-11.

50. Lee MT, Piomelli S, Granger S, et al. Stroke Prevention Trial in Sickle Cell Anemia (STOP): Extended follow-up and final results. Blood 2006;108:847-52.

51. Vichinsky EP, Luban NLC, Wright E, et al. Prospective RBC phenotype matching in a stroke-prevention trial in sickle cell anemia: A multicenter transfusion trial. Transfusion 2001;41:1086-92.

52. Wahl SK, Garcia A, Hagar W, et al. Lower alloimmunization rates in pediatric sickle cell patients on chronic erythrocytapheresis compared to chronic simple transfusions. Transfusion 2012;52:2671-6.

53. Bladon J, Taylor PC. Extracorporeal photopheresis: A focus on apoptosis and cytokines. J Dermatol Sci 2006;43:85-94.

54. Del Fante C, Scudeller L, Viarengo G, et al. Response and survival of patients with chronic graft-versus-host disease treated by extracorporeal photochemotherapy: A retrospective study according to classical and National Institutes of Health classifications. Transfusion 2012;52:2007-15.

55. Barr ML, Baker CJ, Schenkel FA, et al. Prophylactic photopheresis and chronic rejection: Effects on graft intimal hyperplasia in cardiac transplantation. Clin Transplant 2000;14:162-6.

56. Barr ML, Meiser BM, Eisen HJ, et al. Photopheresis for the prevention of rejection in cardiac transplantation. Photopheresis Transplantation Study Group. N Engl J Med 1998;339:1744-51.

57. Dall'Amico R, Montini G, Murer L, et al. Extracorporeal photochemotherapy after cardiac transplantation: A new therapeutic approach to allograft rejection. Int J Artif Organs 2000;23:49-51.

58. Kirklin JK, Brown RN, Huang ST, et al. Rejection with hemodynamic compromise: Objective evidence for efficacy of photopheresis. J Heart Lung Transplant 2006;25:283-8.

59. Jaksch P, Scheed A, Keplinger M, et al. A prospective interventional study on the use of extracorporeal photopheresis in patients with bronchiolitis obliterans syndrome after lung transplantation. J Heart Lung Transplant 2012;31:950-7.

60. Masaki N, Tatami R, Kumamoto T, et al. Ten-year follow-up of familial hypercholesterolemia patients after intensive cholesterol-lowering therapy. Int Heart J 2005;46:833-43.

61. Wang Y, Blessing F, Walli AK, et al. Effects of heparin-mediated extracorporeal low-density lipoprotein precipitation beyond lowering proatherogenic lipoproteins—reduction of circulating proinflammatory and procoagulatory markers. Atherosclerosis 2004;175:145-50.

62. Kobayashi S, Oka M, Moriya H, et al. LDL-apheresis reduces P-Selectin, CRP and fibrinogen—possible important implications for improving atherosclerosis. Ther Apher Dial 2006;10:219-23.

63. Muso E, Mune M, Yorioka N, et al. Beneficial effect of low-density lipoprotein apheresis (LDL-A) on refractory nephrotic syndrome (NS) due to focal glomerulosclerosis (FGS). Clin Nephrol 2007;67:341-4.

64. Silverman GJ, Goodyear CS, Siegel DL. On the mechanism of staphylococcal protein A immunomodulation. Transfusion 2005;45:274-80.

65. Levy R, Pantanowitz L, Cloutier D, et al. Development of electronic record charting for hospital based transfusion and apheresis medicine services: Early adoption perspectives. J Pathol Inform 2010;1:8.

66. Berman K. Therapeutic apheresis: A guide to billing and securing appropriate reimbursement, 2017 ed. Andrzejewski C, Hofmann JC, Arepally GM, et al (eds.). Vancouver, BC: American Society for Apheresis, 2017. [Available at https://www.apheresis.org/?page=Apheresis-Reimbursement (accessed May 1, 2017).]

Chapter 26

The Collection and Processing of Hematopoietic Progenitor Cells

• ● •

Eapen K. Jacob, MD, and Scott A. Koepsell, MD, PhD

HEMATOPOIETIC PROGENITOR CELLS (HPCs) are primitive pluripotent cells capable of self-renewal and differentiation into any cells of hematopoietic lineage (lymphocytes, monocytes, granulocytes, erythrocytes, and platelets), including committed and lineage-restricted progenitor cells, unless otherwise specified, regardless of tissue source [eg, marrow, mobilized peripheral blood, or umbilical cord blood (UCB)].[1(p132)] Clinically, HPCs are able to fully reconstitute marrow function when transplanted into conditioned recipients. For this reason, HPC transplantation is increasingly utilized to treat a diverse array of hematologic and nonhematologic diseases and conditions.

In vivo, HPCs are concentrated in the marrow, where mesenchymal elements—such as osteogenic progenitor cells, osteoblasts, adipocytes, mesenchymal stem/stromal cells, and endothelial cells—interact with hematopoietic precursors to generate a niche that supports and regulates hematopoiesis.[2]

Although the CD34 cell-surface antigen is not specific to HPCs, CD34 is used to identify and quantify HPCs by flow cytometry in cellular products intended for use in transplantation. Historically, CD34 quantification by flow cytometry suffered from significant interinstrument and interprotocol variability, but this limitation has been resolved by more rigorous quality control (QC) procedures and assay standardization.[3]

CLINICAL UTILITY

Myriad indications exist for HPC transplantation, ranging from nonneoplastic immune disorders to malignancies. In general, indications vary with patient age, because immunodeficiencies and inborn errors of metabolism are more common in children, whereas adults more commonly have clonal disorders in their marrow or hematologic malignancies. Ultimately, the decision to perform HPC transplantation requires a complex integration of many variables. These include patient goals, age, prognosis, disease progression, previous therapy, availability of a suitable HPC source (ie, marrow, mobilized peripheral blood, or

26

Eapen K. Jacob, MD, Assistant Professor, Department of Laboratory Medicine and Pathology, Mayo Clinic, Rochester, Minnesota; and Scott A. Koepsell, MD, PhD, Assistant Professor, Department of Pathology and Microbiology, University of Nebraska Medical Center, Omaha, Nebraska

E. Jacob has disclosed no conflicts of interest. S. Koepsell has disclosed a financial relationship with Ortho Clinical Diagnostics.

UCB), and type of transplant (eg, autologous vs allogeneic, myeloablative vs nonmyeloablative).

Autologous Transplantation

In general, autologous HPC transplantation is used for hematopoietic rescue after high-dose antineoplastic therapy. The antitumor effect comes solely from the chemotherapy and radiotherapy used during the conditioning phase of transplantation. For older patients who were not traditional candidates for autologous transplantation, or patients with other significant morbidities, reduced-intensity induction chemotherapy has broadened the clinical utility of HPC transplantation.

Donor requirements for autologous transplants are based on the donor's disease state. The patient must be healthy enough to undergo mobilization (as described below) and HPC procurement, either by peripheral blood apheresis collection or marrow aspiration. Significant levels of prior chemotherapy, radiation, or ongoing marrow disease involvement may make HPC mobilization and collection unfeasible as a result of reduced HPC quality or number.

Eligibility requirements are not mandated by the Food and Drug Administration (FDA) for autologous HPC transplantation [*Code of Federal Regulations* (CFR) Title 21, Part 1271.90], so screening questionnaires to identify relevant communicable disease are not required. However, a general health assessment is needed per AABB *Standards for Cellular Therapy Services (CT Standards).*[1(p86)] AABB *CT Standards* also requires laboratory testing for human immunodeficiency virus types 1 and 2 (HIV-1/2), hepatitis B virus, hepatitis C virus, syphilis, and human T-cell lymphotropic virus types I and II (HTLV-I/II), because autologous products are cryopreserved and stored with other products; thus, the presence of these viruses is a contamination risk.[1(pp45-46)]

Allogeneic Transplantation

Indications for allogeneic HPC transplantation vary. However, in general, allogeneic transplantation is used to treat malignant conditions when both the conditioning antineoplastic therapy and the transplanted cells, because of the graft-vs-neoplasm (GVN) effect, are therapeutic. For patients with inborn errors of metabolism, congenital immunodeficiency, or other diseases and conditions in which germline mutations are present in the patient's cells, allogeneic HPC transplants offer therapeutic benefit by helping to replace the deficient cellular machinery.

In the allogeneic setting, screening and infectious disease testing are mandated in the United States to determine whether transplantation of mobilized peripheral blood or UCB poses a risk for transmitting a relevant communicable disease to the recipient [21 CFR 1271.3(r)]. Screening and testing include administration of a screening questionnaire, a physical examination, a review of the relevant medical records, and applicable testing [21 CFR 1271.3(s) and 21 CFR 1271 Subpart C]. Although marrow products are administered under Sections 375 and 379 of the Public Health Service Act, marrow screening and testing are very similar to mobilized peripheral blood and UCB screening and testing, because all three products are treated similarly under the standards of various accrediting bodies, such as AABB, the Foundation for the Accreditation of Cellular Therapy (FACT), and the National Marrow Donor Program (NMDP).[4] For UCB transplantation, the screening and testing process involves the mother and her samples.

Relevant communicable disease agents that can be transmitted by HPCs to the transplant recipient or to the people who handle the components, and for which there is an FDA-licensed screening test [21 CFR 1271.3(r)], include HIV, hepatitis B and C viruses, *Treponema pallidum*, HTLV-I/II, and cytomegalovirus (CMV). Donor questionnaires have been developed to assist with screening[5] and medical record review for these diseases using FDA guidance documents.[6]

In the United States, infectious disease testing for HPC donors must be performed in a laboratory certified under the Clinical Laboratory Improvement Amendments (CLIA), as mandated by the FDA. If screening or testing detects a risk of a relevant communicable disease, the potential HPC donor is considered ineligible. All parties (the donor, the recipient, and their physicians) are informed of the donor's eligibility status, and a risk/benefit analysis is performed to determine whether the donor's HPCs should be used. If a decision is made to proceed with transplantation of the ineligible donor's HPCs, the urgent medical need, as defined by the FDA [21 CFR 1271.3(u)], is documented. Depending on the institution's accrediting body and the circumstances, such as when the HPCs are from an ineligible donor who is a first- or second-degree relative, the requirement for documenting an urgent medical need may vary. Finally, in addition to screening and testing for infectious diseases, the donor's medical evaluation is used to determine whether the donor is healthy enough to undergo HPC mobilization and collection. (Described below.)

Histocompatibility

In addition to infectious diseases, donor characteristics that may affect transplant outcomes include histocompatibility with the recipient, gender, age, parity, and ABO compatibility. Of these characteristics, histocompatibility is the most important. In general, if a healthy HLA-matched related donor is available, that donor is selected instead of an HLA-matched unrelated donor. However, recent data showed that, in patients with acute myeloid leukemia or myelodysplastic syndrome, an HPC transplant from an HLA-matched unrelated donor may be as effective as a transplant from a sibling.[7,8]

Major histocompatibility antigens were first studied in depth in animal models of skin transplantation.[9(pp97-111)] In humans, these are HLA antigens and are categorized into Class I (HLA-A, -B, and -C) and Class II (HLA-DR, -DQ, and -DP). These highly polymorphic molecules are essential in determining graft survival as well as the likelihood that the recipient will develop graft-vs-host disease (GVHD). As molecular techniques have supplanted serologic methods, the resolution has improved and the number of antigens that can be compared has increased. Matching at the antigen

level has been replaced by allele-level matching for the final selection of peripheral blood and marrow HPC components for a given recipient. *CT Standards* requires that HLA-A, HLA-B, and HLA-DRB1 be determined on living allogeneic donors with DNA-based assays before final selection, but the current standard of care is often more stringent. (See below.)

HLA matching in HPC transplantation has been reviewed in detail elsewhere and is only briefly summarized here.[10] HLA matching has an important impact on outcomes, especially in low-risk patients. Allogeneic transplantation using either mobilized peripheral blood or marrow HPCs with high-resolution (allele-level) mismatching at *HLA-A, -B, -C,* and *-DRB1* is associated with a 5%-10% decrease in survival with each mismatch.[10] The results are similar, although the evidence is a bit less clear, for HPC grafts with mismatches in Class II HLA-DQ and -DP. For mobilized peripheral blood HPC grafts, allele-level mismatching is probably as detrimental to survival as antigen-level mismatching, although these data come from smaller studies. Many centers now match at high resolution for 8 to 10 loci (*HLA-A, -B, -C, -DR,* and *-DQ*). High-resolution 8/8- and 10/10-matched transplants of HPCs from unrelated donors are, at least in part, responsible for the improved outcomes of matched unrelated-donor transplants as compared with matched related donors.[11]

Not surprisingly, HPC transplants in recipients with antibodies against donor HLA [known as donor-specific antibodies (DSAs)] have adverse outcomes.[12] The level at which DSAs have a significant impact is less clear, as is the appropriate course of action when DSAs are detected. Despite the difficulty of predicting graft failure based on the presence of DSAs, screening HPC transplant candidates for DSAs has become more routine as more data emerge.[13]

UCB has several unique characteristics with regard to HLA matching. The level of HLA matching required is less stringent than that required for marrow and mobilized peripheral blood HPCs. Data on UCB indicate that HLA matching at 4 of 6 loci is sufficient for HLA-A and -B at the antigen level and for HLA-DRB1 at the allele level, provided that a sufficient cell dose is achieved.[14] As the number of mismatched alleles increases (from one to two), a higher total nucleated cell (TNC) dose is needed to overcome their deleterious effect, including the use of combined double-cord transplants.[15] In addition, early evidence indicates that noninherited, maternal HLA may be permissive when considering donor-recipient mismatches.[16] Unit-to-unit matching of four to six loci in the setting of double-cord blood transplantation is performed at various institutions; however, firm evidence supporting this practice is not yet available.

Haploidentical transplantation, when the HPC donor is a first-degree relative matched at only half of the HLA loci with the recipient, is becoming more common as a result of advances in GVHD prevention. Advantages of haploidentical HPC transplants include lower upfront costs, fast procurement, and near-universal donor availability because most patients needing an allogeneic HPC transplant have access to one first-degree relative.[17] Haploidentical HPC transplantation presents unique challenges, including overcoming immunologic barriers between donor and recipient with chemotherapy or HPC product manipulation. In addition, because half of the HLA loci are mismatched, potential HPC recipients with DSAs must be carefully screened, as these antibodies can reject or delay HPC engraftment. A large randomized controlled trial comparing UCB and haploidentical transplants is currently being conducted (Blood and Marrow Transplant Clinical Trials Network Protocol 1101).

Other Donor Characteristics

For marrow and mobilized peripheral blood HPC donors, other factors that may have a positive effect on transplant outcomes include male gender, younger age, nulliparity, ABO and CMV status-matching, and greater size of the donor relative to the recipient. Other than HLA compatibility, only donor age appears to be associated with survival.[18] ABO incompatibility has been reviewed extensively with con-

flicting results. The fact that ABH antigens are found on red cells and platelets suggests that ABO incompatibility would affect outcome. However, inconsistent results on outcomes—such as survival, nonrelapse mortality, GVHD, and graft failure—of both major- and minor-ABO-incompatible transplants have been observed.[19] Nonetheless, the risk of delayed red cell engraftment, pure red cell aplasia, increased transfusion requirements, and both immediate and delayed hemolysis is increased following major-ABO-incompatible allogeneic HPC transplants.

Other characteristics specific to UCB HPC donation may affect outcomes, including issues related to maternal history, unit collection, processing, and unit storage.[20] Characteristics of the UCB unit have been utilized in a scoring system, the "Cord Blood Apgar," to determine the utility of the unit by considering the TNC count, CD34 positivity, colony-forming-unit count, mononuclear cell content, and volume.[21]

DETERMINATION OF GRAFT SOURCE

The choice of the source of HPCs for allogeneic transplantation is determined by several variables, including the availability of an adequately matched donor and the clinical stability of the potential recipient. A typical search for an unrelated marrow or peripheral blood donor may take months, whereas a search for UCB takes several days to a few weeks.[22] When a matched donor or a haploidentical donor is not readily available, a UCB transplant may be the best alternative if one- or two-allele-mismatched donor units are available. In addition, for some centers, the relatively rapid availability of UCB units as compared to marrow and peripheral blood products plays a substantial role in graft choice for patients with an immediate need for transplantation.

GVHD and GVN Effect

GVHD and the GVN effect, although linked in terms of their cause, have opposite outcomes. In GVHD, donor lymphocytes attack normal recipient tissues, such as the skin, lung, liver, and gastrointestinal tract. GVHD is categorized as acute or chronic, and occurs in >40% of allogeneic HPC transplant recipients. GVHD is associated with significant morbidity and mortality. Not surprisingly, the risk of GVHD is related to the graft source. Consequently, GVHD risk increases as the lymphocyte content of the HPC product increases. Various techniques have been used to decrease the risk of GVHD, including T-cell depletion, use of antithymocyte globulin, and pharmacologic measures.[23]

The GVN effect is also thought to be driven by donor lymphocytes. In recent years, mobilized peripheral blood has greatly outpaced marrow as an HPC source because of its easier collection and a believed improvement in GVN effect. In the first randomized controlled trial comparing marrow and mobilized peripheral blood HPC grafts in unrelated-donor myeloablative transplantation, the risk of chronic, but not acute, GVHD was higher in patients receiving a peripheral blood HPC transplantation.[24]

Kinetics

The kinetics of engraftment are affected by many variables, such as the degree of HLA matching, HPC dose, DSAs, and the use of granulocyte colony-stimulating factor (G-CSF). In addition, the stem cell source may play a role. For instance, stem cells in UCB appear to have a greater regenerative capacity than those in marrow and peripheral blood.[25] In general, the rate of engraftment is predicted by the number of progenitor cells in each graft. This is greatest in mobilized peripheral blood, followed by marrow, UCB, and other HPC sources.

In a recent meta-analysis of allogeneic related-donor transplantation in which mobilized peripheral blood vs marrow HPCs was analyzed, engraftment was 15 vs 21 days for neutrophils and 13 vs 21 days for platelets, respectively.[26] This was confirmed in a randomized controlled trial[24] in which the time to engraftment was 5 days shorter for neutrophils and 7 days shorter for platelets. A comparison of adult unrelated-donor marrow to UCB HPC grafts showed that engraftment occurred earli-

er with both neutrophils (median of 18 days for matched marrow, 20 for mismatched marrow, and 27 for mismatched UCB) and platelets (median of 29 days for matched marrow and mismatched marrow, and 60 days for mismatched UCB).[27] In the setting of reduced-intensity UCB transplantation, median neutrophil engraftment times approaching those of mobilized peripheral blood and marrow HPC transplants were observed.[25]

Survival

The most important outcome measure for any transplant procedure is patient survival. For recipients of transplants from matched related donors, mobilized peripheral blood may offer an advantage in overall and disease-free survival as compared to marrow HPC grafts, at least in recipients with late-stage hematologic malignancies.[28] In recipients of myeloablative transplants from unrelated donors for hematologic malignancies, a recent randomized controlled trial indicated that marrow and mobilized peripheral blood sources have equivalent effects on survival, with marrow grafts associated with less chronic GVHD but more graft failure.[24]

Based on these findings, the recent rapid increase in the use of mobilized peripheral blood relative to marrow may change. However, this may not be true in nonmyeloablative-treatment patients or transplant recipients at high risk of infection or graft failure. For pediatric transplant recipients, marrow may be preferred over mobilized peripheral blood, although reports differ.[29,30] In addition, when mismatched marrow and mismatched UCB were compared, there was no difference in the rate of overall mortality in adults with leukemia; however, recipients of matched marrow HPC grafts did have a lower overall mortality rate.[27]

Transplant physicians face a complex choice when determining which donor and stem cell source are best for their patients; this is based on numerous factors, including disease type, disease stage, age, and comorbidities. As more data are collected, the choice of HPC graft for a given situation may evolve.

COLLECTION/SOURCES OF HPCs

A medical order is required for procurement and must include procurement goals.[1(p58)] Regardless of the source of HPCs, *CT Standards* requires all institutions that collect HPCs to have a procedure in place to obtain informed consent from the donor or the donor's representative, as dictated by local law.[1(pp18-19,23-25)] The informed consent process should include providing information to the donor regarding the risks and benefits of the procedure, the tests performed on the donor that are designed to protect the recipient, alternative collection methods, and protection of donor health information. In addition, the donor should be given the opportunity to ask questions and to refuse donation. The risks specific to each collection procedure are discussed below.

Another requirement for facilities that collect HPCs is to provide donor access to medical care based on the risks and clinical situation associated with each type of donation. Specifically, procedures should be in place to provide medical or emergency care to donors who experience adverse effects, and criteria for discontinuing the procurement because of medical complications should be specified. Clearance from the donor's physician for HPC collection should be documented.

Marrow HPC Collection

In addition to undergoing relevant donor screening, infectious disease testing, and HLA compatibility testing, marrow donors must also be physically suitable for donation. Marrow harvest is an invasive procedure performed under sterile conditions in the operating room under anesthesia. Therefore, the donor must be able to tolerate the type of anesthesia required to perform the harvest successfully. Another consideration is the donor's medical history. Autologous donors and some allogeneic donors may have had previous radiation therapy to the pelvis, which may limit the amount of marrow available for harvest in the posterior iliac crest. Similarly, previous chemotherapy may limit the number of nucleated cells that can be aspirated from the marrow. For autologous donors, a significant tumor burden in the marrow is a contraindication for collection of HPCs by marrow harvest because tumor cells would contaminate the graft.

Physically, the donor must be able to tolerate the volume loss associated with marrow harvest, which means that young or small donors may not be suitable. The Be The Match Registry limits the volume collected from a marrow donor to 20 mL/kg.[4] Typically, the volume of the harvest requested is dictated by the recipient's weight, with a minimum of 2.0 to 3.0×10^8 nucleated cells/kg needed to facilitate efficient engraftment. Thus, during harvest, checking the TNC count midway through the procedure can help estimate the total volume needed. CD34 quantification midway through the procedure or of the final product for QC may also be performed, depending on institutional policies, and may be used as an alternative to TNC counts.

Marrow harvest techniques vary considerably depending on institutional practice. In general, an 11- to 14-gauge needle on a syringe flushed with anticoagulant is inserted into the posterior iliac crest, and approximately 5 mL of marrow is aspirated. The needle and syringe are then rotated to a different vector, and the aspiration is repeated. Large volume aspiration is avoided to prevent significant peripheral blood contamination of the product. The aspirated marrow is collected into a large collection bag containing anticoagulant and media and/or an infusible-grade electrolyte solution. The process is repeated at different bone sites until the target, based on TNC count or donor volume limit, is reached.

Serious complications of marrow harvest are rare. However, minor complications, such as pain at the site of harvest, fatigue, insomnia, nausea, dizziness, and anorexia, occur frequently but resolve in most donors by 1 month after the procedure.[31] Marrow donors often have significant decreases in hemoglobin concentration after the procedure. As a result, almost all marrow donors donate autologous Red Blood Cells (RBCs) before the procedure, and 76% of donors receive at least 1 autologous RBC unit during or shortly after marrow harvest.[31] If the donor requires an allogeneic

RBC or platelet transfusion before or during the procedure, the units should be irradiated to prevent contamination of the graft by viable leukocytes from these blood components. Marrow donors should be made aware during the informed consent process that they might need a transfusion.

Peripheral Blood HPC Collection

Pharmacologic methods for mobilizing HPCs from the marrow into the peripheral circulation, combined with apheresis technology, have made peripheral HPC collection the most common HPC donation procedure.[32] Because peripheral collection of HPCs requires only vascular access, most apheresis procedures used to collect HPCs are performed on an outpatient basis, with minimal side effects. However, donors with poor vascular access, or who may need multiple apheresis procedures to collect sufficient numbers of HPCs, may require placement of a central line, which imposes additional risks. AABB *CT Standards* requires that correct placement of any central line be confirmed before initiating HPC collection.[1(p57)]

HPCs can be mobilized into the peripheral circulation using various chemotherapeutic agents, hematopoietic growth factors, or receptor antagonists. For most healthy allogeneic HPC donors, sufficient numbers of HPCs can be mobilized with the administration of a hematopoietic growth factor, often G-CSF, alone. G-CSF is administered once per day at a dose of 5 to 20 µg/kg, and doses are often rounded to the nearest vial size.[33] Total white cell count and CD34 percentage can be monitored to determine the optimal collection time, which is usually 3 to 4 days after initiation of G-CSF treatment. The side effects of G-CSF, which are common and mild, include bone pain, myalgia, headache, insomnia, flu-like symptoms, sweating, anorexia, fever, chills, and nausea.[33] Potentially serious complications, such as splenic rupture, are rare. Other growth factor preparations are available, including a pegylated form of G-CSF that allows one-time dosing in most donors.

For some autologous donors and rare allogeneic donors, mobilization of HPCs can be challenging, potentially requiring additional pharmacotherapy to mobilize an adequate number of cells and facilitate efficient engraftment. The minimum number of cells needed for transplantation is commonly cited as 2×10^6 CD34+ cells/kg, although 5×10^6 CD34+ cells/kg is more desirable.[34] Patients who are poor mobilizers may benefit from the addition of plerixafor, a chemokine (C-X-C motif) receptor 4 antagonist, in combination with G-CSF. Various clinical studies demonstrated that plerixafor, in combination with G-CSF, can increase HPC collection yields. Several clinical scenarios where plerixafor may be utilized were described, and patients with multiple myeloma or lymphoma who have difficulty mobilizing HPCs may benefit from plerixafor therapy to collect a sufficient quantity of HPCs.[34]

In autologous donors, a chemotherapy drug, such as cyclophosphamide, can be added to the G-CSF regimen. Although the number of HPCs collected can be increased by using a combination of chemotherapy and G-CSF, complications, such as cytopenias and additional apheresis requirements, may outweigh the potential benefits of this strategy.[35] For adults in many institutions, this mobilization regimen is used only for refractory autologous donors who fail other mobilization methods. If the benefits of adding chemotherapy to G-CSF outweigh the risks, this mobilization strategy may be successful in patients with significant tumor burden or extensive prior chemotherapy.

Peripheral collection of HPCs is performed using an apheresis device according to the manufacturer's instructions. For most allogeneic donors, sufficient numbers of HPCs can be obtained in one to two collections. Up to 20% of donors experience minor apheresis/collection-related adverse events, such as citrate toxicity, nausea, fatigue, chills, hypertension, hypotension, allergic reactions, or syncope.[32] Autologous donors experience similar collection-related side effects, which can be problematic in donors requiring multiple apheresis procedures as a result of poor mobilization. Depending on the donor scenario, large-volume apheresis techniques may be used to limit the number of total procedures.[36] *CT Standards* requires a complete blood count to be performed within 24 hours before the procedure begins for all mobilized donors, and this is especially important for autologous donors, because these apheresis procedures can deplete platelets.[1(p59)]

In both retrospective and prospective series, the absolute lymphocyte count in autologous HPC transplants had a significant effect on outcomes.[37,38] Work first showing that pretransplant lymphocyte counts measured in complete blood counts predicted outcomes was later extended to show that the absolute count of lymphocytes in the product predicted outcome. At this time, it is not possible to change these ratios by manipulating collection parameters. Rather, the simple process of collecting for additional days can allow an absolute count of $>0.5 \times 10^9$ lymphocytes/kg to be achieved.[38] Although it may be possible to perform additional lymphocyte collections without mobilization, the costs of additional days of collection and processing are not inconsequential. As more data are gathered, the financial and survival benefits will need to be evaluated.

PROCESSING HPCs

HPC processing methods can be divided into routine methods, which are usually centrifuge based, and specialized methods involving various technologies. Routine methods include volume (plasma) reduction, red cell reduction, buffy-coat preparation, thawing/washing, and filtration.

Volume reduction is performed in the setting of minor-ABO-mismatched allograft (marrow or peripheral blood) transplantation to reduce the amount of incompatible plasma and prevent fluid balance/overload issues in small patients and/or patients with renal disease or cardiac failure. Volume reduction may also be performed before cryopreservation (eg, for UCB banking where storage space is limited or during cell concentration optimization). (See Method 7-2.)

Classically, red cell reduction employs sedimentation agents such as hydroxyethyl starch to reduce red cell content. This approach is used to prevent hemolytic transfusion reactions when major-ABO-incompatible marrow HPC allografts and allografts with other clinically relevant red cell antigens (eg, Kell, Kidd) are transplanted. Red cell reduction before freezing also limits the amount of lysed red cell fragments and free hemoglobin on infusion and may be particularly important for patients with renal failure. Red cell reduction may also be useful when storage space is limited. Both volume and red cell reduction must be weighed against potential HPC losses during the procedures.

Buffy-coat concentration of marrow involves centrifugation and harvesting of the white cell fraction and can be performed with an apheresis or cell-washing device. Manual centrifugation may be used when product volume is too low for apheresis or cell-washing devices. Buffy-coat preparation is usually used to reduce the unit volume for cryopreservation or as a method of red cell reduction before further manipulation (eg, immunomagnetic selection).

Thawing procedures for all HPCs, regardless of source, are similar. Although it is straightforward, it should be done carefully because frozen plastic containers are prone to break for multiple reasons.[39] The product should be handled with care while it is verified to determine the product's identity and ensure the integrity of the bag. The product is then placed into a clean or sterile plastic bag and submerged in a 37 C waterbath. If the freezing bag breaks, the product may be recovered using this approach, but a risk/benefit discussion with the patient's physician should occur to determine the course of the patient's care.

Gentle kneading allows the thaw procedure to proceed relatively quickly while preventing recrystallization and consequent cell damage/death. A hemostat should be used to prevent loss of the product if the bag breaks, and the contents should be aseptically diverted into a transfer bag. A sample should also be sent for culture.

Washing HPCs removes lysed red cells, hemoglobin, and cryoprotectant [ie, dimethyl sulfoxide (DMSO)], albeit with a potential loss of some HPCs. Although red cells are typically removed from UCB before cryopreservation, UCB remains the primary HPC product that is routinely washed. However, this practice is changing as alternative approaches to UCB preparation for infusion are being adopted. Historically, most institutions based their UCB processing methodology, including the thawing/washing procedure, on the procedure espoused by the New York Placental Blood Program.[40] Briefly, this involves slow, sequential addition of a wash solution (eg, 10% dextran followed by 5% albumin), transfer into an appropriately sized bag for centrifugation, and resuspension of the cell pellet(s) before delivery to the patient care unit for infusion. Many laboratories perform two centrifugation steps, removing the supernatant from the first spin and centrifuging that portion a second time before combining the two cell pellets; this optimizes cell recovery.[41] Alternatively, automated methods can be used.

Marrow harvest typically involves sequential filtration in the operating room or the laboratory to remove bone spicules, aggregates, and debris. However, opinions vary regarding the use of standard blood filters with infusion of HPCs. Whether to use a standard blood filter (>170 microns) is the decision of the individual cell processing laboratory and/or transplant center. If a standard blood filter is used, the laboratory should validate this process.

SPECIALIZED CELL-PROCESSING METHODS

Specialized cell-processing methods can optimize product purity and potency beyond levels obtained by routine methods. Several of these methods, which require unique reagents and instrumentation, are discussed elsewhere; therefore, the descriptions of these methods in this chapter are brief and focus on their application to HPCs.

Elutriation

Counterflow centrifugal elutriation separates cell populations based on two physical characteristics: size and density (sedimentation coefficient). A centrifuge separates the cell populations of a cell product based on density alone. However, if fluid/media is passed through the chamber housing the cells in the direction opposite (counterflow) to the centrifugal force, adjustment of flow rate and/or centrifugation speed also allows separation of cell populations based on size. Through this process, cells with "signature" size/density profiles can be separated from other cells. Historically, this method was used for T-cell depletion of HPC grafts; more recently, it has been used to enrich monocytes for preparing dendritic-cell vaccines.

Cell-Selection Systems

Immunomagnetic cell-selection systems, which incorporate monoclonal antibody-based technologies to target cell-surface antigens [eg, CliniMACS system (Miltenyi Biotec Bergisch, Gladbach, Germany)], have become a widely used method of cell depletion/enrichment. These methods involve isolation of the cell type of interest by either positive selection (ie, target cells retained) or negative selection (target cells depleted). Monoclonal antibodies (eg, anti-CD34 for HPC isolation) are coupled to 50-nm ferromagnetic particles. Magnetically labeled target cells are retained in the process as the cell suspension passes through a column in which a magnetic field is generated. Unlabeled cells pass through the column and are collected in a negative-fraction bag. Bound cells are then released from the column by removal of the magnetic field from the column, which allows passage of the cells into a separate collection bag.

Cell Expansion

Because the dose of nucleated, CD34+, and colony-forming cells is positively correlated with patient outcome, much effort has been focused on ex-vivo expansion of HPCs and progenitors. It is thought that successful expansion enhances hematopoietic engraftment while reducing transfusion dependence, risk of infection, and duration of hospitalization. In recent years, UCB has become the focus of expansion trials because of both the higher proliferative and self-renewal capacity of UCB HPCs and the limited cell quantity in a UCB collection. Most expansion cultures contain a cytokine cocktail that includes stem cell factor, FLT-3 ligand, and thrombopoietin, along with novel and/or proprietary ingredients. The media, culture vessels, and culture duration used vary from protocol to protocol.

CRYOPRESERVATION

Methods for cryopreservation are necessary because HPCs may need to be stored for weeks to years before transplantation.[42] Most cell-processing laboratories use the cryoprotectant DMSO, usually at 10% final concentration, and a source of plasma protein for cryopreserving HPCs. DMSO is a colligative cryoprotectant; it diffuses rapidly into the cell, reducing the osmotic stress on the cell membrane. DMSO prevents dehydration injury by moderating the nonpenetrating extracellular solutes that form during ice formation. It also slows extracellular ice crystal formation. Some laboratories add hydroxyethyl starch (HES), which allows the use of a decreased concentration of DMSO (eg, 5% DMSO plus 6% HES). HES is a nonpenetrating (extracellular), macromolecular cryoprotectant; it likely protects the cell by forming a glassy shell, or membrane, around the cell, retarding the movement of water out of the cell and into the extracellular ice crystals.

HPCs may be frozen at a controlled rate or a noncontrolled rate, in which the HPC product is merely transferred into a freezer bag and placed in a –80 C mechanical freezer. Controlled-rate freezing is favored in the clinical laboratory setting; it uses computer programming to decrease HPC product temperature incrementally in a closely monitored fashion. Controlled-rate freezing protocols vary from institution to institution.

In general, with controlled-rate freezing, the HPC product is placed in the chamber and initially cooled at a rate of 1 C/minute. When the temperature decreases to approximately –14 C to –24 C, the HPC product begins to transition from liquid to solid. At this time, the freezer undergoes a period of supercooling to counteract the latent heat of fusion that is released by the phase change. Following solidification of the HPC product, cooling proceeds at the rate of 1 C/minute until the product has reached –60 C. At this point, the product is cooled at a controlled rate determined by the institution until it reaches –100 C. Following both controlled-rate and noncontrolled-rate freezing, the HPC product is transferred to a storage freezer. Increasing numbers of laboratories store HPCs in the vapor phase of liquid nitrogen (LN$_2$) at temperatures below –150 C; however, some laboratories store cells in the liquid phase of LN$_2$. The required interval between storage temperature recordings changes based on whether products are stored in the vapor or liquid phase.[1(p41)]

QC

QC testing in the clinical cell therapy laboratory serves two purposes: to determine the suitability and safety of the cellular product for the patient, and to monitor overall laboratory practices. QC testing is aimed at characterizing the safety, purity, identity, potency, and stability of the cellular product. The extent of QC testing primarily depends on the complexity of product manufacturing and the nature of the clinical experience (eg, standard practice vs a clinical trial).

Common QC tests for HPCs include cell count and differential, viability, CD34+ cell enumeration, sterility testing, and colony-forming unit assays. Cell count and differential are performed on a hematology analyzer. Cell viability may be determined using various methods, including trypan blue, acridine orange, and 7-aminoactinomycin D (by flow cytometry). Microscope-based methods utilizing vital dyes or fluorescent stains may be particularly useful for quick assessment of overall nucleated cell viability. Flow-cytometry-based analysis is useful when cell-population-specific viability must be determined. Most CD34+ cell-enumeration strategies are based on guidelines of the International Society for Cellular Therapy.[43] Sterility testing is primarily performed using automated microbial detection systems.

The clonogenic assay (most commonly used to count colony-forming units) is the only truly functional assessment of HPCs routinely performed in clinical laboratories. The results of this assay correlate with the speed and likelihood of engraftment of HPCs from marrow, peripheral blood, or UCB.[44-47] However, the similar correlation between results and engraftment speed and likelihood, as well as the more rapid availability of results, have made CD34+ cell enumeration the accepted, albeit surrogate, QC test for graft potency. The clonogenic assay is still useful, despite difficulties in standardization, especially for HPCs that are stored for a long time (eg, UCB banking).[48]

SHIPPING AND TRANSPORTING HPC CELLULAR PRODUCTS

Geographic separation between donors and recipients is possible because of the ability to ship and transport cellular therapy products. These two terms are given specific definitions by accreditation organizations.[1(pp136,138)] With shipping, the product leaves the control of trained personnel in the facilities involved in the distribution and receipt of the product. Conversely, with transport, the transfer of a product between or within facilities occurs under the control of trained personnel.

Three issues are particularly important to ensure the safe delivery of HPC products: product integrity, safety of the personnel involved in the transport, and compliance with applicable regulations and standards. The necessary conditions for shipping and transport vary depending on the type of product, its state (fresh or cryopreserved), and the distance involved. These issues are reviewed in depth elsewhere.[49]

During shipment, products must be placed in secondary containers that can prevent leakage and maintain the temperature range required for the product and the anticipated shipping duration.[1(p38)] For fresh products, several studies showed that shipment at 2 C to 8 C can maintain CD34+ cell viability more effectively than shipment at room temperature, particularly for shipping times of 24 to 72 hours.[50-52] This effect appears to be more pronounced for peripheral blood products than marrow products and for products with higher concentrations of HPCs.

Cryopreserved products are shipped in dry shippers charged with LN_2. These containers maintain temperatures below –150 C for up to 2 weeks, and their temperatures are continuously monitored.[1(p46)] If products are shipped to a noncontiguous facility or on public roads, an appropriately labeled outer container must be used to provide additional protection during transport and shipping. Depending on the mode of transport (eg, air or ground) or destination (eg, international), additional federal government or international requirements must be met. If the recipient has already received high-dose conditioning therapy, shipment using a qualified courier is required. The product should not be x-rayed; instead, it should be manually inspected, if necessary. Appropriate records must accompany the product.

The receiving institution must have protocols in place for the receipt and inspection of the product for acceptability for transplantation.[1(pp43-44)]

PATIENT CARE

Once an HPC product is ready for infusion, it should be delivered to the patient care unit without delay. After the physician approves the product for infusion and proper identification procedures are performed, the product is infused by intravenous (IV) drip directly into a central line, typically without a needle or pump. Some institutions use a standard blood filter at the bedside. To maximize cell dose, the product bag and IV tubing may be flushed with sterile saline after the bag empties. Sterile saline also may be added directly to the bag if the flow rate becomes too slow. (See Method 7-1.)

HPC products are usually infused as quickly as the patient can tolerate, particularly for thawed cells that have not been washed or diluted, to lessen DMSO toxicity to the cells. Although some[53] have concluded that DMSO is not toxic to HPCs at clinically relevant concentrations (ie, 5%-10%) at either 4 C or 37 C for up to 1 hour of incubation, the addition of 1% DMSO to culture dishes suppressed colony-forming units. However, these studies were performed on fresh cells, and studies of the effects of DMSO on previously cryopreserved HPCs are limited. The possible functional defect caused by DMSO coupled with the not-infrequent need to hold clinical products (because of patient-care-related issues) raise concern about possible cell injury from infusing thawed, unwashed HPC products.

The patient's vital signs should be checked, at a minimum, before infusion, immediately after infusion, and 1 hour after infusion. All monitoring information should be captured on an accompanying infusion form. When completed, this form should be returned to the laboratory. If an adverse reaction occurs, more frequent monitoring is required.

Reactions associated with HPC infusion may be very similar to those that occasionally occur with blood transfusion (eg, allergic, hemolytic, and febrile reactions, and those caused by microbial contamination). However, some reactions may be less likely depending on the cell-processing technique used (eg, red cell reduction, plasma reduction, postthaw washing, or dilution). Reactions often attributed to DMSO (eg, nausea, vomiting, cough, and headache) are less common with infusions of smaller volumes and/or washed or diluted products.[54,55] Nonetheless, HPC products are usually well tolerated. Because severe reactions may occur, aggressive IV hydration (eg, 2-6 hours before and 6 hours after infusion, with diuretics, as needed) and the use of prophylactic antiemetics, antipyretics, and antihistamines may be warranted.

The transplant physician and the medical director of the cell therapy laboratory should be notified immediately of an unexpected or moderate-to-severe reaction. An investigation should begin and include laboratory testing (eg, direct antiglobulin test, antibody titer, Gram stain, or culture) that targets the signs/symptoms of the patient.

Data on clinical outcomes (eg, engraftment) and adverse events should be reviewed regularly and discussed with the institutional quality management group. Quarterly reviews are reasonable for engraftment analysis. The medical director's review should include assessment of the HPC product's quality indicators (eg, dose, viability, and colony-forming units), associated deviations, and the presence of infusion reactions, with a focus on potential laboratory-related issues affecting any less-than-optimal outcome.

OTHER REGULATORY CONSIDERATIONS

The relevant regulations regarding HPC collection are discussed above. In general, HPCs that are minimally manipulated and collected for transplantation in an autologous fashion or transplanted to a first- or second-degree relative are regulated solely under Section 361 of the Public Health Service Act and are subject to the jurisdiction of the Center for Biologics Evaluation and Research of the FDA. If HPCs are manufactured in a way that alters their relevant biologic characteristics (eg, genetically modified, expanded ex vivo, or combined with a drug) or they are intended for transplantation into a non-first-or-second-degree relative, then the HPC product is subject to regulation under Title 21, CFR Part 1271 as a drug and/or biologic product and requires licensing or an exemption from licensing from the FDA as part of an investigational new drug (IND) application. HPCs from unrelated donors facilitated through the Be The Match Registry may be administered under its IND (BB-IND 6821) or an institutionally held IND protocol. Similarly, UCB HPCs can now be obtained from FDA-licensed UCB sources or administered under an institutional IND protocol.

CONCLUSION

The indispensable, lifesaving role of HPCs in medicine has been established, especially for patients with hematologic disorders. As HPC biology becomes better understood and the ability to engineer HPC grafts expands, clinical applications of HPCs will continue to grow. Along with the fast-paced growth in the use of HPCs, emerging novel technologies and approaches to manipulate HPCs are adding to the complexity of ensuring that HPCs contin-ue to serve as a safe and effective cellular therapy product for patient use. Addressing this challenge will require regulatory agencies and accrediting bodies to continue to update and modify their applicable rules, regulations, and standards.

KEY POINTS

1. HPCs derived from the patient being treated (autologous) or a donor (allogeneic) can be used to treat multiple malignant and nonmalignant conditions.
2. Autologous HPCs are typically used to rescue marrow function for a patient undergoing high-dose chemotherapy and/or radiotherapy.
3. In addition to the above use, allogeneic HPCs have graft-vs-neoplasm effects and/or the ability to replace defective cellular machinery.
4. Regardless of the HPC donor source, AABB *CT Standards* requires laboratory testing for HIV-1/2; hepatitis B virus; hepatitis C virus; syphilis; and HTLV-I/II. Testing for CMV is required for allogeneic HPC products.
5. Screening and testing for infectious diseases in allogeneic HPC donors is mandated by the FDA; when a risk for a communicable disease is discovered, the donor is ineligible (but may still donate if there is an urgent medical need).
6. Allogeneic HPC donors are chosen with regard to their histocompatibility with the recipient. ABO/Rh compatibility between the donor and recipient, although not required, may offer additional survival benefit.
7. HPCs can be obtained by marrow aspiration, umbilical cord blood collection, or peripheral blood mobilization followed by collection by apheresis.
8. HPCs usually require minimal manipulation and can be stored following cryopreservation with cryoprotectant (dimethyl sulfoxide).
9. Specialized HPC manipulation techniques can reduce HPC product volume, lysed cells, red cells, and cryoprotectant, depending on the recipient's clinical needs.
10. QC is essential for providing safe and efficacious HPC products. Common QC testing includes cell counts (CD34+ cell enumeration, TNC count), microbial contamination testing, and viability testing.

REFERENCES

1. Haspel RL, ed. Standards for cellular therapy services. 8th ed. Bethesda, MD: AABB, 2017.
2. Bianco P. Bone and the hematopoietic niche: A tale of two stem cells. Blood 2011;117:5281-8.
3. Rivadeneyra-Espínoza L, Pérez-Romano B, González-Flores A, et al. Instrument- and protocol-dependent variation in the enumeration of CD34+ cells by flow cytometry. Transfusion 2006;46:530-6.
4. National Marrow Donor Program/Be The Match 23rd edition standards and glossary. Minneapolis, MN: NMDP, 2016. [Available at http://bethematch.org/WorkArea/Download Asset.aspx?id=7711 (accessed April 26, 2017).]
5. Donor history questionnaire—HPC, apheresis and HPC, marrow. Version 1.6. Bethesda, MD: AABB, 2016. [Available at http://www.aabb.org/tm/questionnaires/Pages/dhqhpc.aspx (accessed April 26, 2017).]
6. Food and Drug Administration. Guidance for industry: Eligibility determination for donors of human cells, tissues, and cellular and tissue-based products (HCT/Ps). Silver Spring, MD: CBER Office of Communication, Outreach, and Development, 2007. [Available at

http://www.fda.gov/downloads/Biologics BloodVaccines/GuidanceComplianceRegula toryInformation/Guidances/Tissue/ UCM091345.pdf (accessed April 26, 2017).]

7. Saber W, Opie S, Rizzo JD, et al. Outcomes after matched unrelated donor versus identical sibling hematopoietic cell transplantation in adults with acute myelogenous leukemia. Blood 2012;119:3908-16.

8. National Marrow Donor Program/Be The Match. Unrelated vs. sibling donor outcomes. Minneapolis, MN: NMDP, 2017. [Available at https://bethematchclinical.org/transplant-indications-and-outcomes/additional-outcomes/unrelated-vs--sibling-donor-outcomes/ (accessed April 26, 2017).]

9. Abbas AK, Lichtman AH, Pillai S. Cellular and molecular immunology. 6th ed. Philadelphia: Saunders Elsevier, 2007.

10. Spellman SR, Eapen M, Logan BR, et al. A perspective on the selection of unrelated donors and cord blood units for transplantation. Blood 2012;120:256-65.

11. National Marrow Donor Program/Be The Match. HLA typing and matching. Minneapolis, MN: NMDP, 2017. [Available at https://bethematchclinical.org/Transplant-Therapy-and-Donor-Matching/HLA-Typing-and-Matching/ (accessed April 26, 2017).]

12. Spellman S, Bray R, Rosen-Bronson S, et al. The detection of donor-directed, HLA-specific alloantibodies in recipients of unrelated hematopoietic cell transplantation is predictive of graft failure. Blood 2010;115:2704-8.

13. Brand A, Doxiadis IN, Roelen DL. On the role of HLA antibodies in hematopoietic stem cell transplantation. Tissue Antigens 2013;81:1-11.

14. Barker JN, Byam C, Scaradavou A. How I treat: The selection and acquisition of unrelated cord blood grafts. Blood 2011;117:2332-9.

15. Barker JN, Scaradavou A, Steven CE. Combined effect of total nucleated cell dose and HLA match on transplantation outcome in 1061 cord blood recipients with hematologic malignancies. Blood 2010;115:1843-9.

16. van Rood JJ, Stevens CE, Smits J, et al. Re-exposure of cord blood to noninherited maternal HLA antigens improves transplant outcome in hematologic malignancies. Proc Natl Acad Sci U S A 2009;106:19952-7.

17. Ciurea SO, Bayraktar UD. "No donor"? Consider a haploidentical transplant. Blood Rev 2015; 29:63-70.

18. Kollman C, Spellman SR, Zhang M, et al. The effect of donor characteristics on survival after unrelated donor transplantation for hematologic malignancy. Blood 2016;127:260-7.

19. Rowly SD, Donato ML, Bhattacharyya P. Red blood cell-incompatible allogeneic hematopoietic progenitor cell transplantation. Bone Marrow Transplant 2011;46:1167-85.

20. McCullough J, McKenna D, Kadidlo D, et al. Issue in the quality of umbilical cord blood stem cells for transplantation. Transfusion 2005;45: 832-41.

21. Page KM, Zhang L, Medizabal A, et al. The cord blood apgar: A novel scoring system to optimize the selection of banked cord blood grafts for transplantation. Transfusion 2012;52:272-83.

22. Barker JN, Krepski TP, DeFor TE, et al. Searching for unrelated donor hematopoietic stem cells: Availability and speed of umbilical cord blood versus bone marrow. Biol Blood Marrow Transplant 2002;8:257-60.

23. Giralt S. Graft-versus-host disease: Have we solved the problem? J Clin Oncol 2012;30:360-1.

24. Anasetti C, Logan BR, Lee SJ, Waller EK. Peripheral-blood stem cells versus bone marrow from unrelated donors. N Engl J Med 2012; 367:1487-96.

25. Brunstein CG, Wagner JE Jr. Umbilical cord blood transplantation. In: Hoffman R, Benz E, Shattil SJ, et al, eds. Hematology: Basic principles and practice. 5th ed. Philadelphia: Churchill Livingstone Elsevier, 2009:1643-64.

26. Zhang H, Chen J, Que W. Allogeneic peripheral blood stem cell and bone marrow transplantation for hematologic malignancies: Meta-analysis of randomized controlled trials. Leuk Res 2012;36:431-7.

27. Laughlin MJ, Eapen M, Rubinstein P, et al. Outcomes after transplantation of cord blood or bone marrow from unrelated donors in adults with leukemia. N Engl J Med 2004;351:2265-75.

28. Stem Cell Trialists' Collaborative Group. Allogeneic peripheral blood stem-cell compared with bone marrow transplantation for hematologic malignancies: An individual patient data meta-analysis of nine randomized trials. J Clin Oncol 2005;23:5074-87.

29. Eapen M, Horowitz MM, Klein JP, et al. Higher mortality after allogeneic peripheral-blood transplantation compared with bone marrow in children and adolescents: The Histocompatibility and Alternative Stem Cell Source

Working Committee of the International Bone Marrow Transplant Registry. J Clin Oncol 2004; 22:4872-80.

30. Meisel R, Klingebiel T, Dillo D. Peripheral blood stem cells versus bone marrow in pediatric unrelated donor stem cell transplantation. Blood 2013;121:863-5.

31. Miller JP, Perry EH, Price TH, et al. Recovery and safety profile of marrow and PBSC donors: Experience of the National Marrow Donor Program. Biol Blood Marrow Transplant 2008; 14:29-36.

32. Pulsipher MA, Chitphakdithai P, Miller JP, et al. Adverse events among 2408 unrelated donors of peripheral blood stem cells: Results of a prospective trial from the National Marrow Donor Program. Blood 2009;113:3604-11.

33. Gertz MA. Review: Current status of stem cell mobilization. Br J Haematol 2010;150:647-62.

34. Keating GM. Plerixafor. Drugs 2011;71:1623-47.

35. To LB, Haylock DN, Simmons PJ, Juttner CA. The biology and uses of blood stem cells. Blood 1997;89:2233-58.

36. Abrahamsen JF, Stamnesfet S, Liseth K, et al. Large-volume leukapheresis yields more viable CD34+ cells and colony-forming units than normal-volume leukapheresis, especially in patients who mobilize low numbers of CD34+ cells. Transfusion 2005;45:248-53.

37. Porrata LF, Litzow MR, Inwards DJ, et al. Infused peripheral blood autograft absolute lymphocyte count correlates with day 15 absolute lymphocyte count and clinical outcome after autologous peripheral hematopoietic stem cell transplantation in non-Hodgkin's lymphoma. Bone Marrow Transplant 2004;33: 291-8.

38. Porrata LF, Burgstaler EA, Winters JL, et al. Immunologic autograft engineering and survival in non-Hodgkin lymphoma. Biol Bood Marrow Transplant 2016;22:1017-23.

39. Khuu HM, Cowley H, David-Ocampo V, et al. Catastrophic failures of freezing bags for cellular therapy products: Description, cause, and consequences. Cytotherapy 2002;4:539-49.

40. Rubinstein P, Dobrila L, Rosenfield R, et al. Processing and cryopreservation of placental/umbilical cord blood for unrelated bone marrow reconstitution. Proc Natl Acad Sci U S A 1995;92:10119-22.

41. Laroche V, McKenna D, Moroff G, et al. Cell loss and recovery in umbilical cord blood processing: A comparison of post-thaw and post-wash samples. Transfusion 2005;45:1909-16.

42. Fleming KK, Hubel A. Cryopreservation of hematopoietic and non-hematopoietic stem cells. Transfus Apher Sci 2006;34:309-15.

43. Sutherland DR, Anderson L, Keeney M, et al. The ISHAGE guidelines for CD34+ cell determination by flow cytometry. J Hematother 1996;5:213-26.

44. Spitzer G, Verma DS, Fisher R, et al. The myeloid progenitor cell: Its value in predicting hematopoietic recovery after autologous bone marrow transplantation. Blood 1980;55:317-23.

45. Douay L, Gorin NC, Mary JY, et al. Recovery of CFU-GM from cryopreserved marrow and in vivo evaluation after autologous bone marrow transplantation are predictive of engraftment. Exp Hematol 1986;14:358-65.

46. Schwartzberg L, Birch R, Blanco R, et al. Rapid and sustained hematopoietic reconstitution by peripheral blood stem cell infusion alone following high-dose chemotherapy. Bone Marrow Transplant 1993;11:360-74.

47. Migliaccio AR, Adamson JW, Stevens CE, et al. Cell dose and speed of engraftment in placental/umbilical cord blood transplantation: Graft progenitor cell content is a better predictor than nucleated cell quantity. Blood 2000; 96:2717-22.

48. Pamphilon D, Selogie E, McKenna D, et al. Current practices and prospects for standardization of the hematopoietic colony-forming unit assay: A report by the cellular therapy team of the Biomedical Excellence for Safer transfusion (BEST) collaborative. Cytotherapy 2013;15:255-62.

49. Regan D. Transportation and shipping of cellular therapy products. In: Areman EM, Loper K, eds. Cellular therapy: Principles, methods and regulations. Bethesda, MD: AABB, 2009: 362-74.

50. Antonenas V, Garvin F, Webb M, et al. Fresh PBSC harvests, but not BM, show temperature-related loss of CD34 viability during storage and transport. Cytotherapy 2006;11:158-65.

51. Jansen J, Nolan P, Reeves M, et al. Transportation of peripheral blood progenitor cell products: Effects of time, temperature and cell concentration. Cytotherapy 2009;11:79-85.

52. Kao G, Kim H, Daley H, et al. Validation of short-term handling and storage conditions for marrow and peripheral blood stem cell products. Transfusion 2011;51:137-47.

53. Rowley SD, Anderson GL. Effect of DMSO exposure without cryopreservation on hematopoietic progenitor cells. Bone Marrow Transplant 1993;11:389-93.

54. Davis JM, Rowley SD, Braine HG, et al. Clinical toxicity of cryopreserved bone marrow graft infusion. Blood 1990;75:781-6.

55. Stroncek DF, Fautsch SK, Lasky LC, et al. Adverse reactions in patients transfused with cryopreserved marrow. Transfusion 1991;31:521-6.

Transfusion Support for Hematopoietic Stem Cell Transplant Recipients

● ● ●

Melissa M. Cushing, MD, and Jeanne E. Hendrickson, MD

LLOGENEIC HEMATOPOIETIC STEM cell transplantation (HSCT) recipients are unique patients who present distinct challenges for blood banks and transfusion services. When considering transfusion for an HSCT recipient, one has to consider not only the complexities associated with the patient's underlying condition but also potential problems associated with recipient alloantibodies, donor passenger lymphocytes, and different blood group systems. Over the past two decades, significant growth in transplantation has occurred. Moreover, many patients are now seen in their community hospitals for posttransplant care. Thus, issues regarding the complexity of transfusion support for HSCT recipients are no longer restricted to academic medical centers.

Given the increasing numbers of patients undergoing HSCT from related and unrelated donors, and given the many clinical conditions currently treated with this approach, it is imperative that transfusion medicine specialists be prepared to address the challenges associated with transfusion support for these patients. This chapter addresses the most common and important issues faced by transfusion services in treating HSCT recipients, providing an up-to-date summary for blood bank physicians and other medical practitioners.

Melissa M. Cushing, MD, Associate Professor of Clinical Pathology and Laboratory Medicine, Weill Cornell Medicine, New York, New York, and Medical Director, Transfusion Medicine and Cellular Therapy, and Associate Director of the Clinical Laboratories, New York-Presbyterian/Weill Cornell Medical Campus, New York, New York; and Jeanne E. Hendrickson, MD, Associate Professor of Laboratory Medicine and Pediatrics, Yale University School of Medicine, and Associate Medical Director, Yale Transfusion Medicine Service, New Haven, Connecticut

The authors have disclosed no conflicts of interest.

ABO- AND NON-ABO-RED-CELL-ANTIGEN-INCOMPATIBLE TRANSPLANTATION

The ABO blood group antigen system is not necessarily a barrier to successful HSCT. Unlike solid-organ transplantation, where ABO compatibility may be essential, pluripotent and early committed hematopoietic progenitor cells (HPCs) lack ABO antigens; thus, HPC engraftment is uninhibited, even in the presence of circulating ABO antibodies. Nonetheless, discrepancies in ABO and occasionally non-ABO antigens between donor and recipient do play important roles in transplantation and can become a complicating factor in HSCT recipient transfusion support.

In allogeneic transplantation, the relationship between the ABO types of the donor and recipient falls into one of four categories: compatible, incompatible in the major crossmatch, incompatible in the minor crossmatch, and bidirectional incompatibility.[1,2] Table 27-1 lists potential ABO combinations between donors and recipients, with an indication of the associated compatibility. ABO incompatibilities are present in 25% to 50% of donor/recipient pairs; thus, careful attention to blood component selection for transfusion is necessary.[3,4] Although the terms major, minor, and bidirectional incompatibility are most fre-

quently used in the context of the ABO system, they are also applicable to describe the presence of other red cell alloantibodies, such as anti-K or anti-D, in the plasma of the donor and/or recipient.

Major ABO Incompatibility

Major ABO incompatibility creates two challenges: 1) the potential for acute intravascular hemolysis when ABO-incompatible donor red cells within the graft are infused to a recipient with anti-A and/or anti-B antibodies, and 2) the ongoing production of ABO antibodies by the recipient's immune cells directed against erythroid progenitors and mature red cells produced by the engrafting HPCs. The first challenge is typically addressed during HPC collection and/or processing. Techniques, such as red cell reduction of a marrow graft product, minimize the risk of hemolysis during infusion. Some HPC products, including all cord blood cells, are cryopreserved before administration, and incompatible donor red cells may be lysed during the freeze/thaw process. There is no general consensus about the "threshold" level of incompatible red cells that may be safely infused in adults, although for pediatric recipients, currently acceptable volumes are 10 to 30 mL or 0.4 mL/kg recipient body weight. As suggested by Staley et al,[5] recipient antibody titer may also be used in

TABLE 27-1. Description of Compatibility for HSCT According to ABO Blood Group of Donor and Recipient*

Recipient ABO Status	Donor ABO Status			
	O	**A**	**B**	**AB**
O	Identical	Major	Major	Major
A	Minor	Identical	Bi (major/minor)	Major
B	Minor	Bi (major/minor)	Identical	Major
AB	Minor	Minor	Minor	Identical

*Major incompatibility is due to a naturally occurring antibody (or antibodies) in the recipient (eg, donor is group A, and recipient is group O with naturally occurring anti-A). Minor incompatibility is due to a naturally occurring antibody (or antibodies) in the donor graft product (eg, donor is group O with naturally occurring anti-A, and recipient is group A). "Bi (major/minor)" indicates a bidirectional incompatibility due to naturally occurring antibodies in both the donor and recipient (eg, donor is group A, and recipient is group B).

guiding policy. In the absence of red cell reduction or cryopreservation, therapeutic plasma exchange (TPE) of the recipient immediately before graft infusion may be warranted to reduce the circulating titers of ABO antibodies in extreme cases.

The second challenge, the continuous production of antibodies, is a process that can continue up to 3 to 4 months after HPC infusion. As a result, delays in erythropoiesis are often encountered, with red cell engraftment potentially occurring >40 days after transplantation. Time to red cell engraftment may be prolonged even further with reduced-intensity or nonmyeloablative conditioning regimens.[3,6] In severe cases, pure red cell aplasia (PRCA) can develop. Different treatment options for PRCA include erythropoietin, rapid tapering of calcineurin inhibitors, corticosteroids, rituximab, bortezomib, donor lymphocyte infusion, mesenchymal stem cells, or TPE; no standard of care currently exists. Thus, HSCT involving major ABO incompatibility may render some recipients transfusion-dependent for months following transplantation. Fortunately, major incompatibility tends not to affect early stem cell engraftment or production of other myeloid-lineage cells.

Minor ABO Incompatibility

Analogous to red cell reduction for major incompatibility, plasma reduction of the allograft can decrease donor alloantibodies in the setting of minor ABO incompatibility. Even if antibodies are not completely removed, the ensuing hemolysis is typically mild and self-limited.[2] A more significant problem with minor-incompatible HSCT results from the rapid generation of anti-A and/or -B by donor lymphocytes against residual recipient red cells. This "passenger lymphocyte syndrome" occurs approximately 5 to 16 days after HPC infusion. The patient may experience acute, immune-mediated hemolysis that can result in morbidity and even mortality. In most cases, the hemolysis is not severe and eventually subsides with clearance of recipient red cells.[2] If hemolysis is severe and potentially life-threatening, therapeutic red cell exchange can

be used to replace incompatible recipient red cells with donor-compatible red cells.

Bidirectional ABO Incompatibility

In bidirectional ABO incompatibility, the complications arising from both major- and minor-ABO-incompatible HSCT can be seen in the recipient.

Incompatibility Related to Non-ABO Antigens

Red cell antigens of other blood group systems can present challenges similar to the ones described for ABO-incompatible transplants. Overall, they are less frequently encountered, but the presence of red cell antibodies in the patient (more common) and/or in the donor (less common) require attention and approaches similar to those outlined above. A recent review investigating the importance of the RhD antigen in HSCT concluded that D-antigen incompatibility is not likely to result in serious clinical consequences.[7] As described in more detail below, special consideration may also be needed regarding donor selection in reduced-intensity or nonmyeloablative conditioning regimens involving alloimmunized recipients, so that cognate graft-donor-antigen/recipient-alloantibody pairs can be avoided if at all possible.

BLOOD COMPONENT CONSIDERATIONS

Selection of Blood Components

In determining transfusion requirements for an allogeneic HSCT recipient, it is vital that the blood bank or transfusion service keep detailed records documenting the pretransplant ABO group, recipient ABO antibody titers, and the donor ABO type. It is also imperative to identify the stage of the transplant (ie, preparative period, immediate posttransplant period, or postengraftment period with absence of recipient red cells and/or antibodies).[8] Recommendations for optimal component selection at each point in the transplant process are shown in Table 27-2. With regard to RhD, the

TABLE 27-2. Transfusion Support for Patients Undergoing HSCT According to the Type of ABO Incompatibility and Transplant Stage

Type of Incompatibility	Transplant Stage	ABO Blood Group Selection		
		RBCs	**Platelets***	**Plasma**
Major incompatibility	Preparative regimen	Recipient	Donor	Donor
	Transplantation	Recipient	Donor	Donor
	Recipient antibodies detected	Recipient	Donor	Donor
	Recipient antibodies no longer detected	Donor	Donor	Donor
Minor incompatibility	Preparative regimen	Donor	Recipient	Recipient
	Transplantation	Donor	Recipient	Recipient
	Recipient cells circulating	Donor	Recipient	Recipient
	Recipient cells no longer circulating	Donor	Donor	Donor
Bidirectional incompatibility	Preparative regimen	Group O	Group AB	Group AB
	Transplantation	Group O	Group AB	Group AB
	Recipient antibodies detected/ recipient cells circulating	Group O	Group AB	Group AB
	Recipient antibodies no longer detected/ recipient cells no longer circulating	Donor	Donor	Donor

*Because of the short shelf life and generally limited availability of group AB platelets, it may not always be possible to provide identically matched ABO platelet components, as outlined in this table. In some instances, blood banks and transfusion services may consider providing either a limited number of units of ABO-mismatched platelets per day or ABO-mismatched units that have been volume reduced to diminish plasma content, or demonstrated to have a low titer of anti-A or anti B.

RBCs = Red Blood Cells.

recipient can continue to receive the same type of components transfused before transplantation as long as the HSCT donor and recipient match. However, if the recipient is Rh negative and the donor Rh positive, or vice versa, Rh-negative Red Blood Cells (RBCs) should be considered to prevent alloimmunization to the highly immunogenic D antigen. Given the minimal risk of D alloimmunization from red cells contained in Rh-positive platelet units, selection of Rh-negative platelets is not mandatory.[7]

RBC Support

Most HSCT patients require transfusion support in the peritransplant period, regardless of incompatibilities or blood group antigen mismatches. The transfusion burden after transplantation depends on many factors, including the hemoglobin threshold for transfusion at each institution and ABO incompatibility of the transplant; however, many other variables can also affect transfusion outcomes, including gender, disease state, stem cell source, and conditioning regimen.[9] In one study of 169 HSCT recipients, the median number of RBC units transfused in the first year was 6, and the median time to transfusion independence was 12 days.[10] Posttransplant iron overload is a significant concern, as studies have shown worse outcomes and decreased overall survival with elevated ferritin levels.[11] Symptomatic anemia is one of the most common indications for RBC transfusion in HSCT recipients. Because specific RBC transfusion "triggers" in HSCT populations are lacking, clinicians can rely on general RBC transfusion guidelines. For instance, a threshold hemoglobin level of 7 g/dL is likely appropriate for most stable, nonpostoperative, adult HSCT recipients, whereas a slightly higher threshold of 8 g/dL is likely appropriate for adults with preexisting heart disease, those at risk for end-organ damage, or HSCT recipients in the postoperative setting.[12,13] The Transfusion of Red Cells in Hematopoietic Stem Cell Transplantation (TRIST) study investigated whether a restrictive transfusion strategy (target hemoglobin of 7-9 g/dL) or liberal strategy (target, 9-11 g/dL) improves

outcomes after HSCT.[14] The study found no difference in outcomes between the groups in the two different arms. In addition, an ongoing French randomized controlled trial is attempting to determine whether a single RBC unit transfusion, vs 2 units, is safe using a hemoglobin threshold of 8 g/dL.[15]

The mechanisms underlying anemia and RBC transfusion dependence after HSCT are sufficiently unique to warrant special consideration. After intensive chemotherapy, serum erythropoietin (EPO) levels increase rapidly and peak in the first week after treatment.[16,17] Although autologous HSCT recipients maintain adequate EPO levels throughout the posttransplant course, the situation is different for allogeneic recipients.[18] In this setting, a prolonged period of inappropriately low endogenous EPO levels often necessitates prolonged RBC transfusion support.

Platelet Support

Platelet recovery after allogeneic HSCT has been studied extensively. Several factors are strongly associated with the rate at which patients become platelet-transfusion independent, including 1) the relationship between donor and recipient (related vs unrelated), 2) the conditioning regimen, 3) the presence of graft-vs-host disease (GVHD) or cytomegalovirus (CMV) infection, and 4) the HPC CD34+ cellular source/dose.[19,20] In broad summary, the findings of several studies suggest that slower platelet engraftment tends to be more common in patients receiving unrelated grafts, those with higher-grade GVHD, and patients with viral infections.[20,21] The source of an allogeneic transplant also predicts time to platelet engraftment. Several studies showed that the median time to platelet engraftment for cord blood HPC recipients is significantly longer than for recipients of HPCs from apheresis or marrow.[22-24]

One major consideration for platelet transfusion in HSCT recipients is compatibility. Plasma (a significant volume in platelets) contains variable anti-A and/or anti-B antibody titers.[25] Although transfusion of limited quantities of ABO-incompatible plasma and platelets is common in routine transfusions, it cannot be readily applied to allogeneic HSCT recipients without careful consideration. As such, in ABO-incompatible HSCT, the plasma-containing components should be compatible with both the donor and the recipient whenever possible. Recommendations for component selection are more fully detailed in Table 27-2.

In addition to risks of hemolysis, there are other morbidities associated with ABO-incompatible platelet transfusions. For example, in one pediatric study, such transfusions, when combined with the use of melphalan, correlated with the development of hepatic veno-occlusive disease, possibly as a result of antibody binding to A and/or B antigens on the surface of hepatic endothelial cells.[26] Thus, some centers transfuse only ABO-identical RBCs and platelets to HSCT recipients; at least one group noted that this may improve patient survival.[27]

Several additional areas that require more extensive discussion of platelet transfusion include 1) prophylactic vs therapeutic transfusions, 2) the transfusion threshold, 3) the appropriate transfusion dose, and 4) HLA and platelet antibodies.

Prophylactic vs Therapeutic Platelet Transfusions

Platelet transfusions are frequently administered to prevent bleeding in HSCT recipients, rather than for acute hemorrhage. Two studies reported that, although some bleeding was observed in patients relegated to a therapeutic (rather than a prophylactic) transfusion regimen, there was no evidence of life-threatening hemorrhage. Moreover, when transfusion was limited to therapeutic interventions, there were significant reductions in platelet usage.[28,29] On the other hand, the Trial of Prophylactic Platelets (TOPPS) randomized clinical trial concluded that prophylactic platelet transfusions provided some benefit in preventing hemorrhage in patients with hematologic malignancies, vs a nontransfused control population.[30] However, a prespecified subgroup analysis identified similar rates of bleeding in the two study groups among autologous HSCT patients. In a subsequent event analysis, female gender, treatment plan (chemotherapy/allogeneic hematopoietic stem cell transplant), and fever were also associated with a higher risk of World Health Organization (WHO) Grade 2 to 4 bleeding. These results highlighted the limited role of prophylactic platelet transfusion in reducing the risk of bleeding.[31] Therefore, questions still remain as to appropriate, evidence-based strategies regarding prophylactic transfusion for thrombocytopenic HSCT patients.

Platelet Transfusion Threshold

One of the earliest established thresholds to prevent spontaneous hemorrhage was a platelet count of <20,000/µL for patients undergoing chemotherapy or HSCT.[32] Multiple studies subsequently showed that a platelet count of <10,000/µL in uncomplicated thrombocytopenia (ie, in patients without coexisting conditions such as fever, bleeding, or bacteremia/sepsis) is a reasonable threshold to prevent increased bleeding or hemorrhage-related morbidity.[33] However, one group reported that HSCT patients transfused at a platelet count <10,000/µL demonstrated significantly increased *nonhemorrhagic* mortality and reduced survival when compared to those transfused at counts <20,000/µL.[34]

Platelet Dose

Another question frequently associated with platelet transfusion is the optimal platelet dose per transfusion episode. To date, three large-scale trials have examined the question of platelet transfusion dosing.[35-37] In conjunction with the individual study results, a meta-analysis showed no increased risk for significant bleeding comparing low and standard platelet doses.[38] Further, a subgroup analysis of the Platelet Dosing (PLADO) trial showed no difference in bleeding risk based on platelet dose in pediatric patients.[39] Nonetheless, drawbacks to a lower dosing regimen may include a lower platelet increment after infusion and the potential for a greater number of platelet transfusions over time.[36,38]

HSCT Recipients with HLA and/or HPA Antibodies

Some patients undergoing HSCT have antibodies against HLA and/or human platelet antigens (HPAs), both of which may reduce platelet transfusion efficacy, resulting in lower corrected count increments (CCIs).[40] For a more thorough discussion of the evaluation and treatment of immune-mediated platelet refractoriness, see Chapters 15 and 19. In addition to causing potential problems with platelet transfusion, recipient HLA alloantibodies may affect engraftment.[41,42] Therapeutic plasma exchange can be used to desensitize potential transplant recipients to HLA antigens. (See Chapter 25.)

Plasma, Cryoprecipitated AHF, Factor Concentrates, and Other Support

There are no specific recommendations regarding the usage of plasma, cryoprecipitated antihemophilic factor, or factor concentrates for HSCT patients; as such, adherence to existing guidelines and/or expert recommendations is advised.[43] As discussed above and outlined in Table 27-2, the most important aspects for plasma/cryoprecipitate transfusion relate to the ABO group of the recipient and engrafting HPCs.

Transfusion Support for Autologous Transplant Recipients

Before, during, and after HSCT, autologous recipients should be supported by blood components as needed according to standard protocols applicable to any transfusion recipient. However, because of underlying immunosuppression, autologous HSCT recipients may require specialized products or components needing additional processing steps. Such issues and concerns (applicable to both autologous and allogeneic transplant recipients) are discussed below.

NEUTROPENIC PATIENTS WITH INFECTIONS UNRESPONSIVE TO ANTIMICROBIAL THERAPY

Infusions of fresh granulocytes are used to treat severe, antibiotic-refractory bacterial or fungal infections in patients with absolute neutrophil counts <500/μL. For a more in-depth discussion of granulocyte therapy, see Chapters 15 and 19. A recent multicenter randomized controlled trial, although underpowered, failed to detect a beneficial effect of granulocyte therapy.[44]

SPECIAL PROCESSING OF BLOOD COMPONENTS FOR RECIPIENTS OF HSCT

Irradiation of cellular blood components (eg, RBCs, platelets, and granulocytes) inhibits proliferation of donor lymphocytes, thereby preventing transfusion-associated GVHD (TA-GVHD), which is almost uniformly fatal.[45] Although it is generally accepted that HSCT recipients require irradiated components during and for at least 1 year after transplantation, it is unclear whether these patients require irradiation beyond this point. Despite an absence of evidence indicating that irradiation is essential after this time has elapsed, many institutions indefinitely provide irradiated components to HSCT recipients given the potential for long-term immunosuppression.

The immunocompromised state of HSCT recipients puts them at risk for infections, including CMV. It is generally accepted that prestorage leukocyte-reduced components are as efficacious in CMV risk reduction as components collected from donors lacking antibodies to CMV ("CMV seronegative" donors).[8] Three recent studies in HSCT patients demonstrated no additional risk for transfusing leukocyte-reduced, CMV-unselected components vs CMV-seronegative components, including two prospective observational studies.[46-48] However, in an older meta-analysis of 829 recipients of CMV-seronegative components and 878 recipients of leukocyte-reduced components, the risk of CMV infection was 1.63% and 3.01%, respectively.[49] One major limitation of CMV-seronegative components is their availability (40%-100% of adults are CMV seropositive); in addition, seronegative donors may have recently acquired CMV, with viremia that would not be detected serologically.

Special processing of transfusion units may also be needed for HSCT recipients who repeatedly experience common transfusion reactions.[50] For a more in-depth discussion of the treatment of transfusion reactions, see Chapter 22.

SPECIAL CONSIDERATIONS FOR TRANSFUSING PEDIATRIC HSCT RECIPIENTS

In general, transfusion support of pediatric HSCT recipients is fairly similar to adults.[50] However, indications for transplantation, stem cell source, and donor selection may subtly differ in this patient population. For example, patients with inherited diseases (eg, sickle cell disease, thalassemia major) may be more likely to have transplantation in childhood than adulthood; in addition, high-dose chemotherapy with autologous HSCT rescue may be utilized for some childhood malignancies, including advanced-stage neuroblastoma. Furthermore, umbilical cord blood HPCs may be used for some pediatric recipients, given size considerations (eg, a single dose of cord blood HPCs may be sufficient for a child, but not an adult). A recent web-based survey examining current pediatric transfusion thresholds found that most institutions (60%) use a hemoglobin threshold of 8 g/dL for RBC transfusions in pediatric HSCT recipients, but a significant minority (25%) use 7 g/dL. For platelet transfusions, 47% use 20,000/μL and 44% use 10,000/μL.[51]

Special considerations are necessary for transplantations in children (or adults) with sickle cell disease in both the pre- and peritransplant periods. First, red cell phenotyping of the stem cell donor is recommended in instances of recipient red cell alloimmunization, to help guide both donor selection and product processing. If possible, stem cell donors

negative for cognate red cell antigens against which recipients have existing alloantibodies should be considered. This is particularly important in instances of reduced-intensity or nonmyeloablative conditioning regimens, where long-term mixed chimerism is possible. If antigen-positive donors are used, then red cell reduction of the stem cell product is recommended (even in the absence of ABO incompatibility) to avoid a transfusion reaction during stem cell infusion.[52] Next, because of the association between red cell and HLA/HPA alloimmunization,[53-55] consideration may be given to pretransplant HLA/HPA antibody screening in patients with sickle cell disease. These results should be taken into consideration in developing posttransplant platelet transfusion plans, given general recommendations to keep platelet counts >30,000 to 50,000/μL to prevent cerebrovascular bleeding.[56,57] HLA alloantibody results are also important in HPC donor selection in non-HLA-matched transplant settings.[41,42]

Beta-thalassemia major and severe aplastic anemia may be cured after matched-sibling HSCT in childhood, yet prior transfusion exposure may adversely influence engraftment and outcome.[58-60] The reasons for this association are not well understood, but may include humoral or cellular immunization to transfused antigens (be they defined antigens or other minor histocompatibility antigens) or iron overload, among others. Early transplantation for eligible patients may provide better outcomes.

INFORMATION PORTABILITY FOR HSCT RECIPIENTS

Many patients will undergo HSCT far from their "home" medical institution. Before transplantation, all transfusion history (including red cell, platelet, or leukocyte alloantibody testing) should be communicated to the transplant facility. In addition, the following information should be communicated when patients return from off-site transplant facilities: 1) whether the transplant was autologous or allogeneic and, 2) if allogeneic, the ABO type of the donor and any auto- or alloantibodies developed by the patient during care at that facility. A portable worksheet with these data ideally should be made available to the patient.

KEY POINTS

1. Allogeneic HSCT recipients are unique patients with distinct transfusion challenges because of their immunosuppression, their preexisting diseases, and the potential for changes in their expressed blood group systems.

2. ABO compatibility is not critical in the selection of potential HSCT donors because pluripotent and early-committed HPCs lack ABO antigens. However, ABO incompatibility does influence transfusion decisions in the peritransplant period.

3. ABO incompatibilities, present in 25% to 50% of donor/recipient pairs, fall into one of three categories: major, minor, and bidirectional. Such incompatibilities have the potential to produce acute and, in the case of major incompatibility, ongoing intravascular hemolysis and pure red cell aplasia. They can be partially mitigated by red cell and/or plasma depletion of the graft before infusion.

4. Management approaches for transfusing adult and pediatric HSCT recipients are fairly similar; however, indications for transplantation, stem cell source, and donor selection may subtly differ for pediatric populations.

5. For determining transfusion requirements for allogeneic HSCT recipients, it is vital that the blood bank or transfusion service keep detailed records documenting the pretransplant ABO group of the recipient and the ABO group of the donor.

6. Platelet concentrates are most frequently transfused to HSCT recipients as prophylaxis to prevent acute hemorrhage. A platelet count threshold of 10,000/μL in uncomplicated thrombocytopenia is widely accepted as a safe practice for allogeneic recipients.

7. Cellular blood components are irradiated to inhibit donor lymphocyte proliferation, thereby preventing transfusion-associated graft-vs-host disease. Many institutions indefinitely provide irradiated components to HSCT recipients.

8. Prestorage leukocyte-reduced RBC and platelet components are generally considered equivalent to CMV-seronegative units in terms of CMV transmission risks.

REFERENCES

1. Kaufman R, Sloan S. Transfusion to bone marrow or solid organ transplant recipients. In: Hillyer C, Silberstein L, Ness P, eds. Blood banking and transfusion medicine: Basic principles and practice. 2nd ed. Philadelphia: Churchill Livingstone/Elsevier, 2006:539-50.

2. Worel N, Kalhs P. ABO-incompatible allogeneic hematopoietic stem cell transplantation. Haematologica 2008;93:1605-7.

3. Bolan CD, Leitman SF, Griffith LM, et al. Delayed donor red cell chimerism and pure red cell aplasia following major ABO-incompatible nonmyeloablative hematopoietic stem cell transplantation. Blood 2001;98:1687-94.

4. Kim JG, Sohn SK, Kim DH, et al. Impact of ABO incompatibility on outcome after allogeneic peripheral blood stem cell transplantation. Bone Marrow Transplant 2005;35:489-95.

5. Staley EM, Schwartz J, Pham HP. An update on ABO incompatible hematopoietic progenitor cell transplantation. Transfus Apher Sci 2016; 54:337-44.

6. Dahl D, Hahn A, Koenecke C, et al. Prolonged isolated red blood cell transfusion requirement after allogeneic blood stem cell transplantation: Identification of patients at risk. Transfusion 2010;50:649-55.

7. Cid J, Lozano M, Klein HG, Flegel WA. Matching for the D antigen in haematopoietic progenitor cell transplantation: Definition and clinical outcomes. Blood Transfus 2014;12: 301-6.

8. Schulz WL, Snyder EL. Transfusion support for the oncology patient. In: Simon TL, McCullough J, Snyder EL, et al, eds. Rossi's principles of transfusion medicine. 5th ed. Chichester, UK: Wiley Blackwell, 2016:574-80.

9. Le Viellez A, P'Ng S, Buffery S, et al. Red cell and platelet transfusion burden following myeloablative allogeneic haemopoietic stem cell transplantation. Intern Med J 2015;45:1286-92.

10. Tachibana T, Tanaka M, Numata A, et al. Clinical significance of pre- and 1-year posttransplant serum ferritin among adult transplant recipients. Leuk Lymphoma 2014;55: 1350-6.

11. Meyer SC, O'Meara A, Buser AS, et al. Prognostic impact of posttransplantation iron overload after allogeneic stem cell transplantation. Biol Blood Marrow Transplant 2013;19:440-4.

12. Carson JL, Carless PA, Hébert PC. Transfusion thresholds and other strategies for guiding allogeneic red blood cell transfusion. Cochrane Database Syst Rev 2012;4:CD002042.

13. Carson JL, Grossman BJ, Kleinman S, et al. Red blood cell transfusion: A clinical practice guideline from the AABB. Ann Intern Med 2012;157:49-58.

14. Tay J, Allan DS, Chatelain E, et al. Transfusion of red cells in hematopoietic stem cell transplantation (TRIST Study): A randomized controlled trial evaluating 2 red cell transfusion thresholds (abstract number 1032). Blood 2016;128:1032.

15. Chantepie SP, Mear JB, Guittet L, et al. Transfusion strategy in hematological intensive care unit: Study protocol for a randomized controlled trial. Trials 2015;16:533.

16. Gaya A, Urbano-Ispizua A, Fernandez-Aviles F, et al. Anemia associated with impaired erythropoietin secretion after allogeneic stem cell transplantation: Incidence, risk factors, and response to treatment. Biol Blood Marrow Transplant 2008;14:880-7.

17. Helbig G, Stella-Holowiecka B, Wojnar J, et al. Pure red-cell aplasia following major and bi-directional ABO-incompatible allogeneic stem-cell transplantation: Recovery of donor-derived erythropoiesis after long-term treatment using different therapeutic strategies. Ann Hematol 2007;86:677-83.

18. Sheikh S, Littlewood TJ. Erythropoiesis-stimulating agents for anemic patients with cancer. Expert Rev Hematol 2010;3:697-704.

19. Chang YJ, Xu LP, Liu DH, et al. The impact of CD34+ cell dose on platelet engraftment in pe-diatric patients following unmanipulated hap-loidentical blood and marrow transplantation. Pediatr Blood Cancer 2009;53:1100-6.

20. Pulsipher MA, Chitphakdithai P, Logan BR, et al. Donor, recipient, and transplant characteristics as risk factors after unrelated donor PBSC transplantation: Beneficial effects of higher CD34+ cell dose. Blood 2009;114:2606-16.

21. Jansen J, Hanks SG, Akard LP, et al. Slow platelet recovery after PBPC transplantation from unrelated donors. Bone Marrow Transplant 2009;43:499-505.

22. Kurtzberg J, Prasad VK, Carter SL, et al. Results of the Cord Blood Transplantation Study (COBLT): Clinical outcomes of unrelated donor umbilical cord blood transplantation in pediatric patients with hematologic malignancies. Blood 2008;112:4318-27.

23. Dominietto A, Raiola AM, van Lint MT, et al. Factors influencing haematological recovery after allogeneic haemopoietic stem cell transplants: Graft-versus-host disease, donor type, cytomegalovirus infections and cell dose. Br J Haematol 2001;112:219-27.

24. Pulanic D, Lozier JN, Pavletic SZ. Thrombocytopenia and hemostatic disorders in chronic graft versus host disease. Bone Marrow Transplant 2009;44:393-403.

25. Josephson CD, Castillejo MI, Grima K, Hillyer CD. ABO-mismatched platelet transfusions: Strategies to mitigate patient exposure to naturally occurring hemolytic antibodies. Transfus Apher Sci 2010;42:83-8.

26. Lapierre V, Mahe C, Auperin A, et al. Platelet transfusion containing ABO-incompatible plasma and hepatic veno-occlusive disease after hematopoietic transplantation in young children. Transplantation 2005;80:314-19.

27. Heal JM, Liesveld JL, Phillips GL, Blumberg N. What would Karl Landsteiner do? The ABO blood group and stem cell transplantation. Bone Marrow Transplant 2005;36:747-55.

28. Wandt H, Schaefer-Eckart K, Frank M, et al. A therapeutic platelet transfusion strategy is safe and feasible in patients after autologous peripheral blood stem cell transplantation. Bone Marrow Transplant 2006;37:387-92.

29. Wandt H, Schaefer-Eckart K, Wendelin K, et al. Therapeutic platelet transfusion versus routine prophylactic transfusion in patients with haematological malignancies: An open-label, multicentre, randomised study. Lancet 2012;380:1309-16.

30. Stanworth SJ, Estcourt LJ, Powter G, et al. A no-prophylaxis platelet-transfusion strategy for hematologic cancers. N Engl J Med 2013; 368:1771-80.

31. Stanworth SJ, Hudson CL, Estcourt LJ, et al. Risk of bleeding and use of platelet transfusions in patients with hematologic malignancies: Recurrent event analysis. Haematologica 2015;100:740-7.

32. Beutler E. Platelet transfusions: The 20,000/microL trigger. Blood 1993;81:1411-13.

33. Estcourt LJ, Stanworth SJ, Doree C, et al. Comparison of different platelet count thresholds to guide administration of prophylactic platelet transfusion for preventing bleeding in people with haematological disorders after myelosuppressive chemotherapy or stem cell transplantation. Cochrane Database Syst Rev 2015;(11):CD010983.

34. Nevo S, Fuller AK, Zahurak ML, et al. Profound thrombocytopenia and survival of hematopoietic stem cell transplant patients without clinically significant bleeding, using prophylactic platelet transfusion triggers of $10 \times 10(9)$ or $20 \times 10(9)$ per L. Transfusion 2007;47:1700-9.

35. Heddle NM, Cook RJ, Tinmouth A, et al. A randomized controlled trial comparing standard- and low-dose strategies for transfusion of platelets (SToP) to patients with thrombocytopenia. Blood 2009;113:1564-73.

36. Slichter SJ, Kaufman RM, Assmann SF, et al. Dose of prophylactic platelet transfusions and prevention of hemorrhage. N Engl J Med 2010; 362:600-13.

37. Tinmouth A, Tannock IF, Crump M, et al. Low-dose prophylactic platelet transfusions in recipients of an autologous peripheral blood progenitor cell transplant and patients with acute leukemia: A randomized controlled trial with a sequential Bayesian design. Transfusion 2004;44:1711-19.

38. Estcourt LJ, Stanworth S, Doree C, et al. Different doses of prophylactic platelet transfusion for preventing bleeding in people with haematological disorders after myelosuppressive chemotherapy or stem cell transplantation. Cochrane Database Syst Rev 2015;(10): CD010984.

39. Josephson CD, Granger S, Assmann SF, et al. Bleeding risks are higher in children versus adults given prophylactic platelet transfusions for treatment-induced hypoproliferative thrombocytopenia. Blood 2012;120:748-60.

40. Balduini CL, Salvaneschi L, Klersy C, et al. Factors influencing post-transfusional platelet increment in pediatric patients given hematopoietic stem cell transplantation. Leukemia 2001;15:1885-91.

41. Chang YJ, Zhao XY, Xu LP, et al. Donor-specific anti-human leukocyte antigen antibodies were associated with primary graft failure after unmanipulated haploidentical blood and marrow transplantation: A prospective study with randomly assigned training and validation sets. J Hematol Oncol 2015;8:84.

42. Ciurea SO, Thall PF, Milton DR, et al. Complement-binding donor-specific anti-HLA antibodies and risk of primary graft failure in hematopoietic stem cell transplantation. Biol Blood Marrow Transplant 2015;21: 1392-8.

43. Roback JD, Caldwell S, Carson J, et al. Evidence-based practice guidelines for plasma transfusion. Transfusion 2010;50:1227-39.

44. Price TH, Boeckh M, Harrison RW, et al. Efficacy of transfusion with granulocytes from G-CSF/dexamethasone-treated donors in neutropenic patients with infection. Blood 2015;126:2153-61.

45. Treleaven J, Gennery A, Marsh J, et al. Guidelines on the use of irradiated blood components prepared by the British Committee for Standards in Haematology Blood Transfusion Task Force. Br J Haematol 2011;152:35-51.

46. Hall S, Danby R, Osman H, et al. Transfusion in CMV seronegative T-depleted allogeneic stem cell transplant recipients with CMV-unselected blood components results in zero CMV transmissions in the era of universal leukocyte reduction: A UK dual centre experience. Transfus Med 2015;25:418-23.

47. Kekre N, Tokessy M, Mallick R, et al. Is cytomegalovirus testing of blood products still needed for hematopoietic stem cell transplant recipients in the era of universal leukoreduction? Biol Blood Marrow Transplant 2013;19: 1719-24.

48. Thiele T, Kruger W, Zimmermann K, et al. Transmission of cytomegalovirus (CMV) infection by leukoreduced blood products not tested for CMV antibodies: A single-center prospective study in high-risk patients undergoing allogeneic hematopoietic stem cell transplantation (CME). Transfusion 2011;51: 2620-6.

49. Vamvakas EC. Is white blood cell reduction equivalent to antibody screening in prevent-

ing transmission of cytomegalovirus by transfusion? A review of the literature and meta-analysis. Transfus Med Rev 2005;19:181-99.

50. Luban NL, McBride E, Ford JC, Gupta S. Transfusion medicine problems and solutions for the pediatric hematologist/oncologist. Pediatr Blood Cancer 2012;58:1106-11.

51. Bercovitz RS, Quinones RR. A survey of transfusion practices in pediatric hematopoietic stem cell transplant patients. J Pediatr Hematol Oncol 2013;35:e60-3.

52. Franchini M, Gandini G, Aprili G. Non-ABO red blood cell alloantibodies following allogeneic hematopoietic stem cell transplantation. Bone Marrow Transplant 2004;33:1169-72.

53. McPherson ME, Anderson AR, Castillejo MI, et al. HLA alloimmunization is associated with RBC antibodies in multiply transfused patients with sickle cell disease. Pediatr Blood Cancer 2010;54:552-8.

54. Nickel RS, Hendrickson JE, Yee MM, et al. Red blood cell transfusions are associated with HLA class I but not H-Y alloantibodies in children with sickle cell disease. Br J Haematol 2015;170:247-56.

55. Lo SC, Chang JS, Lin SW, Lin DT. Platelet alloimmunization after long-term red cell transfusion in transfusion-dependent thalassemia patients. Transfusion 2005;45:761-5.

56. Walters MC, Sullivan KM, Bernaudin F, et al. Neurologic complications after allogeneic marrow transplantation for sickle cell anemia. Blood 1995;85:879-84.

57. McPherson ME, Anderson AR, Haight AE, et al. Transfusion management of sickle cell patients during bone marrow transplantation with matched sibling donor. Transfusion 2009; 49:1977-86.

58. Lucarelli G, Clift RA, Galimberti M, et al. Marrow transplantation for patients with thalassemia: Results in class 3 patients. Blood 1996; 87:2082-8.

59. Lucarelli G, Gaziev J. Advances in the allogeneic transplantation for thalassemia. Blood Rev 2008;22:53-63.

60. McCann SR, Bacigalupo A, Gluckman E, et al. Graft rejection and second bone marrow transplants for acquired aplastic anaemia: A report from the Aplastic Anaemia Working Party of the European Bone Marrow Transplant Group. Bone Marrow Transplant 1994; 13:233-7.

Chapter 28

Human Tissue Allografts and the Hospital Transfusion Service

• ● •

Annette J. Schlueter, MD, PhD; Cassandra D. Josephson, MD; and Scott A. Brubaker, CTBS

THE SURGICAL USE of human tissue allografts continues to expand. Every year, member organizations of the American Association of Tissue Banks (AATB) recover tissue from more than 30,000 donors and provide more than 2 million tissue grafts for transplantation.[1] These activities are increasing, in part because of the successful clinical application of tissue allografts from living donors (eg, delivery mothers donating the placenta for grafts derived from the amniotic/chorionic membranes). Many surgical specialties use human tissue allografts: orthopedics, neurosurgery, cardiothoracic surgery, vascular surgery, urology, ophthalmology, burn and other skin wound care, sports medicine, trauma, and cranio/maxillofacial surgery. Increasingly sophisticated grafts continue to be developed by tissue suppliers to meet diverse clinical needs.

Oversight of activities of a tissue service may be managed by an individual, a diverse group, or a department within a hospital, and various departments or surgical specialties may prefer to manage only the tissue their service handles. However, because ordering, receiving, storing, dispensing (issuing), tracking, tracing, investigating adverse events, and managing recalls are functions performed by both transfusion and tissue services, AABB recommends using a centralized tissue service model located within the transfusion service.[2]

TISSUE DONATION AND TRANSPLANTATION

Allografts are selected for transplantation based on intrinsic qualities that meet the surgeon's functional requirements for the patient. Bone (in some form), tendons/ligaments, and corneas are the most frequently implanted human tissues. Others include: skin; amniotic/chorionic membranes;

28

Annette J. Schlueter, MD, PhD, Clinical Professor of Pathology and Medical Director, DeGowin Blood Center Patient Services and Tissue and Cellular Therapies, Department of Pathology, University of Iowa, Iowa City, Iowa; Cassandra D. Josephson, MD, Professor, Pathology and Pediatrics, Emory University School of Medicine, Director of Clinical Research, Center for Transfusion and Cellular Therapies, Program Director, Transfusion Medicine Fellowship, and Medical Director, Children's Healthcare of Atlanta Blood, Tissue, and Apheresis Services, Atlanta, Georgia; and Scott A. Brubaker, CTBS, Senior Vice President of Policy, American Association of Tissue Banks, McLean, Virginia
The authors have disclosed no conflicts of interest.

cartilage/meniscus (with or without bone); certain veins/arteries; soft tissue, such as fascia, pericardium, nerves, rotator cuff, and dura mater; semilunar heart valves; and cardiac conduit grafts. Tissue recovery from deceased donors occurs within 24 hours of death after appropriate consent (also known as "authorization") is obtained from a designated legal authority (eg, the donor's next of kin) or by first-person authorization, if the donor registered his or her wishes before death. Steps taken to minimize tissue contamination include: planning for body cooling after death; use of aseptic surgical recovery techniques, instruments, and supplies; and control of the site where recovery takes place.

Tissue bank personnel responsible for determining donor eligibility do so based on an evaluation of: 1) the validity of the document of authorization (or informed consent for a living donor); 2) answers provided by the donor or other knowledgeable person to questions about the donor's travel, medical history, and behavior that could indicate increased risk; 3) available relevant medical records, including circumstances surrounding death; 4) a physical assessment or physical examination of the donor to identify evidence of high-risk behavior or active communicable disease; 5) relevant infusion and transfusion information to evaluate any blood samples collected for infectious disease testing; and 6) the autopsy report (if an autopsy was performed). High-risk behavior that is considered to increase the possibility of disease transmission leads to a determination that the donor is not eligible. Allografts, similar to blood components and cellular therapy products, are released for use in patients only after the donor has been tested for relevant communicable diseases and the results are determined to be acceptable. (See Table 28-1.)

Types of Transplantable Tissue

Allografts, sometimes referred to as *homografts*, are grafts transferred between the same species. Human allograft tissue may be treated to remove cells and cellular remnants, or carefully preserved to maintain cellular viability. Tissue allografts can be derived from a single tissue or multiple tissues acting as a functional unit. During processing, they may be combined with other biocompatible agents to achieve desired handling and functional characteristics. Depending on the extent of processing and the intended use and effect, human tissue allografts can be regulated by the United States Food and Drug Administration (FDA) as a human tissue, a biological product, a drug, or a medical device.[3]

Autografts are implanted into the individual from whom they were removed.

TABLE 28-1. Required Infectious Disease Testing for Donors of Allograft Tissue[3]

Infectious Agent	Test Performed
Hepatitis B virus (HBV)	HBV surface antigen HBV core antibody (IgM and IgG) HBV nucleic acid testing
Hepatitis C virus (HCV)	HCV antibody HCV nucleic acid testing
Human immunodeficiency virus (HIV)	HIV-1 and HIV-2 antibodies HIV-1 nucleic acid testing
Human T-cell lymphotropic virus (HTLV)*	HTLV-I and HTLV-II antibodies
Syphilis	Nontreponemal or treponemal-specific assay

*Required only for tissues that are rich in viable leukocytes.

Some examples of autograft tissue are bone that has been surgically removed from a patient's ilium, shaped to desired dimensions, and implanted into the vertebral disk space of the same patient, and skull flaps surgically removed after cranial trauma, then reimplanted when cerebral edema recedes. Although autografts are typically not FDA-regulated products, some can be regulated much like allografts, depending on the extent of manufacturing. For example, if the autograft is subjected to steps intended to sterilize it, such as use of irradiation or steam, FDA regulations apply.[4]

Xenografts are transplanted from one species to another. Many medical products have been developed from highly processed, nonviable tissue from nonhuman animals and are regulated as medical devices.

Xenotransplantation products, often confused with xenografts, contain live cells, tissues, or organs from a nonhuman animal, or the products have been exposed during manufacture to live cells, tissues, or organs from a nonhuman animal. Depending on its classification by the FDA, a xenotransplantation product can be a biological product, a drug, or a medical device.

Information concerning certain allografts, such as reproductive tissues (eg, gametes) and cellular therapy products, as well as xenografts and xenotransplantation products, is not provided in this chapter; nonetheless, they might be handled by a transfusion service and tracked and maintained using procedures established for tissue allografts.

Tissue Processing

After tissue has been recovered from a donor, various levels of tissue processing and preservation may be accomplished. The tissue-processing facility and the processing steps (ie, manufacturing) are designed to prevent tissue contamination and cross-contamination. Similar to current good manufacturing practice requirements, current good tissue practice (cGTP) regulations promotes the expectation that temperature, humidity, ventilation, and air filtration will be controlled in critical manufacturing areas to the extent deemed necessary by the tissue establishment and supported by data.

During bone, soft tissue, and connective tissue processing, various solutions may be used to reduce or eliminate bacterial contamination (the bioburden) and to remove lipids and other cellular material. Antibiotics alone or in combination with chemicals such as alcohol, peroxide, and surfactants can be used, and some methods are patented or proprietary. Depending on the type of tissue and its clinical utility or the biomechanical expectations for it, treatment with chemicals and/or graft sterilization may or may not be possible. Allografts containing viable cells or a fragile matrix (eg, fresh or cryopreserved vessels or cardiac grafts) cannot be subjected to chemicals or sterilization without an adverse affect on cellular or matrix integrity. Low-dose electron beam and gamma irradiation are the most frequently used sterilization treatments in the United States; however, the tissue is first treated using proprietary methods. Claims regarding allograft sterility must be supported by validation and, although some methods inactivate viruses, claims of sterility do not include viruses.

Various tissue preservation methods can be used to extend storage of tissue allografts so an inventory (ie, a "bank") can be readily available. Tissue integrity can be maintained through simple freezing and frozen storage or through cryopreservation, a process in which tissues are preserved using a cryoprotectant, such as glycerol or dimethyl sulfoxide, and frozen at a controlled rate to lower subzero temperatures that allow for long-term storage (ie, several years). Refrigerated storage can also be used to preserve cellular viability or slow matrix degradation, but only for short-term storage (days to weeks); examples include corneas, skin for burns, and osteochondral or osteoarticular allografts. The latter two grafts provide bone with a small or large articulating cartilage surface. If the clinical utility of the tissue allows, allografts can be preserved by removing intrinsic water using dehydration, dessication, or, if a very low residual moisture level is desired, lyophiliza-tion (ie, freeze-drying). The storage potential (the expiry) is often predicated on the ability of the packaging configuration to maintain a low level of moisture over time (a year or more).

Clinical Uses of Allografts

Various human tissues are used for transplantation.[5] Examples are listed in Table 28-2. Cadaveric human bone can replace bone lost to degenerative disease, trauma, or malignancy. Allogeneic bone has unique healing characteristics, including osteocon-ductive and osteoinductive properties. In vivo, it acts as a scaffold that allows recipient capillary growth into the graft (osteocon-ductivity) and provides stimulation for the production of new bone (osteoinductivity) by exposing the patient's osteogenic progenitor cells to bone morphogenetic proteins (BMPs), which are growth factors in bone that induce new bone formation. The result is creeping substitution, in which bone remodeling occurs through osteoclastic resorption of the implanted tissue and osteoblastic generation of new bone. Crushed bone, subjected to acid demineralization, can be used alone or sus-pended in a biologically compatible carrier and applied to exposed bone surfaces. BMPs in demineralized bone stimulate osteogenesis, the fusion of adjacent bones, and healing. Precision bone grafts, including a growing array of spinal implants, are shaped using sophisticated, computer-aided cutting devices to fit snugly into surgical instrumentation designed to allow surgeons to place the grafts delicately in the defect. Bone-tendon (eg, Achilles tendon) or bone-ligament-bone (eg, patellar-tibia ligament) grafts are routinely used for anterior cruciate ligament (ACL) repair. The implanted tendon or ligament spans the joint space, and the bone provides an anchor into the femur and/or tibia, thereby restoring joint stability. Surgical techniques for ACL repair were developed using alternative fixation methods with a combination of tendons (without a bony attachment), such as the anterior or posterior tibialis tendons, gracilis, semitendinosus, and peroneus longus. Meniscus and joint allografts are also used to regain mobility after disease or trauma. Skin from a deceased donor can be used as a temporary wound dressing for a severely burned patient, protecting the under-lying tissues from dehydration and infection. Human skin and amniotic/chorionic mem-branes can be preserved and frozen, or pro-cessed to remove cellular elements, producing an acellular matrix that provides a scaffold for revascularization and cellular incorporation in soft tissue reconstructive surgery and wound care. In addition, donor corneal tissues can treat various ocular surface diseases, such as keratoconus, other eye pathologies, and trauma. Scleral, pericardial, and amnion-derived allo-grafts can treat glaucoma, scleral ulcers, and other eye damage.

Although some tissue allografts may provoke an immune response, these are not usually clinically significant, presumably because of a lack of abundant residual cellular material in processed grafts.[6,7] Therefore, it is not necessary to match most allografts to the recipient's HLA or ABO type. Possible exceptions include cryopreserved heart valves, veins, or arteries, for which some clinicians request ABO compatibility, although its significance is unproven. Development of Rh(D), Fy^a, and Jk^b antibodies in recipients following transplantation of unprocessed bone allografts has been documented[8]; however, unprocessed allograft bone is no longer provided in the United States. If unprocessed bone contains marrow elements that cannot be removed mechanically and is intended for use in an Rh(D)-negative female of childbearing potential, her future offspring may be at risk of hemolytic disease of the fetus and newborn. Thus, Rh Immune Globulin prophylaxis can be considered if the Rh type of the allograft donor is positive or unknown.

Disease Transmission through Tissue Transplantation

In the past, rare, sporadic transmission of infectious diseases, including human immuno-deficiency virus (HIV), hepatitis C virus (HCV), hepatitis B virus (HBV), and Creutzfeldt-Jakob

TABLE 28-2. Examples for Clinical Use of Human Tissue Allografts

Allograft Tissue	Clinical Use
Amniotic/chorionic membranes	Leg and foot ulcer/wound care Conjunctiva surface repair Corneal repair Neurosurgery and spine surgery Orthopedic surgery Dental/periodontal surgery Burns
Bone (cortical, corticocancellous, cancellous; powders, pastes, putties, gels, and moldable strips)	Skeletal reconstruction Spinal fusion Dental implant placement Bony defect filler
Bone-tendon (Achilles tendon) Bone-ligament-bone (patellar ligament) Tendons (anterior and posterior tibialis, semitendinosus, gracilis, and peroneus longus)	Anterior cruciate ligament repair Posterior cruciate ligament repair Rotator cuff restoration Biceps tendon rupture repair
Cardiac valves (aortic and pulmonary) and conduits	Replacement for reversal of valvular insufficiency Congenital cardiac defect repairs
Cartilage (costal)	Facial reconstruction
Cornea	Keratoconus correction Fuchs dystrophy repair Traumatic scarring repair Corneal-scleral fistula repair
Decellularized skin (dermal matrix)	Hernia repair Soft tissue reconstruction Gingival restoration
Demineralized bone	Dental implant placement Spinal fusion Bony defect filler
Dura mater	Dural defect/cerebrospinal leak repair
Fascia lata	Soft tissue reconstruction Pelvic floor support
Meniscus	Meniscus replacement
Osteoarticular/osteochondral graft (bone and joint cartilage)	Joint restoration
Pericardium	Dura patch Eyelid reconstruction Soft tissue reconstruction
Sclera	Eye enucleation Scleral ulcer repair Eyelid repair

(Continued)

TABLE 28-2. Examples for Clinical Use of Human Tissue Allografts (Continued)

Allograft Tissue	Clinical Use
Skin	Treatment of burns
	Leg and foot ulcer/wound care
Veins/arteries	Coronary artery bypass grafting
	Tissue revascularization
	Aneurysm repair
	Dialysis access shunts

disease (CJD), was documented following tissue implantation.[9] In addition, bacterial and fungal infections from allografts produced morbidity and mortality. Potential sources of contaminating agents included those that were donor derived or from environmental contaminants introduced at the processing facility. Malignancy was also rarely reported to be transmitted from tissue grafts and is limited to corneal allografts.[9] Currently, disease transmission from transplanted tissue is nearly nonexistent, but vigilance and surveillance are necessary to maintain confidence that controls, such as cGTP, are working. Advances in donor screening, donor testing, and tissue culture and treatment methods, as well as the application of quality assurance and quality control measures, continue to improve the safety profiles of human tissue allografts.

FEDERAL REGULATIONS, STATE LAWS, AND PROFESSIONAL STANDARDS

The FDA regulates the activities of tissue establishments (tissue banks) under Title 21, Parts 1270 and 1271, of the *Code of Federal Regulations* (CFR).[3] Tissue banks engage in one or more manufacturing functions, such as donor screening and testing and tissue recovery, packaging, labeling, processing, storage, and/or distribution for clinical use. These entities manufacture what the FDA classifies as human cells, tissues, and cellular and tissue-based products (HCT/Ps). Table 28-2 lists examples of common nonhematopoietic HCT/Ps. Although a tissue distribution inter-

mediary might perform limited manufacturing functions (eg, storage, distribution), they must follow applicable regulations.

Three subparts of 21 CFR Part 1271 concern: 1) registration of tissue establishments, 2) donor eligibility, and 3) cGTP requirements related to operations and handling HCT/Ps. Compliance with these regulations is required of tissue establishments to control contamination and cross-contamination and avoid disease transmission. Tissue-dispensing institutions, such as hospitals, dental offices, and surgical centers that provide and use tissue within their own facility, are not subject to this oversight except under certain circumstances (eg, redistribution of allografts or autografts to other institutions, including an affiliate located at a different address; application of certain manufacturing steps that could contaminate the tissue).

For a hospital-based tissue service that does not also qualify as a tissue establishment, compliance oversight may be provided by state laws and/or accrediting organizations. The Joint Commission, AABB, the College of American Pathologists (CAP), the Association of periOperative Registered Nurses (AORN), the AATB, and the Eye Bank Association of America (EBAA) all publish standards or guidelines that apply to the practices of tissue services.[10-15] The location of a tissue service in a hospital or medical facility and the scope of its operations dictate which standards are applicable. These standards are updated regularly; therefore, periodic review of the most recent versions is important to guarantee ongoing compliance and to maintain best practices.

Both the AATB and EBAA are voluntary accrediting organizations dedicated to ensuring that human tissues intended for transplantation are safe, available, and of high quality. The AATB's standards pertain to institutional and quality program requirements; donor authorization/informed consent; donor screening and testing; and tissue recovery/acquisition, storage, processing, release, distribution, and dispensing.[14] EBAA's scope encompasses all aspects of eye banking.[15] Accreditation by these organizations is based on verified compliance with established standards and periodic inspections. Both organizations serve as scientific and educational resources for the donation and transplantation communities. A tissue service may find AATB and EBAA accreditation of a supplier to be valuable in assessing that supplier's qualifications. The Joint Commission, CAP, AABB, and AORN all have standards/guidelines that are directed specifically at the activities performed by hospital-based tissue services.

Several states have requirements for tissue banking performed within the state, and these statutes can affect the tissue service of a transfusion service. For example, New York State requires tissue bank licensure when a "tissue service" meets the definition of a "tissue storage facility" or a "tissue transplantation service" as described in Part 52 of Title 10 (Health) of the *Official Compilation of Codes, Rules and Regulations of the State of New York*. In the California Health and Safety Code, Section 1635, a tissue bank licensing provision is included, but for a transfusion service that handles tissue, it depends, in part, on meeting criteria involving the storage of certain tissues.

Finally, other agencies that advise or accredit specific health-care services provide direction that may affect the functions performed by a hospital-based tissue service. For example, the United Network for Organ Sharing (UNOS) has policies for organ donor vessel packaging, labeling, storage, shipping, tracking, and reporting.[16]

HOSPITAL TISSUE SERVICES

There is no requirement for a tissue service to be managed in any particular department or by a specific individual. AABB supports a tissue service within the transfusion service, which has personnel with expertise in providing human-derived products that are perishable, potentially infectious, sometimes in short supply, and require bidirectional traceability between donor and recipient. Ordering, receiving, storing, distributing (issuing), tracking, and tracing products, as well as investigating adverse events, including complaints, recalls, and look-back investigations, are activities that are common to a transfusion service and a tissue service.

Responsibility for Hospital-Based Tissue Services

The Joint Commission requires organizations to assign oversight responsibility for their tissue program, use standardized procedures in tissue handling, maintain traceability of all tissues, and have a process for investigating and reporting adverse events. Either a centralized or a decentralized process is permitted to manage these activities. In either model, designated oversight is required to coordinate tissue-related activities and ensure standardization of practices throughout the organization. The Joint Commission's requirements apply to human and nonhuman cellular-based transplantable and implantable products, including tissue allografts and certain medical devices, as classified by the FDA. Table 28-3 lists the controls a tissue service could support.

Standard Operating Procedures and Policies

Hospital tissue services must have written standard operating procedures (SOPs), either printed or electronic, for all functions pertaining to the acquisition, receipt, storage, issuance, and tracing of tissue grafts, as well as procedures for investigating adverse events and handling recalls. Manufacturers' instructions for handling tissues must be followed.

TABLE 28-3. Overview of Controls a Tissue Service Could Support

1. Tissue supplier (vendor) qualification
2. Tissue graft receipt and inspection
3. Maintenance of graft storage and monitoring, including alarms
4. Promoting tissue recipient informed consent
5. Ensuring that allograft tissue preparation steps (ie, instructions for use) are followed
6. Maintenance of traceability of tissue grafts from receipt through storage, issue (or reissue), and final disposition, including timely tracking to specific tissue recipients
7. Prompt handling of allograft tissue recalls or market withdrawals
8. Recognition and reporting of adverse events in tissue recipients, and participation in investigations
9. Compliance with applicable regulations, statutes, and/or professional standards
10. Oversight of a tissue utilization and safety committee
11. Record-keeping for the above controls

When the blood bank or transfusion service is responsible, AABB requires the medical director to approve all medical and technical policies and procedures.[11(p2)] Establishing policies that address the provision of quality services to support the satisfaction and safety of patients is also helpful.

Tissue Supplier (Vendor) Qualifications and Certification

In contrast to blood banks, tissue processors and distributors often specialize in particular types of products (eg, allografts). Therefore, a hospital tissue service may acquire human tissue products from more vendors than are commonly used by a transfusion service to obtain blood components.

Tissue suppliers should be selected based on their ability to reliably provide high-quality tissues that meet expectations for availability, safety, and effectiveness. The tissue service should establish the minimal criteria for qualifying prospective suppliers. According to the Joint Commission's standards, accredited health care facilities must confirm annually that tissue suppliers are registered with the FDA as a tissue establishment and that they maintain a state license when required. A

written process for review and approval of suppliers is expected and may contain the elements listed in Table 28-4. A list of approved suppliers that includes documentation of each supplier's qualifications, certifications, and appropriate licenses or permits should be developed and maintained. Tissue services should establish procedures to receive or monitor evidence of compliance or noncompliance, such as reviewing FDA warning letters, tissue allograft recalls, and market withdrawals. Accreditation by AATB and/or EBAA may be desirable.

Qualification information for each supplier should be reviewed and approved annually by the hospital tissue service. During these reviews, the performance of suppliers in meeting the transplant facility's needs should be evaluated. Each year, the tissue service should determine whether the supplier remains registered with the FDA. Whether AATB and/or EBAA accreditation is current can also be confirmed; it is best practice to confirm the status of this accreditation by accessing the websites of AATB and EBAA to perform a real-time search. PDF copies or photocopies of accreditation certificates might provide outdated information if the tissue establishment's accreditation has been

TABLE 28-4. Suggested Vendor Qualification Criteria for Suppliers of Human Tissue Allografts

Criterion	Documentation/Performance
FDA registration	Perform an eHCTERS query (https://www.access data.fda.gov/scripts/cber/ CFAppsPub/tiss/index.cfm) for each tissue supplier and print the report
FDA inspection findings	FDA Form 483 findings, if any
	Warning letters and responses, if any
Voluntary accreditation, if available	Proof of current AATB accreditation (as applicable): access www.aatb.org and perform a search for accredited institutions for real-time information and a printout dated the day of the search
	Proof of current EBAA accreditation for ocular tissues: access http://restoresight.org/who-we-are/ find-an-eye-bank/ to perform a search for real-time information
State license, permit, or registration, if required by state laws	Proof of current status (to be reviewed annually)
Reliable supply of tissue types	Adequate notification of tissue shortages
	Ability to meet special requests
	Suitable expiration dates for tissue products
Transparency of the organization	Willingness to provide information regarding donor selection criteria and tissue treatment methods
Medical consultation	Accessibility of the tissue supplier's medical director
Quality assurance/regulatory resources	Accessibility of the tissue supplier's quality program staff
New or trial tissue product support	Willingness to provide information on newly released tissue products
Professionalism of sales representatives	Approval sought by representatives through designated channels before promoting or providing tissue within the hospital

FDA = Food and Drug Administration; AATB = American Association of Tissue Banks; EBAA = Eye Bank Association of America; eHCTERS = electronic Human Cell and Tissue Establishment Registration System.

suspended or withdrawn. FDA web postings should be reviewed for information related to closures, recalls, or MedWatch reports. Inspection reports can be requested from the FDA through the Freedom of Information Act. Complaints from transplanting surgeons concerning the supplier's tissue should be reviewed, along with any report of infection that might have been caused by a tissue allograft. Hospital management may consider establishing a committee of internal stakeholders, including physicians who implant tissue, to provide oversight of the approval of tissue suppliers, as well as tissue utilization and safety monitoring.

Inspection of Incoming Tissue Allografts

Before being placed into inventory, tissue allografts must be inspected upon receipt from a tissue supplier to ensure that packaging remains intact and the label is complete, appears to be accurate, and is adequately affixed and legible. The incoming inspection results should be recorded along with the date, time, and name of the staff person conducting the inspection.

The Joint Commission requires hospitals to verify package integrity and ensure that transport temperature was controlled and acceptable (if applicable). Inspecting the shipping container for evidence of residual coolant (eg, wet ice for refrigerated grafts or dry ice for frozen grafts) may help determine that the required tissue-specific storage environment was maintained during transport.

Many tissue distributors use "validated" shipping containers that are tested to maintain required temperatures for a specified period. If such a container was used, the receiver of the tissue needs to verify only that there is no damage to the container and that it was received and opened within the specified time frame posted on the outside of the shipping container.

Tissues requiring "ambient temperature" (defined as the temperature of the immediate environment) for storage and shipping do not need to have the temperature verified upon receipt. However, the temperature of tissues requiring "room-temperature" storage should be verified and documented if the manufacturer has specified a temperature storage range on the allograft label or in the package insert.

Tissue Storage

As with blood components, tissue grafts are stored under various conditions. (See Table 28-5.) The appropriate storage conditions depend on the nature of the tissue, method of preservation, and type of packaging.

Hospital tissue services should store tissue allografts according to the processor's instructions on the allograft's label or package insert. Storage devices can include "ambient" and/or room-temperature cabinets, refrigerators, mechanical freezers, and liquid-nitrogen storage

TABLE 28-5. Storage Conditions for Commonly Transplanted Human Tissue[14]

Human Tissue	Storage Conditions	Temperature*
Cardiac and vascular	Frozen, cryopreserved	−100 C or colder
Musculoskeletal and osteoarticular	Refrigerated	Above freezing (0 C) to 10 C
	Frozen, cryopreserved (temporary storage for 6 months or less)	-20 C or colder to -40 C (this is warmer than -40 C but colder than -20 C)
	Frozen, cryopreserved (long-term storage)	−40 C or colder
	Lyophilized, dehydrated	Ambient†
Birth tissue	Refrigerated, frozen, cryopreserved, lyophilized, dehydrated	As established and validated by the tissue bank
Skin	Refrigerated	Above freezing (0 C) to 10 C
	Frozen, cryopreserved	−40 C or colder
	Lyophilized, dehydrated	Ambient†

*Warmest target temperature unless a range is listed.
†Ambient temperature monitoring not required for lyophilized tissue.

units. Continuous temperature monitoring of refrigerators and freezers is required. Room-temperature storage equipment should be monitored if the allograft's package insert specifies a storage temperature range. Storage equipment should have functional alarms, and there should be emergency backup capability in case of malfunction or damage to a storage unit. Lyophilized tissues with package insert instructions specifying storage at ambient temperature or colder can tolerate a very broad temperature range, and monitoring during storage is not required.

Storage SOPs should address steps to be taken in the case of excursions from allowable temperature limits or in the event of an equipment or power failure. Emergency backup alternatives, including arrangements for temporary storage, should be described.

Tissue Allograft Traceability and Record-Keeping

Proper management of human allografts requires that the hospital tissue service document all the steps taken in tissue handling as they occur and maintain comprehensive records of these steps. Staff members who have handled the tissue should be identifiable, along with dates and times when the tissue was accepted, issued, and prepared. Records should provide a clear history of all the actions performed. Documentation of the tissue supplier, the unique numeric or alphanumeric identifier(s) of the allograft, its expiration date, and the recipient's name must be maintained for all tissue grafts used. The Joint Commission also requires that documentation of the tissue type and its unique identifier be placed into the recipient's medical record.

Tissue service records need to permit bidirectional traceability of all tissues from the donor and tissue supplier to the recipient(s) or other final disposition, including the discard of tissue. Records should be retained for 10 years, or longer if required by state or federal law, after distribution, transplantation, discard, or expiration (whichever occurs last).

Tissue usage information cards or other systems supplied with the allograft by the tissue bank must be completed and returned to the tissue source facility. This information helps maintain the traceability of the allograft and expedites market withdrawals or recalls should they occur. The tissue supplier may also use this information to understand allograft utilization, obtain positive or negative feedback, and meet customer needs and expectations.

Recognizing and Reporting Adverse Events Possibly Caused by Allografts

Human-derived medical products, such as tissue allografts, carry some risks that must be balanced with clinical benefits. Albeit rarely, human tissue allografts have transmitted disease by bacteria, viruses, and fungi, and one tissue type (dura mater) transmitted a prion disease. In addition, an allograft may have a structural weakness that can lead to an unsuccessful outcome. (See Method 7-3.)

Hospital tissue services are required to have procedures to investigate in a timely fashion any adverse outcome suspected to be caused by a tissue allograft. The Joint Commission requires that allograft-transmitted infections and other severe adverse events be reported immediately to the tissue supplier.

Surgeons play a critical role in identifying allograft-associated adverse outcomes and need to notify the hospital tissue service immediately when they suspect such events. Prompt notification of adverse events enables the hospital tissue service to investigate the cause, report the issue to the tissue supplier, and institute corrective action, including sequestration of any other suspect allografts. Tissue-associated adverse events may also be voluntarily reported directly to the FDA via MedWatch, but this should be done only if an infection is suspected to have been caused by the tissue allograft. The investigation of infections and other adverse events requires cooperation between the tissue service, clinicians, and tissue supplier. Consultation with the hospital infection-control department or an infectious disease specialist may be beneficial. Early notification can prevent complications for potential recipients of other allografts affected by the incident.

State health departments have lists of communicable diseases that must be reported when they are newly diagnosed. For example, a new diagnosis of HIV or viral hepatitis in a tissue allograft recipient where the allograft is suspected as a possible source may need to be reported to the relevant state department of health. An epidemiologic investigation may be needed to establish whether the tissue allograft was the source of the recipient's infection.

Recalls and Look-Back Investigations

A tissue product recall or market withdrawal can occur when a tissue allograft is determined by the tissue supplier to be compromised. The supplier may sequester tissues in inventory not yet distributed, recall all tissues from a specific donor or processing lot, and notify hospitals that received affected allografts. Depending on the nature of the recall, it may be prudent for the hospital to quarantine allografts in inventory, identify recipients, and/or notify the transplanting surgeon(s) of the notification. Surgeons should evaluate the circumstances and notify, if appropriate, each recipient receiving a recalled tissue graft.

Look-back investigation can be triggered when a tissue donor is found, after donation, to have been infected with HIV, human T-cell lymphotropic virus type I or II, HBV, HCV, or other communicable disease known to be transmitted by tissue grafts. Look-back investigations involving tissue grafts are uncommon.

Tissue Autograft Collection, Storage, and Use

Surgical reconstruction using the patient's own tissues has advantages and disadvantages when compared to the use of a tissue allograft. Advantages include faster incorporation/healing and relative safety from transmission of viral disease or immunologic rejection. Disadvantages include morbidity associated with an additional surgical procedure for the patient, including pain and potential surgical-site infection. In addition, the quality (eg, strength) and quantity of autologous tissue may not be adequate for the intended use, and removing the patient's tissue may adversely affect function at the site from which it was removed.

A bone flap removed during decompressive craniectomy is a common type of autograft. In this procedure, a section of skull is excised by the neurosurgeon to reduce intracerebral pressure caused by brain swelling from trauma, stroke, or surgery. After removal, the skull fragment is rinsed, packaged, frozen, and stored for future reimplantation during a procedure known as "cranioplasty."

Written procedures should address the collection, microbial testing, packaging, storage, and issuance of tissue autografts for reimplantation. Appropriate cultures may be obtained after surgical removal and before packaging. Autografts should not be collected from patients with systemic infections or if the tissue is in close proximity to an infected area. Autografts may be stored at the medical facility where they are collected or at an off-site, FDA-registered tissue bank. Procedural recommendations have been published by the AATB and AORN.[13,14]

KEY POINTS

1. Human tissue allografts are obtained from living or deceased donors who must meet stringent donor screening criteria and donor testing requirements similar to those applied to blood donors.
2. Not all tissue allografts are sterile. Depending on the type of allograft, sterilization may not be possible because treatment methods could compromise viability of cellular elements or the structural matrix of the graft and adversely affect performance after transplantation.

Methods to mitigate contamination include the use of antibiotics, proprietary/patented processes, and, to sterilize allografts, ionizing radiation.

3. Human tissue allografts are used for various surgical applications to treat acquired disease, trauma, and other defects.

4. Rarely, viral, bacterial, fungal, and prion-associated diseases have been transmitted by allografts. Like blood components, allografts are released for use only after donor eligibility criteria are met and infectious disease test results are deemed acceptable.

5. In general, bone and soft tissue allografts do not need to be matched for HLA, ABO, or Rh type.

6. Tissue banks are engaged in donor screening and testing and recovery, labeling, processing, storage, and distribution of human tissue for transplantation. They are regulated by the FDA under Title 21, CFR Parts 1270 and 1271 as manufacturers of HCT/Ps; may have a license or permit or be registered in certain states; and may seek voluntary accreditation from the AATB or EBAA.

7. Hospital-based tissue services are not subject to FDA regulatory oversight if their activities are limited to receiving, storing, and dispensing tissue for use within their own facilities. However, The Joint Commission, AABB, CAP, and AORN publish standards and guidelines that apply to tissue services.

8. Functions performed by tissue services that mimic transfusion services include vendor qualification; ordering, receiving, storing, distributing, and tracing products; and investigating adverse events, including complaints, recalls or withdrawals, and look-back investigations.

9. Additional controls that can be undertaken by a tissue service include promoting tissue recipient informed consent and oversight of a tissue utilization and safety committee.

REFERENCES

1. American Association of Tissue Banks. About us. McLean, VA: AATB, 2017. [Available at http://www.aatb.org/?q=about-us (accessed April 30, 2017).]

2. Eastlund DT, Eisenbrey AB, for the Tissue Committee. Guidelines for managing tissue allografts in hospitals. Bethesda, MD: AABB, 2006.

3. Code of federal regulations. Title 21, CFR Parts 1270 and 1271. Washington, DC: US Government Printing Office, 2017 (revised annually).

4. Bashaw MA. Guideline implementation: Autologous tissue management. AORN J 2015; 102:271-80.

5. Warwick RM, Brubaker SA, eds. Tissue and cell clinical use: An essential guide. West Sussex, UK: Wiley-Blackwell, 2012.

6. Malinin TI. Preparation and banking of bone and tendon allografts. In: Sherman OH, Minkoff J, eds. Arthroscopic surgery. Baltimore, MD: Williams and Wilkins, 1990:65-86.

7. Fehily D, Brubaker SA, Kearney JN, Wolfinbarger W, eds. Tissue and cell processing: An essential guide. West Sussex, UK: Wiley-Blackwell, 2012.

8. Cheek RF, Harmon JV, Stowell CP. Red cell alloimmunization after a bone allograft. Transfusion 1995;35:507-9.

9. Eastland T, Warwick, RM. Diseases transmitted by transplantation of tissue and cell allografts. In: Warwick RM, Brubaker SA, eds. Tissue and cell clinical use: An essential guide. West Sussex, UK: Wiley-Blackwell, 2012:72-113.

10. The Joint Commission. Transplant safety (TS). In: Comprehensive accreditation manual for hospitals. Oakbrook Terrace, IL: The Joint Commission, 2017:TS1.

11. Ooley PW, ed. Standards for blood banks and transfusion services. 30th ed. Bethesda, MD: AABB, 2016.

12. College of American Pathologists. Standards for laboratory accreditation. Northfield, IL: CAP, 2015.

13. Association of periOperative Registered Nurses. Standards of perioperative nursing. In: 2015 Guidelines for perioperative practice.

Denver, CO: AORN, 2015. [Available at http://aorn.org/guidelines/clinical-resources/aorn-standards (accessed April 30, 2017).]

14. Osborne JC, Norman KG, Maye T, et al, eds. Standards for tissue banking. 14th ed. McLean, VA: American Association of Tissue Banks, 2016.

15. Eye Bank Association of America. Medical standards. Washington, DC: EBAA, 2016.

16. Organ Procurement and Transplantation Network. Policy 16: Organ and vessel packaging, labeling, shipping, and storage. Rockville, MD: Health Resources and Services Administration, 2017. [Available at https://optn.trans plant.hrsa.gov/governance/policies/ (accessed April 30, 2017).]

Index

●

*Page references in italics
refer to figures or tables*

A

A antigen, 266-267
  biochemistry, 266-267, *268, 269, 279*
  genetics, 270-271
  on platelets, 417-418
  subgroups, 267, 270, 271-272
AABB
  Center for Patient Safety, 102
  Donor History Questionnaire, 112, 116, 119-120
  laboratory accreditation, 86
  patient blood management program, 559
  quality systems, 2
  standards. *See* Standards
A(B) phenotype, 273, 275
ABO compatibility, 476
  of cryoprecipitate, *461, 498,* 626
  of granulocytes, 147, *461, 498,* 519, 626
  in hemolytic transfusion reactions, 577, 579
  of HPC transplants, 670, 684-685, *686,* 687-688
  of organ transplants, 450, 452
  of plasma, *461,* 476, *498,* 626, *686*
  of platelets, 418, *461,* 476, *498,* 514, 624
  of RBCs, *461,* 476, *498, 510, 686*
  of tissue transplants, 698
  of Whole Blood, *461*
ABO discrepancies, *271,* 275-278
ABO hemolytic disease of the fetus and newborn, 273-274, 600
ABO system, 265-278
  antibodies, 266
    anti-A and anti-B, 268, 270, 273-274
    anti-A$_1$, 274, 278
    anti-A,B, 274
  antigens, 265-267, 268, *269,* 417-418
  biochemistry, 265, 266-267, *268, 269, 279*
  in development and aging, 268, 270
  genetics, *233,* 236-237, 247, 270-271
  phenotypes, 266
    A(B), 273, 275
    acquired B, 273, 275

B(A), 273, 275
  cisAB, 270, 273, 275
  subgroups, 267, 270, 271-272, 275, 277
ABO testing
  of blood components, 133, 274-275, 475
  with cold autoagglutinins, 277, 278, 399
  comparison with previous records, 458
  discrepancies in, *271,* 275-278
  hemolysis in, 274
  interpretation of, *267, 271*
  of pediatric patients, 275, 615, 616-617, 629
  in prenatal studies, 601
  reagents for, 274
  of recipients, *267,* 274-275, 460-461
  in transfusion reaction evaluation, 576
  with warm autoagglutinins, 393
ABTI antigen, *343,* 344
Accidents, 39
Accreditation, 22, 77, *78,* 85-86, 701, 702
ACE inhibitors. *See* Angiotensin-converting enzyme inhibitors
Acid-elution stain (Kleihauer-Betke), 604
Acid elutions, *390*
Acquired B phenotype, 273, 275
Activated partial thromboplastin time, 516
Acute disseminated encephalomyelitis, 655
Acute lung injury, 583
Acute normovolemic hemodilution, 532-533
ADAMTS13, 649
Additive solutions, 134, *135,* 618-620
Adsorption, 374-375
  allogeneic, 394-395
  autologous cold, 399
  autologous warm, 393-394
  and elution, 376
  selective, *642,* 643, 659, *659-660,* 662
Adverse reactions/events. *See also* Hemovigilance
  accidents and injuries, 39, 82
  to apheresis, 131, 646-648, 673-674
  in blood donors, 20, 97, 102-105, 129-131
  fatalities (*See* Fatalities)
  to G-CSF, 673
  to HPC infusions, 678
  to marrow harvesting, 672-673
  monitoring and tracking, 565, 569
  related to cellular therapy, 20

I

related to medical devices, 20, 82

related to tissue allografts, 705-706

reporting, 20, 39, 82, *96*, 97, 99-102, 131, 592, *593*

to transfusion (*See* Transfusion reactions)

transfusion-transmitted diseases (*See* Transfusion-transmitted diseases)

AET (2-aminoethylisothiouronium bromide), 278, *369*, 373

Age

  of blood samples, 350-351, 460

  of donors, 113

  effect on antigens and antibodies, 268, 270, 275, 350

  of RBC units, 616, 620, 633

Agency of Healthcare Research and Quality, 99, 102

Agglutination

  false-negative/false-positive results in, 216

  limitations of, 254

  mixed-field, 252, 275, 344, 353-354

  principles of, 215-216, 459

  spontaneous

    in ABO testing, 275, 277, 278, 393

    dispersing with sulfhydryl reagents, 393, 399

    in Rh testing, 312, 392-393

Agreements, 10

AIDS, 164

Air embolism, *573*, 588

Alarm systems, 29, 463

Albumin solutions, *645*

Aliquoting components, 474, 617-618, *619*, 625-626

Alleles, 230-232, 236-238

  frequencies of, 248, 249

  polymorphic, 238

  terminology for, *253*

Allergic reactions

  to apheresis, *130*, 647

  in blood donors, *130*

  to latex, 39

  to transfusions, 492, *571-572*, 581-582

Alliance for Harmonisation of Cellular Therapy Accreditation, 87, 89

Alloantibodies, 349-350. *See also* Antibodies; Antibody detection; Antibody identification

Allografts, 696. *See also* Tissue

Alloimmunization to HLA antigens

  in febrile transfusion reactions, 448, 580

  following pregnancy, 418

  in HPC transplantation recipients, 669, 689, 690

  management of, *574*

  and plasma transfusions, 139

  in platelet refractoriness, 419-420, 447-448, 515-516

  in TRALI, 448, 583, 584

  transfusion-associated, 418

to platelet antigens, 591-592, 605-606, 689

prevention of, 310

to red cell antigens, 349, *574*

  in delayed hemolytic transfusion reactions, 589

  in hemolytic disease of the fetus and newborn, 600

  in sickle cell disease, 257, 308, 310, 477, 508, 630, 690

American Association of Tissue Banks, 701, 702

American Rare Donor Program, 381

Aminocaproic acid, 535, *547-548*

2-aminoethylisothiouronium bromide (AET), 278, *369*, 373

Amotosalen-UV treatment, 151, 152, 194, *195*

Anaphylactic reactions, *572*, 581-582, 647

Anemia

  chronic, 536

  classification of, *506*

  defined, 531

  in delayed transfusion reactions, 588

  fetal, 599-605

  hemolytic (*See* Hemolytic anemia)

  in HPC transplantation, 687

  iatrogenic, 536, 614

  in infants, 614, 620

  iron deficiency, 115, 531, *546*

  pharmacologic agents for, 531

  preoperative, 531

  screening donors for, 114-115

  signs and symptoms of, 505

  tolerance to, 536-537

  transfusions in, 505-507

Anesthesia, 533-534

Angioedema, 581

Angiotensin-converting enzyme inhibitors, *573*, 586, 647

Ankylosing spondylitis, 453

Anti-CD38, 354, 373, 389

Anti-HBc, 164, *171*, 174, 180-181

Antibiotics, in donors, 119

Antibodies, 220-222, 349. *See also* Antibody detection; Antibody identification; *specific types of antibodies*

Antibody-dependent cellular cytotoxicity, 378

Antibody detection

  with autoantibodies, 393-395, 399

  in blood components, 133

  of granulocyte antibodies, 428

of HLA antibodies, 419-420, 447, 516
interpreting results of, 463, *487*
methods for, 215-220, 460, 461
in pediatric patients, 615, 616-617, 629
of platelet antibodies, 217, 416, 422-425
in prenatal evaluations, 601
pretransfusion testing, 461
reagents for, 351-353
with rouleaux, 370-371
specimen requirements for, 351
Antibody identification
   anomalous serum reactions in, 371
   antibodies to high-prevalence antigens,
     312, 367, *368*, 369
   antibodies to low-prevalence antigens, 369-
     370
   with antibodies to reagent components,
     370
   antigen expression in, 350-351
   with autoantibodies, 365-366, 369
   drug-dependent antibodies, 370
   exclusion ("rule-out") in, 356, 358
   factors affecting, 350-351
   immunohematology reference laboratories
     for, 380-381
   interpretation of results, 356, 358-359
   with multiple antibodies, 359, 362, 377
   with no apparent specificity, 362, 364
   patient history in, 353-354, 378
   positive and negative reactions in, 356
   with positive DAT, *361*, 369
   in prenatal evaluations, 601
   probability of accurate identification, 358-
     359
   reagents for, 351-353, *357*
   with rouleaux, 370-371
   and selection of blood, 248, 378-380, 461
   significance of identified antibodies, 378
   specimen requirements for, 351
   test methods, 352, 461
     adsorption, 374-375
     alteration in pH, 372-373
     autologous control, 354, *360-361*
     autologous red cell phenotype, 355-356,
       359, 371-372
     combined adsorption-elution, 376
     DAT, 354-355
     elution, 375-376
     enzymes, *369*, 373
     flowcharts for, *360-361*
     identification panels, 351-352, 355, *357*
     increased incubation time, 372
     increased serum-to-cell ratio, 372
     inhibition techniques, 373-374

LISS and PEG, 372
     selected cells, 358
     sulfhydryl reagents, *369*, 373, 374, 399
     temperature reduction, 372
     titration, 376-377, 601
Antibody-mediated rejection, 655
Antibody screen. *See* Antibody detection
Antibody specificity prediction method, 419-
   420
Anticoagulant medications, 119, 517-518,
   548
Anticoagulant-preservative solutions, 131, *132*
Anticoagulation, in apheresis, 134, 646
Antifibrinolytic agents, 535, *547-548*, 588
Antigen capture assays, 424
Antigen-matching, 379
   DNA-based assays for, 255
   to prevent delayed transfusion reactions,
     590
   in sickle cell disease, 310, 380, 477, 508, 630,
     656
   with warm autoimmune hemolytic anemia,
     397
Antigens. *See also specific blood group antigens*
   granulocyte, 425-427
   platelet, 217, 413-417, 422-424
   red cell
     acquired, 273, 275
     antithetical, 237-238
     of blood group collections, 343
     of blood group systems, 252-253
     changes in storage, 350-351
     chromosomal location of, *233-235*
     detecting, 215-217, 218-219, 253-261
     high-prevalence, 312, 343-344, 367, *368*,
       369, 380
     HLA, 344, 436-438, 439-440
     inactivation of, *369*, 373
     low-prevalence, 344, 369-370
     prevalence of, 248
     terminology for, 252-253
     variations with age, 268, 275, 350
     zygosity and dosage, 238, 350
Antiglobulin test
   in crossmatching, 462
   direct, 386-391
   false-positive/false-negative results, *485-486*
   indirect, 461
   principles of, 459, *460*
   reagents for, 353
Antihistamines, 492, 582
Antiplatelet agents, 119, 145
Antipyretics, 492
AnWj antigen, 340, 343

Apheresis
    complications of, 129-131, 646-648, 673-674
    component collection by, 133
        donor consent, 126
        of granulocytes, *137,* 147-148
        hematopoietic progenitor cells, 673-674
        instrumentation for, 137-138, 141-142,
            145-146, 147-148
        of plasma, *137,* 140-142
        of platelets, *137,* 144-146
        of RBCs, 134, 136-138
    therapeutic (*See* Therapeutic apheresis)
Aplastic anemia, 690
Arterial puncture, in donors, 129, *130*
Aspirin, 145
Assessments
    of blood utilization, 21-22, 538-539, 557-565
    competency, 8
    external, 22, 82-83
    internal, 20-21
    proficiency testing, 22, 85
    quality indicators, 21
    of therapeutic apheresis patients, 643-644,
        645
    of transfusion recipients, 490, 529
At^a antigen, 342-343
Audits, transfusion, 21-22
    concurrent, *560,* 561
    process for, 558-559
    prospective, 538, 559, *560,* 561
    retrospective, *560,* 562
Augustine system, *235, 322,* 342-343
Auto control. *See* Autologous control
Autoagglutination
    in ABO typing, 275, 277, 278
    dispersing with sulfhydryl reagents, 393, 399
    in Rh testing, 312
Autoantibodies
    cold
        in ABO testing, 277, 278, 399
        adsorption of, 399
        antibody identification with, 366, 371
        in cold agglutinin disease, 286, 398-400
        in mixed AIHA, 400
        in paroxysmal cold hemoglobinuria,
            400-401
        in Rh testing, 313, 399
        use of sulfhydryl reagents with, 399
        in warm autoimmune hemolytic
            anemia, 392
    defined, 349
    disease associations with, 354
    distinguishing from alloantibodies, *256,*
        257

    drug-induced, 404
    low-affinity, 398
    in phenotyping problems, 371-372
    platelet, 421, 422, 424-425
    warm
        ABO testing with, 393
        adsorption of, 393-395
        with alloantibodies, 393-395
        antibody identification with, 365, 369
        disease associations with, 354
        mimicking alloantibodies, 395
        in mixed-type AIHA, 400
        in phenotyping problems, 371-372
        Rh testing with, 313, 392-393
        specificity of, 395-396
        transfusion with, 397, 510-511
        in warm AIHA, 391-396
Autografts, 696-697, 706. *See also* Tissue
Autoimmune hemolytic anemia
    classification of, 391
    cold agglutinin disease, 398-400
    DAT-negative, 397-398
    mixed-type, 400
    paroxysmal cold hemoglobinuria, 400-401
    serologic findings in, *392*
    transfusion in, 397, 400, 401, 510-511
    warm, 391-398
Autoimmune neutropenia, 428
Autoimmune thrombocytopenic purpura, 422,
    424-425, 607
Autologous adsorption, 393-394, 399
Autologous blood
    collection of
        by acute normovolemic hemodilution,
            532-533
        by intraoperative blood recovery, 533
        by preoperative blood donation, 532
    donor selection for, 121
    hematocrit of, 131
    infectious disease testing of, 175
    for rare phenotypes, 380
    separation from transfused cells, 371
Autologous control, 354, *360-361, 487*
Autosomal inheritance, 239-241
Autosomes, 230

B

B antigen
    acquired, 273, 275
    biochemistry, 267-268, *279*
    on platelets, 417
    subgroups, 272
B(A) phenotype, 273, 275
Babesiosis, 190-191

Bacterial contamination, 183-185
  detecting, 184-185
  inspecting components for, 134, 474
  during phlebotomy, 126, 184
  of platelets, 143, 183-185, 470-471
  of RBCs, 134, 184
  reactive testing results for, *173*
  of tissue allografts, 700, 705
  in transfusion-associated sepsis, 183-184,
    185, *573*, 580
Band 3 glycoprotein, 334
Be The Match Registry, 672
Benchmarking, 564-565
Bernard Soulier syndrome, 416
Bg antigens, 344, 436, 450
Bilirubin, 600, 602, 621
Bioassays, for radiation monitoring, 55
Biohazardous waste, 47-49
Biological product deviations, 20, 83-84
Biological response modifiers, 583
Biological safety cabinets, 43, *44-45*
Biologics License Application, 81, 82
Biosafety, 41-49
  biohazard storage, 46, 48
  biohazard waste, 47-49
  biological safety cabinets, 43, *44-45*
  biosafety levels, 42, 66
  Bloodborne Pathogens Standard, 41, 43
  decontamination, 43
  in donor room, 46-47
  emergency response plans, 47
  engineering controls, 42-46
  hazard identification and communication, 42
  in laboratory, 46
  personal protective equipment, 46
  safe work practices for, 46-47
  standard precautions, 41-42
  training, 42
Biovigilance, 26, 98, 105-107
Bleeding
  assessing risk of, 532
  microvascular, 587
  pharmaceuticals in control of, *551*
  plasma transfusions for, 516
  platelet transfusions for, 514
  WHO bleeding scale, *512*
Bleeding disorders. *See* Coagulopathy
Blood administration
  assessment of recipient, 490
  blood warmers for, 492-493, 588, 614
  delays in starting transfusion, 494
  documentation of, 499-500
  emergency equipment for, 493
  emergency release, 152, 478, 500, 509-510

errors in, 496, 578-579
filters for, 495-496, *498*, 627
flow rates for, 497, *498*, 627
of granulocytes, 147
identification procedures in, 494, 496
identifying transfusion reactions in, 499,
  569-570
infusion sets for, 495, 627
infusion systems for, 493
IV solutions for, 496
medical history in, 490
medical order for, 490-491, 563, 565
monitoring recipient during, 497, 499
in neonates, 626-627
in operating room and trauma, 500
out-of-hospital, 500-501
postadministration events, 498
premedications for, 492, 581
preparation of units, 491-492
pressure devices for, 493
pretransfusion samples, 458, 491
readiness to transfuse, 494
recipient consent in, 489-490
recipient education in, 490
starting transfusion, 497
syringe infusion pumps for, 493, 618
transportation and dispensing
  components, 494-495
venous access for, 494, 622, 626-627
verifications before starting, 496-497
Blood-Borne Pathogens Standard, 41, 43, 46
Blood clots, in RBCs, 134
Blood collection
  adverse donor reactions in, 129-131
  anticoagulant-preservative solutions for,
    131, *132*
  autologous, 532-533
  blood containers for, 131, 133, 134
  of blood samples, 458, 491
  of components by apheresis
    granulocytes, 147-148
    plasma, 140-142
    platelets, 144-146
    RBCs, 134, 136-138
  donor care after, 127-129
  donor preparation, 125-126, 184
  equipment quality control, 31
  instrumentation for, 137-138, 141-142, 145-
    146, 147-148
  mobile sites, 35
  process of, 127-129
  safety of, 35, 46-47
  storage and transport after, 133
  systems for, 133-134

volume collected, 127
of Whole Blood, 131-133
Blood component selection
  ABO/Rh compatibility in, *461,* 476, *498,*
    510, 514, *686*
  after non-group-specific transfusions, 479
  with clinically significant antibodies, 248,
    378-380, 461, 477
  for exchange transfusions, 616, 622, 656
  for HPC transplantation patients, 685-687
  for intrauterine transfusions, 601-602, 605
  for massive transfusions, 479, 517
  for pediatric patients, 616-617, 620
  of platelets, 419-420, 448, *461,* 514, 624
  rare types, 380
  of red cell components, *461,* 476-477, 509-
    510
  in urgent situations, 478, 479
  in warm autoimmune hemolytic anemia,
    396-397
Blood components. *See also specific components*
  administration of (*See* Blood
    administration)
  aliquoting, 474, 617-618, *619,* 625-626
  bacterial contamination of, 183-185, 474
  CMV-reduced-risk, 175, 601, 689-690
  costs of, 529
  density of, *128*
  expiration of, 463, *464-469,* 497
  identification of, 126, 477, 494, 496-497
  inspection of, 134, 143, 474, 477, 494-495
  irradiated, 149-150, 472, 591, 632
  issuing, 477-479, 494-495
  labeling, 152-153, 477
  leukocyte reduction of, 148-149, 472, 632
  modification by sterile connecting device,
    148
  monitoring use of, 557-565
  ordering, 457-458, 490-491, 563, 565
  pathogen inactivation of, 151-152, 633
  pooling, 150, 473-474
  prepared in open system, 133
  quarantine of, 152, 174
  rare, 380
  receiving into inventory, 475
  records of, 477-478
  regulations regarding, 78-79
  retrieval of prior donations, 170, *171-173,* 174
  return and reissue of, 481
  selection of (*See* Blood component
    selection)
  storage, 463, *464-469,* 470, 509
  temperature requirements for, 463
  testing

ABO/Rh, 133, 274-274, 475
  infectious disease (*See* Infectious disease
    screening)
  phenotyping, 310, 477, 630, 656
traceability of, 475
transporting, 133, 463, *464-469,* 474-475,
  495
volume-reduction of, 151, 473, 624, 632-633
washing, 473, 633
Blood containers
  additive solutions in, 134, *135,* 618-620
  for aliquots, 617-618
  anticoagulant-preservative solutions in,
    131, *132*
  diversion pouch on, 126, 143, 184
  modification by sterile connecting device,
    148
  properties of, 131
Blood donation. *See* Blood collection; Donors
Blood exposure, in employees, 38-39, 46
Blood group genomics, 253-261
  discrepancies between phenotype and
    genotype, 215, 259-261
  to distinguish alloantibody from
    autoantibody, *256,* 257
  to predict donor phenotype, *256,* 259
  to predict phenotype of recently transfused
    patients, 215, 255, *256*
  to predict phenotype when red cells are
    coated with IgG, 255, *256,* 356, 397
  in prenatal practice, *256,* 257-259
Blood group systems. *See also specific blood
  groups*
  clinical significance of antibodies in, *320-
    322, 363-364*
  defined, 229, 252
  genetics of, 229-261
    chimerism, 252
    gene mapping, *233-235,* 251-252
    genomics, 253-261
    inheritance patterns, 239-247
    population genetics, 248-250
    principles of, 230-232, 235-238
    relationship testing, 250-251
  terminology for, *233-235,* 252-253
Blood loss, *506,* 536
Blood management. *See* Patient blood
  management
Blood order schedules, 480, 565
Blood pressure
  of donors, 114
  hypotension
    during apheresis, 647
    associated with ACE inhibitors, *573,* 586

deliberate, 533
in recipients, 577, 585-586
Blood pressure cuffs, 31
Blood recovery, 533, 535-536
Blood samples
age of, 350-351, 460
for antibody identification, 351
from arterial or central lines, 536
collection of, 458, 491
confirming linkage with blood requests,
458
for hemoglobin/hematocrit screening, 114
incompletely clotted, 459-460
labeling, 458, 491
for pretransfusion testing, 351, 459-460, 491
retention and storage of, 476
transportation and shipment of, 57
Blood spills, 47
Blood utilization auditing, 21-22, 557-565
benchmarking in, 564-565
blood order schedules, 565
computerized physician order entry system
in, 563
interventions to change transfusion
practice, 537-539
patterns of blood use by procedure, 565
process for, 558-559
of transfusion-related complications, 565
of transfusions to high-risk patients, 562-563
types of audits
concurrent, *560*, 561
prospective, 538, 559, *560*, 561
retrospective, *560*, 562
Blood volume
of pediatric patients, 614
removed during plasmapheresis, 141
in Whole Blood collections, 127, 131, 136
Blood warmers, 30, 492-493, 588, 614
Bombay phenotype, 267, 270, 280
Bone grafts, 698
Bone marrow. *See* Marrow
Brain natriuretic peptide, 584-585
Bruising, in donors, 129
Buffy-coat concentration of marrow, 674

C

C/c antigens, 308, 310, 311-312, *363*, 603
^{14}C-serotonin release assay, 425
Calcium supplementation, *574*, 586, 646
Calibration, equipment, 8-9, 26
Cancer
in blood donors, 117-118
cytapheresis in, 656
platelet transfusions in, 511-513

CAP. *See* College of American Pathologists
Carboprost, *551*
Cardiac disease, in blood donors, 118-119
Cardiac surgery
fibrinogen concentrates for, 519
point-of-care testing for, 534
transfusions in, 507, 631
Cardiac transplantation, 452
Carriers, of traits, 232
Catheters
for apheresis, 645-646
drawing blood specimens from, 536
for transfusions, 494, 622, 627
CBER. *See* Center for Biologics Evaluation and
Research
CD11a/CD11b, 427
CD34, 667, 676-677
CD36, 418
CD55, 339
CD59 system, *235, 322,* 339, 342
CD99, 335-336
CD109, 417
CD177, 427, 429
Cefotetan, 403
Ceftriaxone, 403
Cell counters, 31
Cell division, 232, *236, 237*
Cell expansion of HPCs, 675-676
Cell selection of HPCs, 675
Cell washers, 29
Cellular therapy. *See also* Hematopoietic
progenitor cell transplantation; Tissue
accreditation of, 87, *88*
regulation of, *78,* 86-89
testing donors, 175-176
Center for Biologics Evaluation and Research
inspections by, 83
regulation of biological products, 78-79
reporting fatalities to, 20, 82, 131, 592,
593
Center for Patient Safety, 102
Centers for Medicare and Medicaid Services,
77, 84-85
Centrifuges, 29, 31
Centromere, 231
Cephalosporins, 403, 404
Cephalothin, 404
Ceppellini effect, 302
cGMP. *See* Current good manufacturing
practice
cGTP. *See* Current good tissue practice
Ch antigens, 338
Chagas disease, 189-190
Change control, 26

Charts
control, 26
pedigree, 239, *240*
Chemical hygiene plan, 49
Chemical/organic solvent elutions, *390*
Chemical safety, 49-53
chemical categories, *50, 69-70*
chemical hygiene plan, 49
chemicals found in blood banks, 67-68
emergency response plan for, 52, 71-75
engineering controls for, 52-53
hazard identification and communication, 50-52
personal protective equipment for, 52
safe work practices for, 52
training for, 49-50
waste disposal, 53
Chemiluminescence assays, 378
Chemotherapy, 673
Chido/Rodgers system, *234, 321,* 338, 374
Chido substance, 374
Chikungunya virus, *173,* 188-189
Children. *See* Neonates; Pediatric patients
Chimerism, 252, 275, 448-450
Chlamydia trachomatis, 176
Chloroquine diphosphate, 373
Chromatids, *231,* 232
Chromosomes, 230-232, *233-235,* 251-252. *See also* Genes
Circular of Information for the Use of Human Blood and Blood Components, 133, 153
Circulatory overload, transfusion-associated, *573,* 584-585
Cis position, 246-247
cisAB phenotype, 270, 273, 275
Citrate toxicity, *130,* 500, *574,* 586, 646-647
Clean rooms, 34
Cleaning and decontamination, 43
Clinical decision support system, 563
Clinical Laboratory Improvement Amendments (CLIA), 77, 84-85
Clocks, 30
Clonogenic assays, 677
Clots, in RBCs, 134
CMS. *See* Centers for Medicare and Medicaid Services
CMV. *See* Cytomegalovirus
Co^a/Co^b antigens, 337, *364*
Coagulation factors
concentrates, *549-550,* 689
in cryoprecipitate, 142, 518
in Thawed Plasma, 471
Coagulopathy
in apheresis, 647-648

in blood donors, 118
in hemolytic transfusion reactions, 577
in massive transfusion, 534, 587-588
in neonates, 625-626
plasma transfusions for, 516-518
in surgical patients, 534
Code of Federal Regulations, 2, 28, 78, *80*
Codominant inheritance, 239
Cold agglutinin disease, 398-400
alloantibody detection in, 399
serologic findings in, *392,* 398-399
specificity of autoantibodies in, 286, 354, 399-400
Cold autoantibodies
ABO typing with, 277, 278, 399
adsorption of, 399
antibody identification with, 366, 371
in cold agglutinin disease, 286, 354, 398-400
in mixed AIHA, 400
in paroxysmal cold hemoglobinuria, 400-401
in Rh testing, 313, 399
use of sulfhydryl reagents with, 399
in warm autoimmune hemolytic anemia, 392
Cold-reactive alloantibodies, 277, 278
Cold stress. *See* Hypothermia
Collections, blood group, 343
College of American Pathologists, 86, 87, *88*
Colton system, *234, 321,* 337, *364*
Column agglutination technology, 352
Compatibility testing. *See* Pretransfusion testing
Competency assessments, 8
Complement
in acute transfusion reactions, 577
in cell opsonization and destruction, 223-224
in DAT testing, 387, 388, *392*
Complement-dependent cytotoxicity, 446
Complications. *See* Adverse reactions/events
Complotype, 442
Computer crossmatching, 397, 458, 462, 479
Computer systems, 13, 17
Computerized provider order entry, 538-539, 563
Concurrent audits, *560,* 561
Confidentiality of information, 17
Consanguineous mating, 240
Consent. See *Informed consent*
Containers
for blood collection, 131, 133
for platelet components, 142
for RBCs, 134

for shipping
    dry shippers, 677
    HPCs, 677
    quality control intervals for, 31
    temperature of, 475, 677, 704
    validation of, 474, 475
Contamination
    bacterial, 183-185
        detecting, 184-185
        inspecting components for, 134, 474
        during phlebotomy, 126, 184
        of platelets, 143, 183-185, 470-471
        of RBCs, 134, 184
        reactive testing results for, *173*
        of tissue allografts, 700, 705
        in transfusion-associated sepsis, 183-
           184, 185, *573*, 580
    fungal, 700, 705
    in polymerase chain reaction, 211
Contracts, 10
Control charts, 26
Controls
    autologous, 354, *360-361, 487*
    for Rh typing reagents, 312
Copper sulfate, 31, 57, 114
Cord blood. *See* Umbilical cord blood
Corrected platelet count increment, 419, 515
Corrective action, 19
Corticosteroids, 147, 492
Cost collection, 343
Costs, health-care, 529
Counterflow centrifugal elutriation, 675
CPOE. *See* Computerized provider order entry
Creutzfeldt-Jakob disease, 192, 698, 700
Cromer system, *234, 321,* 339
Cross-reactive groups, 438
Crossing-over, 244-245, 443-444
Crossmatch-to-transfusion ratios, 480, 565
Crossmatching
    agglutination-based methods, 215-216
    with alloantibodies, 379
    antiglobulin test in, 462
    with autoantibodies, 396-397
    computer, 397, 458, 462, 479
    HLA (lymphocyte), 447, 451
    immediate-spin, 461-462
    interpretation of results, 463, *487*
    in pediatric recipients, 616-617
    platelet components, 420, 448
    in pretransfusion testing, 458-459, 461-463
    virtual, 451
Cryoprecipitated antihemophilic factor, 142
    ABO compatibility of, *461, 498,* 626
    coagulation factors in, 142, 518
    expiration of, 142, 150, *466-467,* 471

in HPC transplantation patients, 689
infusion of, *498*
for pediatric patients, *621, 625,* 626
pooled, 142, 150, *467,* 473-474
preparation of, 142
storage of, 142, *466-467,* 471
thawing, 471
transfusion of, 518-519
transportation of, *466-467,* 475
Cryopreservation
    agents for, 138, 676
    of HPCs, 676, 684
    of RBCs, 138
    of tissue allografts, 697
Cryptic autoantigens, 275
Crystalloids, *645*
Cs^a/Cs^b antigens, 343
Current good manufacturing practice, 2
Current good tissue practice, 2, 697, 700
Customers, 5, 7, 19
Cytapheresis, *642,* 656, *657*
Cytomegalovirus, 174-175
    in neonates, 632
    preventing, with leukocyte reduction, 175,
        632, 689
    screening donors for, *176*
Cytomegalovirus-reduced-risk products, 175,
    601, 632, 689-690

D

D antigen, 302-307
    antibody to (anti-D)
        clinical significance of, *320, 363*
        in hemolytic disease of the fetus and
           newborn, 295, *320,* 600, 603
        and partial D, 307
        passively acquired, 603, 605
        and platelet transfusions, 514
        titrations of, 601
        and weak D, 307
    clinical considerations for, 307
    D epitopes on Rhce, 304, *305*
    D-negative, 299
    D-positive, 303-304
    D_{el}, 304
    elevated D, 304
    in fetus, 257-258
    historical perspective on, 295-298
    nonfunctional RHD alleles, 304
    partial D, *303,* 304, *309,* 313
    in recipients, 306-307, 461
    testing for (*See* Rh testing)
    in tissue transplantation, 698
    weak D, 303-304, *309*

in donors, 259, 306, 307
in prenatal patients, 258, 603
in recipients, 306-307, 461
DAT. *See* Direct antiglobulin test
DAT-negative autoimmune hemolytic
anemia, 397-398
Data collection/data mining, 564
Decontamination procedures, 43, 48-49
Deferrals. *See* Donor deferrals
Deglycerolization, 138, 471-472
Delayed transfusion reactions
hemolytic, 224-225, 366, *574*, 588-590, 630
management of, *574-575*
serologic, 366, 588, 589
Dengue virus, *173*, 188
Density, of blood cells and components, *128*
Derivatives. *See* Plasma derivatives
Designated donations, 120
Desmopressin, 535, *551*
Di^a/Di^b antigens, 334-335, *363-364*
DIC. *See* Disseminated intravascular
coagulation
Diego system, *233, 320,* 334-335, *363-364*
Diethylhexylphthalate (DEHP), 134
Dimethyl sulfoxide, 676, 678
2,3-Diphosphoglycerate (2,3-DPG), 616
Diploid, defined, 232
Direct antiglobulin test, 386-391
false positive/negative results in, *485-486*
method for, 387-388
positive result
after HPC transplantation, 389
in antibody identification, 354-355, *361,*
369
in blood donors, 387
causes of, *386*
in cold agglutinin syndrome, *392*
drug-induced, 389, 401-405, *409-412*
elution with, 389-391
evaluation of, 388-391
medical history in, 388-389
in mixed-type AIHA, *392,* 400
in paroxysmal cold hemoglobinuria,
392, 400
predicting phenotype with, 255
in warm autoimmune hemolytic
anemia, 391, *392*
principles of, 387-388
reagents for, 387-388
specimens for, 387-388
in transfusion reaction evaluation, 387, 576
Directed blood donations, 120-121
Disinfectants, 43, 126, 184
Disposal, waste, 48, 53, 56

Disseminated intravascular coagulation, 577,
578
Dithiothreitol
to disperse autoagglutination, 278, 374,
393, 399
for inactivating blood group antigens, *363-
364, 369,* 373, 374
Diversion pouch, 126, 143, 184
DMAIC (define, measure, analyze, improve,
and control) process, 23
DMSO. *See* Dimethyl sulfoxide
DNA analysis, 207-215
chemistry and structure of nucleic acids,
208-209
clinical applications of, 254-255, *256*
for antigen-negative blood donors, *256,*
259
confirming D status, 311
distinguishing alloantibody from
autoantibody, *256,* 257
fetal genotyping, 257-258, 310, 601, 606
HLA typing, 444-446, 452
HNA typing, 428-429
platelet genotyping, 424
prenatal practice, 257-259, 310
in recently transfused patients, 215, 255,
256, 310
relationship testing, 251
Rh zygosity testing, 310
in sickle cell disease patients, 311
when red cells are coated with IgG, 255,
256, 356, 397
detection of amplification products, 212-215
isolation of nucleic acids, 209
next-generation sequencing, 446
polymerase chain reaction, 209-212, 254,
445-446
reverse-transcriptase PCR, 211
sequence-based amplification, 212
transcription-mediated amplification, 212
Do^a/Do^b antigens, 336-337, *364*
Documents, 14-17. *See also* Records
creation of, 14-15
forms, 16
job aids, 16
labels, 16
maintenance of, 16
policies and processes, 15
quality manual, 15
standard operating procedures, 11, 15, 701-
702
work instructions, 15
Dolichos biflorus lectin, 272, 278
Dombrock system, *234, 320,* 336-337, *364*

Donath-Landsteiner test, 290, 401
Donation identification number, 126, 153, 496
Donor deferrals
    for bleeding conditions or blood diseases, 118
    blood donation intervals for, 141, 145
    for cancer, 117-118
    developing criteria for, 117-119
    for heart and lung conditions, 118-119
    for hemoglobin/hematocrit, 115
    for medications taken by donor, 119, 145
    for reactive infectious screening tests, 169, 170, *171-173*
    records of, 112, 113, 126
    reentry pathways, *171-173*
Donor Hemovigilance Working Group, 103
Donor History Questionnaire, 112, 116, 119-120
Donor room, biosafety in, 46
Donor selection, 111-112
    for autologous donations, 112, 121
    blood-center-defined criteria for, 117-119
    consent of donor in, 113-114, 125-126, 141
    for directed donations, 120-121
    Donor History Questionnaire in, 112, 113, 116
    education of donor, 113-114, 125
    emergency measures, 116-117
    for exceptional medical need, 120
    for frequent donors, 119-120
    hemoglobin or hematocrit in, 114-115, 131
    for HPC transplantation, 668-669, 672
    identification of donor, 112-113, 126
    physical examination in, 114-115
    for plateletpheresis, 145
    registration process in, 112-113
    for tissue donation, 696
Donor-specific antibodies, 669
Donor testing
    ABO, 274-275
    for blood group antigens, 259, 378-379, 477
    for HPC transplantation, 668-669
    for infectious diseases (*See* Infectious disease screening)
    Rh, 259, 306, 307
    silenced or nonexpressed genes in, 259-261
    weak D, 306
Donors
    adverse reactions in, 20, 97, 102-105, 129-131
    age of, 113
    anemia in, 115
    autologous, 121, 175, 532
    bleeding conditions or blood diseases in, 118
    blood pressure of, 114
    blood samples from, 476

    cancer in, 117-118
    care of, after phlebotomy, 127-129
    consent of, 113, 125-126, 141, 672
    deferral of (*See* Donor deferrals)
    designated or directed, 120-121
    disabled, 113
    donation intervals for, 141, 145
    educational materials for, 113-114, 125
    family members as, 380
    frequent or repeat, 119-120
    hearing- or vision-impaired, 113
    heart conditions in, 118-119
    hemoglobin/hematocrit in, 114-115
    hemovigilance, 102-105
    for HLA-matched platelets, 448
    for HPC transplantation, 668, 672-673
    identification of, 112-113, 126
    illiterate, 113
    iron supplementation in, 115
    lung conditions in, 118-119
    medications taken by, 119, 145
    non-English-speaking, 113
    notification of abnormal test results, 174
    phlebotomy of, 126
    physical examination of, 114-115
    plasmapheresis, 126, 140-141
    plateletpheresis, 126, 145
    positive DAT in, 387
    pulse, 114
    with reactive screening tests, 168-169, 170-174
    records of, 113
    registration of, 112-113
    selection of (*See* Donor selection)
    testing (*See* Donor testing)
    of tissue allografts, 696
    and TRALI, 584
    weight of, 114
Dosage effect, 238, 350, 358
Dosimeters, 55, 149
2,3-DPG, 616
Drug-induced immune hemolytic anemia, 401-405
    antibodies in, 401-404
    classification of, 401-404
    drugs associated with, *409-412*
    laboratory investigation of, 404-405
    mechanisms of, 401
Drug-induced thrombocytopenia, 421-422
Drugs
    administered for leukapheresis, 147
    antiplatelet agents, 119, 145
    causing positive DAT, 389, 401-405, *409-412*
    hemostatic agents, 535, *547-548, 550*

interference with antibody identification, 354
platelet antibodies induced by, 421-422
pretransfusion medications, 492, 581
removal of, in apheresis, 648
taken by donors, 119, 145
to treat anemia, 531
Dry ice, 475
Dry shippers, 677
DTT. *See* Dithiothreitol
Duffy system, 330-332
antibodies, *320,* 332, *363*
antigens, *233,* 330-332
Duffy glycoprotein, *331,* 332
and malaria, 332
phenotypes and genotypes, *331*
silenced alleles in, 260

E

E/e antigens, 308, 310, 311-312, *363*
ECMO. *See* Extracorporeal membrane oxygenation
Education
for donors, 113-114, 125
for physicians, 537-538
for recipients, 490
Electrical safety, 40-41
ELISA. *See* Enzyme-linked immunosorbent assay
Elutions, 375-376, 389-391
Elutriation, 675
Embolism, air, *573,* 588
Emergency equipment, 493
Emergency release, 152, 478, 500, 509-510
Emergency response plans, 38
for biohazards, 47
for chemical spills, 52-53, 71-73
for electrical emergency, 41
for fires, 40
for radiation safety, 56
Emm antigen, 343-344
Employees. *See* Personnel
En^a antigen, 326
End-product test and inspection, 26
Engineering controls
for biosafety, 42-46
for chemical safety, 52
for electrical safety, 41
for fire prevention, 40
general guidelines for, 37, 65
for radiation safety, 55-56
Engraftment, in HPC transplantation, 671, 685, 687
Enhancement media, 352-353, 370

Enzyme-linked immunosorbent assay, 217-219, *423,* 424, 425
Enzymes, *363-364, 369,* 373
EPO. *See* Erythropoiesis-stimulating agents
Epsilon-aminocaproic acid, 535, *547*
Equipment
apheresis, 137-138, 141-142, 145-146, 147-148, 642-643
component storage, 463
decontamination of, 43
emergency, 493
failures of, 463, 470
identification of, 9
management of, 8-9
personal protective, 37-38, 46, 63-64
qualification of, 11
quality control of, 29-31
regulations for, 79, *80,* 81-82
selection of, 9
for transfusions, 492-493
validation of, 11
Er^a/Er^b antigens, 343
Ergonomics, 35-36
Errors. *See also* Nonconformances
in ABO and Rh typing, 277, 313
correction of, 17
fatalities due to, 496
identification, 458, 496, 578-579
mislabeled specimens, 458
quarantine release, 177
reporting, 96-97, 99
sources of, in antiglobulin test, *485-486*
wrong blood in tube, 458
Erythroblastosis fetalis, 599
Erythrocytapheresis, *642, 657*
Erythropoiesis, in neonates, 614
Erythropoiesis-stimulating agents, 531, *546-547,* 614
Estrogen, conjugated, *552*
Ethnic groups, differences in
in antibody identification, 358, 367, *368*
in Dombrock system, *336*
in Duffy system, *331*
in Kell system, *328*
in Kidd system, 332-333
in Knops system, *340*
in MNS system, 323, *325*
in Rh system, *296-297, 298,* 303, 304, 306
European Haemovigilance Network, 94
Exchange transfusions
blood warmer for, 614
component choice for, 616, 622, 656
indications for, *642, 657*

hemolytic disease of the fetus and newborn, 602, 627
    hemolytic transfusion reactions, 578
    polycythemia, 627
    sickle cell disease, 508, 629-630, 656
  techniques for, 622
  vascular access for, 622
  volume of, 621, 622
Expiration, of components, 133, 463, *464-469*, 497
Extracorporeal membrane oxygenation, 627-628
Extracorporeal photopheresis, *642*, 656, *658*, 659
Eye Bank Association of America, 700, 701, 702
Eyewashes, 65

F

Face shields, 46, 64
Facilities
  clean rooms in, 34
  design and workflow of, 34
  ergonomic design of, 35-36
  housekeeping in, 34
  licensure of, 81
  mobile sites, 35
  in quality systems, 23
  registration of, 79-81
  regulatory agencies for, 33, 61-62
  restricted areas in, 35
  safety program of, 23, 36-39
Factor VIIa, recombinant, *549*
Factor VIII deficiency, 626
Factor XIII, 518
False-positive/negative test results
  in agglutination tests, 216
  in antiglobulin testing, *485-486*
  in ELISA, 219
  in Rh testing, 313
Fatalities
  during apheresis, 648
  of blood donors, 20, 131
  due to contaminated platelets, 183, 185
  due to identification errors, 496
  due to TRALI, 584
  due to transfusions, 20, 96, 97, 578, 582, 585, 592
  of employees, 39
  related to medical devices, 82
  reporting, 20, 39, 82, 96, 131, 592, *593*
Fc receptors, 222-223, *224*, 426-427
FDA. *See* Food and Drug Administration
FD&C Act, 78, 79
Febrile nonhemolytic transfusion reactions, 448, 492, *571*, 580-581

Fenwal apheresis systems, 137-138, 141, 146
Ferritin, 115
Fetal and neonatal alloimmune thrombocytopenia, 420-421, 506-507
Fetomaternal hemorrhage, 600, 604
Fetus
  genotyping, 257-258, 310, 601, 606
  hemolytic disease in, 599-605
  thrombocytopenia in, 420-421, 605-607
  transfusions in, 601-602
Fever, 448, *571*, 576, 579, 580, 588, 589
FFP. *See* Fresh Frozen Plasma
Fibrin clots, 275
Fibrinogen, 518-519, *550*
Ficin, *363-364*, 373
Filters
  leukocyte reduction, 149, 472, 495-496, *498*
  microaggregate, 495
  standard in-line, 495, *498*, 627
Fire prevention, 39-40
First aid, 38-39
Flow cytometry, 220
  in HLA antibody testing, 447, 451, 516
  to measure fetomaternal hemorrhage, 604
  to measure residual leukocytes, 149
  in platelet antibody detection, 424, 425
  to quantify HPCs, 667
  in red cell survival studies, 378
Flow microarrays, 447
Fluids, replacement, in apheresis, *642, 645*
Focal segmental glomerulosclerosis, 655
Food and Drug Administration
  inspections by, 82-83
  licensure of blood and component manufacturers, 81
  oversight of blood establishments, 77, 78-84
  recalls and withdrawals, 84
  registration by, 79-81
  regulations and guidance, 79
    for blood-related devices, 79, *80*, 81-82
    for cellular therapy, 89, 668, 678
    cGMP, 2, 7
    cGTP, 2, 7, 697, 700
    for infectious disease testing, 165, 168, *171-173*, 174, *176*
    for tissues, *176*, 700
  reporting to
    adverse events, 20, 82
    biological product deviations, 20, 83-84
    fatalities, 20, 82, 131, 592, *593*
  Sentinel BloodSCAN Program, 106
Forensic testing, 452
Forms, 16

FORS system, *235, 289,* 290-291, *322,* 341
Foundation for the Accreditation of Cellular
  Therapy (FACT), 87, *88*
Freeze-thaw elutions, *390*
Freezers, 29, 463, 470
Freezing
  cryoprotective agents for, 138, 676
  Fresh Frozen Plasma, 139
  hematopoietic progenitor cells, 676
  RBCs, 138
Frequency, allele (gene), 248, 249-250
Fresenius AS104 apheresis system, *137,* 147
Fresh Frozen Plasma, 139
  ABO compatibility of, *461, 498,* 626
  aliquoting, 625-626
  expiration of, 139, *467,* 471
  for pediatric patients, *621,* 625-626, 631
  preparation of, 139
  quarantine of, 139
  storage of, 139, *467*
  thawing, 139, 471
  transfusion of, 518
  transportation of, *467,* 475
Fume hoods, 52
Fungal contamination, 700, 705
Fy3, Fy4, Fy5, Fy6 antigens, 331-332
Fy^a/Fy^b antigens, 330-331, 332, *363*

G

G antigen, 308, 603
G-CSF. *See* Granulocyte colony-stimulating
  factor
Ge antigens, 338-339
Gene locus, 230
Genes, 230-232
  of blood group systems, *233-235,* 251-252
  frequencies of, 249-250
  of major histocompatibility complex, 440-
    444
  mapping, *233-235,* 251-252
  mutation of, 238, 344-345
  nucleic acid structure in, 208-209
  position effect, 246-247
  silent or amorphic, 238, 241, 259-261
  suppressor or modifier, 247
  syntenic, 245
Genetic principles
  alleles, 236-238, *253*
  blood group gene mapping, *233-235,* 251-252
  cell division, *231,* 232, *236, 237*
  chimerism, 252
  genes and chromosomes, 230-232
  genotype and phenotype, 235-236, *253*
  inheritance patterns

  autosomal, 239-241
  crossing-over, 244-245, 443-444
  gene interaction and position effect,
    246-247
  independent segregation and
    independent assortment, 244
  linkage, 244-245, 443-444
  linkage disequilibrium, 245-246, 444
  pedigrees, 239, *240*
  sex-linked, 241-243
  of major histocompatibility complex, 440-444
  polymorphism, 238
  population genetics, 248-250
  relationship testing, 250-251
  X chromosome inactivation, 232, 235
Genotype
  defined, 207-208, 235
  DNA-based assays for, 254-255, *256*
    for antigen-negative blood donors, *256,*
      259
    confirming D status, 311
    distinguishing alloantibody from
      autoantibody, *256,* 257
    of fetus, 257-258, 310, 601, 606
    platelet genotyping, 424
    in prenatal practice, 257-259, 310, 603
    in recently transfused patients, 215, 255,
      256, 310, 356
    RHD zygosity, 310
    in sickle cell disease patients, 215,
      311
    when red cells are coated with IgG, 255,
      256, 356, 397
  frequencies of, 249-250
  nomenclature for, *253*
  and phenotypes, 215, 235-236, 259-261
Gerbich system, *234, 321,* 338-339
GIL antigen, 341
Gill system, *234, 321,* 341
Glanzmann thrombasthenia, 416
GLOB collection, 286
Globoside system, 286-290
  antibodies, 289-290, *321*
  antigens, *234,* 286-289
  biochemistry, 287
  genetics, *234,* 287-289
  phenotypes, 286-287
  transfusion practice with, 290
Gloves, 63-64
  and latex allergy, 39
  use for biohazards, 46
  use in donor room, 46-47
Glycerolization of red cells, 138
Glycine-HCl/EDTA, 373

GMP. *See* Current good manufacturing practice
Goggles, safety, 64
GPVI/GPIV platelet antigens, *417,* 418
Graft-vs-host disease
    in HPC transplantation, 670-671
    transfusion-associated, *575,* 590-591
        HLA system in, 448-449, 590
        in neonates, 615
Graft-vs-neoplasm effect, 668, 670, 671
Granulocyte agglutination test, 428
Granulocyte colony-stimulating factor, 147, 673
Granulocyte immunofluorescence test, 428
Granulocytes, 146-148
    ABO compatibility of, 147, *461, 498,* 519, 626
    antigens and antibodies, 425-427, 583-584
    apheresis collection of, *137,* 147-148
    dose of, 626, 631
    expiration of, *466*
    in HPC transplantation patients, 689
    increasing yields of, 146-147
    indications for, 519-520, 626, 631
    infusion of, 147, *498,* 519-520
    irradiation of, 147, *466,* 519
    laboratory testing of, 147
    in pediatric patients, 626, 631
    storage of, 147, *466,* 471, 519
    transportation of, *466,* 475
Growth factors, hematopoietic, 147, 673
Growth hormone, in donors, 119
GTP. *See* Current good tissue practice
Guillain-Barré syndrome, 655
GVHD. *See* Graft-vs-host disease
Gy^a antigen, 336

H

H system, 278-281
    antibodies, 280-281, *321*
    biochemistry and genetics of, *234,* 266-267, *268,* 278, *279*
    Bombay phenotype, 267, 270, 280
    H antigen, 266, 267, *268,* 278
    Para-Bombay phenotype, 280
    transfusion practice for, 281
Haemonetics apheresis systems, *137,* 138, 141-142, 146, 147-148
Hand washing, 46, 65
Haploid, defined, 232
Haplotypes
    ancestral, 444, 453
    defined, 245
    of HLA system, *443,* 444
    of Rh system, 298, 299, *301-302*

Hardy-Weinberg equilibrium, 249-250
Hazardous areas of facilities, 35
Hazardous materials
    biohazards, 41-49
    chemicals, 49-53
    classification of, *50*
    identification and communication of, 37
        for biosafety, 42
        for chemical safety, 50-52
        for electrical safety, 41
        for fire safety, 40
    radioactive, 53-56
    safety plan for, 36
    shipping, 56-57
    waste management of, 47-49, 56
HBsAg. *See* Hepatitis B surface antigen
HBV. *See* Hepatitis B virus
HCT/Ps. *See* Human cells, tissue, and cellular and tissue-based products
HCV. *See* Hepatitis C virus
HDFN. *See* Hemolytic disease of the fetus and newborn
Health history questionnaires. *See* Donor history questionnaire
Heart disease, in blood donors, 118-119
Heart transplants, 452
Heat elutions, *390*
Heating blocks, 30
Hemagglutination. *See* Agglutination
Hematocrit
    of allogeneic donors, 114, 115
    of autologous donors, 131
    of blood in exchange transfusions, 622
    in neonates, 627
    of RBCs, 134
    as transfusion threshold, *617*
    of Whole Blood, 131
Hematologic disorders, in blood donors, 118
Hematoma, in donors, 129, *130*
Hematopoietic growth factors, 147, 673
Hematopoietic progenitor cell transplantation
    ABO typing discrepancies after, 275, 277
    adverse reactions to, 678
    allogeneic, 668-669, 684-685
    autologous, 668, 672, 673, 689
    and CMV, 689-690
    donor requirements for, 668-669
    engraftment kinetics in, 671, 685, 687
    graft source for, 670
    graft-vs-host disease after, 670-671
    graft-vs-neoplasm effect in, 671
    haploidentical, 670
    histocompatibility in, 450, 669-670
    HLA matching in, 669-670

incompatible, 670, 684-685
  bidirectional ABO, *684, 685, 686*
  major ABO, 670, 674, 684-685, *686*
  minor ABO, 670, 674, *684,* 685, *686*
  related to non-ABO antigens, 685
indications for, 667-668
patient care in, 677-678
positive DAT after, 389
records of, 690-691
regulation of, 86-89, 668, 678
sources of cells for (*See* Hematopoietic
  progenitor cells)
survival after, 671
transfusion support for, 683-691
  autologous recipients, 689
  CMV-negative components, 689-690
  cryoprecipitate, 689
  factor concentrates, 689
  incompatible transplants, 684-685,
    686
  information portability, 690-691
  irradiated components, 689
  in patients with HLA/HPA antibodies,
    689, 690
  in patients with neutropenia and
    infection, 689
  in pediatric patients, 690
  plasma, *686,* 689
  platelets, 511-513, *686,* 687-689
  RBCs, *686,* 687
  selection of components, 685-687
  transfusion reactions after, 690
Hematopoietic progenitor cells
  cell expansion, 675-676
  cell selection systems, 675
  collection of, 672-674
  cryopreservation of, 676, 684
  donors of, 668-669
  elutriation of, 675
  infusion of, 677-678
  processing, 674-676
  quality control of, 676-677
  red cell reduction of, 674
  regulation of, 86-89, 678
  shipping and transport of, 677
  sources of, 670, 672-674
  thawing, 674
  volume reduction of, 674
  washing, 675
Hemizygous, defined, 237
Hemochromatosis, hereditary, 442
Hemoglobin
  of apheresis RBCs, 115
  in blood donors, 114-115

decreased, tolerance for, 536-537
  in infants, 613-614, 620, 627
  in RBCs, 136
  testing methods for, 114
  as transfusion threshold, 506-507, 537, 620,
    687, 690
Hemoglobin S, 629
Hemoglobinometers, 31
Hemolysis
  in ABO testing, 274
  extravascular, 224-225, 385, 577, 588
  in hemolytic disease of the fetus and
    newborn, 599
  immune-mediated, 385-386, 387, 388
  intravascular, 224, 225, 385, 576
  nonimmune, *573,* 579, 648
  passenger lymphocyte syndrome, 685
  in patient samples, 576
  in RBCs, 134
Hemolytic anemia
  autoimmune
    classification of, 391
    cold agglutinin disease, 398-400
    mixed-type, 400
    paroxysmal cold hemoglobinuria, 400-
      401
    serologic findings in, *392*
    transfusion in, 397, 400, 511
    warm, 391-398, 510-511
  defined, 385
  drug-induced, 401-405
  immune, 385-386
  microangiopathic, 649
  neonatal, 599-605
  positive DAT in, 387, 388
Hemolytic disease of the fetus and newborn,
  599-605
  ABO, 273-274, 600
  antibodies associated with, *320-322, 363-
    364,* 600
    anti-D, 295, 600
    anti-K, 329, 600
  diagnosis and monitoring, 601
  maternal alloimmunization in, 600
  pathophysiology of, 599-600
  prevention of, 603-605
  red cell selection in, 605
  testing in, 601
    antibody titers, 377, 601
    elutions, 390
    Rh testing, 257-258, 312, 601
  treatment of, 601-602
Hemolytic transfusion reactions
  acute, *571,* 576-579

antibodies associated with, *320-322, 363-364*
clinical evaluation and management of, 570, *571,* 576-577, 578
due to errors, 225, 496, 578-579
elutions in, 390
frequency of, 578
intravascular hemolysis in, 224, 225
pathophysiology of, 577-578
prevention of, 578-579
signs and symptoms of, 225, 570, 576-577
treatment of, 578
delayed, 224-225, *574,* 588-590, 630
nonimmune, *573,* 579
Hemolytic uremic syndrome, 649
Hemorrhage
fetomaternal, 600, 604
intraventricular, 623
postpartum, 518-519
Hemostasis
during massive transfusion, 534, 587-588
in neonates, 624-625
platelets in, 413, 416
tests for, *624*
Hemostatic agents, 535, *547-554*
Hemovigilance, 93-107, 569
international, 94-97
reporting, 20
in United States, 97-107
biovigilance, 98
for blood donors, 102-105
gaps in, 105-107
for recipients, 98-102
Heparin, 425, 646
Heparin-induced thrombocytopenia, 422, 425
Hepatitis, non-A, non-B, 161, 164, 181
Hepatitis B surface antigen, 161, *171,* 174, 180-181
Hepatitis B virus, 180-181
employee exposure to, 38-39
nucleic acid testing for, 169, 181
prophylaxis for, 38
reactive testing results for, *171,* 174
residual transfusion risk of, 177-178, *179,* 181
screening donors for, 161, 164, *166, 176, 181, 696*
supplemental assays for, *166,* 168
transmission through transplantation, 698
Hepatitis C virus, 181
employee exposure to, 38
nucleic acid testing for, 169, 181
reactive testing results for, *172,* 174
residual transfusion risk of, 177-178, *179,* 181
screening donors for, *166, 176,* 181, *696*

supplemental assays for, *166,* 168
transmission through transplantation, 698
Hepatitis E virus, 182-183
Hereditary hemochromatosis, 442
Heredity, genetics of. *See* Genetic principles
Heterozygous, defined, 237-238
HEV. *See* Hepatitis E virus
High-prevalence antigens
901 series, 343-344
antibodies to, 367, *368,* 369, 602
blood selection for, 380
High-titer, low-avidity antibodies, 377
Histocompatibility. *See* HLA system
HIV. *See* Human immunodeficiency virus
Hives, *571,* 581, 582
HLA-matched platelets, 419-420
HLA system
antibodies
detection of, 419-420, 447, 516
donor specific, 669
in febrile transfusion reactions, 448, 580
following pregnancy, 418
in HPC transplantation recipients, 669, 689, 690
management of, *574*
and plasma transfusions, 139
in platelet refractoriness, 419-420, 447-448, 515-516
in TRALI, 448, 583, 584
transfusion-associated, 418
antigens and alleles
absence of antigens, 443
Bg, 344, 436, 450
Class I and Class II, 436-437, 439-440
configuration of, 437
cross-reactive groups, 438
identification of, 444-447
nomenclature for, 437-439
on platelets, *417,* 418
"public," 438
"splits," 438
biochemistry, tissue distribution and structure of, 436-440
biologic function of, 439
and chimerism, 448-449
disease associations with, 452-453
genetics of, 440-444
crossovers, 443-444
finding HLA-identical siblings, 442-443
linkage disequilibrium, 444
organization of genetic regions, 440, 442
patterns of inheritance in, 442-444
in graft-vs-host disease, 448-449, 590
overview of, 435-436

HLA typing
cellular assays for, 446-447
crossmatching, 447, 451, 452
DNA-based assays for, 444-446, 452
in forensic testing, 452
lymphotoxicity assays for, 446
of platelets, 419, *420*, 448, 516
in relationship testing, 452
in transplantation, 450-452, 669-670
HNA. *See* Human neutrophil antigens
Homografts, 696. *See also* Tissue
Homolog, defined, 241
Homozygous, defined, 237-238
Hook effect, 219
Hospitals, regulations for, 85-86
Housekeeping, 34
HPA. *See* Human platelet alloantigens
HPC. *See* Hematopoietic progenitor cells
HTLV. *See* Human T-cell lymphotropic virus
Human cells, tissue, and cellular and tissue-
based products (HCT/Ps), 86-87, 89. *See also*
Tissue
infectious disease testing on donors of, 175-
176, 668-669, *696*
regulation of, 86-89, 678, 700-701
Human immunodeficiency virus, 179-180
employee exposure to, 38-39
nucleic acid testing for, 169, 180
reactive testing results for, *171*, 174
residual transfusion risks for, 177-178, *179*,
180
screening donors for, 164-165, *166*, *176*,
179-180, *696*
supplemental assays for, *166*, 168
transmission through transplantation, 698,
706
Human neutrophil antigens, 425-427, 428-429,
583-584
Human platelet alloantigens, 413-417
Human resources, 7-8
Human T-cell lymphotropic virus, 182
reactive testing results for, *172*, 174
screening donors for, *166*, *176*, 182, *696*
supplemental assays for, *166*, 168
Hydatid cyst fluid, 290, 374
Hydrops fetalis, 599-600
Hydroxyethyl starch, 146-147, 676
Hyperbilirubinemia, 600, 602, 621
Hyperhemolysis, 508, 590, 630
Hyperkalemia, 500, 587-588
Hyperviscosity, 649, 654-655
Hypocalcemia, 500, *574*, 586, 646-647
Hypofibrinogenemia, 518-519
Hypogammaglobulinemia, 277

Hypoglycemia, 622
Hypokalemia, 586-587
Hypotension
in apheresis, 647
associated with ACE inhibitors, *573*, 586
deliberate, 533
in transfusion recipients, 577, 585-586
Hypothermia, 492-493, 533, *574*, 588, 614
Hypovolemia, 647

I

I system, 283-286
antibodies, 285-286, *321*, 399-400
in cold agglutinin syndrome, 286, 354, 399-
400
disease associations with, 285, 354
genetics of, *234*, 285
Ii collection, 283-286
phenotypes, 284-285
transfusion practice with, 286
Iatrogenic anemia, 536
Identification
of blood components
donation identification number, 126,
153
labeling, 152-153, 477-478
prior to administration, 478, 496-497
prior to issue, 477-478, 494
of donors, 112-113, 126, 153
of equipment, 9
errors in, 496, 578-579
of personnel, 17
of phlebotomists, 458, 491
of recipients, 458, 477-478, 494, 496
of tissue allografts, 705
IgA, 222, 581-582
IgD, 222
IgE, 222
IgG, 221-222
in complement activation, 223
in extravascular hemolysis, 225
Fc regions on, 222-223, *224*
structure of, *222*
subclasses of, 221-222, 223, 226
IgM, 221, *222*
cold-reactive autoagglutinins, 398-399
in complement activation, 223, 225
dispersing autoagglutination caused by,
278, 399
in intravascular hemolysis, 225
Immune thrombocytopenic purpura, 422,
424-425, 607
Immunity, 226
antibodies in, 220-222

complement activation in, 223-224
extravascular hemolysis in, 224-225
Fc receptors in, 222-223
in infants, 615
intravascular hemolysis in, 225
Immunoglobulins, 220-222. *See also specific immunoglobulins*
Immunohematology reference laboratories, 380-381
Immunomagnetic cell separation, 675
Immunotherapies, 354, 373, 389
In^a/In^b antigens, 340
Incidence, defined, 248
Incubation time, 372
Incubators, platelet, 29, 463
Independent assortment, 244
Independent segregation, 244
Indian system, *234, 321*, 340
Infants. *See* Neonates; Pediatric patients
Infection, in transplantation patients, 689
Infectious disease screening
    approaches to, *165*
    of autologous donations, 175
    for *Babesia,* 190-191
    for bacterial contamination, 183-185
    for chikungunya virus, 188-189
    of collected Whole Blood, 133
    for cytomegalovirus, 174-175
    for dengue virus, 188
    for hepatitis B virus, 180-181
    for hepatitis C virus, 181
    for hepatitis E virus, 182-183
    historical overview of, 161-165
    in HPC donors, 175-176, 668-669
    for human immunodeficiency virus, 179-180
    for human T-cell lymphotropic virus, 182
    international variations in, 176-177
    logistics of, 168
    for malaria, 191-192
    for new emerging infectious agents, 193
    nucleic acid testing, 169-170
    for parvovirus B19, 193
    for plasma derivatives, 192-193
    for prions, 192
    reactive test results in, 170-174
    regulations and standards for, 165, 170, *171-173*, 174
    residual infectious risks of transfusion, 177-179
    serologic testing, 168-169
    for syphilis, 183
    of tissue donors, *696*
    for *Trypanosoma cruzi,* 189-190
    in the United States, *166-167*

    for West Nile virus, 185-186
    for Zika virus, 186-188
Infectious diseases
    emerging agents, 193, 195
    screening for (*See* Infectious disease screening)
    transmitted by plasma derivatives, 192-193
    transmitted by tissue transplantation, 698, 699
Infectious waste, 48-49
Information management, 17
Informed consent
    for apheresis, 126, 141, 643
    for donation of HPCs, 672
    for transfusion, 489-490
    for Whole Blood donation, 113, 125-126
Infusion pumps, 493
Infusion rates, 497, *498*, 500, 627
Infusion sets, 495, 627
Inheritance patterns
    autosomal, 239-241
    crossing-over, 244-245, 443-444
    gene interaction, 246-247
    independent assortment, 244
    independent segregation, 244
    linkage, 244-245, *246*
    linkage disequilibrium, 245-246, 444
    of major histocompatibility complex, 442-444
    pedigrees, 239, *240*
    position effect, 246-247
    sex-linked, 241-243
Inhibition tests, 373-374
Injuries, 39, 82
Inspections
    of components
        before administration, 474, 477, 494-495
        documentation of, 474
        platelets, 143, 184-185
        prior to release, 474, 477-478, 494-495
        RBCs, 134, 474
        upon receipt, 474-475
    FDA, 82-83
    of incoming supplies, 10-11
    of tissue grafts, 704
Insulin, bovine, 119
Integrins, 416
International Haemovigilance Network, 94
International Normalized Ratio (INR), 516
International Organization for Standardization, 2
International Surveillance of Transfusion-Associated Reactions and Events (ISTARE) database, 94, 96

International Task Force on Biovigilance, 98
Intraoperative blood recovery, 533
Intrauterine transfusions, 601-602
Intravenous immune globulin
    ABO discrepancies with, 277
    in antibody identification problems, 354
    for fetal and neonatal immune
       thrombocytopenia, 606
    in HDFN, 602
    positive DAT result with, 389
Intravenous solutions, 496
Intraventricular hemorrhage, 623
Inventory, blood, 475, 479-481, 529
Iron deficiency anemia, 115, 531, *546*
Iron overload, *575*, 592, 629-630
Irradiated products, 149-150, 472
    expiration of, *464, 465, 466,* 472
    granulocytes, 147, *466*, 519
    indications for, 591
       in HPC transplantation, 689
       for intrauterine transfusions, 601
       for pediatric patients, 622, 632
    platelets, 150, 420, *465, 466*
    potassium leak in, 615-616
    quality control of, 149-150
    RBCs, 150, *464*
    storage of, *464, 465, 466*
    transportation of, *464, 465, 466*
    Whole Blood, *464*
Irradiators, blood, 30, 55-56, 149-150
ISBT (International Society of Blood
   Transfusion)
    128 labeling, 152, 153
    nomenclature, 252-253, *296-297,* 298-299
Isohemagglutinins, 266
Issuing components, 476-479
    delivering blood to patient area, 495
    identification of recipient and component
      before, 477-478, 494
    inspections prior to, 477-478, 494-495
    reissue, 481
    in urgent situations, 152, 478, 500,
      509-510
ITP. *See* Immune thrombocytopenic purpura
IVIG. *See* Intravenous immune globulin

J

Jehovah's Witnesses, 528
Jk^a^/Jk^b^/Jk3 antigens, 332-333, *363*
JMH antigen, *234, 321,* 341
Job aids, 16
Job descriptions, 7
John Milton Hagen system, *234, 321,* 341
The Joint Commission, 85-86, 89, 558-559

JR system, *235, 322,* 341-342
Jr^a^ antigen, 341-342
Js^a^/Js^b^ antigens, 329, *363*

K

K/k antigens, 328, 329, *363*
Karyotype, 230
Kell system, 327-330
    allele frequencies in, 249-250
    antibodies, *320,* 329, *363*
    antigens, *233,* 328-329
    autoantibodies, 329
    functional aspects, 330
    in HDFN, 258, 329, 600, 601, 603
    Kell glycoprotein and KEL gene, *233,* 327-
      328
    K$_{mod}$, 330
    K$_o$ (null) phenotype, 329
    phenotypes, *328*
    position effect in, 246-247
Kernicterus, 600, 602, 621
Kidd system, 332-334
    antibodies, *320,* 333, *363*
    antigens, *233,* 332-333
    genetics, *233*
    Kidd glycoprotein, 333-334
    null phenotype, 332-333
    phenotypes, *333*
    in transfusion reactions, 333
Kidney transplantation, 450-452
Kleihauer-Betke acid-elution test, 604
Knops system, *234, 321,* 339-340
Kp^a^/Kp^b^/Kp^c^ antigens, 328-329, *363*
Kx system, 330
    antigens and antibodies, *321,* 330
    genetics, 232, *234, 235,* 243
    McLeod phenotype, 232, 235, 243, 330

L

Labels
    for biohazardous materials, 42
    for blood components, 152-153, 477-478
    for blood samples, 458, 491
    control of, 16
    for hazardous chemicals, 51
    ISBT 128 system for, 153
    for pooled components, 150
Laboratories, regulations for, 84-85
Laboratory coats, 63
Lan system, *235, 322,* 342
Landsteiner-Wiener system, *234, 321,* 337-338
Latex allergies, 39
Le^a^/Le^b^ antigens, 281-283, *320, 363*

Leadership, organizational, 6-7
Lean Six Sigma, 23
Lectins, 272, 278
Leukemia, 118, 511-513, 656
Leukocytapheresis
    collection of granulocytes by, 146-148
    indications for, *642*, 656, *657*
    instrumentation for, *137*, 147-148
Leukocyte-reduction filters, 149, 472, 495-496, *498*
Leukocytes, in components, 149
Leukocyte-reduced components
    expiration, transportation and storage of, *465*, *466*
    leukocyte content in, 149
    for pediatric patients, 632
    platelets, 148, 149, *465*, *466*
    poststorage filtration, 472
    prestorage filtration, 148-149, 472, 495
    to prevent CMV infection, 175, 632, 689
    RBCs, 149, *465*
    to reduce incidence of posttransfusion
        purpura, 592
Lewis substance, 374
Lewis system, 281-283
    antibodies, 283, *320*, *363*
    antigens, *233*, *279*, 281-282
    biochemistry and synthesis of, *279*, 281-282
    expression in children, 283
    genetics, *233*, 282-283
    phenotypes, 282-283
    saliva testing for, 374
    transfusion practice with, 283
Licensure, of facilities, 81
Likelihood ratio, 251
Linkage, 244-245, *246*
Linkage disequilibrium, 245-246, 444
Lipid apheresis, 659
Liquid nitrogen, 676, 677
Liquid plasma, 140, *468*
LISS, 372
Liver, transplantation of, 452, 534
Liver disease, 534
LKE antigen, 286, 287
Look-back investigations, *171-173*, 174, 706
Low-prevalence antigens, 344, 369-370
Low-volume units, 127, 136
Lu^a/Lu^b antigens, 326, 327, *363*
Lui freeze-thaw elution, *390*
Luke antigen, 286, 287
Luminex system, 220, 428
Lung conditions, in blood donors, 118-119
Lung injury. *See* Transfusion-related acute
    lung injury

Lung transplantation, 452
Lutheran system, 326-327
    antibodies, *320*, 327, *363*
    antigens, *233*, 326-327
    genetics, *233*, 241, 245, *246*, 247, 344-345
LW^a/LW^b antigens, 337-338
Lymphocyte crossmatching, 447
Lymphocytotoxicity assays, *445*, 446, 447
Lyonization, 232, 236

M

M antigen, 323, 325, *363*, 372-373
MACE (modified antigen capture ELISA), *423*, 424
MAIGA (monoclonal antibody-specific
    immobilization of granulocyte antigens), 428
MAIPA (monoclonal antibody-specific
    immobilization of platelet antigens), *423*, 424
Major histocompatibility complex, 435. *See
    also* HLA system
    Class I and Class II antigens in, 436-438, 439-440
    genetics of, 440-444
Malaria, 191-192, 332
MAM antigen, *343*, 344
Management, organizational, 6-7
Manual, quality, 15
Markers, defined, 229
Market withdrawals, 84, 706
Marrow
    adverse reactions to, 678
    allogeneic transplantation of, 668-669
    autologous transplantation of, 668
    buffy-coat concentration of, 674
    collection of, 672-673
    cryopreservation of, 676
    donor requirements for, 668-669
    engraftment kinetics of, 671, 685, 687
    filtration of, 675
    histocompatibility of, 669, 670
    infectious disease testing on donors, 175-176, 668-669
    infusion of, 677-678
    patient survival with, 671
    processing, 674-676
    quality control of, 676-677
    red cell reduction in, 674, 684
    regulation of, 87, *88*, 678
    shipping and transport of, 677
    transplantation outcomes using, 670
Masks, 46, 64
Massive transfusion
    blood utilization review of, 562-563
    complications of, 586-588

defined, 479, 516
in pediatric patients, 633
point-of-care testing for, 534
pretransfusion testing in, 479
protocols for, 516-517, 534, 562-563, 588, 633
Materials management, 9-11
Maximum surgical blood order schedules, 480, 565
McLeod phenotype, 232, 235, 243, 330
2-ME. *See* 2-mercaptoethanol
Medical devices, regulation of, 79, *80*, 81-82
Medical history
in antibody identification, 353-354
in evaluation of positive DAT, 388-389
of recipients, 353-354, 490, 529
Medical waste, 47-49
Medication Deferral List, 119
Medications. *See* Drugs
Meiosis, 232, *237*
Membrane attack complex, 223, *224*, 225
MER2 antigen, 340-341
2-mercaptoethanol (2-ME), 373, 374, 393, 399
Methergine, *551*
Methylene-blue-treated plasma, 151, *195*
Mi^a antigen, 326
Microaggregate filters, 495
Microangiopathic hemolytic anemia, 649
Microarray assays, 219
Microlymphocytotoxicity tests, *445*, 446, 447
Microvascular bleeding, 587
Mirasol system, 151
Misoprostol, *551*
Mitosis, 232, *236*
Mixed-field agglutination, 252, 275, 344, 353-354
Mixed lymphocyte culture, 446-447
Mixed-type autoimmune hemolytic anemia, *392*, 400
MNS CHO collection, 343
MNS system, 319, 323-326
antibodies, *320*, 325-326, *363*, 372-373
antigens, *233*, 323, *325*, 326
effect of enzymes on, 323, *363*
genetics, *233*, 323, *325*
glycoproteins, 323, *324*, *325*
linkage disequilibrium in, 245
phenotypes, *325*
S–s–U– phenotype, 323
Mobilization regimens, 146-147, 673
Molecular immunohematology. *See* Blood group genomics
Monoclonal antibodies, therapeutic, 354, 373, 389

Monoclonal antibody-specific immobilization of granulocyte antigens, 428
Monoclonal antibody-specific immobilization of platelet antigens, *423*, 424
Monocyte monolayer assay, 378
Multiple myeloma, 649, 654-655
Multiple sclerosis, 655
Mur antigen, 326
Mutations, genetic, 238, 344-345

N

N antigen, 323, 325, *363*
Nageotte hemocytometry, 149
Narcolepsy, 453
NAT. *See* Nucleic acid testing
National Healthcare Safety Network, 98-99
National Marrow Donor Program, 87, *88*
Near-miss events, 26
Necrotizing enterocolitis, 628
Neisseria gonorrhea, 176
Neonatal alloimmune neutropenia, 427
Neonatal alloimmune thrombocytopenia, 420-421, 506-507
Neonates (younger than 4 months)
ABO antigens and antibodies in, 268, 270, 275
ABO/Rh typing in, 275, 615, 616-617
anemia in, 614
antibody detection in, 615
antigenic variations in, 268, 350
body size and blood volume, 614
cold stress in, 614
compatibility testing for, 616-617
erythropoietic response in, 614
extracorporeal membrane oxygenation in, 627-628
hemoglobin in, 613-614, 620
hemolytic disease in, 599-605
hemostasis in, 624-625
immunologic status of, 615
Lewis antigens in, 283
metabolic pathways in, 615-616
necrotizing enterocolitis in, 628
neutropenia in, 427
polycythemia in, 627
thrombocytopenia in, 420-421, 605-607, 622-623
transfusion-associated GVHD in, 615
transfusions in
additive solutions in, 618-620
administration of, 626-627
age of units for, 620
aliquots for, 474, 617-618, *619*, 625-626
of cryoprecipitate, *621*, 626

dosing for, *621*
exchange, 602, 621-622, 627
of granulocytes, 626
indications for, 616, *617*, 623-624, *625*
of plasma, *621*, 624-626
of platelets, *621*, 622-624
of RBCs, 616-622
transfusion thresholds for, 620
vascular access for, 494, 622, 626-627
Nerve injury, in donors, 129, *130*
Neutropenia
autoimmune, 428
granulocyte transfusions for, 519-520, 626, 631
in HPC transplantation patients, 689
neonatal alloimmune, 427
Neutrophils. *See* Granulocytes
Next-generation sequencing, 446
Nomenclature
for blood group systems, *233-235*, 252-253
for granulocyte antigens, *426*
for HLA system, 437-439
for human platelet alloantigens, *414-415*
of Rh system, *296-297*, *298-299*
Nonconformances, 17-20, 20, 83-84
Nonimmune-mediated hemolysis, *573*, 579, 648
Nonimmunologic protein absorption, 401, 404, 405
NOR phenotype, 286, 287
Notifications
of nonconformances, 19-20
of reactive screening tests, 113, *171-173*, 174
Nuclear Regulatory Commission, 35, 54
Nucleic acid sequence-based amplification, 212
Nucleic acid testing, 169-170
for hepatitis B virus, 169, 181
for hepatitis C virus, 169, 181
for human immunodeficiency virus, 169, 180
for West Nile virus, 170, 186
for Zika virus, 187-188
Nucleic acids, 208-209
Nucleotides, 208
Null phenotypes, 241, 247, 252, 259-260
of H system, 280
of Kell system, 247, 329
of Kidd system, 332-333
of Lutheran system, *241*, 247, 327
of Rh system, 247, 253, 311

O

Obstetrics, controlling bleeding in, *551*
Occupational Safety and Health Administration
biosafety, 41, 42, 43
chemical safety, 49
electrical safety, 41
employee health services, 38, 39
facility safety, 35, 38
Octreotide, *552-553*
Office of Regulatory Affairs, 79, 83
O$_h$ (Bombay) phenotype, 267, 270, 280
Ok system, *234, 321*, 340
Oligonucleotide probes, 445
Open system, 133
Opsonization, 223, *224*, 225
Orders, physician
auditing, 557-565
computerized provider order entry, 538-539, 563
pretransfusion, 457-458, *459*, 480-481, 490-491
surgical blood orders, 480, 565
verifying prior to transfusion, 496-497
Organ transplantation
ABO compatibility in, 450, 452
HLA testing in, 450-452
kidney, 450-452
positive DAT result after, 389
rejection of, 655, 659
Organizations
in regulation and accreditation, 2, 22, 77, *78*, 85, 701
structure of, 6-7
for workplace safety, 33, 61-62
Orientation programs, 7, 14
OSHA. *See* Occupational Safety and Health Administration
Outpatients, 500-501, 511-512
Oxytocin, *551*

P

P antigen, 286-287, 289, 290
P1 antigen, 286-287, 289-290
P1 substance, 290, 374
P1PK system, 286-290
antibodies, 289-290, *320, 363*
antigens, *233*, 286-289
biochemistry, 287
disease associations with, 354, 401
genetics, *233*, 287-289
phenotypes, 286-287
transfusion practice with, 290
Panel reactive antibody, 451, 516
Panels, red cell, 351-352, 355, *357*
Papain, *363-364*, 373
Para-Bombay phenotype, 280
Paroxysmal cold hemoglobinuria, 290, 354, *392*, 400-401

Partial D, 304, 307, *309,* 313
Parvovirus B19, *173,* 193
Passenger lymphocyte syndrome, 685
Paternal testing, 258-259, 601
Paternity index, 251
Pathogen inactivation, 193-195
   and emerging infectious agents, 179
   for pediatric patients, 633
   of plasma, 151
   of plasma derivatives, 193
   of platelets, 152, 185
Patient blood management
   activity levels of, 539, *555-556*
   acute normovolemic hemodilution, 532-533
   anemia assessment and management, 531
   anesthesia in, 533-534
   bleeding risk assessments, 532
   blood utilization review, 21-22, *530,* 538-539, 557-565
   certification programs for, 559
   changing physician behavior in, 537-538
   coordinators for, 539
   definition of, 527
   increased tolerance of anemia in, 536-537
   intraoperative blood recovery, 533
   limiting phlebotomy in, 536
   medical education in, *530,* 537-538
   patient evaluation, 529
   pharmacologic agents in, 535, *546-554*
   point-of-care testing in, 534-535
   postoperative blood recovery, 535-536
   preoperative autologous blood donation, 532
   program development, *538,* 539
   rationale for, 528-529
   responsibilities for, *555-556*
   scope of, 527-528, *530*
   surgical blood orders in, 480, 565
   surgical techniques in, 533-534
   transfusion algorithms in, 534-535
   transfusion thresholds in, 536-537
Patient Safety and Quality Improvement Act, 99, 102
Patient Safety Organizations, 99, 102
PCR. *See* Polymerase chain reaction
PEDI-PAK system, 618, *619*
Pediatric patients (older than 4 months). *See also* Neonates
   ABO antigens and antibodies in, 268, 270, 275, 277
   CMV prevention in, 632
   Lewis antigens in, 283
   pretransfusion testing in, 629

   thrombocytopenia in, *623*
   transfusions in
      aliquoting, 474, 617-618, *619*
      of CMV-reduced-risk components, 632
      of cryoprecipitate, *621, 623,* 631
      of granulocytes, 631
      in HPC transplantation, 690
      of irradiated components, 632
      of leukocyte-reduced components, 632
      massive, 633
      of pathogen-reduced components, 633
      of plasma, *621, 625,* 631
      of platelets, *621, 623,* 630-631, 690
      of RBCs, *621,* 628-630, 633, 690
      with sickle cell disease, 629-630, 690
      syringe infusion pumps for, 493
      with thalassemia, 630, 690
      vascular access for, 494
      of volume-reduced components, 632-633
      of washed components, 633
      of Whole Blood, 631
Pedigrees, 239, *240*
Peer review, 21-22, 557-565
PEG (polyethylene glycol), 372
PEL antigen, *343,* 344
Penicillin, 403
Peripheral blood hematopoietic progenitor cells
   allogeneic, 668-669
   autologous, 668, 673-674
   collection of, 673-674
   cryopreservation of, 676
   donor eligibility of, 668-669
   donor testing, 175-176, 668-669
   engraftment kinetics of, 671, 685
   infusion of, 677-678
   mobilization of, 673
   patient survival with, 671
   processing, 674-676
   quality control of, 676-677
   regulation of, 87, 678
   shipping and transport of, 677
Personal protective equipment, 37-38, 63-65
   for biosafety, 46
   for chemical safety, 52
   gloves, 39, 46-47, 63-64
Personnel
   accidents and injuries in, 39
   blood exposure in, 38-39, 46
   competency assessment of, 8
   hepatitis prophylaxis for, 38
   hiring, 7
   identification of, 17
   job descriptions for, 7
   latex allergies in, 39

orientation for, 7, 14
protective equipment for, 37-38, 46, 63-64
records, 17
safety monitoring programs for, 38
training (*See* Training)
PF4 ELISA, 425
pH, altering, 350-351, 372-373
pH meters, 30
Pharmacogenetics, 453
Phenotype. *See also specific blood groups*
calculations for, 248
defined, 235
and genetic mutations, 238
and genotypes, 215, 235-236, 259-261
nomenclature for, *253*
prevalence of, 248
rare, *368,* 380
Phenotyping
antigen-matching, 379-380
DNA-based assays for, 255
to prevent delayed transfusion
reactions, 590
in sickle cell disease, 310, 380, 477, 508,
630, 656
with warm autoimmune hemolytic
anemia, 397
autologous red cells, 355-356, 359, 364, 371-
372
with DNA-based assays, 254-255, *256*
for antigen-negative donors, *256,* 259
confirming D type, 259, 311
distinguishing alloantibody from
autoantibody, *256,* 257
in prenatal practice, 257-259, 310
in recently transfused patients, 215, 255,
256, 310
RHD zygosity testing, 310
for sickle cell disease patients, 311
when red cells are coated with IgG, 255,
256, 356, 397
solid-phase assays for, 216-217
Phlebotomy. *See also* Blood collection
adverse reactions to, 129-131
of blood donors, 126-129
blood loss due to, 536
for collection of blood samples, 458
disinfection methods for, 126
donor care after, 127-129
vein selection for, 126
Photopheresis, *642,* 656, *658,* 659
Physical assessment
of apheresis patients, 643-644, *645*
of donors, 114-115
of recipients, 490, 529

Physicians, changing behavior of, 537-539
Physiologic anemia of infancy, 613-614
Piperacillin, 403-404
Pipettes, recalibration of, 30
P^k antigen, 286-287, 289
Plasma, for pretransfusion testing, 459-460
Plasma components, 138-142
aliquoting, 625-626
coagulation factors in, 471
collection by apheresis, *137,* 140-142
donors of, 584
expiration of, 139, 140, *466-469,* 471
pathogen inactivation of, 151, 179, 194, *195,*
518
preparation of, 139-140
as replacement fluid in apheresis, *642, 645*
storage of, 139, 140, *466-469,* 471
thawing, 471
transfusion of (*See* Plasma transfusions)
transportation of, *466-469,* 475
types of
Fresh Frozen Plasma, 139, 518
liquid, 140, *468*
Plasma Cryoprecipitate Reduced, 140,
468, 645
Plasma Frozen Within 24 Hours After
Phlebotomy, 139, *467*
Plasma Frozen Within 24 Hours After
Phlebotomy Held at Room
Temperature Up to 24 Hours After
Phlebotomy, 140, *468*
recovered plasma (for manufacture),
140, *469*
Source Plasma, 140-141
Thawed Plasma, 139, 140, *467,* 471, 518
Plasma derivatives
infectious disease screening for, 192-193
pathogen reduction for, 193, 194
storage, transportation, and expiration, *469*
Plasma exchange. *See* Therapeutic plasma
exchange
Plasma reduction, of HPCs, 685
Plasma transfusions
ABO compatibility of, *461, 476, 498,* 626,
686
allergic reactions to, 582
and HLA antibodies, 139
indications for
HPC transplantation, *686,* 689
invasive procedures, 516
massive transfusion, 516-517, 588, 633
in pediatric patients, *621,* 624-626, 631
treatment of bleeding, 516
warfarin reversal, 517-518

infusion of, *498*
types of plasma for, 138-141, 518
Plasmapheresis, 140-142
    donation intervals for, 140-141
    donor consent for, 126, 141
    instrumentation for, *137,* 141-142
    red cell losses in, 141
    therapeutic plasma exchange, 649-655
        adverse effects of, 646-648
        in hemolytic disease of the fetus and
            newborn, 602
        indications for, 649, *650-654,* 654-655
        replacement fluids for, *642, 645*
    volume of whole blood removed during,
        141
Plasticizers, 134
Platelet antagonists, 119, 145
Platelet antibodies
    anti-HPA, 416-417
    autoantibodies, 421, 424-425
    in autoimmune thrombocytopenic
        purpura, 422, 424-425
    detecting, 217, 416, 422-425, 690
    drug-induced, 421-422, 425
    in fetal and neonatal alloimmune
        thrombocytopenia, 416, 417, 420-421,
        605-606
    in HPC transplantation patients, 689
    in posttransfusion purpura, 421, 591-592
Platelet antigens
    ABO antigens, 417-418
    detecting, 217
    GPIV/CD36, *417,* 418
    GPVI, *417,* 418
    HLA antigens, 418, 436
    human platelet alloantigens, 413-417
Platelet components, 142-146
    agitation of, 142-143, 463, 470
    apheresis, 144-146
    bacterial contamination of, 143, 183-185,
        470-471
    biochemical changes in storage of, 470
    clumping in, 143
    containers for, 142
    crossmatching, 420, 448
    donor selection and monitoring, 145, 584
    expiration of, 143, *465-466,* 470-471
    HLA matched, 419-420, 448, 516
    inspection of, 143
    irradiated, 150, 420, *465, 466,* 632
    leukocyte-reduced, 148, 149, 150, *465, 466,*
        472
    pathogen-reduced, 152, 194, *195*
    pooled, 150, *466,* 473

preparation of, 143-144
red cells in, 143
shipment of, 142, 143
storage of, 142, 143, 463, *465-466,* 470
transfusion of (*See* Platelet transfusions)
transportation of, *465-466,* 475
visual inspection of, 184-185
volume-reduced, 145, 151, 473, 624, 632-
    633
washed, 473, 633
Whole-blood-derived, 143-144
Platelet counts
    corrected platelet count increment, 419,
        515
    fetal and neonatal, 606-607
    maternal, 607
    in plateletpheresis donors, 145
    posttransfusion platelet recovery, 419
    as transfusion threshold, 511, 513, 514, *623,*
        630-631, 688
Platelet disorders
    drug-induced thrombocytopenia, 421-422
    fetal and neonatal alloimmune
        thrombocytopenia, 420-421, 605-607
    immune thrombocytopenia, 422, 424-425,
        607
    in massive transfusion, 587
    platelet transfusion refractoriness, 418-420
    posttransfusion purpura, 421, *575,* 591-592
Platelet factor 4 ELISA, 425
Platelet gel, 472
Platelet genotyping, 424
Platelet incubators, 29, 463
Platelet transfusions
    ABO/Rh compatibility of, 418, *461, 498,* 514
        after HPC transplantation, *686,* 687-688
        in hemolytic transfusion reactions, 579
        in pediatric patients, 624
    allergic reactions to, 582
    dosage of, *621,* 624, 688
    indications for, 623-624
        fetal and neonatal alloimmune
            thrombocytopenia, 606-607
        HPC transplantation, 511-513, *686,* 687-
            689
        invasive procedures, 513
        massive transfusion, 517, 588, 633
        in pediatric patients, *621,* 622-624, 630-
            631
        prophylactic vs therapeutic, 511-514,
            623, 630-631, 688
        therapy-induced thrombocytopenia,
            511-513
        to treat active bleeding, 514

infusion of, *498*
refractoriness to, 418-420, 447-448, 514-516
thresholds for, 511, 513, 514, *623*, 631, 688
Plateletpheresis, 144-146
adverse reactions to, 131
donor consent for, 126
donor selection and monitoring in, 145
instrumentation for, *137*, 145-146
therapeutic, *642*, 656, *658*
volume collected in, 145
Plerixafor, 673
Point-of-care testing, 534-535
Policies, 15
Polyagglutination, 275, 313
Polycythemia, 627
Polyethylene glycol (PEG), 372
Polymerase chain reaction, 209-211
contamination in, 211
in genotyping, 254
in HLA typing, 445-446
inhibitors in, 211
oligonucleotide probes, 445
primer design, 211
real-time, 213, *214*
reverse transcriptase, 211
sequence-based typing, *445*, 446
sequence-specific primers, 445-446
specimen processing in, 210
template degradation in, 210
Polymorphisms, 238, 250-251
Pooled components, 150, 473-474
cryoprecipitate, 142, *467*, 473-474
platelets, 150, *466*, 473
Reconstituted Whole Blood, 474
storage, transportation, and expiration of, *466*, *467*, 473-474
Population genetics, 248-250
Position effect, 246-247
Postoperative blood recovery, 535-536
Posttransfusion platelet recovery, 419
Posttransfusion purpura, 421, *575*, 591-592
Postzone effect, 216
Potassium, 586-587, 615-616
Pregnancy
fibrinogen levels in, 518-519
in patient history, 353
postpartum hemorrhage, 518-519
testing during (*See* Prenatal studies)
Premedication, 492, 581
Prenatal studies
ABO/Rh testing, 601
antibody detection, 601
antibody identification, 370
antibody titration, 377, 601

DNA-based testing, 257-259
fetal, 257-258, 310, 601
maternal, 258, 310
paternal, 258-259, 601
in fetal and neonatal immune thrombocytopenia, 606
in hemolytic disease of the fetus and newborn, 601
Preoperative autologous donation, 121, 532
Pressure devices, 493
Pretransfusion testing
ABO/Rh typing, 460-461
after non-group-specific transfusions, 479
antibody detection, 458-459, 461, *487*
antibody identification (*See* Antibody identification)
antiglobulin test, 459, *460*, 462, *485-486*
with autoantibodies, 392-395, 399
autologous control, *487*
and blood availability, 479-480
blood samples for, 458, 459-460, 491
in cold agglutinin disease, 399
comparison with previous records, 458
component selection, *461*, 476-477
crossmatching, 457, 461-463, *487*
donor unit testing, 475
identification of recipients, 458
interpretation of results, 463
in massive transfusions, 479
methodologies for, 460
in pediatric recipients, 615, 616-617, 629
requests for transfusion, 457-458, *459*, 490-491, 563, 565
serologic testing, principles of, 458-459
turnaround times, 491-492
in urgent situations, 478
Prevalence, of phenotypes, 248
Preventive action, 19
Primed lymphocyte typing, 446-447
Prions, 192
Proband, 239
Procedures, 11, 15
Process documents, 15
Processes
control and management of, 3, 4, 11-14, 26
defined, 4, 26
improvement of, 22-23
monitoring and evaluation of, 20-22
validation of, 11-13
Proficiency testing, 22, 85
Propositus, 239
Prospective audits, 538, 559, *560*, 561
Protamine, *548*

Protein analysis, 215-220
  flow cytometry, 220
  fluid-based assays for, 215-216
  protein microarrays, 219
  solid-phase assays for, 216-219
    for antibody detection, 217
    ELISA, 217-219
    for phenotyping red cells, 216-217
    for platelet testing, 217
  suspension array technology, 220
  Western blotting, 219-220
Protein microarrays, 219
Prothrombin complex concentrates, *549*
Prothrombin time, 516
Proton pump inhibitors, *552*
Prozone effect, 216
Pseudogenes, 440, 442
Psoralen-UV treatment, 151, 152, 194, *195*
Public antigens, 438
Public Health Service Act, 78, 79
Pulmonary disease, in blood donors, 118
Pulmonary edema, 584, 647
Pulse, of donor, 114
Pumps, infusion, 493
Pure red cell aplasia, 685

Q

Quad packs, 617-618
Qualification
  defined, 26
  of equipment, 8, 11
  installation, 11
  operational, 11
  performance, 11
  of suppliers, 9, *10*, 702-703
Quality assurance, 2, 26
Quality control, 14
  defined, 2-3, 26
  of equipment, 9, 29-31
  of HPCs, 676-677
  performance intervals for, 29-31
  unacceptable results for, 14
Quality indicators, 21, 26
Quality management systems
  approach to, 4-5
  background of, 1-2
  Code of Federal Regulations references for, *28*
  concepts of, 2-4
  defined, 1, 3, 26
  elements of, 6
    customer focus, 7
    documents and records, 14-17
    equipment management, 8-9

    evaluation of, 5
    facilities, work environment, and safety, 23
    human resources, 7-8
    information management, 17
    management of nonconforming events, 17-20
    monitoring and evaluation, 20-22
    organization and leadership, 6-7
    process and control management, 11-14
    process improvement, 22-23
    suppliers and materials management, 9-11
  quality control performance intervals, 29-31
  terminology for, 26-27
Quality manual, 15
Quality planning, 4, 27
Quality System Essentials, 2
Quality systems, 3-4
Quarantine, 152, 174
Quarantine FFP, 139
Quarantine release errors, 177

R

Radiation
  biologic effects of, 54
  measurement units for, 53-54
  safety, 53-56
    engineering controls, 55-56
    exposure limits, 54-55
    personal protective equipment, 55-56
    radiation monitoring, 55
    regulations, 54
    safe work practices, 56
    training, 55
    waste management, 56
Raph system, *234, 321*, 340-341
Rare Donor Program, 381
RBCs. *See* Red Blood Cell components
Reagents
  for ABO testing, 274
  antibodies to components of, 275, 277, 370
  antibody detection red cells, 351, 365
  antibody identification red cell panels, 351-352, 355, *357*, 365
  antiglobulin, 353, 387-388
  chloroquine diphosphate, 373
  contamination of, 313
  DTT, *363-364, 369*
  for elutions, *390*
  enhancement media, 352-353, 370
  enzymes, *363-364, 369*, 373
  glycine-HCl/EDTA, 373
  LISS, 372

PEG, 372
for phenotyping, 379
quality control intervals for, 31
for Rh testing, *305,* 306, 312, 313
sulfhydryl, *369,* 373, 374, 393, 399
ZZAP, 373
Recalls, 84, 706
Recipients
ABO/Rh testing, *267,* 274-275, 306-307, 460-461
antibody detection in, 461, 463
assessment of, 490, 529
autonomy and satisfaction of, 529
consent of, 489-490
crossmatching in, 461-463
education of, 490
genotyping
in antibody identification, 355-356, 359, 364
in recently transfused patients, 215, 255, *256,* 310, 356
in sickle cell patients, 215, 311
when cells are coated with IgG, 255, *256,* 356, 397
hemovigilance for, 98-102, 569
identification of, 458, 477-478, 494, 496
immunocompromised, 175
medical history of, 353-354, 490, 529
monitoring during and after transfusions, 497, 499
pediatric patients (*See* Neonates; Pediatric patients)
records of, 458
tracing (look-back), *171-173,* 174, 706
weak D in, 306-307, 461
Recombination, 244-245
Reconstituted Whole Blood, 133, 474
Records
altering or correcting, 17
apheresis, *648, 661,* 662
blood component, 477-478
checking before blood issue, 477-478
comparing testing results to, 458
confidentiality of, 17
donor, 113
electronic, 17
HPC transplantation, 690-691
management of, 16-17
of occupational injuries and illnesses, 39
personnel, 17
storage of, 17
of tissue allografts, 705
transfusion, 477-478, 499-500, 690
Recovered Plasma, 140, *469*

Red Blood Cell components
additive solutions for, 134, *135,* 618-620
age of, 616, 620, 633
aliquoting, 474, 617-618, *619*
anticoagulant-preservative solutions for, 131, *132,* 134
bacterial contamination of, 134, 184
biochemical changes of storage in, 470, 509
blood containers for, 134
clots in, 134
expiration of, 134, *464-465*
hemoglobin/hematocrit of, 134, 136
hemolysis in, 134
inspection of, 134, 494-495
low-volume units, 127, 136
pathogen reduction of, 194-195
phenotyping, 630
preparation of, 136
product types
Apheresis, 115, 134, 136-138, *465*
Deglycerolized, 138, *464, 465,* 471-472
Frozen, 138, *464, 465,* 471-472, 475
Irradiated, 150, *464,* 632
Leukocytes Reduced, 148-149, *465*
prepared from Whole Blood, 136, *464*
Rejuvenated, *465*
Washed, *465,* 473, 633
rare, 380
segments on, 134
shelf life of, 134
storage of, 350-351, *464-465,* 470
survival studies of, 378
transfusion of (*See* Red Blood Cell transfusion)
transportation of, *464-465,* 475
Red Blood Cell transfusion, 505-511
ABO/Rh compatibility of, *461,* 476, *498,* 510, *686*
in emergency release, 478, 500, 509-510
of incompatible units, 226
indications for, 505-511, 616, *617*
anemia, 505-507
autoimmune hemolytic anemia, 397, 400, 401, 510-511
exchange transfusion, 578, 621-622, 627, 629-630, *642,* 656, *657*
in HPC transplantation, 687
intrauterine transfusion, 601-602
massive transfusion, 479, 516-517, 586-588, 633
in pediatric patients, 616-622, 628-630
sickle cell disease, 507-509
thalassemia, 507, 508
infusion of, *498,* 626-627

liberal vs restrictive strategies for, 505-507, 528-529, 537, 620, 687
and RBC storage lesion, 470, 509
Red cell antibodies. *See also specific blood groups*
    associated with HDFN, *320-322, 363-364,* 600
    associated with hemolytic transfusion reactions, *320-322, 363-364*
    with autoantibodies, 393-395
    clinical significance of, *320-322,* 349-350, *363-364,* 378
    defined, 349
    detection of (*See* Antibody detection)
    disease associations with, 354
    distinguishing alloantibodies from autoantibodies, *256,* 257
    dosage effect of, 238, 350, 358
    effect of DTT on, *363-364*
    effect of enzymes on, *363-364, 369,* 373
    to high-prevalence antigens, 367, *368,* 369, 602
    high-titer, low-avidity, 377
    identification of (*See* Antibody identification)
    low-affinity, 398
    to low-prevalence antigens, 369-370
    multiple, 359, 362, 377
    naturally occuring, 349
    nonhemolytic, 225-226
    in selection of units, 378-380, 477
    serologic reactivity of, *363-364*
    in sickle cell disease, 308, 310, 477, 630
    in tissue transplantation patients, 698
    variability of expression, 365
Red cell exchange, 578, 602, *642,* 656, *657*
Red cell losses, in apheresis, 141
Red cell reduction, 674, 684
Red cell survival studies, 378
Reference laboratories, 380-381
Refrigerators, 29, 463, 470
Registration
    of donors, 112-113
    of facilities, 79-81
Regulatory issues
    accreditation, 77, 85-86
    agencies involved in, 77, *78*
    FDA oversight of blood establishments, 78-84
        biological product deviation reporting, 83-84
        blood-related devices, 81-82
        inspections, 82-83
        licensure, 81
        recalls and withdrawals, 84
        registration, 79-81

    for HCT/Ps, 86-87, *88,* 89, 678
    hospital regulations, 85-86
    infectious disease testing, *171-173*
    local laws and regulations, 85
    medical laboratory laws and regulations, 84-85
    for quality systems, 2, 22
    for radioactive materials, 54
    safety, 33, 54, 61-62
    for tissue, 700-701
Reissuing blood products, 481
Rejection, antibody-mediated, 655
Rejuvenated RBCs, *465*
Relationship testing, 250-251, 452
Relative risk, 453
Renal failure, 578, 655
Reports, adverse events
    accidents and injuries in employees, 39, 82
    fatalities, 20, 39, 82, 97, 131, 592, *593*
    hemovigilance, 94-107
    related to blood donation, 20, 97
    related to cellular therapy, 20
    related to medical devices, 82
    related to tissue grafts, 705-706
    related to transfusion, 20, *96,* 97, 99-102
Requests for transfusion, 457-458, *459,* 490-491, 563
Requirement, defined, 27
Respiratory distress, 647
Retrospective audits, *560,* 562
Reverse transcriptase PCR, 211
Rg antigens, 338
Rh compatibility, 476, 514, 685, 687
Rh Immune Globulin, 603-605
    after platelet transfusions, 514
    antepartum administration of, 603
    in antibody identification problems, 354
    development of, 295
    dosage of, 604, *605*
    positive DAT after, 389
    postpartum administration of, 603-605
    with weak D phenotypes, 603
Rh system, 295-313
    antibodies, 311-312, *320, 363*
    antigens, *233, 296-297,* 302-311
        C/c and E/e, 308, 310
        D, 295, 302-307, *309,* 600
        G, 308
    clinical considerations for, 307, 308, 310
    ethnic differences in, *296-297, 298, 305,* 306
    genes and proteins, *233,* 246, 247, 299, *300, 309*
    haplotypes, 298, 299, 302
    historical perspective on, 295, 298

phenotypes, *301-302*
RH locus, 299, *300*
RhAG, *235*, 247, 299, 311, *321*, 341
RHD genotype, 299-302, *309*
Rh$_{null}$, 311
terminology for, *296-297*, 298-299
Rh testing
   with autoagglutinins, 313, 392-393, 399
   of blood components, 133, 259, 306, 307,
      475
   for C, c, E, e antigens, *301-302*
   comparison with previous records, 458
   in component selection, 476, 515
   for D antigen, 306-307, 310-311
   discrepancies in, 307, 313
   false-positive/negative results in, 313
   genotyping
      confirming D status, 311
      fetal *RHD*, 257-258, 310, 601
      in multitransfused patients, 310
      in prenatal evaluation, 257-259, 310,
         601, 603
      RHD zygosity testing, 310
      for sickle cell disease patients, 257, 310,
         311
   in hemolytic disease of the fetus and
      newborn, 312, 601, 603
   in HPC transplantation, 685, 686
   in pediatric patients, 615, 616, 629
   phenotyping, *301-302*
   reagents for, *305*, 306, 312, 313
   of recipients, 306-307, 461
   for weak D, 306, 307, 313, 461, 603
RhAG system, *235*, 247, 299, 311, *321*, 341
Rheopheresis, *642*
Riboflavin/UV-treatment, 151, 152, 194, 195
Risks
   assessment of, 12
   of bleeding, 532
   relative, 453
   of transfusion, 177-179, 528
Rituximab, 655
RNA, 208, 209
Rodgers blood group. *See* Chido/Rodgers
Rodgers substance, 374
Root cause analysis, 18-19
Rosette test, 604
Rotational thromboelastometry, 534-535
Rouleaux
   in ABO testing, 275, 277
   in antibody detection/identification, 370-371
   in Rh testing, 313
   saline replacement technique for, 278, 371

S
S/s antigens, 323, 325, *363*
Safe work practices
   for biosafety, 46-47
   for chemical safety, 52
   for electrical safety, 41
   for fire prevention, 40
   general guidelines for, 38, 63-65
   for radiation safety, 56
Safety data sheets, 49, 50, 51-52
Safety goggles, 64
Safety program
   accidents and injuries, 39
   biosafety, 41-49, 66
   chemical safety, 49-53, 67-73
   electrical safety, 40-41
   emergency response plan, 38
   employee health services, 38-39
   engineering controls, 37-38, 65
   fire prevention, 39-40
   hazard identification and communication,
      37
   latex allergies, 39
   management controls, 36, 38
   personal protective equipment, 37-38, 46,
      63-64
   in quality system, 23
   radiation safety, 53-56
   regulations and recommendations for, 33,
      61-62
   safe work practices, 38, 65
   safety officers, 36, 49, 54
   safety plan, 36
   shipping hazardous materials, 56-57
   training in, 36-37
   waste management, 57
Saline replacement technique, 278, 371
Samples. *See* Blood samples
Sc1/Sc2/Sc3 antigens, 336, *364*
Scianna system, *233*, 320, 336, *364*
SD plasma. *See* Solvent/detergent-treated
   plasma, 151, 179, 193, 194, *195*, 518
Sd^a antigen, *343*, 344
Sd^a substance, 374
Secretors, 245, *246*, 278, *279*, 282
Sedimenting agents, 146-147
Segments, of RBCs, 134
Selective adsorption, *642*, 643, 659, *659-660*, 662
Sentinel BloodSCAN Program, 106
Sepsis
   in neonates, 626
   transfusion-associated, 183, 184, 185, *573*,
      579-580
Sequence-based amplification, 212

Sequence-based typing, *445,* 446
Sequence-specific oligonucleotide probes, 445
Sequence-specific primers, 445-446
Serious Hazards of Transfusion, 96-97
Serotonin release assay, 425
Serum, for pretransfusion testing, 459-460
Serum proteins, in typing discrepancies, 275
Serum-to-cell ratio, 372
Sex-linked inheritance, 241-243
Shelf life. *See* Expiration, of components
Shipping. *See* Transportation
Shock, 577
Short tandem repeat analysis, 251
Showers, emergency, 52
Siblings, 240, 442-443
Sickle cell disease
    alloimmunization in, 308, 310, 477, 508,
        630, 690
    blood selection in, 380, 477, 590, 630, 656
    delayed transfusion reactions in, 590, 630
    genotyping/phenotyping for, 257, 311, 371,
        630
    in HPC transplantation, 690
    hyperhemolytic syndrome in, 508, 590, 630
    iron overload in, 630
    in pediatric patients, 629-630, 690
    red cell exchange in, 508, 629-630, 656
    separation of transfused from autologous
        cells in, 371
    transfusion in, 477, 507-509, 630
Side effects. *See* Adverse reactions/events
Signs, safety, 40, 42, 51
Silent genes, 238, 241, 259-261
Single nucleotide polymorphisms, 215, 238
Six Sigma, 23
Skin appearance, in donors, 115
Skin grafts, 698
Solid-phase red cell adherence testing
    for detection of platelet antibodies, 423-424
    for detection of red cell antibodies, 217
    for phenotyping red cells, 216-217
    for platelet crossmatching, 420
    for platelet testing, 217
    for pretransfusion testing, 352
Soluble substances, 373-374
Solutions
    additive, 134, *135,* 618-620
    anticoagulant-preservative, 131, *132*
    intravenous, 496
Solvent/detergent-treated plasma, 151, 179,
    193, 194, *195,* 518
Source Plasma, 140-141
Specific gravity, of blood cells and
    components, *128*

Specification, defined, 27
Spills
    blood, 47
    chemical, 52-53, 71-75
    radioactive, 56
"Splits," 438
Standard operating procedures, 11, 15, 701-702
Standard precautions, 41-42
Standards
    for biosafety, 41
    for cellular therapies, 87
    for infectious disease testing, 165, *171-173,*
        174
    for tissue transplantation, 700-701
Staphylococcal protein A absorption, 659,
    662
Stem cells. *See* Hematopoietic progenitor cells
Sterile connection devices, 30, 133, 148, 618
Storage
    of biohazardous material, 46, 48
    of blood components, 463, *464-469,* 470
        biochemical changes in, 470, 509
        cryoprecipitate, 142, *466-467,* 471
        granulocytes, 147, *466,* 471, 519
        plasma, 139, 140, *466-469,* 471
        platelets, 142, 143, *465-466*
        RBCs, *464-465,* 470, 509
        Whole Blood, 133, *464*
    of donor samples, 476
    equipment for, 463, 470
    of hazardous chemicals, 52
    liquid nitrogen, 676
    of plasma derivatives, *469*
    of records, 17
    red cell antigen deterioration with, 350-351
    temperature for, 463, *464-469,* 470
    of tissue grafts, *469,* 697, 704-705, 706
Storage lesion, 470, 509
Sulfhydryl reagents, *369,* 373, 374, 393, 399
Suppliers, 9-10, 702-703
Supplies, critical, 10-11
Surgery
    acute normovolemic hemodilution in, 532-
        533
    anemia assessment before, 531
    anesthesia in, 533-534
    assessing bleeding risk in, 532
    blood administration in, 500
    blood ordering practices for, 480, 565
    blood recovery in, 533, 535-536
    patient assessment before, 529
    pharmacologic agents in, 535, *546-554*
    point-of-care testing in, 534-535
    preoperative autologous donation for, 532

surgical techniques in, 533-534
transfusion algorithms in, 534-535
Survey meters, for radiation monitoring, 55
Survival studies of red cells, 378
Suspension array technology, 220
Syncope, 129, 131
Syntenic genes, 245
Syphilis, 183
    reactive testing results for, 170, *172*
    screening blood donors for, *167*, 183
    screening tissue donors for, *176, 696*
Syringe aliquoting devices, 618, *619*
Syringe infusion pumps, 493, 618
System, defined, 27

T

T-activation, 275
TA-GVHD. *See* Transfusion-associated graft-
    vs-host disease
TACO. *See* Transfusion-associated circulatory
    overload
Tc^a/Tc^b/Tc^c antigens, 339
Temperature
    of antibody reactivity, *363-364*, 372, 378
    for component storage, 463, *464-469*,
      470
    monitoring systems for, 463, 470
    of recipients, 490
    regulation of, during surgery, 533
    for shipping containers, 475, 677, 704
    for storing tissue, *704*
    for transporting components, 463
    of Whole Blood after collection, 133
Teratogens, 119
TerumoBCT apheresis systems, 137, 145-146,
    147
Testing. *See also specific testing methods*
    method validation, 13-14
    point-of-care, 534-535
    proficiency, 22, 85
    regulations for, 84-85
Thalassemia, 507, 508, 630, 690
Thawed Plasma, 139, 140, *467*, 471, 518
Thawing
    cryoprecipitate, 471
    devices for, 30
    frozen RBCs, 471-472
    HPCs, 674
    plasma, 139, 471
Therapeutic apheresis
    adverse effects of, 646-648
    anticoagulation in, 646
    cytapheresis, *642*, 656, *657-658*
    documentation of, *648*, 662

extracorporeal photopheresis, *642*, 656,
    658, 659
    indications for, 648-649, *650-654, 657-658,*
    659-660
    modalities of, 642-643
    patient evaluation in, 643-644, 645
    payment for, 662
    principles of, 641-642
    provider credentialing, 662
    records, *648, 661,* 662
    replacement fluids in, *642, 645*
    selective adsorption, *642*, 643, 659-660
    therapeutic plasma exchange, *642*, 649-655
    vascular access in, 645-646
Therapeutic plasma exchange, 649-655
    adverse effects of, 646-648
    indications for, *642*, 649-655
      in hematopoietic progenitor cell
        transplantation, 685
      in hemolytic disease of the fetus and
        newborn, 602
    replacement fluids for, *642, 645*
Thermal amplitude studies, 378, 398-399
Thermometers, 30, 463
Thrombocytapheresis, *642*, 656, *658*
Thrombocytopenia
    drug-induced, 421-422
    fetal and neonatal alloimmune, 420-421,
      605-607
    heparin-induced, 422, 425
    immune, 422, 424-425, 607
    maternal, 607
    in pediatric patients, 622-623, 630-631
    platelet transfusions in, 511-514
    posttransfusion purpura, 421, *575*, 591-592
    therapy-induced hypoproliferative, 511-
      513
    thrombotic thrombocytopenic purpura,
      649
Thrombocytosis, 656
Thromboelastography, 534-535
Thrombotic thrombocytopenic purpura, 649
Time, incubation, 372
Timers, 30
Tissue
    ABO compatibility of, 698
    adverse events caused by, 705-706
    autografts, 696-697, 706
    clinical uses for, 698, *699-700*
    collecting, 696, 706
    disease transmission through, 698, 700
    donation of, 695-696
    donor eligibility for, 696
    expiration of, *469*

hospital-based services for, 701-706
infectious disease testing on donors of, 175-176, *696*
look-back investigations, 706
oversight responsibility of, 695, 701, *702*
preservation of, 697-698
processing, 697-698
recalls of, 706
receipt and inspection of, 704
records of, 705
regulations and standards for, *80*, 700-701
standard operating procedures for, 701-702
storage of, *469*, 697, 704-705, 706
suppliers of, 702-703
traceability of, 705
transplantation of, 695-697, 698, *699-700*
transportation of, *469*, 704
types of grafts for, 696-697
Titration of antibodies, 376-377, 601
Topical hemostatic agents, 535, *550*
TPE. *See* Therapeutic plasma exchange
Traceability, 475, 705
Tracking, in process control, 14
Training
   biosafety, 42
   cGMP and cGTP, 7
   chemical safety, 49-50
   electrical safety, 40
   fire safety, 39
   general safety, 36-37
   new employees, 7, 14
   radiation safety, 55
Traits, 230
   autosomal inheritance of, 239-241
   sex-linked inheritance of, 241-244
TRALI. *See* Transfusion-related acute lung injury
Tranexamic acid, 535, *547-548*, 588
Trans position, 246-247
Transcription-mediated amplification, 212
Transfusion-associated circulatory overload, *273*, 584-585
Transfusion-associated graft-vs-host disease, 448-449, *575*, 590-591, 615
Transfusion-associated sepsis, 183, 184, 185, *573*, 579-580
Transfusion reactions
  acute
    air embolus, *573*, 588
    allergic, 492, *571-572*, 581-582
    anaphylactic, *572*, 581-582
    citrate toxicity, *130*, 500, *574*, 586
    coagulopathy, 587-588

    febrile nonhemolytic, 448, 492, *571*, 580-581
    hemolytic, *571*, 576-579
    hyperkalemia and hypokalemia, 500, 586-587
    hypocalcemia, 500, *574*, 586
    hypotension, *573*, 585-586
    hypothermia, 492-493, *574*, 588
    nonimmune hemolysis, *573*, 579
    transfusion-associated circulatory overload, *573*, 584-585
    transfusion-related acute lung injury, *572*, 582-584
    transfusion-related sepsis, 183, 184, 185, *573*, 579-580
  clinical evaluation and management of, 570, *571-575*
  delayed
    alloimmunization, *574*
    hemolytic, 224-225, 366, *574*, 588-590, 630
    iron overload, *575*, 592, 629-630
    posttransfusion purpura, 421, *575*, 591-592
    transfusion-associated graft-vs-host disease, *575*, 590-591
  in HPC transplantation patients, 690
  identification of, 499, 569-570
  laboratory investigation of, 570, 576
  in massive transfusions, 586-588
  monitoring and tracking, 565, 569
  reporting, 20, 99, *100-101*
  signs and symptoms of, 570, *571-575*
Transfusion-related acute lung injury, 139, 428, 448, *572*, 582-584
Transfusion Requirements in Critical Care trial, 505-506, 507
Transfusion safety officers, 539, 558
Transfusion thresholds
  in pediatric patients, 620, *623*, *625*
  for platelet transfusions, 511, 513, 514, *623*, 630-631, 688
  for red cell transfusions, 506-507, 537, 620, 687, 690
Transfusion-Transmissible Infections Monitoring System, 107
Transfusion-transmitted diseases
  babesiosis, 190-191
  chikungunya virus, 188-189
  dengue virus, 188
  hepatitis B virus, 180-181
  hepatitis C virus, 181
  hepatitis E virus, 182-183
  human immunodeficiency virus, 179-180
  human T-cell lymphotropic virus, 182

malaria, 191-192
parvovirus B19, 193
prions, 192
reducing risks of, 112
screening for (*See* Infectious disease screening)
surveillance of, 107
syphilis, 183
Trypanosoma cruzi, 189-190
West Nile virus, 185-186
Zika virus, 186-188
Transfusions
administration procedures for (*See* Blood administration)
algorithms for, 534-535
auditing, 21-22, 557-565
chimerism after, 448-450
consent for, 489-490
costs of, 529
of cryoprecipitate, 518-519, 626
documentation of, 477-478, 499-500
exchange, 578, 602, 616, 621-622, 627, *642*
fatalities due to, 20, 496, 578, 584, 585, 592
of granulocytes, 147, 519-520, 626
guidelines for, 538, 558, *617, 629*
in HPC transplantation, 685-690
intrauterine, 601-602
massive, 479, 516-517, 534, 562-563, 586-588, 633
in medical history, 353-354, 388-389, 490
mistakes or incidents associated with, 99
monitoring appropriateness of, 557-565
non-group-specific, 479
in operating room and trauma, 500, 633
out-of-hospital, 500-501
in pediatric patients, 616-633
of plasma, 516-518, 624-626
of platelets, 511-516, 622-624
of RBCs, 505-511, 616-622
requests for, 457-458, *459*, 490-491, 563
risks of, 177-179, 528
selection of components for, *461*, 476-477, 605
in urgent situations, 478, 500, 509-510
of Whole Blood, 631
Transmissible spongiform encephalopathy, 192
Transplantation. *See specific types of transplants*
Transportation
of blood components, 133, 463, *464-469*, 474-475, 495
containers for, 31, 474, 475, 677
of frozen components, 475, 677
of hazardous materials, 56-57

of HPCs, 677
monitoring temperature during, 463, 677, 704
of plasma derivatives, *469*
of samples, 56-57
of tissue, *469*, 704
Trauma
blood administration procedures in, 500
massive transfusion in, 516-517, 562-563, 633
point-of-care testing in, 534
Travel, by blood donors, 191
Trending, in quality systems, 14
Treponema pallidum, 176, 183
Trypanosoma cruzi, 189-190
reactive screening tests for, *173, 174*
screening donors for, 189-190
supplemental assays for, *167*, 168
Trypsin, 373
TTP. *See* Thrombotic thrombocytopenic purpura
Type and hold, *459*, 480
Type and screen, *459*, 480-481
Type and screen with crossmatch, *459*

U

U antigen, 323, 325, *363*
UCB. *See* Umbilical cord blood
Ulex europaeus lectin, 272, 278, 280
Umbilical cord blood
antigen expression on, 350
DAT testing on, 388
infectious disease screening, 668-669
for transplantation
cell expansion, 675-676
clinical utility of, 667-668
cryopreservation, 676, 684
donor testing, 668-669, 670-671
engraftment kinetics, 671, 685, 687
HLA matching, 669-670
infusion, 677-678
patient survival, 671
in pediatric patients, 690
processing, 674-676
quality control testing, 676-677
regulations and standards, 87, *88*, 678
shipping and transporting, 677
thawing and washing, 674-675
volume reduction of, 674
Uniforms, 63
Urgent release of blood, 478, 500, 510
Urticaria, *571*, 581, 582
Utilization of blood. *See* Blood utilization auditing

V

Vaccines, 453
Validation
    of computer systems, 13
    defined, 27
    of equipment, 11
    of processes, 11-13
    of shipping containers, 475
    of standard operating procedures, 15
    of test methods, 13-14
Vapors, hazardous, 53
Variable number of tandem repeats, 251
Vascular access
    for apheresis, 645-646
    in pediatric patients, 494, 622, 626-627
    for transfusions, 494
Vasovagal reactions, 129, *130*, 131, 647
Vector-transmitted diseases, 185-192
Vel system, *235, 322*, 342
Venipuncture, 126, 184
Verification, defined, 27
Viability assays for HPCs, 723
View boxes, 30
Viruses
    donor screening for, 179-183, 185-189
    transmitted by tissue transplants, 705
Viscoelastic coagulation testing, 534-535
Viscosity, plasma, 649, 654-655
Vital signs, 490, 497, 499, 678
Vitamin K, *548*
Volume of blood
    in exchange transfusions, 621, 622
    in intrauterine transfusions, 602
    in neonatal transfusions, *621*
    in pediatric patients, 614
    in Whole Blood collections, 127, 131
Volume overload. *See* Transfusion-associated
    circulatory overload
Volume reduction
    of HPCs, 674
    of platelets, 145, 151, 473, 624, 632-633
    of RBCs, 473
von Willebrand disease, 118, 626

W

Waldenström macroglobulinemia, 655
Warfarin reversal, 517-518, *548*
Warm autoantibodies
    ABO testing with, 393
    adsorption of, 393-395
    with alloantibodies, 393-395
    antibody identification with, 365, 369
    disease associations with, 354
    mimicking alloantibodies, 395

    in mixed-type AIHA, 400
    in phenotyping problems, 371-372
    Rh testing with, 313, 392-393
    specificity of, 395-396
    transfusion with, 397, 510-511
    in warm AIHA, 391-396
Warm autoimmune hemolytic anemia, 391-
398
    allogeneic adsorption, 394-395
    autologous adsorption, 393-394
    blood selection in, 396-397
    DAT-negative, 397-398
    serologic characteristics of, 391-392
    serologic problems in, 392-393
    specificity of autoantibody in, 395-396
    testing adsorbed serum, 395
    transfusions in, 397, 510-511
Warmers, blood, 30, 492-493, 588, 614
Washed components, 473
    HPCs, 675
    for pediatric patients, 615-616, 633
    platelets, 473, 633
    RBCs, *465*, 473, 633
Waste management, 57
    biohazardous, 47-49
    chemical, 53
    disposal, 48, 53, 56
    radioactive, 56
    treating waste, 48-49
Waterbaths, 30
Weak D, 303-304, *309*
    in donors, 259, 306, 307
    in prenatal patients, 258, 603
    in recipients, 306-307, 461
    testing for, 306, 307, 313, 461, 603
Weight
    of donors, 114
    of neonates, 614
WES^a/WES^b antigens, 339
West Nile virus, 185-186
    nucleic acid testing for, 170
    reactive testing results for, *173*, 174
    screening donors for, *167*, 170, *176*, 186
Western blotting, 219-220
Whole Blood
    ABO compatibility of, *461*
    collection of, 125-131
        adverse donor reactions in, 129-131
        anticoagulant-preservative solutions
            for, 131, *132*
        containers for, 131, 133
        donor care after, 127-129
        donor preparation, 125-126
        handling after, 133

process of, 127-129
volume collected, 127, 131
expiration of, *464*
hematocrit of, 131
irradiated, *464*
pathogen inactivation of, *195*
processing, 136
reconstituted, 133, 474
storage of, *464*
temperature for, 133, 136
testing, 133
transfusion of, 631
transportation of, 133, *464*, 475
Wipe tests, 55
Withdrawals, market, 84
WNV. *See* West Nile virus
Work environment, 23, 34-36
Work instructions, 15
World Health Organization, 96
World Marrow Donor Association, 87, *88*
Wr^a/Wr^b antigens, 335
Wrong blood in tube, 458

X

X-borne genes, 241-243
X chromosome inactivation, 232, 236
Xenografts, 697
Xenotransplantation products, 697
Xg system, 335-336
antibodies, *320*, 335-336, *364*
genes and antigens, *233*, 335
inheritance pattern of, 232, 242
Xg^a antigen, 335, *364*
XK gene, 232, *234*, 243, 330

Y-Z

Yt system, *233*, *320*, 335, *364*
Yt^a/Yt^b antigens, 335, *364*
Zika virus, 186-188
reactive screening tests for, *173*, 174
screening donors for, *167*, 187-188
Zone of equivalence, 215-216
Zygosity, 237-238, 350
ZZAP, 373, 399

USING YOUR USB FLASH CARD

The USB flash card that accompanies this edition of the AABB *Technical Manual* contains the Methods Sections and the book's general appendices in a convenient storage format. The card's longevity will be enhanced through proper handling, data retrieval, and storage when not in use.

Directions for Safe Handling

- As you remove the flash card from its protective sleeve, avoid placing your finger on the metal portion of the tab that swings out for insertion into the USB socket of your device.

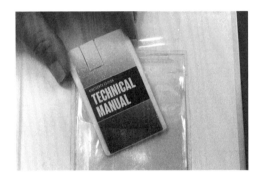

- The tab on a new flash card may be stiff, but will be easier to handle after use. The hinge is along the outer edge of the card, so apply gentle pressure to the hinge. It swings in one direction only; do not force it.

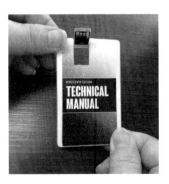

- The tab is designed to be inserted into device sockets in one direction only. If it does not glide easily on the first try, do not force it. Try changing the direction of the tab. You may need to look closely at the both the device socket and the flash card tab to be sure that you have lined up the connection properly.

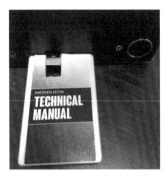

- Do not leave the flash card in the socket while it is not in use. Damage to the flash card and/or the device socket may occur if the card is accidently bumped or jarred roughly.

- After all operations are completed, remove the flash card from the host device gently. Swing the tab back into its original position, again avoiding skin contact with the metal portion.

- Place the flash card back in its protective sleeve.